# Primary Care Pediatrics for the Nurse Practitioner

**Theresa Kyle, DNP, APRN, CPNP-PC, CNE,** earned a Bachelor of Science in Nursing from the University of North Carolina at Chapel Hill, a Master of Science in Nursing (Child Health) from Emory University, and a Doctor of Nursing Practice in Educational Leadership from American Sentinel University. She is a certified pediatric nurse practitioner and certified nurse educator. Having been in pediatric nursing for over 36 years, she has had the opportunity to serve children and their families in a variety of diverse settings. She has experience as a pediatric nurse practitioner in pediatric specialty clinics, primary care, and juvenile justice. She currently teaches remotely in the nurse practitioner program at the University of West Florida, and AdventHealth University. She is a fellow in the National Association of Pediatric Nurse Practitioners and a member of Sigma Theta Tau International Honor Society of Nursing, the National League for Nursing, and the Society of Pediatric Nurses.

# Primary Care Pediatrics for the Nurse Practitioner

## A Practical Approach

Theresa Kyle, DNP, APRN, CPNP-PC, CNE

EDITOR

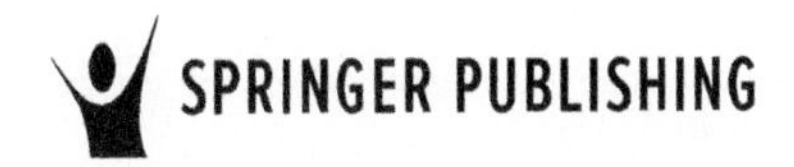

Springer Publishing Company, LLC
11 West 42nd Street, New York, NY 10036
www.springerpub.com
connect.springerpub.com/

*Acquisitions Editor*: Elizabeth Nieginski
*Compositor*: Amnet Systems

*ISBN*: 978-0-8261-4094-4
*ebook ISBN*: 978-0-8261-4095-1
*DOI:* 10.1891/9780826140951

**SUPPLEMENTS:**
**Instructor Materials:**

***Qualified instructors may request supplements by emailing textbook@springerpub.com***

Instructor's Manual ISBN: 978-0-8261-6021-8
Instructor's Test Bank ISBN: 978-0-8261-6022-5
Instructor's PowerPoints ISBN: 978-0-8261-6023-2
Image Bank ISBN: 978-0-8261-6024-9

**Student Materials:**

***A supplementary Online Prescribing Guide and Patient Educational Downloads are available at connect.springerpub.com/content/book/978-0-8261-4095-1***

Online Prescribing Guide ISBN: 978-0-8261-6025-6
Patient Education Downloads ISBN: 978-0-8261-6026-3

22 23 24 / 5 4 3 2



**Library of Congress Cataloging-in-Publication Data**

Names: Kyle, Terri, editor.
Title: Primary care pediatrics for the nurse practitioner : a practical approach / [edited by] Theresa Kyle.
Description: New York, NY : Springer Publishing Company, LLC, 2021. | Includes bibliographical references and index.
Identifiers: LCCN 2021012452 | ISBN 9780826140944 (paperback) | ISBN 9780826140951 (ebook) | ISBN 9780826160218 (instructor's manual) | ISBN 9780826160225 (instructor's test bank) | ISBN 9780826160232 (instructor's PowerPoints) | ISBN 9780826160249 (image bank) | ISBN 9780826160256 (student resources) | ISBN 9780826160263 (patient education downloads)
Subjects: MESH: Primary Health Care—methods | Pediatric Nursing—methods | Nurse Practitioners | Infant | Child | Adolescent
Classification: LCC RJ245 | NLM WY 159 | DDC 618.92/00231—dc23
LC record available at https://lccn.loc.gov/2021012452



Printed in the United States of America.

*This textbook is dedicated to*
*all of the infants, children, and adolescents who are our future.*

# Contents

# Contributors

**Jamie H. Andre, MS, PA-C**
Section of Critical Care Medicine
Department of Pediatrics
Baylor College of Medicine
Texas Children's Hospital
Houston, TX

**Megan Arnold, PA-C**
Faculty
Baylor College of Medicine
Texas Children's Hospital
Houston, TX

**Nicole Lynne Audritsh, DNP, CNM**
Graduate Specialty Coordinator, Clinical Instructor
School of Nursing
Wayne State University
Detroit, MI

**Melody M. Avila, DNP, FNP-C**
Assistant Professor
College of Nursing
University of New Mexico
Albuquerque, NM

**Janine M. Bamberger, MS, RDN, CD**
Adjunct Instructor, Dietetics Department
School of Natural & Health Sciences and Education
Mount Mary University
Milwaukee, WI
Adjunct Instructor, Exercise Science
Department of Human Movement Sciences
College of Health Sciences
Carroll University
Waukesha, WI

**Paula Barbel, PhD, CPNP-PC**
Associate Professor
Department of Nursing
SUNY Brockport
Brockport, NY

**Pamela Biernacki, DNP, FNP-C**
Assistant Professor
School of Nursing and Health Studies
Georgetown University
Washington, DC

**Shelby R. Boone, MSN, APRN, CPNP-AC, CPN**
Instructor, Nurse Practitioner
Baylor College of Medicine
Texas Children's Hospital
Houston, TX

**Lai Brooks, DNP, FNP-BC**
Le Bonheur Children's Hospital
Comprehensive Neuroscience Institute
Assistant Professor
College of Nursing
University of Tennessee Health Science Center
Memphis, TN

**Pamela Bryant, DNP, CRNP, AC-PC**
Assistant Professor, Specialty Track Coordinator for Pediatric Primary Care Program
School of Nursing
University of Alabama at Birmingham
Birmingham, AL

**Stacy B. Buchanan, DNP, RN, CPNP**
Adjunct Clinical Faculty
School of Nursing
Georgia State University
Atlanta, GA

**Mandi Cafasso, DNP, APRN, CPNP**
Assistant Professor, Doctor of Nursing Practice Program
University of Cincinnati
Pediatric Nurse Practitioner, Endocrinology
Cincinnati Children's Hospital Medical Center
Cincinnati, OH

**Vivianna Carter, BSN, RN, TNS, TCRN**
Registered Nurse, Emergency Department
SSM Health Cardinal Glennon Children's Hospital
St. Louis, MO

**Tracey Cobb-Scully, MSN, RN, CEIS**
Doctoral Candidate
School of Nursing
University of Connecticut
Storrs, CT

**Samantha Colbert, MS, PA-C**
Baylor College of Medicine
Texas Children's Hospital
Houston, TX

**Elizabeth Coleman, MSN, CRNP, CPNP-PC**
Nursing Instructor
School of Nursing
The University of Alabama at Birmingham
Birmingham, AL

**Sylvia Cooper, DNP, APRN, CPNP-AC**
Instructor
Baylor College of Medicine
Pediatric Critical Care
Texas Children's Hospital
Houston, TX

**E. Allison F. Crabtree, DNP, CRNP, FNP-C**
Assistant Professor
School of Health Professions and Wellness
Jacksonville State University
Jacksonville, AL

**Daniel Crawford, DNP, ARNP, CPNP-PC, CNE**
Associate Professor (Clinical)
Director, Pediatric Primary Care Nurse Practitioner Program
College of Nursing
The University of Iowa
Iowa City, IA

**Shauna di Bari, MSN, APRN, CPNP-AC**
Instructor, Baylor College of Medicine
Texas Children's Hospital
Houston, TX

**Elizabeth P. Elliott, MS, PA-C**
Associate Professor
School of Health Professions, Department of Pediatrics
Baylor College of Medicine
Houston, TX

**Donna Lisa Evans, MSN, APRN, CPNP AC/PC**
Instructor
Department of Pediatrics
Critical Care Medicine
Baylor College of Medicine
Houston, TX

**Rebecka Evans, CPNP, PMHCNS-BC, RN**
Bedford Pediatrics
Bedford, MA
Cambridge Eating Disorder Center
Cambridge, MA
Clinical Preceptor
School of Nursing
Boston College
Chestnut Hill, MA

**Vicky Fan, MPAS, PA-C**
Pediatric Critical Care Medicine
Baylor College of Medicine
Texas Children's Hospital
Houston, TX

**Jennifer B. Frank, DNP, RN, PCNS, BC**
Assistant Professor
School of Health Professions and Wellness
Department of Nursing
Jacksonville State University
Jacksonville, AL

**Megan Gentry, MHS, PA-C**
Instructor Faculty
Department of Pediatrics
Section of Critical Care Medicine
Baylor College of Medicine
Houston, TX

**Sara Gerrie, DNP, CPNP, CPON**
Instructor, Pediatrics
University of Colorado Health Sciences Center
Children's Hospital Colorado, Center for Cancer and Blood Disorders
Denver, CO

**Brandi Guyton, MSN, CPNP-AC/PC**
Instructor
Baylor College of Medicine
Texas Children's Hospital
Houston, TX

**Keeley A. Harding, DNP, APRN, CNS, CPNP-AC/PC**
Adjunct Faculty, Doctor of Nursing Practice Program
College of Nursing
University of Cincinnati
Cincinnati, OH

**Kelly M. Henson, DNP, CPNP-AC, IBCLC**
Major, United States Air Force
Ramstein Air Base, Germany

**Beth Heuer, DNP, CPNP-PC, PMHS**
Mitochondrial Medicine Frontier Program
Children's Hospital of Philadelphia
Philadelphia, PA

**Lani A. Kajihara-Liehr, DNP, FNP**
Assistant Associate
Monroe Carell Jr. Children's Hospital at Vanderbilt
Instructor
Vanderbilt School of Nursing
Vanderbilt University
Nashville, TN

**Chrisla Key, DNP, NP-C**
Assistant Professor
College of Nursing
University of Tennessee Health Science Center
Le Bonheur Children's Hospital
Memphis, TN

**Meredith Kopp, MSN, APRN, CPNP-AC**
Instructor/Faculty
Baylor College of Medicine
Houston, TX

**Lacey L. Kruse, MD**
Assistant Professor of Pediatrics and Dermatology
Northwestern University Feinberg School of Medicine
Chicago, IL

**Theresa Kyle, DNP, APRN, CPNP-PC, CNE**
Adjunct Faculty
School of Nursing
Advent Health University
Orlando, FL
Nova Southeastern University
Ft. Lauderdale, FL
University of West Florida
Pensacola, FL

**Michaela Lewis, DNP, ARNP, CPNP, CPN, CPEN, CNE, CNE-cl, PMHS**
Assistant Professor
College of Nursing
University of Colorado, Anschutz Medical Campus
Aurora, CO

**Lindsey Locke, MSN, CPNP-PC**
Pediatric Nurse Practitioner
Division of Orthopaedic Surgery
Le Bonheur Children's Hospital
Adjunct Faculty
College of Nursing
University of Tennessee Health Science Center
Memphis, TN

**Holly Lydigsen, DNP, CPNP-PC, CNL**
Pediatric Genetics
UT Le Bonheur Pediatric Specialists
Assistant Professor
College of Nursing
The University of Tennessee Health Science Center
Memphis, TN

**Thuy Lynch, PhD, RN**
Nursing Faculty
College of Nursing
The University of Alabama in Huntsville
Huntsville, AL

**Kari Lyn Martin, MD, FAAD**
Associate Professor of Dermatology & Child Health
Columbia School of Medicine
University of Missouri
Columbia, MO

**Sara Rose McClelland, MSN, CPNP-AC**
Instructor, Baylor College of Medicine
Texas Children's Hospital
Houston, TX

**Jenna N. McDonald, MSN, RN, CPNP**
Instructor of Nursing
School of Health Professions and Wellness
Jacksonville State University
Jacksonville, AL

**Steadman McPeters, DNP, CPNP-AC, CRNP, RNFA**
Assistant Professor
School of Nursing
University of Alabama at Birmingham
Birmingham, AL

**Exie Meredith, DNP, CPNP-AC**
Instructor
Baylor College of Medicine
Texas Children's Hospital
Houston, TX

**Mariah Morris, DNP, APRN, CPNP-PC**
Clinical Assistant Professor
School of Nursing
University of West Florida
Pensacola, FL

**Tammy Morrow, DNP, RN**
Assistant Professor
School of Health Professions and Wellness
Department of Nursing
Jacksonville State University
Jacksonville, AL

**Priscila Nakano, MSN, APRN, CPNP-AC**
Instructor
Baylor College of Medicine
Nurse Practitioner, Critical Care Medicine
Texas Children's Hospital
Houston, TX

**Wendy Quiroz Nasser, DNP, APRN, CPNP-AC/PC**
Critical Care Medicine Associate Chief
Director of Critical Care Medicine Advanced Practice Providers, Main Campus
Assistant Professor
Baylor College of Medicine at Texas Children's Hospital
Department of Pediatrics
Houston, TX

**Cynthia S. Nelson, PA-C, MS, MPH**
Instructor
Baylor College of Medicine
Texas Children's Hospital
Houston, TX

**Elizabeth Neptune, MS, PA-C**
Instructor, Pediatric Critical Care Medicine
Baylor College of Medicine
Texas Children's Hospital
Houston, TX

**Melissa Nunn, DNP, APRN, CPNP-PC/AC**
Director of Advanced Practice
Children's Hospital, New Orleans
Instructor of Clinical Nursing, PNP Program Coordinator
School of Nursing
Louisiana State University Health Sciences Center
New Orleans, LA

**Elizabeth A. Paton, DNP, RN-BC, PNP-AC, PPCNP-BC, CPEN, FAEN**
Assistant Professor
College of Nursing
University of Tennessee Health Science Center
Director of Advanced Practice Nursing
Le Bonheur Children's Hospital
Nurse Practitioner, Pediatric Surgery
Memphis, TN

**Imelda Reyes, DNP, MPH, FNP-BC, CPNP-PC, CNE, FAANP**
Clinical Associate Professor
Emory Nell Hodgson Woodruff School of Nursing
Emory University
Atlanta, GA

**Leslie N. Rhodes, DNP, PPCNP-BC**
Pediatric Nurse Practitioner
LeBonheur Children's Hospital
Assistant Professor
College of Nursing
University of Tennessee Health Science Center
Memphis, TN

**Paige Ricca, DNP, MS, MBA, RN**
Clinical Assistant Professor
College of Nursing
University of Illinois at Chicago
Chicago, IL

**Jennifer Ridgway, DNP, APRN, CPNP**
Instructor of Nursing
School of Nursing
Vanderbilt University
Nashville, TN

**Claire M. Rizk, CPNP-PC/AC**
Instructor, Critical Care Medicine
Baylor College of Medicine
Texas Children's Hospital
Houston, TX

**Morgan Rockwell, MS, PA-C**
Instructor, Department of Pediatrics
Baylor College of Medicine
Pediatric Critical Care
Texas Children's Hospital
Houston, TX

**Laura Roettger, PhD, APRN, CPNP-PC**
Assistant Professor
Director of the Pediatric Nurse Practitioner Program
College of Nursing
Philadelphia University, Thomas Jefferson University
Philadelphia, PA

**Kristine Ruggiero, PhD, MSN, RN, CPNP**
Nurse Scientist, Department of Medicine
Boston Children's Hospital
Faculty, School of Nursing
MGH Institute of Health Professions
Boston, MA

**Brandi M. Runnels, MS, MMS, PA-C**
Instructor/Physician Assistant
Baylor College of Medicine
Texas Children's Hospital
Houston, TX

**Graciela Sanabria, PA-C**
Instructor
Pediatrics Critical Care Medicine
Baylor College of Medicine
Texas Children's Hospital
Houston, TX

**Allison Sindle, MD**
Resident Physician
Department of Dermatology
University of Missouri
Columbia, MO

**Jacquelyn Sink, MD, FAAD**
Dermatologist
Northwestern Medicine Regional Medical Group
Winfield, IL

**Sonia A. Smith DNP, CPNP/CNS, AE-C**
Pediatric Nurse Practitioner
Pulmonology and Sleep Medicine
Ascension Sacred Heart
Pensacola, FL

**Tedra S. Smith, DNP, CPNP-PC, CNE, CHSE**
Associate Professor
School of Nursing
The University of Alabama at Birmingham
Birmingham, AL

**Patricia M. Speck, DNSc, CRNP, FNP-BC, DF-IAFN, FAAFS, DF-AFN, FAAN**
Professor, Coordinator of Advanced Forensic Nursing
Department of Family, Community, and Health Systems
School of Nursing
The University of Alabama at Birmingham
Birmingham, AL

**Danielle R. Stratton, DNP, RN, PPCNP-BC**
Assistant Professor
Department of Nursing
SUNY Brockport
Brockport, NY

**Katherine Taylor, MSN, APRN, CPNP-AC/PC**
Nurse Practitioner, Instructor
Critical Care Medicine
Baylor College of Medicine
Texas Children's Hospital
Houston, TX

**Kathleen P. Thompson, MPAS, PA-C**
Assistant Professor
Physician Assistant Program
Department of Pediatrics, Section of Critical Care Medicine
School of Health Professions
Baylor College of Medicine
Texas Children's Hospital
Houston, TX

**Jill Travis, MSN, FNP-C**
Nurse Practitioner, Division of Pediatric Urology
UT Le Bonheur Pediatric Specialists
Assistant Professor, Health Promotion and Disease Prevention
College of Nursing
University of Tennessee Health Science Center
Memphis, TN

**John West, MSN, APRN, CPNP-AC**
Instructor, Nurse Practitioner
Department of Pediatrics, Critical Care Medicine
Baylor College of Medicine
Texas Children's Hospital
Houston, TX

**Maria Fatima G. Westry, MSPAS, PA-C**
Associate Director of Critical Care Advanced Practiced Practitioners
Pediatric Critical Care Medicine
Baylor College of Medicine
Texas Children's Hospital
Houston, TX

**Brittany Williams, DNP, CPNP-PC, CNL**
Assistant Professor
College of Nursing
University of Tennessee Health Science Center
Memphis, TN

**Terry Witherington, DNP, APRN, PNPC**
Assistant Professor
Vanderbilt University
Nashville, TN

**Elke Jones Zschaebitz, DNP, APRN, FNP-BC**
Assistant Professor, Advanced Practice Department, FNP Program
School of Nursing and Health Studies
Georgetown University
Washington, DC

# Chapter Reviewers

**Christina Aplin-Snider, DNP, FNP-BC**
Assistant Professor
School of Nursing
University of Michigan
Flint, MI

**Nicole Boucher, PhD, CPNP-PC**
Certified Adverse Childhood Experiences Trainer
Clinical Assistant Professor
School of Nursing
University of Michigan
Ann Arbor, MI

**Kathleen Bradbury-Golas, DNP, RN, FNP-C, ACNS-BC**
Associate Clinical Professor
College of Nursing and Health Professions
Drexel University
Philadelphia, PA

**Adelita G. Cantu, PhD, RN**
Associate Professor
School of Nursing
UT Health San Antonio
San Antonio, TX

**Jennie Choe, MSN, CPNP-AC**
University of Maryland SON- DNP candidate
Baltimore, MD

**Christine M. Cogil, DNP, MPS, RN, FNP-BC**
Associate Professor
College of Nursing
University of New Mexico
Albuquerque, NM

**Beth Condley, DNP, CPNP-AC**
Clinical Faculty
College of Nursing
University of South Alabama
Mobile, AL

**Alicia Cook, MNSc, CPNP-AC**
Faculty
University of Arkansas Medical Sciences
Little Rock, AR
Adjunct Faculty
School of Nursing
University of South Alabama
Mobile, AL

**Karen G. Duderstadt, PhD, RN, CPNP, FAAN**
Clinical Professor Emerita
Department of Family Health Care Nursing
School of Nursing
University of California San Francisco
San Francisco, CA

**Ann Marie Felauer, DNP, CPNP-AC/PC**
Director, Pediatric Nurse Practitioner Specialties
Assistant Professor
School of Nursing
University of Maryland
Baltimore, MD

**Susan D. Fernbach, RN, BSN**
Co-Director, Office of Community Engagement and Diversity
Assistant Professor, Dept. Molecular and Human Genetics
Baylor College of Medicine
Texas Children's Hospital
Houston, TX

**Angela Fetty, DNP, CRNP, PNP-AC**
Assistant Professor of Nursing Education
School of Nursing
Shepherd University
Shepherdstown, WV

**Gloria Galloway, MD, MBA, FAAN, FACNS, FAANEM**
Professor, Neurology
Wexner Medical Center
Ohio State University
Columbus, OH

**Angela R. Gethers, MSN, RN, CPNP-PC, CPN**
APRN Assistant Director
Urgent Care Services
Children's Mercy Hospitals & Clinics
Kansas City, MO

**Amy S. Hamlin, PhD, APRN, FNP-BC**
Professor
School of Nursing
Austin Peay State University
Clarksville, TN

**Cindy Sue Herrera, DNP, APRN, PPCNP-BC**
College of Nursing
University of Toledo
Toledo, OH

**Judy W. Herrman, RN, PhD, CNE, ANEF, FAAN**
Consultant
NurseTim, Inc.
Emerita Professor
University of Delaware
Lewes, DE

**Samantha Hoffman, MS, CPNP-PC**
Clinical Simulation Training Specialist and Nursing Skills Coordinator
School of Nursing
University of Maryland
Baltimore, MD

**Stephanie N. Hosley, DNP, APRN-CNP, CNE**
Assistant Professor of Clinical Practice
College of Nursing
The Ohio State University
Columbus, OH

**Beth Heuer, DNP, CPNP-PC, PMHS**
Mitochondrial Medicine Frontier Program
Children's Hospital of Philadelphia
Philadelphia, PA

**Amanda Kotowski, DNP, RN, CPNP-PC/AC, CLC**
Clinical Faculty
College of Nursing
Marquette University
Milwaukee, WI

**Kun Lu, DNP, PNP**
UCSF Benioff Children's Hospital
San Francisco, CA

**Rachel Mahas, PhD, MS, MPH**
Program Director, Master of Public Health
Assistant Professor of Nursing and Health
Madonna University
College of Nursing and Health
Livonia, MI

**Christiana Makinde, DNP, PNP-BC**
Adjunct Associate Professor, Graduate Nursing Program
Lehman College, CUNY
Pediatric Nurse Practitioner, Division of Neonatology
Maimonides Medical Center
New York, NY

**Amelia Malcom, DNP, FNP-BC**
Assistant Professor, NP Coordinator
Mary Inez Grindle School of Nursing
Brenau University
Gainesville, GA

**Ashley Marass, DNP, CPNP, SANE-A**
Associate Professor
Chair, Maternal Child Department
College of Nursing
University of South Alabama
Mobile, AL

**Bethany McClean, RN, MSN, FNP-BC**
Assistant Clinical Professor
College of Nursing and Health Innovation
University of Texas at Arlington
Arlington, TX

**Kari McDonald, PhD, RN**
Clinical Assistant Professor
School of Nursing
University of Texas
Austin, TX

**Angela N. Morehead, DNP, FNP-BC**
Assistant Professor
School of Nursing
Middle Tennessee State University
Murfreesboro, TN

**Nicole S. Murry, PhD, RN**
Clinical Assistant Professor
School of Nursing
University of Texas at Austin
Austin, TX

**Yeow Chye Ng, PhD, CRNP, CPC, AAHIVE, FAANP**
Associate Professor
College of Nursing
The University of Alabama in Huntsville
Huntsville, AL

**Nicole (Nico) Osier, PhD, RN**
Assistant Professor
School of Nursing
University of Texas at Austin
Austin, TX

**Amrish Patel, MD**
Atlanta Hand Specialist
Atlanta, GA

**Kathleen Pitts, PhD, APRN, PNP-BC, MPH**
Instructor, Department of Pediatrics
Baylor College of Medicine
Section of Allergy, Immunology & Retrovirology
Texas Children's Hospital
Houston, TX

**Tracey Power, DNP, RN, CNE, CCRN, CPN**
Clinical Assistant Professor
Loewenberg College of Nursing
University of Memphis
Memphis, TN

**Anna Richmond, DNP, FNP-C, CPNP**
Assistant Professor
School of Nursing
Vanderbilt University
Nashville, TN

**Julie Schreiner, DNP, PMHNP, FNP, RN**
Sterling Psychiatric Group
Surfside Pediatrics
Ventura County, CA

**Allison Scott, DNP, CPNP-PC, IBCLC**
Associate Professor
Eleanor Mann School of Nursing
University of Arkansas
Fayetteville, AR

**Abigail Smith, PA-C, MPH**
Children's Healthcare of Atlanta
Atlanta, GA

**Katelynn Socha, MSN, APRN, PPCNP-BC**
Blackstone Valley Pediatrics
Cumberland, RI

**Andrew Storer, PhD, DNP, FNP-C, ACNP-BC, FAANP**
Executive Director, Professional Practice, Nursing Education, and Nursing Research
Roswell Park Comprehensive Cancer Center
Buffalo, NY

**Taylor Swing, DNP, CPNP-PC**
Assistant Professor
School of Nursing
University of Maryland
Baltimore, MD

**Theresa Turick-Gibson, candidate - Ed.D.program, MA, PPCNP-BC, RN-BC**
Professor Emerita, Curriculum Chair
Department of Nursing
Hartwick College
Oneonta, NY

**Aimee Vael, DNP, APRN, FNP-BC**
Professor, FNP Program Coordinator
Columbus State University
Columbus, GA

**Alejandra B. Valenzuela, DNP, APRN, CPNP-AC/PC**
Clinical Assistant Professor
School of Nursing Graduate Education
The University of Texas at El Paso
El Paso, TX

**Barbara Wise, PhD, RN, CPNP- AC/PC**
Assistant Professor
School of Nursing
University of Maryland
Baltimore, MD

**Catherine Witt, PhD, APRN, NNP-BC**
Associate Professor, Dean
Loretto Heights School of Nursing
Regis University
Denver, CO

**Donna R. Wyly, MSN, RN, CPNP-AC, PPCNP-BC, ONC**
APRN Education Coordinator
Division of Urgent Care
Children's Mercy Kansas City
Kansas City, MO

# Foreword

Like a Maestro who orchestrates multiple virtuosos to perform an exquisite musical symphony, Dr. Kyle and her editorial team have united a remarkable group of national pediatric clinicians, educators, scientists, advocates, and thought-leaders to share their expertise in this textbook dedicated for nurse practitioner students. Their work offers a clear, harmonious, and practical resource destined to inspire future clinicians poised to support families, mentor youth, promote interprofessional partnerships, and deliver expert primary care services. Using a wealth of evidence-based, multifaceted tools to cultivate competence and confidence, this textbook offers a refined approach toward successful certification and professional credentialing in pediatric primary care. Chapters and study tools are coordinated to educate and inspire students' agency to meet the unique challenges and responsibilities emerging in pediatric and adolescent primary care settings across the nation. No singular authors' voice could have achieved this goal, especially in a dynamic and evolving healthcare environment; we needed visionary orchestration to create this resource uniquely designed for pediatric primary care providers and nurse leaders of the future. I am delighted to congratulate this symphony of authors, and welcome this textbook as an academic tool to promote excellence among our future pediatric providers who will undoubtedly recall this resource as a foundation in their development.

*Anne Derouin, DNP, APRN, CPNP, PMHS, FAANP*
Professor, Assistant Dean, MSN Program
Duke University School of Nursing
Durham, North Carolina

# Preface

The contemporary primary healthcare system is complex and challenging, and children are a particularly special population. The intricacies of child development, and the influences of genetic, epidemiologic, and environmental factors must be understood when providing pediatric primary care. Clinicians working with children and their families need an in-depth understanding of necessary approaches to working with children, normal child development, the health promotion process for children, and disease management. The text is laid out in a bulleted user-friendly fashion, making it simple for the experienced clinician to quickly reference a topic, and for the student nurse practitioner to thoroughly learn a particular concept. The emphasis of this text is on health supervision and promotion, as well as disease prevention and management from the primary care provider's standpoint. The text focuses on the nurse practitioner's level of diagnosis and management. Referral and consultation recommendations are provided for those health problems residing in the acute or specialty care realm.

Organized in four units, each chapter within a unit is structured similarly to ease the learning process for the reader. The distinct layout provided in Units II, III, and IV, improves readability and learner understanding of the content. Chapters begin with a list of student learning outcomes, an introduction, and a chapter map linking content areas with the Pediatric Nursing Certification Board CPNP-PC® exam outline (lettering and numbering within the map matches the exam outline items precisely). Pro Tips and Alerts are featured throughout the chapter and a list of key points summarizes the content at the end. Current evidence-based guidelines, useful decision-making algorithms, and procedures are referenced throughout the text. Resources for families and nurse practitioners are provided with online links included as appropriate, such as Bright Futures and Mass General Pediatric symptom checklists, CDC immunization schedules, and other tools. A robust art program features four-color original figures and tables essential to understanding each condition specific to pediatrics.

Unit I focuses on general information related to the provision of primary care to children and provides the nurse practitioner with the necessary foundation for caring for children. Concepts covered in Unit I include the role of the nurse practitioner, influences on child health, health assessment, laboratory and diagnostic testing and interpretation, pediatric prescribing, and pain management. The emphasis in Unit II covers the expected development for each of the main age groups. In addition to developmental milestones, activity, nutrition, sleep, and safety are included in each age-appropriate development chapter, creating a seamless approach to caring for a child of a particular age. Management of common developmental concerns is included in Units II and III. Health supervision and anticipatory guidance are emphasized in Unit III. Comprehensive well-child visit information is provided based on the Bright Futures recommendations.

Commonly occurring health disorders frequently seen in primary care are addressed in Unit IV. The information concerning each disease or health concern is presented consistently in a problem-oriented format allowing for development of the diagnostic reasoning process. Pathophysiology of the disease or disorder is followed by subjective data (including risk factors and review of systems), objective findings, laboratory or diagnostic testing (listed with positive results), the differential diagnosis, and the treatment or management plan including family education and information on when to refer outside of primary care. This problem-oriented focus emphasizes diagnostic reasoning used within the scope of the nurse practitioner's role.

To even further enhance the educational content in the text itself, a comprehensive ancillary resource bundle includes an instructor's manual with WHAT-WHY-APPLY case studies, a test bank that mirrors the PNCB's CPNP-PC® Certification Exam, PowerPoints corresponding with each chapter, an image bank replete with dermatologic photos and other pediatric figures, as well as student resources containing an online prescribing guide for the top 10 pediatric disorders, and patient education downloads covering parent or caregiver interactions, preventions, immunizations, referrals, and other necessary information.

*Theresa Kyle*

**Qualified instructors may obtain access to supplemental materials, including an Instructor Manual, Test Bank, PowerPoints, and Image Bank, by emailing textbook@springerpub.com.**

**A supplementary Online Prescribing Guide and Patient Educational Downloads are available at connect.springerpub.com/content/book/978-0-8261-4095-1**

# Acknowledgments

I would like to express my deepest gratitude to Elizabeth Nieginski, nursing publisher, for once again believing in my vision for educating nursing professionals for the purpose of improving the health and well-being of children and their families. Special thanks are given to Hannah Hicks and Robin Bushing for their talented and persistent editorial efforts in the development of this manuscript. I am especially grateful to this team at Springer who tirelessly supported my efforts, and persevered with me throughout the creation of this text. This project also could not have been completed without the love and support of my family: my husband, John, who tirelessly champions me, and my children, Christian and Caitlin, who inspire me to reach higher. Motivated by the anticipation of her arrival and now inspired by the joy of her presence, my granddaughter, Sophia, is my daily example of the importance of high quality pediatric primary care.

# UNIT I

# Foundations of Child Health

# CHAPTER 1

# The Role of the Nurse Practitioner

Kristine Ruggiero

## Student Learning Objectives

1. Identify the role of the nurse practitioner (NP) when caring for children and families.
2. List the educational, certification, and licensure requirements for becoming a NP.
3. Discuss the concept of family-centered care.
4. Describe the role of the NP in the medical home, including the role of billing and coding.
5. Recognize the key components of employment negotiation.

## INTRODUCTION

Florence Nightingale wrote in 1860, "Were there none who were discontented with what they have, the world would never reach anything better" (Nightingale, n.d.). This text was designed for the NP student caring for pediatric patients, specifically, the pediatric nurse practitioner (PNP) and the family nurse practitioner (FNP) student. Being a NP student in the health professions in today's current climate is not easy. Students must contend with rapid changes in technology, difficulties with insurance coverage, and the challenge of new diseases such as coronavirus disease 2019 (COVID-19). This timeless dilemma reflects the need to continuously advance and advocate for the role of the NP. Learning goes beyond the pages of this text and our nursing programs; it continues in our roles as clinicians and future mentors.

Remember, you had a life before this NP program. You probably had a job, personal relationships, and family and friends. The point is, before you entered this NP program you had lived experiences. Consciously, or more likely unconsciously, these lived experiences may affect your approach to some clinical encounters as a NP student. It is important to not forget this and, more importantly, to incorporate these past lived experiences into the care you will be providing. At the same time, it is important to acknowledge that these past experiences could have a potential negative impact on care. In clinical medicine, answers and approaches to different clinical questions and family circumstances yield varied approaches to pediatric patients and families. Any implicit bias from your past experiences should be acknowledged and addressed, but the art of medicine and our approach to patient care affords us diverse opportunities to incorporate all we have learned from other sources, and all of this influences our diverse philosophies on patient care.

According to the American Association of Nurse Practitioners (AANP, n.d.-a), NPs are educated at the graduate level to provide primary, acute, chronic, and specialty care to patients of all ages, depending on their field of practice. Advanced practice registered nurses (APRNs) have the knowledge to assess patient needs, order and interpret diagnostic and laboratory tests, diagnose disease, and formulate and prescribe treatment plans as well as provide basic disease prevention, coordination of care, and health promotion. Essential members of the healthcare workforce, APRNs provide increased access to care in a cost-effective manner (NAPNAP, 2017).

## HISTORY OF THE ROLE OF THE NURSE PRACTITIONER

To honor the 200th birthday of the nursing pioneer Florence Nightingale, the World Health Organization (WHO) declared 2020 the Year of the Nurse and

Midwife. Coincidentally, 2020 celebrates the centennial birthday of another nursing maverick, Loretta C. Ford, supporter and activist of the role of the NP (Brennan, 2020). Historically, the NP role first emerged shortly after the implementation of Medicare and Medicaid. With this expansion of healthcare financing on a national scale, specifically primary care, and the need for rural health care, Loretta Ford saw an opportunity and partnered with a pediatrician to develop the first NP program out of the University of Colorado in 1965, focusing on pediatric primary care. The first master's level NP program was established two years later at Boston College. In 1967, the National Association of Pediatric Nurse Practitioners (NAPNAP) was established. This was the first professional organization dedicated to the needs of the PNP. In 1974, the American Nurses Association (ANA) helped legitimize the role of the NP by establishing the Council of Primary Care Nurse Practitioners, which created an early description of an NP's duty. To further standardize the duties of NPs, the ANA began offering NP certification examinations in 1977. In 1985, the American Academy of Nurse Practitioners was established (AANP, n.d.-b).

Over the next decade, the 101st Congress expanded reimbursement to NPs through the Omnibus Reconciliation Act of 1989. Direct reimbursement was granted to NPs through the Balanced Budget Act of 1997, which increased the care they were providing to patients on a national level (105th Congress, 1997). By 2000, NPs were legally able to practice in all 50 states (Dellabella, 2015). In 2004, the American Association of the Colleges of Nursing (AACN) issued a statement on the practice doctorate in nursing, sparking an initiative to require a Doctor of Nursing Practice (DNP) degree for the advanced practice role (AACN, 2020). While this ultimately did not occur by the year 2015 as planned, the impetus for a move to transition from NP master's programs to DNP programs continues to build.

# EDUCATION REQUIREMENTS

Most NPs, also known as advanced practice nurses (APNs) and APRNs receive their education primarily through one of two ways. As an RN, the student completes either a master of science in nursing (MSN) degree or a doctor of nursing practice degree with a focus on the particular specialty area. Education for NPs centers around a holistic approach to care, and education for those seeking primary care certification is largely focused on health promotion and disease prevention. This is in contrast to traditional medical education, which is problem-focused, emphasizing cause and effect. For example, exposure to a microbe (cause) will result in an infection (effect), thus in the medical model the healthcare provider seeks to treat the cause specifically.

There is no single national accreditation agency for NP programs. Rather, PNP and FNP education programs are housed within graduate programs accredited by AACN's Commission on Collegiate Nursing Education (CCNE) or the Accreditation Commission for Education in Nursing (ACEN).

## Role Competencies

NP education is competency-based. A competency is focused on performance integrating knowledge, skills, abilities, and clinical judgment. The National Organization of Nurse Practitioner Faculties (NONPF) sets the standard requirements for NP education programs. Whether education is obtained at the master's or doctoral level, the NP must demonstrate competency in:

- Scientific foundation
- Leadership
- Quality
- Practice inquiry
- Technology and information literacy
- Policy
- Health care delivery system
- Ethics
- Independent practice (NONPF, 2017)

Additional population-focused competencies have also been identified. They correlate with the NP core competencies and more specifically delineate the NP's focus of care for children. Both the primary care PNP and the family NP demonstrate a commitment to family-centered care. The population-focused competencies may be accessed at https://cdn.ymaws.com/www.nonpf.org/resource/resmgr/competencies/populationfocusnpcomps2013.pdf.

# SCOPE OF PRACTICE

The scope of practice of NPs is regulated by state boards of nursing and the state nurse practice acts. The scope of practice for the NP includes health promotion and disease prevention; health education and counseling to individuals, families, and communities; the diagnosis and management of acute, chronic, and complex health problems; healthcare research; interdisciplinary consultation; and patient advocacy. The NP performs health assessments, initiates and interprets diagnostic and laboratory tests, makes diagnoses, initiates and manages treatment (including prescribing medication and nonpharmacologic treatments), and coordinates care (AANP, 2019). The NP's role within the pediatric population includes caring for children from birth to young adulthood, thus necessarily it includes a focus on age-appropriateness. The NP's provision of care to children is performed within a framework of respect for the child's and family's needs and values.

The role of NPs has become even more invaluable under the Affordable Care Act (ACA) with the expansion of access to primary care services. Currently, NPs have full scope of practice in 21 states and the District of Columbia, while the remainder of states permit reduced or restricted practice requiring either collaboration with or supervision by another healthcare provider (AANP, 2021). Presently, more than 290,000 NPs are licensed to practice in the United States (AANP, 2020). NPs should have a sound knowledge and understanding of the limitations or restrictions placed on the NP's ability to engage in elements of NP practice, particularly in reduced or restricted access states.

A PNP is qualified to provide comprehensive care to all children, beginning at birth and continuing until young adulthood. The PNP certified in primary care will screen, evaluate, diagnose, and treat children in primary care settings (e.g., clinics, private practices, schools) (NAPNAP, Society of Pediatric Nurses, & American Nurses Association, 2015). When children with special health care needs or chronic pediatric conditions reach 21 years of age, they may be transitioned to adult care, though some children may not successfully achieve that transition until slightly older (NAPNAP, 2019). Family NPs are educated to provide family-centered primary care to all ages of patients from birth through old age (Population-Focused Competencies Task Force, 2013).

## Certification

To become a NP, the first step is to be licensed as a registered nurse, then complete an appropriate program of study and pass a national certifying examination. The NP must then maintain that certification or recertify periodically in certain cases, in order to remain licensed and continue to practice. The certifying bodies require the examinee to have graduated from a nationally accredited program. In 1975, the Pediatric Nursing Certification Board (PNCB) came into being and began providing a certification examination for the primary care PNP just two years later. Historically, the PNCB has certified the majority of primary care PNPs (PNCB, n.d.). While the American Nurses Credentialing Center (ANCC) formerly offered the primary care PNP certification, they ceased doing so in 2018 (ANCC, n.d.-b). ANCC and the American Academy of Nurse Practitioners Certification Board (AANPCB) both offer a certification examination for the family NP (AANPCB, n.d.; ANCC, n.d.-a). Each of these certification examinations and their corresponding provider are recognized by all state boards of nursing.

## Licensure

Currently, APRNs are granted licensure by the individual state boards of nursing. When the APRN moves to another state, they must receive endorsement of their current license and be issued an APRN license in the new state. Not yet adopted, the Consensus Model for APRN Regulation: Licensure, Accreditation, Certification & Education (APRN Consensus Model) is a uniform model of regulation for the future of advanced practice nursing that is designed to align the interrelationships among licensure, accreditation, certification, and education. The Consensus Model provides guidance for states to adopt uniformity in the regulation of APRN roles. According to the National Council of State Boards of Nursing (NCSBN), many states have adopted portions of the Consensus Model, but not completely. If regulatory requirements differ from state to state, this represents a potential obstacle that would potentially prevent access to care. The Consensus Model for APRN Regulation has the potential to improve access to care and ease APRN transition across states by outlining regulatory requirements in licensure, accreditation, certification, and education that should be adopted by every state (NCSBN, n.d.).

## Family-Centered Care

The PNP or FNP employs family-centered care. Children's care focuses on their changing developmental, emotional, and physical needs; this care should be continuous and comprehensive. Families exhibit varied cultural, ethnic, and religious backgrounds and their valuable input into the child's care should be respected. Parents and caregivers perform a significant role in the well-being and health of children of all ages, serving as sources of support and strength, as well as serving as experts on their children (American Academy of Pediatrics [AAP], Committee on Hospital

Care, & Institute for Patient and Family-Centered Care, 2012). As a mutually beneficial partnership between the APRN, the child, and the family, parents'/caregivers' confidence in their skills will be increased and children will also participate in care and decision-making. The core concepts of family- centered care include dignity and respect, information sharing, participation, and collaboration (Institute for Patient- and Family-Centered Care [IPFCC], n.d.). Additional information may be found on the IPFCC website at https://www.ipfcc.org. These core concepts align with the Institute for Healthcare Improvement's (IHI) explanation of person- and family-centered care (IHI, n.d.-a). Along with person- and family-centered care, the patient experience is a central component of one of the three prongs of the Triple Aim for Populations. Along with the patient experience, population health improvement and reduction in per capita cost form the Triple Aim (IHI, n.d.-b). NPs are particularly well suited to contribute to the success of the Triple Aim.

### Medical Home

To build trust and a comprehensive relationship with the family, the PNP or FNP establishes themselves as provider for the medical "home" for the child. This promotes a high level of supervision, resulting in coordinated, comprehensive, and cost-effective care. As a medical home, the care is local, accessible, culturally effective, and family-centered. The partnership in the medical home is built on an atmosphere of mutual trust. Within the security of the medical home, the NP is able to share any concerns that may arise longitudinally in relation to the child's physical, emotional, or developmental status. Additionally, immunization rates are improved when children have a medical home (AAP, n.d.-b).

### Coding and Billing

Not only will the NP have the competencies to provide high-quality, family-centered care to children, they will also need to document, code, and bill appropriately. Codes decide the reimbursement rates for an encounter and several factors affect the code, including patient status (new versus established), health history, the physical examination, and complexity of medical decision making. Current procedural terminology sets specific guidelines for the codes (numbers) assigned to medical, procedural, and diagnostic services delivered by healthcare providers and then reimbursed either through Medicaid or by private insurance. Evaluation and management charges are determined by the amount of time spent counseling the child and/or family in addition to obtaining the history and physical examination (AAP, n.d.-a).

Appropriate coding is necessary not only for the financial success of the pediatric or family practice, but also for the avoidance of fraud. Billed codes must match the documentation provided in the health record. A selection of a more complex visit code may flag insurance companies to investigate for fraud, whereas a lower code will result in not being appropriately compensated for the services provided. Having correct knowledge of coding practices is extremely important for the NP. Numerous updated publications are available from the AAP in relation to coding (https://shop.aap.org/coding/#sort=relevance&topic=12074&page=1). Additionally, the NP is responsible for correctly coding for health conditions. These conditions are coded according to the International Diseases Classification, 10th edition, Clinical Modification (ICD-10, CM) guidelines. The Health Information Portability and Accountability Act (HIPAA) requires that the guidelines be adhered to for all encounters (Centers for Disease Control and Prevention, 2020).

## EMPLOYMENT NEGOTIATIONS

As a new NP graduate beginning a new job, contract negotiations may be complicated. It is important not to sell oneself short in employment negotiations. Common themes when speaking with recent NP graduates about their first job after NP school is they "will take what I can get" or "want to get my foot in the door." Having this perspective may sell oneself short; therefore, it is important to perform adequate research prior to contract negotiations. Employment contracts can provide many perks if properly negotiated. For example, know your worth including your own skill set (i.e., another language, other special skills, certifications, publications, research, or other unique types of experiences you possess). In addition to this it is important to know your specific desires. For example, what hours per day do you want to work? Do you want to be salaried or paid hourly? Are there loan-repayment options? Nonmonetary contributions should also be considered, including: Are you willing to travel? Will you take on-call or weekend coverage? What will your commute to work be? All of these questions should help develop your specific wants/needs before you sit down to negotiate.

The NP working with children and families plays a vital role in their health promotion and disease treatment. Educated at the master's or doctoral level, the NP is certified within a particular specialty in order to receive licensure in any state in the U.S. Providing family-centered care within the medical home is the expected mode of practice for NPs working with children and their families.

## KEY POINTS

- Pediatric and family NPs are qualified to provide primary, acute, chronic, and specialty care to children of all ages.
- NPs assess the needs of children and families; order and interpret diagnostic and laboratory tests; diagnose disease; formulate and prescribe treatment plans; and provide basic disease prevention, coordination of care, and health promotion.
- The education level required to practice as a NP is currently a master's degree, though currently the movement is toward a doctoral degree for entry into practice.
- The NP working with children and families provides family-centered care within the medical home.
- Consider the benefits and risk requirements of the NP profession prior to negotiating employment.

## REFERENCES


101st Congress. (1989). *H.R.3299—Omnibus Budget Reconciliation Act of 1989.* https://www.congress.gov/bill/101st-congress/house-bill/3299

105th Congress. (1997). *H.R.2015—Balanced Budget Act of 1997.* https://www.congress.gov/bill/105th-congress/house-bill/2015

American Academy of Nurse Practitioners Certification Board. (n.d.). *Family nurse practitioner.* https://www.aanpcert.org/certs/fnp

American Academy of Pediatrics. (n.d.-a). *Coding tips for pediatricians: Evaluation and management coding strategies.* https://www.aap.org/en-us/professional-resources/practice-transformation/getting-paid/Coding-at-the-AAP/Pages/Coding-Tips-for-Pediatricians-Evaluation-and-Management-Coding-Strategies.aspx

American Academy of Pediatrics. (n.d.-b). *What is medical home?* https://www.aap.org/en-us/professional-resources/practice-transformation/managing-patients/Pages/what-is-medical-home.aspx

American Academy of Pediatrics, Committee on Hospital Care, & Institute for Patient and Family-Centered Care. (2012). Policy statement: Patient and family-centered care and the pediatrician's role. *Pediatrics, 129*(2), 394–404. http://pediatrics.aappublications.org/content/129/2/394

American Association of Colleges of Nursing. (2020). *DNP fact sheet.* https://www.aacnnursing.org/News-Information/Fact-Sheets/DNP-Fact-Sheet

American Association of Nurse Practitioners. (n.d.-a). *All about NPs.* https://www.aanp.org/about/all-about-nps

American Association of Nurse Practitioners. (n.d.-b). *Historical timeline.* https://www.aanp.org/about/about-the-american-association-of-nurse-practitioners-aanp/historical-timeline

American Association of Nurse Practitioners. (2019). *Scope of practice for nurse practitioners.* https://www.aanp.org/advocacy/advocacy-resource/position-statements/scope-of-practice-for-nurse-practitioners

American Association of Nurse Practitioners. (2020). *NP fact sheet.* https://www.aanp.org/about/all-about-nps/np-fact-sheet

American Association of Nurse Practitioners. (2021). *State practice environment.* https://www.aanp.org/advocacy/state/state-practice-environment

American Nurses Credentialing Center. (n.d.-a). *Our certifications.* https://www.nursingworld.org/our-certifications

American Nurses Credentialing Center. (n.d.-b). *Pediatric Primary Care Nurse Practitioner Certification (PPCNP-BC).* https://www.nursingworld.org/our-certifications/pediatric-primary-care-nurse-practitioner

Brennan, C. (2020). Tracing the history of the nurse practitioner profession in 2020, the year of the nurse. *Journal of Pediatric Healthcare, 34*(2), 83–84. https://doi.org/10.1016/j.pedhc.2019.12.005

Centers for Disease Control and Prevention. (2020). *ICD-10-CM official guidelines for coding and reporting.* https://www.cdc.gov/nchs/data/icd/10cmguidelines-FY2021.pdf

Dellabella, H. (2015). *50 years of the nurse practitioner profession.* https://www.clinicaladvisor.com/home/web-exclusives/50-years-of-the-nurse-practitioner-profession

Institute for Healthcare Improvement. (n.d.-a). *Person- and family-centered care.* http://www.ihi.org/Topics/PFCC/Pages/Overview.aspx

Institute for Healthcare Improvement. (n.d.-b). *Triple aim for populations.* http://www.ihi.org/Topics/TripleAim/Pages/Overview.aspx

Institute for Patient- and Family-Centered Care. (n.d.) *Patient- and family-centered care.* https://www.ipfcc.org/about/pfcc.html

National Association of Pediatric Nurse Practitioners. (2017). NAPNAP position statement on access to care. *Journalof Pediatric Health Care, 31,* A13–A16. http://doi.org/10.1016/j.pedhc.2016.08.013

National Association of Pediatric Nurse Practitioners. (2019). NAPNAP position statement on age parameters for pediatric nurse practitioner practice. *Journal of Pediatric Health Care, 33,* A11–A13. https://doi.org/10.1016/j.pedhc.2018.10.007

National Association of Pediatric Nurse Practitioners, Society of Pediatric Nurses, & American Nurses Association. (2015). *Pediatric nursing: Scope and standards of practice* (2nd ed.). American Nurses Association.

National Council of State Boards of Nursing. (n.d.). *APRN consensus model.* https://www.ncsbn.org/aprn-consensus.htm

National Organization of Nurse Practitioner Faculties. (2017). *Nurse practitioner core competencies content.* https://cdn.ymaws.com/www.nonpf.org/resource/resmgr/competencies/2017_NPCoreComps_with_Curric.pdf

Nightingale, F. (n.d.). *Notes on nursing: What it is, what it is not* (commemorative ed.). J. B. Lippincott.

Pediatric Nursing Certification Board. (n.d.). *About us.* https://www.pncb.org/about

Population-Focused Competencies Task Force. (2013). *Population-focused nurse practitioner competencies.* https://cdn.ymaws.com/www.nonpf.org/resource/resmgr/competencies/populationfocusnpcomps2013.pdf

# Factors Influencing Child Health

Thuy Lynch, Michaela Lewis, and Vivianna Carter

## Student Learning Outcomes

**Upon completion of this chapter the reader should be able to:**

1. Distinguish unique family situations such as blended, communal, extended, single-parent, binuclear, and LGBTQ+.
2. Define culture, culture humility, and cultural awareness.
3. Describe the social influences on child development.
4. Differentiate the effects of prenatal substance use on infants' health.
5. Characterize the influence of environmental and physical hazards as well as social media on child health.

## INTRODUCTION

Child health and the care of children and their families are multifactorial and varying. Family structure and functioning, culture, genetics, and the environments in which children are nurtured, born, grow, and live influence a child's overall well-being. Children and families are integral partners of the healthcare team; the perspectives and information they offer are essential components of high-quality clinical reasoning and decision making. Nurse practitioners must be informed by the history, trends, and issues affecting contemporary practice, and the ethical and legal frameworks within which pediatric nursing care is provided. Assessing and capitalizing on the strengths of the family unit, maximizing genetic potential, recognizing and respecting the confluence of cultural factors, and optimizing the physical and emotional spaces that children occupy are the essence of family-centered care. This chapter explores prominent influences on child health and their implications for the child, family, and society at large.

The content in this chapter maps to the following areas on the Pediatric Nursing Certification Board (PNCB) Pediatric Nurse Practitioner—Primary Care certification examination:

CONTENT AREAS:

### I. Health Promotion and Maintenance

**A. Partner with patients/caregivers to support growth and development from infancy to young adulthood.**

**E. Advise patients/caregivers about age appropriate injury prevention and safety including but not limited to:**

1. Environmental exposure
3. Social situations

### III. Management

**D. Collaboration and Referral**

3. Refer children, adolescents or caregivers to community resources as indicated

### IV. Professional Role and Responsibilities

**A. Leadership and Evidence-Based Practice**

1. Serve as a clinical resource for other healthcare professionals

**C. Legal and Ethical Issues**

2. Incorporate cultural awareness and inclusiveness into all aspects of practice
3. Maintain ethical practices

## FAMILY

A family is a fundamental unit of a society. A family is a unit of two or more individuals that identify themselves to be related whether through marriage, birth, adoption, or other arrangement as defined by the individuals within the unit. Different types of families exist, and families can include people who are related biologically as well as people who bond together through circumstance. A functional family unit is one in which everyone mutually respects, supports, and cares for each other. It is imperative to remain cognizant that families present in many different structures and functions, and that they shape a child's personality as it pertains to mental and emotional well-being.

There are three different theories to identify how a family structure responds to internal and external events: family systems theory, family stress theory, and family development theory (Johnson & Ray, 2016). Family systems theory classifies the family structure not only as one entire unit, but also as the individuals within the family being separate parts that regularly interact with each other. The family stress theory acknowledges stress as an unavoidable experience for any family and explores healthy and unhealthy ways in which the family reacts to stress (Walsh, 2016). The family stress theory and family development theory are closely related theoretical frameworks (or consist of similar concepts). The family development theory explores the ways in which a family can grow and change as one singular unit over time (Martin, 2018). Family theories should be utilized as an adjunct to a thorough history and physical examination to guide appropriate family-centered care.

## TYPES OF FAMILIES

*Family structure* is a term referring to a group of individuals living and interacting with each other based on roles that each person in the group has mutually defined. Roles and designations can be determined and agreed upon by all members of that group, or they can be influenced by societal customs and traditions. Family roles and structures can change based on life events, experiences, and circumstances that can include marriage, divorce, cohabitation, birth, death, abandonment, or incarceration. According to the American Academy of Pediatrics (AAP, 2020), there are several different types of families, including traditional nuclear, blended, extended, single-parent, binuclear, polygamous, communal, and LGBTQ+. A family's structure has an impact on the child's growth and development, and the nurse practitioner should take this into consideration when developing an individualized patient care plan.

### Traditional Nuclear Family

A traditional nuclear family includes a married man and woman and their biological offspring. A child born from this type of marriage lives with both of their biological parents in the same household and, if there are multiple children, they are full siblings. Extended family members are separated from the nuclear family and this may contribute to fragmentation of the family (AAP, 2015).

### Blended Family

A blended family (also known as a reconstituted family or stepfamily) includes at least one individual designated as a stepparent, who is the spouse of a child's biological parent. Unique challenges are faced by blended families., and they differ greatly from challenges in nuclear families (Kumar, 2017). The stepparent may also have a child from a previous relationship. In this case, the two children would be considered stepsiblings. In addition, the children involved need time to learn and adapt to a new life with new people.

### Extended Family

There are two instances in which a family can be considered an extended family. The first instance includes at least one parent, at least one child, and at least one member of the extended family (e.g., grandparent, aunt, uncle, cousin) living in the same household. When a grandparent lives with their child and grandchildren, they may become an integral part of the family (AAP, 2015). The second instance involves at least one child living with at least one extended family member where the extended family member primarily assumes care and guardianship of the child in the absence of the biological parent. About 6% of children are being raised by the grandparents (Md-Yunus, 2017).

### Single-Parent Family

A single-parent family includes only one parent and at least one child. The single parent may have chosen not to marry or live with the parent of the child(ren). Or it could result from divorce, death, abandonment, or incarceration. An individual may also have personally chosen to be a single parent through artificial insemination, assisted reproductive technology, or adoption through the foster care system. Approximately 32% of children live in a single-parent family (Livingston, 2018). Single parents more often receive financial assistance and practical help (such as looking after the children, cooking, cleaning) from the child's grandparents than do two-parent households (Rabindrakumar, 2018). A larger percentage of children living with single mothers live in poverty as compared to those living with single fathers or in two-parent families (Livingston, 2018).

### Binuclear Family

A binuclear family includes at least one child who spends a designated amount of time between one biological parent and the other biological parent. When parents divorce or separate, the family dynamics shift and with shared custody, parents must redefine their roles. Children then move between two separate households, each headed by one of their parents (Ferraro, 2016). In this case, both parents mutually agree on a set schedule that helps to determine when and how long the child or children stay with each parent. The parents are not married or in a relationship together, but they are maintaining active parenting roles for the child or children between them.

### Polygamous Family

In a polygamous family structure, there is either one man who has two or more wives, or one woman who has two or more husbands. The former of the two is more common, and in this circumstance, each child has the same father, with the potential for half-siblings. Potentially many children can exist in these families, which can have a significant impact on child growth and development when considering the child's need for love and connection from both parents (Al-Sharfi et al., 2015). A polygamous family, while not legally recognized in the United States, is still a family structure that one may come across as a nurse practitioner.

### Communal Family

A communal family is one in which a group of nonrelated individuals live together and interact with each other in a nonnuclear construct. Individuals in a communal family may share possessions and responsibilities, and there are not always clearly defined roles within these communities. Or individual families may each live in a separate home but eat multiple meals together each week and make goods and services available to all members in the community. Children from these types of communities have the opportunity to learn skills from adults other than their parents and benefit from the close-knit physical support (Martin, 2019). This type of family structure values mutual respect and interdependence among its members.

### LGBTQ+ Families

Same-sex couples are able to have families if they so desire. The possibility for having children in these unions may come from a variety of methods (Ferrara et al., 2016), including previous relationships, adoption, surrogacy, and artificial fertilization and insemination. A nonjudgmental approach is imperative when caring for LGBTQ+ families; families exist across a continuum and all families should be recognized as such and treated similarly. It is also important to be aware of families in which the child or adolescent may identify as part of the LGBTQ+ community. Identify this individual as they wish to be identified, and exercise respect and professionalism in all encounters with them. Prejudice and discrimination against the LGBTQ+ child or family members can deter that child's willingness to participate and follow the individualized care plan.

### Foster Care

A child can be placed in foster care for several reasons. If biological parents cannot adequately care for a child, the corresponding state's foster care system typically looks to extended family to assume care of the child. If this cannot be done, then the child may be placed into nonkinship foster care. Sometimes children are placed into a communal home with other children of similar circumstances. Each state has its own set of rules and regulations regarding who can adopt a child and regulations for the adoption process. Care is taken not to separate siblings, but this is a possibility when considering the financial resources and household space that adopting multiple children can entail.

### Adoptive Families

Children may be adopted into any type of family structure. Couples considering adoption should thoroughly research the process in their state and assess their own home situation before beginning the adoption process to ensure that the child or children they are planning to adopt can thrive. When adoption occurs internationally or across states, records review, waiting periods, concerns about fetal exposure, and additional recommended screenings and/or tests can be discussed with the adoptive parent(s) (Yogman et al., 2018). Refer to chapter 44 for additional information. Knowledge of these parameters can aid in the development of an appropriately individualized care plan.

## INTERACTION WITH THE FAMILY

Caring for the pediatric population includes caring not only for children, but also for their family members. The family needs to be viewed as a unit in its entirety because family dynamics play an important role in the growth and development of the child. Additionally, it is important to use effective communication and incorporate appropriate decision-making when addressing the care of the child and family. In order to be active participants in decision-making related to the health and comfort of the child, parents/caregivers will need clear, truthful, and complete information (Richards et al., 2017). Parents are most appreciative when healthcare providers explain all aspects of the child's care in an easy-to-understand manner. Consider utilizing teach-back methods, providing written material that is easy to read and understand, and incorporating the use of images and videos to encompass all ways in which one can learn and comprehend.

Positive outcomes can be attained when the child of appropriate age and developmental level is encouraged to actively participate in their own care. This includes allowing the child to ask questions and voice concerns. Give the child the opportunity to make choices and offer choices that are simple and clear. Take into consideration that children are emotionally connected to and influenced by their family. The concept of family-centered care focuses on acknowledging that the family is the child's most consistent means of self-identification and self-awareness within their world. Family-centered care involves fostering a sustainable professional partnership together with the child and family. Effective communication that includes answering questions truthfully in terms that the child can understand will build and maintain rapport, which is crucial to the child's willingness to participate and follow the individualized care plan.

### Family Support

Family support plays an important role in child growth and development. Families should support children mentally, physically, and emotionally. The ability of a family to financially support a child is also a factor in access to care and healthcare outcomes. Regardless of the type of family, children thrive in a family structure that provides unconditional love, stability, and consistency.

Provide parents of chronically ill children with resources such as access to parent support groups and counseling. This can aid in minimizing caregiver role strain, which will optimize the care the parents will be able to provide to the child or children. A strong family support system can help to guide a child not only in maintaining health, but also in managing acute and chronic illness.

Parents look to healthcare providers to have an appropriate knowledge base with which they can provide the best possible care for the child. The nurse practitioner is often in the unique position to listen to family experiences. With this comes the opportunity to use therapeutic communication to provide real-time, nonjudgmental feedback and education. Recognition and acknowledgment of the needs of the community and reinforcement of the safety initiatives within that community is another facet of family-centered care. Proactively taking the initiative to ensure that children and their families have the necessary resources to adequately participate in and contribute to the individualized care plan effectively promotes patient satisfaction and positive patient care outcomes.

## CULTURE

Culture is rich and deeply rooted, an organ of sustenance that gives rise to ways of belief and knowing within social and organizational constructs. It consists of the material (e.g., physical objects, resources and spaces) and nonmaterial (e.g., values, language, norms, symbols, organization, and institutions) traits that influence how humans view the world, experience it emotionally, and behave in relation to their environments and others (Andrews & Boyle, 2020).

Cultural practices inform inherent views of well and ill states and the significance attributed to them; they shape the standards from which principles of growth and development emerge and directly influence the invisible constructs of attitudes, cultural norms, and expectations that are responsible for the observed behaviors of child rearing (Yildiz et al., 2018). The health of the child cannot be separated from the culture and status of the family unit, the condition of the environments into which children are born and inhabit, and the political and social climates of the day. Child health is the foundation of the health and well-being of future societies, having widespread short- and long-term sociological and economic implications.

Caregivers of different cultures play a crucial role in shaping children's behavior, temperament, and thinking patterns (Slobodskaya et al., 2019). They are credited with the responsibility of preparing their children to interact with a broader society. Caregiver–child interactions serve as a model for future relationships and social interactions, teaching a variety of sociocultural rules, expectations, and taboos. For instance, young children typically develop a conversational style resembling their parents', and that often depends on culture. Cultural differences in interactions between adults and children also influence how a child behaves socially. For example, in Chinese culture, where parents often assume much responsibility and authority over children, parents may interact with children in a more authoritative manner and expect deference from their children. Children growing up in such environments are more likely to adhere to their parents' requests, even when they are reluctant to do so. While children are unique and develop at individual rates, the cultural influence on their development is clearly significant.

Globalization and technology have eliminated ethnic silos and encouraged the intermingling of distinctive cultural elements that retain their essence, rather than a melting or assimilation of heterogeneous parts into one homogenous whole. According to the Pew Research Center analysis of United Nations data from 2017, there are more than 250 million migrants worldwide (Cilluffo & Cohn, 2018). Foreign-born United States (U.S.) citizens account for a near record 14% of the U.S. population, with 2065 projections attributing 88% of the future U.S. population to immigrants and their descendants if current demographic trends continue (Pew Research Center, 2015).

Cultural diversity is rapidly increasing and demands the attention of those who are tasked with meeting the needs of an evolving society, particularly stewards of healthcare. From a quality and safety perspective, quantitative and anecdotal evidence support the linkage between membership of a cultural minority group and healthcare disparities, namely access barriers, decreased quality of rendered healthcare services, and suboptimal outcomes. Racial and ethnic minorities are more likely to be uninsured, have higher rates of mortality (e.g., infant mortality and deaths from accidents), and suffer at disproportionate rates from chronic disease (e.g., obesity, asthma, cancer, cardiovascular disease) when compared with their White/Caucasian counterparts (Carratala & Maxwell, 2020).

The untoward consequences of cultural stagnancy include but are not limited to the perpetuation of ethnocentric healthcare delivery systems that are intimidating and increasingly difficult to navigate, systems whose structural policies and procedures miss the marks of equity and inclusion that are the lifeblood of caring professions. An effort must be made to create culturally competent healthcare systems that empower individuals to make informed decisions about health maintenance and illness and injury prevention behaviors within the context of their own cultures, while recognizing the undeniable influence of culture on the attitudes, beliefs, and practices of minority populations and healthcare delivery alike. Many conceptual models exist that address the provision of culturally competent care. Among the most prominent models are themes of cultural humility, cultural awareness, cultural knowledge, cultural encounter, and cultural desire.

## CULTURAL COMPETENCY

Child primary care providers should develop the skills related to cultural competency. Cultural competency begins with examination of one's own beliefs and values. It includes the development of cultural humility and awareness. In addition, obtaining cultural knowledge is a major component in the establishment of cultural competency.

### Cultural Humility and Awareness

Cultural competence is a continuous process of self-examination, one that calls for an in-depth exploration and recognition of one's own cultural and professional biases, prejudices, and assumptions about other groups through the lens of cultural humility (Alizadeh & Chavan, 2015). To develop cultural humility, practitioners must let go of preconceived notions and labels formerly applied to individuals, groups, places, and circumstances (Rosa, 2017). An understanding of diverse cultural backgrounds may lead practitioners to evaluate their own cultural and religious beliefs, which may in turn influence their practices.

### Cultural Knowledge

The process of obtaining cultural knowledge is active and veracious; it entails, first, procuring factual information that pertains to the material and nonmaterial cultural traits of diverse groups. In the theoretical sense, it is the act of wearing another's shoes and empathetically examining how their worldview informs their way of being and their lived experiences. From a healthcare perspective, it includes examining the intersection of culture and health-related behaviors and the influence that each exerts on healthcare outcomes, particularly as it relates to genetic and social determinants of health and patterns of disease incidence and prevalence among diverse groups. It is a process that may begin in the classroom but must extend beyond, to incorporate experiences with diverse groups over time and reflection on those experiences.

## GENETICS

Genetics plays an important role in a child's ability to grow and develop. The term *genetics* refers to the study of hereditary constructs and their influence on varying traits and attributes as they are passed from parent to offspring and from generation to generation. Recall that genes and traits have long been identified using what is widely known as Mendelian inheritance, which categorizes them as either dominant or recessive. *Genes* are the units of heredity passed from parents to children, containing all of the material required to specify traits, as well as pass on certain disease. "The genome is an organism's complete set of deoxyribonucleic acid (DNA) ... that contains the genetic instructions needed to develop and direct the activities of every organism" (National Human Genome Research Institute, n.d., line 1).

Family history directly influences whether a child might develop certain genetic disorders, disease processes, and conditions. A genetic disorder is a disease process that is caused by a variation in the DNA sequence due to a mutation in one or more genes, either acquired at birth or over the course of a person's life. Individuals directly descended from family members with specific genetic disorders have a high likelihood of also being born with or developing the same conditions. Innovations in healthcare have created opportunities for individuals to test their genetics for abnormalities before reproduction. With these opportunities, families can properly engage in family planning and be aware of all possible reproductive outcomes. A thorough history and physical examination is essential in identifying any genetic disorders or disease processes a child may have, as well as identifying conditions they are at greater risk of developing later in life.

## SOCIAL AND COMMUNITY INFLUENCES

Children are certainly influenced by their surroundings and their immediate environment. Communities serve as a mechanism of opportunity, development, and growth for children and families. Community influences can originate in neighborhoods, schools, or other organizations and can function through children's peer groups, the adults with whom children come into contact, or the larger set of social and cultural practices in neighborhoods. The child's community may have a positive or negative affect on the child's health and development. When the community is able to provide high-quality early childhood education, socioemotional and cognitive development in young children are promoted. High-quality preschool education has a positive long-term effect on academic performance and occupational outcome (AAP, Council on Community Pediatrics, 2016). Conversely, communities can also contribute to toxic stress if violence and poverty are pervasive. Toxic stress responses damage child development and have lifelong effects on learning, behavior, and overall health (Center on the Developing Child, 2016).

Humans are innately social beings and need social interaction to maintain mental and emotional well-being. Although social influences are important for children of all ages, their nature and form change over the progression of childhood. Community conditions can adversely affect children's development, especially in the case of children growing up in dangerous and socially disorganized communities (Gratale et al., 2020).

### SOCIOECONOMIC CHARACTERISTICS

The socioeconomic characteristics of a community have strong associations with certain individual health outcomes such as birth weight, infant mortality, mental health, and cardiovascular risks (Gratale et al., 2020). Neighborhood and community processes may affect children's development in certain ways. The neighborhood's institutions and systems (e.g., schools, quality of food markets, healthcare facilities, public health, and law enforcement agencies) rather than individual neighbors can make a difference in influencing health behaviors and outcomes.

Poverty is a highly prevalent risk factor for children in the United States and is linked to a host of negative health risks and delays in development. Even as the poverty rate rises, it does not reflect the number of families who do not have sufficient resources to meet their basic needs for housing, childcare, food, transportation, healthcare, or other expenses. Food insecurity is more prevalent among low socioeconomic households and negatively affects children, particularly infants. In food-insecure households, infants face negative health outcomes including poor motor skills, age-normed growth stunting (low length-for-age), and wasting (low weight-for-age). Poverty is also associated with higher rates of childhood obesity. Childhood obesity rates are highest in communities that lack access to healthy fruits and vegetables and full-service grocery stores.

## SCHOOLS AND EARLY EDUCATION PROGRAMS

Daycare programs, preschools, and schools should be places for children to play, learn, and grow. When children are in these settings, they expand their relationships and connections with peers and authority figures other than their parents or caregivers. Schools play a major role in the process of a child's socialization and the shaping of a child's development (Wentzel, 2015). While in school, children are taught based on a curriculum, and throughout the school day they are influenced by their teachers and peers. Characteristics of the school, teachers, and peer groups all influence the socialization of children within school settings. Although the family continues to be a primary part of children's socialization, children will have other important people in their lives from whom they will learn the skills of social interaction. The school setting is where the learning of the new role as a student occurs. When children begin school, they are socialized to respect authority and how to be a citizen within society.

The overall socialization of children, as theorized by Bronfenbrenner (1979), is disseminated into various realms that focus on the different areas of social context that children experience in their lives. Families and schools are key contributors to socialization, but there are other systems of socialization within ecological systems theory. The child interacts with many aspects of the environment, all of which contribute to the child's social development. The overall outcome of socialization is theorized to be the result of how all the systems interact with one another.

A major objective of socialization in the school setting is to make a child socially competent. Children must develop skills that allow them to function socially, emotionally, and intellectually within the school environment. Within the school setting, social competence is achieved when students adopt and achieve socially approved goals. These goals (e.g., learning to share, participating in lessons, working in groups), when embraced, also serve to integrate the child into social groups at school. Social approval is obtained when children accept the goals of the school setting, and they are acknowledged and reinforced on a consistent basis through social acceptance by teachers and other peers.

## COMMUNITY RESOURCES

Parents play a key role in educating and supporting their children. However, parents also rely on resources within their community—including teachers, healthcare providers, and other key members (e.g., spiritual leaders, family, friends)—to fulfill their parenting role. The degree of cohesion among members of the community (measured, for example, by the presence or absence of community organizations or community activism) influences the nature of these relationships. Communities characterized by high levels of cohesion, such as those with active community groups, provide valuable opportunities for individuals to become involved in and develop richer connections within their community.

# ENVIRONMENTAL INFLUENCES

A child's environment can include the different sights and experiences the child encounters each day and can influence early learning, growth, and development. The child's environment encompasses the mood and setting that occur at home, at school, at daycare, in the neighborhood, and in other areas where the child spends a significant amount of time. The child's behaviors may also be affected by the home environment and by relationships formed with neighbors. If the child lives in an environment that is overcrowded or chaotic, it can have a negative impact on a child's personality and behavior. Too many people living in the same house can reduce the time spent with the child, as the parents' time and attention are occupied elsewhere in the household. These distractions may result in the child resorting to other ways of keeping busy and distancing themself mentally and emotionally early in life. Parents have the responsibility of establishing a suitable environment for the child, as it will affect personality development, learning, and behavior.

Early home environment has a profound effect on a child's health and well-being. Beginning in infancy, a difficult home environment can disrupt the brain's stress response system, reduce the quality of caregiving a child receives, and interfere with healthy development. Brain imaging research suggests that growing up in a poorly resourced environment may be associated with disruptions in brain development (Hair et al., 2015). For example, living in an environment surrounded by chaos and poverty can lead to changes in the brain's stress system that increase a child's vulnerability to chronic diseases that may develop in childhood or adolescence, and persist throughout the lifespan.

## PRENATAL EXPOSURE

Safety promotion is important throughout a woman's pregnancy because the prenatal period is a critical timeframe for the developing fetus. Exposing the fetus to harmful substances during the gestational period has the possibility of causing great damage to neuromuscular and cognitive development and function of the fetus through birth, infancy, and throughout the lifespan. A thorough history of the mother's health should include inquiry about prescription medications that may negatively affect fetal development. The most commonly abused substances during pregnancy include alcohol, cocaine, tobacco, and marijuana. Additionally, it is important not only to be aware of the effects on the fetus from methamphetamine exposure, but also to acknowledge that opiate use has skyrocketed in recent years in the American population. It is important to recognize the signs and symptoms of substance exposure in infancy and be able to assess the need to conduct effective screening and education for expectant mothers of all ages across the lifespan.

### Alcohol Exposure

Alcohol misuse during pregnancy has the potential to delay cognitive processing as it pertains to infant growth and development, potentially resulting in fetal alcohol spectrum disorder (FASD). FASD refers to a group of conditions that have the potential to develop in an infant whose mother has consumed alcoholic beverages of any amount during the pregnancy. These conditions are irreversible and have no cure. Currently, there is no particularly safe amount of alcohol or timeframe in which alcohol can be consumed during the gestational period (Dejong et al., 2019). Because of this, those of childbearing age who are pregnant or planning to become pregnant should not consume alcohol at any point within the first three months prior to conception and should be encouraged to avoid drinking alcohol at any time during the gestational period after conception to promote positive fetal outcomes. Refer to chapter 39 for additional information related to FASD.

### Cocaine Exposure

Cocaine is a central nervous system (CNS) stimulant and peripheral sympathomimetic drug that usually comes in the form of a fine, white powder, and when attained illicitly can be mixed with a plethora of other addictive and nonaddictive substances. Cocaine has the potential to induce fetal hypoxemia by impairing uterine circulation. It can also impair cardiac and immune function for the developing fetus. Infants born to mothers who use cocaine during pregnancy are at risk for lower birth weights, shorter birth lengths, and smaller head circumferences. According to the National Institute on Drug Abuse (NIDA, 2016a, 2016b), cocaine ingestion and consumption during fetal development can lead to later deficits in some children, including behavior regulation problems, cognitive deficits, difficulty with information processing, and decreased attention span.

### Tobacco Exposure

The nicotine in cigarettes and tobacco products is a potent vasoconstrictor, and thus can cause decreased oxygen and nutrient circulation through the mother's bloodstream and reduce the supply to the fetus. Without adequate oxygenation and nutrition from the mother, the fetus is at risk for adverse conditions at birth, including low birth weight and physical defects of the mouth and lip (NIDA, 2020). In addition, tobacco can decrease neurological development, negatively affecting memory and cognition, altering behavior regulation capacities, and lessening hearing ability from infancy and into adulthood (NIDA, 2020). It is necessary to educate pregnant patients about the possibility of adverse birth events related to the use of e-cigarettes. E-cigarettes and any other form of vaping are capable of transferring nicotine from mother to baby just as readily as traditional smoking does.

### Marijuana Exposure

Marijuana is a plant-based substance smoked or ingested by individuals. Δ-9-tetrahydrocannabinol (THC) and other cannabinoids cross the placenta when a mother smokes during pregnancy. THC disturbs normal functioning of the endocannabinoid system in the brain and other parts of the body and may have long-term effects on prenatal development (NIDA, 2019a). Of greatest concern is the possibility of marijuana use in combination with other harmful substances, as this can compound negative effects for the fetus. It is recommended that those of childbearing age who are pregnant or looking to become pregnant should avoid marijuana use for the entire pregnancy. Further research must be conducted to determine short-term effects of marijuana use on the fetus, as well as long-term effects in infancy and across the lifespan.

### Methamphetamine Exposure

Methamphetamine is a CNS stimulant that has a white, odorless powder consistency and easily dissolves in alcohol- or water-based solutions. Methamphetamine use during pregnancy is associated with preterm delivery and low birth weight (Wright et al., 2015). Exposed infants are at increased risk for lethargy and neuromuscular changes with regard to extremity movement. Other physiological effects to the infant after birth can potentially include changes in heart rate and rhythm, vomiting, poor weight gain, and recurrent infections (NIDA, 2019b). Infants should be closely monitored if it is known or suspected that the mother used methamphetamines during the gestational period.

### Opioid Exposure

Opiate and narcotic medications are generally prescribed to individuals to treat pain. However, an individual can become addicted to these medications. Examples of narcotics that are commonly abused are heroin and fentanyl. Opiates and narcotics have a low molecular weight, which means that they can easily advance across the placental barrier and flow into fetal circulation (Anand & Campbell-Yeo, 2015). Other chemical substances in the opiate and narcotic classification that may cause neonatal withdrawal include caffeine, methadone, and PCP. Neonatal abstinence syndrome (NAS) is a group of symptoms that describe an infant experiencing withdrawal related to any particular substance ingested or consumed by the mother. Clinical manifestations of NAS may include irritability, seizures, trouble sleeping, tremors, rhinorrhea, dyspnea, poor feeding and poor weight gain, vomiting, diarrhea, and fevers (Anand & Campbell-Yeo, 2015). The reversal agent of choice for opiates and narcotics is naloxone (Narcan). Refer to chapter 42 for additional information related to NAS.

### Radiation Exposure

Pregnant women potentially may be exposed to radiation either occupationally or from diagnostic imaging. Typically, these are low-dose exposures and are less likely to negatively affect the health of the fetus because several layers of protection are provided by the uterus and placental tissues (Centers for Disease Control and Prevention [CDC], 2020). Exposure above the regulatory limits, however, can cause harm to the developing fetus. Based on the stage of fetal development, doses greater than 0.5 grey (Gy) can be dangerous and result in severe health consequences (CDC, 2020). These health consequences can include growth restriction, malformations, impaired brain function, and cancer (CDC, 2020). Essentially, exposure to radiation is less likely than other substances to cause infant harm, although it pose possible risk to the developing fetus.

## SOCIAL MEDIA

As never witnessed before, the information superhighway has formed a web of global connectivity facilitating the often uninhibited and instantaneous exchange of knowledge, mass media communications, entertainment, and social correspondence. Online platforms that make possible the sharing of information, ideas, electronic communications, and personal branding in synchronous and/or asynchronous formats are the basis of social media and social networking.

The advantages associated with the use of social media are accompanied by notable negatives. The social media paradox is that connectivity often breeds disconnection. Networking is accomplished through artificial means outside of the context of human interface. Instant access and gratification limit the capacity for patience and attention. Limited experiences of mindful, therapeutic communication inhibit language acquisition and command and hinder the development of interpersonal skills. There is a steady assault of images, advertisements, and media ploys designed to pique the most primal of instincts. Misinformation, security breaches, the presentation of false narratives and idealistic facades have demonstrable connections to fraud, anxiety, depression, loneliness, disrupted images of self, and egocentrism.

### Cyberbullying

Cyberbullying has emerged as a formidable foe. A single, unified definition of cyberbullying does not exist, but cyberbullying is thought to encompass the following components: intentionality, an act of aggression, and an imbalance of power (Giumetti & Kowalski, 2019). The cloak of anonymity and the withdrawal of proximity provided by the online environment encourage the exercise of free agency, sometimes to the detriment of society. Recent research suggests high variability in cyberbullying prevalence rates, ranging from 2.8% to 50% for reports of cyberbullying victimization and 5% to 33% for cyberbullying perpetration (Giumetti & Kowalski, 2019). The degree of variability may be attributed to the lack of consensus on a formal definition of *cyberbullying*, which contributes to the inconsistent documentation of the observed phenomenon and the lack of longitudinal research that incorporates the use of a representative sample. Additional studies that examine the link between race/ethnicity and sexual orientation and cyberbullying are needed (Giumetti & Kowalski, 2019). This information is integral to the development of anti-cyberbullying initiatives that are especially efficacious for children and adolescents.

## FIREARM-RELATED INJURIES

Firearm-related injuries accounted for 15% of deaths among children and adolescents in 2016; with respect to intent, the data specify that 59% of firearm deaths were homicides, 25% were suicides, and 4% were unintentional injuries (Cunningham et al., 2018). The rate of firearm deaths among children and adolescents in the United States is higher than all other countries with available data; 90% of firearm-related deaths in children under 15 years old occur in the United States (Flaherty & Klig, 2020). A staggering 28% increase in the rate of firearm deaths was observed between 2013 and 2016 (Cunningham et al., 2018). Differences in the observed rates may be attributed to laws governing the purchase of firearms and ammunition, storage practices, geographical location, and adolescent developmental considerations. While the firearm mortality rates of children and adolescents in rural and urban settings were comparable, the firearm homicide rate was 2.3 times as high among urban youth as among rural youth, and the firearm suicide rate was 2.1 times as high among rural youth as among urban youth (Cunningham et al., 2018).

The growing and developing bodies of children and adolescents lack the natural protective mechanisms that the adult client possesses; developing skin, bone, and muscle tissues lack the ability to absorb the kinetic energy of penetrating forces, predisposing children to increased rates of more severe injury (Flaherty & Klig, 2020). Commonly observed primary firearm-related injuries include penetrating head trauma, intra-abdominal wounds, and extremity trauma; common secondary complications include acute respiratory distress syndrome (ARDS), pneumonia, and cardiac arrest (Flaherty & Klig, 2020). Unfortunately, up to half of children who survive hospitalization for firearm-related injuries are discharged with a disability, including ongoing psychological consequences (Flaherty & Klig, 2020).

Reduced pediatric firearm-related injuries have been associated with the enforcement of laws that require universal background checks and permits to purchase firearms, a minimum purchasing age of 21 years, and safe firearm and ammunition storage efforts (Flaherty & Klig, 2020). In addition, communities have firearm safety initiatives in place at local businesses and hospitals, and parents who own firearms are encouraged to become familiar with these initiatives to promote child safety within the home.

## WATER AND AIR POLLUTION

Long-term exposure to chemicals in the water and air can potentially damage or delay both physical and neurological development in children. Pollution is associated with several noncommunicable diseases in children, such as low birth weight, asthma, cancer, and neurodevelopmental disorders (Landrigan et al., 2019). Exposures to pollution in the water and air, at times, are unavoidable owing to home environment and geographical location, which are both generally out of the child's control. Positive outcomes may be influenced by effective communication and good rapport with children and their families. Thus, the nurse practitioner can learn about the family's external environment and how it may influence the health of the child.

Water can become polluted when chemicals from littered trash, landfill waste, and agricultural pesticide use are absorbed into the nearby water supply. Most of the time, water gets filtered and then distributed within the community. However, at times, water has to go under a "boil order" because of an unexpected circumstance where water was contaminated in a particular area, such as when a natural disaster occurs. Water contamination can adversely affect the integumentary system, exacerbating conditions such as eczema and psoriasis, as well as the gastrointestinal system, commonly causing abdominal pain, nausea, vomiting, and diarrhea (Walker et al., 2019). Potential parasitic infections can occur, which can further damage the circulatory and nervous systems, leading to more serious conditions such as seizures, sepsis, and meningitis. Drinking, bathing, or swimming in water that is contaminated can make people sick and can negatively affect child growth and development. Information related to the safety of drinking water may be found on the Environmental Protection Agency website at https://ofmpub.epa.gov/apex/sfdw/f?p=108:200.

When toxic chemicals are emitted and dispersed into the atmosphere, they begin to negatively change the quality of the air. Some sources of air pollution include gas emissions from vehicles, chemical residuals from factories and other industrial buildings, and smoke from wildfires and volcanoes. Air pollution can affect the function of many different body systems. Impairment may occur in brain-related functions such as perceptual and sensory information processing, intellectual and cognitive development, memory and executive functions, and emotion and self-regulation (D'Angiulli, 2018). Air pollution exacerbates asthma by increasing dyspnea and adventitious lung sounds and irritates eczema by increasing inflammation and subsequent pruritis. Air pollution also aggravates many autoimmune diseases due to increased cellular inflammation and tissue damage. A thorough history and physical examination can identify premature infants, as well as children with respiratory disorders and autoimmune diseases, as being at risk for serious secondary effects from exposure to toxic chemicals in the air within their community.

## HEAVY METALS

Heavy metals are naturally existing elements that have fairly high atomic weight and a minimum density five times the density of water (Osman et al., 2019). Heavy metals include mercury, lead, chromium, cadmium, barium, aluminum, and copper. Environmental and public health concerns have been raised due to the dangerous effects of exposure. Heavy metals can be found in industries, homes, agriculture, and medicine, leading to their widespread presence in the environment. Most heavy metals are considered highly toxic. They also have numerous exposure routes, including ingestion, inhalation, and dermal absorption, subsequently producing some health effects resulting from human contact with heavy metals. The implications of heavy metals with regard to children's health have been noted to be more severe compared with adults' health. The elements' harmful consequences for children include neurocognitive disorders, behavioral disorders, respiratory problems, cancer, and cardiovascular diseases.

## MANMADE CHEMICALS

Manmade chemicals can adversely affect growth and development of the child. Examples of these chemicals include pesticides, pool chemicals, and endocrine disruptors. Many of these chemicals can be found in common household products. Frequent education to parents is required to ensure that all pesticide chemicals are kept out of reach of children. The national hotline phone number for the Poison Control Centers is 1-800-222-1222. It is important as a provider to know or have access to this number as a means to help guide the plan of care for parents who are concerned that their children may have come in contact with harmful substances. Additionally, the website www.healthychildren.org, created by the AAP, has a full list of exposure prevention strategies. It is updated regularly and has proven to be an invaluable resource that can be shared with parents to promote child safety at home.

### Pesticides

Pesticides are divided into several different categories:

- Insecticides for insects and mites. They can be found in insect repellents, garden and orchard sprays, flea and tick collars, and mothballs.
- Herbicides are used for weeds in the yard. They can be found in weed killers and other lawn care products.
- Rodenticides are used for all rodents, including mice and rats. They are used in any mouse and rat bait products.
- Fungicides are used for mold and mildew. They can be found in flower sprays and paint additives.
- Disinfectants are used for mold and mildew as well, but they also are used for any bacteria. They can be found in bleach and ammonia, kitchen and bathroom cleaners, and pool and spa cleaners.
- Pesticide chemicals can also be found in some wood preservatives and protectants.

Pesticide exposure can have dangerous consequences for all individuals, but children especially. Children are at higher risk for health effects from exposure to pesticides than adults, because their internal organs are still developing and maturing (AAP, 2020). Education on preventive measures is paramount, and parents should be provided with resources on how to reduce exposure. Organic produce, though more costly, has been determined to have fewer pesticides and drug-resistant bacteria than regular produce items. A more cost-effective intervention with produce involves washing fruits and vegetables before eating them, especially when bought from farmer's markets.

### Pool Chemicals

As previously mentioned, pool and spa cleaners are disinfectants. Chlorine and bromine are two chemicals used to disinfect pools; however, the chemical most commonly used to clean pools is chlorine. Obtain a thorough history and physical examination because chlorine can have a drying effect on skin, which can potentially exacerbate eczema for some children. Encourage these children and their family members to incorporate showering immediately after swimming in a chlorinated pool to avoid skin irritation. Urge children to avoid drinking and swallowing swimming pool water whenever possible, to prevent ingestion of chlorine. According to Geisenger Health (2017), a child that may have been exposed to or ingested too much chlorine may experience symptoms such as vision changes, decreased blood pressure, dyspnea, dysphagia, abdominal pain, hematochezia, and vomiting. Educate parents to properly store cleaning products away from areas that are easily accessible to children, and stress that children should not take part in setup of pool-cleaning processes.

### Endocrine Disrupters

Endocrine-disrupting chemicals (EDCs) can be found in a variety of everyday objects and materials. EDCs are chemicals that block or disable proper function of the glands in the endocrine system. Many EDCs have effects on the pituitary gland and thereby exert influence on various endocrine axes. The results are concerns such as precocious or delayed puberty and circadian disruption (Lauretta et al., 2019). Recall that the pituitary gland is one of the most essential glands in the endocrine system and is responsible for a multitude of body functions because it is the glandular control center of the entire body. EDCs can cause serious adverse effects on child growth and development.

According to the National Institute of Environmental Health Services (2020), common EDCs include bisphenol A (BPA), found in many plastic products and food storage containers; perchlorate, found in drinking water and fireworks; phthalates, found in food packaging, cosmetics, children's toys, and medical devices; phytoestrogens, which have hormone-like activity and are found in soy products like tofu or soy milk; and triclosan, found in some antimicrobial and personal care products, such as body washes. Consider the increased risk of exposure in the pediatric population from infancy to young adult ages regarding the use of some of the preceding products. A thorough history and physical examination are paramount when children present with symptoms after recently handling common materials.

Effects of EDCs on the pituitary gland were mentioned earlier, but that is not the only component of the endocrine system that is at risk. The glands of the reproductive system are, arguably, the most vulnerable to EDCs. According to Lauretta et al. (2019), it is possible that EDCs can play a role in decreasing male and female fertility and damaging androgenic function for testicular and ovarian health, but more research must be conducted to determine specific trends and correlations. Little research is available with regard to the effects of EDCs on the adrenal glands. EDCs may also alter iodine absorption, negatively affecting the thyroid gland's structure and function with the potential to cause hypothyroidism (Lauretta et al., 2019). The nurse practitioner should maintain awareness of EDCs, as they have been linked to the development of reproductive, brain, and immune dysfunctions.

## PHYSICAL HAZARDS

Physical hazards (such as motor vehicle accidents, firearms, and lack of use of recommended safety equipment) also exert an influence on child health. Amid a global society that has no shortage of public health crises, the issue of unintentional injury continues to rise above others demanding urgent attention. Consistently, unintentional injury monopolizes annual childhood morbidity and mortality rates. In 2016, the most recent year with published national data in the United States, there were 20,360 deaths among children and adolescents (1–19 years of age); "more than 60% resulted from injury-related causes" (Cunningham et al., 2018). Equally troubling are the emotional and psychological sequelae that emerge and the undeniable economic burden, stretching into the billions of dollars annually, incurred as the result of costly medical treatment and lost productivity. The most prominent mechanisms of injury among children and adolescents originate from physical hazards.

The term *physical hazards* describes an existing or potential danger that can cause serious bodily harm or death through contact, encompassing chemicals that can perpetuate harm through skin or eye contact rather than inhalation (Occupational Safety and Health Administration [OSHA], 2015). Injury, disability, or death due to falls, fire or burns, drug overdose or poisoning, drowning, and suffocation are not uncommon. However, morbidity and mortality rates are categorically dominated by motor vehicle crashes (MVCs), which account for 20% of deaths among children and adolescents (Cunningham et al., 2018). Of overall deaths, 15% are attributed to the second leading cause of death among this population, firearm-related injuries (Cunningham et al., 2018).

Motor vehicle and roadway usage present countless opportunities for physical injury on a daily basis. Distracted, reckless, or inebriated driving, environmental hazards, the use of excessive traveling speeds, and the poor or noncompliant use of safety devices pose a threat to safe roadways and their occupants alike. Children, who are innately curious, self-willed, and not yet in full control of their personal faculties, are especially vulnerable to physical hazards in their immediate and frequented environments. When considering MVC involvement, certain innate qualities of the developing child make fertile the grounds for developing head, neck, spine, and thoracic injuries. In infants and young children, the disproportionate size and weight of the head in relation to the rest of the body, a thin skull allowing for easy deformation, weak neck ligaments and muscles, and poorly protected thoracic and abdominal organs pose threats when encountering significant external acceleration and deceleration forces (Figaji, 2017). The most recent report issued by the U.S. Department of Transportation, National Highway Traffic Safety Administration (NHTSA, 2010) says that the most common injuries sustained by children ages 1 to 8 years in MVCs include head injuries (e.g., concussions, lacerations, and contusions), thoracic injuries (lung contusions or lacerations, rib fractures), abdominal injuries (liver, spleen, small and large bowel injury, and kidney injury), upper extremity injuries (clavicular, humeral, radial, and ulnar fractures), and lower extremity injuries (fractures of the pelvic, femur, tibia, and fibula).

Steps should be taken to mitigate the risk factors associated with the prevalence of unintentional injury, while considering highly influential factors such as age, developmental level, the interplay of societal norms and values, governmental regulation, health disparities and global comparisons in mortality and morbidity data. Unintentional injury, disability, and death resulting from physical hazards are preventable and require widespread vigilance and the development and adoption of evidence-based health promotion and injury preventative measures to lessen their impact at the individual, local, and national levels.

## BEHAVIORAL AND SOCIAL HAZARDS

A child's social environment is mainly determined by where the parents live and enroll children in school. Children form social connections within their environment, and the quality of these social connections or relationships is important. As such, parents' decisions about where to live, work, and have their children attend school can ultimately affect the health and well-being of their children.

Growing up in a positive social environment is associated with less risk-taking behavior. Children who grow up in positive environments are less likely to experience accidents requiring treatment than those who do not. There is also a reduced risk of developing a substance use disorder among children who have positive social relationships compared with those who do not. A higher level of social organization in a neighborhood is associated with better family and child outcomes. Neighborhoods in which parents frequently come into contact with one another and share values are more likely to monitor the behavior of and potential dangers to children (Health Engine, 2010; McDonell & Sianko, 2020).

Social organization is affected by the degree of sprawl in a community; increased sprawl restricts the time and energy people have available for civic involvement and reduces the opportunities for spontaneous, informal social interactions. Sprawl is also associated with decreased use of public facilities, reducing opportunities to mingle with other people, segregating people, and disrupting continuity of community across the lifespan. There is evidence supporting the idea that mixed-use, walkable neighborhoods contribute to social capital, as measured by knowing one's neighbors and being socially active (Oidjarv, 2018).

## THE ROLE OF THE NURSE PRACTITIONER

Every healthcare encounter presents an opportunity to maximize health promotion and injury and illness prevention for the child, family, and community. Screening measures and anticipatory guidance should be facilitated in a way that acknowledges the influence of genetic factors, family structure and function, culture, and the environment on a child's overall well-being, as they capitalize upon individual, family, and community strengths. Nurse practitioners are well positioned to identify risk and protective factors that have the potential to influence childhood growth and development through skillful observations of the child and family in the context of their immediate environment and society at large and authentic, informed, ethical patient–provider interactions.

## KEY POINTS

- Child health cannot be separated from genetic influences, the culture and status of the family unit, the condition of the environments in which children are born and inhabit, and the political and social climates of the day.
- Cultural awareness, cultural humility, and cultural competence across pediatric healthcare settings are important in delivery of family-centered care.
- Family structure and function have a strong influence on child growth and development.
- Prenatal exposure to harmful substances can cause lasting negative effects on children throughout the lifespan.
- Provision of equitable healthcare services to children and families relies upon a comprehensive consideration of factors that influence child health and the optimization of community and education-based resources.

## REFERENCES


Alizadeh, S., & Chavan, M. (2015). Cultural competence dimensions and outcomes: A systematic review of literature. *Health and Social Care in the Community, 24*(6), e117–e130. https://doi.org/10.1111/hsc.12293

Al-Sharfi, M., Pfeffer, K., & Miller, K. A. (2015). The effects of polygamy on children and adolescents: A systematic review. *Journal of Family Studies, 22*(3), 272–286. https://doi.org/10.1080/13229400.2015.1086405

American Academy of Pediatrics. (2015). *The "perfect" family.* https://www.healthychildren.org/English/family-life/family-dynamics/Pages/The-Perfect-Family.aspx

American Academy of Pediatrics. (2020). *Protecting children from pesticides: Information for parents.* https://www.healthychildren.org/English/safety-prevention/all-around/Pages/Protecting-Children-from-Pesticides-Information-for-Parents.aspx

American Academy of Pediatrics, Council on Community Pediatrics. (2016). Poverty and child health in the United States. *Pediatrics, 137*(4), e20160339. https://doi.org/10.1542/peds.2016-0339

Anand, K. J., & Campbell-Yeo, M. (2015). Consequences of prenatal opioid use for newborns. *Acta Paediatrica, 104*(11), 1066–1069. https://doi.org/10.1111/apa.13121

Andrews, M. M., & Boyle, J. S. (2020). Chapter 1: Theoretical foundations of transcultural nursing. In M. M. Andrews, J. S. Boyle, & J. W. Collins, *Transcultural concepts in nursing care* (8th ed., pp. 3–29). Wolters Kluwer Health.

Billings, D. M., & Halstead, J. A. (2020). *Teaching in nursing: A guide for faculty* (6th ed.). Elsevier.

Bronfenbrenner, U. (1979). *The ecology of human development: Experiments by nature and design.* Harvard University Press.

Carratala, S., & Maxwell, C. (2020). *Fact sheet: Health disparities by race and ethnicity.* https://cdn.americanprogress.org/content/uploads/2020/05/06130714/HealthRace-factsheet.pdf

Center on the Developing Child. (2016). *Applying the science of child development in child welfare systems.* http://www.developingchild.harvard.edu

Centers for Disease Control and Prevention. (2020). *Radiation and pregnancy: Information for clinicians.* https://www.cdc.gov/nceh/radiation/emergencies/prenatalphysician.htm

Cilluffo, A., & Cohn, D. (2018). *7 demographic trends shaping the U.S. and the world in 2018.* https://www.pewresearch.org/fact-tank/2018/04/25/7-demographic-trends-shaping-the-u-s-and-the-world-in-2018

Cunningham, R. M., Walton, M. A., & Carter, P. M. (2018). The major causes of death in children and adolescents in the United States. *The New England Journal of Medicine, 379*(25), 2468–2475. https://www.nejm.org/doi/10.1056/NEJMsr1804754

D'Angiulli, A. (2018). Severe urban outdoor air pollution and children's structural and functional brain development, from evidence to precautionary strategic action. *Frontiers in Public Health, 6*, 1–7. http://doi.org/10.3389/fpubh.2018.00095

Dejong, K., Olyaei, A., & Lo, J. O. (2019). Alcohol use in pregnancy. *Clinical Obstetrics and Gynecology, 62*(1), 142–155. https://doi.org/10.1097/GRF.0000000000000414

Ferrara, P., Corsello, G., Sbordone, A., Cutrona, C., Ehrich, J., & Pettoello-Mantovani, M. (2016). The role of pediatricians in caring for the well-being of children living in new types of families. *The Journal of Pediatrics, 176*, 226–228. https://doi.org/10.1016/j.jpeds.2016.06.064

Ferraro, A. J. (2016). Binuclear families. *Encyclopedia of Family Studies.* https://doi.org/10.1002/9781119085621.wbefs024

Figaji, A. (2017). Anatomical and physiological differences between children and adults relevant to traumatic brain injury and the implications for clinical assessment and care. *Frontiers in Neurology, 8*(685), 1–15. https://doi.org/10.3389/fneur.2017.00685

Flaherty, M. R., & Klig, J. E. (2020). Firearm-related injuries in children and adolescents: An emergency and critical care perspective. *Current Opinion in Pediatrics, 32*(3), 349–353. https://doi.org/10.1097/MOP.0000000000000905

Geisenger Health. (2017). *Gulp—Don't drink the pool water!* https://www.geisinger.org/health-and-wellness/

wellness-articles/2017/06/20/20/26/gulp-dont-drink-the-pool-water
Giumetti, G., & Kowalski, R. (2019). *Cyberbullying in schools, workplaces, and romantic relationships: The many lenses and perspectives of electronic mistreatment*. Routledge. https://doi.org/10.4324/9781315110554
Gratale, D. J., Counts, N., Hogan, L., Hewitt, A., Chang, D., Wong, C., Davis, M., Schoessow, G., McCabe, M. A., Johnson, K., Goldfinger, J., & Gionfriddo, P. (2020). Accountable communities for health for children and families: Approaches for catalyzing and accelerating success. *NAM Perspectives*. https://doi.org/10.31478/202001b
Hair, N. L., Hanson, J. L., Wolfe, B. L., & Pollak, S. D. (2015). Association of child poverty, brain development, and academic achievement. *JAMA Pediatrics, 169*(9), 822–829. https://doi.org/10.1001/jamapediatrics.2015.1475
Health Engine. (2010). *Parenting, the social environment, and its effects on child development*. https://healthengine.com.au/info/parenting-the-social-environment-and-its-effects-on-child-development
Johnson, B. E., & Ray, W. A. (2016). *Family systems theory*. https://doi.org/10.1002/9781119085621.wbefs130
Kumar, K. (2017). The blended family life cycle. *Journal of Divorce and Remarriage, 58*(2), 110–125. https://doi.org/10.1080/10502556.2016.1268019
Landrigan, P. J., Fuller, R., Fisher, S., Suk, W. A., Sly, P., Chiles, T. C., & Bose-O'Reilly, S. (2019). Pollution and children's health. *Science of the Total Environment, 650*, 2389–2394. http://doi.org/10.1016/j.scitotenv.2018.09.375
Lauretta, R., Sansone, A., Sansone, M., Romanelli, F., & Appetecchia, M. (2019). Endocrine disrupting chemicals: Effects on endocrine glands. *Frontiers in Endocrinology, 10*, 178. https://doi.org/10.3389/fendo.2019.00178
Livingston, G. (2018). *About one-third of U.S. children are living with an unmarried parent*. https://www.pewresearch.org/fact-tank/2018/04/27/about-one-third-of-u-s-children-are-living-with-an-unmarried-parent
Martin, C. E. (2019). *Coming of age in co-housing*. https://archive.curbed.com/2019/2/13/18194960/cohousing-families-communities-united-states-muir-commons
Martin, T. F. (2018). Family Development Theory 30 years later. *Journal of Family Theory and Review, 10*, 49–69. https://doi.org/10.1111/jftr.12237
McDonell, J.R., & Slanko, N. (2020). Neighborhood, neighborliness, and family and child well-being. *American Journal of Orthopsychiatry*. Advance online publication. https://doi.org/10.1037/ort0000496
Md-Yunus, S. (2017). *Development of well-being in children raised by grandparents*. https://www.childresearch.net/papers/rights/2017_02.html
National Human Genome Research Institute. (n.d.). *Human Genome Project FAQ*. https://www.genome.gov/human-genome-project/Completion-FAQ
National Institute of Environmental Health Services. (2020). *Endocrine disruptors*. https://www.niehs.nih.gov/health/topics/agents/endocrine/index.cfm
National Institute on Drug Abuse. (2016a). *Principles of substance abuse prevention for early childhood*. U.S. Department of Health and Human Services, National Institutes of Health. https://www.drugabuse.gov/publications/principles-substance-abuse-prevention-early-childhood/chapter-3-intervening-in-early-childhood
National Institute on Drug Abuse. (2016b). *What is cocaine?* https://www.drugabuse.gov/publications/research-reports/cocaine/what-cocaine
National Institute on Drug Abuse. (2019a). *Is marijuana safe to use while pregnant or breastfeeding?* https://www.drugabuse.gov/publications/marijuana-safe-to-use-while-pregnant-or-breastfeeding
National Institute on Drug Abuse. (2019b). *What are the risks of methamphetamine misuse during pregnancy?* https://www.drugabuse.gov/publications/research-reports/methamphetamine/what-are-risks-methamphetamine-misuse-during-pregnancy
National Institute on Drug Abuse. (2020). *What are the risks of smoking during pregnancy?* https://www.drugabuse.gov/publications/research-reports/tobacco-nicotine-e-cigarettes/what-are-risks-smoking-during-pregnancy
Occupational Safety and Health Administration. (2015). *Definitions*. https://www.osha.gov/laws-regs/regulations/standardnumber/1926/1926.1202
Oidjarv, H. (2018). The tale of two communities: Residents' perceptions of the built environment and neighborhood social capital. *SAGE Open, 8*, 1–20. https://doi.org/10.1177/2158244018768386
Osman, M., Yang, F., & Massey, I. (2019). Exposure routes and health effects of heavy metals on children. *Biometals, 32*, 563–573. https://doi.org/10.1007/s10534-019-00193-5
Pew Research Center. (2015). *Modern immigration wave brings 59 million to U.S., driving population growth and change through 2065: Views of immigration's impact on U.S. society mixed*. https://www.pewresearch.org/hispanic/wp-content/uploads/sites/5/2015/09/2015-09-28_modern-immigration-wave_REPORT.pdf
Rabindrakumar, S. (2018). *Family portrait: Single parent families and transitions over time*. https://www.greenmebrasil.com/wp-content/uploads/2019/01/Sheffield_Solutions_Modern_Families.pdf
Richards, C. A., Starks, H., O'Connor, M. R., & Doorenbos, A. Z. (2017). Elements of family-centered care in the pediatric intensive care unit: An integrative review. *Journal of Hospice and Palliative Nursing, 19*(3), 238–246. https://doi.org/10.1097/NJH.0000000000000335
Rosa, W. (2017). Immersing in context: A requisite for socially responsible transcultural nursing. *Journal of Transcultural Nursing, 28*(2), 117–118. http://doi.org/10.1177/1043659616689291
Slobodskaya, H., Kozlova, E., Han, S., Gartstein, M., & Putnam, S. (2019). Cross-cultural differences in temperament. In M. Gartstein & S. Putnam (Eds.), *Toddlers, parents, and culture: Findings from the joint effort toddler temperament consortium* (1st ed., pp. 38–45). Routledge.
United States Department of Transportation, National Highway Traffic Safety Administration. (2010). *Children injured in motor vehicle traffic crashes*. https://crashstats.nhtsa.dot.gov/Api/Public/ViewPublication/811325
Walker, D. B., Baumgartner, D. J., Gerba, C. P., & Fitzsimmons, K. (2019). Chapter 16—Surface water Pollution. In M. L. Brusseau, I. L. Pepper, & C. P. Gerba (Eds.), *Environmental and pollution science* (3rd ed., pp. 261–292). https://doi.org/10.1016/B978-0-12-814719-1.00016-1
Walsh, F. (2016). Family resilience: A developmental systems framework. *European Journal of Developmental Psychology, 13*(3), 313–324. https://doi.org/10.1080/17405629.2016.1154035
Wentzel, K. R. (2015). Socialization in school settings. In J. E. Grusec & P. D. Hastings (Eds.), *Handbook of socialization: Theory and research* (2nd ed., pp. 251–275). Guilford Press.

Wright, T. E., Schuetter, R., Tellei, J., & Sauvage, L. (2015). Methamphetamines and pregnancy outcomes. *Journal of Addiction Medicine, 9*(2), 111–117. https://doi.org/10.1097/ADM.0000000000000101

Yildiz, S., Toruner, E. K., & Altay, N. (2018). Effects of different cultures on child health. *Journal of Nursing Research and Practice, 2*(2), 6–10. https://www.pulsus.com/scholarly-articles/effects-of-different-cultures-on-child-health.pdf

Yogman, M., Lavin, A., Cohen, G., & Committee on Psychological Aspects of Child and Family Health. (2018). The prenatal visit. *Pediatrics, 142*(1), e20181218. https://doi.org/10.1542/peds.2018-1218

# Health Assessment

Pamela Bryant and Patricia M. Speck

## Student Learning Outcomes

**Upon completion of this chapter, the reader should be able to:**

1. Adjust elements of the health history depending on the age of the child.
2. Distinguish the physical and developmental changes in growth occurring during the infant, toddler, preschool, school-age, and adolescent periods of development.
3. Identify the appropriate physical examination sequence and health assessment approaches that relate to the child's developmental stage.
4. Discriminate normal health assessment variations from findings indicating potentially serious health alterations.
5. Evaluate the secondary sex characteristics of females and males to determine sexual maturity.

## INTRODUCTION

Dramatic changes occur to children's bodies and minds from infancy through adolescence. The advanced practice provider (APP) must be attentive to the normal changes occurring throughout childhood when obtaining the health history and performing the physical examination. The health history and physical examination are the windows into variations from normal expectations of growth and development and minor disease states. Variations from normal tell the provider what system to follow as well as if it is a normal variant, delayed expression, or actual serious complication of congenital, genetic, or environmental exposure to elements or disease. Approaches to the health history and physical examination of children are different from those used with an adult; one must remember that children are not little adults.

The content in this chapter maps to the following areas on the Pediatric Nursing Certification Board (PNCB) Pediatric Nurse Practitioner—Primary Care certification examination:

CONTENT AREAS:

**II. Assessment and Diagnosis**

**A. Growth and Development**

1. Evaluate and interpret growth parameters
2. Perform developmental surveillance

**B. History and Physical Examination**

1. Obtain history of present illness
2. Obtain a comprehensive health history for new patients
3. Complete an interval history for established patients
4. Perform a review of systems
5. Perform a complete physical examination

**C. Diagnostic Testing and Screening**

1. Order and interpret office/clinic based screening tests

**D. Analyzing Information**

1. Integrate health history and physical examination findings into the plan of care
2. Assimilate findings from screening and diagnostic testing into plan of care

**E. Diagnosis**

1. Establish a diagnosis based on evaluation of patient data

### III. Management

**A. Child and Caregiver Counseling and Education**

1. Provide condition-specific counseling and education, including treatment options

**B. Therapeutic Interventions**

5. Utilize communication techniques and brief cognitive interventions, including motivational interviewing and joint decision-making, to develop health care goals and facilitate change

**C. Collaboration and Referral**

2. Refer to specialists as indicated for evaluation, counseling, and/or treatment
3. Refer children, adolescents, or caregivers to community resources as indicated

**D. Care Coordination**

1. Facilitate patient and family-centered care for children of all ages with acute and chronic conditions

**E. Evaluation and Follow-up**

2. Establish a plan for follow-up care

## COMMUNICATING EFFECTIVELY

A child will adapt very easily to a provider who is at ease, calm, and unhurried. The skilled APP learns that maintaining eye contact with a friendly child and talking softly in an unhurried manner are key to making a child feel relaxed. If the child is avoiding eye contact and clings to the parent or guardian, they are more than likely fearful and will need to be approached slowly while gently talking to them. Also talk with the parent while they are holding the child as the child adapts to the unfamiliar environment. It is best if the parent can hold the child in their lap while you are performing the assessment.

Always establish rapport in conversation with the parent/guardian while maintaining safety, privacy, and confidentiality. Use a slow, nonjudgmental approach. Establishing rapport with the infant or young child may be achieved through play. Always use direct communication in the context of the developmental stage of the child. Children are more comfortable when they know what to expect. With a preschool or school-age child or adolescent, explain what you're going to do during the assessment before you do it. This will help to alleviate any fear or anxiety that they might have and will also give them an opportunity to ask you any questions. As you are conducting the examination, explain what you are doing as you are doing it and why.

## HEALTH HISTORY

The health history is structured to meet the needs of the child and their family and moves through a stepwise analysis. The accuracy of the physical examination and, ultimately, the diagnosis depends heavily on the historian's information. It is important that the APP does not use any medical terminology that may cause confusion. If the historian does not speak English, an interpreter should be provided. The key to obtaining a high-quality health history is to be courteous, provide comfort, connect, and confirm your understanding (Teall & Gawlik, 2021).

A developmental history consists of data that are collected about when the child met his or her developmental milestones. The episodic or focused health history is used to collect data about a specific problem the child is having. Questions should be focused on eliciting information based on the chief concern. This history is generally limited to one or two systems.

The interval history does not require a past, medical, family, or social history. It is the data collection that occurs at a visit subsequent to one in which a comprehensive history and physical examination were completed. It also notes the general condition of the child during the period between the visits. An interval history would be needed for a subsequent hospital visit. The comprehensive health history is discussed later in this chapter.

### PATIENT-IDENTIFYING INFORMATION

The first information to be collected in the health history is the patient-identifying information. The APP collects the name, birth date, sex/gender, address, record number, and name of historian, along with the relationship to the child. If the institutional culture allows and as part of the trust-building process, the child should be asked which personal pronoun they prefer. As a provider, we should share our own pronouns so that we may encourage the child to be comfortable with opening up to us.

### CHIEF CONCERN

Elicit the chief concern from the child and/or parent/caregiver. The chief concern is why the child came to the healthcare facility and is documented in the child's or guardian's own words (e.g., subjective narrative; Duderstadt, 2019). The chief concern often is reported by the adult in the room who may not be custodial, so ensure the identity of the adult, and presence of proper consent as necessary.

## HISTORY OF PRESENT ILLNESS

Next, the provider elicits the history of the present illness. The history of present illness elaborates on the chief concern. It includes onset, location, duration, characteristics, aggravating factors, relieving factors, timing, and severity (OLDCARTS) in relation to the presenting symptom(s). Ask about the child's and/or caregivers' thoughts and feelings about the illness. Culture, gender, and developmental issues may also be identified during this part of the health history. Keep in mind that somatic or developmental concerns may occur independently or be related to issues within the family.

### Past Medical History

The past medical history provides significant events that inform the APP about the well-being of the child and unresolved issues from previous visits, such as illness resolution or safety in the home. Examples include physical status of the particular illness or family environments that prevent supervision and failing to protect the child from normal developmental curiosity and untoward outcomes. For example, a toddler opens a pill container when it is documented that safety caps were recommended at the previous visit when the child ingested medication. The past medical history includes information about the child's prenatal, birth, and neonatal history, developmental history, acute or chronic illness, allergies, medications, past surgeries, injuries or hospitalizations, immunizations, and health promotion.

#### Developmental History

When obtaining the developmental history, ask the parent or guardian at what ages developmental milestones were met. These milestones include gross motor, fine motor, and language skills, as well as functional skills such as self-feeding, sleep habits, and urine/bowel continence. You may also ask the parent to compare the development with that of any siblings and the parents. Ask about parental relationships and relationships with friends. For the school-age child or adolescent, inquire about school performance.

#### Prenatal, Birth, and Neonatal History

When eliciting the prenatal history, begin with neutral questions about the parents' partners and activities during pregnancy (be culturally sensitive and tolerant of lifestyle choices). Ask about maternal age, prenatal care, maternal health during pregnancy (including infections), medications, exposures, smoking, alcohol use or prescribed and illicit drug use during pregnancy. For the birth history, note duration of pregnancy, length of labor, type of delivery, and any complications associated with it for either the mother or the infant. When determining the neonatal history, note gestational age, birth weight, length, and head circumference. Was the infant born with any congenital or genetic abnormalities? Did the infant encounter any medical problems at birth or experience difficulties with feeding? How long was the infant hospitalized after birth? Determine if the infant experienced any illnesses in the first two months of life (Duderstadt, 2019).

#### Acute or Chronic Illness

Inquire about the child's history of common acute illness (such as infections, diarrhea, vomiting, dehydration) or childhood disease (measles, mumps, rubella, varicella, pertussis). Determine if the child has a congenital anomaly, a vision or hearing deficit, or other disorders with a genetic predisposition. Ask about chronic illnesses such as cancer, diabetes, cystic fibrosis, asthma, eczema, or sickle cell disease. For all illnesses, ascertain age of onset, treatment prescribed, and the child's response to treatment (Chiocca, 2020).

#### Allergies

Parents and children often do not know what an allergy is, so it is important for the APP to define the serious allergies to food or medication. Determine allergy to food, medication, animals, environmental irritants, insect bites or sting, and latex. Ask what type of reaction the child has to the allergen. Does it result in a rash or hives? Is there itching or respiratory distress? Parents may confuse routine side effects of medication with allergy, so be sure to probe into the response to the perceived allergen in order to accurately document the child's allergies. If the child has experienced anaphylaxis, the parent needs to understand the seriousness of the allergy as compared with a simply troublesome contact rash, which is not an emergency.

## Medications

Ask about all prescribed or over-the-counter medications the child is taking. Inquire about the dose and frequency, and when the last dose was given. Also, include information about any herbal treatments, use of alternative medicines, or supplements.

## Past Surgeries, Injuries, and Hospitalizations

Determine whether the child has experienced any surgical procedures or intentional and/or unintentional injuries. If the child has ever been hospitalized, include reason, length of stay, and disposition.

## Immunizations

Determine the child's immunization history. Include immunizations received and age of receipt. Review the official immunization record for this information. Parental recall is not sufficient for immunization documentation. If immunizations are delayed, inquire as to the circumstances for the delay. Understanding the circumstances (such as personal or religious beliefs, or lack of insurance coverage) provides an opportunity for education and possible referral for resources (Chiocca, 2020).

## Health Promotion

Ask about currency of well-child visits and obtain details about the most recent well-child visit. Inquire about health screenings and their results.

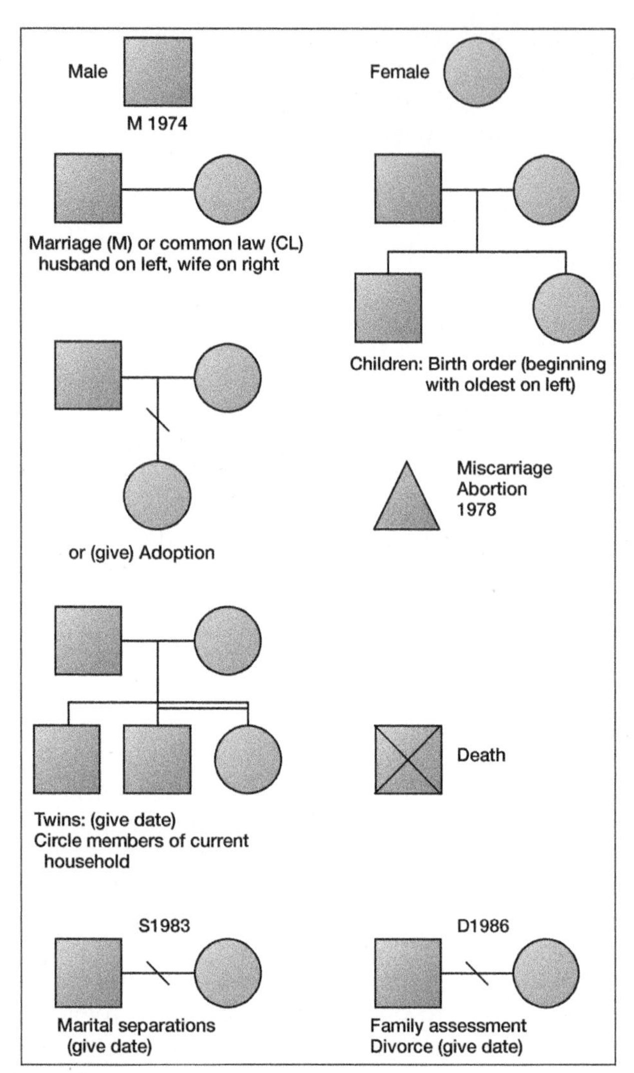


FIGURE 3.1 Genogram symbols.

*Source*: Reproduced from Chiocca, E. M. (2020). *Advanced pediatric assessment* (3rd ed.). Springer Publishing Company.

## Family History

Determine the family history to reveal patterns of disease. Assess three generations (the child's, the parents', and the child's grandparents). Ask about consanguinity, hereditary and other health conditions, and cause of death for deceased family members (Chiocca, 2020; Quinlin & Gawlik, 2021). Construct a genogram to visually depict a gathering of information about family health and causes of death. Use symbols with a legend to depict family members, relationships, health issues, and causes of death. Refer to Figure 3.1 for examples of symbols commonly used in the genogram. Figure 3.2 depicts an example of a three-generation genogram.

## Social History

Determine if the caregiver is the biological parent or legal guardian. Ask about parents' or guardian's education level and occupations. Does the family have adequate resources to ensure food security? Inquire about the child's living arrangement, home conditions, neighborhood safety, and exposure to violence. Determine the extent of the family's social support system. What are the family's or child's religious or spirituality ideals? Are particular practices followed? Document if the child attends day, preschool, or school, or if the child is home-schooled. Inquire if the child is exposed to cigarette smoke in the home or car. For older children and adolescents, ask about tobacco, e-cigarette, alcohol, and illicit drug use as well as sexual history (Chiocca, 2020; Quinlin & Gawlik, 2021).

## Functional Assessment

The functional assessment includes information about elimination, nutrition, sleep, and safety.

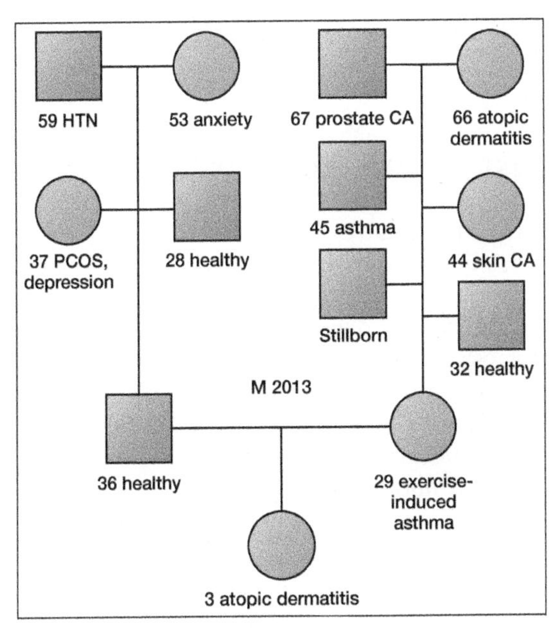


FIGURE 3.2 Three-generation genogram.

Determine the child's elimination patterns, recognizing differences depending upon the child's age. The infant should have at least six to eight wet diapers per day. The infant's stool consistency and pattern will vary according to intake. Breastfed infants tend to have frequent loose, seedy stools, whereas formula-fed infants tend to have less frequent, drier stools. As the infant begins to eat solid foods, the stools change. For the infant or preschooler, determine progress or success with toilet teaching. The school-age child should demonstrate urinary and bowel continence.

## Nutrition History

The infant's/young child's brain is undergoing tremendous growth, so appropriate nutrition is required for this growth. In the breastfeeding infant, determine frequency of feeding, satiation, number of wet diapers and stools per day, and whether the infant is being supplemented with water (not advised) or formula. In addition, for the bottle-fed infant, determine type of formula and volume per feeding. Inquire about details related to progression to solid foods. For the young child, ask about self-feeding with fingers or utensils and avoidance of foods with a high risk of choking. For children and adolescents of all ages, determine intake of sugar-containing beverages (including fruit juice), nutrient-poor foods, and high-fat foods.

Culture also plays a role in how and what the child is fed, such as whether or not breastfeeding is an acceptable practice, when to advance the infant's diet, and what types of foods are fed to the infant or child (Duderstadt, 2019). Family, racial, and ethnic considerations also contribute to nutrition and growth patterns in infants. A 24-hour diet recall may be helpful in any child with poor or excess growth.

## Sleep History

Sleep is essential for the optimal health and growth of children and adolescents. It is associated with improved memory, attention and learning, behavior and emotional regulation, better immune function, and better overall health outcomes (Duderstadt, 2019). Gather information regarding:

- usual time the child goes to bed
- bedtime routine (particularly for younger children)
- problems going to bed
- whether the child sleeps all night (or wakes during the night)
- hours of sleep
- if the child takes naps.

The American Academy of Pediatrics (AAP) recommends the guidelines in Table 3.1 for sleep hours for optimal health. .

## Safety Assessment

When obtaining information about maintaining the child's safety, consider safety in the home, in the water, in the car, and while at play. Answers given related to safety provide an opening for the provider to further educate the family about safety. Regarding the child's home, ask about:

- Working smoke and carbon monoxide detectors
- Hot water heater temperature (should be set at less than 120 °F)

**TABLE 3.1 Recommended Sleep Hours for Children**

| Age | Hours of Sleep |
|---|---|
| 4 months to 12 months of age | 12 to 16 hours per 24 hours (including naps) |
| 1 to 2 years of age | 11 to 14 hours per 24 hours (including naps) |
| 3 to 5 years of age | 10 to 13 hours per 24 hours (including naps) |
| 6 to 12 years of age | 9 to 12 hours per 24 hours |
| 13 to 18 years of age | 8 to 10 hours per 24 hours |

*Source*: Data from American Academy of Pediatrics. (2018). *Healthy sleep habits: How many hours does your child need?* https://www.healthychildren.org/English/healthy-living/sleep/Pages/Healthy-Sleep-Habits-How-Many-Hours-Does-Your-Child-Need.aspx

- Firearms (locked up, unloaded, with ammunition stored separately)
- Safe crib (for infants and young toddlers), or do they co-sleep?
- Poisons, cleaning products, and various personal care products stored in a high, locked cabinet

Considering safety in the water, ask about the presence of a swimming pool at the home and about a locked door to the pool area and/or a locked fence around the pool area. Determine use of age-appropriate child safety restraints used in automobiles and trucks. Inquire about the use of helmets with wheeled vehicles and other safety equipment associated with physical activities such as wrist guards for skating or roller blading.

### Review of Systems

The review of systems (ROS) provides an opportunity to obtain subjective data from the parent or caregiver and child (as age permits) about the past and present symptoms the child has experienced per body system. Table 3.2 provides information per age group that should be asked about in the ROS.

# PHYSICAL EXAMINATION

The physical examination of a child of any age always begins with the general appearance. The sequence of the remainder of the physical examination will be determined by the child's developmental age and level of cooperation. The newborn or infant may lie in the caregiver's lap or be assessed on the examination table with the caregiver close by. Toddlers should be permitted as much freedom of movement as possible. Auscultate the heart and lungs while the infant or young child is quiet. With a parent close by, the preschooler may cooperate with the examination while seated on the examination table. School-age children and adolescents are comfortable on the examination table. Adolescents will likely prefer for the parent to exit the room while the examination is performed (to protect their privacy).

Always plan the physical assessment in such a way as to minimize trauma to the child or adolescent. For infants and younger children, explain all steps of the examination to the parents or caregiver. Toddlers and preschoolers may be responsive to play throughout the assessment and often like to handle the equipment prior to it being used on them. Always perform the most invasive examinations, such as the ear, mouth, and throat assessment, last in the infant or young child. For the school-age child or adolescent, conduct the physical examination in a head-to-toe fashion, reserving the genitalia and anus examination for last.

## GENERAL APPEARANCE

Observe the child's overall general appearance while they are being held by the parent or caregiver and/or walking around or playing. Include observations about the child's demeanor, behavior, level of consciousness, facies (facial appearance typical of a particular syndrome), social skills, motor coordination, mobility, hygiene, nutritional status, and interpersonal interactions with the parent/caregiver and provider (Chiocca, 2020).

## ANTHROPOMETRIC MEASUREMENTS

Accurate measurement of growth parameters in children is essential in determining the child's health status (Chiocca, 2020). A child who is failing to grow as expected, or who is trending toward being overweight or obese, likely will need additional assessment and/or intervention. The Centers for Disease Control and Prevention (CDC) published revised growth charts in 2000. These charts provide a more accurate representation of current diversity among children in the United States (CDC, 2010). Weight, length or height, and head circumference (until age 24 months) are obtained at each well-child visit (Tanski & Garfunkel, 2010). Weight for length is compared among younger children, whereas body mass index (BMI) is assessed in older children. These measurements are plotted on the gender- and age-appropriate growth charts and maintained in the child's health record. Normal growth ranges are generally considered to be:

- World Health Organization (WHO) growth charts (age birth to 2 years)—2nd to 98th percentile
- CDC growth charts (age 2–20 years)—5th to 95th percentile (CDC, 2013)

The clinical growth charts may be found in the appendix and at https://www.cdc.gov/growthcharts/clinical_charts.htm.

**PRO TIP** Additional anthropometric measurements include the chest circumference, mid-upper arm circumference, and skinfold measurement at the triceps, abdomen, or subscapular regions. These are usually used only with a nutritionist consultation.

**TABLE 3.2 Review of Systems Across Developmental Stages**

| Review of Systems | Neonate/Infant | Toddler/Preschool | School Age/Adolescent |
|---|---|---|---|
| **Constitutional** | State of health, growth (recent weight loss or gain), fever, fatigue or weakness, malaise, pain | State of health, growth (recent weight loss or gain), fever, fatigue or weakness, malaise, pain | State of health, growth (recent weight loss or gain), fever, fatigue or weakness, malaise, pain |
| **Integumentary** | Birth marks or pigmentation, skin changes | Birth marks, rashes or lesions, pruritis, hives, changes in moles, changes in body hair, problems with nails, infestation | Birth marks, rashes or lesions, pruritis, hives, changes in moles, changes in body hair, problems with nails, infestation |
| **Head and neck** | Changes in head shape, soft spot (fontanel) | Head injury | Head injury, loss of consciousness, headache, dizziness |
| **Eyes** | Strabismus, excessive tearing, discharge, redness, eyelid edema | Squinting, sitting very close face-to-face, 3 years and over: date of last visual acuity testing and results | Double or blurry vision, sitting close to blackboard or computer screen, holding book close to face, use of glasses or contact lenses |
| **Ears** | Hearing test result at birth, ear pain, drainage, concerns re: hearing loss | Delayed speech | Tinnitus |
| **Nose** | Frequent rhinorrhea, stuffiness, or nasal congestion | Allergies, mouth breathing, snoring, epistaxis, altered sense of smell | Allergies, mouth breathing, snoring, epistaxis, altered sense of smell |
| **Mouth and throat** | Pattern of tooth eruption, teething, sores or white coating in mouth or tongue | Pattern of tooth loss, tooth pain, tooth trauma, gum bleeding, sore throats, hoarseness, voice changes | Pattern of tooth loss, tooth pain, tooth trauma, gum bleeding, sore throats, hoarseness, voice changes |
| **Chest** | Extra nipple, nipple drainage, breast tissue enlargement | Extra nipple, nipple drainage, breast tissue enlargement | Female thelarche, male gynecomastia |
| **Respiratory** | Breathing problems, cough, stridor, cyanosis | Wheeze, sputum expectoration, dyspnea at rest or with activity | Wheeze, sputum expectoration, dyspnea at rest or with activity |
| **Cardiovascular** | Poor feeding, murmur, cyanosis | Murmur, fatigue, night sweats | Chest pain, syncope, racing heart |
| **Gastrointestinal** | Change in appetite, vomiting, diarrhea, constipation, increased crying | Nausea, soiling with stooling, belching, flatulence, anal itching, blood in stool | Nausea, soiling with stooling, belching, flatulence, anal itching, blood in stool |
| **Genitourinary** | Circumcised/noncircumcised, male urine stream, swelling of scrotum with crying | Urinary frequency, urgency, dysuria, scrotal swelling | Enuresis, menarche, date of last menstrual period, length and quality of periods, sexually active |
| **Musculoskeletal** | Hip disorder | Exercise tolerance, knock-kneed, pigeon-toed, limp, fractures | Curved spine, sprains, lack of coordination, joint or muscle pain |
| **Neurologic** | Developmental milestone achievement, social interactivity, tremors | Tics, uncontrolled movements, fears, nightmares, unusual habits | Headache, nervousness, dizziness, tingling, sensory changes, memory loss |
| **Endocrine** | Growth disturbance, thyroid disease | Excessive thirst, excessive voiding, excessive eating, signs of early puberty, excessive sweating, temperature change intolerance | Delayed puberty, abnormal hair distribution |
| **Hematologic** | Pale color, bruising in nonwalker, or excess bruising, bleeding gums | Pale color, bruising in nonwalker, or excess bruising, bleeding gums | Pale color, bruising in nonwalker, or excess bruising, bleeding gums |
| **Lymphatic** | Frequent fever | Swollen lymph nodes | Swollen lymph nodes |
| **Psychosocial** | Developmental delay, irritability | Behavior changes, tantrums, breath-holding spells | Bedwetting, school failure, social withdrawal, depression, substance abuse |

*Source*: From Chiocca, E. M. (2020). *Advanced pediatric assessment* (3rd ed.). Springer Publishing Company.

### Weight

Weigh all children at each health maintenance visit. Weigh infants completely nude on a zeroed digital or balanced-beam scale intended for use in infants. The toddler may also be weighed similarly to the infant until the toddler is able to stand well. Record the measurement to the nearest 10 g or 0.5 ounces. When children are able to stand well (by 2–3 years of age), weigh them on an upright scale wearing only underpants or dry diaper and a gown, with shoes removed. Record the measurement to the nearest 100 g or 0.25 pounds.

### Length/Height

Measure recumbent length in children under 2 years of age. The birth to 24 months growth charts are reflective of recumbent length. When the child is able to stand well, measure the height utilizing a stadiometer with the child's back to the wall or upright post, feet flat, facing forward, and chin perpendicular to the floor. The 2 to 20 years growth charts are reflective of standing height.

▶ ALERT: Use caution with cloth or paper measuring tapes, as they may stretch over time and affect accuracy of measurement.

### Weight for Length

When the birth to 24 months growth charts are being used, plot the child's weight for the child's recumbent length. This result is compared with BMI in older children and may be used to determine underweight or overweight in children up until age 24 months. Weight for length determinations include:

- Normal weight for length: between the 2nd and 98th percentile
- Underweight: weight for length <2nd percentile
- Overweight: weight for length >98th percentile

### Body Mass Index

BMI provides the standard by which to determine healthy weight in children age 2 to 20 years. Online electronic calculators are available for determining BMI (CDC, 2020; Gavin, 2020). Manual calculations are made by the following:

- English Method: {weight (lb)/height (in)/height (in)} × 703
- Metric Method: {weight (kg)/height (cm)/height (cm)} × 10,000

Instructions for manual calculation of BMI may also be found on the clinical growth charts. Plot the child's BMI on the gender-appropriate clinical growth charts based on the child's age to the nearest quarter-year:

- Normal BMI is between the 5th and 85th percentile
- BMI <5th percentile is considered underweight
- BMI between the 85th and 95th percentile is overweight
- BMI >95th percentile indicates obesity

### Head Circumference

The occipito-frontal head circumference is an indirect measure of brain growth, which is very rapid during the first 2 years of life, particularly in infancy. The head circumference is measured by placing the tape measure around the largest point of the occipito-frontal circumference. Measure the head circumference at birth, at each health maintenance visit until age 24 months, and whenever there is a concern. Plot the head circumference on the birth to 24 months growth chart. The head circumference is considered within normal range if it plots between the 2nd and 98th percentile for age and gender, and steadily maintains the approximate percentile curve over time.

**PRO TIP** If problems with brain growth (such as microcephaly or macrocephaly) are present at age 24 months, the head circumference should be measured at the annual well-child visit until 6 years of age.

## INTEGUMENTARY SYSTEM

When assessing the skin, adequate lighting is essential and the room should be at a comfortable temperature. Inspect and palpate the skin. Note the child's skin color, which should be pink, as appropriate for race. Refer to Table 3.3 for an explanation of differences in skin color. Quickly scan the child's or adolescent's body before removing any clothes or drapes to inspect all areas of the body. Inspect the skin for hair distribution, the presence of any birthmarks or freckles, areas of differing pigmentation, moles, rashes, lesions, piercings, or tattoos. Palpate the skin for temperature, turgor, texture, and moisture.

**PRO TIP** In infants and toddlers, closely inspect small freckles to insure they are not petechiae, which can be a sign of hemorrhagic disease or child maltreatment.

**TABLE 3.3 Causes of Differences in Skin Color**

| Variation/Description | Cause |
|---|---|
| Pallor: in light-skinned children, a decrease in pinkness; in dark-skinned children, ashy-gray color | Fever, anemia, syncope, or shock |
| Central cyanosis: blue color of the perioral region, lips, tongue, oral mucosa, or trunk | Hypoxia, circulatory collapse |
| Yellowing of nose, palms, or soles | Excess intake of yellow vegetables |
| Jaundice (overall yellow color) | Physiologic in the newborn; liver or hematopoietic disease in any age child |
| Redness | Blushing, localized inflammation, hyperthermia, cold exposure, alcohol ingestion |
| Lack of color in skin, hair, and eyes | Albinism |

*Source*: Data from Bickley, L. S., Szilagyi, P. G., Hoffman, R. M., & Soriano, R. P. (2021). *Bates' guide to physical examination and history taking* (13th ed.). Wolters Kluwer; Jarvis, C., & Eckhardt, A. (2020). *Physical examination and health assessment* (8th ed.). Elsevier.

The newborn may have lanugo (fine, downy hair) covering the back and extremities. Beyond infancy, delayed or precocious appearance of body hair may indicate a hormonal imbalance. Birthmarks are also called café-au-lait spots. Document their size, shape, and number (if the child has six or more café-au-lait spots, an evaluation for neurofibromatosis is warranted). The newborn (especially darker-skinned infants) may have macular areas of bluish pigmentation particularly over the lumbar/sacral area, the lower extremities, and posterior shoulders. Commonly called Mongolian spots, these areas of congenital dermal melanocytosis usually fade and/or disappear entirely by 4 weeks to 4 months of age (Kibbi & Bergqvist, 2019). Document their size and locations, so as not to confuse them with bruises in the future. When other skin areas of concern are identified during the inspection, palpate the area and classify by size, color, morphology, texture, firmness, configuration, location, and distribution (Chiocca, 2020; Duderstadt, 2019).

▶ ALERT: Mongolian spots not receding by 1 year of age or that are extensive may be associated with inborn errors of metabolism and other rare genetic disorders (Kibbi & Bergqvist, 2019).

Inspect and palpate the hair and scalp, noting hair distribution, hair texture, and condition of the scalp. If present, document lesions, flaking, or infestation. Observe the nails for cleanliness and general condition as well as color, contour, texture, and thickness. White or yellow nails may indicate infection, while nail pallor may occur with anemia. Furrows or spooning in the nail may occur with nutritional disorders.

▶ ALERT: Bruising in the infant who is not yet cruising is a concerning finding. It may be indicative of a bleeding disorder or nonaccidental trauma (abuse).

## HEAD AND FACE

Assessment of the head and face begins when you first see the child. In all children, observe face for symmetry of movement and organ placement. Inspect the head for size, shape, and symmetry. Variations in head size include macrocephaly (larger than normal) and microcephaly (smaller than normal). Macrocephaly may be a normal variation or associated with intracranial hemorrhage, tumor, or hydrocephalus. Microcephaly may be associated with a genetic syndrome, Zika virus infection, or fetal alcohol spectrum disorder. Variations in head shape and/or symmetry (with significance) are listed in Table 3.4.

In infants, assess head control, which is usually achieved by 4 months of age. Lack of head control after 6 months of age is abnormal and may be the result of an anoxic brain injury or neuromuscular disorder. Also inspect and palpate the fontanels. The posterior fontanel closes sometime between birth and 2 months of age. The anterior fontanel is open and flat, closing between 9 and 12 months of age. It may be pulsatile. When the infant cries, the anterior fontanel may bulge slightly or feel more tense. A truly tense or bulging fontanel may indicate increased intracranial pressure. A depressed or sunken fontanel is indicative of dehydration or severe malnutrition. Also palpate the head for the presence of lymph nodes (usually nonpalpable).

## NECK

Assessment of the neck includes inspection, palpation, and auscultation. Assess the infant's and toddler's neck while they are in the parent's arms. Note range of motion, jugular vein pulsation, and tracheal alignment. The trachea should be midline; a deviation in the trachea's position may indicate a foreign body, neoplasm, or pneumothorax. Look

**TABLE 3.4 Head Shapes**

| Head Shape Variation | Illustration | Significance |
|---|---|---|
| Brachiocephaly | | Wide shape of cranium (appears shorter in relation to width). The back of the head is flattened with resultant bulging of the front of the head. May result from infant positioning. |
| Dolichocephaly (Scaphocephaly) | | Common in premature infants. Narrow shape of the cranium (appears longer in relation to the width). |
| Plagiocephaly | | Misshapen head related to infant positioning; flattening on one side of the back of the head often results in contralateral bulging of the forehead. Usually benign. |
| Trigonocephaly | | Bulging down center of forehead resulting from a fused metopic suture. |

for webbing, masses, lymph node presence, lesions, or scars.

Palpate the neck for tenderness, the presence of lymph nodes, and to assess the thyroid and jugular vein. The thyroid gland is usually not palpable in infants and young children. In school-age children and adolescents, palpate the thyroid gland using an approach from the front of the neck, although the posterior approach may also be used in the adolescent. When palpating the thyroid, note size, shape, tenderness, and the presence of any nodules. Palpate the anterior and posterior cervical lymph node chains noting size, location, temperature, and mobility. Auscultate the thyroid and jugular veins in the older child and adolescent. No bruit should be noted in either and the jugular vein pulse should be soft and nonbounding.

## EARS

Physical examination of the ears includes inspection and palpation of the external ear as well as inspection of the external auditory canal and tympanic membrane (TM). Begin the examination by inspecting the external ear. The ears should be placed similarly on both sides of the head with the top of the pinna no lower than an imaginary line from the outer canthus of the eye. Low-set ears are often associated with chromosomal anomalies or other genetic conditions. The size and shape of both ears should be symmetrical and the color of the auricles should be close to the facial color. Note deformity of the ear and the presence of preauricular pits or skin tabs. Redness or bruising may be indicative of trauma (possibly nonaccidental). Palpate the auricle for any masses, pain, or tenderness.

Inspect the external auditory canal for color, and presence of discharge or odor. Utilizing the otoscope, further inspect the internal auditory canal. The presence of cerumen is an expected finding. Inspect the TMs for color (gray, silver or pink, or red after crying), translucency, intactness, contour, and foreign body. Note the light reflex (cone of light) between the 4 and 6 o'clock positions on the right TM and the 6 to 8 o'clock positions on the left TM. Assess TM mobility with the pneumatic bulb attachment on the otoscope. TM mobility indicates appropriate middle ear pressure.

### Screening Hearing Tests

To grossly screen hearing, use the whisper test, the Weber test, and the Rinne test (the child must be developmentally able to cooperate with these tests). For the whisper test, the child places the hand over the ear not being tested. The examiner stands a few feet behind the child and whispers a word with two distinct syllables (such as football). The child then says the word. Repeat the process with the opposite ear. For the Weber test, gently strike the tuning fork and place on top of the child's head or middle of the forehead. Ask the child if the sound is heard in the right ear, left ear, or the middle. A normal response is equal hearing in both ears. For the Rinne test, gently tap the tuning fork to create vibration. Place the tuning fork on the child's mastoid process (bone conduction [BC]) and ask the child to note when the sound is no longer heard. Then move the tuning fork with tines toward the external auditory canal (air conduction [AC]), asking the child to note when the sound is no longer heard. AC time is twice as long as BC time with normal hearing (Table 3.5).

TABLE 3.5 **Weber and Rinne Results With Conduction and Sensorineural Hearing Loss**

| Test | Conductive Hearing Loss | Sensorineural Hearing Loss |
|---|---|---|
| Weber | Sound will be better heard on the affected side | Sound will not be heard in the affected ear |
| Rinne | BC is greater than AC or BC = AC | AC is greater than BC |

AC, air conduction; BC, bone conduction

## EYES

A complete examination of the eye in children includes inspection and palpation of ocular structures, assessment of visual fields and extraocular movement, and visual acuity testing. Inspect the external eye, noting symmetry of the eyebrows and eyelids, and whether or not the eye lashes are evenly distributed. The palpebral fissures are normally symmetrical. In children of African or European descent, the palpebral fissure is ordinarily horizontal, whereas in Asian children or those with Down syndrome, the palpebral fissure slants slightly upward (Chiocca, 2020). Inspect the conjunctiva for irritation, which should be absent. Check the lid margins for erythema, crusting, cysts, or lesions (which should also be absent). Observe the sclerae, which should be white, smooth, and clear. Young infants' sclerae may have a slightly bluish undertone, but blue sclerae may be indicative of osteogenesis imperfecta (Snell & Gardner, 2017). The sclerae of children with a darker skin tone may have a yellowish tinge, but truly yellow sclerae occur with jaundice (Snell & Gardner, 2017).

▶ ALERT: Ocular injury emergencies associated with nonaccidental trauma (abuse) include hyphema, conjunctival, or hemorrhagic petechiae and may be associated with strangulation or suffocation (look for neck or trunk bruising above the pressure line) in infants.

Next inspect the cornea, lens, iris, and pupils. Note symmetry of the corneal light reflex (Hirschberg test) when the child looks at the light from a penlight held 18 to 24 inches away. The light reflex (a small white dot of light) should fall on the same place on the pupil in both eyes. An asymmetric corneal light reflex occurs with amblyopia and strabismus. Using a penlight, examine the cornea. The cornea is normally clear, round, and smooth, without obscurities; opacity of the lens occurs with cataracts. Note the color and shape of the iris. In the first six months of life, the iris is usually blue to grayish in light-skinned infants and dark brown in darker-skinned infants. The iris should be circular. Variations of the iris include different colors (heterochromia), which may be an abnormal finding or associated with Horner syndrome. Brushfield spots are tiny white spots on the iris arranged in a circle around the pupil and may occur with Down syndrome or tuberous sclerosis. A coloboma is a keyhole appearance to the pupil and is often associated with genetic syndromes.

Inspect the pupils' size, shape, symmetry, and reaction to light and accommodation. The pupil size in children is 2 to 6 mm. With anisocoria (pupil asymmetry), if the difference in size is less than 1 mm, document the finding to establish a baseline. If the difference in size is greater than 1 mm, refer the child to a pediatric neurologist, as a neurologic disease may be present. In a darkened room, shine a penlight directly into each eye. The pupils should constrict briskly. Sluggish constriction may indicate a neurologic problem.

▶ ALERT: Pupillary lack of responsiveness to light or a unilateral pupil reaction indicates eye trauma or a serious neurologic injury. Refer the child immediately to a pediatric neurologist.

To examine for a red reflex, in a darkened room shine the ophthalmoscope's beam of light toward each pupil, from about 12 to 15 inches away. The red reflex should be present in both eyes, and equal in size, brightness, and color. In light-skinned children, the pupils will appear reddish orange and in darker-skinned children it will be brownish-red. A red reflex that is white in color (leukocoria) is associated with retinoblastoma and an absent red reflex may occur with cataract, glaucoma, or retinopathy of prematurity.

▶ ALERT: Refer infants and children with an absent red reflex in either or both eyes to pediatric ophthalmology immediately, in order to preserve future vision.

Check pupil accommodation by holding an object about 12 inches away from the child's face in midline and asking the child to follow the object as it is moved. Moving the object toward the child's nose should result in bilateral, equal pupillary constriction as well as convergence (moving together) of the eyes. When the object is moved approximately 12 inches away from the face, the pupils should dilate equally bilaterally.

▶ ALERT: When pupils are asymmetric, if the difference is greater than 1 mm, neurological disease may be present. Refer the child to a pediatric neurologist.

At age 6 months, the infant should be able to fix on and follow a light or small toy. Begin extraocular movement testing when the child is developmentally able to cooperate (usually age 4 or 5 years). Extraocular movement testing assesses the function of the oculomotor nerve (CN II), trochlear nerve (CN IV), and abducens (CN VI). To conduct extraocular movement testing, stand approximately 12 inches in front of the child. Instruct the child not to move the head, but to follow the examiner's finger as it is moved through the six cardinal fields of gaze. Move the finger through this path: left and right lateral gaze, left and right lateral inferior gaze, and left and right lateral superior gaze. The child's eyes should move smoothly and equally. A few beats of nystagmus may be noted during the superior, lateral gaze and are considered normal. Begin visual acuity testing at 3 years of age (see chapters 4, 12).

▶ ALERT: Marked nystagmus should be investigated, as it may be associated with a neurological problem.

## NOSE AND SINUSES

First assess the child's nose while the child is in the parent's arms or sitting quietly to observe any nasal flaring. Inspect the external nose for midline placement on the face, and for shape and symmetry. To determine nasal patency, first occlude one side of the nose by pressing with the pad of the finger. Observe the child evenly and quietly breathing through the open nostril. Repeat on the other side. To inspect the internal nose, use a penlight or nasal speculum. Observe the nasal septum for alignment, perforation, bleeding, or lesions. View inferior and middle turbinates, noting color and the presence or absence of swelling.

**PRO TIP** Infants and toddlers often resist the nose, mouth, and throat examination. Save this portion of the examination for last, following the ear examination.

To assess the sinuses, begin with inspecting the facial area over the sinus for edema or erythema. In the school-age and older child, palpate the maxillary and frontal sinuses. Place the thumbs along the orbital ridge on the forehead and press gently upward to determine if tenderness is present. Palpate the maxillary sinuses by pressing upward under both zygomatic arches. A normal examination will reveal no edema, erythema, or tenderness.

## MOUTH AND THROAT

Examination of the oral cavity includes assessing the lips, buccal mucosa, gums, teeth, tongue, palate, uvula, pharynx, and tonsils. Inspect the lips' color, moisture, texture, fissures, swelling, symmetry, lesions or clefts. Note breath odor; foul or offensive breath odor may be due to bacteria accumulation between the teeth or on the tongue related to inadequate oral hygiene or may occur with tooth decay. Inspect the buccal mucosa for color, moisture, lesions, and ulcers, and the gums for color, swelling, and lesions. Bleeding of the gums may occur with poor oral hygiene, gingivitis, malnutrition, or oral infection. Inspect the teeth for number, type, and condition. Examine the tongue for movement, color, texture, moistness, size, and ulcerations. Observe the hard and soft palate color, shape, intactness, and lesions. Evaluate symmetric upward movement of the soft palate and uvula when the child says "ah." Inspect the pharynx for color, swelling, drainage, and lesions. Observe the tonsils for size, color, exudate, pitting or enlarged crypts, or membranous coverings. The tonsils may ordinarily be quite large in the young child. Document the tonsillar size (Table 3.6).

## CHEST AND LUNGS

Assessment of the chest and lungs involves inspection, auscultation, palpation, and percussion. Begin by inspecting the child's chest at rest. With the child's head in the midline position, inspect the chest size, shape, symmetry, and movement. Infants normally have a round thorax, with the anterior-posterior (A-P) and transverse diameters being equal. By the age of 6 years, the thorax is that of an adult ratio 1:2 (A-P to transverse diameter). Evaluate the respirations for rate, rhythm, and pattern. The effort should be smooth and symmetrical, without the use of accessory muscles. Count the child's respirations while calm and at rest. Normal respiratory rate ranges are listed in Table 3.7.

▶ ALERT: Nasal flaring and significant retractions in the infant indicate greatly increased work of breathing, which may lead to apnea when the infant runs out of energy.

**TABLE 3.6 Assessing Tonsillar Size**

| 1+: Tonsils Slightly Visible | 2+: Tonsils Halfway Between Tonsillar Pillars and Uvula | 3+: Tonsils Almost Touch Uvula | 4+: Tonsils Touch Each Other in Midline ("Kissing Tonsils") |
|---|---|---|---|
| 1+ 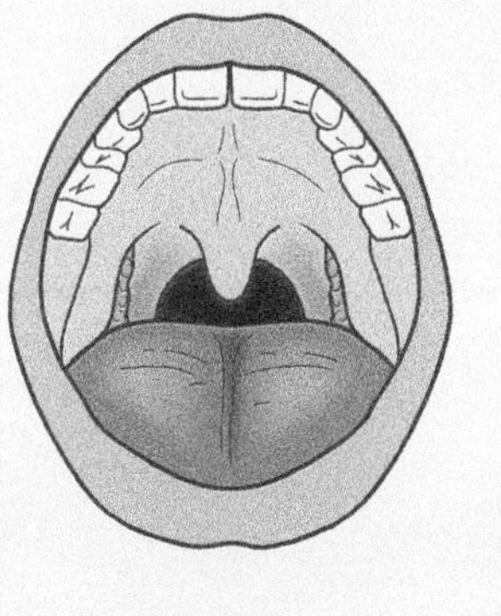 | 2+ 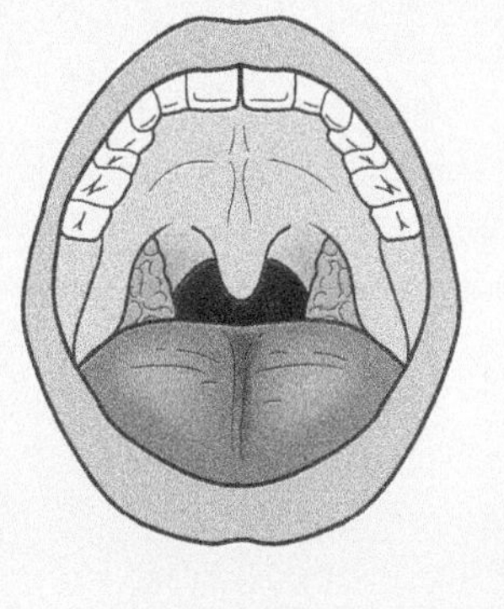 | 3+ 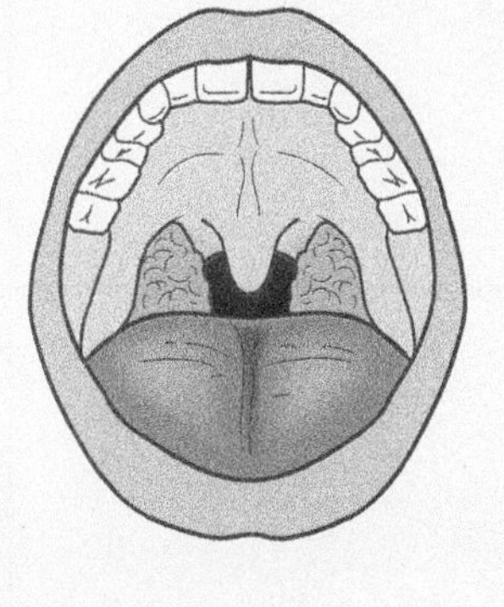 | 4+ 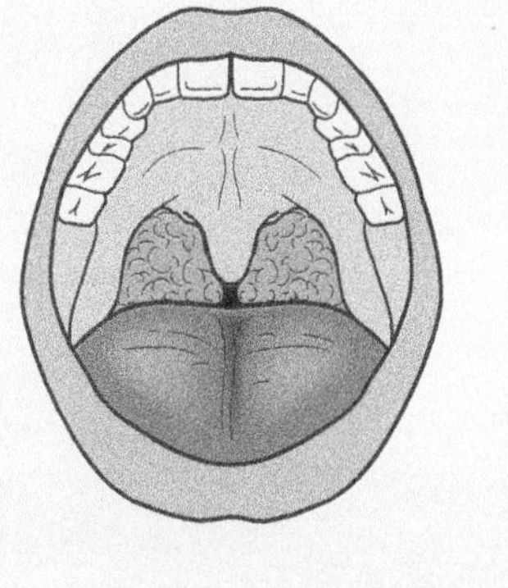 |

**TABLE 3.7 Respiratory Rates by Age Ranges**

| Age Range | Normal Range for Respiratory Rate (breaths per minute) |
|---|---|
| Newborn | 30–50 |
| 1–12 months | 30–45 |
| 1–4 years | 20–30 |
| 5–7 years | 20–25 |
| 8–11 years | 14–22 |
| Over 12 years | 12–20 |

Auscultate all lung fields in a systematic fashion (Table 3.8). Listen in each area for one full respiratory cycle, comparing with the opposite side. Note quality of breath sounds. To decrease any anxiety or fear that the child might have, perform auscultation of the infant's or toddler's breath sounds while the child is in the parent's arms. Place the diaphragm of the stethoscope directly on the child's skin. Do not auscultate over the clothing. Both the anterior and posterior chest should be auscultated. Normal breath sounds include bronchial, bronchovesicular, and vesicular. Abnormal breath sounds are discussed in Table 3.9. Qualities of normal breath sounds are as follows:

- Bronchial—high-pitched, harsh/hollow, heard over the trachea
- Bronchovesicular—moderately-pitched, mixed type of sound, heard between first and second intercostal space (bifurcation of the trachea)
- Vesicular—low-pitched blowing sound heard throughout the peripheral lung fields

Palpate the chest systematically while having the child say "99" or "blue moon." Tactile fremitus is revealed as palpated vibrations while the child is speaking. Fremitus is found between the scapula and near the bronchi and clavicles in the upper chest. It is not normally present in the lower chest. Also palpate the chest and neck for crepitus (a grating sensation of friction between cartilage and bone), normally absent. Palpate the supraclavicular and axillary areas for the presence of lymph nodes.

## BREASTS

At each health maintenance visit, examine the breasts of all children for size, symmetry, masses, and nipple discharge. Abnormal findings include infection, pain, or premature thelarche. Normal findings include:

- Newborn males and females—asymmetry, presence of thin, milky discharge (witch's milk), both of which are related to the influence of maternal hormones
- Prepubertal males—gynecomastia (Banikarim & De Silva, 2020)

**TABLE 3.8 Positions for Auscultation**

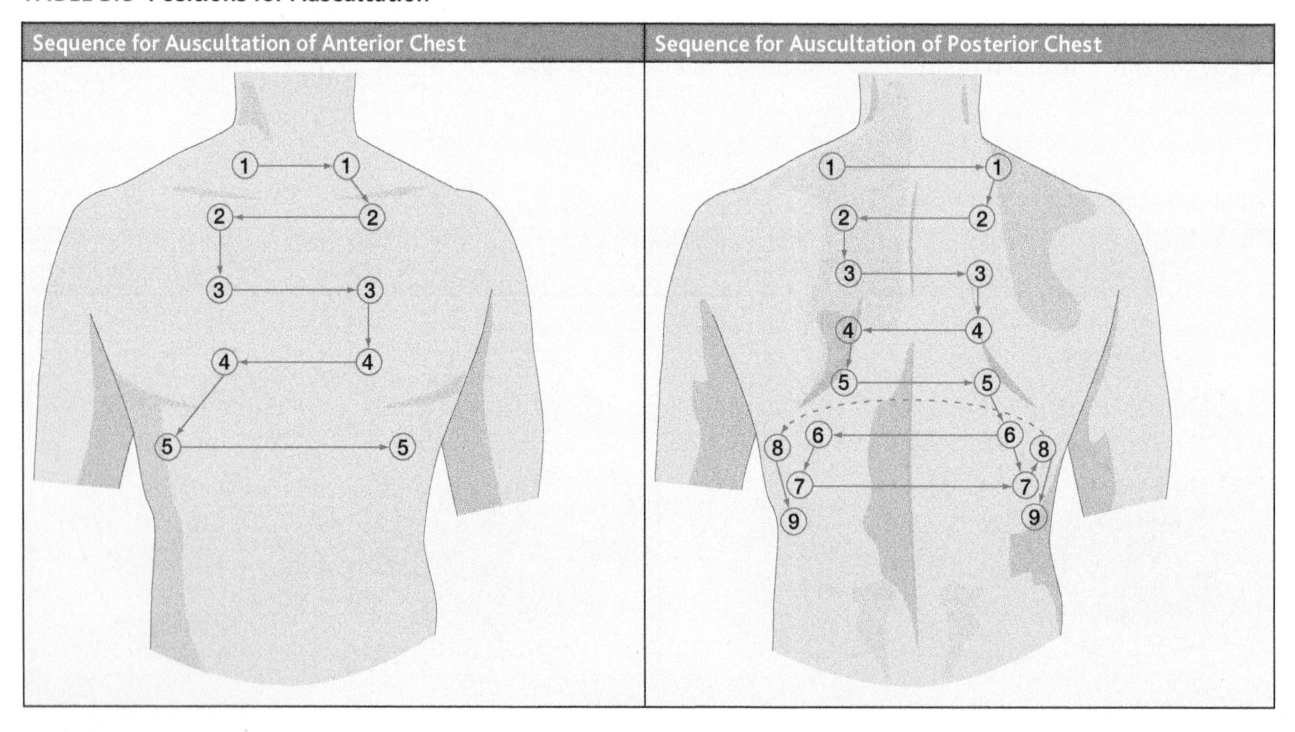

TABLE 3.9 **Description of Abnormal Breath Sounds**

| Breath Sound | Description |
|---|---|
| Crackles (rales) | Soft, high-pitched, crackling, or popping (fine crackles) or low-pitched gurgling (coarse crackles)—do not clear with coughing |
| Diminished breath sounds | Less audible breath sounds over a particular area |
| Pleural friction rub | Low-pitched, creaking, or grating sound, greatest on inspiration |
| Rhonchi | Low-pitched, loud, rattly, or bubbly—may clear with coughing |
| Stridor | Loud, high-pitched, coarse inspiratory sound heard without stethoscope |
| Wheeze | High-pitched, whistling or squeaky, musical sound occurring more often on expiration, but can be inspiratory |

*Source*: Adapted from Chiocca, E. M. (2020). *Advanced pediatric assessment* (3rd ed., p. 329, Table 17.5). Springer Publishing Company.

Begin sexual maturity rating of the female breast at age 11 years; the clinical breast examination does not begin until age 20 years. Refer to chapter 11 for an illustration of the breast sexual maturity rating scale (Tanner stage).

Palpate the breasts in a systematic fashion, noting that breast tissues should feel smooth, firm, and elastic. Note nodules or masses if present. A tender nodule just under the nipple results from pubertal changes, although it may be difficult to assess in girls with excessive adipose tissue. Palpate for axillary lymph nodes with the child's arms slightly abducted yet relaxed, noting size and texture of nodes if present.

## CARDIOVASCULAR

The cardiovascular examination begins with observation of the child's color, and inspection and palpation of the chest. Note the child's general appearance and activity level. Determine the child's color, which should be pink or appropriate for race. Assess the nailbeds for absence of clubbing. View the chest to determine presence of a heave and palpate for a thrill (both unusual in children). Observe and palpate for the point of maximal impulse (PMI), often visible in thinner children. The PMI is located in the fourth intercostal space just medial to the left midclavicular line in infants and young children. As the child grows, it usually reaches the fifth intercostal space at the left

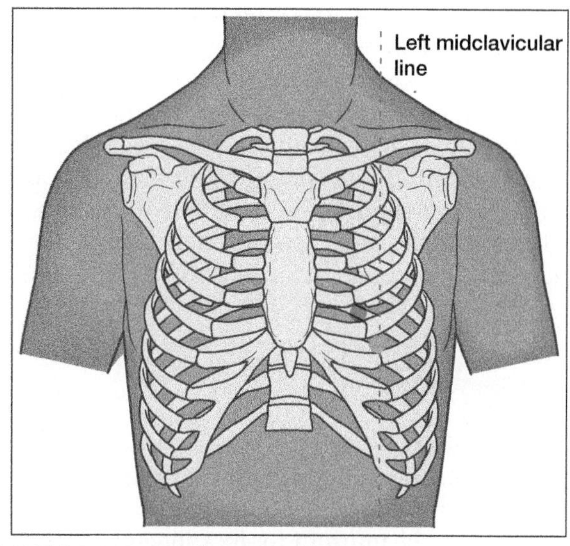


FIGURE 3.3 Point of maximal impulse.

midclavicular line (similar to adults) by school age (Figure 3.3).

Palpate the chest using the fingertips for the presence of lifts and heaves or thrills (all abnormal). Evaluate the apical pulse by palpating in the area of the PMI. Assess the pulses throughout. Note strength and quality of pulses while comparing the upper body to lower body pulses, as well as the left to the right, all of which should be equal. The pedal, brachial, and femoral pulses are usually easily palpated in children of all ages. In children younger than 2 years of age, the radial pulse is very difficult to palpate. Note warmth of the distal extremities and determine capillary refill time (perfusion adequacy is present with a capillary refill time of less than 3 seconds). Compare finger capillary refill time with that of the toes.

▶ ALERT: The presence of pallor, cyanosis, or mottling may indicate a cardiovascular problem.

Auscultate the heart in a stepwise fashion using both the diaphragm (to pick up high-frequency sounds) and the bell (to pick up low-frequency sounds) of the stethoscope. Auscultate all four valvular areas anteriorly. Determine $S_1$, $S_2$, extra heart sounds, or murmurs. In children, $S_1$ is usually loudest in the tricuspid and mitral areas, increasing in intensity with fever, exercise, and anemia, while $S_2$ is usually most intense in the pulmonic and aortic areas. Splitting of the second heart sound ($S_2$), varying with inspiration and expiration, is a normal finding in children. In healthy children, an $S_3$ is considered normal, although in the child with a chronic cardiac condition an $S_3$ may develop when congestive heart failure is present. Sinus arrhythmia is an irregular heart rhythm in which the heart rate increases with inhalation and decreases with exhalation. It is a common and normal finding in children and adolescents. To differentiate sinus arrhythmia, ask the child to hold their breath, during which time the rhythm becomes regular.

▶ ALERT: $S_4$ is considered abnormal (usually occurring with cardiac disease).

Listen closely for the presence of a murmur. In the infant or younger child, certain murmurs radiate to the axilla or posteriorly; auscultate in those areas as well. Evaluate the murmur for location, intensity, timing, and duration. Auscultate for murmurs, noting location (where heard loudest or most easily best), timing, and duration of the murmur:

- Systolic murmurs occur in association with $S_1$ (closure of the atrioventricular valves)
- Diastolic murmurs occur in association with $S_2$ (closure of the semilunar valves)
- For the murmur's duration, note occurrence early or late in diastole or systole, or if it occurs all the way across systole (holosystolic)

Table 3.10 discusses grading of murmur intensity.

The child has a more dynamic circulation, thin chest wall, and angulated vessels, resulting in the frequent occurrence of innocent murmurs (Jone et al., 2018). Most often heard at the second or fourth intercostal space, an innocent murmur is systolic in timing, medium-pitched, and musical. It will often disappear when the child changes position. One type of innocent murmur is the venous hum (heard in the supraclavicular area with possible radiation down the chest). Additional information on murmurs may be found in chapter 25. Palpate the pulses, comparing upper with lower, and right side with left side, noting regularity, strength, and equality.

**TABLE 3.10 Heart Murmur Intensity**

| Grade | Sound |
|---|---|
| 1 | Barely audible (usually heard only with intense concentration0); sometimes heard, sometimes not |
| 2 | Quiet, soft; heard each time the chest is auscultated |
| 3 | Audible, has an intermediate intensity |
| 4 | Audible, with a palpable thrill |
| 5 | Loud, audible with edge of the stethoscope lifted off the chest |
| 6 | Very loud, audible with the stethoscope placed near but not touching the chest |

*Source*: Data from Jone, P., VonAlvensleben, J., Burkett, D., Darst, J. R., Collins, K. K., & Miyamoto, S. D. (2018). Cardiovascular diseases. In W. W. Hay, M. J. Levin, R. R. Deterding, & M. J. Abzug (Eds.), *Current pediatric diagnosis and treatment* (24th ed, Chapter 20). McGraw-Hill Education.

▶ ALERT: Refer any child with a noninnocent murmur to a pediatric cardiologist for further evaluation.

## GASTROINTESTINAL

Allow infants, toddlers, and young children to sit on their parent's or caregiver's lap while facing the APP. Begin assessment of the abdomen by inspecting for contour, symmetry, pulsations, lesions, any visible masses, surface motion, rashes, bruising, and signs of injury (Chiocca, 2020). Auscultate the abdomen before percussion and palpation. Determine the frequency and character of the bowel sounds in all four quadrants. Beginning auscultation in the right lower quadrant (RLQ), in proximity to the ileocecal valve, will allow for any hypoactive bowel sounds to be heard (Chiocca, 2020). Percuss the abdomen to assess for air, fluid, or a mass, and to define the size of abdominal organs.

Palpation of the abdomen is very important and is used to identify tender areas, masses, or enlarged organs. Palpate the abdomen systematically in all four quadrants. For an infant or toddler, sit knee-to-knee with the parent or caregiver so the child may lie supine across your laps. This may allow abdominal palpation without upsetting the infant or toddler. An older child can lie supine and flex their knees so that palpation of the abdomen can be performed. Use light palpation first (the pad of the fingers, not the fingertips) to determine areas of tenderness. Closely observe the child's reactions during palpation. For deep palpation, use gentle but firm and steady pressure. To determine the presence of rebound tenderness (indicative of inflammation), remove the palpating hand quickly and the child will note tenderness.

To palpate the liver, place the fingertips below the right costal margin in the midclavicular line and palpate toward the liver until a bump is felt on inspiration. The liver border in infants and children may be palpable 1 to 2 centimeters below the costal margin. The spleen is difficult to feel upon palpation unless enlarged. Place the fingertips along the left posterior costal margin, palpating inwardly and upwardly during the child's inspiration. In the constipated child, a sausage-like mass may be felt in the left lower quadrant. In the infant with pyloric stenosis, an olive-like mass may be felt in the right upper quadrant (more easily palpable if the infant is sucking on a pacifier dipped in sugar water).

**PRO TIP** To decrease ticklishness during abdominal palpation, encourage the child to place his or her hand over your hand to "help" you.

## FEMALE GENITALIA

Assessment of the genitalia can make a child nervous, anxious, or upset. Because this examination can cause discomfort or embarrassment, the parent or caregiver should be present, although the adolescent should be provided the opportunity for privacy if desired. Examination of the genitalia is very important because it can help to identify infection or sexual abuse (Chiocca, 2020). Before starting the examination, explain to the child what you are going to do as well as what to expect. Maintain eye contact with the child as much as possible during the examination.

Inspect the vulva for symmetry, as well as for redness, swelling, lesions, drainage, foul odor, or tearing that may be indicative of sexual abuse. Observe the mons pubis for skin discoloration, lesions, and pubic hair distribution, checking for infestation. Rate the sexual maturity using the Tanner stages found in chapter 11. Inspect the labia for edema, irritation, tenderness, or erythema, all of which should ordinarily be absent. Determine that the labia are not adhered. Observe the clitoris for size and position. Note any erythema, discharge, or swelling of the urinary meatus. Palpate the labia majora and minora for edema, tenderness, or lesions.

## MALE GENITALIA

Inspect the penis and scrotum, then palpate the pubic area, inguinal canals, penis, and scrotum. Determine sexual maturity using the Tanner stages found in chapter 11. Inspect the penis for foreskin status, lesions, size, and curvature. Evaluate the prepuce for phimosis. In uncircumcised males, gently retract the foreskin. Observe the urinary meatus for position (should be centered on glans penis) and note discharge, redness, or warts (which should not be present). Inspect the scrotum for size, redness, or swelling. Palpate the scrotum for consistency, mass, or pain, determining presence of bilateral testes.

**PRO TIP** If the testicles are retractile or difficult to palpate, have the young boy sit tailor-style (with legs crossed) or instruct the older boy to squat in a baseball catcher's position, which may force the testicles to come down. It may also be helpful to press the opposite fingers over the inguinal area to prevent testis retraction.

Inspect and palpate the inguinal area for lymphadenopathy, mass, or bulge. If a bulge is present, palpate it to determine if it is a hernia, which should be reducible into the inguinal canal.

▶ ALERT: If an inguinal hernia is nonreducible or hard, refer the child to a pediatric surgeon.

## ANUS AND RECTUM

Inspect the anal area, which should appear moist and tightly closed, with dark folds and absence of fissures or visible hemorrhoids. Briefly touching the anal area with a cotton-tipped applicator or the gloved finger should result in a reflex tightening action called the anal wink. Rectal examinations are not routinely performed on infants and children except in the case of constipation, other stooling concerns, or potential child abuse. If indicated, gently insert the gloved finger (or little finger for an infant) into the rectal vault, using adequate lubrication. Assess for tone, hemorrhoids, and the presence or absence of stool. Test the stool for occult blood.

## MUSCULOSKELETAL

Begin the musculoskeletal examination by observing the child's body position, limb symmetry, posture, tone, and for any obvious deformities while lying or sitting. Also observe the toddler or child walking around and playing. While observing a child's gait, look for genu varum (bowlegs), genu valgum (knock knees), in-toeing, or out-toeing. Remove shoes and socks to evaluate posture and symmetry of the limbs while standing. Evaluate the upper and lower extremities for strength, size, and range of motion (flexion, extension, adduction, abduction, internal and external rotation). Assess grip, forearm, shoulder, thigh/hip, and ankle strength. Pull the infant from supine into a sitting position, evaluating head lag, which is significant in the newborn and lessens over time, disappearing by 4 months of age. To assess the infant's muscle tone, evaluate the infant in vertical suspension and horizontal suspension. In vertical suspension, the normotonic infant will remain hanging from the axillae in the examiner's hands, while the hypotonic infant will slip through the hands. In horizontal suspension, the normotonic infant will slightly flex and the head will rise, while the hypotonic infant will flop downward (like a rag doll). Refer to Figure 3.4(A, B).

Palpate the joints for tenderness, unusual prominence, pain, and thickening. Examine the infant for the presence of developmental dysplasia of the hip (DDH) until 9 months of age or until walking independently. DDH is screened utilizing the Ortolani and Barlow maneuvers (see chapter 34 for additional information). Assess the spine for range of motion, congenital abnormalities, and curvatures. In the infant, check for a sacral dimple or sinus, hair tuft, or hemangioma. To determine range of motion, ask the child to bend forward, side to side, and backward (Chiocca, 2020). Begin scoliosis screening in the preadolescent. Refer to chapter 34 for additional information regarding scoliosis screening.

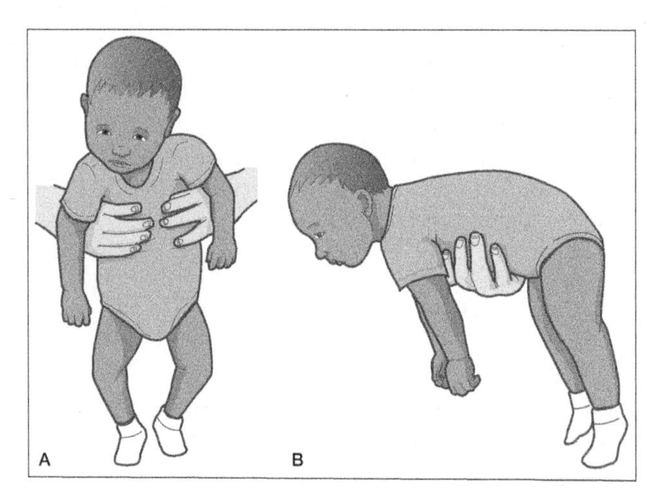


FIGURE 3.4 Vertical and horizontal suspension. (**A**) Vertical suspension: place the hands under the axillae and suspend the infant vertically, taking care not to grip the thorax. (**B**) Horizontal suspension: with palm up, under the infant's abdomen/thorax, suspend the infant.

**PRO TIP** The infant may demonstrate internal tibial torsion (Figure 3.5). To differentiate the normal finding of internal tibial torsion, grasp the infant's knees and attempt to straighten the legs, sliding the hands down to the ankles, rotating the ankles and the feet into a straightened position. Internal tibial torsion is related to in utero position, and resolves over time, but may not do so until after a period of time of weight-bearing.

## NEUROLOGIC

To evaluate the infant or child's neurologic status, assess mental status, speech and language, cranial nerve (CN) function, sensation, motor function, muscle strength, gait, balance and coordination, deep tendon reflexes (DTRs), and in the infant, primitive and postural reflexes (Chiocca, 2020). When determining neurologic status, always take into consideration the

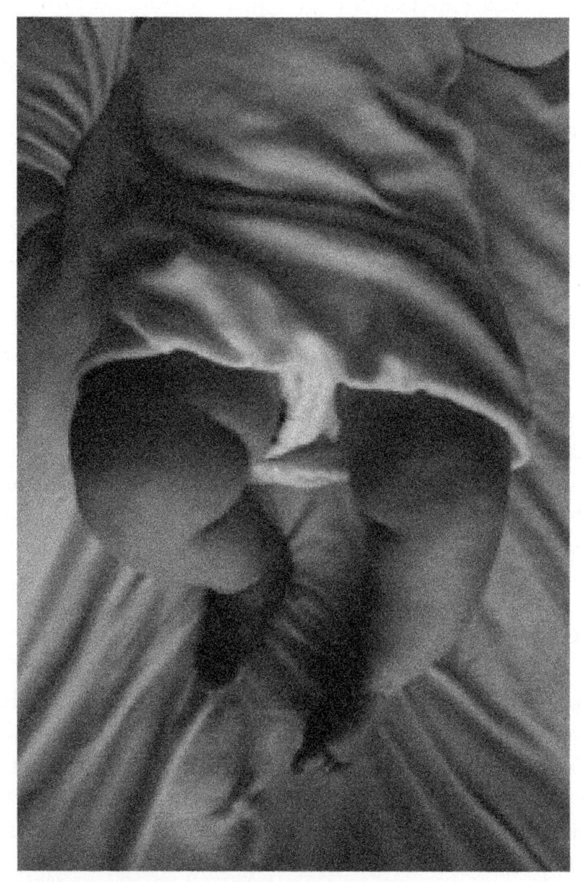

FIGURE 3.5 Internal tibial torsion.

child's developmental level. To assess mental status, first note the child's level of consciousness and presence or absence of irritability. How are the child's thought processes? In the younger child, are they able to follow simple directions or identify common objects? Can the older child adequately converse about their life (family, school, friends, activities)? Ask older children about their mood, and how happy they are feeling. In younger children, observe their affect. When assessing speech and language, keep in mind that children 5 years and younger may often have normal articulation difficulties, but older children and adolescents should not (Chiocca, 2020). Observe for impulse control and attention span. Ask questions to assess memory. Remember that abstract reasoning does not occur until adolescence.

**PRO TIP** If the infant or young child is lethargic or extremely irritable, the ability to be consoled by the parents can be a reassuring sign.

Assess CN function (CN I is rarely tested in infants and young toddlers, and taste is also not assessed in infants). Some of the assessments occur while assessing other parts of the body and may be incorporated elsewhere in the examination. Refer to Table 3.11 for assessment methods by age group (infants, children) for the CNs.

Assess balance by watching the child's gait while walking and movements when climbing or sitting. Keep in mind that the early walker displays the typical toddler gait of a widened base with moderate in-toeing and the presence of physiologic lordosis. In the older child or adolescent, determine cerebellar function with the Romberg test, having the child hop in place (age 4 years), tandem-walk (heel-to-toe, age 6 years), use rapid-alternating movements (age 8 years), finger-to-nose (age 8 years), and heel-to-shin (age 8 years).

Assess the infant's and child's DTRs. The newborn's DTRs are typically brisker, decreasing to normal by 4 months of age. Additionally, the newborn may exhibit 4 to 5 beats of clonus and the older child,

TABLE 3.11 **Cranial Nerve Assessment Methods**

| Cranial Nerve | Infants | Children |
|---|---|---|
| **CN I (olfactory)** | Not tested | Starting at preschool age, ask child to identify a familiar scent such as chocolate, soap, or bubble gum |
| **CN II (optic)** | Pupillary reaction (through age 3 years) | Pupillary reaction, visual acuity |
| **CN III (oculomotor), CN IV (trochlear), CN VI (abducens)** | Blink reflex, pupillary response to light | Pupillary size, accommodation, consensual response; extraocular movements |
| **CN V (trigeminal)** | Touch cheek with cotton wisp, suck and swallow | Test for sharp and dull, observe chewing and swallowing, ask child to make a mean face |
| **CN VII (facial)** | Taste not tested, observe facial movement for symmetry | Identify familiar flavor, observe facial movement for symmetry |
| **CN VIII (acoustic—vestibulocochlear)** | Startle response to sound (up to 4 months), acoustic blink reflex, objective hearing test | Whisper, Weber, Rinne tests, audiometric test, Romberg |
| **CN IX (glossopharyngeal), CN X (vagus)** | Gag reflex, suck and swallow, pitch of cry | Identify familiar flavor, gag reflex, child says "Ah," voice quality |
| **CN XI (spinal accessory)** | Turn infant's head from side to side while infant lying supine | Turn head side to side, lower chin, and shrug shoulders against resistance |
| **CN XII (hypoglossal)** | Suck and swallow; while infant is crying, check for absence of lateral deviation of tongue | Stick out tongue, move side to side, pronunciation of letter "R" |

CN, cranial nerve

*Source*: Adapted from Chiocca, E. M. (2020). *Advanced pediatric assessment* (3rd ed., pp. 502–506, Tables 22.6 and 22.7). Springer Publishing Company.

1 to 2 beats of clonus, which in either instance if symmetric may be considered normal (Schor, 2020). Rate the DTR response as follows:

- 0—Absent
- +1—Hypoactive
- +2—Normal
- +3—Hyperactive without clonus
- +4—Hyperactive with clonus (note number of beats of clonus)

When DTRs are +1 or +3, they may be considered normal if they are symmetric (Schor, 2020).

In the newborn and younger infant, assess primitive reflexes. The primitive reflexes are intact in the neurologically healthy newborn. Refer to Table 3.12 for a description and age of disappearance of the primitive reflexes. In the older infant, assess protective reflexes. As the primitive reflexes are integrated (disappear), the protective reflexes emerge. These motor responses are related to equilibrium, are necessary for appropriate motor development, and once present remain so throughout life. Refer to Table 3.13 for a description and age of appearance of the protective reflexes. Lastly, refer to Table 3.14 for common abnormal findings by age group.

**PRO TIP** Children often find it difficult to relax during assessment of the DTRs. When assessing upper extremity DTRs, distract the child by asking them to look at the ceiling and count the dots in the ceiling tile (or something similar). When assessing lower extremity DTRs, distract the child by asking them to grasp the fingertips of the hand together and pull hard without the hands separating.

**TABLE 3.12 Primitive Reflexes**

| Reflex | Description | Expected Response | Age of Disappearance |
|---|---|---|---|
| **Step** | Hold the infant with one foot down on a flat surface. | The infant automatically places other foot down as if initiating walking | 6–8 weeks |
| **Root** | Stroke the infant's cheek (on one side) | The infant turns to that side with mouth open. | 3 months |
| **Suck** | Insert a nipple or gloved finger in the infant's mouth | The infant automatically initiates sucking motion | 2–5 months |
| **Tongue extrusion** | Place a tongue blade or spoon on the infant's tongue | The infant's tongue thrusts forward | 4 months |
| **Palmar grasp** | Place the index finger in the infant's palm | The infant reflexively grasps the finger | 4–6 months |
| **Moro (startle, embrace)** | With infant supine, pull infant's arms upward until shoulders slightly off table, then release | The arms abduct, moving upward with the fingers forming a 'C' | 4–6 months |
| **ATNR** | With infant supine, turn the infant's head to one side | Extremities on the side the head is turned to extend, while extremities on the opposite side flex (also called fencing position) | 4–6 months |
| **Plantar grasp** | Hold the infant's lower leg with one ~~had~~ hand taking care not to touch the foot or ankle. Press the pad of the index finger onto the bottom of the infant's foot below the toes | The infant's foot and toes flex, as if grasping with the bottom of the foot | 9 months |
| **Babinski** | Hold the infant's lower leg with one hand taking care not to touch the foot or ankle. With one finger, stroke the lateral aspect of the sole, moving up and across the plantar surface | The infant's toes fan out and hyperextend. | 12 months |

ATNR, asymmetric tonic neck reflex

*Source*: Data from Chiocca, E. M. (2020). *Advanced pediatric assessment* (3rd ed.). Springer Publishing Company; Kyle, T., & Carman, C. (2021). *Essentials of pediatric nursing* (4th ed.). Wolters Kluwer Health; Schor, N. F. (2020). Neurologic evaluation. In R. M. Kliegman, J. St. Geme, N. J. Blum, S. S. Shah, R. C. Tasker, K. M. Wilson, & R. E. Behrman (Eds.), *Nelson textbook of pediatrics* (21st ed., Chapter 608). Elsevier.

**TABLE 3.13 Protective Reflexes**

| Reflex | Description | Expected Response | Age of Appearance |
|---|---|---|---|
| **Neck righting** | Hold infant in support sitting position, then tilt body slightly. | Infant's neck keeps the head in an upright position | 4–6 months |
| **Protective extension** | In a supported sitting position, apply gentle sideward force to the infant's center of gravity | Arms will abduct, involuntary extension of the arm outward to the side of the fall with palm open | 5–7 months |
| **Forward or downward Parachute** | Suspend the infant prone, firmly supported, then quickly lower the infant toward a flat surface | Infant extends arms forward in a protective manner | 8 months |
| **Backward parachute** | With infant in sitting position and legs out in front, slightly push infant backward. | Infant extends arms backward in a protective manner | 9–10 months |

*Source*: Data from Chiocca, E. M. (2020). *Advanced pediatric assessment* (3rd ed.). Springer Publishing Company; Kyle, T., & Carman, C. (2021). *Essentials of pediatric nursing* (4th ed.). Wolters Kluwer Health; Schor, N. F. (2020). Neurologic evaluation. In R. M. Kliegman, J. St. Geme, N. J. Blum, S. S. Shah, R. C. Tasker, K. M. Wilson, & R. E. Behrman (Eds.), *Nelson textbook of pediatrics* (21st ed., Chapter 608). Elsevier.

**TABLE 3.14 Common Abnormal Physical Examination Findings by Age Group**

| System | Neonate/Infant | Toddler/Preschool | School Age/Adolescent |
|---|---|---|---|
| **Integumentary** | Laguna, cradle cap, birth marks or pigmentation, skin changes (jaundice, cyanosis, mottling, rashes/lesions), dermatitis; if bruising/petechiae in noncruiser = mandatory reporting for suspected child abuse | Birth marks, rashes or lesions, pruritis, hives (urticaria), contact dermatitis, atopic dermatitis, seborrhea/eczema, acne, changes in moles (neoplasm melanoma), changes in body hair (excessive/loss hair growth), nail disorders, infestation (pediculosis, scabies). | |
| **Lymphatics** | Fever | Fever, pallor, lymphadenopathy | |
| **HEENT** | Early fontanel closure, eye drainage, rhinorrhea | Glasses or contacts, decreased hearing associated with ear infections, rhinorrhea, dental caries, malocclusion, erythematous pharynx | |
| **Respiratory** | Grunting, increased respiratory rate, retractions, cyanosis | Increased respiratory rate, retractions, cough, sputum expectoration, wheeze | |
| **Cardiac** | Murmur, cyanosis, tachycardia | Murmur, cyanosis, tachycardia | Chest pain, cyanosis, tachycardia, syncope, night sweats |
| **Gastrointestinal** | Vomiting, diarrhea, constipation, increased crying | Vomiting, diarrhea, constipation, abdominal pain | Nausea, vomiting, diarrhea, constipation, abdominal pain, anorexia |
| **Genitourinary** | Vaginal discharge in newborn may be normal—beyond newborn period, discharge or bleeding may indicate abuse, labial adhesion, undescended testicle | Hematuria, dysuria, polyuria, pyuria, vaginal discharge (prepubertal girl) | |
| **Musculoskeletal** | Genu varum | Genu valgum, genu varum, limp | Scoliosis, joint swelling, abnormal gait, limp |
| **Neurologic** | Developmental delay, uncontrolled movements | | Headache, nervousness, dizziness, tingling |

HEENT, head, eyes, ears, nose, throat.

# PREPARTICIPATION PHYSICAL EVALUATION

While the preparticipation physical evaluation (PPE) has been and continues to be used to determine medical eligibility for youth participation in sports, the evidence is unclear as to its value. Research has yet to determine the validity of the PPE or provide standardization of the process (Bernhardt & Roberts, 2019). Nevertheless, advanced providers are routinely called upon to determine medical eligibility and clear children for sports participation.

## HEALTH HISTORY

Ideally, the PPE is performed by the primary care provider in the child's medical home. The health history is focused on determining the child's risk related to sports participation. The child should be asked which sport(s) they intend to participate in. Past and current medical conditions are then explored, noting allergies, medications and supplements used, and past surgeries. Questions are then asked related to the child's psychosocial status. General questions are explored, and a variety of medical issues are inquired about. An important question to explore in detail relates to history of previous concussion, particularly if the child is interested in playing a contact sport. The remainder of the health history is focused on heart health, bone and joint issues, and female menstruation. The PPE also provides a time for the provider to explore more sensitive issues with the child or adolescent, such as stress; feeling safe at home; tobacco, alcohol, drug, or anabolic steroid use; car and bicycle safety; and the use of condoms.

### Heart Health

The provider asks about the child, noting if there is a history of:

- Syncope during or after exercise
- Chest pain, heart flutters, palpitations, lightheadedness or shortness of breath during exercise
- Any heart problems or tests related to the heart
- Seizures

Next the provider determines the family history, inquiring about a history of:

- Unexpected/unexplained sudden death before age 35 (genetic heart problem)
- Pacemaker or implanted defibrillator before age 35

### Bones and Joints

Determine if the child or adolescent has ever had a stress fracture or an injury to a joint, ligament, tendon, or bone that prevented a child from practicing or playing in a game. Additionally, determine if the child currently has any joint, ligament, tendon, or bone that is currently bothering the child.

### Menstruation

For females, determine age at menarche or note that menarche has not yet occurred. Ask when the last menstrual period was and how many periods have occurred in the past 12 months.

## PHYSICAL EXAMINATION

Perform a comprehensive physical examination including height, weight, vital signs, and visual acuity testing. When observing the child's appearance, note if Marfan stigmata are present. Upon heart auscultation, listen for murmurs while the child is standing, sitting, and performing the Valsalva maneuver. For the musculoskeletal system, determine full range of motion of each joint and perform the double-leg squat test, single-leg squat test, and box drop or step drop test.

## PROVIDING MEDICAL CLEARANCE

If the health history or the physical examination reveals any abnormal heart findings, consider ordering an electrocardiogram and echocardiogram and referring the athlete to a pediatric cardiologist. Other abnormal findings during the health history and physical examination should be evaluated in the context of the desired sport, paying particular attention to whether the sport is considered contact, minimal contact, or noncontact. Many school districts and schools have a standardized form to be completed for medical clearance, while others utilize the form produced by the AAP. Preparticipation PE forms are available for download on the AAP's website (www.aap.org/en-us/advocacy-and-policy/aap-health-initiatives/Pages/PPE.aspx):

- Medical History (available in English and Spanish)
- Physical Evaluation
- Medical Eligibility Form

A supplemental history form for athletes with disabilities is also available on the website.

## KEY POINTS

- All children are on a developmental trajectory in which physical, psychological, and social elements have normal ranges.
- The assessment of a child may vary depending on genetics and life or environmental experiences.
- The health history in children also includes the perinatal history and developmental milestones.
- Utilize the chief concern to guide in-depth investigation into particular parts of the health history.
- Developmental history requires more attention in the younger child, while school performance and adjustment become more important during the school-age and adolescent periods.
- Encourage the young verbal child to answer questions during the health history as appropriate.
- Direct health history questions to the school-age child and adolescent, seeking clarification from the parents as needed.
- Provide confidentiality and privacy for the adolescent during the health history.
- Weight and length or height should be assessed at each well-child visit to determine adequacy of growth.
- Normal vital sign ranges depend upon the child's age.
- Base the sequencing of the physical examination on the child's developmental age and level of cooperation.

## REFERENCES


American Academy of Pediatrics. (2018). *Healthy sleep habits: How many hours does your child need?* https://www.healthychildren.org/English/healthy-living/sleep/Pages/Healthy-Sleep-Habits-How-Many-Hours-Does-Your-Child-Need.aspx

Banikarim, C., & De Silva, N. K. (2020). Breast disorders in children and adolescents. *UpToDate.* https://www.uptodate.com/contents/breast-disorders-in-children-and-adolescents

Bernhardt, D. T., & Roberts, W. O. (2019). *PPE preparticipation physical evaluation* (5th ed.). American Academy of Pediatrics.

Bickley, L. S., Szilagyi, P. G., Hoffman, R. M., & Soriano, R. P. (2021). *Bates' guide to physical examination and history taking* (13th ed.). Wolters Kluwer.

Centers for Disease Control and Prevention. (2010). *WHO growth standards are recommended for use in the U.S. for infants and children 0 to 2 years of age.* https://www.cdc.gov/growthcharts/who_charts.htm

Centers for Disease Control and Prevention. (2013). *Use and interpretation of the WHO and CDC growth charts for children from birth to 20 years in the United States.* https://www.cdc.gov/nccdphp/dnpa/growthcharts/resources/growthchart.pdf

Centers for Disease Control and Prevention. (2020). *BMI percentile calculator for child and teen.* https://www.cdc.gov/healthyweight/bmi/calculator.html

Chiocca, E. M. (2020). *Advanced pediatric assessment* (3rd ed.). Springer Publishing Company.

Duderstadt, K. G. (2019). *Pediatric physical examination: An illustrated handbook* (3rd ed.). Elsevier.

Gavin, M. L. (2020). *Body mass index (BMI).* https://kidshealth.org/en/parents/bmi-charts.html

Jarvis, C., & Eckhardt, A. (2020). *Physical examination and health assessment* (8th ed.). Elsevier.

Jone, P., VonAlvensleben, J., Burkett, D., Darst, J. R., Collins, K. K., & Miyamoto, S. D. (2018). Cardiovascular diseases. In W. W. Hay, M. J. Levin, R. R. Deterding, & M. J. Abzug (Eds.), *Current pediatric diagnosis and treatment* (24th ed., Chapter 20). McGraw-Hill Education.

Kibbi, A.-G., & Bergqvist, C. M. (2019). Congenital dermal melanocytosis (Mongolian spot). In D. M. Elston (Ed.), *Medscape.* Retrieved November 3, 2020 from https://emedicine.medscape.com/article/1068732-overview

Kyle, T., & Carman, C. (2021). *Essentials of pediatric nursing* (4th ed.). Wolters Kluwer Health.

Quinlin, L., & Gawlik, K. (2021). Evidence-based history-taking approach for wellness exams, episodic visits, and chronic care management. In K. S. Gawlik, B. M. Melnyk, & A. M. Teall (Eds.), *Evidence-based physical examination: Best practices for health and well-being assessment* (pp. 17–42). Springer Publishing Company.

Schor, N. F. (2020). Neurologic evaluation. In R. M. Kliegman, J. St. Geme, N. J. Blum, S. S. Shah, R. C. Tasker, K. M. Wilson, & R. E. Behrman (Eds.), *Nelson textbook of pediatrics* (21st ed., Chapter 608). Elsevier.

Snell, B. J., & Gardner, S. L. (2017). *Care of the well newborn.* Jones & Bartlett Learning.

Tanski, S., & Garfunkel, L. C. (2010). Physical examination: Assessing growth and nutrition. In S. Tanski, L. C. Garfunkel, P. M. Duncan, & M. Weitzman (Eds.), *Performing preventive services: A Bright Futures handbook* (pp. 51–56). American Academy of Pediatrics.

Teall, A. M., & Gawlik, K. (2021). Approach to implementing and documenting patient-entered, culturally sensitive evidence-based assessment. In K. S. Gawlik, B. M. Melnyk, & A. M. Teall (Eds.), *Evidence-based physical examination: Best practices for health and well-being assessment* (pp. 43–54). Springer Publishing Company.

# Laboratory and Diagnostic Testing Interpretation

Katherine Taylor, Megan Arnold, Sylvia Cooper, and John West

## Student Learning Outcomes

**Upon completion of the chapter the reader should be able to:**

1. Describe the role and responsibility of the pediatric nurse practitioner in coding and billing for diagnostic testing.
2. Describe risks and common errors in blood sampling and identify reduction strategies.
3. Describe needle-fear and identify interventions to decrease needle-related pain.
4. Identify, order, and interpret office/clinic-based screening tests.
5. Identify, order, and interpret common office/clinic-based diagnostic laboratory and imaging tests.
6. Assimilate findings of common screening and diagnostic testing into the patient's plan of care.

## INTRODUCTION

Health screenings are a routine part of well-child care and are essential in early recognition and intervention of developmental delays or chronic medical conditions. Diagnostic laboratory and imaging data can be valuable sources of information in both preventive care and sick care. In order for the information gleaned from these screenings and tests to be useful, the healthcare provider must understand the utility of the tests and order them appropriately. Ordering unnecessary testing or conducting ill-timed screenings can lead to over- or underdiagnosis of medical or developmental problems and unnecessary pain and anxiety for the child and their caregivers. The nurse practitioner must also be able to accurately interpret the findings of screenings and diagnostic tests to avoid diagnostic errors and ensure that the information can be appropriately incorporated into the child's plan of care. This chapter will focus on best practices for laboratory collection and diagnostic testing, common childhood screenings, and common laboratory testing and diagnostic imaging for the advanced practice nurse in the primary care setting.

The content in this chapter maps to the following areas on the Pediatric Nursing Certification Board (PNCB) Pediatric Nurse Practitioner—Primary Care certification examination:

### CONTENT AREAS:

#### II. Assessment and Diagnosis

**C. Procedures**

1. Perform procedures in accordance with diagnostic guidelines and plan of care

#### IV. Professional Role and Responsibilities

**B. Practice Management**

1. Document patient encounters in a manner which supports applicable diagnostic and procedure codes
2. Utilize appropriate billing and coding to facilitate reimbursement

## BLOOD COLLECTION

Blood has many functions in both physiological and pathophysiological processes, and the resulting biomarkers within the blood make it an ideal specimen for diagnostic sampling (Baskin et al., 2019). Collection of blood for testing is a common diagnostic procedure used throughout the healthcare system (Normandin & Benotti, 2018; World Health Organization [WHO], 2010). *Phlebotomy* is the use of a hollow-bore needle to remove blood for testing or donation purposes. Some tests that require only small quantities of blood can utilize capillary blood, which is obtained via finger prick or, in the case of young infants (up to 6 months of age), heel prick. However, while capillary sampling is possible, even for term neonates the preferred method of sampling is venipuncture (WHO, 2010). Both venous sampling and capillary sampling should be performed by well-trained professionals to decrease risks to the child and healthcare provider, child pain, and possibility of diagnostic error.

## Risks in Blood Sampling

As with any procedure, informed consent in which risks and benefits are explained to the child and/or caregiver should be obtained when performing phlebotomy. The collection of blood involves risks to both the patient and the healthcare worker, but following infection control best practices can effectively reduce these risks. The WHO's publication *WHO guidelines on drawing blood: Best practices in phlebotomy* (2010) outlines these risks and reduction strategies that can be employed:

- Risks to the child:
  - Infection at sampling site
    - Risk of infection can be greatly reduced by performing proper hand hygeine, ensuring appropriate antisepsis of sampling site, and always using sterile needles and syringes.
  - Pain at sampling site
    - Phlebotomy should always be performed by well trained personnel and utilizing the least painful site (studies show venipuncture is less painful than a heel prick in neonates).
  - Thrombus, hematoma, excessive bleeding
    - Risk of hematoma or thrombus can be reduced by ensuring that the catheter gauge is appropriately sized and enters the vessel at 30 degrees or less. Also, healthcare worker should apply pressure for 3–5 minutes after the blood draw.
    - Take a thorough history from all children (or their parents) to identify any persons who have a history of bleeding disorders or are taking anticoagulant medications.
  - Nerve damage
    - The antecubital vessels should be utilized whenever possible, and avoid probing for the vessel.
    - Avoid finger pricks in children; opt for phlebotomy instead.
  - Vasovagal reaction or syncope
    - Be sure the child is well hydrated and allow them to lie down if they desire.
    - Provide measures to reduce anxiety, such as audiovisual distraction.
- Risks to the healthcare worker:
  - Sharps injury
    - Always use safety devices such as needleless systems, needle covers, and safety lancets
    - Keep sharps containers within arm's reach and dispose of used sharps immediately
  - Blood exposure
    - Vaccination against blood-borne pathogens should be encouraged and gloves should be worn anytime there is risk of body fluid exposure.
    - Use transfer devices when drawing for multiple tubes.
    - If there is an exposure, be sure the institution's reporting protocol is followed.

## Errors in Blood Sampling

There are three phases of laboratory testing: preanalytical, analytical, and postanalytical. The majority of errors occur in the preanalytical phase and are preventable with proper training (Emergency Nurses Association [ENA], 2016). The most frequently recognized preanalytical error is poor specimen quality, with the most common causes being inappropriate patient preparation, specimen contamination, and hemolysis (Baskin et al., 2019; Kazmierczak, 2019; Normandin & Benotti, 2018).

### Proper Patient Preparation and Timing

Proper preparation includes ensuring the correct timing of all tests. Fasting samples can be typically be drawn 2 hours after a meal without excessive increases in serum glucose, triglycerides, aspartate aminotransferase (AST), and bilirubin (Baskin et al., 2019). Therapeutic drug monitoring is necessary for several classes of pharmaceuticals in order to optimize treatment. Effective therapeutic drug monitoring is necessary for increased desirable effects, or efficacy, and decreased negative effects, or toxicity (McMillin & Johnson-Davis, 2019). The timing of therapeutic drug monitoring is variable depending on the drug being monitored, so it is essential to follow manufacturer guidelines for timing of collection. The primary care provider should always consult with a specialist when conducting therapeutic drug monitoring to ensure that all changes to medication doses are appropriate and follow-up is scheduled.

### Contamination

Contamination of blood samples can be due to improper site preparation or poor site selection. Antisepsis of the skin is usually accomplished with an isopropyl alcohol, chlorhexidine gluconate (CHG), or iodine solution, depending upon skin condition and institutional protocol (Baskin et al., 2019; WHO, 2010). Adequate drying time is essential to ensure removal of local skin flora and minimize the risk of alcohol interference with testing. Iodine solutions should be avoided when performing skin puncture due to false elevation of uric acid, potassium, and phosphorus (Baskin et al., 2019; WHO, 2010). Poor site selection can lead to samples that are contaminated or diluted with intravenous (IV) fluid. Care should be taken that phlebotomy is never performed proximal to an infusing peripheral IV line, and when samples are drawn from an existing IV or central line it is recommended that specific amounts of blood be discarded prior to sampling depending upon the length of the catheter (Baskin et al., 2019).

### Hemolysis

Hemolysis is a disruption of the erythrocyte membrane resulting in intracellular components (i.e., hemoglobin, AST, lactate dehydrogenase, and electrolytes such as potassium and magnesium) being released into the surrounding plasma or serum (Kazmierczak, 2019). Hemolysis can be from in vivo or in vitro causes, with in vitro hemolysis accounting for the majority of samples received at the laboratory and deemed unsuitable for testing (Kazmierczak, 2019). In vivo causes of hemolysis include hemoglobinopathies, infection, autoimmune disorders, transfusion reactions, or enzyme deficiences. In vitro hemolysis can occur during phlebotomy (e.g., with excessive force or vacuum or small catheter size); during sample handling and processing due to mechanical damage or shaking; or during sample storage, as with delayed time to centrifugation or freezing of the sample (ENA, 2016; Kazmierczak, 2019). Evidence-based research identifies measures that may decrease in vitro hemolysis including low-fill vacuum tubes, direct venipuncture instead of sampling from an IV, and staff education (ENA, 2016). If in vitro hemolysis is suspected, a new sample should be obtained immediately to verify the results.

## Needle-Related Pain and Needle Fear

Many needle-related procedures, such as phlebotomy, IV insertion, and vaccination, are common in childhood and can be a significant source of pain, fear, and anxiety for children and their caregivers (Bergomi et al., 2018; Birnie et al., 2018; Stoltz & Manworren, 2017). The fear associated with needles exists on a wide continuum. The more mild "needle fear" comprises general anxiety and fear, while the more extreme "needle phobia" is a psychiatric disorder that can be associated with complete visual avoidance and vasovagal response (McLenon & Rogers, 2019; McMurtry, Noel et al., 2015). Needle fear can extend beyond childhood and have serious repercussions, including avoidance of preventive medical care such as vaccinations, delays in obtaining necessary treatment for acute and chronic conditions, and delays in obtaining dental care (McLenon & Rogers, 2019; McMurtry, Riddell et al., 2015). Studies also show that needle fear contributes to vaccine hesitancy among parents, a growing global public health crisis, and the effective management of needle-related procedure pain has implications for enhancing public health (McLenon & Rogers, 2019; McMurtry, Noel et al., 2015; McMurtry, Pillai Riddell et al., 2015). There are both pharmacological and nonpharmacological interventions to help ameliorate needle-related pain. Naturally, the method used will depend not only on the training and resources available to the healthcare worker, but also the child's cognitive development and subsequent understanding of the context of the pain (McMurtry, Pillai Riddell et al., 2015).

### Pharmacologic Interventions

The use of topical, local anesthetics can effectively decrease pain associated with venipuncture, and the method selected will depend on the urgency of the situation (Hsu, 2020; Stoltz & Manworren, 2017). A topical liposomal agent will have to remain in place for 30 to 60 minutes, depending on the medium selected, while needle-free lidocaine delivery systems provide pain relief in 1 to 3 minutes (Hsu, 2020; Normandin & Benotti, 2018). For neonates and young infants, effective control for episodic pain can be accomplished with an oral sucrose solution delivered via oral syringe or pacifier dipped in the solution. Studies suggest that oral sucrose has an onset of about two minutes and will provide pain relief for approximately three to five minutes (Anand, 2020; Normandin & Benotti, 2018).

▶ ALERT: The use of lidocaine is contraindicated in children with G6PD deficiency.

### Nonpharmacologic Interventions

Nonpharmacologic pain interventions, such as topical cold and vibration therapy and psychological interventions, are appealing for many reasons. They often require little or no specialized training, can be employed by many healthcare providers and parents, and can be used across a broad range of settings (Birnie et al., 2018). A study by Bergomi and others (2018) found that the use of nonpharmacologic interventions during venipuncture decreased pain and anxiety for both the child and their parents when compared with standard practice. Buzzy® (MMJ Labs, Atlanta, GA) is a bee-shaped device that that has been shown to decrease pain during venipuncture, vaccination, and subcutaneous injection (Ballard et al., 2019; Bergomi et al., 2018; Redfern et al., 2018). It combines cold therapy with vibration, stimulating A-beta nociceptive fibers and decreasing the transmission of pain information to the spinal cord (Ballard et al., 2019; Bergomi et al., 2018). Passive distraction interventions such as watching cartoons were found to be more effective than active distraction interventions, such as playing a video game (Bergomi et al., 2018). Cognitive behavioral therapy is a psychological intervention using a combination of techniques that draw on the child's own coping tendencies (Birnie et al., 2018). Child-life specialists, if available, can help with cognitive behavioral therapy, which includes preparation prior to the event, relaxation and deep breathing exercises, distraction, positive reinforcement, and coaching (Birnie et al., 2018; Normandin & Benotti, 2018).

## SCREENING TESTS

Screening tests commonly performed in the pediatric population include vision and hearing screening, newborn screening, and tests for dyslipidemia, hypertension, anemia, lead poisoning, and hyperbilirubinemia.

### Vision Screening

Visual screens identify children who have structural ocular abnormalities or impaired vision. These visual screens should include both instrument-based screening and direct visual acuity testing with age-appropriate symbols. Appropriate visual screening can detect abnormalities in vision and also detect retinal abnormalities, cataracts, glaucoma, retinoblastoma, strabismus, and/or neurologic disorders (American Academy of Pediatrics [AAP], 2016).

#### Timing of Vision Screening

Ocular history, external inspection of eyes, red reflex testing, and pupil examination should be performed at the first newborn visit and all subsequent well-child checks. Instrument-based screening, if available, can take place starting at the 12-month visit, and every year until the child is able to participate in visual acuity age-appropriate symbol assessment. If the child is developmentally appropriate and cooperative, this should start by age 3 (Donahue & Baker, 2016).

#### Referral

Premature infants or infants with a family history of ocular abnormalities such as congenital cataracts, retinoblastoma, or metabolic disease should all be referred to a pediatric ophthalmologist.

### Hearing Screening

Hearing loss in newborns and young children can be associated with speech and language delay, and delay in cognitive development. Early detection and intervention are the goals of hearing screens. Hearing loss can be congenital, progressive, or delayed onset, which is why screening is recommended throughout childhood and into adolescent years. Hearing loss occurs in approximately 15% of children 6 to 19 years of age (Centers for Disease Control and Prevention [CDC], 2020).

#### Timing of Hearing Screening

The first hearing screen should occur no later than 1 month of age. If the infant fails, they should have a comprehensive audiological evaluation no later than 3 months of age (Joint Committee on Infant Hearing [JCIH], 2019). At each well-child check, observation of auditory behavior and developmental milestones should be noted and discussed with the family. Parental concerns about language and hearing should be assessed at every well-child check. If risk assessment is positive in the young child, hearing screening should occur. Hearing screen with audiometry is recommended routinely at 4, 5, 6, 8, and 10 years, then once between 11 and 14 years, once between 15 and 17 years, and once between 18 and 21 years of age (AAP, 2020b). Audiometry determines the softest decibel threshold (dB) at which the child can hear a sound

50% of the time for each tested frequency. Normal hearing threshold is between -10 to 15 dB (American Speech-Language-Hearing Association, 2020).

Earlier and more frequent assessments are indicated for infants with perinatal infections, syndromes associated with progressive hearing loss, neurodegenerative disorders, and infants who are receiving chemotherapy and who experience trauma.

### Referral

Any child who fails a hearing screening should be referred to a pediatric audiologist, pediatric otolaryngologist, and speech-language pathologist, with early intervention as soon as possible.

## Newborn Screening

Newborn screening is a program that screens all newborns within the first few days of life for certain conditions that may not be apparent at birth or tested during the prenatal period, and that only become symptomatic later. It was designed to reduce morbidity and mortality, and also initiate interventions early in certain conditions that may not be evident at the time of birth (Kemper, 2019). In addition to hearing screening and critical congenital heart disease screening, there is newborn screening via blood sampling tests for congenital, genetic, and metabolic disorders. The U.S. Department of Health and Human Services (USDHHS) has published a Recommended Uniform Screening Panel, yet each state determines what conditions to include in newborn screening (Kemper, 2019). Conditions included in the Recommended Uniform Screening Panel may be found at www.hrsa.gov/advisory-committees/heritable-disorders/rusp/index.html.

### Timing of Newborn Screening

Initial newborn screens should be completed after the first 24 hours following birth and prior to the newborn leaving the hospital or birth center (Kemper, 2019). Some states require a secondary screening because of the risk of false negatives and/or positives, which should be sent when the infant is between 1 to 2 weeks old. Approximately 25% of newborns in the United States receive secondary screening (CDC, 2019). Results from the initial screening should be communicated to the primary care office within 2 to 4 weeks per state programs. Primary care practitioners should note that certain factors can alter newborn screening results, such as gestational and postnatal age, diet, transfusions, and total parenteral nutrition. These newborns may need additional screening if their first newborn screening was abnormal (Kemper, 2019).

Be aware that there is a risk of false-positive and/or false negative results associated with newborn screenings. All out-of-range results should be confirmed. Additionally, although newborn screens are mandated in most states, parental refusal may occur. In these cases, parents should sign a waiver documenting their refusal (CDC, 2019).

### Referral

If a newborn screening contains out-of-range results, referrals to specific specialists based on the results may be indicated due to the lifelong implications and the management needed. Also, genetic counseling for families should be offered.

## Anemia Screening

Anemia screening is most commonly used to detect iron deficiency anemia. *Anemia* is defined as hemoglobin level <11 g/dL in children 6 months to 5 years and pregnant females over 15 years of age, <11.5 g/dL in children 5 to 11 years, <12 g/dL in children 12 to 15 years and females older than 15 years, and <13 g/dL in males older than 15 years of age (Powers, 2020). Laboratory findings of microcytic anemia support a diagnosis of iron deficiency anemia. A confirmatory test of a low serum ferritin level can support the diagnosis.

The recommended screening method is a complete blood count (CBC). If not available, a hemoglobin concentration (Hgb) can be used to screen children for anemia.

### Timing of Anemia Screening

All infants should have a risk assessment completed at 4 months of age and should be screened at 12 months of age. If a child has risk factors such as prematurity or low birth weight, screening should be done as early as 4 months old. After 1 year of age, risk assessments should be performed at well child visits. Children with low iron diets (i.e., vegetarian), limited access to food, or those with special needs may require screening past 1 year of age (Kelly, 2020).

### Referral

Education on dietary changes and initiation of iron supplementation can be done in the primary care setting. If not resolved, or if other abnormalities are seen on screening labs, referral to a pediatric hematologist is recommended.

## Dyslipidemia Screening

Lipid screening is used for early identification, evaluation, and treatment of pediatric dyslipidemia which, in turn, decreases the risk of cardiovascular disease in the future. A full lipid panel includes total cholesterol, high-density lipoprotein cholesterol (HDL-C), and triglycerides. These values are used to calculate low-density lipoprotein cholesterol (LDL-C), and non-high-density lipoprotein cholesterol (non-HDL-C). If the results are abnormal (Table 4.1), the official diagnosis requires confirmation testing of a fasting lipid panel on two separate occasions, 2 to 12 weeks apart (de Ferranti & Newburger, 2020).

### Timing of Dyslipidemia Screening

Cardiovascular disease risk should be assessed annually in children. If the child has one or more risk factors, lipid screening should be performed. Risk factors include family history of cardiovascular disease or high cholesterol, hypertension, diabetes mellitus, chronic kidney disease, certain congenital heart defects, and obesity. If the child does not have any risk factors, screening should occur between ages 9 and 11 years (de Ferranti & Newburger, 2020).

### Referral

If lipid values are abnormal, the first step is diet and lifestyle modifications, which can be managed in a primary care setting. If values continue to be abnormal, prescribing a statin medication is the next step. If repeat lipid levels remain elevated, a referral to a pediatric cardiologist is recommended.

**PRO TIP** Lipid screening can be completed fasting or nonfasting, but whether it is one or the other should be documented.

**TABLE 4.1 Abnormal Lipid Values**

| | |
|---|---|
| Total Cholesterol | ≥200 |
| LDL-C | ≥130 |
| Non-HDL-C | ≥145 |
| Triglycerides | |
| Ages: 0 to 9 years | ≥100 |
| Ages: 10 to 19 years | ≥130 |

LDL-C, low-density lipoprotein cholesterol; Non-HDL-C, non-high-density lipoprotein cholesterol.

## Lead Screening

The goal of lead screening is to prevent neurodevelopmental effects caused by lead poisoning. Lead poisoning is diagnosed if the blood lead level is ≥5 mcg/dL (Kelly, 2020).

### Timing of Lead Screening

It is recommended that screening should occur at 12 months and 24 months of age, because these ages are identified as the highest risk of exposure. Risk assessments should also be performed at 6, 9, 12, 18, and 24 months of age, and annually until age 6 years (AAP, 2020b). Risk factors that require additional screening include:

- Child lives in a home or attends childcare in a building with an identified lead hazard.
- Child lives in a home or attends childcare in a building that was built before 1978 and is in poor condition or recently renovated (Kelly, 2020).

Children and adolescents between 6 months and 16 years of age who enter the United States as immigrants, refugees, or international adoptees should be tested for blood lead concentration at the time of arrival (Kelly, 2020). Most states require that elevated blood lead levels be reported to the state health department.

**PRO TIP** Also check state lead screening requirements, as some states have additional requirements.

### Referral

Blood lead levels >15 mcg/dL should be evaluated and treated in conjunction with an expert. Contact the local Pediatric Environmental Health Specialty Unit for consultation and recommendations.

## Hypertension Screening

Pediatric hypertension is defined as blood pressure readings on three separate occasions that are greater than the 95th percentile for the age, sex, and height of the child, or ≥130/80 mmHg. Hypertension screening is recommended to identify and prevent cardiovascular disease secondary to hypertension in children (Mattoo, 2020).

### Timing of Hypertension Screening

It is recommended to begin hypertension screening annually in children with no risk factors starting at age 3 years. Risk factors include, but are not limited to, prematurity, low birth weight, renal disease, organ transplant, malignancy, obesity, diabetes mellitus, or congenital heart disease. Children 3 years and older with risk factors should be screened at every encounter with their primary care practitioner (Kelly, 2020). If elevated blood pressure or hypertension is diagnosed, additional screening should be ordered, e.g., urinalysis (UA), chemistry panel, and lipid profile (Flynn et al., 2017).

### Referral

If the child has elevated blood pressure (≥90th percentile to <95th percentile or 120/80 mm Hg), the primary care practitioner should counsel child and family on lifestyle modifications that include dietary and weight management. If the child has stage 1 hypertension (≥95th percentile to <95th percentile + 12 mmHg, or 130–139/80–89 mmHg), medication initiation along with lifestyle modifications are recommended. Children with stage 2 hypertension (≥95th percentile + 12 mmHg, or ≥140/90 mmHg) should be referred to pediatric nephrology or cardiology for additional evaluation and management (E/M; Flynn et al., 2017).

▶ ALERT: Any child presenting with a blood pressure reading 30 mmHg or more above the 95th percentile should receive immediate evaluation and treatment with IV antihypertensive due to potentially life-threatening effects (Flynn et al., 2017).

### Bilirubin Screening

Newborns with severe hyperbilirubinemia (total bilirubin level >25 mg/dL) are at risk of developing bilirubin-induced neurologic dysfunction (Wong & Bhutani, 2020). Screening of bilirubin levels is recommended to identify infants with hyperbilirubinemia and provide treatment if needed. Screening includes physical examination, assessment, and measurement of bilirubin levels. Risk factors for hyperbilirubinemia include prematurity of 35 to 36 weeks, being exclusively breastfed, hemolytic disease, family history of hyperbilirubinemia requiring phototherapy, jaundice observed in the first 24 hours, and East Asian race (Wong & Bhutani, 2020).

#### Timing of Bilirubin Screening

It is recommended that a risk assessment and total bilirubin level be obtained prior to discharge from the birth center or hospital after birth. Newborns should have follow-up with their primary care provider within 72 to 96 hours after birth for reassessment. Total bilirubin levels should peak within this time and repeat levels may be indicated (Wong & Bhutani, 2020).

### Referral

The primary care practitioner should be familiar with and utilize nomograms that provide guidelines on determining a child's risk of severe hyperbilirubinemia, and guidelines on phototherapy and exchange transfusion initiation. Refer to chapter 42.

## COMMON LABORATORY AND DIAGNOSTIC TESTS

Common blood tests used in the pediatric population include the CBC and chemistry panels. The rapid strep test is a commonly used point-of-care test. Other frequently used tests include respiratory viral panels, chest radiograph, and UA.

### Complete Blood Count

The CBC with or without differential (Table 4.2) gives data on white blood cell (WBC) count, red blood cell (RBC) count, hemoglobin, hematocrit, platelet count, mean corpuscular volume (MCV), mean corpuscular hemoglobin (MCH), mean corpuscular hemoglobin concentration (MCHC), and red cell distribution width (RDW). The WBC count can be further differentiated into neutrophil, leukocyte, monocyte, eosinophil, and basophil count with an absolute neutrophil count (ANC; Corbett & Banks, 2019).

#### Timing of Complete Blood Count Screening

The CBC is collected via blood draw, either from a venous or finger/heel stick. A CBC is done to detect or monitor various health conditions, including clotting disorders, anemia, infection, leukemia, RBC production or destruction or loss from bleeding, or as part of a routine checkup.

#### Accuracy

Reference points will vary slightly from laboratory to laboratory. Quality control is set by the manufacturer of the machine and as long as machine calibration is maintained, outside of extrinsic factors such as hemodilution or hemoconcentration, the results can be assumed to be accurate (Vis & Huisman, 2016).

TABLE 4.2 **Complete Blood Count Reference Ranges**

| Test | Range |
|---|---|
| WBC | Newborn: 9000–30000/mm$^3$<br><2 yr: 6200–17000/mm$^3$<br>>2 yr: 5000–10000 |
| RBC (× 10$^6$/uL) | Newborn: 4.8–7.1<br>2–8 weeks: 4–6<br>2–6 months: 3.5–5.5<br>6 mo–1 yr: 3.5–5.2<br>1–6 yr: 4–5.5<br>6–18 yr: 4–5.5 |
| Hemoglobin (g/dL) | Newborn: 14–24<br>0–2 weeks: 12–20<br>2–6 months: 10–17<br>6 mo–1 yr: 9.5–14<br>1–6 yr: 9.5–14<br>6–18 yr: 10–15.5 |
| Hematocrit (%) | Newborn: 44–64<br>2–8 weeks: 39–59<br>2–6 months: 33–50<br>6 mo–1 yr: 29–43<br>1–6 yr: 30–40<br>6–18 yr: 32–44 |
| Platelets | Newborn: 150000–300000/mm$^3$<br>Infant: 200000–475000/mm$^3$<br>Child: 150000–400000/mm$^3$ |
| MCV | Newborn: 96–108 um$^3$<br>Child: 80–95 um$^3$ |
| MCH | Newborn: 32–34 pg<br>Child: 27–31 pg |
| MCHC | Newborn: 32–33 g/dL<br>Child: 32–36 g/dL |
| RDW | 11–14.5% |
| Neutrophil (%) | 55–70 |
| Lymphocytes (%) | 20–40 |
| Monocytes (%) | 2–8 |
| Erythrocytes (%) | 1–4 |
| Basophils (%) | 0.5–1 |
| ANC (WBC × [% neutrophils + % bands]) | >1000 |

ANC, absolute neutrophil count; MCH, mean corpuscular hemoglobin; MCHC, mean corpuscular hemoglobin concentration; MCV, mean corpuscular volume; RBC, red blood cell; RDW, red cell distribution width; WBC, white blood cell

TABLE 4.3 **Chemistry Reference Ranges**

| Test | Range |
|---|---|
| Sodium (mEq/L) | Newborn: 134–144<br>Infant: 134–150<br>Child: 136–145 |
| Potassium (mEq/L) | Infant: 4.1–5.3<br>Child: 3.5–4.7 |
| Chloride (mEq/L) | Infant: 96–106<br>Child: 90–110 |
| $CO_2$ (mEq/L) | 20–28 |
| BUN (mg/dL) | Newborn: 3–12<br>Infant/Child: 5–18 |
| Creatinine (mg/dL) | Infant: 0.2–0.4<br>Child: 0.3–0.7<br>Adolescent: 0.5–1.0 |
| Glucose (mg/dL) | Infant: 40–90<br>Child < 2 yr: 60–100<br>Child > 2 yr: 70–105 |
| ALP (U/L) | < 2 yr: 85–235<br>2–8 yr: 65–210<br>9–15 yr: 60–300<br>16–21 yr: 30–200 |
| Albumin (g/dL) | Newborn: 3.5–5.4<br>Infant: 4.4–5.4<br>Child: 4–5.9 |
| Protein total (g/dL) | Newborn: 4.6–7.4<br>Infant: 6–6.7<br>Child: 6.2–8 |
| Bilirubin total (mg/dL) | 0.3–1 |
| ALT (U/L) | 4–36 (infants may be twice as high) |
| AST (U/L) | Newborn/Infant: 15–60<br>Child: 0–35 |
| Magnesium (mEq/L) | Newborn: 1.4–2<br>Child 1.4–1.7 |
| Phosphorus (mg/dL) | Newborn: 4.3–9.3<br>Child: 4.5–6.5 |
| Calcium (mg/dL) | 10 days–2 yrs: 9–10.6<br>Child: 8.8–10.8 |

ALP, alkaline phosphatase; ALT, alanine aminotransferase; AST, aspartate aminotransferase; BUN, blood urea nitrogen; $CO_2$, bicarbonate

## Chemistry Panel

A chemistry panel is a group of tests ordered to evaluate the body's electrolyte balance and/or the status of major body organs (Table 4.3). Panels include:

- Basic metabolic panel (BMP): 8 tests, also known as a chem 7, it contains sodium, potassium, chloride, bicarbonate (reported as $CO_2$), glucose, calcium, blood urea nitrogen (BUN), and creatinine.
- Chem 10: contains the 8 tests from the BMP with the addition of magnesium and phosphorus.
- Complete metabolic panel (CMP): usually contains 14 tests—the 8 included in the BMP, as well as liver function (alkaline phosphatase [ALP], alanine aminotransferase [ALT], AST, bilirubin), albumin, and total protein—but *does not include* magnesium and phosphorus

### Timing of the Chemistry Panel

The chemistry panel is obtained by blood draw, either from a venous puncture or a heel stick. It may be ordered as part of the examination to determine if dehydration, hyperglycemia, metabolic acidosis, or other electrolyte imbalances are present, or to evaluate kidney and liver function (American Association of Clinical Chemistry [AACC], 2020a).

### Accuracy

Typically, these tests are accurate as long as the machine has been calibrated per the manufacturer's guidelines; however, there are extrinsic factors that can lead to false results. These include hemolysis falsely elevating the potassium level (too much force during collection is a common cause), hemodilution, or over-the-counter medications/herbs/vitamins that can interfere with laboratory results (AACC, 2020b).

## Rapid Antigen Detection Test

The rapid antigen detection test (RADT), sometimes commonly known as the rapid strep test, is based upon enzyme or acid extraction of antigen from throat swabs.

### Timing of the Rapid Strep Test

Testing is suggested in children with evidence of acute tonsillopharyngitis or scarlatiniform rash and absence of signs and symptoms of viral infections, or those with exposure to an individual with group A streptococcal infection (GAS) at home or school, or high prevalence of GAS infections in community *and* symptoms of GAS, or those with suspected acute rheumatic fever (ARF) or poststreptococcal glomerulonephritis. Testing should not be performed in children with evidence of viral illness. Specimens should be obtained before initiation of antimicrobial therapy, as a single dose can result in a negative RADT or culture (Wald, 2020).

> **PRO TIP** Two swabs should be obtained simultaneously, so that if RADT is negative, a confirmation culture can be sent.

### Accuracy

RADT has a specificity of ≥95% and a sensitivity averaging 85% (Cohen et al., 2016). Given this, a positive RADT is useful in diagnosing GAS pharyngitis, but a negative RADT does not rule out GAS. A study of 300 children suggests a false positive rate of 11.5% in children who were treated in the 28 days previously for strep, indicating that a culture alone should drive antibiotic treatment in this subgroup (Barakat et al., 2019).

## Respiratory Viral Panel

The respiratory viral panel is a point-of-care test (POCT) that may be done in the office for influenza and/or respiratory syncytial virus (RSV). In the United States, only a POCT rapid test is available for influenza and RSV, although a laboratory "sendout" can be completed for adenovirus, human metapneumovirus, parainfluenza viruses 1–3, influenza A-subtypes H1 and H3, influenza B, and rhinovirus. POCT is typically antigen testing or nucleic acid detection, whereas laboratory sendouts are polymerase chain reaction (PCR) testing. Turnaround time for laboratory sendouts will vary on laboratory choice. MariPOC (a Finnish company) has developed a respiratory POCT for 11 viruses/bacteria, although it is not yet commercially available in the United States.

### Timing of Respiratory Virus Panel

Testing is suggested in children with upper respiratory symptoms (cough, sore throat, runny nose, and/or congestion) and with fever, to determine if medication is needed. This is especially important during influenza season when treatment with antivirals should be commenced within 48 hours of onset of symptoms. The main impact of POCT for primary care is to direct the plan of care, with positive rapid testing increasing the appropriate prescription of antiviral therapy and reducing unnecessary antibiotic prescriptions in pediatrics (Basile et al., 2018).

### Accuracy

To maximize detection of respiratory viruses in the upper respiratory tract, the sample should be obtained from the nasopharynx. This will require either a swab, wash, or aspirate. A nasal swab can result in lower overall sensitivity when compared with samples from the nasopharynx (Pinsky & Hayden, 2019).

Rapid influenza tests have suboptimal sensitivity, with false negative results common, but sensitivity for influenza B is lower than that of influenza A (CDC, 2016). Specificity is high but false positive results can also occur, most notably during times when influenza activity is low. Sensitivity for antigen testing is estimated to be 50% to 70%; however, sensitivity with PCR testing is >95%, leading to higher antiviral prescribing in children tested via PCR who were positive and decreased use in children who were negative when compared with antigen testing (Benirschke et al., 2019). Rapid RSV testing, in comparison, has a sensitivity of 80% and specificity of 97%, leading to confidence in diagnosis based on test results in pediatrics. Sensitivity drops to 29% in adults, however, which means that it is not a valuable test for adults (Chartrand et al., 2015).

## Chest Radiograph (X-ray)

A chest radiograph is a fast and painless imaging test of the chest, using electromagnetic waves to create a picture of the skeleton and organs held in the thorax.

### Timing of Chest Radiographs

This test can be used to help diagnose and monitor conditions of the lungs (pneumonia, tuberculosis, sarcoidosis, and fibrosis), the heart (evaluate heart size, heart failure, positioning), and bones (fractures, dislocations, growths). Chest x-rays are performed with as little covering the chest as possible (National Heart, Lung, and Blood Institute, n.d.). One view (anterior-posterior, or AP) or two views (AP/lateral) can be performed, depending on what the provider is searching for, but other views may also be accomplished.

### Accuracy

Technique, patient cooperation, and interfering clothing/jewelry items can affect the accuracy of a chest x-ray. In diagnosing pneumonia, chest x-rays hold a sensitivity of 93%, but no specificity in one study (Taghizadieh et al., 2015). Multiple studies have found poor accuracy in chest x-ray interpretation by less experienced physicians, so it can be suggested that an x-ray should be reviewed by a radiologist for improved accuracy (Cheung et al., 2018).

## Urinalysis

The most common biochemical test done in infancy and early childhood, the UA, evaluates urine for the presence of hematuria, proteinuria, leukocyturia, nitrituria, and uropathogenic bacteria (Table 4.4). It is a basic component of the evaluation of diseases of the kidneys and urinary tract, most commonly performed to diagnose or rule out a urinary tract infection (UTI) or renal disease. It may be performed by either a dipstick or microscopy. Both dipstick and microscopy test for pH, RBCs, protein, glucose, ketones, nitrites, leukocyte esterase, and bacteria; however, microscopic UA further analyzes cells for WBCs, RBCs, epithelial cells, casts, and crystals (Corbett & Banks, 2019).

TABLE 4.4 **Urinalysis Reference Ranges**

| Test | Range |
|---|---|
| Blood | Negative |
| Bilirubin | Negative |
| Clarity | Clear to slightly hazy |
| Color | Light yellow to amber |
| Glucose | Negative |
| Ketones | Negative |
| Leukocyte esterase | Negative |
| Nitrite | Negative |
| pH | 5–8 |
| Protein | Negative |
| Specific gravity | 0–1 yr 1.001–1.02<br>>1 yr 1.003–1.03 |
| Casts | None present |
| Crystals | Negative |
| WBC | 0–4 per low power field |
| RBC | <5 |
| Squamous epithelial cells | <10 per low power field |

RBC, red blood cell; WBC, white blood cell

### Timing of the Urinalysis

In children who have achieved urinary continence, midstream urine should be obtained after cleaning the genitals and perineum with soap and water or CHG wipes to lessen the likelihood of contamination. In infants and children who are not continent, urine can be obtained in four other ways:

- Bag urine: Bag is placed after genitals have been inspected and cleaned; however, due to the high likelihood of contamination, this method is unsuitable for culture
- Clean catch urine: Child is held on adult's lap with genitals exposed, and urine that is spontaneously voided is caught in a sterile vessel
- Catheter urine: Suitable urine sample is obtained after cleansing the genitals and a one-time catheterization obtains urine directly from the bladder. This is ideal for sending for culture
- Suprapubic bladder puncture: Simple but rarely performed, slightly invasive procedure used to acquire a urine sample if pyelonephritis is suspected (Tosif et al., 2012; Utsch & Klaus, 2014).

### Accuracy

Leukocyturia as an isolated finding is highly sensitive (83%) for a UTI, but specificity is low (78%). Dipstick tests for leukocyte esterase can be made positive for many reasons (lysed leukocytes or subpreputial material), thus microscopy for leukocytes is recommended. Nitrite testing has a sensitivity in dipstick testing of only 30% to 50% in infants, but in girls ages 3 years and older is as high as 98%.

**PRO TIP** Simultaneous demonstration of nitrituria and leukocyturia is 93% sensitive for a UTI.

Urine dipstick tests mainly disclose the presence of albumin; however, the Biuret reaction gives a quantitative measure of all urinary proteins. Hematuria has a 74% sensitivity rate for diagnosing UTIs, with a range of 73% to 89% sensitivity and 81% to 93% specificity for hematuria on dipstick (Utsch & Klaus, 2014). Sensitivity and specificity for proteinuria on dipstick were 90% and 95% in adults in one study; for glucosuria in the same study sensitivity was 100%, specificity 98.5% (Zamanzad, 2009). Most laboratories will run a microscopy on an abnormal dipstick for more information.

## BILLING AND CODING FOR LABORATORY AND DIAGNOSTIC TESTING

Once the pediatric nurse practitioner (PNP) has ordered and interpreted the appropriate screening and diagnostic examinations and a plan of care has been formulated for the child, attention must be turned to proper coding and billing for services rendered. The process of coding, billing, and reimbursement is complex and encompasses an entire professional field in its own right. Numerous organizations, such as the American Academy of Professional Coders (AAPC), offer professional certifications to medical coders and reimbursement specialists (AAPC, 2020). While the PNP is not expected to become an expert in this field, the PNP does have legal and professional obligations to submit accurate and timely documentation of care delivered. Inaccurate coding can lead not only to inaccurate identification of the child's diagnosis and incorrect data collection, but also to inappropriate payment and charges of fraud and abuse (Tuli, 2020).

In order to submit documentation for reimbursement in the primary care setting, the PNP, in addition to educational and professional certification standards, must have a national provider identifier (NPI). The NPI requirement is mandated by the Health Insurance Portability and Accountability Act (HIPAA) of 1996, and is a standard, unique identifier for each healthcare provider (Centers for Medicare and Medicaid Services, 2019). Another element required to be authorized to submit documentation for reimbursement is credentialing and privileging by the hiring institution (McMullen & Howie, 2020).

### Elements of Documentation

There are three primary entities through which the PNP will be reimbursed for care provided: Medicaid, which is administered in the pediatric population through the Children's Health Insurance Program (CHIP); private insurance such as Blue Cross/Blue Shield or Aetna; and direct payments from noninsured/self-paying individuals. Regardless of coverage, the elements of accurate and thorough documentation remain the same. According to the Center for Medicaid and Medicare Services (2020) *Evaluation and Management Services Guide*, in addition to the regular elements of documentation of a patient visit (chief complaint, health history, physical examination, etc.), documentation for reimbursement must include the following elements:

- Selection of the proper Common Procedural Terminology (CPT) code
- Selection of the proper International Classification of Diseases, 10th revision, Clinical Modification/Procedure Coding System (ICD-10-CM) codes

It is not necessary for the PNP to memorize CPT codes or ICD-10-CM codes, but the professional PNP will have a familiarity with the system and a working knowledge of codes commonly used in their practice.

### Common Procedural Codes

CPT codes are standardized numbers assigned to every task and service a healthcare practitioner may provide to a patient, including medical, surgical, and diagnostic services. CPT codes are typically 5-digit numbers without a decimal and will occasionally have a letter in the place of a digit. Selection of CPT codes is based on three factors: patient type, setting of service, and level of E/M performed. For example, the CPT code for an illness-based visit by an established patient (a patient who has established care in your office) will use the code 99213 or 99214 based on the severity of illness and the complexity of medical decision making involved. If a diagnostic examination (e.g., a rapid strep test) is performed, that will call for an additional CPT code, in this case 87880.

Preventive care will use different CPT codes as outlined in the Coding for Pediatric Preventative Care -2020 published by the AAP (2020a). For example, the CPT code for a new patient well child visit for an infant less than 1 year old is 99381.

### ICD-10-CM Codes

In addition to CPT codes that describe the service that a PNP may provide, ICD-10-CM codes are diagnostic codes for describing the conditions that a PNP may treat. The Center for Medicare and Medicaid Services (2020) provides examples of some common pediatric ICD-10 codes:

- H66.003 Acute suppurative otitis media without spontaneous rupture of ear drum, bilateral
- J45.20 Mild intermittent asthma, uncomplicated
- J02.0 Streptococcal pharyngitis

### Fraud and Abuse in Medical Documentation and Billing

While most medical offices will employ medical coders or a reimbursement specialist or contract with a billing and coding service, it is the responsibility of the PNP to correctly identify and document the services provided by the PNP. Chronic over- or underbilling may be construed as fraud or abuse by reimbursement agencies. *Fraud* is submission of claims for services not provided. *Abuse* is the systemic submission of such claims, whether intentional or inadvertent. Red flags indicating potential fraudulent/abusive documentation include:

- Coding for all E/M at one or two levels
- Billing for nonallowed services
- Excessive charges
- Services not provided as claimed
- Routine waiver of co-pays
- Advertising for free services/underbilling
- Billing for no-shows
- Unbundling services – split billing/return visit for procedure
- Billing established patient as new (Tuli, 2020)

**PRO TIP** Remember: Proving personal financial benefit is not a prerequisite for prosecution.

## KEY POINTS

- The collection of blood for diagnostic testing is a common procedure that has inherent risks to both the patient and the healthcare worker. The PNP should be aware of these risks and take appropriate steps to ensure the highest level of safety and comfort for the patient and the provider.
- Frequent exposure to needle-related procedures in childhood, such as routine vaccination and lab collection, can lead to the development of needle-fear. Needle-fear can be severe and cause children to avoid necessary medical care, dental care, and preventative vaccinations. Measures should be taken by the medical team to decrease procedure-related pain and lessen the likelihood of developing needle-fear.
- Health screenings are performed at specific ages/intervals in order to assist in early recognition of chronic conditions.
- Diagnostic laboratory and imaging tests are used in conjunction with the health history and physical examination to develop the most appropriate plan of care and follow-up for the patient. If a test result does not correlate with the history or examination findings, it should be repeated to confirm the result. If the result is still out of the expected range, then consult with the physician or refer to a specialist to determine the next steps in diagnosis.
- Clinic and office-based POC testing can be a cost-effective and quick way to confirm or rule out a diagnosis and can assist in determining if antibiotics are necessary.
- It is not necessary for the PNP to memorize individual CPT or ICD-10 codes, but the PNP should develop a working knowledge of the billing/reimbursement system and the codes that are common to their practice.
- It is the sole responsibility of the PNP to submit accurate and timely documentation for services provided. Although coding of services may be done by office or support personnel, the responsibility for the accuracy of documentation submitted for reimbursement rests solely with provider of those services.

## REFERENCES

American Academy of Pediatrics. (2016). Visual system assessment in infants, children, and young adults by pediatricians [Position statement]. *Pediatrics, 137*(1), 28–30. https://doi.org/10.1542/peds.2015-3596

American Academy of Pediatrics. (2020a). *Coding for pediatric preventative care—2020*. https://www.aap.org/en-us/documents/coding_preventive_care.pdf

American Academy of Pediatrics. (2020b). *Recommendations for pediatric preventive health care—Periodicity schedule*. https://downloads.aap.org/AAP/PDF/periodicity_schedule.pdf

American Academy of Professional Coders. (2020). *About AAPC*. https://www.aapc.com/aboutus

American Association of Clinical Chemistry. (2020a). *Chemistry panels*. https://labtestsonline.org/tests/chemistry-panels

American Association of Clinical Chemistry. (2020b). *How reliable is laboratory testing?* https://labtestsonline.org/articles/laboratory-test-reliability

American Speech-Language-Hearing Association. (2020). *Hearing loss—Beyond early childhood*. https://www.asha.org/Practice-Portal/Clinical-Topics/Hearing-Loss/#Degree_of_Hearing_Loss

Anand, K. (2020). Prevention and treatment of neonatal pain. *UpToDate*. https://www.uptodate.com/contents/prevention-and-treatment-of-neonatal-pain

Ballard, A., Khadra, C., Adler, S., Doyon-Trottier, E., & Le May, S. (2019). Efficacy of the Buzzy device for pain management during needle-related procedures: A systematic review and meta-analysis. *The Clinical Journal of Pain, 35*(6), 532–543. https://doi.org/10.1097/AJP.0000000000000690

Barakat, A., Evans, C., Gill, M., & Nelson, D. (2019). Rapid strep testing in children with recently treated streptococcal pharyngitis. *Pediatric Investigation, 3*(1), 27–30. https://doi.org/10.1002/ped4.12109

Basile, K., Kok, J., & Dwyer, D. (2018). Point-of-care diagnostics for respiratory viral infections. *Expert Review of Molecular Diagnostics, 18*(1), 75–83. https://doi.org/10.1080/14737159.2018.1419065

Baskin, L., Chin, A., Abdullah, A., & Naugler, C. (2019). Errors in patient preparation, specimen collection, anticoagulation, and preservative use: How to avoid such pre-analytical errors. In A. Dasgupta & J. L. Sepulveda (Eds.), *Accurate results in the clinical laboratory: A guide to error detection and correction* (2nd ed., pp. 11–25). Elsevier. https://doi.org/10.1016/B978-0-12-813776-5.00002-9

Benirschke, R., McElvania, E., Thomson, Jr., R., Kaul, K., & Das, S. (2019). Clinical impact of rapid point-of-care PCR influenza testing in an urgent care setting: A single-center study. *Journal of Clinical Microbiology, 57*(3), e01281-18. https://doi.org/10.1128/JCM.01281-18

Bergomi, P., Scudeller, L., Pintaldi, S., & Dal Molin, A. (2018). Efficacy of non-pharmacological methods of pain management in children undergoing venipuncture in a pediatric outpatient clinic: A randomized controlled trial of audiovisual distraction and external cold and vibration. *Journal of Pediatric Nursing, 42*, e66–e72. https://doi.org/10.1016/j.pedn.2018.04.011

Birnie, K., Noel, M., Chambers, C., Uman, L., & Parker, J. (2018). Psychological interventions for needle-related procedural pain and distress in children and adolescents. *Cochrane Database of Systematic Reviews*. https://doi.org/10.1002/14651858.CD005179.pub4

Centers for Disease Control and Prevention. (2016). *Rapid influenza diagnostic tests*. https://www.cdc.gov/flu/professionals/diagnosis/clinician_guidance_ridt.htm

Centers for Disease Control and Prevention. (2019). *CDC newborn screening portal*. https://www.cdc.gov/newbornscreening/index.html

Centers for Disease Control and Prevention. (2020). *Data and statistics about hearing loss in children*. https://www.cdc.gov/ncbddd/hearingloss/data.html

Centers for Medicare and Medicaid Services. (2019, December 12). *National provider identifier standard*. https://www.cms.gov/Regulations-and-Guidance/Administrative-Simplification/NationalProvIdentStand

Center for Medicare and Medicaid Services. (2020). *Evaluation and management services guide*. https://www.cms.gov/outreach-and-education/medicare-learning-network-mln/mlnproducts/downloads/eval-mgmt-serv-guide-icn006764.pdf

Chartrand, C., Tremblay, N., Renaud, C., & Papenburg, J. (2015). Diagnostic accuracy of rapid antigen detection for respiratory syncytial virus infection: Systematic review and meta-analysis. *Journal of Clinical Microbiology, 53*(12), 3738–3749. https://doi.org/10.1128/JCM.01816-15

Cheung, T., Harianto, H., Spanger, M., Young, A., & Wadhwa, V. (2018). Low accuracy and confidence in chest radiograph interpretation amongst junior doctors and medical students. *Internal Medicine Journal, 48*(7), 864–868. https://doi.org/10.1111/imj.13946

Cohen, J. F., Bertille, N., Cohen, R., & Chalumeau, M. (2016). Rapid antigen detection test for group A streptococcus in children with pharyngitis. *Cochrane Database of Systematic Reviews, 2016*(7). https://doi.org/10.1002/14651858.CD010502.pub2

Corbett, J. V., & Banks, A. (2019). *Laboratory tests and diagnostic procedures with nursing diagnoses* (9th ed.). Pearson.

de Ferranti, S., & Newburger, J. (2020). Dyslipidemia in children: Definition, screening, and diagnosis. *UpToDate*. https://www.uptodate.com/contents/dyslipidemia-in-children-definition-screening-and-diagnosis

Donahue, S., & Baker, C. (2016). Procedures for the evaluation of the visual system by pediatricians. *Pediatrics, 137*(1), e20153597. https://doi.org/10.1542/peds.2015-3597

Emergency Nurses Association. (2016). *Clinical practice guideline: Prevention of blood specimen hemolysis in peripherally-collected venous specimens*. https://www.ena.org/docs/default-source/resource-library/practice-resources/cpg/hemolysiscpg.pdf?sfvrsn&Site=ENA2015

Flynn, J., Kaelber, D., Baker-Smith, C., Blowey, D., Carroll, A., Daniels, S., Ferranti, S., Dionne, J., Falker, B., Flinn, S., Gidding, S., Goodwin, C., Leu, M., Powers, M., Rea, C., Samuels, J., Simasek, M., Thaker, V., & Urbina, E. (2017). Clinical practice guideline for screening and management of high blood pressure in children and adolescents. *Pediatrics, 140*(3), e20171904. https://doi.org/10.1542/peds.2017-1904

Hsu, D. (2020). Clinical use of topical anesthetics in children. *UpToDate*. https://www.uptodate.com/contents/clinical-use-of-topical-anesthetics-in-children

Joint Committee on Infant Hearing. (2019). Year 2019 position statement: Principles and guidelines for early hearing detection and intervention programs. *The Journal of Early Hearing Detection and Intervention, 4*(2), 1–44. https://doi.org/10.15142/fptk-b748

Kazmierczak, S. (2019). Interferences of hemolysis, lipemia, and high bilirubin on laboratory tests. In A. Dasgupta & J. L. Sepulveda (Eds.), *Accurate results in the clinical laboratory: A guide to error detection and correction* (2nd ed., pp. 57–67). Elsevier. https://doi.org/10.1016/B978-0-12-813776-5.00005-4

Kelly, N. (2020). Screening tests in children and adolescents. *UpToDate*. https://www.uptodate.com/contents/screening-tests-in-children-and-adolescents

Kemper, A. R. (2019). Newborn screening. *UpToDate*. https://www.uptodate.com/contents/newborn-screening

Mattoo, T. (2020). Definition and diagnosis of hypertension in children and adolescents. *UpToDate*. https://www

.uptodate.com/contents/definition-and-diagnosis-of-hypertension-in-children-and-adolescents

McLenon, J., & Rogers, M. A. M. (2019). The fear of needles: A systematic review and meta-analysis. *Journal of Advanced Nursing, 75*(1), 30–42. https://doi.org/10.1111/jan.13818

McMillin, G., & Johnson-Davis, K. (2019). Issues of interferences in therapeutic drug monitoring. In A. Dasgupta & J. L. Sepulveda (Eds.), *Accurate results in the clinical laboratory: A guide to error detection and correction* (2nd ed., pp. 215–231). Elsevier. https://doi.org/10.1016/B978-0-12-813776-5.00013-3

McMullen, P. C., & Howie, W. O. (2020). Credentialing and privileging: A primer for nurse practitioners. *The Journal for Nurse Practitioners, 16*(2), 91–95. https://doi.org/10.1016/j.nurpra.2019.10.015

McMurtry, C., Noel, M., Taddio, A., Antony, M., Asmundson, G., Riddell, R., Chambers, C., & Shah, V. (2015). Interventions for individuals with high levels of needle fear: Systematic review of randomized controlled trials and quasi-randomized controlled trials. *The Clinical Journal of Pain, 31*(10S), S109–S123. https://doi.org/10.1097/AJP.0000000000000273

McMurtry, C., Pillai Riddell, R., Taddio, A., Racine, N., Asmundson, G., Noel, M., Chambers, C., & Shah, V. (2015). Far from "just a poke": Common painful needle procedures and the development of needle fear. *The Clinical Journal of Pain, 31*(10S), S3–S11. https://doi.org/10.1097/AJP.0000000000000272

National Heart, Lung, and Blood Institute. (n.d.). *Chest X-ray.* https://www.nhlbi.nih.gov/health-topics/chest-x-ray

Normandin, P., & Benotti, S. (2018). Pediatric phlebotomy: Taking the bite out of Dracula. *Journal of Emergency Nursing, 44*(4), 427–429. https://doi.org/10.1016/j.jen.2018.03.017

Pinsky, B., & Hayden, R. (2019). Cost-effective respiratory virus testing. *Journal of Clinical Microbiology, 57*(9), e00373-19. https://doi.org/10.1128/JCM.00373-19

Powers, J. (2020). Iron deficiency in infants and children <12 years: Screening, prevention, clinical manifestations, and diagnosis. *UpToDate.* https://www.uptodate.com/contents/iron-deficiency-in-infants-and-children-less-than12-years-screening-prevention-clinical-manifestations-and-diagnosis

Redfern, R., Chen, J., & Sibrel, S. (2018). Effects of thermomechanical stimulation during vaccination on anxiety, pain, and satisfaction in pediatric patients: A randomized controlled trial. *Journal of Pediatric Nursing, 38*, 1–7. https://doi.org/10.1016/j.pedn.2017.09.009

Stoltz, P., & Manworren, R. (2017). Comparison of children's venipuncture fear and pain: Randomized controlled trial of EMLA® and J-Tip needleless injection system®. *Journal of Pediatric Nursing, 37*, 91–96. https://doi.org/10.1016/j.pedn.2017.08.025

Taghizadieh, A., Ala, A., Rahmani, F., & Nadi, A. (2015). Diagnostic accuracy of chest x-ray and ultrasonography in detection of community acquired pneumonia: A brief report. *Emergency, 3*(3), 114–116. https://www.ncbi.nlm.nih.gov/pmc/articles/PMC4608340/

Tosif, S., Baker, A., Oakley, E., Donath, S., & Babl, F. (2012). Contamination rates of different urine collection methods for diagnosis of urinary tract infections in young children: An observational cohort study. *Journal of Paediatrics and Child Health, 48*(8), 659–664. https://doi.org/10.1111/j.1440-1754.2012.02449.x

Tuli, S. (2020, April 29). *Coding for pediatrics 2016.* Lecture.

Utsch, B., & Klaus, G. (2014). Urinalysis in children and adolescents. *Deutsches Arzteblatt International, 111*(37), 617–626. https://doi.org/10.3238/arztebl.2014.0617

Vis, J., & Huisman, A. (2016). Verification and quality control of routine hematology analyzers. *International Journal of Laboratory Hematology, 38*(S1), 100–109. https://doi.org/10.1111/ijlh.12503

Wald, E. (2020). Group A streptococcal tonsillopharyngitis in children and adolescents: Clinical features and diagnosis. *UpToDate.* https://www.uptodate.com/contents/group-a-streptococcal-tonsillopharyngitis-in-children-and-adolescents-clinical-features-and-diagnosis

Wong, R., & Bhutani, V. (2020). Unconjugated hyperbilirubinemia in term and late preterm infants: Screening. *UpToDate.* https://www.uptodate.com/contents/unconjugated-hyperbilirubinemia-in-term-and-late-preterm-infants-screening

World Health Organization. (2010). *WHO guidelines on drawing blood: Best practices in phlebotomy.* https://apps.who.int/iris/bitstream/handle/10665/44294/9789241599221_eng.pdf;jsessionid=15D61B54BF5EED950F80FF96D10A8615?sequence=1

Zamanzad, B. (2009). Accuracy of dipstick urinalysis as a screening method for detection of glucose, protein, nitrites, and blood. *Eastern Mediterranean Health Journal, 15*(5), 1323–1328.

# Pediatric Prescribing

Pamela Biernacki, E. Allison F. Crabtree, Jennifer B. Frank, Jenna N. McDonald, and Tammy Morrow

## Student Learning Outcomes

**Upon completion of this chapter, the reader should be able to:**

1. Describe pharmacodynamics and pharmacokinetics in children.
2. Determine accurate pediatric dosing of medications.
3. Write prescriptions for children accurately.
4. Demonstrate an understanding of antibiotic stewardship and its importance.

The content in this chapter maps to the following areas on the Pediatric Nursing Certification Board (PNCB) Pediatric Nurse Practitioner—Primary Care certification examination:

CONTENT AREAS:

**III. Management**

**A. Child and Caregiver Counseling and Education**

2. Educate about benefits and potential adverse reactions of pharmacological interventions
5. Review the risks of non-adherence to recommended treatment

**B. Therapeutic Interventions**

1. Prescribe pharmacologic agents

**IV. Professional Role Responsibilities**

**A. Leadership and Evidence-based Practice**

4. Develop, implement, and/or modify clinical practice guidelines

**B. Practice Management**

1. Document patient encounters in a manner which supports applicable diagnostic and procedure codes

**C. Legal and Ethical Issues**

1. Practice in accordance with regulatory guidelines (e.g., Health Insurance Portability and Accountability Act [HIPAA], scope of practice)
4. Prepare and maintain materials for licensure, credentialing and privileging

## INTRODUCTION

Prescribing medication for children is an important responsibility. The prescriber must have an understanding of pharmacodynamics and pharmacokinetics in children. Pediatrics encompasses a broad range of ages and sizes from neonatal to adolescent, and this variability must be taken into consideration. Although most drug research has occurred in adults, in recent years it has begun to be undertaken in children, yet is a relatively new area. Medication dosing in children is most often based on weight and prescriptions are written utilizing current recommendations for weight. The nurse practitioner (NP) must understand their prescriptive authority, elements of prescription writing, and accurately prescribe medications. Additionally, the NP should be thoughtful of avoiding contributing to antibiotic resistance and practice antibiotic stewardship.

## PHARMACOKINETICS AND PHARMACODYNAMICS

Understanding the basic pharmacologic principles of pharmacokinetics and pharmacodynamics is imperative when dosing pediatric medications. For practical purposes, *pharmacokinetics* is the means by which the body processes the drug, the movement of drug into, through, and out of the body. The drug disposition through the body is divided into four stages that are recognized by the acronym ADME:

- Absorption from the site of administration
- Distribution within the body
- Metabolism throughout the body
- Excretion from the body.

*Pharmacodynamics* refers to the drug's effect on the body, the biochemical and physical effects along with the mechanisms of drug actions. Further, the effects of drugs on the body involve receptor binding (and receptor sensitivity), post-receptor effects, and chemical interactions. The pharmacologic response depends on the drug binding to its target, the concentration of the drug and the drug's effect at the receptor site. In addition, a specific drug's pharmacodynamics can be affected by physiologic changes due to a disease or disorder, the aging process, and/or interactions with other drugs. Examples of disorders affecting the pharmacodynamics of a drug include genetic mutations, insulin-resistant diabetes mellitus, malnutrition, myasthenia gravis, and thyrotoxicosis. In summary, pharmacokinetics and pharmacodynamics help to explain a drug's effects, i.e., the relationship between dose and response.

### DIFFERENCES IN CHILDREN

Pediatric pharmacokinetics and pharmacodynamics are very different from those for adults. The pharmacokinetics of many drugs vary with age. Challenges exist when prescribing safe, effective doses of therapeutic agents to children because of the rapid changes in size, body composition, and organ function, especially during the first year of life. Pediatric doses cannot be scaled down proportionally from an adult using weight (i.e., mg/kg); this results in a dose too small in infants and children because elimination does not change in direct proportion to weight, and a dose too large in neonates whose drug elimination pathways are immature. Further, differences in drug metabolism in adolescents and between the sexes also adds to the complexity of prescribing. Understanding the differences in pharmacokinetics across the lifespan assists with prescribing; considering several developmental factors aids in the ability to better understand the dose, the concentration, and the effect profile for a specific drug in children of various ages (Koren, 2018).

Factors affecting pharmacokinetics in pediatrics include the level of maturation of organ function and body composition. The capacity of the end organ, such as the brain, heart, kidney, or skeletal muscle to respond to medications may also differ in children compared with adults (pharmacodynamics effects). Modifying the dosage to achieve an optimal clinical response or target effect and avoiding toxicity is required for pediatric prescribing. In addition, dosage calculations are needed and are based on knowledge of pharmacokinetics and pharmacodynamics (Koren, 2018).

## PEDIATRIC DOSING

The importance of correct dosing for children cannot be overstated. More than 200,000 medication adverse events are reported to the poison control center annually, with 30% of those occurring in children (Wu, 2019). The pharmacokinetics of many drugs are different in children compared with those for adults, leading to very specific dosage calculations. Finding the correct doses for children is complicated by a lack of pharmacokinetic studies. Pediatric doses cannot always be extrapolated directly from adult studies (Yao, 2018). In a 2018 study, at least 38% of pediatric prescriptions were considered off-label (meaning they had not been studied in children (Allen et al., 2018).

Most pediatric dosing is calculated based on body weight (mg/kg) or body surface area (mg/m$^2$). Chemotherapeutic drugs are commonly dosed according to body surface area. Pediatric doses based on a child's weight require continued adjustment depending on the child and the clinical response. Dosing also varies by indication; therefore, diagnostic information is helpful when calculating doses. Medications are available in multiple concentrations such as mL (volume) or mg (weight). It is important to double-check dose calculations. The calculated pediatric dose usually should not exceed the adult dose. Care must be taken to properly convert body weight from pounds to kilograms (1 kg = 2.2 lb) before calculating doses based on body weight. Doses are often expressed as mg/kg/day or mg/kg/dose; therefore, orders must be clearly written. The prescriber must note the amount per dose and the frequency of dosing per day.

Prescriptions must be written in a manner that conveys accurate information to the pharmacist, the parent or caregiver, and the child, and in the child's health record. Among the most common errors in prescriptions are illegible handwriting, misplaced or ambiguous decimal points, omitted information, and inappropriate choice of medications (Lofholm & Katzung, 2018). An electronic health record (EHR) assists with eliminating these errors. Online resources are also available to help decrease prescribing errors. Electronic prescribing or e-prescribing via an EHR has greatly reduced prescribing errors by allowing the primary care provider to avoid legibility errors, cross-check the prescription for drug-drug interactions and known allergies, calculate appropriate drug dosing based upon weight and/or body surface area, and note dosage limits (Lofholm & Katzung, 2018).

## DOSAGE CALCULATION

The following examples are typical of drug dosing for the pediatric population (Tables 5.1 and 5.2).

## PRACTICAL PEDIATRIC PRESCRIBING

Three practical considerations are used when prescribing to children to maximize the likelihood of adherence: taste and drug form, frequency of administration, and cost of medications.

### Taste and Drug Form

Many medications have a bitter taste (especially the penicillin agents) with flavorings that often poorly mask the taste and are not tolerated by young children. There are exceptions, but these medications tend to be more costly. In addition to taste, it is helpful to

**TABLE 5.1 Calculation for Amoxicillin Suspension in Milliliters (mLs) for a Child Weighing 24 lbs**

| | |
|---|---|
| Step 1. Convert pounds to kg: | 26 lb × 1 kg/2.2 lb = 11.8 kg |
| Step 2. Calculate the total daily dose in mg: | 11.8 kg × 40 mg/kg/day = 472 mg/day |
| Step 3. Divide the dose by the daily frequency: | 472 mg/day ÷ 2 (twice daily) = 236 mg/dose twice daily |
| Step 4. Convert the mg dose to mL: | 236 mg/dose × 400 mg/5 mL = 2.95 mL<br>At this point round up to 3 mL twice daily. |

*The dosage required is 40 mg/kg/day given twice per day and the liquid suspension is available in a concentration of 400 mg/5 mL.

**TABLE 5.2 Calculation for Acetaminophen in Milliliters (mLs) for a Child Weighing 18 kg**

| | |
|---|---|
| Step 1. Calculate the dose in mg: | 18 kg × 10 mg/kg/dose = 180 mg/dose |
| Step 2. To check within maximum daily dosage; multiple the dose by the frequency: | 75 mg/kg maximum = 1350 mg/kg is max/daily<br>Every 4 to 6 hours = 4 to 6 times per day<br>180 mg/dose × 6 doses/day = 1080 mg/max daily, so this is a maximum daily safe dose to recommend |
| Step 3. Convert the mg dose to mL: | 180 mg/dose ÷ 160 mg/5 mL = 5.6 mL/dose |

*The dosage required is 10 mg/kg/dose given every 4 to 6 hours as needed, not to exceed the maximum daily dose of 75 mg/kg. Oral suspension of acetaminophen is available in 160 mg/5 mL.

ask the child and parent about the form of medication. Children often prefer liquid over tablet until around the age of seven; younger children do not have the developmental capabilities to safely swallow a tablet. However, children are very different in their willingness to accept unpleasant-tasting medicine or a tablet. Some children will take anything, whereas others need careful administration by the parents. Parents usually know how well the child accepts medications; this information should be sought from them and used to help select the form and the taste of a liquid. For antibiotics, in studies using children as tasters, antibiotics ranked as good-tasting were azithromycin (Zithromax), amoxicillin and clavulanate (Augmentin), loracarbef (Lorabid), and cefixime (Suprax); lower-ranking in taste were clarithromycin (Biaxin), erythromycin and sulfisoxazole (Pediazole), ceprozil (Cefzil), and cefpodoxime (Vantin). In addition, inform the parents that it is best to use a calibrated syringe or dropper, as household teaspoons are not accurate for measuring medication doses.

### Frequency of Administration

Minimizing the frequency with which medication is given increases the likelihood and ability of the parent to adhere to the regimen. Medications with a short half-life, which must be given often, should be reconsidered. Samples of antibiotics requiring only once-a-day dosing are azithromycin, ceftibuten, and cefixime; those requiring twice-daily dosing are trimethoprim/sulfamethoxazole, amoxicillin, amoxicillin and clavulanate, ceprozil, loracarbef, cefuroxime, and clarithromycin. When it is necessary to dose more frequently and improve adherence, educate the parents to administer the medication around daily events such as meals or bedtime.

### Medication Cost

Before prescribing an antibiotic, the nurse practitioner (NP) should ask the parent/guardian how payments for prescriptions are covered. Insurance companies and Medicaid generally pay for or require a copayment for prescription medications; parents without insurance/prescription plan may have to pay for the entire prescription out of pocket. Newer brand name medications tend to be more costly; the older medications that are available as generics are often less expensive. Online resources for many insurance plans regarding the out-of-pocket or co-pay cost are readily available.

## PEDIATRIC MEDICATION SAFETY

Annually, approximately 30% of all medication errors that are reported involve children. These errors include prescribing, dispensing, and administering these medications (Mueller et al., 2019). However, the most common medication error is related to medication dosing, specifically during hospitalization (Wu, 2019). Medication errors directly affect patient safety but are ultimately preventable.

## PRESCRIBING AND DISPENSING MEDICATIONS

Children can incur higher rates of medication errors because their medications are most often prescribed based on weight (Mueller et al., 2018). Clinicians must ensure that they have access to an accurate weight and note that most medicines are calculated using kilograms. Pharmacists and pharmacy technicians should ascertain weight of the child before dispensing medication (Wu, 2019). It has been documented that most prescriptions have not included the weight of the child; therefore, pharmacists cannot double-check the weight (Schuman, 2017).

Prescribing errors may also include illegible handwriting, misplaced decimal points, calculation errors, and misunderstood abbreviations (Schuman, 2017). The American Academy of Pediatrics (AAP, 2020) recommends that when writing prescriptions, abbreviations should be avoided. Following general prescribing rules such as adding the zero before a number less than one and never using a trailing zero should also be practiced (AAP, 2020). Also, the use of generic names is preferred and spelling out the units provides more clarity (Schuman, 2017). Attention to the diagnosis that the prescriber is treating will affect the dose that is required. There are recommendations based on diagnosis and adult versus pediatric usage (Schuman, 2017). Also, caution must be exercised to avoid prescribing a dose that is not therapeutic (Wu, 2019). Prescriptions that are omitted or delayed are also a concern as this could lead to adverse events (Cousins et al., 2019).

## ADMINISTERING MEDICATIONS

Children are also dependent on a caregiver to administer the correct dosage (Mueller et al., 2019). The ability and understanding of the caregiver should be considered. If there is a concern about a learning or language barrier that may affect their ability to understand the instructions, then educate the caregiver, including on how to draw up the correct amount of medication and what device they should use. One approach is to have them validate using a syringe to demonstrate how much medicine to administer and have them take that syringe home to use with the medication. In a study of 100 pediatric experiences, the teaspoon used by caregivers at home varied from between 1.5 mL to 5 mL, and thus should not be used to measure medication (Schuman, 2017). Prescribers must also ensure that the concentrations associated with the medications are evident. Caregivers may inadvertently administer the wrong concentration of an over-the-counter drug (OTC) if the directions are not clear. An example would be OTC ibuprofen that is available in concentrations of 50 mg/1.25 mL and 100 mg/5 mL (Schuman, 2017). Low-cost options may include a summary of these OTC medications in chart format for patients in the office. Some prescribers recommend that families use apps for dosing on OTC medications (Schuman, 2017), but not all families have access to these technologies. Overall, there are many new resources available to ensure that the caregiver receives the appropriate education necessary to administer the correct drug and dose.

## SECURITY CONCERNS

Safety precautions should be taken when writing, handling, and storing prescriptions and prescription pads, whether handwritten on paper or by using electronically printed or electronic prescribing systems. Prescription pads or printer paper should be tamper-proof. The state pharmacy laws follow federal guidelines in the adoption of the required elements for tamper-proof paper and inks. Spelling out the desired quantity to be dispensed using an Arabic numeral (e.g., "twenty [20]") is a useful deterrent toward unwanted alterations in the intended amount. Faxing prescriptions directly to the pharmacy can also serve as an added precaution. Electronic transmission via a digital process or facsimile of a prescription to the pharmacy adds convenience and is especially helpful with controlled substances except for those in Schedule II. A facsimile for a Schedule II controlled substance is not considered original except in cases of drugs dispensed to nursing homes, hospice agencies, or for parenteral medications for home intravenous administration. Prescription pads or prescription printer paper should have designated areas of locked storage with limited access. Prescriptions should never be signed in advance; doing so constitutes fraud and subjects the provider to state or federal penalties. Security measures serve as effective mechanisms to minimize fraud and potential drug diversion.

## Electronic Health Record

Medication errors may result anywhere along the continuum from writing the prescription to administration of the drug, so it is important for the NP to be aware of the entire process. EHRs are most commonly the mainstay of medical charting. With most clinics and agencies using strictly EHRs, it is imperative to be cautious and properly skilled in each system. EHRs offer many benefits including convenience, safety parameters, and continuity of care for patients. The EHR system has also been extremely helpful in reducing errors, such as decreasing the illegible handwriting errors, and providing safety features for dosing (Mueller et al., 2019). Most EHRs aid the practitioner in the medication reconciliation of the patient, keeping information concise and organized, yet it is still vital to update these medicines at every visit. Each prescribed drug should be listed with dosage, duration, and indication, as well as noting any over-the-counter or herbal medications used by the patient. Any drug or food allergies should be documented along with any associated effects. It is important to obtain information on any other medical visits in the interim of patient visits to verify any additional drugs prescribed by another provider.

Although it offers significant advantages, there are many precautions that providers should employ while writing patient prescriptions (Schiff et al., 2018). EHRs can increase errors when used to prescribe medication for children if the parameters are *not* adjusted to reflect the settings to support weight-based dosing (Mueller et al., 2019). The use of technology, such as computerized provider order entry systems, decreases the risk of drug diversion and medication errors. Human errors still prevail when prescribers become overly reliant on prepopulated fields (Woo & Robinson, 2020). The NP should be mindful to consider individual patient circumstances when prescribing in electronic systems, especially if using templates or copy-forward features. Ultimately, it is the responsibility of the NP prescriber to verify the accuracy of a prescription before providing a written or printed copy or before transmitting it to the dispensing pharmacy via an electronic method. It is of utmost importance that the clinician is familiar with the electronic prescribing system and undergoes specialized training to enhance safety features and avoid any electronic pitfalls.

## Family Education and Adherence

One of the biggest hurdles of prescribing a medication is to ensure understanding by the family as well as to promote adherence. Fortunately, thorough education about each drug may improve overall adherence to therapy. Prescribers should spend considerable time to educate each child (as age permits) and their caregiver about the drug, indication, usage, and duration. The family should be provided with any available instructions by verbal, written, or demonstration methods to suit the appropriate learning preferences of the individual. Increased educational time spent with the family, quality communication, and addressing any concerns or barriers greatly affects child and caregiver adherence to the recommended plan of care (Woo & Robinson, 2020). In pediatrics, it is appropriate to speak to the child, and/or the caregiver if the child is nonverbal, about factors for medication administration such as flavored medicines, texture aversions, and the ability to swallow pills.

Other crucial considerations are factors that may inhibit adherence to therapy, such as monetary expenses and insurance drug formularies. Samples from pharmaceutical representatives may help a family in need; giving a one-dose medication during the visit may be an option for aiding with medication expenses or even adherence. However, the prescriber must be cognizant of rules and regulations in regard to dispensing of samples to patients (Stewart & Denisco, 2019). Some families may not feel they can request generic drug options or question the prescriber's decision.

A beneficial practice is to ensure that the caregiver knows to contact the prescriber should any question arise at the pharmacy regarding cost, availability, formulary, etc.

## WRITING A PRESCRIPTION

Writing a prescription is an essential role of the advanced practice nurse. In pediatrics, it is especially important to be knowledgeable and conscientious when issuing a medication to a child. Careful attention to detail, understanding the elements of a prescription, and proper collaboration ensures that the correct therapy reaches the child.

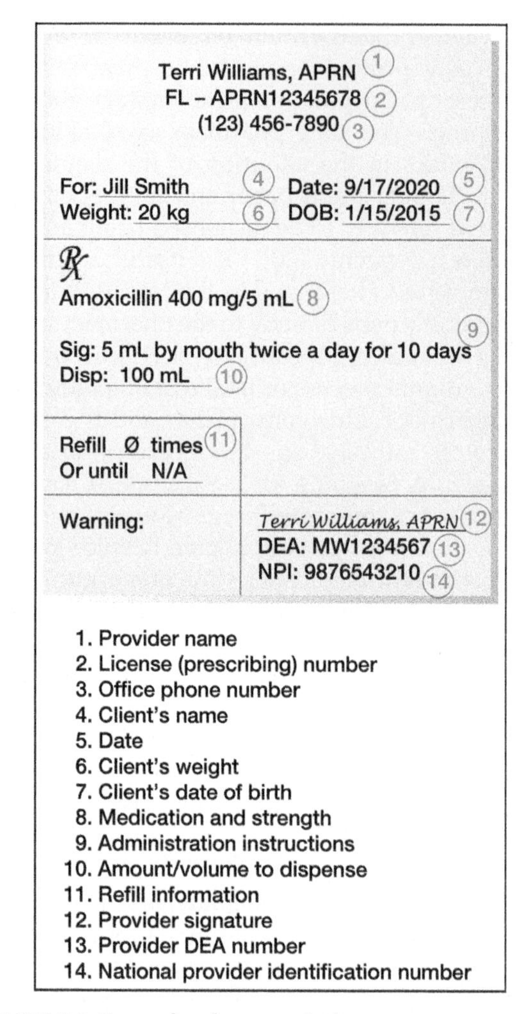

Terri Williams, APRN (1)
FL – APRN12345678 (2)
(123) 456-7890 (3)

For: Jill Smith (4) Date: 9/17/2020 (5)
Weight: 20 kg (6) DOB: 1/15/2015 (7)

℞
Amoxicillin 400 mg/5 mL (8)

Sig: 5 mL by mouth twice a day for 10 days (9)
Disp: 100 mL (10)

Refill Ø times (11)
Or until N/A

Warning:

Terri Williams, APRN (12)
DEA: MW1234567 (13)
NPI: 9876543210 (14)

1. Provider name
2. License (prescribing) number
3. Office phone number
4. Client's name
5. Date
6. Client's weight
7. Client's date of birth
8. Medication and strength
9. Administration instructions
10. Amount/volume to dispense
11. Refill information
12. Provider signature
13. Provider DEA number
14. National provider identification number

FIGURE 5.1 Example of a prescription.

## ELEMENTS OF THE PRESCRIPTION

Written or verbal directions must be communicated to the pharmacist to dispense a prescription properly. Many states require specific elements to be present on a prescription pad or may require specific drugs to be written on duplicate or triplicate copy pads. It is imperative that prescribing NPs familiarize themselves with the state requirements. At a minimum, the NP prescriber's name, address, and telephone number should be printed on the prescription pad to allow verification by the dispensing pharmacist. Prescriptions should have the date of the day written, include an indication of authorized refills, and feature a legible order that contains the complete drug name, strength, dosage, and form to dispense. Although not as common as in the past, including the indication of the prescription for the patient may help with compliance and safety of administration (Schiff et al., 2018). Furthermore, it may aid in pharmacist collaboration for appropriate dosing and family education. Other requirements include the quantity to distribute, indication for use using terms such as "for nausea," or any special dosing considerations related to potentially concerning side effects or dietary considerations. An example of these might include "caution sedation" or "take with food." The use of metric units of measure, such as milligrams and milliliters, is preferred over apothecary units. The NP prescriber should avoid using abbreviations and avoid terms such as "take as directed" or "take as needed." The prescription pad should have clear indications for instructions, such as "dispense as written" or "may substitute." Including the weight of a child is an added safety precaution for weight-based dosing. It is imperative for all prescribers to ensure transmission of complete and unambiguous prescription instructions for the safety and understanding of each child and family (Schiff et al., 2018). See Figure 5.1 for an example of a prescription.

Other elements commonly required on a prescription pad are the NP prescriber's state-issued prescribing license number and name of the collaborative physician if indicated. The state-issued prescribing number is uniquely associated with the prescriber and may or may not be the same as the provider's advanced practice license number. Other elements that could be optional or may be required are the National Provider Identification (NPI) number and the U.S Drug Enforcement Administration (DEA) registration number, if applicable. An NPI number is a unique number associated explicitly with the provider and is used for all prescriptions billed through insurance as well as for other billable services. This number should be obtained by the NP as soon as feasibly possible after obtaining licensure. Applying for an NPI number is free and can be completed conveniently online. Other items that may be prescribed by a NP are durable medical equipment and devices and needles and syringes.

## STATE-ISSUED PRESCRIPTIVE AUTHORITY

Federal law establishes whether a drug requires a prescription but does not dictate who may prescribe. State law determines who has the authority to prescribe. Prescriptive authority for NPs varies from state to state as well as by clinical setting (Stewart & Denisco, 2019). Some states grant prescriptive authority to NPs solely through the board of nursing, whereas others require a collaborative process through a state board of medicine or pharmacy. The NP's prescriptive authority is either dependent or independent. Dependent prescribing occurs when a primary prescriber delegates prescriptive authority to another through a collaborative practice or supervisory agreement. NPs with independent prescriptive authority act autonomously within the confines of the state scope of practice and board regulations. Most NPs have the privilege to prescribe legend drugs; however, the authority to prescribe controlled substances varies widely. Some states may restrict an NP from prescribing specific legend drugs as well. The term *legend drug* describes a drug that requires a prescription from a licensed provider and is not available over the counter. It is the responsibility of the NP to familiarize themself with the regulations of the state in which they practice.

The NP should be knowledgeable regarding the classification of individual drugs, both by the DEA and the state in which they practice. States have controlled substance acts patterned after federal law but may have allowable differences in drug scheduling. For example, a state may make a controlled substance more, not less, restrictive than the federal designation. NPs who have authority in a state to prescribe controlled substances must apply for state prescriptive authority before applying for a DEA number. Applying for a DEA number can be completed online through the DEA website (U.S. DEA, n.d.). Applications for statewide prescriptive privilege should be with the governing bodies responsible for controlling the prescriptive authority of providers. Before applying for a DEA number, the NP should verify with the state board of nursing or, in some cases, the state board of pharmacy if a state-issued prescribing license number or certification is issued separately from the NP's advanced practice license. Often, the state-issued prescribing number correlates with the NP's state license for advanced practice. Another consideration in prescribing controlled substances is the state-mandated collaborative practice requirement. In states that mandate a collaborative practice agreement, the state-issued certificate for prescribing controlled substances is bound to the supervising physician agreement, and a separate agreement and certificate must be in place for each collaborating or supervising physician. Requirements and regulations vary widely from state to state.

## ANTIBIOTIC RESISTANCE

Antibiotics are an effective tool used to treat life-threatening infections. However, any time antibiotics are used, there is an increase in healthcare cost, exposure to unnecessary side effects for patients, and enhancement of antibiotic resistance. Overprescribing antibiotics has created increased antibiotic resistance and led to insufficient antibiotic choices for multidrug resistant organisms (Zetta et al., 2018). At least 30% of antibiotic prescriptions are unnecessary (Centers for Disease Control and Prevention [CDC], 2019a). Of antibiotics prescribed to children, 29% were unnecessary (Fleming-Dutra et al., 2018). Up to 46% of the time, depending upon the outpatient setting, antibiotics are prescribed for respiratory tract illnesses when not needed (Palms et al., 2018). Furthermore, another study found that azithromycin, a commonly prescribed antibiotic in children, is often prescribed when it is not recommended or not the recommended drug of choice by clinical guidelines. That same study reported that amoxicillin (35%) and azithromycin (18%) were the most common of the 67 million prescribed antibiotics in the pediatric population (Fleming-Dutra et al., 2018). Antibiotic resistance develops as a result of inappropriate use of antibiotics for viral illnesses, inappropriate dosing or drug selection, or increased use of empiric or repeat regimens.

## INAPPROPRIATE PRESCRIBING OF ANTIBIOTICS

Upper respiratory infections (URIs) or common colds are the most common presenting chief complaints in clinical practice. Preschool children, on average, experience three to eight URIs a year, with infants experiencing up to six to seven. Common colds are typically self-limiting, with the aim of treatment being symptomatic relief (CDC, 2017). Despite the benign course, many children and their caregivers place undue pressure on prescribers for antibiotic prescriptions. It is important for the NP prescriber to be mindful that antibiotics are ineffective in treating viral illnesses, such as the common cold. The use of antibiotics for viral infections places the child at risk for a multitude of reasons.

First, the unnecessary use of antibiotics increases the likelihood of antibiotic resistance to secondary bacterial infections. While secondary bacterial infections may develop and complicate the common cold, a practical symptomatic treatment period and watchful waiting approach may be prudent in treating the viral URI. Second, inappropriate use of antibiotics places the child at risk for adverse drug reactions. Adverse drug reactions range from minor to life-threatening fatal reactions. At every encounter in which a medication is prescribed or recommended, the child or caregiver should be given either verbal or written advice regarding the signs and symptoms of adverse drug effects, with clear instructions for reporting concerning findings. Lastly, adding unnecessary medications, especially antibiotics, increases the risk of drug-drug interactions. Many viral illnesses respond to OTC treatments; therefore, the addition of an unnecessary antibiotic increases the risk of drug-drug interactions, placing the child at risk for ineffective treatment, added side effects, or potentially serious adverse reactions.

## INAPPROPRIATE DOSING OR DRUG SELECTION

The first consideration for selection of a drug is to determine whether treatment with an antibiotic is indicated. NP prescribers should develop a practice of determining if the benefits of using antibiotics outweigh the risks in each child. The decision to prescribe an antibiotic should only be made after this determination has occurred and child-specific factors have been considered. The NP prescriber's decision to treat should be made with a clear purpose in mind and free from the pressure of parents or other individuals. For self-limiting infections, such as URIs with a viral etiology, symptomatic treatment rather than treatment with antibiotics should be the mainstay. Research has found that 17.6% to 18.6% of women's health and pediatric providers prescribed antibiotics in the absence of diagnostic uncertainty (Yox & Scudder, 2014). If the determination is made that an antibiotic is indicated, selection of the most appropriate drug is crucial. This is optimally accomplished by a culture-derived selection, but in some cases empiric treatment may be necessary as an initial intervention. The NP prescriber should strive as much as feasibly possible to narrow and determine the clinical diagnosis. Collection of specimens for culture and sensitivity testing is indicated in a wide variety of clinical conditions. The NP should be mindful that, in some cases, bacterial colonization of sites limits the usefulness of a culture. In other clinical situations, obtaining a culture would be impossible without invasive testing; therefore, in the outpatient setting, cultures are not typically obtained. Limitations to consider when relying on culture for clinical decision making and drug selection choice include possible misinterpretation of infection due to bacterial colonization; risks of laboratory errors due to mislabeling, mishandling, and quality control issues; and issues related to costs of microbial testing (Woo & Robinson, 2020).

If definitive diagnosis can be made through laboratory testing, the most appropriate antibiotic should be selected for the targeted organism, taking into consideration individual factors such as the child's drug-allergy history and other considerations such as drug cost, ease of use, and potential child or caregiver adherence. In cases where a definitive diagnosis cannot be made, empirical treatment may be necessary. With empirical treatment, microbial diagnosis and drug selection are determined by epidemiological studies. NP prescribers should familiarize themselves with sources that compile and continuously update the results of large epidemiological studies, such as:

- *The Sanford Guide to Antimicrobial Therapy* (Gilbert et al., 2019)
- *The Medical Letter on Drugs and Therapeutics* (The Medical Letter, 2020; an annual subscription is available)
- Readily available material on the CDC website at https://www.cdc.gov/antibiotic use.

The goal of treating a condition empirically is to select the most narrow-spectrum antibiotic available that covers the most likely organism for the specific clinical condition in question. Other sources of reference for prescribing NPs include local sources in the form of antibiograms, as trends in susceptibility have an impact on local rates of resistance. The CDC's Active Bacterial Core Surveillance data provides practical guidance in determining ongoing surveillance that is active and population-based (CDC, 2020).

Prescribers are more likely to change antibiotic prescription writing habits if rapid results of laboratory tests and knowledge of community patterns of antibiotic resistance are available.

## INCREASED USE OF EMPIRIC BROAD-SPECTRUM ANTIBIOTICS/REPEATED USE OF ANTIBIOTICS

The use of broad-spectrum antibiotics or repeated therapy with any antibiotics can result in bacterial or fungal overgrowth (i.e., superinfection) or an antibiotic-resistant organism. One of the most common, and potentially lethal, superinfections is *Clostridium difficile* infection (CDI). CDI manifests as diarrhea during antibiotic use or up to several weeks after discontinuation of the medication. The diarrhea may be watery or bloody and be associated with abdominal cramps, pain, fever, or (in severe cases) pseudomembranous colitis. Children on broad-spectrum antibiotics or those treated repeatedly with antibiotics should be monitored for signs and symptoms of CDI, with prompt treatment after definitive diagnosis.

Other patient safety concerns related to use of broad-spectrum antibiotics or repeated use of antibiotics is risk of hepatotoxicity or renal toxicity. Children especially should be monitored due to the immaturity of developing organs. Maintaining adequate hydration during periods of antibiotic treatment is imperative; clear instructions should be provided to the child or caregiver, including actions to take if symptoms of dehydration develop or the child is unable to maintain oral intake.

## DEVELOPMENT OF ANTIBIOTIC STEWARDSHIP

In 2019, the CDC published *Antibiotic Resistance Threats in the United States*, a report updated from the previous 2013 report, which outlines the burden and threats posed by antibiotic-resistant organisms and highlights the impact on health in the United States. This updated report notes that 2.8 million people are infected with resistant bacteria and 35,000 people die annually in the United States from resistant bacteria (CDC, 2019b). These statistics are alarmingly high and increased from the prior report, which estimated a prevalence of 2 million people infected with antibiotic-resistant infections responsible for causing as many as 23,000 deaths (CDC, 2019b). The 2019 report is intended to serve as a reference for information on antibiotic resistance. The report's resistance burden estimates and highlights emerging areas of concern and action needed (CDC, 2019b).

*Antibiotic stewardship* refers to an organized effort to enhance appropriate prescribing, "by promoting the selection of optional drug regimen, dose, route, and duration of therapy" (Hamdy et al., 2019, p. 10). Therefore, professional societies and organizations such as the CDC have developed guidelines for the management of infectious diseases that include recommendations for antibiotic prescribing and antibiotic stewardship principles. Continued research and evidence-based guidelines will play critical roles in effectively treating infections and reducing side effects caused by unnecessary antibiotic use (CDC, 2019a).

### Elements of Antibiotic Stewardship

Following CDC guidance, many healthcare systems have implemented antibiotic stewardship programs. At the core, these programs promote using the most appropriate antibiotic at best dose, route, and duration for each patient. Components of antibiotic stewardship programs include strategies such as treatment pathways for specific infectious diseases, formulary restrictions, dosage optimization, prescription audits, and continued education for prescribers.

The CDC Core Elements of Antibiotic Stewardship (CDC, 2019c) is a comprehensive approach to address the burden of antibiotic resistance, and includes frameworks for stewardship programs in outpatient settings, nursing homes, and hospitals. These core elements include:

- **Education:** Ensure educational resources are available for providers and patients on antibiotic prescribing.
- **Commitment:** Demonstrate dedication to and accountability for optimizing antibiotic prescribing for patient safety.
- **Action for policy and practice:** Implement policies and practices to improve antibiotic prescribing; assess and modify as necessary to ensure success.
- **Tracking and reporting:** Monitor prescribers' antibiotic prescribing habits and offer feedback and support for clinician self-improvement in prescribing practices.

The Joint Commission (TJC), the accrediting body for hospitals across the United States, in collaboration with the CDC and the Centers for Medicare and Medicaid Services (CMS), approved a regulatory requirement in 2017 for hospitals and nursing care centers to develop and implement antibiotic stewardship programs. Per the CDC recommendations for core elements, this program includes education for providers and patients about the benefits and harms of antibiotic use, tracking of antibiotic use, and use of evidence-based protocols to guide patient care (Woo & Robinson, 2020). The goal of these regulations is to improve appropriate use of antibiotics, reduce emergence of drug-resistant organisms, and decrease risks of patient harm from antibiotic use.

### Other Factors Influencing Antibiotic Selection

In consideration of the many factors influencing the NP's decision to prescribe an antibiotic, patient-specific factors have an impact on the final product selection. Some case-specific items to consider include the child's allergy history, age and genetic factors, current state of immunity, and drug considerations such as affordability and convenience of dosage.

## PEDIATRIC PHARMACOLOGIC RESEARCH

Historically there is a lack of research to support the efficacy and safety of medicines for use in the pediatric population (U.S. Food and Drug Administration [FDA], 2016). Most medicines have not been tested on children from neonates through adolescents, which has proven to have detrimental outcomes. Dating back to the early 1900s, elixirs were used to help children with sleep disturbances, which caused tragic deaths (National Institutes of Child Health and Human Development [NICHHD], n.d.). Again, in the 1950s the drug thalidomide, prescribed to pregnant women for nausea, resulted in maternal deaths as well as birth defects and limb deformities in the infant (NICHHD, n.d.). The FDA's Pediatric Rule of 1994 allowed the labeling of drugs if the medications had a similar response in children as adults. This rule resulted in a small number of appropriate studies that improved pediatric labeling (NICHHD, n.d.). With the efforts of the NICHHD and the Pediatric Pharmacology Units (PPRU), the network created change for 20 drugs and contributed to more than 250 publications to benefit children (Balevic & Cohen-Woklowiez, 2018). In 1997, the FDA Modernization Act began providing incentives to pharmaceutical companies that increased medicines used for pediatrics (NICHHD, n.d.). In 2002, the NICHHD enacted The Best Pharmaceuticals for Children Act (BPCA), which became a law. The BPCA encouraged the pharmaceutical industry to perform studies to improve labeling for patented drugs used in children and allowed longer for these patents to persist (NICHHD, n.d.). Over the past five years, data indicate there have been more studies conducted to benefit children than in the previous years combined (U.S. FDA, 2016). The National Institutes of Health has increased the sponsorship for clinical trials in areas for off-patent drug products that require research (NICHHD, n.d.).

## RESEARCH LIMITATION AND IMPORTANCE

There are multifactorial reasons for the lack of pediatric drug testing. Pharmaceutical companies recognize that pediatric research will not bring large financial benefits (U.S. FDA, 2016). To successfully market a drug, it can take up to 15 years of research, trials, and approval, which can be costly (Balevic & Cohen-Woklowiez, 2018). Pharmaceutical companies consider the costs and the fact that 42% of recent pediatric trials failed due to the inability to establish safety and drug efficacy in children (Balevic & Cohen-Woklowiez, 2018). Drugs that are more often prescribed that would bring a larger revenue have already been studied (U.S. FDA, 2016). Also, many physician-scientists are not supported financially or allowed time to research at their academic centers (Stoll & Taegtmeyer, 2018). There is now support that research would go beyond the health of children but also would affect outcomes as the child ages into adulthood (Stoll & Taegtmeyer, 2018). Most researchers feel that it is more difficult to perform research on children due to their developmental needs and differences (U.S. FDA, 2016). Children require research environments that are appropriate for their developmental needs and a scientist who can relate to them (U.S. FDA, 2016). Procedures such as obtaining blood or urine samples from children can be more difficult than with adults. There are also multiple layers of informed consent when working with children, which include the legal caregiver and child (U.S. FDA, 2016). When conducting research that involves children, the researcher must comply with the National Institute of Health (NIH) guidelines, specifically the Common Rule at 45 C.F.R. 46, Subparts A and D.

## KEY POINTS

- Understanding the basic pharmacologic principles of pharmacokinetics and pharmacodynamics is imperative when dosing pediatric medications.
- Pediatric doses cannot be scaled down proportionally from an adult using weight.
- Care must be taken when properly calculating doses based on body weight.
- Practical considerations when prescribing to children are taste and drug form, frequency of administration, and the cost of medications.
- Prescribing medication safely for children is vital for the advanced practitioner.
- Careful attention should be paid when choosing medications for children.
- Education for parents and caregivers is of utmost importance and increases the likelihood of adherence to therapy.
- All prescribers should be properly trained with prescription protocols or EHR used in the clinical setting. Although providing great convenience and security, the EHR should not be considered error proof.
- A prescription is a verbal message conveyed to the pharmacist. It is important to communicate prescriptions clearly to the pharmacist to ensure that the proper instructions reach the caregiver and child.
- Adherence to best-practice recommendations decreases risks of medication errors and increases medication compliance.
- The practitioner is responsible for obtaining information necessary from certifying agencies and state boards regarding prescriptive authority.
- The practitioner should be properly educated on any electronic system before starting in clinical practice and should be aware of insurance drug formularies, financial consideration of the family, and regulations on sample drugs from pharmaceutical representatives.
- Overprescribing antibiotics persists, producing antibiotic resistance and insufficient antibiotic choices.
- The use of antibiotics in treating self-limiting, acute viral illnesses is ineffective and should be avoided.
- Inappropriate use of antibiotics poses a significant risk to individual and global health.
- Drug selection and dosing require careful consideration on the part of the prescriber.
- Use of broad-spectrum antibiotics or prolonged treatment regimens significantly increases risks of adverse drug reactions, treatment complications, and antibiotic resistance patterns.
- Antibiotic stewardship programs provide a framework for prescribers and organizations to address the burden of antibiotic resistance and threats to patient safety.
- There continues to be great controversy over pediatric drug research due to ethics and safety concerns.
- The FDA ensures that researchers comply with specific regulations when studying drug effects on children.

## REFERENCES


Allen, H. C., Garbe, M. C., Lees, J., Aziz, N., Chaaban, H., Miller, J. L., Johnson, P., & DeLeon, S. (2018). *Journal of the Oklahoma State Medical Association, 111*(8), 776–783. https://www.ncbi.nlm.nih.gov/pmc/articles/PMC6677268/

American Academy of Pediatrics. (2020). *Preventing prescribing errors*. https://pediatriccare.solutions.aap.org/drug.aspx?resultClick=1&gbosid=172028

Balevic, S., & Cohen-Woklowiez, M. (2018). Innovative study designs optimizing clinical pharmacology research in infants and children. *The Clinical Journal of Pharmacology, 58*(10), S58–S72. https://doi.org/10.1002/jcph.1053

Centers for Disease Control and Prevention. (2017). *Antibiotic prescribing and use in doctor's office: Pediatric treatment recommendations.* https://www.cdc.gov/antibiotic-use/community/for-hcp/outpatient-hcp/pediatric-treatment-rec.html

Centers for Disease Control and Prevention. (2019a). *Antibiotic prescribing and use in the U.S.* https://www.cdc.gov/antibiotic-use/stewardship-report/index.html

Centers for Disease Control and Prevention. (2019b). *Antibiotic resistance threats in the United States, 2019.* https://www.cdc.gov/drugresistance/biggest-threats.html

Centers for Disease Control and Prevention. (2019c). *The core elements of outpatient antibiotic stewardship.* https://www.cdc.gov/antibiotic-use/community/pdfs/16_268900-A_CoreElementsOutpatient_508.pdf

Centers for Disease Control and Prevention. (2020). *Active bacterial core surveillance (ABCs): Surveillance reports.* https://www.cdc.gov/abcs/reports-findings/surv-reports.html

Cousins, D., Crompton, A., Gell, J., & Hooley, J. (2019). The top ten prescribing errors in practice and how to avoid them. *The Pharmaceutical Journal, 302*(7922). https://doi.org/10.1211/PJ.2019.20206123

Fleming-Dutra, K. E., Demirjian, A., Bartoces, M., Roberts, R. M., Taylor, T. H., & Hicks, L. A. (2018). Variations in antibiotic and azithromycin prescribing for children by geography and specialty—United States, 2013. *Pediatric Infectious Disease Journal, 37*(1), 52–58. https://doi.org/10.1097/INF.0000000000001708

Gilbert, D. N., Eliopoulos, G. M., Chambers, H. F., Saag, M. S., & Pavia, A. T. (Eds.). (2019). *The Sanford guide to antimicrobial therapy: 50 Years: 1969-2019.* Antimicrobial Therapy.

Hamdy, R. F., Neal, W., Nicholson, L., Ansusinha, E., & King, S. (2019). Pediatric nurses' perceptions of their role in antimicrobial stewardship: A focus group study. *Journal of Pediatric Nursing, 48*, 10–17. https://doi.org/10.1016/j.pedn.2019.05.020

Koren, G. (2018). Chapter 59: Special aspects of perinatal & pediatric pharmacology In B. G. Katzung (Ed.), *Basic and clinical pharmacology* (14th ed.). McGraw-Hill Education.

Lofholm, P. W., & Katzung B. G. (2018). Chapter 65: Rational prescribing and prescription writing. In B. G. Katzung (Ed.), *Basic and clinical pharmacology* (14th ed.). McGraw-Hill Education.
The Medical Letter on Drugs and Therapeutics. (2020). Medical Letter, Inc. https://secure.medicalletter.org/aboutus
Mueller, B. U., Neuspiel, D. R., Stucky Fisher, E. R., & Council on Quality Improvement and Patient Safety, Committee on Hospital Care. (2019). Principles of pediatric patient safety reducing harm due to medical care. *Pediatrics, 143*(2), e20183649. https://doi.org/10.1542/peds.2018-3649
National Institutes of Child Health and Human Development. (n.d). *Best Pharmaceuticals for Children Act.* https://www.nichd.nih.gov/research/supported/bpca/history
Palms, D. L., Hicks, L. A., Bartoces, M., Hersh, A. L., Zetts, R., Hyun, D. Y., & Fleming-Dutra, K. E. (2018). Comparison of antibiotic prescribing in retail clinics, urgent care centers, emergency departments, and traditional ambulatory care settings in the United States. *JAMA Internal Medicine, 178*(9), 267–1269. https://doi.org/10.1001/jamainternmed.2018.1632
Schiff, G., Mirica, M. M., Dhavle, A. A., Galanter, W. L., Lambert, B., & Wright, A. (2018). A prescription for enhancing electronic prescribing safety. *Health Affairs, 37*(11), 1877–1883. https://doi.org/10.1377/hlthaff.2018.0725
Schuman, A. (2017). Safety first: How to avoid missteps when prescribing medications. *Contemporary Pediatrics.* https://www.contemporarypediatrics.com/pediatric-practice-improvement/safety-first-how-avoid-missteps-when-prescribing-medications
Stewart, J., & Denisco, S. (2019). *Role development for the nurse practitioner* (2nd ed.). Jones & Bartlett Learning.
Stoll, B. J., & Taegtmeyer, H. (2018). Challenges for today's pediatric physician-scientists. *JAMA Pediatrics, 172*(3), 220–221. https://doi.org/10.1001/jamapediatrics.2017.4954
U.S. Drug Enforcement Administration. (n.d.). *How to apply.* https://www.dea.gov/how-apply
U.S. Food and Drug Administration. (2016). *Drug research and children.* https://www.fda.gov/drugs/drug-information-consumers/drug-research-and-children
Woo, T. M., & Robinson, M. V. (2020). *Pharmacotherapeutics for advanced practice nurse prescribers* (5th ed.). F. A. Davis.
Wu, A. (2019). Minimizing medication errors in pediatric patients. *US Pharmacist, 44*(4), 20–23. https://www.uspharmacist.com/article/minimizing-medication-errors-in-pediatric-patients
Yao, L. (2018, September 13). *Extrapolation in pediatric drug development: An evolving science.* U.S. Food and Drug Administration. https://www.fda.gov/media/100571/download
Yox, S., & Scudder, L. (2014). *Too many antibiotics! Patients and prescribers speak up.* https://www.medscape.com/features/slideshow/public/antibiotic-misuse#1
Zetta, R. M., Stoesz, A., Smith, B. A., & Hyun, D. Y. (2018). Outpatient antibiotic use and the need for increased antibiotic stewardship efforts. *Pediatrics, 141*(6), e20174124. https://doi.org/10.1542/peds.2017-4124

# Pain Assessment and Management

Elizabeth A. Paton and Lindsey Locke

## Student Learning Outcomes

**Upon completion of this chapter the reader should be able to:**

1. Identify appropriate pain scales to use for children of various age groups.
2. List pharmacologic agents that may be used to control pediatric pain, including dosing, route, and typical indications.
3. Describe nonpharmacologic methods to manage pain in children.

## INTRODUCTION

Assessment of pain is considered to be the fifth vital sign. The assessment of pain in the pediatric population can be challenging. However, it is essential to recognize that children do experience pain and that their demonstrations of pain may differ significantly from those of adults. Assessment tools exist to specifically aid in assessing pain in various age groups from neonates to adolescents.

Pain is categorized into different types with varying sources. Types of pain include nociceptive, neuropathic, and functional. Nociceptive pain may be a result of inflammation or tissue injury and is delineated into either somatic and visceral. The sensation of pain occurs through four specific processes: transduction, transmission, modulation, and perception. Transduction is the initiation of pain in the nociceptor fibers caused by a noxious stimulus, then the pain impulses are transmitted through the sensory nervous system. Next, the pain sensation is modulated by endogenous mechanisms that determine the duration and intensity of the pain based on several factors. The final process is perception, which is how the brain processes the pain based on sensory and emotional experiences (Bolick et al., 2021).

Neuropathic pain results from damaged sensory nerves (Hauer & Jones, 2020). Functional pain is a result of the triggering of abnormal pain pathways (Bolick et al., 2021). The majority of pain experienced by children is acute and the result of an injury or illness. Chronic pain is more often a result of functional pain, the most frequent of which is functional abdominal pain.

Chronic pain can be defined in two different ways. One definition is related to precisely how long the pain has been present, with mention made of time frames greater than one month and greater than three months (Lee et al., 2017). A second definition is pain that outlasts the expected period of healing (Olson, 2013).

The content in this chapter maps to the following areas on the Pediatric Nursing Certification Board (PNCB) Pediatric Nurse Practitioner—Primary Care certification examination:

### CLINICAL PROBLEMS: PAIN

CONTENT AREAS:

**II. Assessment and Diagnosis**

**A. History and Physical Examination**

1. Obtain history of present illness
2. Obtain a comprehensive health history for new patients

3. Complete an interval history for established patients
5. Perform a complete physical examination

**D. Analyzing Information**

1. Integrate health history and physical examination findings into the plan of care

**E. Diagnosis**

2. Establish a diagnosis based on evaluation of patient data

## III. Management

**A. Child and Caregiver Counseling and Education**

1. Provide condition-specific counseling and education, including treatment options
2. Educate about benefits and potential adverse reactions of pharmacological interventions
3. Discuss non-pharmacological interventions
4. Counsel regarding the threshold for seeking follow-up care
5. Review the risks of non-adherence to recommended treatment

**B. Therapeutic Interventions**

1. Prescribe pharmacologic agents
2. Recommend the use of over-the-counter pharmacologic agents
3. Order or recommend non-pharmacologic treatments for the management of symptoms
4. Discuss use of complementary and alternative therapies as appropriate

**E. Care Coordination**

1. Facilitate patient and family-centered care for children of all ages with acute and chronic conditions

**F. Evaluation and Follow-up**

1. Evaluate the plan of care and modify based on patient response or outcomes
2. Establish a plan for follow-up care

## IV. Professional Role Responsibilities

**A. Leadership and Evidence-based Practice**

4. Develop, implement, and/or modify clinical practice guidelines

# DIFFERENCES AMONG CHILDREN RELATED TO PAIN

Pain assessment and management varies based on age and development. It is essential to address pain based on the child's age and cognitive status. In primary care, the practitioner needs to be knowledgeable about pain management interventions, as pain is exhibited for a variety of reasons. Children may present with acute pain due to an injury, infectious process (e.g., otalgia due to otitis media), or acute manifestation of a chronic disease state. Chronic pain may be manifested as headache, abdominal pain, and musculoskeletal pain (Friedrichsdorf et al., 2016).

Failure to treat pain in children can have physiologic and psychologic complications. The physiologic responses often seen in the primary care setting include tachycardia and tachypnea. Other physiologic responses may also be observed. Long-term complications may include behavioral changes such as nocturnal enuresis, poor sleep patterns, behavioral outbursts, and post-traumatic stress disorder. Assessment of pain should include not only a measure of severity (mild, moderate, severe) using an age and cognitively appropriate pain scale, but also the impact of pain on daily function. Inquire about interference with activities such as school attendance, playing with peers, and sleep patterns.

Procedures commonly performed in pediatric primary care may cause pain. These procedures include heel or finger sticks for blood sampling, injections (e.g., immunizations), suturing of lacerations, immobilization of injured extremities, urethral catheterization, and infant circumcision. Pain assessment and management should be tailored to the child's developmental and cognitive age, availability of medications and supplies, and the duration of time that the pain will be experienced.

## Pain Assessment

When assessing pain in children, determine the onset, location, duration, character, aggravating factors, relieving factors, timing, and severity (OLDCARTS). Additionally, various tools have been developed and validated to quantify pain in children. These tools span several age groups from premature infants and neonates to adolescents and have also been developed to aid in assessing pain in children with special health care needs. Measurements may be primarily observational for the nonverbal child or self-reporting for the verbal child, often using some type of visual scale. While many tools exist to measure pain, the most common are discussed here.

### Neonatal Infant Pain Scale

The Neonatal Infant Pain Scale (NIPS) has been validated for assessment of procedural pain in neonates and infants up to 12 months of age. Facial expression, breathing pattern, relaxation or flexion of arms and legs, and state of arousal are scored either zero (0) or one (1). Crying is measured as 0, 1, or 2 (Gouin et al., 2018).

### CRIES

The CRIES measurement is based on five areas, each receiving a score of 0 to 2: crying, requiring increased oxygen administration, increased vital signs, expression, and sleeplessness. It has been validated in infants up to 6 months of age in the intensive care unit, though it is widely used for older infants as well (Beltramini et al., 2017).

### Faces, Legs, Activity, Crying, and Consolability

The Faces, Legs, Activity, Crying, and Consolability (FLACC) tool (Table 6.1) is used and has been validated for children who are unable to communicate verbally. Scores are from 0 to 2 for each of the five categories: face, legs, activity, crying, and consolability (Choueiry et al., 2020). Resultant measures included relaxed and comfortable, mild discomfort, moderate pain, and severe discomfort or pain.

### Wong-Baker FACES® Pain Rating Scale

The Wong-Baker FACES® Pain Rating Scale is reliable and valid in children as young as 3 years of age. It is a visual tool allowing children to indicate their level of pain based on a series of faces expressing increasing amounts of pain or distress (Wong-Baker FACES® Foundation, 2016). The scale is widely available at institutions and medical offices/clinics throughout the country. Refer to https://wongbakerfaces.org to view the scale. To use the scale, instruct the child to choose a face indicating how much pain they have. Face zero is smiling; it does not hurt at all. Face five hurts the most. It may be beneficial to explain one of the faces for some children.

### Numeric Pain Scale

The numeric pain scale may be used in children 6 to 8 years of age and older. Ask the child to rate the intensity of their pain on a numeric scale, typically from a range of 0 (no pain) to 10 (severe pain). See Figure 6.1.

### Visual Analog Scale

Children 6 to 8 years of age and older are developmentally able to use a visual analog scale to rate their pain (Figure 6.2). On a horizontal line 10 centimeters in length, the child notes a place on the line between "no pain" (at the left end of the scale) and "worst pain" (on the right end of the scale).

## Pain Management

Both nonpharmacologic and pharmacologic methods may be used to manage pain in children (Table 6.2). The goal of treatment is to decrease, stop, or limit pain using both nonpharmacologic and pharmacologic methods (Hauer & Jones, 2020). Complementary and alternative methods include distraction, positions of comfort, music therapy, pet therapy, relaxation

**TABLE 6.1 FLACC Scale***

| | Scoring | | |
|---|---|---|---|
| **Categories** | **0** | **1** | **2** |
| **Face** | No particular expression or smile | Occasional grimace or frown, withdrawn, disinterested | Frequent to constant quivering chin, clenched jaw |
| **Legs** | Normal position or relaxed | Uneasy, restless, tense | Kicking, or legs drawn up |
| **Activity** | Lying quietly, normal position, moves easily | Squirming, shifting back and forth, tense | Arched, rigid or jerking |
| **Cry** | No cry (awake or asleep) | Moans or whimpers, occasional complaint | Crying steadily, screams or sobs, frequent complaints |
| **Consolability** | Content, relaxed | Reassured by occasional touching, hugging, or being talked to, distractable | Difficult to console or comfort |

*Each of the five categories (F) Face, (L) Legs, (A) Activity, (C) Cry, (C) Consolability is scored from 0–2, which results in a total score between 0 and 10.

*Source*: Reproduced with permission from Merkel, S. I., Voepel-Lewis, T., Shayevitz, J. R., & Malviya, S. (1997). The FLACC: A behavioral scale for scoring postoperative pain in young children. *Pediatric Nursing, 23*(3), 293–297.

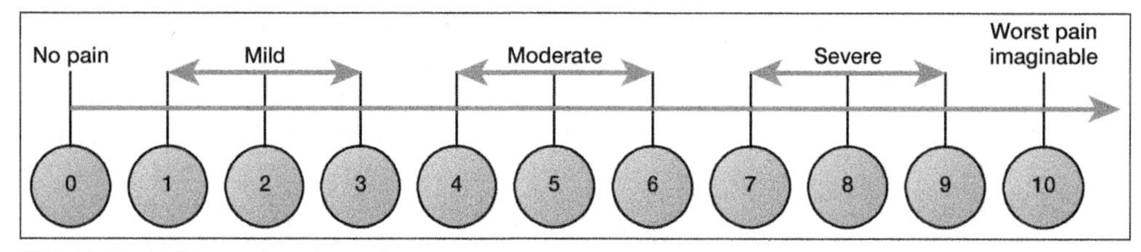


FIGURE 6.1 Numeric pain scale.

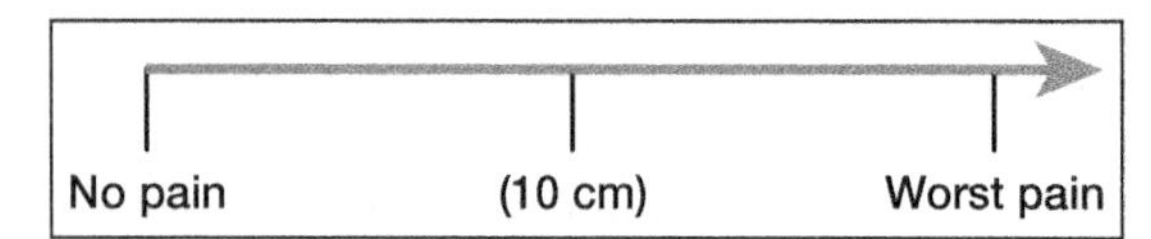


FIGURE 6.2 Visual analog pain scale.

techniques, and hot or cold therapy. Pharmacologic management of pain may be achieved with over-the-counter (OTC) or prescription medications.

## Nonpharmacologic Pain Management

Distraction is appropriate for use with the toddler, preschooler, school-age child, and adolescent. Interventions are based on the child's developmental age and may include blowing bubbles, looking at books, counting, playing with toys, watching videos, or playing video games (Figure 6.3). It may be helpful to engage the caregiver when possible. Holding the child in a position of comfort is effective for infants, toddlers, and preschool-age children.

Music therapy has been shown to significantly reduce pain, particularly in the postoperative period and during painful procedures. Methods include live music therapy, recorded music, and the opportunity for children to participate in actual music sessions (Boric et al., 2017; Nilsson et al., 2009; van der Heijden et al., 2018). Pet therapy has been shown to improve coping skills and decrease anxiety (Sampson & Allbright, 2018). It is appropriate for use with the toddler, preschool, and school-age child. Relaxation techniques such as guided imagery or hypnosis are appropriate for school-age children and adolescents.

Heat therapy (thermotherapy) is particularly useful for visceral pain and pain associated with exacerbations of sickle cell disease. Warm baths, hot compresses, heating pads, or water bottles may be used. Cold therapy's primary use is for acute injuries (soft tissue or musculoskeletal). It is most beneficial during the inflammatory phase of injury (up to 7 days after injury). The recommendation is crushed ice in water in a cloth-covered ice bag applied directly to the

**TABLE 6.2 Summary of Pain Assessment and Management Techniques in Pediatrics**

| Age Group | Pain Score | Common Sources of Pain | Nonpharmacologic Interventions | Pharmacologic Interventions |
|---|---|---|---|---|
| Infants (0–6 months) | NIPS<br>CRIES<br>FLACC | Circumcision<br>Heel stick<br>Immunizations<br>Injuries | Swaddling<br>Facilitated tucking<br>Non-nutritive sucking<br>Breastfeeding<br>Skin-to-skin contact<br>Holding child in position of comfort | Acetaminophen<br>Oral sucrose |
| Older infants and toddlers (6 months–3 years) | FLACC | Immunizations<br>Injuries | Holding a security object<br>Distraction<br>Blowing bubbles<br>Watching videos/cartoons<br>Playing games<br>Looking at books<br>Pet therapy<br>Music therapy | Acetaminophen<br>Ibuprofen (>6 months) |

(continued)

**TABLE 6.2 Summary of Pain Assessment and Management Techniques in Pediatrics *(continued)***

| Age Group | Pain Score | Common Sources of Pain | Nonpharmacologic Interventions | Pharmacologic Interventions |
|---|---|---|---|---|
| Preschool | FLACC<br>FACES | Immunizations<br>Injuries | Distraction<br>Blowing bubbles<br>Watching videos/cartoons<br>Looking at books<br>Playing with toys<br>Pet therapy<br>Music therapy | Acetaminophen<br>Ibuprofen<br>May add hydrocodone for severe, acute pain |
| School age | FACES<br>Numeric | Trauma<br>Headache<br>Somatic or visceral<br>Functional | Distraction<br>Games (video, board)<br>Tablets<br>Looking at books<br>Counting<br>Virtual reality goggles<br>Pet therapy<br>Music therapy<br>Relaxation techniques<br>Ice packs/warm compresses | Acetaminophen<br>Ibuprofen<br>May add hydrocodone for severe, acute pain |
| Adolescent | Numeric | Trauma<br>Headache<br>Somatic or visceral<br>Functional | Relaxation techniques<br>Games (video, board)<br>Tablets<br>Counting<br>Virtual reality goggles<br>Pet therapy<br>Music therapy<br>Ice packs/warm compresses | Acetaminophen<br>Ibuprofen<br>May add hydrocodone for severe, acute pain |

FLACC, faces, legs, activity, crying, and consolability; NIPS, Neonatal Infant Pain Scale

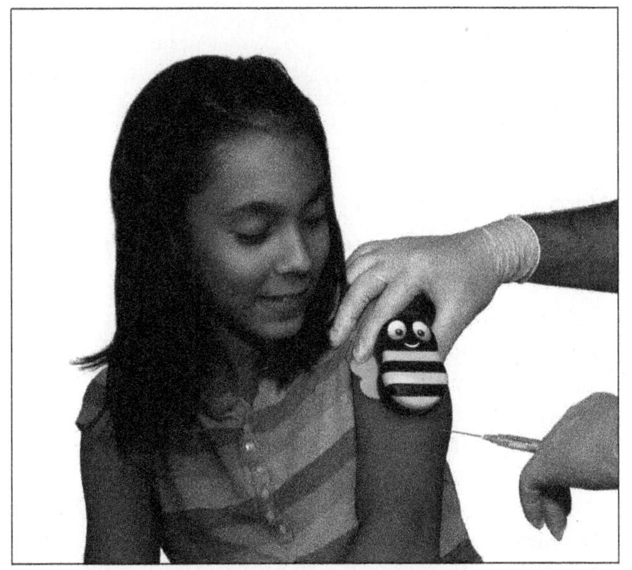

FIGURE 6.3 Distraction (such as with the Buzzy® device shown here) may assist with procedural pain.

skin for either set intervals (20 minutes every hour, 10 minutes on followed by 10 minutes off) or three to four times per day. In cases of acute injury with edema, cold therapy is most effective when used in conjunction with compression. Contraindications to the use of cold therapy include Raynaud phenomenon, impaired sensation, and cold urticaria.

### *Specific Interventions for Infants*

Procedures in the primary care setting that could induce a pain reaction in infants include heel sticks, circumcision, and injections (immunizations) (McNair et al., 2019). Interventions that have been found to reduce pain include:

- Swaddling or facilitated tucking: Wrap or hold infant with limbs flexed close against the body (Figure 6.4). It is most effective when used in conjunction with oral sucrose (Erkut & Yildiz, 2017).

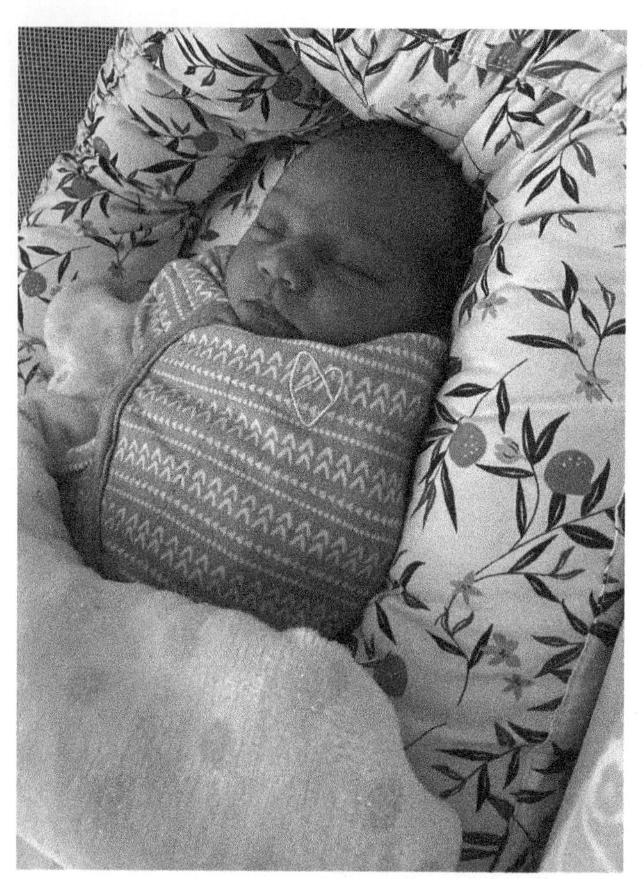

FIGURE 6.4 Swaddling.

- Non-nutritive sucking on pacifier with or without sucrose: Sucrose is effective for a single procedural event in infants up to 42 weeks (e.g., heel stick, blood draw). It has not been shown to be effective as a single agent in longer procedures such as circumcision which is also associated with post-procedural pain. Sucrose may be administered as 0.5 to 2.0 mL of 24% solution directly on tongue or pacifier dipped in sucrose solution 1 to 2 minutes before the procedure (Stevens et al., 2016).
- Skin to skin contact (Kangaroo care) (Johnston et al., 2017; Thrane et al., 2016).
- Breastfeeding (Shah et al., 2012)

## Pharmacologic Pain Management

Pharmacologic pain management consists of either non-narcotic medications, narcotic medications, or a combination of both. Whenever possible, combine pharmacologic and non-pharmacologic measures to manage pain in children, as this has been shown to be the most effective approach.

**PRO TIP** Consider duration and severity of pain when recommending pharmacologic interventions.

### *Non-Narcotic Medications*

Non-narcotic pain medications include acetaminophen and nonsteroidal anti-inflammatory drugs (NSAIDs). Acetaminophen may be administered orally, rectally, or intravenously at a dose of 10 to 15 mg/kg/dose every 4 to 6 hours (not to exceed 75 mg/kg/day). It should be used with caution in children with liver failure. NSAIDs used for pain management in children include ibuprofen, naproxen, and ketorolac.

Ibuprofen may be given orally at a dose of 10 mg/kg/dose every 6 hours (not to exceed 40 mg/kg/day). In children weighing less than 60 kg, naproxen may be administered orally at a dose of 5 to 6 mg/kg/dose twice a day (maximum dose: 1000 mg/day). Children weighing more than 60 kg may take 250 to 375 mg of naproxen orally twice a day. Ketorolac may be given orally at a dose of 1 mg/kg every 6 to 8 hours or intramuscularly/intravenously 0.5 mg/kg/dose every 6 to 8 hours. Do not use ketorolac for longer than 5 days (Hauer & Jones, 2020; Lexicomp Online, 2020). NSAIDs should not be used in children younger than 6 months of age and should be avoided in children with gastrointestinal bleeding or renal impairment.

**PRO TIP** If parents report no pain relief with over-the-counter pain medications, verify dosage and frequency of administration. Caregivers often undermedicate their children.

### *Narcotic Medications*

The recommended doses for narcotic medictions are:

- Acetaminophen/HYDROcodone 0.1 to 0.2 mg/kg/dose orally every 4 to 6 hours
- Acetaminophen/OXYcodone 0.1 to 0.2 mg/kg/dose orally every 6 hours
- Oxycodone
  - <6 months of age: 0.025 to 0.05 mg/kg/dose orally every 4 to 6 hours
  - 6 months of age & <50 kg: 0.1 to 0.2 mg/kg/dose orally every 4 to 6 hours
  - >6 months of age & >50 kg: 5 to 10 mg orally every 4 to 6 hours (Lexicomp Online, 2020).

Morphine sulfate and hydromorphone may be given either orally or intravenously and are used for severe and/or chronic pain.

▶ ALERT: Acetaminophen and codeine should NOT be used in children younger than 12 years of age or in any child who has undergone a tonsillectomy and adenoidectomy between the ages of 12 and 18. It is not a preferred medication for the treatment of pain in pediatrics due to its variability in metabolism, which increases the risk of overdose. *Avoid use* (Hauer & Jones, 2020; Lexicomp Online, 2020).

## KEY POINTS

- To adequately control the child's pain, the provider must determine the onset, location, duration, characteristics, aggravating factors, relieving factors, and the appropriate treatment plan (OLDCARTS).
- Utilization of the most appropriate pain assessment tool based on age and cognitive function is essential.
- Pain management in pediatrics may include nonpharmacologic and pharmacologic interventions.
- Nonpharmacologic interventions should be first-line therapy for pain management in the outpatient setting.
- Acetaminophen and ibuprofen are the most common non-narcotic medications used to treat pediatric pain.

## REFERENCES

Beltramini, A., Milojevic, K., & Pateron, D. (2017). Pain assessment in newborns, infants, and children. *Pediatric Annals, 46*(10), e387–e395. https://doi.org/10.3928/19382359-20170921-03

Bolick, B., Reuter-Rice, K., Madden, M., & Severin, P. (2021). *Pediatric acute care: A guide for interprofessional practice* (2nd ed.). Elsevier.

Boric, K., Dosenovic, S., Kadic, A. J., Batinic, M., Cavar, M., Urlic, M., Markovina, M., & Puljak, L. (2017). Interventions for postoperative pain in children: An overview of systematic reviews. *Paediatric Anaesthesia, 27*(9), 893–904. https://doi.org/10.1111/pan.13203

Choueiry, J., Reszel, J., Hamid, J. S., Wilding, J., Martelli, B., & Harrison, D. (2020). Development and pilot evaluation of an educational tool for the FLACC pain scale. *Pain Management Nursing, 21*(6), 523–529. https://doi.org/10.1016/j.pmn.2020.06.002

Erkut, Z., & Yildiz, S. (2017). The effect of swaddling on pain, vital signs, and crying duration during heel lance in newborns. *Pain Management Nursing, 18*(5), e328–e336. https://doi.org/10.1016/j.pmn.2017.05.007

Friedrichsdorf, S., Giordano, J., Dakoji, K. D., Warmuth, A., Daughtry, C., & Schulz, C. (2016). Chronic pain in children and adolescents: Diagnosis and treatment of primary pain disorders in head, abdomen, muscles and joints. *Children, 3*, 42. https://doi.org/10.3390/children3040042

Gouin, S., Gaucher, N., Lebel, D., & Desjardins, M. P. (2018). A randomized double-blind trial comparing the effect on pain of an oral sucrose solution vs. placebo in children 1 to 3 months old undergoing simple venipuncture. *The Journal of Emergency Medicine, 54*(1), 33–39. https://doi.org/10.1016/j.jemermed.2017.08.015

Hauer, J., & Jones, B. L. (2020). Evaluation and management of pain in children. In D. G. Poplack (Ed.), *UpToDate*. Retrieved September 3, 2020, from https://www.uptodate.com/contents/evaluation-and-management-of-pain-in-children

Johnston, C., Campbell-Yeo, M., Disher, T., Benoit, B., Fernandes, A., Streiner, D., Inglis, D., & Zee, R. (2017). Skin-to-skin care for procedural pain in neonates. *Cochrane Database of Systematic Reviews*. https://doi.org/10.1002/14651858.CD008435.pub3

Lee, R. R., Rashid, A., Ghio, D., Thomson, W., & Cordingley, L. (2017). Chronic pain assessments in children and adolescents: A systematic literature review of the selection, administration, interpretation, and reporting of unidimensional pain intensity scales. *Pain Research and Management, 2017*, Article ID 7603758. https://doi.org/10.1155/2017/7603758

Lexicomp Online. (2020). *Pediatric and Neonatal Lexi-drugs online*. Wolters Kluwer Clinical Drug Information.

McNair, C., Yeo, M. C., Johnston, C., & Taddio, A. (2019). Nonpharmacologic management of pain during common needle puncture procedures in infants: Current research evidence and practical considerations: An update. *Clinics in Perinatology, 46*(4), 709–730. https://doi.org/10.1016/j.clp.2019.08.006

Merkel, S. I., Voepel-Lewis, T., Shayevitz, J. R., & Malviya, S. (1997). The FLACC: A behavioral scale for scoring postoperative pain in young children. *Pediatric Nursing, 23*(3), 293–297.

Nilsson, S., Kokinsky, E., Nilsson, U., Sidenvall, B., & EnskÄr, K. (2009). School-aged children's experiences of postoperative music medicine on pain, distress, and anxiety. *Paediatric Anaesthesia, 19*(12), 1184–1190. https://doi.org/10.1111/j.1460-9592.2009.03180.x

Olson, K. A. (2013). History of pain: A brief overview of the 19th and 20th centuries. *Practical Pain Management, 13*(7). https://www.practicalpainmanagement.com/treatments/history-pain-brief-overview-19th-20th-centuries

Sampson, J., & Allbright, R. (2018). Distracting pediatric patients during painful procedures. *Nursing, 48*(7), 56–57. https://doi.org/10.1097/01.NURSE.0000534109.96519.25

Shah, P. S., Herbozo, C., Aliwalas, L. L., & Shah, V. S. (2012). Breastfeeding or breast milk for procedural pain in neonates. *Cochrane Database of Systematic Reviews*. https://doi.org/10.1002/14651858.cd004950.pub3

Stevens, B., Yamada, J., Ohlsson, A., Haliburton, S., & Shorkey, A. (2016). Sucrose for analgesia in newborn infants undergoing painful procedures. *Cochrane Database of Systematic Reviews*. https://doi.org/10.1002/14651858.CD001069.pub5

Thrane, S. E., Wanless, S., Cohen, S. M., & Danford, C. A. (2016). The assessment and non-pharmacologic treatment of procedural pain from infancy to school age through a developmental lens: A synthesis of evidence with recommendations. *Journal of Pediatric Nursing, 31*(1), e23–e32. https://doi.org/10.1016/j.pedn.2015.09.002

van der Heijden, M. J. E., Jeekel, J., Rode, H., Cox, S., van Rosmalen, J., Hunink, M. G. M., & van Dijk, M. (2018). Can live music therapy reduce distress and pain in children with burns after wound care procedures? A randomized controlled trial. *Burns, 44*(4), 823–833. https://doi.org/10.1016/j.burns.2017.12.013

Wong Baker FACES Foundation. (2016). *Wong-Baker Faces® Pain Rating Scale*. https://wongbakerfaces.org

# UNIT II

## Child Development

# Growth and Development During Infancy

Theresa Kyle

## Student Learning Outcomes

**Upon completion of this chapter the reader should be able to:**

1. Examine physical developmental changes and growth occurring during the period of infancy.
2. Differentiate among gross motor, fine motor, and language milestones expected during infancy.
3. Identify expected psychosocial, cognitive, and moral development changes for various ages throughout the period of infancy.
4. Describe appropriate sleep, rest, and nutrition for infants.
5. Discuss typical developmental issues occurring during infancy.

## INTRODUCTION

Infancy is defined as the period from birth to 12 months of age, with the newborn or neonatal period of infancy occurring from birth until 28 days of age. Throughout infancy and childhood, growth and development are interrelated, ongoing processes. While growth denotes an increase in physical size, development is the sequential process by which infants and children acquire various abilities. Growth and development are influenced by heredity, as it determines the child's potential, while the degree of achievement is significantly influenced by the infant's environment.

Over the first year of life, growth and development progress at a rapid pace. Physical growth, body system maturation, and gross and fine motor skills progress in an orderly and somewhat consecutive fashion. Timing of skill acquisition may vary from infant to infant. In the psychosocial and cognitive, language and communication, and social/emotional domains, infants also demonstrate a vast amount of change in the first 12 months. Appropriate growth and development generally indicate health in the infant. Familiarity with normal developmental milestones permits the nurse practitioner (NP) to adequately assess the infant's development as well as provide age-appropriate anticipatory guidance to the parents.

The content in this chapter maps to the following areas on the Pediatric Nursing Certification Board (PNCB) Pediatric Nurse Practitioner—Primary Care certification examination:

### CONTENT AREAS:

**I. Health Promotion and Maintenance**

**A. Partner with patients/caregivers to support growth and development from infancy to young adulthood**

**II. Assessment and Diagnosis**

**A. Growth and Development**

1. Evaluate and interpret growth parameters

**III. Professional Role Responsibilities**

**A. Leadership and Evidence-based Practice**

1. Serve as a clinical resource for other health care professionals
2. Critically evaluate and synthesize research and apply findings to clinical practice

## GROWTH

Infants and children who demonstrate growth within the average range over time are generally healthy, whereas poor growth may be an indicator of a physical illness or mental/emotional issue. Inadequate or excessively rapid growth can be identified and addressed with interventions early when demonstrated by ongoing assessments. Early intervention will provide for maximization of the potential for further appropriate growth. Growth is fastest during the period of infancy, and weight, length, and head circumference are the parameters demonstrating that growth.

### WEIGHT

At birth, the average full-term newborn weighs 3.400 kg (7.5 lb); boys are often slightly heavier than girls. Over the first week of life, newborns may lose up to 10% of their body weight. Average weight gain in the newborn period is about 20 g to 30 g per day, with birth weight being regained by about 2 weeks of age. Birth weight doubles by 4 to 5 months of age and triples by the age of 12 months old (Levine, 2019).

### LENGTH

At birth, the average full-term newborn's length is 50 cm. During the first 6 months of life, gains in length occur more rapidly than during month 7 through the end of the first year. An increase of length by 50% is expected by 12 months of age (Levine, 2019).

### HEAD CIRCUMFERENCE

At birth, the average full-term newborn's head circumference is 35 cm (13.5 inches). Brain growth is very rapid during the first year of life, particularly the first 6 months. Infants will experience a total increase in head circumference of about 10 cm from birth to 12 months of age (Levine, 2019).

**PRO TIP** Infants born prematurely may demonstrate delays in physical growth and attainment of developmental milestones. For premature infants, always use the infant's adjusted age to evaluate growth and development. Adjusted age is calculated by subtracting the number of weeks the infant was premature from the infant's chronologic age. For example, an infant born at 30 weeks' gestation was born 10 weeks early. When 4 months old, subtract 2. 5 months (10 weeks) from 4 months. This infant should demonstrate the growth and developmental skills of a 1 ½ month old baby, rather than those of a 4-month-old.

### CULTURAL INFLUENCES ON GROWTH

Cultural feeding practices in some cultures may lead to overweight or underweight in some children. Vegetarianism is advocated by certain religions and in some cultures. Infants on vegetarian diets can demonstrate adequate growth, but may need nutritional assessment to ensure they are consuming enough protein. Because of their genetic makeup, particular ethnic groups tend to be shorter than others (Sinha, 2019). These infants' lengths may naturally be shorter than those of other ethnic backgrounds.

## PHYSICAL CHANGES

As the infant grows, the organ systems undergo tremendous changes. Significant changes occur in the neurologic, cardiovascular, respiratory, gastrointestinal, genitourinary, hematopoietic, immunologic, and integumentary systems.

### NEUROLOGIC SYSTEM

Substantial changes in the neurologic system occur over the first 12 months of life. The brain grows significantly, more neurons are added, and continued myelination of the spinal cord occurs. The changes allow for involuntary movement to progress to voluntary control, and for crying and immature vocalizations to progress to the ability to speak. Although the newborn's brain is immature, when the newborn is able to move through states of consciousness in sequence, the parents and providers may be reassured that the neurologic system is intact. The progression through these states is usually slow; the newborn does not usually go from deep sleep immediately into outright crying. The six states of consciousness of the normal newborn are:

- Deep sleep: No movement and sleeping with eyes closed
- Light sleep: Rapid eye movements and irregular movements occur while sleeping with eyes closed

- Drowsiness: Appearing to be dozing, the infant's eyes may close or be half-lidded
- Quiet alert state: The infant's body is calm and the eyes are wide open
- Active alert state: Body movements occur and the infant's eyes are open
- Crying: The infant is crying or screaming; it is difficult to engage the infant's attention (Leigh, 2016)

### Brain and Spinal Cord

As the neurologic system continues to mature throughout infancy, the brain undergoes substantial growth. By 12 months of age, the brain weighs about 2.5 times more than it did at birth. The anterior fontanel remains open to accommodate this rapid brain growth. The fontanel usually closes by 12 to 18 months of age but may close as early as 9 months of age in an infant with age-appropriate growth and development.

The multiple and varied developmental skills acquired in the first 12 months of life are possible because of the maturation of the neurologic system and ongoing myelination of the spinal cord and nerves. Infants demonstrate reflexive behavior at birth; with neurologic maturation the behavior is replaced with purposeful action. Reflexive behavior is subcortical and often involves a whole-body response, resulting in the primitive reflexes. Primitive reflexes, primarily integrated over the first 4 to 6 months of life, give way to the protective reflexes (postural responses or reflexes). Protective reflexes are gross motor responses related to maintenance of equilibrium and are necessary for appropriate gross motor development; these remain throughout life once they are established. Age-appropriate primitive reflexes and their disappearance, as well as the emergence of protective reflexes, indicate a healthy neurologic system. An abnormality of the neurologic system may result in persistence of primitive reflexes beyond the usual age of disappearance. Refer to chapter 3 for additional information on the specific reflexes.

## RESPIRATORY SYSTEM

The full-term newborn has about 150 million alveoli (one-half that of the healthy adult). The respiratory system continues to mature over the first year of life, thus requiring a higher respiratory rate for ventilation to occur. The newborn has an average respiratory rate of 30 to 60 breaths per minute (bpm), slowing to a rate of about 20 to 30 bpm in the 12-month-old. Additionally, the newborn breathes in an irregular pattern with periodic pauses. Over the first 12 months, the respiratory pattern becomes more regular and rhythmic. The infant also has smaller and shorter airways throughout the entire respiratory system, a larger tongue relative to the airway size, and a highly compliant chest wall and trachea, all of which places the infant at increased risk of respiratory compromise. Additionally, the mucosal lining of the upper respiratory tract lacks immunoglobulin A (IgA), contributing to higher risk for respiratory problems in infancy.

## CARDIOVASCULAR SYSTEM

During the first 12 months of life, the heart will double in size. The average newborn heart rate is 120 to 140 bpm and will decrease to about 100 bpm by 12 months of age. The average newborn blood pressure of 60/40 will increase steadily to an average 100/50 in the 12-month-old. The newborn and young infant is more susceptible to heat loss because the peripheral capillaries are closer to the surface of the skin. Thermoregulation becomes more effective over the first 12 months as the peripheral capillaries become better able to constrict in response to a cold environment and dilate in response to heat.

## GASTROINTESTINAL SYSTEM

The typical newborn does not have teeth. The first deciduous (primary) teeth begin to erupt between the ages of 6 and 8 months on average, although gum swelling around the impending tooth eruption begins earlier. Usually, the lower central incisors are the first to appear, followed by the upper central incisors (Figure 7.1). By 12 months of age, babies usually have four to eight teeth (Gandhi, et al., 2020).

> **PRO TIP** Occasionally an infant may be born with one or more teeth (natal teeth). *Neonatal teeth* is the term used to describe teeth appearing in the first 30 days of life. Refer infants with natal or neonatal teeth to pediatric dentistry for evaluation and potential treatment (American Academy of Pediatric Dentistry, 2015).

In the first 3 months of life, the infant has only small amounts of saliva, with ptyalin being present only in small amounts in that saliva, and thus must rely on hydrochloric acid and rennin for gastric digestion. The stomach capacity of the newborn is only about

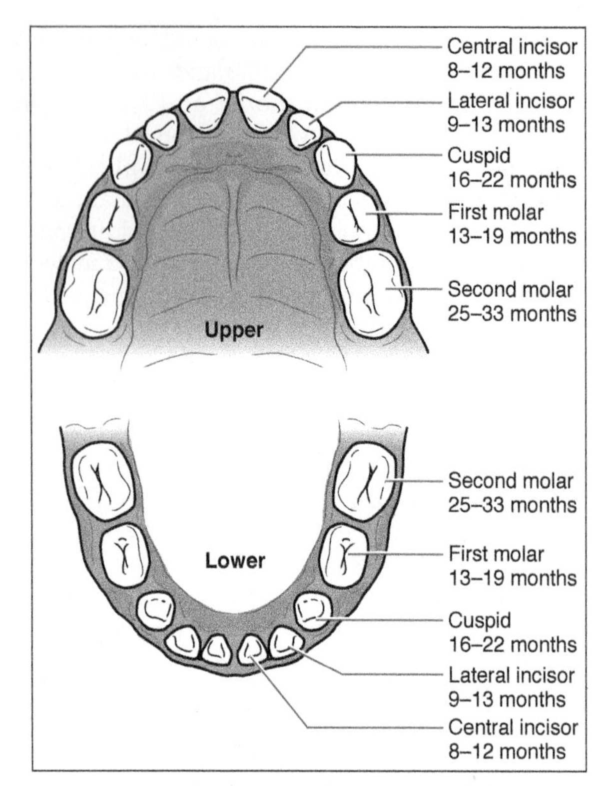


**FIGURE 7.1 Usual sequence of primary teeth eruption.**

*Source*: Chiocca, E. M. (2020). *Advanced pediatric assessment*. Springer Publishing Company.

15 to 30 mL, increasing in capacity to allow for three full infant-sized meals and several snacks per day by the age of 12 months. The small intestine is about 270 cm long at birth, significantly shorter than the older child's and adult's (Maqbool & Liacouras, 2016). The stomach capacity is relatively small at birth, holding about one-half to 1 ounce. In the duodenum, trypsin exists in sufficient quantities for protein digestion after birth, yet amylase (necessary for complex carbohydrate digestion) and lipase (required for appropriate fat digestion) do not reach adult levels until about 5 months of age.

The liver is also immature at birth, yielding immature gluconeogenesis, vitamin storage, and protein metabolism (refer to chapter 42 for additional information).

Stools in the first day or two of life are the result of amniotic fluid swallowed in utero and are greenish-black and sticky (meconium). Over the next several days, the stools transition to tan or yellowish in color, being looser and seedy in breastfed babies and the consistency of peanut butter in formula-fed infants. Newborns may produce stools eight to 10 times per day; after the newborn period frequency decreases. Some infants may have a bowel movement only once every several days, which may be considered normal if the stool is soft. Newborns and young infants frequently strain and grunt when having a bowel movement, due to the immaturity of the gastrointestinal tract. Stool color and texture may change depending on the foods that the infant is ingesting (Swanson & Cohen, 2020).

▶ ALERT: The infant's stools should not be red, white, or black; mucous-like or frothy; frequent and watery; foul-smelling; or pellet-like (hard, dry, formed). Instruct parents to call the primary care provider if these types of stools occur or if the infant is vomiting.

## GENITOURINARY SYSTEM

The infant has a higher percentage of total body water relative to weight than does the older child or adult, placing the infant at increased risk for dehydration. During infancy, intracellular fluid volume increases while extracellular fluid (lymph, interstitial fluid, and blood plasma) decreases, reaching the adult levels of 20 to 25%, and 30 to 40%, respectively, by 12 months of age (Karp & Greenbaum, 2019). Infants' urine has a relatively low specific gravity. and infants urinate frequently as the glomerular filtration rate, tubular secretion, reabsorption, and renal perfusion rate are reduced. The renal structures mature over the first 24 months of life.

## HEMATOPOIETIC SYSTEM

Over the first 12 months of life, substantial changes occur in the infant's hematopoietic system. Relatively low hemoglobin and hematocrit occur around 2 to 3 months of age (physiologic anemia of infancy) due to significant decrease in erythrocyte production after birth (Wang et al., 2020). Maternal iron stores are transferred to the fetus during the last 3 months of gestation, with healthy newborns typically being born with sufficient iron stores. The newborn's high hemoglobin concentration decreases over the first 2 to 3 months, during which iron is reclaimed and stored. Iron stores are usually adequate for the first 6 to 9 months of life, but if iron supplementation does not occur, stores will become reduced (Powers & Mahoney, 2020).

**PRO TIP** Premature infants will miss all or at least a portion of the maternal-fetal iron store transfer during the last trimester of pregnancy, placing them at increased risk for iron deficiency anemia as compared with term infants.

## IMMUNOLOGIC SYSTEM

IgG transfers in large amounts through the placenta from the mother to the fetus, conferring immunity during the first 3 to 6 months of life for antigens to which the mother has been previously exposed. After birth, with exposure and immunization, infants synthesize their own IgG, and by 12 months of age reach approximately 60% of the adult level (Cherry et al., 2019). Infant IgA, IgD, and IgE production increases very gradually, while IgM is produced in substantial amounts after birth, reaching adult levels by the age of 9 months (Cherry et al., 2019).

## INTEGUMENTARY SYSTEM

In utero, the fetus is covered with vernix caseosa, which protects the developing infant's skin, but production ceases at birth. Less gestationally mature newborns may be covered with vernix, or it may be found only in the folds of the skin, axilla, and groin areas in newborns of a later gestational age. Lanugo covers the body of many newborns, with darker-skinned races tending to have more lanugo present at birth than those with lighter skin. Lanugo is lost over time.

Acrocyanosis, normal in the newborn, occurs as a result of circulatory immaturity, decreasing over the first few days of life. Mottling of the skin also occurs due to circulatory immaturity and decreases over the first few months of life. The newborn and young infant's skin is relatively thin, with the peripheral capillaries being closer to the surface, resulting increased absorption of topical medications.

## SENSORY DEVELOPMENT

Unless there is a problem, hearing is fully developed at birth and is of adult acuity. Newborns demonstrate a preference for human voices over nonhuman sounds. The 1-month-old infant is able to recognize the sounds of those they know best. As the infant grows, the other senses (sight, smell, taste, and touch) continue to develop, maturing at different rates.

The newborn is myopic and prefers to view objects at a distance of 20 to 38 cm (8–15 inches). The newborn's preference for viewing is the human face and objects with contrasts such as black-and-white graphic designs. The 1-month-old infant recognizes the people they know best, by sight. Binocularity (ability to meld two ocular images into one cerebral picture) begins developing at 6 weeks of age and is well established by 4 months of age. Distance vision, the ability to track objects, and full color vision develop by age 7 months.

A 7-day-old infant preferentially turns toward the mother's smell and can differentiate the smell of their mother's breast milk from that of another woman. Newborns prefer sweet tastes to all others, which persists for many months, with eventual acceptance of nonsweet flavors. Infants prefer soft sensations over coarse sensations and may cry with rough handling. The upset infant may calm with rocking, stroking, or cuddling and the drowsy infant may alert with those actions. The caregiver's mood is interpreted by the infant by the way the infant is touched by the caregiver.

▶ ALERT: Warning signs indicating sensory development issues include:

- young infant is unresponsive to loud noises
- infant does not focus on a near object
- not making sounds or babbling by 4 months of age
- not turning to locate sound at age 4 months of age
- persistent strabismus at age 6 months of age

# DEVELOPMENTAL MILESTONES

Infants progress through various stages of development in a predictable fashion. Motor and language milestones are usually achieved in a sequential and orderly manner, although some infants may develop at a faster rate than others. Culture also influences health promotion behaviors and parenting styles. Some cultures may "baby" their infants for longer periods, whereas others that highly value independence encourage or expect their infants to develop quickly.

## MOTOR SKILL DEVELOPMENT

Infants exhibit phenomenal increases in their gross and fine motor skills over the first 12 months of life. *Gross motor skills* refers to those skills utilizing large muscles (e.g., head control, rolling, sitting, and walking). Gross motor skills develop in a cephalocaudal fashion with the infant learning to lift the head before learning to roll over and sit (Goldson et al., 2020). At birth, babies have poor head control and need to have their necks supported when being held. Maturation of hand and finger use results in the development of fine motor skills that develop in a proximodistal fashion. The infant will first bat with the whole hand, then progress to gross grasping, and eventually develop a fine pincer grasp (Goldson et al., 2020). Refer to Table 7.1 for examples of gross motor and fine motor skills according to age.

▶ ALERT: Warning signs indicating problems with motor development include:

- extremities are stiff or floppy
- infant cannot support head at 4 months of age
- infant reaches with one hand only
- infant cannot sit with assistance at 6 months of age
- infant does not crawl by 12 months of age
- infant cannot stand with support by 12 months of age

## LANGUAGE AND COMMUNICATION

For the first few months of life, the infant's the only means of communication is crying, the basic reason for which is unmet needs. For the infant to learn communication skills, it is very important for the parent or caregiver to talk to the infant. Communication progresses from crying to cooing, making other vocalizations, and to differentiated crying (Table 7.2). Next, true sounds are made and the infant progresses to using words by 12 months of age. When the infant is focusing energy on other skills, such as crawling or walking, a brief regression in language development may occur. If the infant's hearing is normal, language acquisition will later continue to progress. Infants in bilingual families may use some words from each

TABLE 7.1 **Gross and Fine Motor Skills in Infancy**

| Age | Gross Motor Skills | Fine Motor Skills |
|---|---|---|
| 1 month | In prone position, lifts and turns head to side<br>When pulled to sit, the newborn infant shows significant head lag 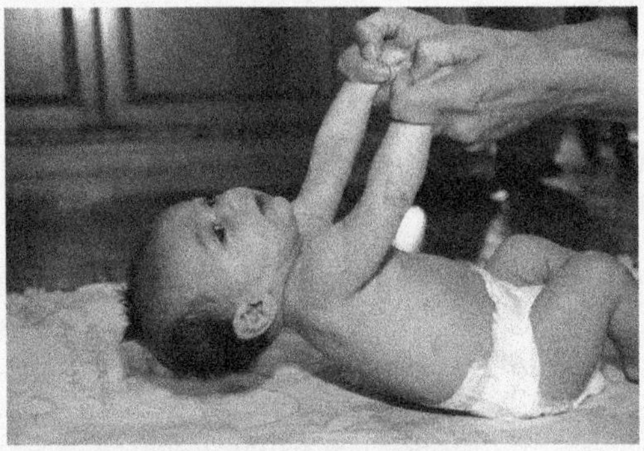<br>In supported sitting, back is rounded | Fists are mostly clenched<br>Hand movements are involuntary |
| 2 months | Can raise head and chest, then hold the position<br>At 2 months old, the following shows improving head control 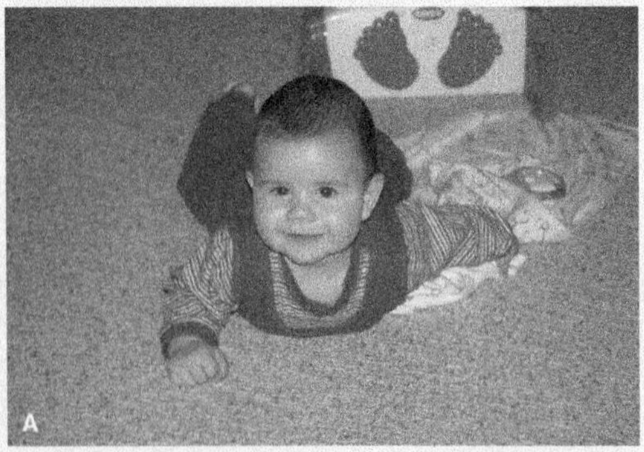<br>A | |

(continued)

TABLE 7.1 **Gross and Fine Motor Skills in Infancy** *(continued)*

| Age | Gross Motor Skills | Fine Motor Skills |
|---|---|---|
| 3 months | In prone positions, raises head to 45 degrees<br>When pulled to sit, has slight head lag | Hands open<br>Holds hand in front of face |
| 4 months | Able to roll from prone position to supine position<br>The 4-month-old infant demonstrates no head lag<br>When pulled to sit, head leads body<br>In the prone position, lifts head and looks around 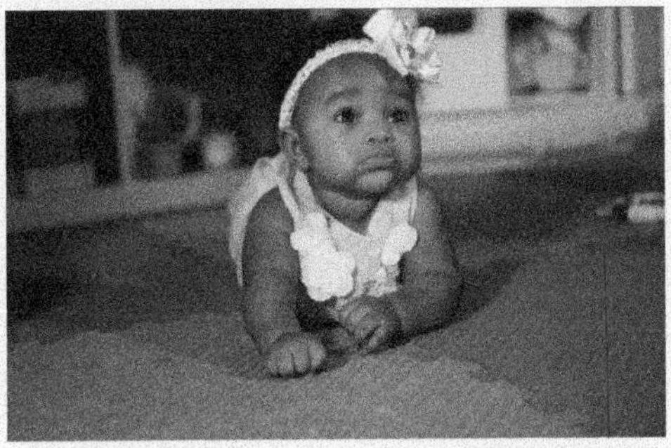 | Bats at objects (whole hand) |
| 5 months | Able to roll from supine position to prone position, then back again<br>When supported, sits with back upright | Able to grasp a rattle |
| 6 months | Average 6-month-old infant sits in the tripod position (legs out, hand out front on floor for support) 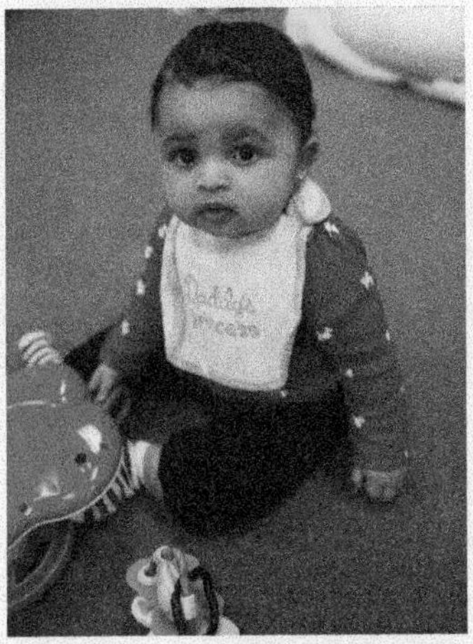 | Is able to release an object in one hand to take another object in the same hand |
| 7 months | With use of hands for support, sits alone | Is able to transfer an object from one hand to the other |
| 8 months | The 8-month-old sits well independently and unsupported 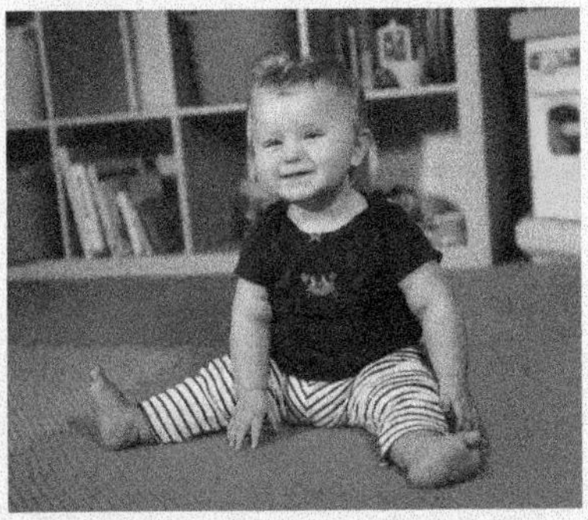 | Rakes small objects with whole hand (gross pincer grasp) |

*(continued)*

**TABLE 7.1 Gross and Fine Motor Skills in Infancy** *(continued)*

| Age | Gross Motor Skills | Fine Motor Skills |
|---|---|---|
| 9 months | The 9-month-old infant crawls with the abdomen off of the floor | Is able to bang objects together with both hands |
| 10 months | Pulls to stand<br>The 10-month-old infant cruises (walks while holding on to furniture) 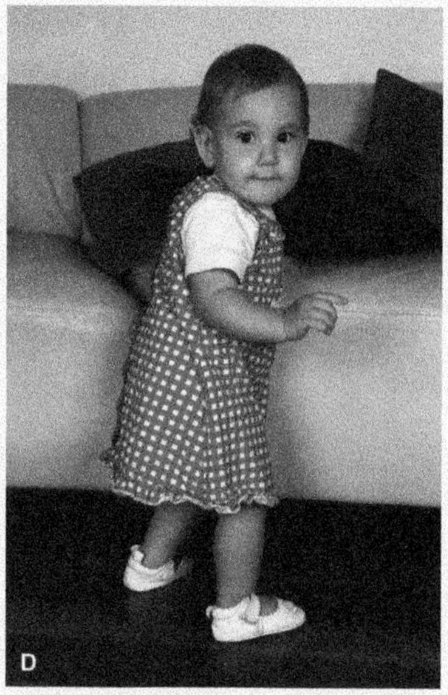<br>D | Picks up small objects with index finger and thumb (fine pincer grasp)<br>Is able to put objects into a container and take them out again |
| 11 months | | Will offer an object to others and release the object |
| 12 months | Able to sit from a standing position<br>Walks independently 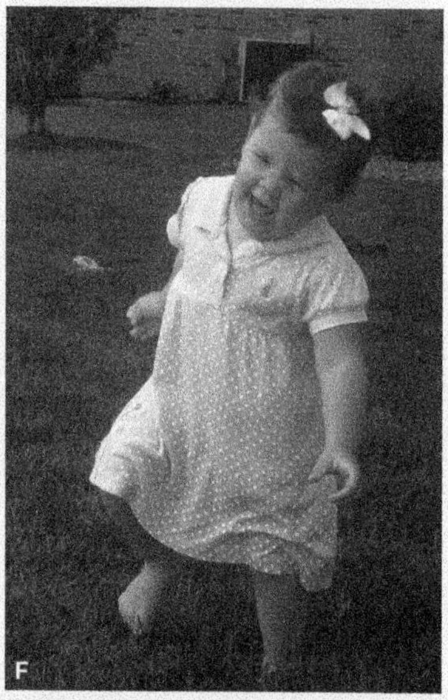<br>F | Able to feed self with cup and spoon<br>With a crayon, is able to make a simple mark on paper<br>Pokes with index finger |

*Sources*: Data from Centers for Disease Control and Prevention. (2020). *Developmental milestones.* http://www.cdc.gov/ncbddd/actearly/milestones/index.html; Goldson, E., Angulo, A. S., Raz, D. M., & Reynolds, A. (2020). Child development and behavior. In W. W. Hay, M. J. Levin, M. J. Abzug, & M. Bunik (Eds.), *Current diagnosis & treatment: Pediatrics* (25th ed., Chapter 3). McGraw Hill Education; Levine, D. A. (2019). Growth and development. In K. J. Marcdante & R. M. Kliegman (Eds.), *Nelson's essentials of pediatrics* (8th ed., Section 2). Elsevier.

Photographs 4–8 months courtesy of Centers for Disease Control and Prevention; Photographs 1–2 months, and 11–12 months from Chiocca, E. M. (2020). *Advanced pediatric assessment*. Springer Publishing Company.

**TABLE 7.2 Language and Communication Skills in Infancy**

| Age | Language/Communication Skills |
|---|---|
| 1 to 3 months | Coos<br>Makes other vocalizations<br>Has different cries for different reasons (differentiated crying) |
| 4 to 5 months | Simple vowel sounds<br>Laughs aloud<br>Makes "raspberries"<br>Vocalizes in response to voices<br>Responds to own name<br>Begins to respond to "no" |
| 4 to 7 months | Starts to distinguish emotions based on the tone of voice |
| 6 months | Squeals<br>Yells<br>(either may be used to express joy or displeasure) |
| 7 to 10 months | Begins to babble<br>Progresses to strings without meaning (e.g., bababa, mamama, dadada)<br>Responds to simple commands |
| 9 to 12 months | Starts to attach meaning to "mama" and "dada"<br>Begins imitating other speech sounds |
| 12 months | Uses two or three recognizable words with meaning<br>Able to recognize objects by name<br>Begins to imitate animal sounds<br>Pays increasing attention to speech and tries to imitate words<br>May also say "uh-oh"<br>Babbles with inflection (with the rhythm and timing of spoken language, but few of the words make sense) |

*Sources*: Data from Goldson, E., Angulo, A. S., Raz, D. M., & Reynolds, A. (2020). Child development and behavior. In W. W. Hay, M. J. Levin, M. J. Abzug, & M. Bunik (Eds.), *Current diagnosis & treatment: Pediatrics* (25th ed., Chapter 3). McGraw Hill Education; Levine, D. A. (2019). Growth and development. In K. J. Marcdante & R. M. Kliegman (Eds.), *Nelson's essentials of pediatrics* (8th ed., Section 2). Elsevier.

language (language mixing), a normal progression in language development for these children (Lowry, 2016).

ALERT: Warning signs indicating a problem in language development include:

- Not making sounds at 4 months of age
- Not laughing or squealing by 6 months of age
- Not babbling by 8 months of age
- Not using single words with meaning at 12 months of age (mama, dada)

## COGNITIVE DEVELOPMENT

An infant's cognitive development occurs through their emerging sensory and motor capacities. Most of the cognitive development occurring in infancy is guided by cause and effect. The first stage of cognitive development is described as the sensorimotor stage and occurs from birth to 2 years of age (Piaget, 1969). Cognitive development in infancy is divided into four substages within the sensorimotor stage: reflexes, primary circular reaction, secondary circular reaction, and coordination of secondary schemes. Refer to Table 7.3 for activities related to the first four substages of the sensorimotor stage of cognitive development.

The concept of object permanence begins to develop between 4 and 7 months of age and is solidified by about 8 months of age (Piaget, 1969). If an object is hidden from the infant's sight, they will search for it in the last place it was seen, knowing it still exists. This development of object permanence is essential for the development of self-image. By age 12 months the infant knows he or she is separate from the parent or caregiver. Self-image is also promoted through the use of mirrors. By 12 months of age, infants can recognize themselves in the mirror. The 12-month-old will explore objects in different ways, such as throwing, banging, dropping, and shaking, and learn about

**TABLE 7.3 Cognitive Development in Infancy**

| Substage | Activities |
|---|---|
| Substage 1:<br>Use of reflexes<br>(birth to 1 month) | Using senses and motor skills to learn about the world<br>Reflexive sucking leads to the pleasure of satiety<br>Begins gaining control over reflexive actions and recognizes familiar objects, sounds, and odors. |
| Substage 2:<br>Primary circular reactions<br>(1 to 4 months) | Thumb sucking happens by chance; it is then purposefully repeated to bring pleasure<br>Imitation begins<br>Affect is shown by infant |
| Substage 3:<br>Secondary circular reactions<br>(4 to 8 months) | Object permanence begins at some point in this time period; infant begins to repeat an action to achieve desired results (shaking a rattle to hear the noise)<br>Actions are purposeful but the infant does not always have an end goal in mind |
| Substage 4:<br>Coordination of secondary schemes<br>(8 to 12 months) | Object permanence fully present at about 8 months of age. Previously learned schemes are coordinated with previously learned behaviors (grasp *and* shake a rattle intentionally, or crawls across room to reach a toy)<br>Can anticipate events by associating symbols with them (waving goodbye means someone is leaving) |

*Sources*: Data from Goldson, E., Angulo, A. S., Raz, D. M., & Reynolds, A. (2020). Child development and behavior. In W. W. Hay, M. J. Levin, M. J. Abzug, & M. Bunik (Eds.), *Current diagnosis & treatment: Pediatrics* (25th ed., Chapter 3). McGraw Hill Education; Piaget, J. (1969). *The theory of stages in cognitive development*. McGraw-Hill.

themselves and the world. They may imitate gestures and know how to use certain objects correctly (e.g., put phone to ear, turn up cup to drink, attempt to comb hair; Piaget, 1969).

## SOCIAL AND EMOTIONAL DEVELOPMENT

The psychosocial crisis of infancy is trust versus mistrust (Erikson, 1963). It is crucial for infants to develop of a sense of trust in the first year. This sense of trust is the underpinning for later acquisition of other psychosocial tasks. Trust is developed when the infant's needs are consistently met (feeding, changing diapers, cleaning, holding, or touching, talking to the infant). Yet when those needs are inconsistently met, the infant develops a sense of mistrust. By about 2 months of age, the infant is ready to start socializing and truly smiles for the first time. The infant often watches and observes what goes on the environment. To engage the caregiver, the 3-month-old will smile widely and possibly gurgle. The caregiver is then prompted to smile in return and talk to the infant. This reciprocal interaction continues as the infant smiles more, coos, gurgles, and moves the arms and legs. Mimicking the parent's facial movements (widening the eyes, sticking out the tongue), the 3- to 4-month-old may hesitate at first, but once a pleasant response is noted, the infant engages and participates in the interaction. If the pleasant interaction stops, then the infant may cry. Socially interactive games (pat-a-cake, peek-a-boo) are enjoyed by the 6- to 8-month-old infant (Goldson et al., 2020).

Stranger anxiety may develop around the age of 8 months. The previously very friendly and happy infant may cling and whine when approached by strangers or other people not well known. With nervous system maturation, infants begin realizing they are separate from their caregivers and others. Becoming more aware of new people and new places, the infant may perceive an interaction with a stranger as threatening and start crying, even if the parent is close by (Goldson et al., 2020; Levine, 2019). Separation anxiety may also start in the last few months of infancy, with the infant becoming quite distressed when the parent leaves. Eventually, the infant will calm down and engage with the current caregiver.

### Temperament

Temperament refers to an individual's nature. The child's inborn traits determine how they interact with the world (Child Development Institute [CDI], 2019). Normal along a continuum, temperament ranges from low or moderately active, regular, and predictable, to highly active, more intense, and less adaptable. This innate temperament affects the way the infant responds to the environment. Parents will start to learn about their infant's temperament as they notice how intensely the infant reacts with others and the environment, and how stimulated the infant becomes with interactions. Parents will eventually be able to describe how adaptable, flexible, predictable, and/or persistent their baby is (CDI, 2019).

▶ ALERT: Warning signs of possible problems with social/emotional development include:

- Does not smile at people at 3 months of age
- Infant refuses to cuddle
- Does not seem to enjoy people
- Shows no interest in peek-a-boo at 8 months of age.

## SLEEP AND REST

Newborns sleep approximately 16 to 19 hours a day, waking every 1½ to 2½ hours to feed and quickly returning to sleep. By 4 months of age, most infants are able to sleep 6 hours per night without waking, sleeping a total of 9 to 17 hours per day including daytime naps. By 6 months of age the infant is more active and alert, does not require a night feeding, and may sleep as long as 8 hours during the night with total daily sleep averaging 13 hours including daytime naps. The same is true for the remainder of infancy (Barry, 2020).

## NUTRITION

Infants experience tremendous growth in the first year as well as a great amount of development. They need diets supporting these rapid changes. The National Association of Pediatric Nurse Practitioners (NAPNAP) suggests breastfeeding as the natural and preferred method of infant feeding, with exclusive breastfeeding in the first 6 months (NAPNAP, 2019). Breast milk provides complete infant nutrition. The American Academy of Pediatrics (AAP), the American Academy of Family Physicians (AAFP), the Association of Women's Health, Obstetrics, and Neonatal Nurses (AWHONN), and the Academy of Nutrition and Dietetics (AND) make a similar recommendation (AAFP, 2015; AAP, Section on Breastfeeding 2012; AND, 2015; AWHONN, 2015). Bottle-feeding of commercially prepared formulas is chosen by some families. Infant formulas are created to imitate human milk. Standard infant formulas based on cow's milk provide 20 kcal/ounce, use lactose as a source for carbohydrates, vegetable as the source of fat, and whey or casein to provide protein (Buchanan & Marquez, 2019). Keep in mind that dietary practices are often affected by culture, including progression of infant feeding and types of food consumed. The newborn's daily caloric requirement is 105–108 kcal/kg, the 1- to 6-month-old infant's is 108 kcal/kg, and the 6- to 12-month-old requires 98 kcal/kg. The daily fluid requirement is:

- Newborn: 140 to 160 mL/kg/day
- Infant: 100 mL/kg/day for the first 10 kg and 50 mL/kg/day for the next 10 kg (Kleinman et al., 2021)

After 6 months of age, in addition to their breast milk or formula, infants usually require the nutrients available in solid foods. Successful solid food consumption best occurs when the tongue extrusion reflex is disappearing or has disappeared. In the newborn and young infant, the tongue automatically extrudes to latch on when a nipple is placed in the mouth, triggering sucking. With disappearance of this reflex around 4 to 6 months of age, the spoon may be successfully introduced (Duryea & Fleisher, 2020). The infant should also be capable of sitting up (even if supported). Additionally, the ability to swallow solid food does not become completely functional until 4 to 6 months of age, at which time the enzymes necessary for digestion and absorption of food other than breast milk and formula become available. At 6 to 8 months of age, the cup may be introduced.

▶ ALERT: Ordinary cow's milk is not recommended for the first year of life, as it is lacking in iron and does not provide the carbohydrate/fat/protein balance required by infants for optimal growth.

# COMMON DEVELOPMENTAL ISSUES

Commonly occurring developmental issues may raise concern among parents and caregivers of infants. These include spitting up, colic, and pacifiers, thumb sucking, and security items.

## SPITTING UP

All infants spit up (regurgitate small amounts of stomach contents), and many perfectly normal infants seem to spit up excessively. Spitting up after feeding may create concern in parents, although the vast majority of infants do it. Those infants who are more likely to spit up are those who do not burp well or who are overfed based on a parent-designed feeding schedule, rather than an infant on-demand schedule. When the infant is wetting at least six diapers per 24 hours and gaining weight, parents should be reassured that the spitting up is normal (AAP, 2019). Refer to chapter 18 for additional guidance related to spitting up.

## COLIC

Colic refers to a period of inconsolable crying lasting 3 hours or longer per day for 3 to 7 days per week, beginning as early as 2 weeks of age, resolving by 3 months of age, and for which there is no physical cause. The crying period most often occurs in the evening. Colic may be related to gastrointestinal or neurologic system immaturity, infant temperament, or parenting style of the mother or father. An overly anxious or overly attentive parenting style, as well as not giving the infant the attention needed, may contribute to an infant's fussing and crying (Zeifman & St. James-Roberts, 2017). By 3 months of age, infants are better able to soothe themselves and colic usually resolves. Chapter 14 provides strategies for the management of colic.

## PACIFIERS, THUMB SUCKING, AND SECURITY ITEMS

A need for nonnutritive sucking exists in all infants to a certain extent (even fetuses suck their thumbs or fingers in utero). Nonnutritive sucking is a healthy, self-comforting activity, and infants who suck their thumbs or pacifiers are better able to self-soothe. Pacifier use should stop by age 1 year, and thumb sucking should be discontinued by 4 or 5 years of age in order to void dental complications (Altmann et al., 2019). Hygiene is a concern with pacifier use, as is the increased incidence of otitis media (Goldson et al., 2020). Similarly, infants may also become attached to a security item such as a blanket, stuffed animal, or doll. Access to the attachment item gives the infant the security to self-soothe when he or she is uncomfortable. Additional information about self-soothing and security items is found in chapter 14.

## KEY POINTS

- Tremendous growth occurs during infancy, with doubling of the birthweight by 6 months of age and tripling the birthweight by 12 months of age.
- Most organ systems are immature at birth, continuing to develop and mature over the first year of life.
- Infant developmental skill acquisition is generally orderly, sequential, and predictable, progressing in a cephalocaudal and proximodistal fashion.
- Cognitive development in infancy is achieved by the infant's use of their senses, progressing to the use of motor skills to explore and master the environment.
- The infant is mastering the psychosocial task of trust, becomes increasingly social over time, and may experience stranger anxiety and separation anxiety during the latter part of infancy.
- The 12-month-old uses two or three words with meaning and is able to babble expressively.
- While breastfeeding is the preferred method for infant feeding, both breastfed and bottle-fed infants should both be fed on demand rather than on a parent-designed schedule.
- The spoon may be used to introduce solid foods at the age of 4 to 6 months, while the cup may be introduced at 6 months of age.
- Spitting up, colic, and teething occur as a part of normal development in the otherwise thriving infant and do not require medical intervention.

## REFERENCES


Academy of Nutrition and Dietetics. (2015). *Position of the Academy of Nutrition and Dietetics: Promoting and supporting breastfeeding*. https://www.eatrightpro.org/-/media/eatrightpro-files/practice/position-and-practice-papers/position-papers/promotingbreastfeeding.pdf

Altmann, T., Hill, D. L., Shelov, S. P., & Hannemann, R. E. (2019). *Caring for your baby and young child* (7th ed.). Bantam Books.

American Academy of Family Physicians. (2015). Breastfeeding policy statement. *American Family Physician, 93*(6), 368–376. https://www.aafp.org/afp/2018/0915/p368.html

American Academy of Pediatric Dentistry. (2015). *Management considerations for pediatric oral surgery and oral pathology*. https://www.aapd.org/globalassets/media/policies_guidelines/bp_oralsurgery.pdf

American Academy of Pediatrics. (2019). *Why babies spit up*. https://www.healthychildren.org/English/ages-stages/baby/feeding-nutrition/Pages/Why-Babies-Spit-Up.aspx

American Academy of Pediatrics, Section on Breastfeeding. (2012). Breastfeeding and the use of human milk—Policy statement. *Pediatrics, 129*(3), e827–e841. https://doi.org/10.1542/peds.2011-3552

Association of Women's Health, Obstetric, and Neonatal Nurses. (2015). *Breastfeeding support: Preconception care through the first year* (3rd ed.).

Barry, E. S. (2020). What is "normal" infant sleep? Why we still do not know. *Psychological Reports*. https://doi.org/10.1177/0033294120909447

Buchanan, A. O., & Marquez, M. L. (2019). Section 6, Pediatric nutrition and nutritional disorders. In K. J. Marcdante & R. M. Kliegman (Eds.), *Nelson's essentials of pediatrics* (8th ed.). Elsevier.

Centers for Disease Control and Prevention. (2020). *Developmental milestones*. http://www.cdc.gov/ncbddd/actearly/milestones/index.html

Cherry, J., Harrison, G. J., Kaplan, S. L., Steinbach, W. J., & Hotez, P. (2019). *Feigin and Cherry's textbook of pediatric infectious diseases* (8th ed.). Elsevier, Saunders.

Child Development Institute. (2019). *Temperament and your child's personality*. http://childdevelopmentinfo.com/child-development/temperament_and_your_child/

Chiocca, E. M. (2020). *Advanced pediatric assessment*. Springer Publishing Company.

Duryea, T. K., & Fleisher, D. M. (2020). Patient education: Starting solid foods during infancy (Beyond the basics). In K. J. Motil & J. E. Drutz (Eds.), *UpToDate*. Retrieved October 31, 2020, from https://www.uptodate.com/contents/starting-solid-foods-during-infancy-beyond-the-basics#H3

Erikson, E. H. (1963). *Childhood and society* (2nd ed.). New York: W. W. Norton.

Gandhi, R. P., Puranik, C. P., Wilson, A., & Chin, K. L. (2020). Chapter 17, oral medicine and dentistry. In W. W. Hay, M. J. Levin, M. J. Abzug, & M. Bunik (Eds.), *Current diagnosis & treatment: Pediatrics* (25th ed.). McGraw Hill Education.

Goldson, E., Angulo, A. S., Raz, D. M., & Reynolds, A. (2020). Chapter 3: Child development and behavior. In W. W. Hay, M. J. Levin, M. J. Abzug, & M. Bunik (Eds.), *Current diagnosis & treatment: Pediatrics* (25th ed.). McGraw Hill Education.

Karp, A. M., & Greenbaum, L. A. (2019). Chapter 32, fluids and electrolytes. In K. J. Marcdante & R. M. Kliegman (Eds.), *Nelson's essentials of pediatrics* (8th ed.). Elsevier.

Kleinman, K., McDaniel, L., & Molloy, M. (Eds.). (2021). *The Harriet Lane handbook: A manual for pediatric house officers* (22nd ed.). Elsevier.

Leigh, B. (2016). *Six states of alertness for newborns*. https://www.centreforperinatalpsychology.com.au/states-of-alertness

Levine, D. A. (2019). Section 2, growth and development. In K. J. Marcdante & R. M. Kliegman (Eds.), *Nelson's essentials of pediatrics* (8th ed.). Elsevier.

Lowry, L. (2016). *Bilingualism in young children: Separating fact from fiction*. http://www.hanen.org/helpful-info/articles/bilingualism-in-young-children--separating-fact-fr.aspx

Maqbool, A., & Liacouras, C. A. (2016). Chapter 354: Normal development, structure, and function of the stomach and intestines. In R. M. Kliegman, J. W. St. Geme, N. J. Blum, S. S. Shah, R. C. Tasker, K. M. Wilson, & R. E. Behrman (Eds.), *Nelson textbook of pediatrics* (21st ed.). Elsevier.

National Association of Pediatric Nurse Practitioners. (2019). NAPNAP position statement on breastfeeding. *Journal of Pediatric Health Care, 33*(1), A11–A15. https://doi.org/10.1016/j.pedhc.2018.08.011

Piaget, J. (1969). *The theory of stages in cognitive development*. McGraw-Hill.

Powers, J. M., & Mahoney, M. H. (2020). Iron deficiency in infants and children <12 years: Screening, prevention, clinical manifestations, and diagnosis. In K. J. Motil, J. E. Drutz, & S. A. Abrams (Eds.), *UpToDate*. Retrieved October 27, 2020, from https://www.uptodate.com/contents/iron-deficiency-in-infants-and-children-less-than12-years-screening-prevention-clinical-manifestations-and-diagnosis

Sinha, S. K. (2019). *Short stature*. http://emedicine.medscape.com/article/924411-overview

Swanson, W. S., & Cohen, M. (2020). *The scoop on poop: What's normal, what's not*. http://www.parents.com/baby/diapers/dirty/baby-bowel-movement/?page=2

Wang, M., McKinney, C., Nuss, R., & Ambruso, D. R. (2020). Chapter 30, hematologic disorders. In W. W. Hay, M. J. Levin, M. J. Abzug, & M. Bunik (Eds.), *Current diagnosis & treatment: Pediatrics* (25th ed.). McGraw Hill Education.

Zeifman, D. M., & St. James-Roberts, I. (2017). Parenting the crying infant. *Current Opinion in Psychology, 15*, 149–154. https://doi.org/10.1016/j.copsyc.2017.02.009

# Growth and Development During Toddlerhood

Theresa Kyle

## Student Learning Outcomes

**Upon completion of this chapter the reader should be able to:**

1. Examine physical developmental changes and growth occurring during toddlerhood.
2. Differentiate gross motor, fine motor, and language milestones expected during toddlerhood.
3. Distinguish expected psychosocial, cognitive, and moral development changes for various ages throughout toddlerhood.
4. Describe appropriate sleep, rest, and nutrition for toddlers.
5. Discuss typical developmental issues that occur during toddlerhood.

## INTRODUCTION

Toddlerhood includes the second 2 years of life, from age 1 year to age 3 years. During this time, significant advancement in growth and development occurs. Toddlerhood is often a challenging time for parents. The toddler constantly tests their environment and their own power by struggling with holding on and letting go. Toddlers learn that parents are reliable and predictable, then learn that their own behavior may also have a reliable, predictable effect on others. Toddlers will take risks and make many mistakes. As compared with the time of intense growth and development during infancy, both physical growth and acquisition of new motor skills slow somewhat during the toddler years. During toddlerhood, continued cognitive growth, acquisition of appropriate language skills, and refinement of motor skills are of prime importance. These years are active and trying years; the challenge is to encourage independence and autonomy while keeping the curious toddler safe.

The content in this chapter maps to the following areas on the Pediatric Nursing Certification Board (PNCB) Pediatric Nurse Practitioner—Primary Care certification examination:

CONTENT AREAS:

**I. Health Promotion and Maintenance**

**A. Partner with patients/caregivers to support growth and development from infancy to young adulthood**

**B. Provide patients/caregivers with age/developmentally appropriate anticipatory guidance**

**F. Counsel about age-appropriate social, behavioral, and mental health concerns**

**II. Assessment and Diagnosis**

**A. Growth and Development**

1. Evaluate and interpret growth parameters

**IV. Professional Role Responsibilities**

**A. Leadership and Evidence-based Practice**

1. Serve as a clinical resource for other health care professionals
2. Critically evaluate and synthesize research and apply findings to clinical practice

## CULTURAL INFLUENCES

The toddler's ability to grow adequately may be directly influenced by poverty or homelessness because resources for the purchase and preparation of appropriate food may be lacking. Those situations may also lead to lack of availability of appropriate, safe toys. The child's diet and ability to ingest appropriate nutrients continue to be affected by the family's food customs. Additionally, the toddler's development may be influenced by the individual family's value system. Some families highly value independence and encourage the toddler to walk everywhere on his or her own rather than carrying the child. Other families may delay weaning or continue to feed the child baby food or puréed food for a longer period, as they desire for their child to remain a baby longer. Culture also has an impact on emotional development. Some families discourage crying in boys beginning at a very young age and encourage them to "be a man" or to "act like a big boy." The toddler's self-concept may be harmed if the toddler is ridiculed for crying at this age. A balance must be achieved when educating families about normal growth and development while continuing to support and value the family's cultural practices (Martorell, 2019).

**PRO TIP** As grandparents are increasingly taking on the role of primary caregivers for their grandchildren, be alert to the possibility of increased stress on the older caregiver.

# GROWTH

After the extremely rapid growth experienced during infancy, growth during the toddler period slows somewhat in velocity, although it does increase steadily. Gains in weight and length/height tend occur in spurts during toddlerhood, rather than steadily. The average toddler gains 1.36 to 2.27 kg (3–5 lb) per year. Reaching about half of their adult height by 2 years of age, the toddler's length/height increases by an average of 7.62 cm (3 inches) per year. The toddler's head circumference increases about 2.54 cm (1 inch) in the second year of life, then increases an average of 1.27 cm (a half inch) per year until age 5. The anterior fontanel closes by the time the toddler is 18 months old. Closer to age 3 years, the toddler's head size becomes more proportional to the rest of the body (Carter & Feigelman, 2020a, 2020b; Goldson et al., 2020).

# PHYSICAL CHANGES

The toddler's organ systems continue to grow and mature in their functioning, although these changes are not as pronounced as the changes that occur during infancy. The respiratory, cardiovascular, and musculoskeletal systems continue to undergo changes, and important changes in function occur within the neurologic, gastrointestinal, and genitourinary systems.

## RESPIRATORY AND CARDIOVASCULAR SYSTEMS

The respiratory structures continue to grow and mature throughout toddlerhood, with the trachea and lower airways continuing to grow but remaining small as compared with the airways of the adult. While the alveoli continue to increase in number, they do not reach the adult number until about 7 years of age. The tongue remains relatively large in comparison with the size of the mouth, as do the tonsils. The adenoids are also somewhat relatively large, and the eustachian tubes remain short and straight, rather than downward angled as in later childhood. During toddlerhood, the blood vessels remain close to the skin surface and are easily compressed when palpated. The heart rate continues to decrease while the blood pressure increases in toddlerhood.

## NEUROLOGIC SYSTEM

Increases in head circumference reflect growth in the brain, which reaches about 90% of its adult size by 2 years of age (Carter & Feigelman, 2020b; Zero to Three, 2020). The brain and spinal cord continue to myelinate in a process that is complete around 24 months of age. With completed myelination comes the ability to exercise sphincter control (important for bowel and bladder mastery), as well as improved coordination and equilibrium. Integration of the primitive reflexes occurs in infancy, allowing for the emergence of the protective reflexes near the end of infancy or early in toddlerhood. As the child starts to toddle, the forward or downward parachute reflex is particularly helpful while numerous falls occur. Continued progression of cognitive development is evidenced in the rapid increase in language skills during the toddler period.

## GASTROINTESTINAL SYSTEM

The toddler consumes three regular meals per day as the stomach continues to increase in size, with pepsin production maturing by 2 years of age. While the small intestine continues to grow in length, it does not reach the maximum length of 2 to 3 meters until adulthood (Maqbool & Liacouras, 2020). Frequency of stool passage decreases in toddlerhood to one or more per day. The toddler is able to gain control over bowel elimination by the end of this period. Depending on the toddler's diet, the color of the stool may change (brown, green-yellow, or orange). The toddler's intestines remain somewhat immature, and will often pass whole pieces of difficult-to-digest food such as corn.

## GENITOURINARY SYSTEM

During toddlerhood the bladder capacity increases, allowing the toddler to retain urine for increased periods of times and gain control over urinary elimination by the end of the toddler period. Urine output is about 1 mL/kg/hour, and bladder and kidney function reach adult levels by 16 to 24 months of age. The urethra remains short in both the male and female toddler, making them more susceptible to urinary tract infections compared with adults.

## MUSCULOSKELETAL SYSTEM

The toddler's bones increase in length and the muscles mature and become stronger. In early toddlerhood, the abdominal musculature remains weak, resulting in the appearance of a swayback with a potbelly. By about 3 years of age, as the abdominal musculature strengthens, the abdomen becomes flatter in appearance.

## SENSORY DEVELOPMENT

Toddler visual acuity continues to progress and should be 20/50 to 20/40 in both eyes. Depth perception also continues to mature. Hearing is fully developed at birth. As the sense of smell matures, toddlers may comment if they do not care for the way something smells. Toddlers may exhibit preferences for certain flavors of foods, although taste discrimination is not completely developed. Thus, the toddler is more likely to try a new food if its smell or appearance is familiar. As noted earlier, the toddler is at risk of accidental ingestion due to the lack of complete taste discrimination. To thoroughly explore the world around them, toddlers use all of their senses. They examine new items by looking at them, feeling them, smelling them, shaking them to hear what sound they make, and placing them in their mouths.

# DEVELOPMENTAL MILESTONES

Mastery over many tasks is achieved during toddlerhood. As the toddler masters a new task, they gain confidence to conquer the next challenge. The toddler's sense of self-esteem continues to grow as each new skill is mastered. Some toddlers are eager to face challenges and will likely develop more quickly than toddlers who are more reluctant. The senses of hearing, sight, and touch are useful in helping to coordinate gross and fine motor movement. Toddlers use language to organize their world and make sense of it. The use of thoughtfully planned language can provide behavior guidance and contribute to the avoidance of power struggles during the toddler period.

## MOTOR SKILL DEVELOPMENT

During toddlerhood the child refines some motor skills and gains many other new ones. The toddler's large muscle groups are strengthened as gross motor skills are mastered and then used repeatedly. While the toddler will progress from walking to running, climbing, and jumping, initially their gait is not smooth. The new walker displays the classic toddler gait with legs planted widely apart, toes pointed forward, and apparent swaying from side to side while moving forward. Speeding along and pitching forward, the toddler appears ready to topple over at any moment (Figure 8.1). The toddler falls often and uses outstretched arms to catch themselves (parachute reflex). After about 6 months of practice walking, the toddler's gait is smoother, feet are closer together, and by 3 years of age, the toddler walks in a heel-to-toe fashion similar to that of adults. The toddler also accomplishes pushing or pulling a toy, throwing a ball, and pedaling a tricycle. Physical actions such as running, jumping, and hitting are often used by toddlers to express their emotions because they are only just beginning to learn language.

Fine motor skills progress rapidly from simply holding and pinching to the abilities of managing utensils, holding a crayon, stringing a bead, and using

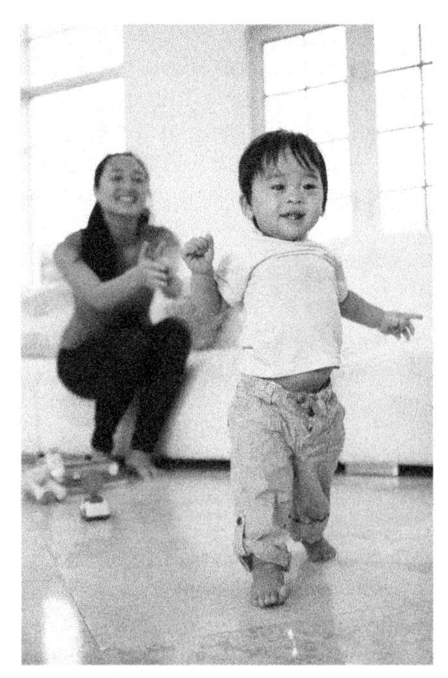

FIGURE 8.1 Toddler gait.

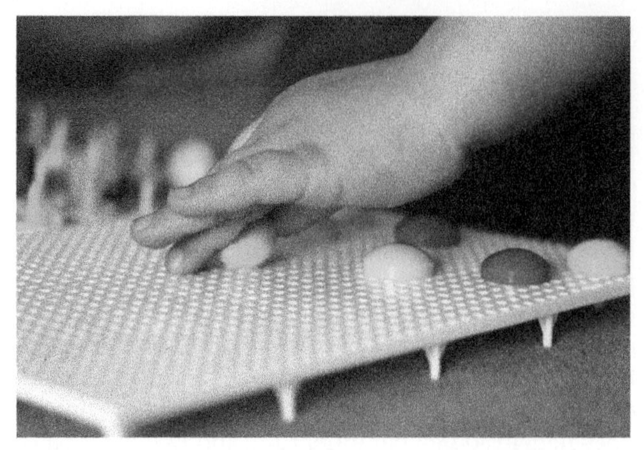

FIGURE 8.2 Hand-eye coordination is needed for inserting pegs into boards.

a computer. All of these skills require control and agility, and fine motor skills become refined, and some perfected, during toddlerhood. Adequate vision and the development of eye-hand coordination are necessary for this refinement (see Figure 8.2). As the curious toddler increases mobility and the ability manipulate items, they are better able to explore and learn from their environment. Refer to Table 8.1 for the average ages at which gross and fine motor skills are attained during toddlerhood.

▶ ALERT: Warning signs indicating problems with motor development include:

- After independent walking for several months: persistent tiptoe walking, failure to develop a mature walking pattern
- 18 months: Not walking
- 2 years: Cannot push a toy with wheels
- 3 years: difficulty with stairs, frequent falling, cannot build tower of more than four blocks, difficulty manipulating small objects, cannot copy a circle

## LANGUAGE AND COMMUNICATION

Language acquisition is a dynamic and complex process, occurring rapidly during the toddler years. The types of language the child is exposed to, as well as age and social interactions, influence language development. Typically, receptive language (the ability to understand what is being said or asked) is far more advanced than expressive language (the ability to communicate one's desires and feelings; Carter & Feigelman, 2020b; Goldson et al., 2020). In toddlers younger than 30 months of age, a common occurrence is echolalia, the repetition of words and phrases without understanding. Young children exposed to more than one language may experience simultaneous acquisition of both languages. In potentially bilingual children, the first word may be slightly delayed as compared with single-language speakers, but still occurs within the normal range (Lowry, 2016). Language mixing in potentially bilingual children may make it more difficult for the provider to identify a language delay. Early identification and referral of any toddler with a potential speech delay is critical, as early intervention may increase the child's potential to acquire age-appropriate receptive and expressive language skills. Table 8.2 provides an overview of receptive and expressive language development in the toddler.

▶ ALERT: Warning signs indicating a problem in language development include:

- 18 months: not speaking 15 words, does not understand function of common household items
- 2 years: does not use two-word sentences, imitate actions, or follow basic instructions
- 3 years: cannot communicate in short phrases, presence of echolalia, does not understand simple instructions, unclear speech, persistent drooling

**TABLE 8.1 Motor Skill Development in Toddlerhood**

| Age | Gross Motor Skills | Fine Motor Skills |
|---|---|---|
| **12–15 months** | Walks independently | Feeds self finger foods<br>Uses index finger to point |
| **18 months** | Pulls toys while walking<br>Climbs stairs with assistance | Masters reaching, grasping, and releasing: stacks blocks, puts things in slots<br>Removes shoes and socks<br>Stacks four cubes<br>Turns book pages (singly with board book, multiple if paper) |
| **24 months** | Can stand on tiptoe<br>Carries several toys, or a large toy while walking<br>Climbs onto and down from furniture without assistance<br>Kicks ball<br>Runs | Builds tower of six or seven cubes<br>Imitates circular and vertical strokes<br>Puts round pegs into holes<br>Right- or left-handed<br>Scribbles and paints<br>Starting to turn knobs |
| **36 months** | Bends over easily without falling<br>Climbs well<br>Pedals tricycle<br>Runs easily<br>Walks up and down stairs with alternate feet | Builds tower of nine or ten cubes<br>Copies circle<br>Holds a pencil in writing position<br>Screws/unscrews lids, nuts, bolts<br>Turns book pages one at a time<br>Undresses self |

*Sources*: Data from Altmann, T., Hill, D. L., Shelov, S. P., & Hannemann, R. E. (2019). *Caring for your baby and young child: Birth to 5.* Bantam Books; Carter, R. G., & Feigelman, S. (2020a). The preschool years. In R. M. Kliegman, J. W. St. Geme III, N. J. Blum, S. S. Shah, R. C. Tasker, K. M. Wilson, & R. E. Behrman (Eds.), *Nelson textbook of pediatrics* (21st ed., Chapter 24). Elsevier; Carter, R. G., & Feigelman, S. (2020b). The second year. In R. M. Kliegman, J. W. St. Geme III, N. J. Blum, S. S. Shah, R. C. Tasker, K. M. Wilson, & R. E. Behrman (Eds.), *Nelson textbook of pediatrics* (21st ed., Chapter 23). Elsevier; Centers for Disease Control and Prevention. (2020). *Developmental milestones.* http://www.cdc.gov/ncbddd/actearly/milestones/index.html; Goldson, E., Angulo, A. S., Raz, D. M., & Reynolds, A. (2020). Child development and behavior. In W. W. Hay, M. J. Levin, M. J. Abzug, & M. Bunik (Eds.), *Current diagnosis & treatment: Pediatrics* (25th ed., Chapter 3). McGraw-Hill Education; Levine, D. A. (2019). Growth and development. In K. J. Marcdante & R. M. Kliegman (Eds.), *Nelson's essentials of pediatrics* (8th ed., Section 2). Elsevier.

## COGNITIVE DEVELOPMENT

Toddlers move through the last two substages of the first stage of cognitive development, the sensorimotor stage, between 12 and 24 months of age (Piaget, 1969). Young toddlers engage in tertiary circular reactions, progressing to mental combinations. This means that, rather than just repeating a behavior, the toddler experiments with a behavior to determine what happens. Toddlers are capable of using symbols allowing for imitation by 24 months of age. As cognitive abilities increase, toddlers display delayed imitation (e.g., imitating a household task that they observed a parent doing several days ago).

The second stage of cognitive development is the preoperational stage, occurring in children between ages 2 and 7 years (Piaget, 1969). Symbolic thought becomes more sophisticated during this stage; the older toddler's thinking is far more advanced than that of the infant or young toddler, who views the world as a series of objects. During the preoperational stage, the toddler understands that objects have characteristics making them unique from one another (large or small, a particular color or shape, having a unique texture). It is in this stage that cognitive thought moves beyond the connection of sensory information and physical action: words and images allow the toddler to begin development of symbolic thought by providing a label for the objects' characteristics (Piaget, 1969).

ALERT: Be alert to the mental status of a toddler's mother; maternal depression is a risk factor for poor cognitive development, as the depressed mother may not be as sensitive to their child (Viguera, 2020).

Symbols are also used in dramatic play. Initially, toddlers imitate life with appropriate toy objects, and then become able to substitute objects in their play. A play broom may be used for sweeping, but then later it can be ridden like a horse. Toddlers also may attribute human feelings and characteristics to objects (animism; Martorell, 2019). See Table 8.3 for examples of cognitive development in toddlerhood.

TABLE 8.2 **Communication and Language Development in Toddlers**

| Age | Receptive Language | Expressive Language |
|---|---|---|
| **12 months** | Follows a one-step command accompanied by gesture<br>Understands common words independent of context | Communicates desires with word and gesture combinations<br>First word with meaning<br>Imitates or uses gestures such as waving goodbye<br>Uses a finger to point to things<br>Vocal imitation |
| **15 months** | Follows a one-step command without gesture<br>Looks at adult when communicating<br>Understands 100–150 words | Babbles in what sound like sentences<br>Repeats words that he or she hears |
| **18 months** | Comprehends 200 words<br>Sometimes answers the question, "What's this?"<br>Understands the word "no" | Uses at least 5–20 words<br>Uses names of familiar object |
| **24 months** | Begins to use "my" or "mine"<br>Enjoys listening to simple stories<br>Names a variety of objects in the environment<br>Points to named body parts<br>Points to pictures in books | Asks questions ("what that?")<br>Repeats overheard words<br>Sentences of two or three words ("me up," "want cookie" [telegraphic speech])<br>Two-thirds of what child says should be understandable<br>Uses simple phrases<br>Uses descriptive words (hungry, hot)<br>Vocabulary of 40–50 words |
| **30 months** | Follows a series of two independent commands | Vocabulary of 150–300 words |
| **36 months** | May follow a three-part command<br>Participates in short conversations<br>Understands most sentences<br>Understands physical relationships (on, in, under) | Asks "why?" and "what?" (a lot)<br>Can say name, age, and gender<br>Speech usually understood by those who know the child, about half understood by those outside family<br>Talks about something that happened in the past<br>Three- to four-word sentences<br>Uses pronouns and plurals<br>Vocabulary of 1,000 words |

*Sources*: Data from Altmann, T., Hill, D. L., Shelov, S. P., & Hannemann, R. E. (2019). *Caring for you baby and young child: Birth to 5*. Bantam Books; Carter, R. G., & Feigelman, S. (2020a). The preschool years. In R. M. Kliegman, J. W. St. Geme III, N. J. Blum, S. S. Shah, R. C. Tasker, K. M. Wilson, & R. E. Behrman (Eds.), *Nelson textbook of pediatrics* (21st ed., Chapter 24). Elsevier; Carter, R. G., & Feigelman, S. (2020b). The second year. In R. M. Kliegman, J. W. St. Geme III, N. J. Blum, S. S. Shah, R. C. Tasker, K. M. Wilson, & R. E. Behrman (Eds.), *Nelson textbook of pediatrics* (21st ed., Chapter 23). Elsevier; Centers for Disease Control and Prevention. (2020). *Developmental milestones*. http://www.cdc.gov/ncbddd/actearly/milestones/index.html; Goldson, E., Angulo, A. S., Raz, D. M., & Reynolds, A. (2020). Child development and behavior. In W. W. Hay, M. J. Levin, M. J. Abzug, & M. Bunik (Eds.), *Current diagnosis & treatment: Pediatrics* (25th ed., Chapter 3). McGraw-Hill Education; Levine, D. A. (2019). Growth and development. In K. J. Marcdante & R. M. Kliegman (Eds.), *Nelson's essentials of pediatrics* (8th ed., Section 2). Elsevier.

## SOCIAL AND EMOTIONAL DEVELOPMENT

Toddlerhood is a time of exerting independence, with the chief psychosocial task being achieving a sense of autonomy versus shame and doubt. Having developed a sense of trust in infancy, the toddler is ready to abandon dependence and to assert their sense of control (Erikson, 1963). During toddlerhood the child separates from the parent/caregiver, spontaneously shows affection, and imitates adults and playmates. Although able to withstand delayed gratification and becoming increasingly enthusiastic about playmates, the toddler cannot take turns in games until age 3 years.

The toddler struggles for self-mastery, learning to do for self what others have been doing them. This struggle results in ambivalence and emotional lability. The toddler experiences rapid changes from happy and smiling, to crying and screaming. Negativism abounds during this period and as an exertion of independence, the toddler's favorite response becomes "no," whether or not the toddler means no or yes. Although

TABLE 8.3 **Cognitive Development in Toddlerhood**

| Stage/Substage | Activities |
|---|---|
| Sensorimotor<br>Substage 5: tertiary circular reactions<br>Age: 12–18 months | Uses ALL senses to explore environment<br>Differentiates self from objects<br>Increased object permanence (knows that objects that are out of sight still exist [e.g., cookies in the cabinet])<br>Places items in and out of containers |
| Sensorimotor<br>Substage 6: Mental combinations<br>Age: 18–24 months | Imitation is more symbolic<br>Imitates domestic chores (domestic mimicry)<br>Starting to think before acting<br>Understands requests and is capable of following simple directions |
| Preoperational<br>Age: 2–7 years | Has a sense of ownership (my, mine)<br>Uses mental trial and error rather than physical<br>Makes mechanical toys work<br>Plays make-believe with dolls, animals, and people<br>Increased use of language for mental representation<br>Time, space, and causality understanding is increasing<br>Understands concept of "two"<br>Starting to make connections between an experience in the past and a new one that is currently occurring<br>Sorts objects by shape and color<br>Completes puzzles with four pieces |

*Sources*: Data from Altmann, T., Hill, D. L., Shelov, S. P., & Hannemann, R. E. (2019). *Caring for your baby and young child: Birth to 5*. Bantam Books; Goldson, E., Angulo, A. S., Raz, D. M., & Reynolds, A. (2020). Child development and behavior. In W. W. Hay, M. J. Levin, M. J. Abzug, & M. Bunik (Eds.), *Current diagnosis & treatment: Pediatrics* (25th ed., Chapter 3). McGraw-Hill Education; Piaget, J. (1969). *The theory of stages in cognitive development*. McGraw-Hill.

negativism is a normal part of healthy toddler development, it can become frustrating for parents.

Toddler emotional development focuses on separation and individuation (Martorell, 2019). While the toddler is seeing themselves as separate from the parent or primary caregiver (separation), they are also forming a sense of self and learning to exert control over their environment (individuation). Egocentrism, or focus on self, is displayed by the toddler because they need to feel in control of their world, further contributing to emotional lability (Lieberman, 2018). While identifying the boundaries between themselves and the parent or primary caregiver, the toddler is learning to negotiate a balance between independence and attachment, initially relying on the parents' signals and communication to initiate appropriate behavior or inhibit undesirable behavior. The toddler has a difficult time choosing between sets of behaviors as they occur in different situations, resulting in frequent power struggles. Parents should intentionally and thoughtfully develop the rituals and routines providing stability and security for the toddler (Carter & Feigelman, 2020b). Many toddlers rely on a security item such as blanket, doll, or stuffed animal to comfort themselves in stressful situations. This ability to self-soothe is a function of autonomy.

During the toddler period, the child also begins to learn about gender differences, observing the differences between male and female body parts if exposed to them. The toddler may question parents about these body differences and may begin to explore their own genitals. Toddlers are also beginning to understand and mimic social gender differences. Their observations about gender-specific behaviors are dependent upon their exposure to behaviors.

## SEPARATION ANXIETY

Toddlers become increasingly skilled at mobility, realizing that if they have the capability to leave, then so does the parent. Continued conflicts over closeness versus exploration and increasing development of self-awareness may lead to re-emergence of separation anxiety around the ages of 18 to 24 months (Lieberman, 2018). Increased distress at separation from the parent occurs and power struggles may escalate. Having a predictable routine with appropriate limit setting helps the toddler feel more secure and safe during this period. Separation anxiety again eases from the age of 24 to 36 months. Object constancy is present in the older toddler. The child has an internal representation of the parent or caregiver so is better able to tolerate separation, knowing that a reunion will occur.

### TEMPERAMENT

The biologic basis for personality is temperament, that emotional and motivational core around which the personality develops over time (Child Development Institute, 2019). Temperament affects how the toddler responds to and interacts with the environment. The easygoing toddler is more adaptable and accepting of changes in routine than other toddlers. The easygoing toddler usually demonstrates predictable and regular behaviors, and sleeps and eats well. However, temper tantrums still occur as the toddler expresses frustration. This is in contrast with the difficult toddler, who is more likely to have intense reactions, whether negative or positive, with more frequent and intense temper tantrums, and is the most active of the three temperament types. Without structure and routine for security, the child feels insecure and as a result is more likely to behave inappropriately. To avoid temper tantrums in the difficult toddler, suggest to the parent to be especially diligent about maintaining structure and routine, as well as avoiding tantrum triggers such as fatigue and hunger. The difficult toddler is also the most active of the three temperament types. The slow-to-warm-up toddler is a bit of a loner, may be very shy, and may experience more difficulty with separation anxiety. Parents will want to exercise additional patience with new activities, as extra time may be needed by this child. This toddler is very watchful, sometimes withdrawn, may take longer to mature, yet not as upset by changes in routine because they are more passive in nature (Lieberman, 2018).

▶ ALERT: Warning signs of possible problems with social/emotional development include, at age 3, extreme difficulty separating from the parent or caregiver, not engaging in make-believe play, and little interest in other children.

## SLEEP AND REST

The daily sleep requirement for toddlers varies by age:

- 18-month-old—13.5 hours
- 24-month-old—13 hours
- 3-year-old—12 hours (Carter & Feigelman, 2020a, 2020b).

Typically, the toddler is capable of sleeping through the night and takes one daytime nap. Around 3 years of age, most children discontinue daytime napping. When the toddler is physically capable of climbing over the rails of the crib, it becomes unsafe. At that time, the toddler must make the transition to a youth or toddler bed, or even a full-size bed. Some families practice bedsharing; the children sleep in the parents' bed. Some professionals believe that bedsharing may interfere with the toddler's struggle for independence, yet this theory has not been shown to be true. It is important to support the family's choice for sleep arrangements unless bedsharing becomes unsafe, either physically or psychologically (SafeBedSharing, 2020). Refer to http://www.safebedsharing.org for bed-sharing safety guidelines.

## NUTRITION

Breastfeeding may continue during the toddler years, but for adequate growth the toddler requires nutritients found in food as well. The toddler should be weaned from the bottle in early toddlerhood if not done so already. Toddlers are developmentally capable of drinking from the cup, chewing soft foods in early toddlerhood, and eating firmer foods as they get a little older. Developmentally they may finger feed and utilize utensils to eat. The expected weight gain in toddlerhood is 35 g/day for boys age 12 to 24 months, 30 g/day for girls age 12 to 24 months, 28 g/day for boys age 24 to 36 months, and 25 g/day for girls age 24 to 36 months. While fat accounts for about 40% of weight gain in infants, it accounts for only 3% of weight gain in the 2- to 3-year-old. Protein contributes to 11% of weight gain in infants, whereas by 24 months of age it is contributing to 21% of weight gain. Nutrient requirements for age may be found in Table 8.4.

## COMMON DEVELOPMENTAL ISSUES

Commonly occurring developmental issues may raise concern among parents and caregivers of toddlers. These include temper tantrums and aggressive behaviors.

### TEMPER TANTRUMS AND AGGRESSIVE BEHAVIORS

Even the most easygoing of infants may lose their temper frequently during the toddler period. Toddlers

TABLE 8.4 **Nutrient Requirements in Toddlerhood**

| Nutitional Component | 12 to 24 months | 24 to 36 months |
|---|---|---|
| **Energy requirements** | 90 kcal/kg/day | 90 kcal/kg/day |
| **Protein** (35% being from essential amino acids) | 1.2 g/kg/day | 1.1 g/kg/day |
| **Fat** (no more than 10% from saturated fat) | Up to 35% of calories per day | |
| **Carbohydrates** (no more the 10% as simple sugar) | 50% to 60% of calories per day | 45% to 65% of calories per day |
| **Calcium** | 500 mg/day | |
| **Iron** | 7 mg/day | |

*Sources*: Data from Buchanan, A. O., & Marquez, M. L. (2019). Pediatric nutrition and nutritional disorders. In K. J. Marcdante & R. M. Kliegman (Eds.), *Nelson's essentials of pediatrics* (8th ed., Section 6). Elsevier; Haemer, M. A., Diab, L. K., Primak, L. E., & Krebs, N. F. (2020). Normal childhood nutrition & its disorders. In W. W. Hay, M. J. Levin, M. J. Abzug, & M. Bunik (Eds.), *Current diagnosis & treatment: Pediatrics* (25th ed., Chapter 11). McGraw-Hill Education.

with more intense temperaments may have more temper tantrums. Toddlers experience frustration with their continued efforts at learning new things and their inability to expressively communicate their desires. Temper tantrums are a natural result of that. Toddlers do not behave badly intentionally; they simply need to mature, master new skills over time, and develop the cognitive capability to understand the rules. Negative behavior and temper tantrums are promoted when fatigue, hunger, or stress limit the toddler's coping abilities. Because toddlers are only just beginning to learn how to verbalize feelings and desires, they tend to commit alternative actions and aggressive behaviors. Temper tantrums vary from simple screaming and crying to a full-scale episode with the toddler throwing themselves on the floor kicking, pounding, screaming, and possibly breath-holding. Toddlers also typically display aggressive behaviors by grabbing other children's toys, or even pushing, hitting, or biting another child (Altmann et al., 2019; Brazelton & Sparrow, 2015).

## KEY POINTS

- Growth slows during toddlerhood as compared with infancy, while the toddler's organ systems are continuing to mature.
- Visual acuity continues to progress and reaches at least 20/50 by the end of the toddler period.
- During toddlerhood, cognitive development continues to develop through exploration with the senses and progressing motor skills, transitioning to becoming preoperational in nature.
- Social development for the toddler is focused on becoming independent and attaining a sense of autonomy as the toddler experiences separation and individuation.
- For the toddler, refinement of gross motor skills is the focus after achieving the ability to walk. Fine motor skills are marked by use of utensils and the improved ability to manipulate toys.
- The 12-month-old has limited expressive language capabilities and advances to a vocabulary of 900 words by age 3 years.
- As toddlers experience frustration while learning about their environment and struggling with independence, aggressive behaviors, temper tantrums, and negativism occur.

## REFERENCES


Altmann, T., Hill, D. L., Shelov, S. P., & Hannemann, R. E. (2019). *Caring for your baby and young child: Birth to 5*. Bantam Books.

Brazelton, T. B., & Sparrow, J. (2015). *Discipline: The Brazelton way* (2nd ed.). Capo Press.

Buchanan, A. O., & Marquez, M. L. (2019). Pediatric nutrition and nutritional disorders. In K. J. Marcdante & R. M. Kliegman (Eds.), *Nelson's essentials of pediatrics* (8th ed., Section 6). Elsevier.

Carter, R. G., & Feigelman, S. (2020a). The preschool years. In R. M. Kliegman, J. W. St. Geme III, N. J. Blum, S. S. Shah, R. C. Tasker, K. M. Wilson, & R. E. Behrman (Eds.), *Nelson textbook of pediatrics* (21st ed., Chapter 24). Elsevier.

Carter, R. G., & Feigelman, S. (2020b). The second year. In R. M. Kliegman, J. W. St. Geme III, N. J. Blum, S. S. Shah, R. C. Tasker, K. M. Wilson, & R. E. Behrman (Eds.), *Nelson textbook of pediatrics* (21st ed., Chapter 23). Elsevier.

Centers for Disease Control and Prevention. (2020). *Developmental milestones*. http://www.cdc.gov/ncbddd/actearly/milestones/index.html

Child Development Institute. (2019). *Temperament and your child's personality*. http://childdevelopmentinfo.com/child-development/temperament_and_your_child/

Erikson, E. H. (1963). *Childhood and society* (2nd ed.). W. W. Norton.

Goldson, E., Angulo, A. S., Raz, D. M., & Reynolds, A. (2020). Child development and behavior. In W. W. Hay, M. J. Levin, M. J. Abzug, & M. Bunik (Eds.), *Current diagnosis & treatment: Pediatrics* (25th ed., Chapter 3). McGraw-Hill Education.

Haemer, M. A., Diab, L. K., Primak, L. E., & Krebs, N. F. (2020). Normal childhood nutrition & its disorders. In W. W. Hay, M. J. Levin, M. J. Abzug, & M. Bunik (Eds.), *Current diagnosis & treatment: Pediatrics* (25th ed., Chapter 11). McGraw-Hill Education.

Levine, D. A. (2019). Growth and development. In K. J. Marcdante & R. M. Kliegman (Eds.), *Nelson's essentials of pediatrics* (8th ed., Section 2). Elsevier.

Lieberman, A. (2018). *The emotional life of a toddler.* Simon & Schuster.

Lowry, L. (2016). *Bilingualism in young children: Separating fact from fiction.* http://www.hanen.org/helpful-info/articles/bilingualism-in-young-children--separating-fact-fr.aspx

Maqbool, A., & Liacouras, C. A. (2020). Normal development, structure, and function of the stomach and intestines. In R. M. Kliegman, J. W. St. Geme III, N. J. Blum, S. S. Shah, R. C. Tasker, K. M. Wilson, & R. E. Behrman (Eds.), *Nelson textbook of pediatrics* (21st ed., Chapter 354). Elsevier.

Martorell, G. (2019). *Life: The essentials of human development.* McGraw-Hill.

Piaget, J. (1969). *The theory of stages in cognitive development.* McGraw-Hill.

SafeBedSharing. (2020). *Bed-sharing or co-sleeping.* http://www.safebedsharing.org

Viguera, A. (2020). Postpartum depression: Risks of abnormal child development. *In P. P. Roy-Byrne & C. J. Lockwood (Eds.), UpToDate.* Retrieved November 12, 2020, from https://www.uptodate.com/contents/postpartum-depression-risks-of-abnormal-child-development

Zero to Three. (2020). *Frequently asked questions about brain development.* http://main.zerotothree.org/site/PageServer?pagename=ter_key_brainFAQ

# Growth and Development During the Preschool Years

Theresa Kyle

## Student Learning Outcomes

Upon completion of this chapter the reader should be able to:

1. Examine physical developmental changes and growth occurring during the preschool years.
2. Differentiate gross motor, fine motor, and language milestones expected during the preschool years.
3. Distinguish expected psychosocial, cognitive, and moral development changes for various ages throughout the preschool years.
4. Describe appropriate sleep, rest, and nutrition for preschoolers.
5. Discuss typical developmental issues that occur during the preschool years.

## INTRODUCTION

The preschool period is the time between ages 3 and 6 years. Although physical growth continues much more slowly as compared with the toddler and infant years, advances in cognitive, language, and psychosocial development are substantial during the preschool years. During this time, mastering and perfecting many tasks begun during toddlerhood occur. With a longer attention span and toleration of separation from parents, the preschool child continues learning skills leading to later success during the school-age years. Most children enter elementary school by the end of the preschool period, so preparation for school success is ongoing during this time.

The content in this chapter maps to the following areas on the Pediatric Nursing Certification Board (PNCB) Pediatric Nurse Practitioner—Primary Care certification examination:

CONTENT AREAS:

**I. Health Promotion and Maintenance**

**A. Partner with patients/caregivers to support growth and development from infancy to young adulthood**

**B. Provide patients/caregivers with age/developmentally appropriate anticipatory guidance**

**F. Counsel about age-appropriate social, behavioral, and mental health concerns**

**II. Assessment and Diagnosis**

**A. Growth and Development**

1. Evaluate and interpret growth parameters

**IV. Professional Role Responsibilities**

**A. Leadership and Evidence-based Practice**

1. Serve as a clinical resource for other health care professionals
2. Critically evaluate and synthesize research and apply findings to clinical practice

## GROWTH

The healthy preschooler has an upright posture and appears more slender than the toddler. Growing 6.5 to 7.8 cm (2.5–3 inches) per year, the average preschool child is 96.2 cm (37 inches) tall at 3 years of age, 103.7 cm (40.5 inches) tall at 4 years of age, and 118.5 cm (43 inches) tall when 5 years old. On average, the preschool child gains about 2.3 kg (4–5 lb) per year during this time (Carter & Feigelman, 2020). The average

3-year-old weighs about 14.5 kg (32 lb), and by age 5, the average child's weight is 18.6 kg (41 lb).

## CULTURAL INFLUENCES ON GROWTH

As with infants and toddlers, feeding practices in some cultures may contribute to the development of overweight or obesity in some preschool-age children. Certain religions and cultures advocate the practice of vegetarianism, and although preschoolers can demonstrate adequate growth on vegetarian diets, their intake should be assessed to determine need for any supplementation. Keep in mind that persons of certain ethnic backgrounds tend to be shorter than those of others; this will also be reflected in the preschool child's height (Sinha, 2019).

# PHYSICAL CHANGES

By the preschool years, most of the body systems have matured, although the eustachian tubes remain relatively short and straight rather than angled downward. Twenty deciduous teeth should be present in the preschool-age child. While the number of alveoli continues to increase, the respiratory structures are also continuing to grow in size. During the preschool years, the heart rate decreases and the blood pressure increases slightly. Splitting of the second heart sound may become evident during this time and an innocent heart murmur may be heard upon auscultation for the first time. The small intestine continues to grow in length and the average preschool-age child usually passes stool once or twice per day. Spinal cord myelination allows for bowel and bladder control to be achieved by most children by age 3 years.

The 4-year-old generally has adequate bowel control. As the urethra remains short in both boys and girls, they continue to be more susceptible to urinary tract infections than adults. The 4- and 5-year-old child usually has adequate bladder control, but may occasionally have a wetting accident if absorbed in an interesting activity or if undergoing stress.

During the preschool years, baby fat is lost and muscle growth occurs, giving the preschool-age child a more mature appearance. The 3- to 5-year-old also becomes stronger and more agile as the bones lengthen and the muscles continue to mature. While appearing clumsy as a toddler, the child is now able to run more smoothly. The lower jaw becomes more pronounced and the skull length increases slightly. In preparation for the emergence of permanent teeth (usually starting around age 6), the upper jaw widens during the preschool years.

Hearing should remain intact at full acuity throughout the preschool years. Color vision is intact and visual acuity is continuing to progress and should do so equally, bilaterally. The average 5-year-old has a visual acuity of 20/40 or 20/30. As compared with older children, the young preschooler has less taste discrimination, placing them at increased risk for accidental ingestion. The senses of smell and touch continue to develop throughout the preschool years.

# DEVELOPMENTAL MILESTONES

The preschool child's musculoskeletal system is continuing to mature, allowing for refinement of existing motor skills and development of new ones. The preschooler has more voluntary control over their movements and is less clumsy than the toddler. Significant refinement in fine motor skills occurs during the preschool period.

Major development occurs in the area of fine motor coordination. Psychosocial development is focused on the accomplishment of initiative. Preconceptual thought and intuitiveness dominate cognitive development. The preschooler is an inquisitive learner and absorbs new concepts like a sponge absorbs water.

## MOTOR SKILL DEVELOPMENT

The preschool-age child demonstrates agility while standing, walking, running, and jumping and seems to be moving constantly. The child is able to walk forward and backward easily, as well as ascend and descend stairs. With extra concentration, the preschooler is also able to stand on the tiptoes or on one foot. The 3-year-old moves each finger independently, and by 5 years of age the child can demonstrates increasingly refined fine motor skills. Refer to Table 9.1 for motor skills expected at various ages.

▶ ALERT: Warning signs indicating a problem with motor development include:

- By 4 years of age:
  - Cannot throw a ball overhand, jump in place, or ride a tricycle
  - Cannot stack four blocks or copy a circle
  - Does not grasp crayon with thumb and fingers, or has difficulty with scribbling
- By 5 years:
  - Cannot build tower of six to eight blocks
  - Cannot brush teeth, wash and dry hands, or undress efficiently

TABLE 9.1 **Expected Motor Skill Development for Age**

| Age | Expected Gross Motor Skills | Expected Fine Motor Skills |
|---|---|---|
| **3 years** | Bends over easily without falling<br>Climbs well<br>Pedals tricycle<br>Runs easily<br>Walks up and down stairs with alternate feet | Builds a tower of 9 or 10 cubes<br>Copies a circle<br>Holds a pencil in writing position<br>Screws/unscrews bolts, lids, nuts<br>Turns pages in book one at a time<br>Undresses self |
| **4 years** | Alternates feet going up and down steps<br>Catches bounced ball<br>Hops on one foot<br>Kicks ball forward<br>Moves forward and backward with agility<br>Stands on one foot up to 5 seconds<br>Throws ball overhand | Copies capital letters<br>Draws a person with two to four body parts<br>Draws circles and squares<br>Laces shoes<br>Traces a diamond or cross<br>Uses scissors successfully |
| **5 years** | May learn to skate and swim<br>May skip<br>Somersaults<br>Stands on one foot 10 seconds or longer<br>Swings and climbs well | Can learn to tie laces<br>Cares for own toileting needs (most of the time)<br>Copies triangle and other geometric patterns<br>Draws person with body and at least six parts<br>Dresses/undresses without assistance<br>Prints some letters<br>Uses fork, spoon, and knife well |

*Sources*: Data from Altmann, T., Hill, D. L., Shelov, S. P., & Hannemann, R. E. (2019). *Caring for your baby and young child: Birth to 5*. Bantam Books; Carter, R. G., & Feigelman, S. (2020). The preschool years. In R. M. Kliegman, J. W. St. Geme III, N. J. Blum, S. S. Shah, R. C. Tasker, K. M. Wilson, & R. E. Behrman (Eds.), *Nelson textbook of pediatrics* (21st ed., Chapter 24). Elsevier; Goldson, E., Angulo, A. S., Raz, D. M., & Reynolds, A. (2020). Child development and behavior. In W. W. Hay, M. J. Levin, M. J. Abzug, & M. Bunik (Eds.), *Current diagnosis & treatment: Pediatrics* (25th ed., Chapter 3). McGraw-Hill Education; Levine, D. A. (2019). Growth and development. In K. J. Marcdante & R. M. Kliegman (Eds.), *Nelson's essentials of pediatrics* (8th ed., Section 2). Elsevier.

## LANGUAGE AND COMMUNICATION

During the preschool years, language skills are refined, with expressive language capabilities catching up to receptive language abilities. This acquisition of language skills allows the preschool-age child to express their thoughts and demonstrate their creativity by talking about their dreams and fantasies. The 3-year-old often uses telegraphic speech, which is very short sentences containing only the essential information. Then by 5 years of age, the child uses about 2,000 words with sentences that are more adult-like in structure (Carter & Feigelman, 2020). Box 9.1 lists language and communication skills at various ages during the preschool period.

The preschooler may stutter or demonstrate nonfluent language, although 80% of children have spontaneous resolution of stuttering by 8 years of age (Carter & Feigelman, 2020). Teach parents to provide the child time to get their thoughts out with language by not interrupting or rushing them. The ability to smoothly link sounds, syllables, and words when speaking (fluency) improves over time. By age 5 years, most children master difficult-to-enunciate sounds such as *f*, *v*, *s*, and *z* sounds, with some children not mastering *sh*, *l*, *th*, and *r* sounds until age 6 years or later. By the end of the preschool period, the potentially bilingual child will be able to differentiate and use both languages, but lags slightly behind the single-language speaker early in the preschool years (Lowry, 2016).

▶ **ALERT**: Warning signs indicating a problem in language development include:

- At 4 years of age:
  - Does not use sentences with three or more words
  - Cannot use the words "me" and "you" appropriately
- By 5 years of age:
  - Cannot use plurals or past tense

## COGNITIVE DEVELOPMENT

The preschool child's cognitive development continues to be in the preoperational stage (Piaget, 1969).

**BOX 9.1 Communication Skills by Age**

**4 years:**
- 75% of speech understood by others outside of family
- Asks many questions; especially "who," "how," "how many"
- Counts a few numbers
- Follows a three-part command
- Knows at least one color
- Knows names of familiar animals
- Names common objects in magazines or books
- Stays on topic in a conversation
- Tells a story that is easy to follow
- Understands the concepts of "different" and "same"
- Vocabulary of 1,500 words

**5 years:**
- Persons outside of the family can understand most of the child's speech
- Answers questions that use "why" and "when"
- Counts to 10
- Explains how an item is used
- Generally uses correct grammar
- Participates in long, detailed conversations
- Recalls part of a story
- Says name and address
- Talks about past, future, and imaginary events
- Vocabulary of 2,100 words

*Sources*: Data from Carter, R. G., & Feigelman, S. (2020). The preschool years. In R. M. Kliegman, J. W. St. Geme III, N. J. Blum, S. S. Shah, R. C. Tasker, K. M. Wilson, & R. E. Behrman (Eds.), *Nelson textbook of pediatrics* (21st ed., Chapter 24). Elsevier; Centers for Disease Control and Prevention. (2020). *Developmental milestones.* http://www.cdc.gov/ncbddd/actearly/milestones/index.html; Levine, D. A. (2019). Growth and development. In K. J. Marcdante & R. M. Kliegman (Eds.), *Nelson's essentials of pediatrics* (8th ed., Section 2). Elsevier.

Preoperational thought is based on a self-centered understanding of the world and is dominant during this stage. In the preconceptual phase of preoperational thought, the child remains egocentric and is able to approach a problem from a single point of view only. The young preschooler may understand the concept of counting and begins to engage in fantasy play. Table 9.2 lists activities demonstrating the stages of cognitive development during the preschool year.

Vocabulary expansion allows the preschool child to progress further with symbolic thought. The preschool child normally displays magical thinking, believing that their thoughts are all-powerful. Magical thinking allows the preschooler to participate in fantasy, making room in the world for the actual or the real as well. Along with make-believe, magical thinking helps the preschooler satisfy their curiosity about everything around them. Also, the preschooler may have an imaginary friend, existing only in the child's imagination, which allows the child to experiment with various activities and behaviors as well as practice conversational skills (Altmann et al., 2019; Goldson et al., 2020). Despite their imagination, the preschool child easily switches between reality and fantasy. During the preschool period, the child cannot completely understand the concept of death or its permanence, possibly inquiring when their pet or grandparent who died is coming back.

▶ ALERT: Warning signs indicating a problem in cognitive development include:

- At 4 years of age:
  - Does not engage in fantasy play
  - Resists using toilet, dressing, sleeping
- By 5 years of age:
  - Distracts very easily (difficulty concentrating on one activity for 5 minutes)
  - Has difficulty with eating, sleeping, or using the toilet
  - Rarely engages in fantasy play

TABLE 9.2 **Cognitive Development in the Preschool Years**

| Stage/Substage | Activities |
|---|---|
| Preoperational substage: Preconceptual phase<br>Age: 2–4 years | Attention span is short<br>Demonstrates animism (attributing life-like qualities to inanimate objects)<br>Displays an active imagination<br>Egocentric thinking diminishes as the child approaches age 4<br>Learning occurs through observing and imitating<br>Makes simple classifications<br>Understands the concept of opposites (hot/cold, soft/hard) by age 4 |
| Preoperational substage: Intuitive phase<br>Age 4–7 years | Better understands the concept of time<br>Classifies and relates objects<br>Counts 10 or more objects<br>Demonstrates a more realistic sense of causality<br>Displays much curiosity about facts<br>Knows about items used in everyday life (appliances, food, money)<br>Knows acceptable cultural rules<br>Names at least four colors<br>Thought processes are more intuitive (knows if something is right or wrong, but may not be able to state why)<br>Tolerates others' differences while not understanding them<br>Uses words appropriately but often does not have a true understanding of their meaning<br>When reasoning, uses transduction (generalizes from one situation to another, even though they may be unrelated) |

*Sources*: Data from Altmann, T., Hill, D. L., Shelov, S. P., & Hannemann, R. E. (2019). *Caring for your baby and young child: Birth to 5*. Bantam Books; Carter, R. G., & Feigelman, S. (2020). The preschool years. In R. M. Kliegman, J. W. St. Geme III, N. J. Blum, S. S. Shah, R. C. Tasker, K. M. Wilson, & R. E. Behrman (Eds.), *Nelson textbook of pediatrics* (21st ed., Chapter 24). Elsevier; Goldson, E., Angulo, A. S., Raz, D. M., & Reynolds, A. (2020). Child development and behavior. In W. W. Hay, M. J. Levin, M. J. Abzug, & M. Bunik (Eds.), *Current diagnosis & treatment: Pediatrics* (25th ed., Chapter 3). McGraw-Hill Education.

## SOCIAL AND EMOTIONAL DEVELOPMENT

The psychosocial task of the preschool years is for the child to establish a sense of initiative rather than guilt (Erikson, 1963). An inquisitive learner, the preschool child demonstrates much enthusiasm about learning new things. Feeling a sense of accomplishment when succeeding in these new activities and pride in their own accomplishment helps the child develop this sense of initiative. Yet the child may extend themselves beyond their current capabilities and thereby be unsuccessful, which may result in guilt. As the preschool child develops a sense of identity, the child should be encouraged to do simple things for themselves, e.g., dressing and washing their hands and face. It is important for parents to give the child the time needed to complete the task, contributing to the child's sense of accomplishment. Identity development also includes gender identity as well as belonging to a particular community, culture, or family.

Strong emotions are common in the preschool child, who may demonstrate excitement and giddiness one moment, and extreme disappointment the next. With a vivid imagination, fears are very real to preschoolers. Older preschoolers have learned to control their behaviors, and are capable of naming their feelings rather than acting on them. Parents can help the child give a name to the emotion that is being experienced, validate the feeling or emotion, and discuss with the child alternatives for dealing with the emotion. The preschool child will take pride in the use of self-control rather than giving in to impulses.

When the child enters kindergarten, the child should have a useful set of social skills to help with success in school and life in general. These skills include display of affection, conversation, cooperation, expression of feelings, kindness, generosity, helping others, making friends, and sharing. To encourage the child to develop the social and emotional skills needed upon school entry, the parent should spend one-to-one communication time with the child (who will thrive on it). This interactive communication helps the child learn to express feelings and ideas; fosters cognitive, emotional, and moral development; and builds self-esteem. When asked questions, the child is required to think out intentions or motivations. Interactive communication can also be used to explore right and wrong, while encouraging vocabulary development. The preschool child feels valued when the parent listens to the child's answers. Being listened to while answering parents' questions gives preschoolers a sense that they are valued.

▶ ALERT: Warning signs indicating a problem in social or emotional development include:

- At age 4 years:
  - Clings or cries if parents leave
  - Does not show interest in interactive games
  - Ignores other children
  - Will not respond to people outside the family
- By 5 years of age:
  - Cannot separate from parent without major protest
  - Has little interest in playing with other children
  - Is often unhappy or sad, or extremely aggressive, fearful or timid, or unusually passive

## MORAL DEVELOPMENT

During the preschool period the superego or development of a conscience is completed, forming the basis for moral development (understanding right and wrong). The inner voice, warning or threatening, is developing during this time period. The preconventional stage of moral development occurs in children 2 to 7 years of age, and is demonstrated by a punishment-obedience orientation (Kohlberg, 1984). The child sees morality as existing outside of self, with the child deferring to adult authority. Children learn to determine good versus bad dependent upon an associated punishment. Standards set by the parents or caregivers are adhered to in order to gain a reward or avoid a punishment. When punishment occurs, the preschooler will experience guilt rather than initiative. For example, the child needs to learn the socially acceptable limits of behavior, but also the rewards of good manners.

At this age, the child's imagination allows for the possibility of any and all things, and the child does not yet have a logical view of the world. As such, the child's concept of faith is intuitive and projective in nature (Adams et al., 2016). With limited life experiences, the child may project a feeling onto a new person or situation, using it to help them understand what is going on around them. The child may also impose the parent's feelings or characteristics onto "God" (if mommy is mad, then God is mad too probably).

### TEMPERAMENT

When the child reaches 3 years of age, they are able to recognize that what they do actually matters. The child's temperament can indicate how the child might react in a certain situation. For task orientation, temperament ranges from highly attentive and persistent to more distractible and active (Child Development Institute, 2019). Parents who tune in to their child's temperament have an easier time finding ways to ease transitions and changes for that child. The child can demonstrate social flexibility, but may need the parent's support. It helps if the parent views the child as an active participant in the parent–child relationship. The 4-year-old's language skills allow them to be more capable of considering complex ideas, temper tantrums should be easing off, and the child should be better at learning self-control. Also, the 4-year-old is capable of visualizing the rewards of growing up and demonstrates more awareness of self-power, which may lead to additional fears. By age 5 years, the child's temperament may be more of a vulnerable as opposed to a confident type, leading to an increased likelihood of experiencing fears.

## SLEEP AND REST

Some preschool-age children will continue to take a nap during the day. The daily total sleep requirement for preschool-age children is 10 to 13 hours (American Academy of Pediatrics, 2020). Some children may require a security item for sleep and others may experience fear of the dark, requiring a nightlight. The vivid imagination of the preschool-age child stays with them through bedtime, so a structured bedtime routine is usually needed.

## NUTRITION

The average preschool-age child gains about 20 grams per day. To meet the average requirements, the preschooler's daily diet should include 19 grams of protein and 25–35 grams of fat per day. The remaining calories should be obtained from complex carbohydrates. Particular nutrient requirements include:

- Iron 10 mg daily
- Calcium 1,000 mg daily
- Zinc 5 mg daily (Maqbool et al., 2020; Phillips & Jensen, 2020)

Adequate fiber intake is needed for lowering the risk for the development of chronic diseases such as cardiovascular disease, diabetes, and obesity. The preschool child should consume 14 g of fiber for every 1,000 kcal per day (Haemer et al., 2020).

# COMMON DEVELOPMENTAL ISSUES

Commonly occurring developmental issues may raise concern among parents and caregivers of preschool-age children. These include lying, sex education, and masturbation.

## LYING

Preschool children commonly lie. Perhaps the child fears punishment, or possibly has gotten carried away with the imagination, or is even imitating what the child sees the parent do. With an extremely vivid imagination, the preschool child may need assistance with how to appropriately use that imagination. When the lying occurs simply as a result of the imagination getting out of control, parents can help guide the child to distinguish myth from reality (Sears & Sears, 2020). Because preschool children often imitate their parents, parents must serve as role models: if the child hears the parents lie, the child may think it is acceptable.

## SEX EDUCATION

With ample curiosity, the preschool child demonstrates excellent observation skills but does not yet have the capability to correctly interpret everything they see. Being very inquisitive and wanting to learn about everything around them, the child is likely to ask questions about where babies come from and about sexual activity. It must first be determined what the child is really asking and what the child is already thinking about that subject. The child only needs the information being requested in a simple, direct, honest fashion. Additional questions are certain to arise in the future and can be addressed at that point.

## MASTURBATION

Normal curiosity during the preschool years often leads to self-genital exploration (Carter & Feigelman, 2020). Despite being upsetting to some parents, masturbation is a natural and healthy part of normal preschool development if it occurs in moderation. The excess attention received if the parent overreacts to the behavior may encourage it to occur more frequently. Parents should treat masturbation as a normal but personal part of life matter-of-factly, while teaching the child that nudity and masturbation, while unacceptable in public, are private behaviors. Additionally, the child should also be taught safety: no other person should be permitted to touch the private parts unless it is the parent, doctor, or nurse checking to see when something is wrong.

# KEY POINTS

- Growing at a slower rate, the preschool child presents a more upright appearance than the toddler.
- During the period from 3 to 6 years of age, the child gains additional motor skills and displays significant refinement of fine motor abilities.
- Acquiring cognitive and language skills in the preschool years helps prepare the child for school success.
- Dysfluency or hesitancy in speech is a normal finding in the preschool period, improving as the child gets older.
- The vocabulary of the preschool child increases at a rapid rate and the child is able to use tenses and prepositions appropriately while speaking in full sentences.
- The preschool child moves away from an egocentric approach to the world toward a more empathetic understanding of what happens outside of the self.
- Developing a sense of initiative is the primary psychosocial task of the preschool period.
- The preschool child requires a well-balanced diet with fat content between 25% and 35% of calories consumed.
- Preschoolers need about 10–13 hours of sleep per day and benefit from a structured bedtime routine.
- Lying, questions about sex, and masturbation occur as normal parts of preschool development.

# REFERENCES

Adams, K., Bull, R., & Maynes, M.-L. (2016). Early childhood spirituality in education: Towards an understanding of the distinctive features of young children's spirituality. *European Early Childhood Education Research Journal, 24*(5), 760–-774. https://doi.org/10.1080/1350293X.2014.996425

Altmann, T., Hill, D. L., Shelov, S. P., & Hannemann, R. E. (2019). *Caring for your baby and young child: Birth to 5.* Bantam Books.

American Academy of Pediatrics. (2020). *Healthy sleep habits: How many hours does your child need?* https://www.healthychildren.org/English/healthy-living/sleep/Pages/Healthy-Sleep-Habits-How-Many-Hours-Does-Your-Child-Need.aspx

Carter, R. G., & Feigelman, S. (2020). The preschool years. In R. M. Kliegman, J. W. St. Geme III, N. J. Blum, S. S. Shah, R. C. Tasker, K. M. Wilson, & R. E. Behrman (Eds.), *Nelson textbook of pediatrics* (21st ed., Chapter 24). Elsevier.

Centers for Disease Control and Prevention. (2020). *Developmental milestones.* http://www.cdc.gov/ncbddd/actearly/milestones/index.html

Child Development Institute. (2019). *Temperament and your child's personality.* http://childdevelopmentinfo.com/child-development/temperament_and_your_child

Erikson, E. H. (1963). *Childhood and society* (2nd ed.). W. W. Norton.

Goldson, E., Angulo, A. S., Raz, D. M., & Reynolds, A. (2020). Child development and behavior. In W. W. Hay, M. J. Levin, M. J. Abzug, & M. Bunik (Eds.), *Current diagnosis & treatment: Pediatrics* (25th ed., Chapter 3). McGraw-Hill Education.

Haemer, M. A., Diab, L. K., Primak, L. E., & Krebs, N. F. (2020). Chapter 11: Normal childhood nutrition & its disorders. In W. W. Hay, M. J. Levin, M. J. Abzug, & M. Bunik (Eds.), *Current diagnosis & treatment: Pediatrics* (25th ed.). McGraw Hill Education.

Kohlberg, L. (1984). *Moral development.* Harper & Row.

Levine, D. A. (2019). Growth and development. In K. J. Marcdante & R. M. Kliegman (Eds.), *Nelson's essentials of pediatrics* (8th ed., Section 2). Elsevier.

Lowry, L. (2016). *Bilingualism in young children: Separating fact from fiction.* http://www.hanen.org/helpful-info/articles/bilingualism-in-young-children--separating-fact-fr.aspx

Maqbool, A., Parks, E. P., Shaikhkhalil, A., Panganiban, J., Mitchell, J. A., & Stallings, V. A. (2020). Nutritional requirements. In R. M. Kliegman, J. W. St. Geme III, N. J. Blum, S. S. Shah, R. C. Tasker, K. M. Wilson, & R. E. Behrman (Eds.), *Nelson textbook of pediatrics* (21st ed., Chapter 55). Elsevier.

Phillips, S. M., & Jensen, C. (2020). Dietary history and recommended dietary intake in children. In K. J. Motil (Ed.), *UpToDate.* Retrieved December 3, 2020, from https://www.uptodate.com/contents/dietary-history-and-recommended-dietary-intake-in-children

Piaget, J. (1969). *The theory of stages in cognitive development.* McGraw-Hill.

Sears, W., & Sears, M. (2020). *Lying: 5 reasons kids lie—What to do.* http://www.askdrsears.com/topics/parenting/discipline-behavior/morals-manners/why-do-kids-lie

Sinha, S. (2019). *Short stature.* http://emedicine.medscape.com/article/924411-overview

# Growth and Development During the School-Age Years

Theresa Kyle

## Student Learning Outcomes

Upon completion of this chapter the reader should be able to:

1. Examine physical developmental changes and growth occurring during the school-age years.
2. Differentiate gross motor, fine motor, and language milestones expected during the school-age years.
3. Distinguish expected psychosocial, cognitive, and moral development changes for various ages throughout the school-age years.
4. Describe appropriate sleep, rest, and nutrition for school-age children.
5. Determine a counseling plan for the family for common developmental concerns experienced during the school-age years.

## INTRODUCTION

The school-age period is the time between the ages of 6 and 12 years. Slow progressive physical growth is occurring, while social and developmental growth accelerates and becomes more complex. The focus of the school-age child's world expands from the family to teachers, classmates, and other outside influences such as the media, coaches, and club leaders. Increasing independence occurs during this stage as the child is participating more frequently in activities outside the home.

The content in this chapter maps to the following areas on the Pediatric Nursing Certification Board (PNCB) Pediatric Nurse Practitioner—Primary Care certification examination:

CONTENT AREAS:

**I. Health Promotion and Maintenance**

**A. Partner with patients/caregivers to support growth and development from infancy to young adulthood**

**II. Assessment and Diagnosis**

**A. Growth and Development**

1. Evaluate and interpret growth parameters

**IV. Professional Role Responsibilities**

**A. Leadership and Evidence-based Practice**

1. Serve as a clinical resource for other health care professionals
2. Critically evaluate and synthesize research and apply findings to clinical practice

## GROWTH

During the school-age period, the child grows an average of 6 to 7 cm (2.5 in) per year, which increases the height by at least 1 foot. Weight is gained at an average of 3 to 3.5 kg (7 lb) per year (Finkelstein & Feigelman, 2020). During the early school-age years, boys and girls appear more graceful and thinner than in previous years, and are also similar in weight and height. Most girls begin to be taller and heavier than boys in the later school-age years. It is important to remember that physical maturity is not necessarily associated with emotional and social maturity. A 9-year-old who is the size of a 12-year-old will continue to act like and think like a 9-year-old.

## PHYSICAL CHANGES

Organ maturation remains fairly consistent until late school age. During the late school-age years, boys gain height slowly yet experience increased weight gain, which may lead to obesity, whereas girls undergo changes in the body that begin to soften the body lines. In the school-age years, the brain and skull continue to grow very slowly, with brain growth complete by the time the child is 10 years old. The shape of the head becomes longer, while growth of the facial bones changes facial proportions. The respiratory system continues to mature, with the alveoli reaching adult numbers by about 7 years of age. The respiratory rate decreases and abdominal breathing transitions to diaphragmatic breathing. The tonsils are decreased in size as compared with the preschool years, yet they remain larger than adolescents' tonsils even in the absence of infection. By 7 years of age, the frontal sinuses are developed. The heart is smaller in size in relation to the rest of the body than at any other developmental stage, as it grows more slowly during the middle years. During the school-age years the pulse rate decreases and the blood pressure increases. During this period, all 20 primary deciduous teeth are lost, being replaced by 28 of the 32 permanent teeth. The stomach capacity increases and caloric needs are lower than in the earlier years. Bladder capacity increases during the school-age years, permitting longer periods between voiding.

### PREPUBESCENCE

The late school-age years are also part of a time period referred to as preadolescence (between middle childhood and the 13th birthday). During this time period, prepubescence occurs (the 2 years before the beginning of puberty). In the prepubescent period, the secondary sexual characteristics develop, girls grow rapidly, and boys experience continued growth. Girls usually begin prepubescence about 2 years earlier than boys. Differences in sexual development as compared to peers may result in negative self-concept in boys not yet developing, and embarrassment, low self-esteem, and concerns about physical changes in girls (particularly when developing early). These negative feelings may lead to risk-taking behaviors in both boys and girls. These differences in development between boys and girls are most apparent toward the end of the school-age period.

## DEVELOPMENTAL MILESTONES

During the school-age years the child's physical, social, and psychological characteristics continue to mature. Eye-hand-muscle coordination improves, allowing the child to participate in organized sports. The child moves toward abstract thinking and seeks approval of peers, teachers, and parents, as well as learning to cooperate with others. Typically, the school-age child will value school attendance and school activities.

### MOTOR SKILL DEVELOPMENT

During the school-age years, gross and fine motor skills continue to refine, and speed and accuracy increase. Balance, coordination, and rhythm improve, facilitating the opportunity to dance, jump rope, ride a two-wheeled bike, and participate in various other sports. As they become older, school-age children may become awkward as their bodies grow faster than their ability to compensate. Gross motor activities are enjoyed greatly by children between the ages of 6 and 8, who remain in constant motion. Between 8 and 10 years of age, children's energy levels remain high, but they are less restless and exhibit more graceful muscular movements and improved rhythm. This allows them to participate in physical activities such as soccer or baseball that require longer periods of increased concentrated attention and effort. Energy levels remain high but are more controlled and focused in the 10- to 12-year-old, with physical skills being similar to those of the adult. Fine motor skills continue to become more refined with hand usage improving and becoming more steady, allowing children success in activities requiring increased precision such as writing, building models, and sewing. Between 10 and 12 years of age, the child's manipulative skills become comparable to those of an adult.

### LANGUAGE AND COMMUNICATION

The school-age child's vocabulary expands with continued acceleration of language skills. Bilingual children often speak English in school and a second language at home. All children use culturally specific words. Learning to read occurs during this time, and improves language skills. More complex grammatical forms such as plurals and pronouns are used by the school-age child. The child also develops metalinguistic awareness: the ability to think about language and comment on its properties. Metalinguistic awareness enables the child to enjoy jokes and riddles and comprehend metaphors as they understand double meanings and plays on words and sounds.

## COGNITIVE DEVELOPMENT

From the age of 7 to 11 years, the stage of cognitive development is the period of concrete operational thoughts (Piaget, 1969). The development of concrete operations permits the child to integrate and organize information about the world from different dimensions. Stored memories of past experiences are used to evaluate and interpret present situations. The school-age child is able to see another person's point of view and think through an action before taking it while anticipating its consequences. Classification is a cognitive skill refined during the school-age years. The child is able to divide things into different sets based on a variety of characteristics and relationships to each other. The child is capable of classifying members of four generations while also understanding that one person can be a mother, daughter, aunt, and granddaughter. An interest in collecting objects begins at this age, with younger school-age children collecting multiple objects and older school-age children demonstrating increased selectivity. A key concept achieved during concrete operational thinking is the understanding of the principle of conservation, that matter does not change when its form changes. The classic example of conservation, shown in Piaget's preoperational stage, is the understanding that pouring one cup of water into a tall, thin glass is the same amount of water when poured into a short, wide glass, despite the taller glass appearing to hold more (Figure 10.1). Box 10.1 provides additional information about activities demonstrated by the child during the period of concrete operation.

## SOCIAL AND EMOTIONAL DEVELOPMENT

The psychosocial task during the school-age years is the development of a sense of industry rather than one of inferiority (Erikson, 1963). Children this age are interested in knowledge and are particularly interested in how things are made and how they work or run. They are increasingly involved in interactions with peers and activities outside of the home, such as sports, clubs, and other group activities. These interactions and activities provide them with an opportunity to demonstrate success in personal and social tasks. During the school-age years, peer relationships are developed and questioning of parents may begin, especially in the later school-age years. Parental conflict may occur with testing of parental or family values.

The older school-age child may show a decreased interest in family functions, often preferring to be in the company of peers, requiring an adjustment for parents. As this is a normal developmental trend, parents should continue to support the child while continuing to enforce restrictions. The school-age child's beginning search for independence may be supported, but parental authority and controls continue to have an impact on choices and values.

The influence of school is secondary only to the influence of the family in the school-age child's life, serving as a means to transmit societal values and for the child to establish peer relationships. School is an

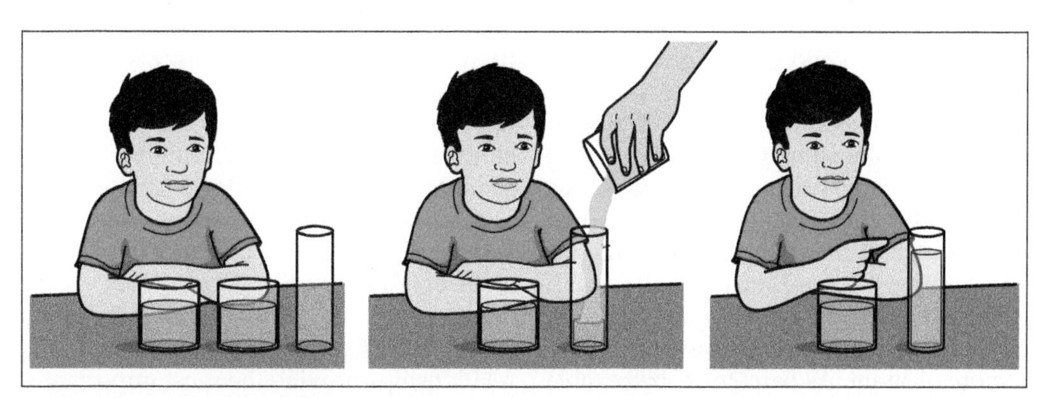

FIGURE 10.1 The concept of conservation.

**BOX 10.1 Activities Occurring in the Concrete Operational Stage**

- Begins collections of items
- Capable of reversing thought process
- Classifies items based on their commonalities
- Comprehends relationships among objects
- Knows that certain characteristics of objects remain constant
- Lacks abstract thinking ability
- Learns through concrete object manipulation
- Participates in serial ordering, addition, subtraction
- Understands the concept of time

*Sources*: Data from Finkelstein, L. H., & Feigelman, S. (2020). Middle childhood. In R. M. Kliegman, J. W. St. Geme III, N. J. Blum, S. S. Shah, R. C. Tasker, K. M. Wilson, & R. E. Behrman (Eds.), *Nelson textbook of pediatrics* (21st ed., Chapter 25). Elsevier; Piaget, J. (1969). *The theory of stages in cognitive development*. McGraw-Hill.

environment in which structured group activities are directed by an adult other than the parent, and conformity is required of the child. Positive, supportive parents may promote a smooth school entry, while parents encouraging clinging behaviors may inadvertently delay a successful school transition. Systems of rewards and punishments utilized by teachers affect the child's self-concept; thus, teachers have a role not only in the intellectual development and socialization of the child, but also in development of their self-esteem.

## Temperament

Temperament continues to influence the school-age child's social and emotional development. Patterns identified in infancy may continue, providing clues to how the child may react to new or different situations, although these reactions may change over time with the child's abilities and experiences. Commonly noted temperaments are:

- easy and adaptable
- slow to warm up
- difficult and easily frustrated (Levine, 2019).

Not every child can be placed into one of these groups, and variations of combinations of these categories also occur. Understanding the child's temperament may help the parent to understand the child's behavior, actions, and how the child relates to the world. The child who adapts easily may transition to school entry and other experiences smoothly, with little or no stress. The slow-to-warm-up child may exhibit discomfort when placed in new or different situations, and may have a more difficult transition to school entry. The child with a more difficult temperament may require patience, firmness, and understanding to make the transition to school entry more pleasant. As parents are better able to understand their child's temperament, they may adapt or modify their parenting style to better fit the child, helping limit emotional and behavioral problems (Finkelstein & Feigelman, 2020).

## Self-Esteem

Self-esteem is the child's view of their individual self-worth, consisting of both negative and positive qualities. By this time the child has continually received feedback from perceived authorities (parents, daycare workers, teachers) and the child's opinion of their own self-worth has been influenced by this feedback, leading to the development of either self-confidence or self-doubt. The child who mastered the earlier psychosocial tasks of autonomy and initiative is able to face the world with feelings of pride rather than shame (Erikson, 1963). When the school-age child regards themselves as worthwhile, the resulting higher self-esteem has an impact on the child's future success.

### Peer Relationships

The school-age child's concept of self is also influenced by peer relationships. Peers approve and critique the skills of school-age children. Younger school-age children most often choose to associate with peers of the same sex. Valuable lessons are learned from interactions with other children of their own age and the child learns to respect differing points of view represented in their groups. Peers form groups with rules and values, and these groups establish norms and standards signifying acceptance or rejection. Thus, the child may modify behavior to gain acceptance. Peer relationships may help to support the school-age child by providing security in some instances; continuing relationships provide the most important social interaction for the school-age child.

### Body Image

Body image also influences self-esteem. The school-age child is interested in their peers' acceptance of their clothing, body, and body changes. Modeling themselves after a parent, peer, or celebrity helps the child to deal with body image. Often, the child may require additional support if they feel their body or style is not comparable to the chosen role model. The child seeks acceptance, and self-esteem may be damaged if the child feels different or is teased, which often has lasting effects.

## MORAL DEVELOPMENT

The child's sense of morality continues to be developed during the school-age years. The conventional stage of moral development is experienced by the school-age child (Kohlberg, 1984). The 7- to 10-year-old will usually follow rules in order to be a "good" person. The 10- to 12-year-old is able to determine if an action is good or bad based on the reason for the action, not just on the possible consequences of the action. Refer to Table 10.1 for additional information related to the conventional stage of moral development.

During the school-age years, children remain concrete thinkers and will usually simply follow the parent's religious lead, conforming to the family's spiritual or religious practices (Therivel & Schub, 2019). While comforted by the beliefs and rituals of their religion, the school-age child is only initially starting to comprehend the differences between natural and supernatural. The school-age child may desire to learn more about their religion and incorporating religious practices in daily life may help the school-age child to cope with stressors.

## SLEEP AND REST

School-age children require 9 to 12 hours of sleep daily to promote adequate growth and development, with the younger school-age child requiring more and the older school-age child less (American Academy of Pediatrics [AAP], 2020). After being in school for most of the day, the young school-age child may be tired, occasionally requiring a brief nap after school to boost energy. A consistent schedule with bedtime ritual remains important throughout the school-age years. Bedtime expectations should be set as well as methods for waking up at the scheduled time (alarm clock, parent calling out). In the 6- to 8-year-old, night terrors or sleepwalking may occur, but these usually resolve by 8 to 10 years of age. The 11- to 12-year-old child may benefit from a regular sleep schedule on weekdays, with variation permitted on weekends.

## NUTRITION

To prevent the development of obesity, the school-age child's diet should limit fatty meats, high-fat dairy products, hydrogenated oils, and processed sugars. The average 6- to 9-year-old gains about 15 grams of weight per day, while the average 9- to 12-year-old gains about 12 grams per day. To meet the average requirements, the school-age child's daily diet should include:

- Protein 19 g daily calories until age 8, then 34 g daily thereafter
- Fat 25 to 35 g daily
- Carbohydrates 45% to 65% of daily calories (limiting to less than 10% from added or concentrated sugars)

**TABLE 10.1 The Conventional Stage of Moral Development**

| Stage | Explanation |
|---|---|
| Stage 3: Interpersonal conforming 7 to 10 years of age | "Good child, bad child"<br>Behavior viewed as either completely right or wrong<br>An act is considered to be wrong if it brings punishment<br>Adult is viewed as being right (when child and adult differ in opinions, the adult is right)<br>Child to be a good person to parents, friends, and teachers as well as to self<br>Lacks complete understanding of the reason behind the rules |
| Stage 4: Law and order<br>10 to 12 years of age | Behavior is guided by child's desire to cooperate and by child's respect for others<br>Child understands the golden rule (treat others as you would like to be treated)<br>Incorporates own behavior into the golden rule<br>Is able to put self into another's position<br>Acts judged based on intention, rather than on reward or punishment |

*Sources*: Data from Finkelstein, L. H., & Feigelman, S. (2020). Middle childhood. In R. M. Kliegman, J. W. St. Geme III, N. J. Blum, S. S. Shah, R. C. Tasker, K. M. Wilson, & R. E. Behrman (Eds.), *Nelson textbook of pediatrics* (21st ed., Chapter 25). Elsevier; Kohlberg, 1984.

Particular nutrient requirements include:

- Iron 10 mg daily through age 8 years, then 8 mg daily ages 9 to 12
- Calcium 1,300 mg daily
- Zinc 5 mg daily through age 8 years, then 8 mg daily ages 9 to 12 (Maqbool et al., 2020; Phillips & Jensen, 2020)

The school-age child should consume 14 g of fiber for every 1,000 kcal per day to lower the risk for the development of chronic diseases such as cardiovascular disease, diabetes, and obesity (Haemer et al., 2020).

## COMMON DEVELOPMENTAL ISSUES

Commonly occurring developmental issues may raise concern among parents and caregivers of school-age children. These include fears, school refusal, lying, and stealing.

### FEARS

The school-age child continues to demonstrate fears as a normal part of development. As the school-age child's thinking matures, fears shift away from pretend things, like monsters, to things that could actually really happen, such as natural disasters, others hurting them, or the death of a loved one, as older school-age children have a more adult-like understanding of death (Lyness, 2018). Although less fearful of harm to their body than the preschool child, the school-age child may fear being kidnapped or undergoing surgery. Fear of the dark may continue, but fears of animals and loud noises diminish. Reassure the child that these fears are normal for the child's age. Parents should recognize the child's fears without catering to them. Teach the child coping strategies such as positive self-statements and relaxation techniques (deep breathing or visualization) to help the child face their fears (Lyness, 2018).

### SCHOOL REFUSAL

School refusal (also termed school phobia or school avoidance) is defined as either difficulty remaining in school for an entire day or outright refusal to attend school; it occurs in approximately 5% of children (AAP, 2017). Typical behaviors include severe misbehavior before school, chronic school tardiness, frequent absences, or attending school with great fear. Fears expressed by children refusing to attend school include parental separation, bus riding, tests, teacher reprimands, anxieties over toileting in a public bathroom, bullying or physical harm, or undressing in the locker room. These fears may cause significant emotional distress in the child and result in reports of stomachache or headache in the younger child, with the addition of palpitations or feelings of faintness in the older child. School refusal may be an symptom of a deeper problem, thus should be investigated.

### LYING AND STEALING

During the school-age years, lying and stealing are inappropriate behaviors that may occur. These behaviors usually disturb parents, which may cause them difficulty in appropriately addressing them. Usually the child will outgrow these behaviors, and learn a good lesson when they do occur. While common in the preschool period due to vivid imaginations, lying is not a normal developmental finding in the school-age years. See chapter 9 for additional information about lying. Parents usually have difficulty in addressing these issues and need help in providing appropriate interventions.

The 6- to 8-year-old child does not fully understand the concept of property rights and ownership. The child may steal an item simply because they like the look of it, because of peer pressure, or in relation to low self-esteem. By the age of 9 years, the child should understand that stealing is wrong and respect other persons' possessions and property. Stealing is a concern if the child steals without remorse, steals continuously, or if the stealing is accompanied by other behavior problems (Johns Hopkins Medicine, n.d.).

## KEY POINTS

- During the school-age years of 6 to 12, physical growth is slow and steady, while cognitive and social development are progressing rapidly.
- Prepubescence may begin in the later school-age years.
- In the school-age period, refinements in motor skills permit the child to successfully participate in sports as well as increase activities requiring improved fine motor skills.
- The school-age child's cognitive ability permits classification of objects, the ability to identify relationships among objects, and an understanding of the concept of conservation.

- While school-age children are capable of concrete operations, solving problems, and making decisions, parents need to continue to provide guidance, direction, and rules.
- The psychosocial task for the school-age child is to develop a sense of industry.
- With school entry, children begin to be influenced by peers and teachers.
- The school-age child develops a conscience, can understand and obey rules, and comprehends cultural and social values.
- The incorporation of religious practices into the school-age child's life may be a source of comfort.
- Typical development concerns in the school-age period include fears, school refusal, lying, and stealing.

## REFERENCES

American Academy of Pediatrics. (2017). *School avoidance: Tips for concerned parents*. http://www.healthychildren.org/English/health-issues/conditions/emotional-problems/pages/School-Avoidance.aspx

American Academy of Pediatrics. (2020). *Healthy sleep habits: How many hours does your child need?* https://www.healthychildren.org/English/healthy-living/sleep/Pages/Healthy-Sleep-Habits-How-Many-Hours-Does-Your-Child-Need.aspx

Erikson, E. H. (1963). *Childhood and society* (2nd ed.). W. W. Norton.

Finkelstein, L. H., & Feigelman, S. (2020). Middle childhood. In R. M. Kliegman, J. W. St. Geme III, N. J. Blum, S. S. Shah, R. C. Tasker, K. M. Wilson, & R. E. Behrman (Eds.), *Nelson textbook of pediatrics* (21st ed., Chapter 25). Elsevier.

Haemer, M. A., Diab, L. K., Primak, L. E., & Krebs, N. F. (2020). Normal childhood nutrition & its disorders. In W. W. Hay, M. J. Levin, M. J. Abzug, & M. Bunik (Eds.), *Current diagnosis & treatment: Pediatrics* (25th ed., Chapter 11). McGraw-Hill Education.

Johns Hopkins Medicine. (n.d.). *Lying and stealing*. https://www.hopkinsmedicine.org/health/conditions-and-diseases/lying-and-stealing

Kohlberg, L. (1984). *Moral development*. Harper & Row.

Levine, D. A. (2019). Growth and development. In K. J. Marcdante & R. M. Kliegman (Eds.), *Nelson's essentials of pediatrics* (8th ed., Section 2). Elsevier.

Lyness, D. (2018). *Normal childhood fears*. https://kidshealth.org/en/parents/anxiety.html

Maqbool, A., Parks, E. P., Shaikhkhalil, A., Panganiban, J., Mitchell, J. A., & Stallings, V. A. (2020). Nutritional requirements. In R. M. Kliegman, J. W. St. Geme III, N. J. Blum, S. S. Shah, R. C. Tasker, K. M. Wilson, & R. E. Behrman (Eds.), *Nelson textbook of pediatrics* (21st ed., Chapter 55). Elsevier.

Phillips, S. M., & Jensen, C. (2020). Dietary history and recommended dietary intake in children. In K. J. Motil (Ed.), *UpToDate*. Retrieved December 3, 2020, from https://www.uptodate.com/contents/dietary-history-and-recommended-dietary-intake-in-children

Piaget, J. (1969). *The theory of stages in cognitive development*. McGraw-Hill.

Therivel, J., & Schub, T. (2019). *Spiritual care: Providing to children and their families*. https://www.ebscohost.com/assets-sample-content/SWRC-Spiritual-Care-Providing-to-Clildren-Families-Practice-Skill.pdf

# Growth and Development During Adolescence

Tedra S. Smith and Elizabeth Coleman

## Student Learning Outcomes

**Upon completion of this chapter, the reader should be able to:**

1. Describe the physical growth and development of adolescents.
2. Explain variations between early, middle, and late adolescence.
3. Discuss common risk behaviors and developmental red flags.

## INTRODUCTION

Adolescence generally covers the age from 11 to 21 years, and is a period of enhanced development and rapid changes. This stage emulates infancy in terms of the amount of physiologic growth and development. Parents often struggle to know what is "normal" and what is "abnormal." The adolescent generally feels confused and misunderstood. Reassurance for parents and the adolescent is an essential component of annual well-child appointments during this time. The pace of adolescent development may vary from child to child, yet remains sequential. Monitoring for appropriate growth and development over this wide age range is important. This chapter highlights the normal growth and development of adolescents and presents healthcare providers with strategies for interaction with the adolescent patient. It is important to note that adolescent growth patterns are greatly influenced by genetics. The healthcare provider is encouraged to show interest in the adolescent and their concerns during the health assessment. The adolescent should always be interviewed by the healthcare provider both with and without the caregiver present.

The content in this chapter maps to the following areas on the Pediatric Nursing Certification Board (PNCB) Pediatric Nurse Practitioner—Primary Care certification examination:

CONTENT AREAS:

**I. Health Promotion and Maintenance**

**A. Partner with patients/caregivers to support growth and development from infancy to young adulthood**

**B. Provide patients/caregivers with age/developmentally appropriate anticipatory guidance**

**F. Counsel about age-appropriate social, behavioral, and mental health concerns**

**II. Assessment and Diagnosis**

**A. Growth and Development**

1. Evaluate and interpret growth parameters

**IV. Professional Role Responsibilities**

**A. Leadership and Evidence-based Practice**

1. Serve as a clinical resource for other health care professionals
2. Critically evaluate and synthesize research and apply findings to clinical practice

## GROWTH

During early adolescence growth is rapid due to the hormonal changes of puberty, but it decreases in middle and late adolescence. Girls and boys experience changes not only in size, but also in appearance.

### WEIGHT

The average weight increase in adolescent boys is 7 to 30 kg (15–65 lb). Female adolescents will demonstrate a weight increase of 7 to 25 kg (15–55 lb) over the course of this period.

### HEIGHT

The growth trend may be characterized by a period of rapid growth (the growth spurt), then slow growth, then another period of rapid growth. Girls experience a rapid increase in height before menarche and full height is usually reached 2 to 2½ years after menarche. The average increase in height for girls is 5 to 20 cm (2–8 in). Boys start their growth spurt between the ages of 10½ and 16 years and it ends between the ages of 13½ and 17½ years. The average increase in height for boys is 10 to 30 cm (4–12 in).

### BODY MASS INDEX

Throughout adolescence, body mass index (BMI) is calculated based on the person's weight and height. The BMI is then evaluated on the gender-appropriate growth chart to determine if it falls within the normal range of the 5th to the 85th percentile for age. If BMI is less than the 5th percentile the adolescent is considered underweight, between the 85th and 95th is considered overweight, and obesity is defined by a BMI greater than the 95th percentile for age (Hagan et al., 2017).

### PHYSICAL CHANGES

During adolescence, all organ systems reach full adult maturation. The head, neck, and hands reach adult proportions, and the percentage of body fat is increased. The brain's size does not increase further, but faster neural processing occurs in response to myelinization of the neurons. The heart rate decreases, systolic blood pressure increases, and the respiratory rate decreases, all reaching adult norms by the end of the adolescent period. During the adolescent's growth spurt, strength and muscle mass increase in both boys and girls. Additionally, the adolescent's skin becomes tougher and thicker, and the sweat glands function at adult levels.

#### Puberty

Puberty generally refers to the biological process of developing adult-like hormonal regulatory systems. There are five stages that define puberty. Although all adolescents move through each stage in order, the progression rate varies per individual adolescent. The sexual maturity ratings (SMR) also known as Tanner stages are used to stage (assess) adolescent development from prepubertal to adult. The SMR are based on sexual characteristics. It is helpful to have a picture diagram during the health supervision visit so that the adolescent can visualize what changes to expect.

#### Female Sexual Maturity Ratings

Female adolescents typically begin pubertal changes a year or two earlier than boys. Over the past 10 years, the age of onset of puberty has decreased from age 11 to 9 and it varies with ethnicity. Most girls will complete physical pubertal changes by the age of 15. The pattern of development is as follows:

- *Ovaries*: During puberty, the ovaries enlarge in size and produce estrogen and progesterone. Estrogen is the hormone responsible for breast growth as well as the development of the vagina, uterus, and fallopian tubes.
- *Breast development*: Breast budding begins to occur around age eight for most females. Breast development is complete between ages 12 and 18. See Table 11.1. Soreness and tenderness of the breast specifically around the nipple are common complaints during puberty by boys and girls.
- *Linear growth*: Females usually see their body get curvier during puberty. There is an increase in fat production especially around the breast and hip, which is a normal process.
- *Pubic hair*: Pubic hair begin to develop prior to adolescence but reaches adult patterns by age 18 years. The pubic hair typically develops in a triangular pattern. See Table 11.1.
- *Menarche*: The first menstrual period typically begins during the time of linear growth deceleration (11–12 years of age). Breast budding is often noted about 2 years prior to menarche. The average age of menarche in the United States is 12 years.

**TABLE 11.1 Sexual Maturity Rating**

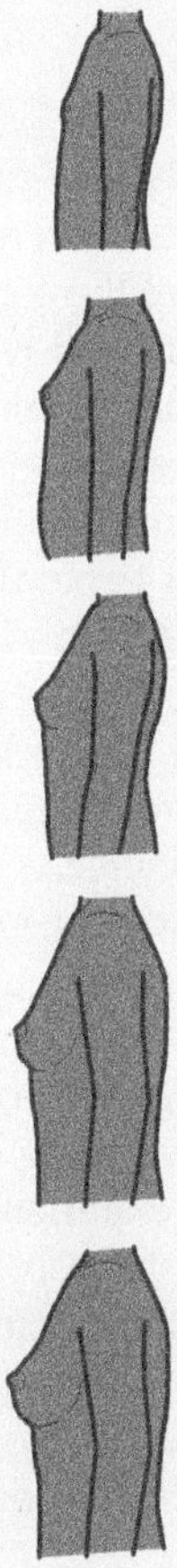

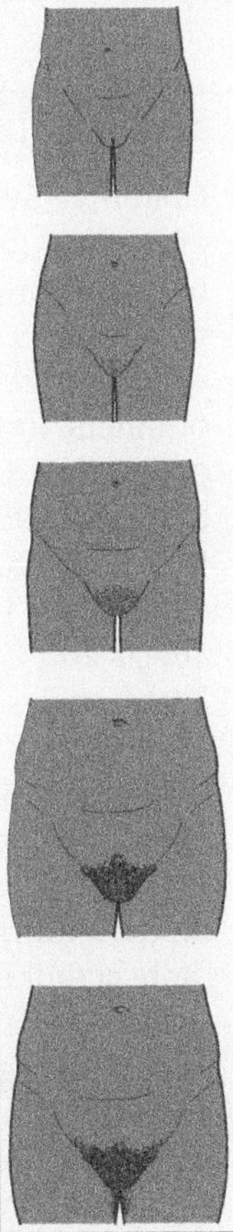

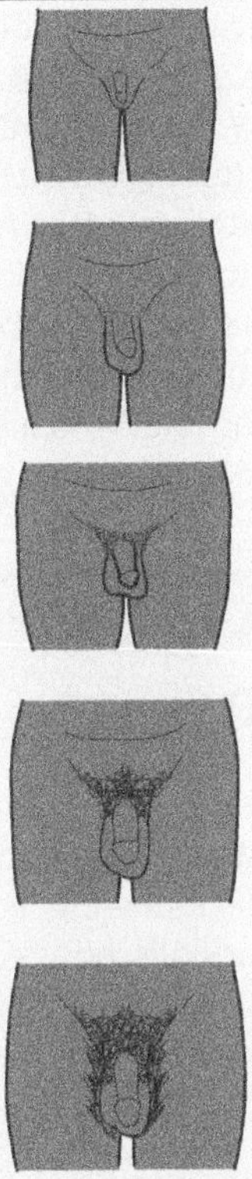

| Breast Development | Female Pubic Hair Development | Male Genitalia Development |
|---|---|---|
| **Stage 1: Prepubertal** Nipple elevation begins. | **Stage 1: Prepubertal** No pubic hair | **Stage 1: Preadolescent** No pubic hair; penis and testes are same size and proportion as in childhood |
| **Stage 2: Breast budding** Breast and nipple elevation appears as a small mound with areolar enlargement. | **Stage 2:** Sparse, long, straight hair | **Stage 2:** Sparse pubic hair; slight enlargement of penis and testes |
| **Stage 3: Continued enlargement** The breast and areola enlarge without distinct evidence of separation between them. | **Stage 3:** Darker, coarser, curly, sparse hair over the mons pubis | **Stage 3:** Darker, coarser pubic hair; further enlargement of penis and testes |
| **Stage 4: Secondary mound** A secondary mound forms beyond the original breast mound as the areola and nipple project. | **Stage 4:** Darker, curly, abundant hair over the mons pubis | **Stage 4:** Coarse and curly pubic hair covering more area; further enlargement of penis and testes |
| **Stage 5: Breast maturity** The nipple projects and the areola becomes part of the breast contour | **Stage 5:** Adult triangle pattern with hair growth on medial thighs | **Stage 5:** Hair spread to medial surface of the thighs and adult in quality and quantity; penis and testes reach adult size and proportion |

*Source*: From Chiocca, E. M. (2019). *Advanced pediatric health assessment* (3rd ed., pp. 437–438, Figures 20.7 and 20.8). Springer Publishing Company.

## Male Sexual Maturity Ratings

Male adolescents typically enter into puberty between age 10 and 14 years, with the majority reaching completion by age 16 years. Musculature and the brain will continue to grow and develop. The adolescent male pattern of development is as follows:

- *Testicular enlargement*: The enlargement of testicles and the scrotal sac is the first sign of puberty in males. The color of the scrotum gets darker, the skin begins to thin, and tiny bumps (hair follicles) appear as the testicles enlarge. Most males will have one testicle (commonly the left) hanging lower than the other does. The penis (shaft and glans) also increase in size.
- *Pubic hair*: The second sign of puberty in males is the development of pubic hair, which appears shortly after the increased testicular size. Hair development first appears near the base of the penis in a diamond shape. As the hair grows, it becomes coarse in texture, curly, and turns darker. Over the next few years, the hair covers the entire pubic area and begins to extend to the thigh area on both sides. The appearance of hair on the face, legs, arms, and chest starts to occur about 2 years after pubic hair development.
- *Length and width of penis*: The penis grows in length, then in width. It is not uncommon for a 13-year-old to have genitals the size of an adult. The average range for penile maturation is 13 to 18 years of age. At this point in sexual development, it is common for boys to frequently assess their penis and compare their size with others in their developmental age group (Table 11.1).
- *Fertility/Spermarche*: About one year after the testicles begin to enlarge, boys are able to reproduce. The

testicles are now able to produce sperm as well as testosterone. The Cowper's glands and the prostate (two seminal vesicles) combine with the sperm to produce semen during ejaculation. Each ejaculation has approximately 200 million to 500 million sperm. It is common for the first ejaculation to occur during masturbation. Nocturnal emissions, also known as wet dreams, are not uncommon with the development of sexual maturation.

- *Vocal changes*: The larynx and vocal cords enlarge shortly after the growth spurt. The first noticeable sign is the voice cracking, which later turns into a deeper voice. The Adam's apple gets larger.

## DEVELOPMENTAL MILESTONES

### GROSS MOTOR SKILLS

By adolescence, coordination, general motor ability, physical endurance, and strength increase. Adolescents can participate in the following activities to facilitate strengthening of motor skills: bowling, walking or climbing, swimming, riding a bike, dancing, and playing on wobble bridges and rope ladders. Adolescent males typically make significant gains in their gross motor skills before age 14 years, whereas most adolescent females only make minimal gains until age 14 years. Gross motor skill development continues until the early 20s.

### FINE MOTOR SKILLS

Fine motor skills develop at the same pace as gross motor skills. During adolescence, increased coordination of small movements of the hands occurs. Adolescents are more equipped to move with precision. Specific activities may assist the adolescent with building fine motor skills. Such activities include cooking (e.g., chopping vegetables or kneading pizza dough), playing a musical instrument (woodwind and guitar), juggling, blocks, handiwork, crafts, artistic endeavors, and solving 3D puzzles.

### LANGUAGE SKILLS

Most adolescents are able to read on an adult level unless there are developmental delays. During adolescence, language begins to include a higher use of words, in part because of more abstract thinking. Adolescents are more inclined to analyze the function of words and their meaning. The ability to compare and contrast two concepts and understand the use of metaphor increases during adolescence. They begin to mature in their use of irony, wit, and humor.

## COGNITIVE DEVELOPMENT

Cognitive development during adolescence is often referenced as the time one moves from childlike thinking to adult thinking. Adolescents begin to think and reason in a more complex manner. They are able to think about different possibilities and consider the thoughts of others, indicating a maturation of skills in empathy and caring. Overall, cognitive development generally occurs between ages 12 to 18; however, the rate varies with each adolescent. During this period of growth, adolescents form their own worldview and it directly affects and is affected by their cognitive development. Early adolescence is characterized by an increase in challenging of societal rules and standards. Adolescents may be highly idealistic and see the value of changing the status quo and challenging "how things are." They may be influenced by both positive and negative role models, affirming the need for parental monitoring of daily activities and contacts. Life issues and experiences also influence how the adolescent moves from concrete thinking to formal operations. This includes being able to think logically through situations and become less self-centered. By late adolescence, there are more thoughts on issues that affect the world, the situations of others, and the future as an adult.

Healthy cognitive development may occur with positive reinforcement and targeted strategies by caregivers and healthcare providers. Adolescents should be included in discussions about various issues, topics, and events affecting the world. Caregivers should be encouraged to allow the adolescent to share their thoughts and opinions as well as participate in goal setting with the adolescent. Adolescents need to make decisions and have space to self-evaluate good and bad decisions without harsh punishment.

## PSYCHOSOCIAL DEVELOPMENT

Adolescents experience rapid physical changes, which may lead to more self-awareness and self-judgment of external characteristics. In contrast, it may engender uncomfortable thoughts of self-criticism and comparing personal status with others. During the period of rapid growth, adolescents assume that everyone is looking at them and internally wonder if they are "normal." One of the main goals of an adolescent well-child examination is assurance that the adolescent is normal. It is imperative to include that growth occurs in a sequence. However, the timing is very individualized. The major tasks related to psychosocial development during this period are attainment of independence, body image awareness and acceptance, the ability to build healthy peer relationships, and identity development. See Table 11.2 for a list of developmental red flags.

Freud characterizes the adolescent period as the genital stage. This stage lasts throughout adulthood. During the genital stage, adolescents begin to venture into romantic relationships. Adolescents begin to explore sexual interests. The overall goal is to learn how to balance the various areas of life that affect relationships.

Adolescents progress through the fifth and sixth stages of psychosocial development according to Erikson's stages of development: identity vs. role confusion (12–18) and intimacy vs. isolation (18–40). During the fifth stage, adolescents are attempting to identify their own personal values, morals, and goals. The main objective is to answer the question "Who am I?" The adolescent begins to develop a sense of self.

## Early Adolescence (11–14 years of age)

The first stage of puberty begins in early adolescence with a period of rapid physical changes. The changes often cause increased anxiety related to what is normal. At this age, the adolescent has concrete thinking, which means they think more in terms of black and white (e.g., right or wrong). See chapter 18 for more information related to health promotion.

## Middle Adolescence (15–17 years of age)

Physical growth is usually complete by middle adolescence, but the brain continues to grow and develop. During middle adolescence, boys are generally better at physical activities than girls. This is a period when adolescents establish their own personal identity and seek autonomy. See chapter 18 for more information on health promotion.

## Late Adolescence (18–21 years of age)

Late adolescence is a period known for frequent life changes that involve home, school, work, and personal identity. At this point males and females are gaining a sense of self and acceptance of their physical

**TABLE 11.2 Adolescent Developmental Red Flags**

| Age | Physical | Cognitive | Social/Emotional |
|---|---|---|---|
| Early Adolescence (11–14) | Puberty beginning in females before age 8; in males before age 9<br>Delayed puberty (boy 14 years or older or girl 13 years or older with no signs of puberty)<br>Delayed/decreased rate of growth<br>Sudden weight loss or gain<br>Accelerated growth/tall for family | Abnormal headaches<br>Failing classes<br>Problems paying attention in class | High-risk behaviors<br>Increased anxiety<br>Abnormal HEADSSS screening[a]<br>Positive screening from modified PHQ-9 questionnaire for depression[a] |
| Middle Adolescence (15–17) | Girls who have not progressed with menarche within 5 years of breast buds<br>Males who are not at Tanner 5 within 4.5 years of start of puberty<br>Sudden weight loss or gain<br>Delayed/decreased rate of growth<br>Report of unsafe sex | Abnormal headaches<br>Failing classes<br>Problems paying attention in class | High-risk behaviors<br>Abnormal HEADSSS screening[a]<br>Positive screening from modified PHQ-9 questionnaire for depression[a] |
| Late Adolescence (18–21) | Delayed/decreased rate of growth<br>Sudden weight loss or gain<br>Reports of unsafe sex | Abnormal headaches<br>Unable/unwilling to plan for the future<br>Problems paying attention in class | High-risk behaviors<br>Abnormal HEADSSS screening[a]<br>Positive screening from modified PHQ-9 questionnaire for depression[a] |

[a] Refer to Chapter 18 for additional information.

HEADSSS, home, education/employment, activities, drugs, sexuality, suicide/depression/self-image, safety; PHQ-9, Patient Health Questionnaire.

appearance. Males may continue to develop physically until the age of 21. See chapter 18 for more information on health promotion.

## MORAL DEVELOPMENT

Adolescents are better able to understand that there may not be a definite answer to every question. As they develop, adolescents are increasingly able to understand why some people make one choice while another group of people makes a different choice. Adolescents have a greater appreciation for logical thinking and value conversation around various topics with the adults they trust. Adolescents can better understand rules once those rules are explained and they are allowed to ask questions. The rule, then, is clear from their perspective.

## SLEEP/REST

The National Sleep Foundation (NSF) recommends that an adolescent get at least 8 to 10 hours of sleep per night (NSF, 2020). Adolescents are known to skip sleeping to attend social activities, e.g., school sports, social media participation, and video game playing. Physiological changes during the adolescent stage, including further brain development, require that the adolescent get sufficient sleep. The lack of a sufficient amount of sleep can contribute to illness, acne, short temper, aggressive behavior, and a limitation in the ability to concentrate and solve problems.

Sleep hygiene is essential for the adolescent population. This includes going to sleep and waking up at the same time every day, keeping a relaxing bedtime routine each night, and avoiding any screen time within one hour of bedtime. In fact, it is best to encourage parents to provide a *technology-free* bedroom for their child, with no electronics of any kind allowed in the room at night (NSF, 2020). Bedtime routines can involve reading a book, taking a bath or shower, listening to calm music, or journaling. Poor sleep hygiene not only results in a tired adolescent, but also can affect brain development. Telzer et al. (2015) found that changes in sleep duration could have long-term consequences on the development of the adolescent brain.

Increased screen time during the day can also affect the sleep patterns of teenagers. Screen time is linked to insomnia and even symptoms of depression in the adolescent population (NSF, 2020). The blue light that is emitted from electronic devices suppresses the release of melatonin, thus disturbing the sleep-wake cycle (NSF, 2020). This can cause issues in adolescents not being able to fall asleep and can make it more difficult for them to stay asleep. With a shortened sleep duration, this can result in depressive symptoms (NSF, 2020).

Additionally, adolescents with shortened sleep duration are at increased risk for lower insulin sensitivity, hyperglycemia, poor diet, and obesity (Gohil & Hannon, 2018). When adolescents are sleeping for a shorter amount of time, they spend less time in rapid-eye movement (REM) sleep, which is also linked to increased weight gain. Part of the hormonal link to sleep involves leptin and ghrelin. In patients with shorter sleep duration, ghrelin levels are increased and leptin levels decrease, which causes an increase in hunger (Gohil & Hannon, 2018).

One important aspect to keep in mind while discussing sleep patterns of the adolescent is to assess for sleep apnea. Consider sleep apnea as a diagnosis when an adolescent not only snores at night, but also gasps, wakes up, chokes, moves around in bed, or has labored breathing. Additional signs and symptoms might include troubling behavior at school, falling asleep in classes, and bedwetting. Children who are obese are at higher risk as well (NSF, 2020).

## NUTRITION

During adolescence, the body demands more energy and protein (2,200–3,000 calories/day) due to rapid growth and development. On average, boys require 2,800 calories per day while girls require 2,200 calories per day. Adolescents who participate in sports will need more calories per day due to increased energy needs. To begin a nutritional assessment, the healthcare provider is encouraged to obtain a 24-hour diet recall and question the adolescent about foods eaten in various food groups. The 24-hour diet recall provides a typical day's food intake overall when assessing the nutritional status.

Healthy eating is essential to growth and development of the adolescent population. It also prevents several health conditions. Adolescents should use a healthy eating pattern that includes a variety of fruits, vegetables, whole grains, fat-free or low-fat dairy products, protein foods, and oils. Adolescents should also limit calories from solid fats as well as added sugars. They should also reduce their sodium intake (Centers for Disease Control and Prevention [CDC], 2019a).

Furthermore, adolescents need to eat a healthy breakfast each morning. This can improve cognitive function, including memory, and reduce absenteeism (CDC, 2019a). Eating a healthy breakfast is also positively associated with improved mood. Adequate hydration is important as well, as it is also associated with improved cognitive function (CDC, 2019a). Encouraging water consumption is a critical health promotion and development strategy.

According to Lassi et al. (2017), micronutrient supplementation, especially with iron, can decrease the prevalence of anemia in the adolescent population. In pregnant adolescents, improvement in nutrition can decrease low birth weight and preterm birth. In addition, because of the increased rate of growth during this extended period of puberty, the nutritional resources needed can be greater than at any other point in life (Das et al., 2017).

Another important aspect of nutrition to consider is metabolism. The components of metabolism are energy cost of growth, basal metabolic rate, and activity energy expenditure. Issues arise when the caloric intake of adolescents is greater than the energy cost of growth and activity energy expenditure. This leads to increased weight gain and obesity. When caloric intake decreases to become less than the basal metabolic rate, then this can cause issues as well. The energy cost of growth and activity energy expenditure are affected, causing decreased growth rate, delay in puberty, amenorrhea, and issues with bone mass (Das et al., 2017).

Male adolescents will need higher caloric intake than female adolescents, due to the larger increases in height, weight, and lean body mass. This intake should include 50% or more from carbohydrates, and less than 10–25% from sugar sources. Females ages 11 to 14 should have increased protein intake, and males ages 15 to 18 should increase their protein intake, due to faster velocities of growth (Das et al., 2017).

# COMMON DEVELOPMENTAL ISSUES

## RISK-TAKING BEHAVIORS

As adolescents begin to self-identify and create a life outside of their family unit, they begin to participate in more risky behavior. Adolescents are known to experiment by testing the limits and breaking parental and societal rules. Independence displayed by the adolescent is a natural occurrence and a positive growth factor, but requires self-management. Parents begin to feel conflicted about when to intervene and how to address their cautions and concerns with the adolescent. The healthcare provider becomes a parental and adolescent resource.

### Tobacco Use

The use of tobacco typically starts during adolescence. There has been an increased usage of tobacco products with the emergence of vaping and e-cigarettes. Current data indicates that 67% of adolescents in high school and 49% of adolescents in middle school have used flavored tobacco (within the past 30 days; CDC, 2019b).

### Alcohol Use

Alcohol is the most widely used substance among adolescents and is a nationwide concern.

According to the CDC (2020), alcohol is the drug used and abused most often by adolescents. In a 2019 survey, 8% of eighth-graders reported drinking within the past 30 days, with the percentage increasing to 29% in 12th-graders (Johnston et al., 2020). Everyone feels the effects of behaviors and consequences that occur because of underage drinking. Underage drinking is known to cause physical and mental injuries, personal damage, violence, and death.

### Opioid and Illicit Substance Use

While adolescent alcohol use is a significant concern, adolescents are also involved in the use of opioids and illicit substances. The adolescent's brain is maturing and is particularly vulnerable to substance use, placing the adolescent at increased risk for substance misuse and addiction (Inman et al., 2020). One-third of adolescents report having access to opioids, two-thirds report access to stimulants, and 13% to 26% of adolescents use marijuana (Garofoli, 2020; Inman et al., 2020). Of particular concern is that 5% to 9% of adolescents report using synthetic cannabinoids, which exert a more toxic and potent effect than natural marijuana, in an unpredictable fashion (Inman et al., 2020). An additional concern is the potential contamination of illicit drugs such as heroin with substances such as fentanyl in toxic quantities. A large percentage (65%) of adolescents report wanting to discuss their substance use with a healthcare provider, although only 35% report having done so (Garofoli, 2020).

## ACNE

Several hormonal changes occur during the adolescent period for males and females. The body grows rapidly and produces hormonal stimulation that prompts the sebaceous glands to produce more sebum. The extra sebum creates an overproduction of dead cells, which leads to acne on the face, neck, chest, and upper back. Acne is an issue that affects the majority of adolescents. It is not a serious health issue; however, severe cases can cause significant scarring and have a negative effect on self-esteem. See chapter 19 for more information on acne.

## DATING AND SEXUALITY

During middle adolescence, adolescents begin to become intrigued with dating. However, it is common for some adolescents not to date until late adolescence. Adolescents begin to identify with their sexual identities, which allows for the formation of adult relationships. The word *dating* is not used as often as it was in the past. The new terminology is now "going out" (with someone, possibly romantically involved) or "hanging out" (typically with friends). Most experiences begin with "going out" with a group and advance to couples-only outings toward the end of late adolescence. Although adolescents are going out, the age of sexual intercourse initiation has decreased. In 2011, 47% of adolescents reported having sexual intercourse while in high school as compared with 54% in the early 1900s (Wildsmith et al., 2013).

### Health Issues Related to Sexuality

Selected health issues related to sexuality include pregnancy and contraception (covered in chapter 29), and sexually transmitted infections (STIs) and human immunodeficiency virus (HIV; covered in chapter 31). Conversations about sexuality may be difficult for some providers and for adolescents, but the provider must always place the adolescent's safety first. Discuss with the adolescent that consent is always required for any type of sexual activity. The following are selected healthcare provider principles of care for the preceding health issues related to sexuality:

- Sex education
- Confidentiality
- Emotional support
- Normalization
- Respect the patient's preference
- Direct questioning—Conversations on sexual behavior are often avoided by healthcare providers but are imperative to providing holistic care to the adolescent. Asking specific questions will help improve patient participation in the discussion.

## SUICIDE PREVENTION

Suicide prevention is a topic that is essential to address at every adolescent visit, whether for a well-child check or a sick visit.

The first aspect to assess is the availability of firearms in the household. It is important to ensure that if there are firearms in the home, they are unloaded *and* in a locked safe that is inaccessible to children. Access to firearms increases the risk of suicides and accidental deaths associated with firearms (Zalsman et al., 2016). Access to large amounts of analgesics, pesticides, and other toxic substances should also be limited. The adolescent should not have unlimited access to these substances, as this can also increase the risk of suicide (Zalsman et al., 2016).

Healthcare providers in primary care should refer patients with mental health issues to a specialist who can provide pharmacologic treatment. The treatment of these conditions can also decrease the risk of suicide (Zalsman et al., 2016). Lithium can decrease the risk of suicide in patients with mood disorders, and clozapine can reduce the risk of suicide in patients in psychosis (Zalsman et al., 2016). Adolescents with depression may have increased suicide ideation when taking antidepressants, but the risk of suicide attempts due to having untreated depression is higher; thus pharmacologic treatment is recommended. Adding cognitive behavioral therapy (CBT) can decrease this side effect (Zalsman et al., 2016). Selective serotonin reuptake inhibitors (SSRIs), specifically fluoxetine, are the first-line recommended pharmacologic treatments. Additionally, multisystemic therapy can help reduce suicide attempts. This therapy includes the improvement of parenting skills, community involvement, school involvement, peer support, and encouragement of social activities (Zalsman et al., 2016).

The education of primary care providers regarding recognition of depression and treatment is extremely helpful in decreasing suicide rates and the morbidity associated with depression. Screening for depression and suicide ideation in adolescents in the primary care setting can help to identify those at risk (Zalsman et al., 2016). The modified Patient Health Questionnaire (PHQ-9) is ideal for this screening technique (https://www.uspreventiveservicestaskforce.org/Home/GetFileByID/218).

## SOCIAL MEDIA USE

Social media use in the adolescent population continues to be an area of concern among healthcare providers. However, adolescents use social media as a way to increase their social connections and learn technical skills. Adolescents have also reported that social media is used to strength peer relationships, allows them to support others their age on specific issues, and provides them with a different viewpoint on various social issues. According to the Pew Research report, adolescents report that social media makes them feel self-confident and included rather than excluded (Anderson & Jiang, 2018). Social media has a tremendous effect on the mental status on the developing brain of the adolescent. The increased use has been linked to low self-esteem as well as increased anxiety. Adolescents struggle with self-regulation of screen time. They often spend a significant amount of time online, which increases their exposure to peer pressure, cyberbullying, and sexting. There are pertinent health issues that can develop through the use of social media, such as depression, anxiety, communication issues, envy, and oppositional defiant disorder (see Chapter 18).

## KEY POINTS

- Early adolescence marks a period of rapid growth, due to the hormonal changes of puberty, followed by slower growth in middle and late adolescence.
- The average weight increase in adolescent males is 7 to 30 kg. Female adolescents increase in weight by approximately 7 to 25 kg.
- Pubertal development in females typically follows the pattern of breast bud formation, rapid linear growth, pubic hair, and then menarche.
- Pubertal development in males typically begins with testicular enlargement, pubic hair development, spermarche, elongation and widening of the penis, rapid linear growth, vocal changes, and facial hair development.
- Cognitive development of the adolescent should include thinking and reasoning in a more complex manner.
- Psychosocial development includes attainment of independence, body image awareness and acceptance, the ability to build healthy peer relationships, and identity development.
- Adolescents need 8–10 hours of sleep per night and need to maintain good sleep hygiene.
- Adolescent males require 2,800 calories per day; females require 2,200 calories per day.
- Suicide prevention is a topic that is essential to address at every adolescent visit, whether for a well-child check or a sick visit.

## REFERENCES


Anderson, M., & Jiang, J. (2018, November 28). *Teens' social media habits and experiences*. Pew Research Center. https://www.pewresearch.org/internet/2018/11/28/teens-social-media-habits-and-experiences

Centers for Disease Control and Prevention. (2019a). *CDC healthy schools: Childhood nutrition facts*. https://www.cdc.gov/healthyschools/nutrition/facts.htm

Centers for Disease Control and Prevention. (2019b). *Youth and tobacco use*. https://www.cdc.gov/tobacco/data_statistics/fact_sheets/youth_data/tobacco_use/index.htm

Centers for Disease Control and Prevention. (2020). *Fact sheets—Underage drinking*. https://www.cdc.gov/alcohol/fact-sheets/underage-drinking.htm

Chiocca, E. M. (2019). *Advanced pediatric health assessment* (3rd ed.). Springer Publishing Company.

Das, J. K., Salam, R. A., Thornburg, K. L., Prentice, A. M., Campisi, S., Lassi, Z. S., Koletzko, B., & Bhutta, Z. A. (2017). Nutrition in adolescents: Physiology, metabolism, and nutritional needs. *Annals of the New York Academy of Sciences, 1393*, 21–33. https://doi.org/10.1111/nyas.13330

Garofoli, M. (2020). Adolescent substance abuse. *Primary Care: Clinic in Office Practice, 47*, 383–394. https://doi.org/10.1016/j.pop.2020.02.013

Gohil, A., & Hannon, T. S. (2018). Poor sleep and obesity: Concurrent epidemics in adolescent youth. *Frontiers in Endocrinology, 9*, 364. https://doi.org/10.3389/fendo.2018.00364

Hagan, J. F., Shaw, J. S., & Duncan, P. M. (Eds.). (2017). *Bright futures: Guidelines for health supervision of infants, children, and adolescents* (4th ed.). American Academy of Pediatrics.

Inman, D., El-Mallakh, P., Jensen, L., Ossege, J., & Scott, L. (2020). Addressing substance use in adolescents: Screening, brief intervention, and referral to treatment. *The Journal for Nurse Practitioners, 16*(1), 69–73. https://doi.org/10.1016/j.nurpra.2019.10.004

Johnston, L. D., Meich, R. A., O'Malley, P. M., Bachman, J. G., Schulenberg, J. E., & Patrick, M. E. (2020). *2019 overview: Key findings on adolescent drug use*. Institute for Social Research, The University of Michigan. http://www.monitoringthefuture.org//pubs/monographs/mtf-overview2019.pdf

Lassi, Z. S., Moin, A., Das, J. K., Salam, R. A., & Bhutta, Z. A. (2017). Systematic review on evidence-based adolescent nutrition interventions. *Annals of the New York Academy of Sciences, 1393*, 34–50. https://doi.org/10.1111/nyas.13335

National Sleep Foundation. (2020). *Children, teens, and sleep*. https://www.sleepfoundation.org/sleep-topics/children-teens-sleep

Telzer, E. H., Goldenberg, D., Fuligni, A. J., Lieberman, M. D., & Gálvan, A. (2015). Sleep variability in adolescence is associated with altered brain development. *Developmental Cognitive Neuroscience, 14*, 16–22. https://doi.org/10.1016/j.dcn.2015.05.007

Wildsmith, E., Barry, M., Manlove, J., & Vaughn, B. (2013). Dating and sexual relationships. *Child Trends*. https://www.childtrends.org/wp-content/uploads/2013/10/2013-04DatingSexualRelationships.pdf

Zalsman, G., Hawton, K., Wasserman, D., van Heeringen, K., Arensman, E., Sarchiapone, M., Carli, V., Höschl, C., Barzilay, R., Balazs, J., Purebl., G., Kahn, J. P., Sáiz, P. A., Lipsicas, C. B., Bobes, J., Cozman, D., Hegerl, U., & Zohar, J. (2016). Suicide prevention strategies revisited: 10-year systematic review. *The Lancet Psychiatry, 3*(7), 646–659. https://doi.org/10.1016/S2215-0366(16)30030-X

# UNIT III

# Pediatric Health Promotion

# Health Supervision: Well-Child Visits

Theresa Kyle

## Student Learning Outcomes

**Upon completion of this chapter the reader should be able to:**

1. Describe the purpose of health supervision in the pediatric population.
2. Identify the components included in each health supervision visit.
3. Discuss developmental surveillance, screening, and evaluation.
4. Determine universal or selected screening recommended at each age.
5. Select immunizations appropriate for the child's age.
6. Integrate findings surveillance and screening into the child's plan of care.

## INTRODUCTION

The goal of health supervision, beginning at birth and continuing through adolescence, is the provision of proactive services to optimize each child's level of functioning. The health supervision visit may occur in any publicly accessible setting having appropriate equipment for health supervision such as a private office, clinic, community health department, day care center, school, or homeless shelter. The goals of the health supervision visit are disease detection (through physical examination, surveillance, and screening), health promotion, and anticipatory guidance (Hagan et al., 2017). Collaboration between the American Academy of Pediatrics (AAP) and the Maternal Child Health Bureau has resulted in the Bright Futures' recommendation for pediatric health supervision. The goals of health supervision visits are to promote:

- Lifelong health for families and communities
- Family support
- Health for children and youth with special health care needs
- Healthy development
- Mental health
- Healthy weight
- Healthy nutrition
- Physical activity
- Oral health
- Healthy sexual development and sexuality
- Healthy and safe use of social media
- Safety and injury prevention (Hagan et al., 2017)

The Bright Futures program utilizes evidence-based information as the basis for their published guidelines. In instances where the evidence is lacking or inconclusive, expert opinion has been utilized. Recent changes to the guidelines emphasize working collaboratively with families, integrating mental health care into the primary care setting, gaining cultural competence, addressing complementary and alternative care, and recognizing the need for attention toward children with special health care needs. The guidelines are meant to be individualized to the particular child's needs (Treitz et al., 2020).

The content in this chapter maps to the following areas on the Pediatric Nursing Certification Board (PNCB) Pediatric Nurse Practitioner—Primary Care certification examination:

CONTENT AREAS:

**I. Health Maintenance and Promotion**

**A. Partner with patients/caregivers to support growth and development from infancy to young adulthood**

**B. Provide patients/caregivers with age/developmentally appropriate anticipatory guidance**

**C. Recommend and prescribe immunizations according to current CDC guidelines**

**D. Educate about illness prevention and early warning signs of pediatric illness and emergencies**

**E. Advise patients/caregivers about age appropriate injury prevention and safety (environmental exposure, risk taking behaviors, social situations, sports and recreation, and vehicle safety)**

**F. Counsel about age-appropriate social, behavioral, and mental health concerns (e.g., substance abuse, social media use, grief and loss, and sexual orientation/LGBTQ)**

**II. Assessment and Diagnosis**

**A. Growth and Development**

1. Evaluate and interpret growth parameters
2. Perform developmental surveillance

**B. History and Physical Examination**

1. Obtain history of present illness
2. Obtain a comprehensive health history for new patients
3. Complete an interval history for established patients
4. Perform a review of systems
5. Perform a complete physical examination

**C. Diagnostic Testing and Screening**

1. Order and interpret office/clinic based screening tests
4. Select, utilize, and interpret developmental, behavioral and mental health screening and assessment tools

**D. Analyzing Information**

1. Integrate health history and physical examination findings into the plan of care
2. Assimilate findings from screening and diagnostic testing into plan of care

**IV. Professional Role and Responsibilities**

**B. Practice Management**

1. Document patient encounters in a manner which supports applicable diagnostic and procedure codes
2. Utilize appropriate billing and coding to facilitate reimbursement

## THE WELL-CHILD VISIT

During the well-child visit, attending to parental concerns is of prime importance.

The development of a trusting provider-child-parent relationship is remarkably important if the child and parent are to confide their concerns effectively. Building this relationship takes time, and is facilitated by continuity of visits with a particular provider. In addition to trust-building, the child and parent need to view the provider's advice as effective and valid. Skills important for relationship building include:

- Showing respect in all areas
- Committing time and attention to the particular concern
- Utilizing vocabulary that communicates understanding and competence
- Maintaining confidentiality
- Demonstrating empathy (Treitz et al., 2020).

Surveillance, screening, and evaluation are components of the health supervision visit. Surveillance considers overall health and social risk factors that put the child at risk for illness or developmental delays. Screening uses testing to determine physical health (or lack thereof) and standardized checklists to determine achievement of developmental milestones. Further evaluation is warranted when surveillance or screening identifies a concern in relation to physical health development. The well-child visit includes developmental surveillance, observation of the parent-child interaction, determination of adequate growth, a complete health assessment, universal and selective screenings, immunizations, and anticipatory guidance (Hagan et al., 2017). The schedule for recommended health supervision visits in childhood and adolescence (AAP, Bright Futures, 2020).

During the health supervision visit, it is important to take into account the family's health beliefs and cultural values. Primary responsibility for caring for the child falls to the mother in most cultures. In some cultures, however, it is the father or grandparents who are responsible for major health-related decisions. A family's religious or spiritual background can strongly influence their health beliefs, sometimes creating conflict when the health provider has a different belief system than that of the child's family. Family practices related to growth and development may also vary according to culture. Many times, the practices are not harmful and should be supported by provider, as long as they are safe for the child. Never make assumptions about a family's cultural practices based on their name, accent, or skin color; rather assess each family individually to ensure an adequate assessment (Marion et al., 2017).

## DEVELOPMENTAL SURVEILLANCE

Through developmental surveillance at the health supervision visit, children who may have or may be at risk for a developmental delay are identified. When performing developmental surveillance determine and turn your attention to parental concerns. Ask parents if they have any concerns about the child's behavior, development, or learning. Also ask what new things they have noticed the child doing (Lipkin et al., 2020). Maintain a developmental history in the child's health record, as reviewing the history over time may reveal abnormalities or deviations in development (Aites & Schonwald, 2020). The developmental history should include information about social skills, self-help, receptive and expressive verbal language, and attainment of gross and fine motor skills (Hagan et al., 2017). Refer to chapters 7 through 11 for additional information related to ages for expected developmental milestones.

Also identify child risk and protective factors. Child risk factors for developmental delay or issues with behavior include:

- Perinatal infections or other exposures
- Birth complications
- Medical or genetic conditions
- Adverse childhood or family experiences (Aites & Schonwald, 2020). Adverse childhood experiences (ACES) are potentially traumatic events occurring during childhood.

Parental factors placing the child at risk for developmental or behavioral concerns include:

- Unemployment
- Mental health problems
- Limited education or low literacy level
- Teenage parents (Aites & Schonwald, 2020)

Protective factors for development and behavior that also promote resilience include:

- Active parent-child engagement
- Strong connections in a supportive, loving family
- Opportunities for interaction with other children
- The chance to grow in independence in a safe environment with appropriate structure (Aites & Schonwald, 2020).

Always record the findings of developmental surveillance as well as specific actions and plans so the child's progress can be tracked across visits. As needed, collaborate with other professionals working with the child and family. Refer to chapters 13 through 18 for specific developmental information according to the child's age.

## PARENT-CHILD INTERACTION OBSERVATION

Observe the child and parent-child interaction noting the level of warmth, caring, and responsiveness of the parent to the child's cues. Determine the extent to which the child looks to the parent for support and comfort (Aites & Schwartz, 2020). Note reciprocity between the infant or toddler and the parent. Determine the emotional tone of the parent and child, noting if the child is anxious or calm and if the parent is overly controlling or critical. Observe whether the parent shares positive information about the child or responds to the child in a positive manner. Note if the parent permits the older child to communicate with the provider directly (Hagan et al., 2017).

## DETERMINATION OF ADEQUATE GROWTH

At each health supervision visit plot each of the child's growth measurements on the appropriate growth chart for age and gender. Growth measurements include weight, recumbent length (2 years and under) or height, head circumference (through age 2 years), and weight for stature (2 years and under) or body mass index (over age 2 years). For typically growing infants, length and weight measures commonly cross over a percentile line. After approximately 18 months of age, one percentile curve for each measurement is generally followed for most healthy children (Treitz et al., 2020). Chapter 3 provides additional information about growth measurements. The clinical growth charts for age and gender may be found at:

- World Health Organization (WHO) growth charts (birth to 2 years; Centers for Disease Control and Prevention [CDC], 2010)
- CDC clinical growth charts (2 to 20 years; CDC, 2017)

**PRO TIP** Developmental surveillance, screening, and evaluation, as well as plotting of growth measurement of former premature infants should be based on the child's adjusted age, rather than the chronological age, until at least 2 years. Health supervision visits and their other components should occur at the recommended chronological age.

# COMPLETE HEALTH ASSESSMENT

The health supervision visit allows for comprehensive assessment of the child and an opportunity to provide further evaluation if there are concerns related to development or the child's physical health status (Turner, 2018). The complete health assessment includes a thorough health history and comprehensive physical examination.

## HEALTH HISTORY

A unique feature of the pediatric health history is that it represents a combination of parents' objective reporting of facts, parents' subjective interpretation of their child's symptoms or skills, and in the older child, their self-reported history of events. The history provide by the child and parents may be very specific and detailed or it may be somewhat vague, in which case more focused probing is required. Working with the family to truly understand their concerns about the child will help to distinguish organic, emotional, and/or behavioral conditions, thereby minimizing unneeded testing and intervention (Treitz et al., 2020). Again, the provider-family relationship is a crucial component for obtaining an accurate and thorough health history. The pediatric historical database should include:

- Demographic information
- Allergies
- Routine medications
- Birth history
- Results of prior screenings
- Immunizations
- Current concerns
- Medical history
- Diet
- Family history
- Social history (including childcare or school attendance/performance)
- Attainment of developmental milestones
- Sexual history
- Review of systems (Treitz et al., 2020)

Refer to chapter 3 for a thorough discussion of the pediatric health history.

## PHYSICAL EXAMINATION

Conduct a comprehensive physical examination at each health supervision visit (Drutz et al., 2020). Refer to chapters 13–18 for specific assessments typically revealed at certain ages.

# UNIVERSAL AND SELECTIVE SCREENINGS

Screening refers to testing for disease or delay in a child or population that otherwise appears to be healthy. The goal of screening is to identify children at increased risk of development delay, behavioral disorder, or disease who warrant additional testing. Universal screening refers to the screening of every child at a particular age. Selective screening refers to screening children having a characteristic or characteristics leading the provider to believe that the screening may be positive. The positive predictive value of a test is increased with selective screening (Kelly, 2020). Bright Futures recommends both universal screening for particular items at certain ages and selective screening at certain ages based on risk factors.

## NEWBORN SCREENING

Newborn screening includes testing for inborn errors of metabolism, certain inherited disorders, critical congenital heart disease of the newborn, and hearing acuity. Refer to chapter 13 for additional information.

## BLOOD PRESSURE SCREENING

The AAP recommends screening blood pressure annually beginning at age 3.

## VISION SCREENING

Vision screening is performed at every health supervision visit until age 30 months. This screening includes inspection of the eyes and lids, assessment for presence of bilateral red reflex, determination of fixating and following (beginning at 2 months of age), corneal light reflex for strabismus assessment (2 months to 5 years), and cover testing for strabismus assessment (6 months to 5 years). Beginning at age 3 years, begin fundoscopic examination and visual acuity testing with a preliterate chart (Treitz et al., 2020). Vision screening is then recommended annually in the 3- to 6-year-old, and at the 8, 10, 12, and 15 year visits (AAP, Bright Futures, 2020).

## HEARING SCREENING

If the newborn hearing evaluation is normal, conduct a hearing risk assessment at each health supervision visit. The risk assessment includes auditory skills monitoring, developmental surveillance, and assessment of parental concern. Determine if the following risk factors for hearing loss are present:

- Parental concern regarding hearing, speech, language, or development
- Family history of permanent childhood hearing loss
- Chronic or recurrent otitis media with effusion
- Adenoid hypertrophy, cleft palate
- Neonatal intensive care unit (NICU) stay of ≥5 days
- NICU stay (regardless of duration) requiring extracorporeal membrane oxygenation, assisted ventilation, exchange transfusion for hyperbilirubinemia, or exposure to loop diuretics
- Congenital or central nervous system infections
- Ototoxic drug exposure, including chemotherapy
- Head trauma or congenital head and neck deformities
- Syndromes associated with hearing loss
- Neurodegenerative disorders
- Exposure to loud noises over extended periods of time

## ANEMIA

Universally screen for anemia with a hemoglobin level at 12 months of age. Selectively screen at other visits based on risk assessment (Kleinman & Greer, 2020).

## DYSLIPIDEMIA SCREENING

Screen all children for dyslipidemia once between 9 and 11 years of age, and once between 17 and 21 years of age. Selectively screen at other visits based on risk assessment.

## LEAD SCREENING

Obtain serum lead levels on all children at 12 and 24 months of age if in a high prevalence area for lead poisoning or if the child is on Medicaid. Selectively screen at other visits from 6 months to 6 years of age based on risk assessment.

# IMMUNIZATIONS

One of the greatest public health achievements of modern times, immunization in the United States, has resulted in the annual incidence of diphtheria, paralytic poliomyelitis, measles, mumps, rubella, and Haemophilus influenzae type b (Hib) falling by more than 99% compared with the 20th century (Daley et al., 2020). Herd immunity resulting from childhood immunization is also responsible for significant decreases in pneumococcal, rotavirus, and varicella infections in adults. Immunization coverage rates in 2017 for children age 19 to 35 months were more than 90% for poliovirus, measles-mumps-rubella, varicella, and hepatitis B, while more recently recommended vaccines such as rotavirus and hepatitis A demonstrate coverage rates of around 75% (CDC, 2020a).

While previously generally positive, public perceptions surrounding routine childhood immunization have resulted in recent parental concerns about vaccine safety. These concerns were partly fueled by unfounded speculation about an association between immunizations and autism (Daley et al., 2020). Current vaccines demonstrate a high degree of safety, and immunization benefits strongly outweigh the very rare risks of serious adverse events. Families may also have concerns related to religious or other beliefs.

**PRO TIP** When discussing the risks and benefits of immunizations, provide factual information clearly in an empathetic and nonjudgmental manner.

## TYPES OF IMMUNIZATIONS

The current recommended childhood and adolescent immunization schedule provides protection against (administration route follows each listed:

- Hepatitis B (intramuscular [IM])
- Diphtheria, tetanus, and pertussis (IM)

- Haemophilus influenzae type b (IM)
- Pneumococcus (IM)
- Polio (IM or subcutaneous [SC])
- Rotavirus (oral)
- Influenza (IM or intranasal)
- Measles, mumps, rubella (SC)
- Varicella (SC)
- Hepatitis A (IM)
- Human papilloma virus (IM)
- Meningococcal meningitis (IM) (CDC, 2020b)

The schedule may be downloaded from www.cdc.gov/vaccines/schedules/hcp/imz/child-adolescent.html. The CDC recommends the following strategies to increase immunization rates:

- Recommend immunizations to parents and reinforce when to return to receive the vaccines
- Send reminder messages to parents
- Keep accurate immunization records
- Flag health records with immunization reminders
- Reduce missed opportunities for immunizations (know the true contraindications, otherwise, provide the immunization)
- Reduce office barriers to immunization
- Assess and provide feedback on provider/practice immunization rates

## VACCINE INFORMATION STATEMENTS

It is the provider's responsibility to educate the parents about the benefits and risks of the immunizations, as well as obtain their consent for administration. All immunizations covered under the Vaccine Injury Compensation Program must be accompanied the corresponding Vaccine Information Statement (VIS), given to the parent each time the particular vaccine is given (CDC, 2020c). The current VISs may be retrieved from www.cdc.gov/vaccines/hcp/vis/current-vis.html.

## ADMINISTRATION AND DOCUMENTATION

Use a separate syringe for each vaccine and only sterile needles for administration of immunizations. Alcohol (70% solution) may be used to cleanse the top of the immunization vial and to cleanse the child's skin prior to administration. Provide IM injection at a 90-degree angle to the skin, using a needle that is sufficiently long to reach the muscle tissue (see Table 12.1). Administer a SC injection at a 45-degree angle. Aspiration is neither recommended nor required for either route.

Documentation required for each immunization in the health record includes:

- Date of administration
- Site and route of administration
- Vaccine manufacturer
- Lot number
- Expiration date
- VIS version

A sample immunization record created by the Immunization Coalition is available at www.immunize.org/catg.d/p2022.pdf/.

**TABLE 12.1 Recommended Injection Sites and Needle Sizes**

| Age | Needle Gauge | Needle Length | Site |
|---|---|---|---|
| **Intramuscular** | | | |
| **Birth–28 days** | 25 gauge | 5⁄8 inch | Anterolateral thigh |
| **1–12 months** | 23–25 gauge | 1 inch | Anterolateral thigh |
| **1–2 years** | 23–25 gauge | 1–1.25 inch<br>5⁄8–1inch | Anterolateral thigh Deltoid |
| **3–18 years** | 22–25 gauge | 1–1.25 inch<br>5⁄8–1inch | Anterolateral thigh Deltoid |
| ***Subcutaneous*** | | | |
| **1–12 months** | 23–25 gauge | 5⁄8 inch | Anterolateral thigh in the fatty tissue |
| **>12 months** | 23–25 gauge | 5⁄8 inch | Anterolateral thigh or triceps area in the fatty tissue |

*Sources*: Data from Daley, M. F., O'Leary, S. T., Nyquist, A. C., & Cataldi, J. R. (2020). Immunization. In W. W. Hay, M. J. Levin, M. J. Abzug, & M. Bunik (Eds.), *Current diagnosis & treatment: Pediatrics* (25th ed., Chapter 10). McGraw-Hill Education; Immunization Action Coalition. (2020). *Administering vaccines: Dose, route, site, and needle size.* http://www.immunize.org/catg.d/p3085.pdf

**PRO TIP** To promote atraumatic care, apply a topical emulsion of 5% lidocaine-prilocaine to the administration site 30 to 60 minutes prior to the injection.

## ANTICIPATORY GUIDANCE

Anticipatory guidance is defined as proactive or preventive counseling addressing the significant physical, emotional, psychological, and developmental changes that will occur in children during the time between health supervision visits. Areas covered include health promotion, developmental and behavioral issues, diet, and safety/injury prevention. In order for anticipatory guidance to be most helpful, it must be age-appropriate and timely (Treitz et al., 2020).

Anticipatory guidance helps to avoid future problems. Educating parents about what to expect in the next phase of development gives parents the tools needed to support child's development safely. It is necessary to address issues in depth, rather than touching on them superficially. The information should be reviewed orally, providing the child and parent the opportunity to have questions answered. Written information should also be provided, keeping in mind the parent's literacy level and primary language. Bright Futures provides a wide selection of handouts at https://brightfutures.aap.org/clinical-practice/Pages/default.aspx. Additional handouts created by the Children's Hospital of Philadelphia are available at www.chop.edu/primary-care/well-child-visits-what-expect

### SOCIAL DETERMINANTS OF HEALTH

Social determinants of health are conditions in the environment in which the child lives, learns, plays, or worships. The determinants may affect a wide range of health outcomes and contribute to risk. Social engagement and sense of well-being or security are also considered social determinants of health (U.S. Department of Health and Human Services [USDHHS], 2020). Bright Futures recommends assessing social determinants of health at each health supervision visit (Hagan et al., 2017). Some examples of resources considered to be social determinants include:

- Safe housing
- Healthy food availability
- Education access
- Local health and emergency services
- Absence of life-threatening toxins
- Social norms or attitudes in the local community
- Crime or violence in the area
- Social support
- Language and literacy
- Social norms and attitudes (Hagan et al., 2017; USDHHS, 2020)

### NUTRITION

Children's nutrient requirements are influenced by their body composition, the composition of new growth, and by their growth rate, all of which vary over time (Haemer et al., 2020). Growth rates are highest during infancy, followed by adolescence. Nutritional requirements for each age group are presented in corresponding chapters 6 through 11. Anticipatory guidance related to nutrition according to age is covered in chapters 13 through 18.

### SLEEP

Sleep requirements vary according to the child's age and activity. Refer to chapters 13 through 18 for anticipatory guidance for sleep according to age.

### TEMPERAMENT, BEHAVIOR, DEVELOPMENT, AND DISCIPLINE

A large component of anticipatory guidance is includes the topics of development, behavior, temperament, and discipline. Always provide counseling related to the child's current status or the parents' concerns, as well as guidance related to the upcoming stages. Additional information is found in chapters 13 through 18.

### DENTAL HEALTH

The promotion of oral health is critically important to the infant and child's overall health. Provision of anticipatory guidance related to oral health is provided in chapter 18. Once the infant's first tooth has erupted, the child should have the first dental visit. Stress to the parents the importance of the dental home. The ongoing relationship of the dentist and the child/family provides for optimal, accessible, family-centered oral health and the optimum outcome for the child (Hagan et al., 2017). Resources related to oral health may be found at:

- National Maternal and Child Oral Health Resource Center: www.mchoralhealth.org
- AAP: www.aap.org/en-us/advocacy -and-policy/aap-health-initiatives/Oral-Health/Pages/Oral-Health.aspx
- American Academy of Pediatric Dentistry: www.aapd.org/resources/resources/

### Fluoride Varnish

In young children at high-risk for dental caries, particularly those not visiting the dentist regularly, fluoride varnish applied by the primary care provider is recommended. Risk factors for dental caries include:

- Low socioeconomic status
- Lack of access to dental care
- Suboptimal parental knowledge regarding oral health
- Inadequate tooth brushing or inadequate use of fluoride-containing toothpastes Risk factors for low community water fluoride levels
- Tooth enamel defects
- Cariogenic diet (frequent exposure to refined carbohydrates and dietary sugar)
- Inappropriate bottle feeding
- Maternal caries or maternal poor oral hygeine

Varnish application is well tolerated by infants and young child. Begin varnish treatments upon eruption of the first tooth and continue 4 times annually throughout early childhood. The unit does package provides a disposable brush, and a premeasured amount of 5% fluoride solution. Dry the teeth and quickly apply the varnish to tooth surfaces one quadrant at the time. Having the young child drink some water immediately after the application assists with setting the varnish. Instruct the family to withhold toothbrushing until the following day (Boulter, 2010; Clark et al., 2014).

## SAFETY

Age-appropriate topics for anticipatory guidance related to safety that should be covered at each health supervision visit include environmental exposure, risk-taking behaviors, social situations, sports and recreation, and vehicle safety, at a minimum. Additional topics may also be addressed according to the child's age. Refer to chapters 13 through 18 for specific safety information guidance per age.

## KEY POINTS

- The well child visit is comprised of observation of the parent-child interaction, growth measurement, developmental surveillance, and a comprehensive history and physical examination.
- Screen blood pressure annually beginning at age 3 years.
- A screening hemoglobin is obtained and 12 months of age and at other visits depending upon the risk assessment.
- Hearing, vision, dyslipidemia, and lead level are also screening according to the child's age and the AAP recommendations.
- Utilize the current recommended immunization schedule to provide immunizations based on the child's age.
- Provide anticipatory guidance relative to the child's age on social determinants of health, nutrition, sleep, dental health, and safety, as well as temperament, behavior, development and discipline.

## REFERENCES

Aites, J., & Schonwald, A. (2020). Developmental-behavioral surveillance and screening in primary care. In M. Augustyn (Ed.), *UpToDate*. Retrieved December 4, 2020, from https://www.uptodate.com/contents/developmental-behavioral-surveillance-and-screening-in-primary-care

American Academy of Pediatrics, Bright Futures. (2020). *Recommendations for preventive pediatric health care*. https://downloads.aap.org/AAP/PDF/periodicity_schedule.pdf

Boulter, S. (2010). Fluoride varnish application tips. In S. Tanski, L. C. Garfunkel, P. M. Duncan, & M. Weitzman (Eds.), *Performing preventive services: A Bright Futures handbook*. American Academy of Pediatrics.

Centers for Disease Control and Prevention. (2010). *WHO growth standards are recommended for use in the U.S. for infants and children 0 to 2 years of age*. https://www.cdc.gov/growthcharts/who_charts.htm

Centers for Disease Control and Prevention. (2017). *Clinical growth charts*. https://www.cdc.gov/growthcharts/clinical_charts.htm

Centers for Disease Control and Prevention. (2020a). *2016–2017 childhood vaccination coverage combined birth year dashboard*. https://www.cdc.gov/vaccines/imz-managers/coverage/childvaxview/interactive-reports/dashboards/2016-2017.html

Centers for Disease Control and Prevention. (2020b). *Immunization schedules: Recommended child and adolescent immunization schedule for ages 18 years or younger, United States, 2020*. https://www.cdc.gov/vaccines/schedules/hcp/child-adolescent.html

Centers for Disease Control and Prevention. (2020c). *Vaccine information statements (VISs)*. https://www.cdc.gov/vaccines/hcp/vis/index.html

Clark, M. B., Slayton, R. L., & the Section on Oral Health. (2014). Fluoride use in caries prevention in the primary care setting. *Pediatrics, 134*(3), 626–633. https://doi.org/10.1542/peds.2014-1699

Daley, M. F., O'Leary, S. T., Nyquist, A. C., & Cataldi, J. R. (2020). Immunization. In W. W. Hay, M. J. Levin, M. J. Abzug, & M. Bunik (Eds.), *Current diagnosis & treatment: Pediatrics* (25th ed., Chapter 10). McGraw-Hill Education.

Drutz, J. E. (2020). The pediatric physical examination: General principles and standard measurements. In T. K. Duryea (Ed.), *UpToDate*. Retrieved December 4, 2020, from https://www.uptodate.com/contents/the-pediatric-physical-examination-general-principles-and-standard-measurements

Haemer, M. A., Diab, L. K., Primak, L. E., & Krebs, N. F. (2020). Normal childhood nutrition & its disorders. In W. W. Hay, M. J. Levin, M. J. Abzug, & M. Bunik (Eds.), *Current diagnosis & treatment: Pediatrics* (25th ed., Chapter 11). McGraw-Hill Education.

Hagan, J. F., Shaw, J. S., & Duncan, P. M. (2017). *Bright futures: Guidelines for health supervision of infants, children, and adolescents*. American Academy of Pediatrics.

Immunization Action Coalition. (2020). *Administering vaccines: Dose, route, site, and needle size*. http://www.immunize.org/catg.d/p3085.pdf

Kelly, N. R. (2020). Screening tests in children and adolescents. In J. E. Drutz (Ed.), *UpToDate*. Retrieved December 4, 2020, from https://www.uptodate.com/contents/screening-tests-in-children-and-adolescents

Kleinman, R. E., & Greer, F. R. (2020). *Pediatric nutrition* (8th ed.). American Academy of Pediatrics.

Lipkin, P. H., Macias, M. M., & the Council on Children with Disabilities, Section on Developmental and Behavioral Pediatrics. (2020). Promoting optimal development: Identifying infants and young children with developmental disorders through developmental surveillance and screening. *Pediatrics, 145*(1), e20193449. https://doi.org/10.1542/peds.2019-3449

Marion, L., Douglas, M., Lavin, M. A., Barr, N., Gazaway, S., Thomas, E., & Bickford, C. (2017). Implementing the new ANA standard 8: Culturally congruent practice. *Online Journal of Issues in Nursing, 22*(1). http://ojin.nursingworld.org/MainMenuCategories/ANAMarketplace/ANAPeriodicals/OJIN/TableofContents/Vol-22-2017/No1-Jan-2017/Articles-Previous-Topics/Implementing-the-New-ANA-Standard-8.html

Treitz, M., Nicklas, D., & Fox, D. (2020). Ambulatory & office pediatrics. In W. W. Hay, M. J. Levin, M. J. Abzug, & M. Bunik (Eds.), *Current diagnosis & treatment: Pediatrics* (25th ed., Chapter 9). McGraw-Hill Education.

Turner, K. (2018). Well-child visits for infants and young children. *American Family Physician, 98*(6), 347–353. https://www.aafp.org/afp/2018/0915/p347.html

U.S. Department of Health and Human Services. (2020). *Social determinants of health*. https://www.healthypeople.gov/2020/topics-objectives/topic/social-determinants-of-health

# Well-Child Visits During the Newborn Period

Daniel Crawford, Steadman McPeters, and Paige Ricca

## Student Learning Outcomes

**Upon completion of this chapter the reader should be able to:**

1. Determine adequacy of growth of newborns.
2. Evaluate developmental milestones of newborns.
3. Choose appropriate screening tests based on current recommendations for child's age and risk status.
4. Select immunizations based on current recommendations for child's age and risk status.
5. Determine applicable anticipatory guidance for each scheduled visit during the newborn period.

## INTRODUCTION

The newborn period provides an opportunity for the healthcare provider and family to establish a relationship and work collaboratively to support the newborn's health. This serves as the foundation for the lasting parent-child-provider relationship that will support the health of the child and family throughout childhood. Establishing trust and supporting new parents are vital elements of the relationship-building process and should be considerations for framing the interactions that take place during the newborn period.

During this period, Bright Futures recommends two standard outpatient well visits (Hagan et al., 2017). The first newborn visit should take place at 3 to 5 days of life and within 48 to 72 hours of discharge from the hospital (American Academy of Pediatrics [AAP], 2010, reaffirmed 2015; Hagan et al., 2017). Newborns who are born via cesarean delivery and with a hospitalization that lasts greater than 96 hours should be seen within the first week of life (Hagan et al., 2017). The second newborn visit should take place by 1 month of age (Hagan et al., 2017).

The content in this chapter maps to the following areas on the Pediatric Nursing Certification Board (PNCB) Pediatric Nurse Practitioner—Primary Care certification examination:

CONTENT AREAS:

**I. Health Maintenance and Promotion**

**A. Partner with patients/caregivers to support growth and development from infancy to young adulthood**

**B. Provide patients/caregivers with age/developmentally appropriate anticipatory guidance**

**C. Recommend and prescribe immunizations according to current CDC guidelines**

**D. Educate about illness prevention and early warning signs of pediatric illness and emergencies**

**E. Advise patients/caregivers about age appropriate injury prevention and safety (environmental exposure, risk taking behaviors, social situations, sports and recreation, and vehicle safety)**

**F. Counsel about age-appropriate social, behavioral, and mental health concerns (e.g., substance abuse, social media use, grief and loss, and sexual orientation/LGBTQ)**

**II. Assessment and Diagnosis**

**A. Growth and Development**

1. Evaluate and interpret growth parameters
2. Perform developmental surveillance

**B. History and Physical Examination**

1. Obtain history of present illness
2. Obtain a comprehensive health history for new patients
3. Complete an interval history for established patients
4. Perform a review of systems
5. Perform a complete physical examination

**C. Diagnostic Testing and Screening**

1. Order and interpret office/clinic based screening tests
4. Select, utilize, and interpret developmental, behavioral and mental health screening and assessment tools

**D. Analyzing Information**

1. Integrate health history and physical examination findings into the plan of care
2. Assimilate findings from screening and diagnostic testing into plan of care

**IV. Professional Role and Responsibilities**

**B. Practice Management**

1. Document patient encounters in a manner which supports applicable diagnostic and procedure codes
2. Utilize appropriate billing and coding to facilitate reimbursement

## PARENT-CHILD INTERACTION

Bringing a newborn home from the hospital can be one of the most significant transitions in the life of the family and is characterized by new role development. This initial transition is often marked by a combination of physical and emotional responses ranging from joy to sadness, hope to fear, readiness to embark on this new adventure to uncertainty and feelings of inadequacy, as well as the gamut of excitement to exhaustion. In this initial newborn visit, it is important for the healthcare provider to assess the family's transition to the home environment. This transition period can set the stage for bonding and the building of family relationships, which have significant implications for the health of the child, so it is important that the transition be assessed.

Specific questions should be asked at this visit regarding the newborn's adjustment to the new home environment, as well as the family's adjustment experience and role delineation including parents, siblings, or others in the home. Families should be assured that the range of physical and emotional responses they are experiencing is expected and encouraged to care for themselves while also caring for the infant. This transition period can be difficult for siblings to adjust to, so the provider should be sure to ask questions related to the sibling experience for households where sibling(s) are present in the home. Parents should be encouraged to ensure dedicated time spent with the sibling(s), to reassure them that they are loved and secure, and to provide a safe environment for the sibling(s) to express their emotions to the parents.

There are a number of factors that can affect attachment between the newborn and family and the newborn's transition to the home environment. Variation in infant behaviors such as a newborn with colic or fussiness, parental factors such as postpartum depression (PPD), or misalignment between parent and newborn attachment styles can affect this process. There are also cultural factors that must be understood as to their effects on the attachment process. It is important for the healthcare provider to both understand and account for these when supporting newborn and family attachment.

## CULTURALLY HUMBLE APPROACH TO ASSESSING ATTACHMENT AND TRANSITION TO HOME

The profession of nursing was one of the first healthcare professions to emphasize the importance of a culturally competent or culturally humble approach to care of individuals and their families (American Nurses Association, 2019). Cultural humility can be distinguished from the idea of cultural competence as an approach to culturally sensitive care. Cultural humility was originally proposed in the context of care for people from racial/ethnic minority backgrounds and should be extended to the care of all newborns (Tervalon & Murray-Garcia, 1998). Instead of using the term *cultural competence*, which suggests specific endpoints, cultural sensitivity may be a more appropriate term to reflect a type of cultural humility, as it reflects self-evaluation, self-critique, and attempts to display awareness of dominant versus nondominant cultural practices within a community setting. To ensure the provision of culturally humble care, the healthcare provider should approach the interaction by being open to new ideas, ensuring self-awareness, demonstrating humility toward others, creating a positive interaction with the infant and family, and reflecting on their own experience and feelings related to the encounter (Foronda et al., 2016). With increased globalization, the practice of cultural humility results in increased accuracy of assessments and decreases in health disparities.

TABLE 13.1 **Newborn Developmental Milestones**

| | Gross Motor | Fine Motor | Language | Social |
|---|---|---|---|---|
| Birth to 1 month | Reflexive extremity movement<br>Turns head to side<br>Lifts chin when lying prone | Holds hands/fingers closed, near face<br>Reflexive palmar grasp<br>Visually tracks objects to midline | Cries<br>Startles to sounds<br>Calms to voice<br>Begins to recognize mother's voice<br>Makes limited, short vowel sounds | Makes limited eye contact when held<br>Calms when picked up<br>Will look at objects in visual fields briefly, prefers black & white objects/patterns |

*Sources*: Data from Hagan, J. F., Shaw, J. S., & Duncan, P. M. (Eds.). (2017). *Bright futures* (4th ed.). American Academy of Pediatrics; Scharf, R. J., Scharf, G. J., & Stroustrup, A. (2016). Developmental milestones. *Pediatrics in Review, 37*(1), 25–47. https://doi.org/10.1542/pir.2014-0103.

# DEVELOPMENTAL SURVEILLANCE

The newborn acquires the emergence of developmental skills across all domains. The acquisition of these skills serves as the foundation for ongoing growth and development. Developmental surveillance for acquisition of expected developmental milestones is performed at all newborn well-child visits. Recognition of delayed milestone acquisition in the newborn period is imperative and requires further investigation to determine the need for intervention. Early intervention supports superior developmental outcomes for the newborn. Expected milestones developing over the first month of life in the gross motor, fine motor, language, and social domains are outlined in Table 13.1.

**PRO TIP** Early identification and intervention with developmental delays support superior outcomes.

# HEALTH ASSESSMENT

Each newborn visit will include a comprehensive health assessment. The assessment includes developmental surveillance, as noted earlier, as well as health history and physical examination data and anticipatory guidance.

## SUBJECTIVE DATA

An important component in caring for the newborn is ensuring that a comprehensive health history (CHH) has been performed. If the provider has examined the newborn in the inpatient setting, the CHH is completed at that time, but should be reviewed in the context of this visit. For those cases where this is the first time the newborn is evaluated by the healthcare provider, it is important to take the time to ensure that a CHH is performed. At the one-month visit, the healthcare provider completes an interval history that reviews pertinent information from the initial comprehensive history as well as events that have occurred/changed in the interim. Components of the newborn comprehensive history are outlined in Table 13.2.

▶ ALERT: Developmental warning signs in the newborn include:

- young infant is unresponsive to loud noise
- stiff or floppy extremities
- excessive sleepiness, difficulty awakening to feed
- excessive irritability

## OBJECTIVE DATA

For all newborns, it is important to include a comprehensive physical examination during both of the newborn outpatient visits. This physical examination should mirror that completed in the inpatient setting. Details related to the components of the comprehensive physical examination of the newborn are reviewed in Table 13.3.

# PREVENTION

Primary and secondary prevention are important components of the newborn visits.

## IMMUNIZATIONS

According to the Advisory Committee on Immunization Practices (ACIP) vaccine schedule, newborns should receive the hepatitis B vaccine within 24 hours of birth (Centers for Disease Control and Prevention [CDC], 2020; Schillie et al., 2018). If the hepatitis B immunization

**TABLE 13.2 Newborn Comprehensive History**

| | Items to Address |
|---|---|
| Maternal Health History | General health<br>Conditions that can affect pregnancy (hypertension, diabetes, epilepsy, infectious disease, thyroid disorder, metabolic disorder)<br>Medications and/or supplements taken routinely or during pregnancy<br>Tobacco, alcohol, or illicit drug use |
| Pregnancy History | Gravida and parity<br>Prenatal care<br>Method of conception<br>Results of prenatal tests<br>Complications during pregnancy |
| Birth History | Gestational age<br>Delivery method (e.g., vaginal, cesarean)<br>Use of assistive devices<br>Medications during labor<br>Length of labor<br>Fetal distress<br>Rupture of membranes and appearance of amniotic fluid |
| Neonatal History | Anthropometric measurements (weight, length, orbital frontal cortex)<br>Vital signs<br>APGAR scores<br>Complications after delivery during hospitalization<br>Resuscitation and thermoregulation |
| Family History | Chronic conditions and/or inherited disorders<br>Neonatal deaths<br>Unexplained deaths<br>Consanguinity |
| Social History | People living in the home<br>Details of home setting (e.g., type of housing, housing stability, location)<br>People responsible for caring for the child<br>Access to food—screening for food insecurity |
| Newborn-Specific History | Feeding<br>Sleep<br>Elimination<br>Development and adaptation to new home environment |

is not administered during hospitalization, it should be administered at the initial newborn visit. At the one-month visit, the healthcare provider discusses the standard immunization schedule and reviews vaccines to be administered at the 2-month well child visit. Providers should answer questions that the family has related to vaccines and be willing to discuss the rationale for the prescribed immunization schedule. Immunization status for parents, siblings, and caregivers should be reviewed (Hagan et al., 2017). Vaccines for influenza and pertussis should be up to date for those who come in contact with or are involved in caregiving for the newborn.

## SCREENINGS

During the newborn period, order and/or review results from hearing, critical congenital heart disease, and state newborn screening for metabolic and/or certain inherited disorders (Hagan et al., 2017). Typically, these screenings are completed in the hospital or birth place setting. However, it is important that the healthcare provider ensures that these screenings are completed. If the hearing screening is not completed prior to discharge, the screen is ordered during the initial clinic visit. Infants that fail the initial hearing

**TABLE 13.3 Newborn Physical Examination**

| Body System | Physical Examination Findings | Abnormal Physical Findings |
|---|---|---|
| Vital Signs/Growth Measurement<br>15–30 gm/day | Vital signs—temperature, respiratory rate (30–60 breaths/min), heart rate (80–100 beats/min; 70–80 during sleep; 120–160 awake), blood pressure (57–69 systolic; 44–52 diastolic)<br>Occipitofrontal head circumference (32–38 cm)<br>Recumbent length (44–55 cm)<br>Weight (2500–3900 g)<br>Chest circumference (30–36 cm; ~ 1–3 cm < OFC w/average 2 cm < than OFC)<br>Abdominal circumference (32–36 weeks' gestation equal to OFC; after 36 weeks gestation, > OFC) | Temperature instability—<97.7 °F (36.5 °C) after 4 hours of discharge<br>Low birth weight infants—<2500 g<br>Small for gestational age—birth weight below the 10th percentile for age<br>Large for gestational age—birth weight greater than the 90th percentile for age |
| General Observations | New Ballard Score (shortly after birth)<br>APGAR Score (at delivery)<br>Assess for alertness and any signs of distress<br>Assess for posture, tone, and self-symmetry<br>Assess for self-soothing measures<br>Observe for congenital anomalies | Heart defects, neural tube defects, and Down syndrome<br>Abnormal posturing, floppy or very jittery, abnormal cry<br>Moro reflex<br>Poor sucking<br>Poor rooting |
| Skin | Assess the color and note any skin lesions, birthmarks<br>**Common skin conditions:**<br>Acrocyanosis<br>Accessory tragi<br>Cavernous hemangiomas<br>Clinical jaundice<br>Cutis marmorata<br>Erythema toxicum 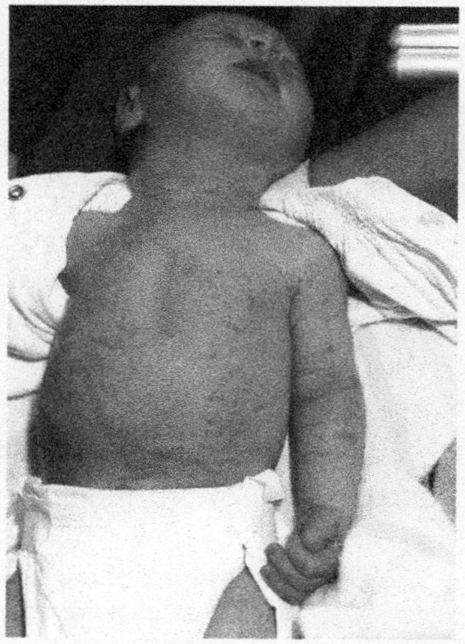 | Jaundice occurring in the first 24 hours of life with associated hyperbilirubinemia resulting from hemolysis |

(continued)

**TABLE 13.3 Newborn Physical Examination** (*continued*)

| Body System | Physical Examination Findings | Abnormal Physical Findings |
|---|---|---|
| | Miliaria rubra (prickly heat rash)<br>Nevus simplex, nevus flammeus<br>Sturge-Weber Port Wine nevi<br>Transient neonatal pustular melanosis<br>Assess skin turgor | |
| Head | Observe shape (sutures, molding), size, and fontanels (anterior and posterior)<br>Assess scalp hair<br>Assess the symmetry of the face | Unusual or dysmorphic features of the face—hyper or hypotelorism, epicanthal folds<br>Evidence of birth trauma (molding, caput succedaneum, cephalhematoma) (A) Caput results from diffuse swelling. (B) Cephalohematoma results from bleeding beneath the periosteum.<br>Severe microcephaly with partially collapsed skull<br>Macrocephaly |

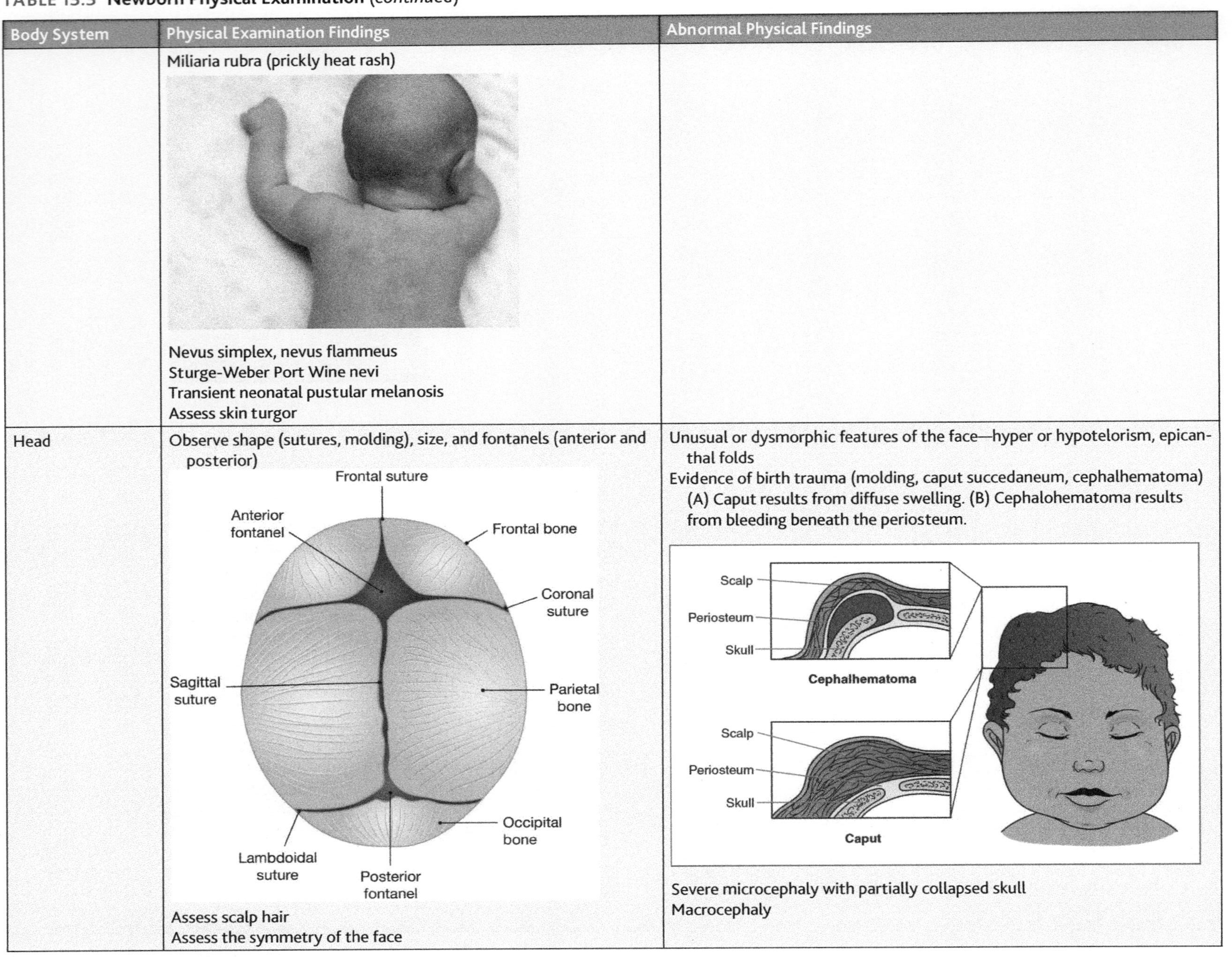

| | | |
|---|---|---|
| Eyes | Inspect eyes and eyelids regarding shape, edema, and drainage<br>Assess the sclera, conjunctiva for color and scleral hemorrhages<br>Examine pupils for opacification and red reflexes<br>Assess visual acuity using fixate and follow response | Absent red reflex<br>Unequal pupillary sizes<br>Scarring and pigment changes to the back of the eye |
| Ears | Observe the shape and position of the pinnae<br>Note the patency of auditory canals<br>Assess the visualization of the tympanic membrane<br>Inspect for the presence of pits or tags | External ears with tags or pinhole openings |
| Nose | Observe for patency, discharge, and nasal flaring | Septal deviation<br>Choanal atresia |
| Oral | Note the symmetry of the mouth and throat<br>Assess for cyanosis and inspect the hard and soft palate<br>Inspect for the presence of teeth, cysts, Epstein pearls, thrush<br>Note the size of the chin<br>Note the size and position of the tongue<br>Inspect for moist mucous membranes | Clefts of lip or palate<br>Mouth with teeth<br>Hypoglossia/Macroglossia<br>Excessive oral secretions |
| Neck | Assess for range of motion | Presence of webbing or masses (e.g., cystic hygroma)<br>Presence of lymph nodes<br>Evidence of fractured clavicle<br>Exaggerated tonic neck |
| Heart | Auscultate rate, rhythm, heart sounds—identify S1 and S2<br>(Soft III/IV systolic murmur normal for first 12–24 hours because ductus arteriosus may not yet be closed)<br>Note the apical pulse location and quality<br>Assess for the brachial, femoral, pedal pulses, noting symmetry, quality | Presence of murmurs and/or extra heart sounds<br>Irregular rate/rhythm <100 or >180 bpm<br>Absent or decreased femoral pulses (coarctation of the aorta)<br>Slow capillary refill |
| Chest/Lungs | Observe respiratory rate, rhythm, and retractions<br>Note the shape, size, and symmetry of movement<br>Auscultate breath sounds<br>Note the amount of breast tissue, engorgement, nipples—symmetry and discharge | Chest shape with pectus excavatum/carinatum<br>Supernumerary nipples<br>Moist and grunting/retractions of breath sounds after 4 hours of age<br>Apnea and respirations <30 or >60 per minute |
| Abdomen | Inspect the shape, size, symmetry<br>Auscultate bowel sounds in all four quadrants and note the characteristic of the bowel sounds (normoactive, hypoactive, hyperactive, absent) (Auscultate prior to palpation)<br>Palpate for liver, spleen, kidneys, evidence of diastasis recti<br>Examine the umbilical cord for the number of vessels, color, drainage, odor, and presence of hernia | Abdominal skin thin or missing, asymmetrical, or distended<br>Discharge, redness, or odor from umbilical cord<br>Absence of bowel sounds or hyperactive bowel sounds<br>Lower liver edge 3 cm+ below costal margin<br>Palpable spleen<br>Enlarged bladder (1–4 cm above symphysis pubis) |

(*continued*)

TABLE 13.3 **Newborn Physical Examination** (*continued*)

| Body System | Physical Examination Findings | Abnormal Physical Findings |
|---|---|---|
| Genitalia/rectum | *Male*<br>Observe the position of the urethral meatus, passage of urine<br>Inspect testes—descended or undescended<br>Observe for penile anomalies<br>*Female*<br>Observe the size of the labia majora, labia minora, vaginal discharge, skin tags<br>Note any labial masses, passage of urine<br>Observe for labial or vaginal anomalies<br>Rectum<br>Assess the position and patency of the anus<br>Note the passage of meconium | *Ambiguous genitalia*<br>If gender is uncertain, prompt karyotype or other genetic evaluation is warranted<br>Anus absent or not patent<br>Imperforate anus<br>Dimples or asymmetry of the buttocks<br>*Male*<br>Meatal opening on penis placed abnormally (hypospadias or epispadias)<br>Absence of testes in either inguinal canals or scrotal sac, hydrocele, bifid scrotum, discoloration, bruising<br>*Female*<br>Masses in labia (i.e., hernia, enlarged Bartholin gland, vesicles)<br>Labial adhesions |
| Musculoskeletal | Extremities<br>Note the symmetry, shape, strength, range of motion, number of digits of the extremities<br>Note the texture and color of the nails<br>Note the creases in the palms and soles<br>Note any foot or arm/hand abnormalities<br>Abduct hips for dislocation—perform Barlow and Ortolani maneuvers (see chapter 34)<br>Back<br>Note the spinal contour<br>Inspect for presence of cysts, sinuses, dimples, and tufts of hair<br>Note any uneven skin folds<br>Note presence of any nevi<br>Note deformities of the back and spine<br>Palpate the clavicles for crepitus | More/fewer than five fingers/toes on each hand/foot<br>Dislocation/pain/fracture of clavicle(s)<br>Abnormal Barlow or Ortolani sign<br>Bowing of extremities<br>Abnormal foot positions<br>Flaccid upper extremity<br>Lesions or dimpling of lower spine<br>Limited flexibility of joints with clubfeet<br>Increased muscle tone |

| | | |
|---|---|---|
| Neurological | Assess posture, muscle tone, movement<br>Assess head control<br>Note quality of cry<br>Note response to light and sound<br>Assess primitive reflexes | Observation of ankle clonus<br>Seizure activity<br>High-pitched cry<br>Asymmetric movements or reflexes |
| Screening Tests & Labs | Passage of urine and meconium<br>Critical congenital heart disease screening passed?<br>Newborn screening test, newborn hearing screening results<br>Point-of-care glucose testing<br>Complete blood cell count<br>Hematocrit<br>Blood type<br>Coombs<br>Bilirubin | |

*Sources*: Data from Ballard, J. L., Khoury, J. C., Wedig, K., Wang, L., Eilers-Wlasman, B. L., & Lippo, R. (1991). New Ballard score, expanded to include extremely premature infants. *Journal of Pediatrics, 119*(3), 417–423. https://doi.org/10.1016/S0022-3476(05)82056-6; Carley, A., & Duderstadt, K. (2019). Newborn assessment. In K. Duderstadt (Ed.), *Pediatric physical exam: An illustrated edition* (3rd ed., pp. 67–88). Elsevier; Gooding, J. R., & McClead, R. E., Jr. (2015). Initial assessment and management of the newborn. *Pediatric Clinics of North America, 62*(2), 345–365. https://doi.org/10.1016/j.pcl.2014.12.001; Hagan, J. F., Shaw, J. S., & Duncan, P. M. (Eds.). (2017). *Bright futures* (4th ed.). American Academy of Pediatrics; Salandy, S., Rai, R., Gutierrez, S., Ishak, B., & Tubbs, R. S. (2019). Neurological examination of the infant: A comprehensive review. *Clinical Anatomy, 32*(6), 770–777. https://doi.org/10.1002/ca.23352; Zickler, C. F. (2020). Making newborn rounds. In B. Richardson (Ed.), *Pediatric primary care: Practice guidelines for nurses* (4th ed., pp. 27–38). Jones & Bartlett Learning.

Clinical jaundice photograph courtesy of CDC, Public Health Image Library, 1967.

Erythema toxicum photograph courtesy of CDC, Dr. James R. Allen, Public Health Image Library, 1976.

Miliaria rubra (prickly heat rash) source Aisylu Ahmadieva

Caput and cephalohematoma. (A) Caput results from diffuse swelling. (B) Cephalohematoma results from bleeding beneath the periosteum. From Gawlick, K. S. (2020). *Evidence-based physical examination*. Springer Publishing Company.

screening in the hospital are rescreened as soon as possible but no later than 3 months of age. State newborn screening results may be processed by the time the newborn is being seen for the first outpatient visit and should be reviewed if available. If not available, the healthcare provider should contact the state laboratory for results prior to the next clinic appointment. A second metabolic screen is recommended between 7 and 30 days of life. Other screenings include follow-up for hyperbilirubinemia and congenital heart disease (Hagan et al., 2017; Warren & Phillipi, 2012). For newborns determined to be at risk for vision conditions, screening should be completed at this time.

### Screening for Postpartum Depression

Screening for anxiety and depression during pregnancy and the postpartum period is recommended by the American College of Obstetrics and Gynecologists (ACOG), the United States (U.S.) Preventive Services Task Force (USPSTF), the Association of Women's Health, Obstetric, and Neonatal Nurses (AWHONN), and the AAP (ACOG, 2018b; AWHONN, 2015a; Siu & USPSTF, 2016; Sriraman et al., 2017). Approximately 8 to 20% of women experience PPD without psychosis (Isley, 2021). However, actual occurrence is likely greater than reported because it is often unrecognized and undiagnosed (ACOG, 2018b). In addition to maternal PPD, it should be noted that fathers can also experience paternal PPD, which often goes unaddressed (Sriraman et al., 2017). When PPD is identified early, it is highly treatable and has a direct impact on family attachment and improved clinical outcomes for the newborn. Hence, it is important for providers to screen for PPD during the one-month and subsequent visits (Sriraman et al., 2017).

The Edinburgh Postnatal Depression Scale (EPDS) is a widely used and validated screening tool for PPD (Cox et al., 2014). This tool has been validated in the screening of both mothers and fathers (Sriraman et al., 2017). In a crosscultural study of the EPDS, investigators found that level of education and continent (Europe or United States), more than ethnicity/race, influenced the expression of PPD on the EPDS. This highlights the importance of a culturally sensitive approach to clinical care, including screening for PPD as an important part of providing effective care to the newborn (Di Florio et al., 2017).

**PRO TIP** Screen mothers and fathers for PPD using the EPDS at each newborn visit.

## ANTICIPATORY GUIDANCE

Bright Futures has established anticipatory guidance priorities for the newborn period (Hagan et al., 2017). These priority areas include the following:

- **Social determinants of health** (e.g., living situation, food security/insecurity, tobacco exposure, family support structure)
- **Parent and family health and well-being** (e.g., adjustment for siblings, transition to the home environment for family members)
- **Newborn behavior and care** (e.g., brain development, transition to home for the newborn, bathing and dressing, how to manage newborn crying, managing health concerns, sun safety, and minimizing illness exposure)
- **Newborn nutrition** (e.g., managing feedings, nutritional requirements, breastfeeding, expected weight changes)
- **Safety** (e.g., heat exposure, car seat safety, safe sleeping practices, and limiting hot water exposure in the home; Hagan et al., 2017)

With each of these categories, questions should be asked related to each topic. Evidence-based guidance should be provided to families. It is common for new parents to have many questions related to these categories. The healthcare provider should structure the dialogue in a way that answers parents' questions, gathers the necessary information, and provides up-to-date recommendations for care.

## SAFETY

Newborn safety is key for the well-being and optimal health of the newborn at home. Well-intentioned efforts are needed by all members of the family to promote safety of the newborn. It is important that all safety labels are read, understood, and implemented prior to use as directed on all items used in the home (e.g., toys). A happy and healthy newborn is a safe newborn.

### General Considerations

#### Smoking

Educate parents, guardians, relatives, and friends about the risk of secondhand smoke or the use of vapor devices around the newborn. Studies have shown that secondhand smoke exposure increases newborn risk of respiratory disease, ear infections, tooth decay, and sudden infant death syndrome (SIDS) death (Pineles et al., 2016; Snodgrass et al., 2016).

### Pacifiers

One-piece pacifiers are recommended as they are less likely to break into multiple pieces, which can cause an increased choking hazard. Encourage families to inspect the pacifier regularly, as they deteriorate over time. In exclusively breastfed infants, avoid introducing a pacifier until the infant is 3 to 4 weeks of age. Pacifiers can be cleaned with mild soap and water or intermittently be cleaned in the dishwasher.

### Constipation

Constipation is a common problem experienced in the newborn due to increased feedings, a change in formula, and/or the transition from breastmilk to formula. Breastfed infants may have 4 to 8 stools per day compared with formula-fed infants, who may have 1 to 2 stools/day. Management of constipation with prune or pear juice may be done after 30 days of age, but families should limit the volume of juice to encourage calories from breast milk or formula. The AAP does not recommend the use of branded Karo syrup in newborns less than 1 month of age due to the possibility of *Clostridium botulinum* spores being present.

### Water Safety

Newborns should NEVER be left unattended around water of any source. The use of infant bathtubs is appropriate; however, supervision of the infant is required when water is present. A newborn can drown in less than one inch of water. Set the hot water heater temperature at 120° or less.

### When to Call the Healthcare Provider

Call the healthcare provider when any of the following occur:

- Difficulty in breathing: too fast or too slow and/or color changes (i.e., pale or a blue hue in color)
- Temperature 100.4 °F (38 °C)
- Increased irritability/unable to be consoled
- Poor feeding
- Projectile vomiting
- Decreased urination (e.g., no wet diapers in 12 hours)
- Black or decreased bowel movements
- Reddened or draining umbilicus
- Jaundice that does not improve with prescribed therapy
- Any concerns that increase anxiety of the caregiver

### Safe Sleep

Sleep and rest are vital elements for the newborn period as it differs from the sleep and rest of children and adults. Newborns sleep approximately 16 to 17 hours a day in either "active-sleep" or stage rapid-eye-movement (REM) sleep (Wielek et al., 2019). The activity of sleep is essential for mental/behavioral, emotional and physical health, as well as improved immune response leading to healthy outcomes during the first 30 days of life.

The implementation of safe sleep and rest is crucial to the well-being of the newborn. However, when educating parents about safe sleep and rest for the newborn, the provider must be culturally sensitive and aware while providing information that is evidence-based regarding practices of both safe sleep practices and environments (Hagan et al., 2017). Examples of safe sleep practices are outlined in Box 13.1.

In regard to sleep and feedings, the infant should wake for feedings every 2 to 4 hours. The infant should be awake and alert to feed robustly (breastfed or bottle fed). Once the feeding is complete, the infant should then fall back to sleep. Note that the infant's respirations could be irregular during and after feeding, a normal finding (Zickler, 2020). Lastly, the provider will need to teach safe sleep implementation practices to engage family, friends, and other childcare providers to ensure that the newborn will experience safety and continuity of sleep (Hagan et al., 2017).

### Car Safety

The use of car seats is mandated across all 50 states in the United States. Providers need to educate families and/or guardians to purchase the Federal Motor Vehicle Standards (FMVSS) tested and approved car seats (Zickler, 2020). The car seat must be installed in the rear-facing position for newborns in the back seat of a vehicle. Families and/or guardians can follow the specific car seat instructions regarding installation, height, and weight mandates. The car seat should always be placed in the middle of the back seat away from the door and never placed in the front seat while the newborn or child is in a rear-facing position. Implementing car seat safety will assist in promoting safety for the newborn during travel.

**PRO TIP** Local hospitals, fire departments, and other organizations can assist with car seat evaluation and installation.

### Nutrition

A very important first task for parents during their newborn's first week is learning how much their infant needs, either breast milk or formula. The first-week

**BOX 13.1 Safe Sleep Practices**

During the newborn period (0–30 days of life):

- Newborns should sleep on their back on firm, flat surface in crib for up to 1 year of age. No pillows/toys/blankets/wedges or positioning devices in crib, to avoid having the infant get their face against it and be smothered.
  - Side-sleeping is a risk factor for Sudden Infant Death Syndrome (SIDS) until the infant is able to roll over on their own.
- Infant sleep clothing, such as wearable blankets, is preferred to swaddling or blankets. No head coverings should be attached to sleep clothing. Avoid overheating the infant when preparing for sleep.
- Infants should sleep in their own cribs—not with parents—to minimize potential for rollovers, suffocation, and falls. Having the infant sleep in the same room with the parent is encouraged up to 1 year of age—at least until 6 months of age.
- Preterm infants should sleep supine and follow the same guidelines as term infants. Parents should be counseled on the increased risk of SIDS with preterm infants.
- Avoid use of commercial devices that claim to reduce SIDS risk, such as wedges and positioners.

*Sources*: Data from Hagan, J. F., Shaw, J. S., & Duncan, P. M. (Eds.). (2017). *Bright futures* (4th ed.). American Academy of Pediatrics; Zickler, C. F. (2020). Making newborn rounds. In B. Richardson (Ed.), *Pediatric primary care: Practice guidelines for nurses* (4th ed., pp. 27–38). Jones & Bartlett Learning.

visit can provide parents with reassurance that their baby is getting the appropriate amount of feeding, as evidenced by gaining weight or a return to the birth weight. It is not uncommon for newborns, particularly those who are breastfed, to lose up to 10% of their body weight during the first few days of life (Flaherman et al., 2015). It should be expected that breastfed newborns return to birthweight within the first 2 to 4 weeks of life. Newborns with jaundice may be more difficult to arouse for feedings, which can make it more difficult to achieve adequate feeding amounts, particularly with breastfeeding.

Careful assessment is required to determine to what extent parents are waking their newborn for feeding to ensure adequate nutrition and hydration. Providing parents with guidance to recognize the newborn's signals for hunger and satiation will help them find an appropriate feeding amount and frequency, including the risk of overfeeding. The infant will slow or stop sucking when it is time to burp, which should occur several times per feeding to allow release of air and decrease spitting up. Discuss the benefits of holding the newborn during feeding and observing the newborn feeding to assess for signs of reflux or other abnormalities that may have a negative impact on feeding success. Gastrointestinal reflux can cause the infant to arch their back and pull away, which can leave a parent with the wrong impression that the baby does not like the breast milk, formula, or being held for feedings. The provider should reinforce that introduction of complementary foods should be delayed until after 6 months of age.

## Guidance on Breastfeeding

Exclusive breastfeeding continues to be the ideal source of nutrition for at least the first 6 months of life, and healthcare provider support is essential for breastfeeding success (AAP, 2012; ACOG, 2018a; American Academy of Family Physicians, 2021; American College of Nurse Midwives [ACNM], 2018; AWHONN, 2015b; Chantry et al., 2015; National Association of Pediatric Nurse Practitioners, 2019; Webber & Serowoky, 2017; World Health Organization [WHO], 2019). The healthcare provider should advocate for breastfeeding and ensure appropriate community support or referral to a lactation consultant when working with newborns and their families. Establish a breastfeeding family office; recommendations may be found at www.aap.org/en-us/advocacy-and-policy/aap-health-initiatives/Breastfeeding/Documents/Breastfeeding_Friendly Practice.pdf.

Breastfeeding on demand is recommended during the first few weeks to establish adequate milk supply and promote infant growth. Assess breastfeeding support, infant latch, and overall breastfeeding experience during the first month. Avoid the use of supplements that are not medically indicated. Newborns need to breastfeed at least 8 to 12 times during a 24-hour period (AAP, 2012). Further, a baby should be wetting their diaper 6 to 8 times per day. Additionally, provide Vitamin D supplementation to all breastfed infants (400 international units once daily). Mothers who breastfeed can often receive breast pumps, breast shells, or nursing supplements from their health insurance, Women, Infants, and Children (WIC), or similar agencies to help support the initiation of breastfeeding. Encourage skin-to-skin contact (kangaroo care) in the delivery room until after the initial breastfeeding and continue to promote at home to support breastfeeding and bonding. Breastfed infants have a more stable microbiome compared with formula-fed infants, which modulates brain development and acts as a barrier to pathogens. Discuss pumping and appropriate storage of breast milk.

ALERT: Warning signs related to breastfeeding include:

- Extreme maternal breast or nipple pain
- Poor latch
- Flutter sucking
- Fewer than six to eight wet or dirty diapers per day
- Infant choking or gagging with nursing
- Inconsolable crying

### *Lactation and LGBTQ+ Families*

Members of the lesbian, gay, bisexual, transgender, queer/nonbinary, intersex (LGBTQ+) community are increasingly parents who provide human milk to their infants. They face lactation and family adjustment concerns similar to those of cis-gender mothers, but may also require unique adaptations to offer human milk (Farrow, 2015). For example, a lesbian couple may have one woman give birth and breastfeed, and the female coparent may choose to induce lactation so that she can also feed the baby. Transgender men may provide human milk through chest feeding (chest feeding is often the preferred term rather than breastfeeding). The coparent may also breastfeed by induced lactation or by using a supplementary feeding device (Wolfe-Roubatis & Spatz, 2015).

## Formula Feeding

There are infrequent cases where breastfeeding is contraindicated due to health (e.g., certain metabolic disorders) or social factors (e.g., maternal medication or substance use). Additionally, some families simply make the choice not to breastfeed. In these cases, formula feeding should be encouraged. Newborns who are formula-fed often have different feeding patterns. It is important to discuss formula safety issues. A typical formula feeding should not take more than 30 minutes. If the newborn is too sleepy to take an adequate amount of formula, it may be an indication of some underlying condition that requires further investigation.

Commercially produced, iron-fortified formula should always be used, unless otherwise indicated for certain rare infant conditions. Soy formulas are not routinely recommended, and infants should not be fed evaporated milk or standard cow's milk. Formula may be purchased as ready-to-feed, or as powder or liquid requiring further dilution or mixing. Teach families to mix the formula according to the manufacturer's instructions and never to dilute it further or make it more concentrated. Formula that has been heated and has been out of the refrigerator for more than 1 hour should be discarded. Unused portions should be discarded after 48 hours. Parents should discuss changing formulas with their healthcare provider because further questions are needed to investigate the reasons why the parents feel that a different formula is indicated.

## KEY POINTS

- The healthcare provider is in a unique position to support the new family as they adjust to caring for their newborn. Utilizing cultural humility, the provide supports the family as mutual attachment occurs.
- Obtain a CHH on the first newborn visit, and interval history on subsequent visits.
- Perform a full physical examination with each newborn visit.
- Note developmental alterations or deficiencies, referring them for early intervention.
- Newborn visits include hepatitis B vaccination, hearing screening, state newborn screening for inherited and metabolic disorders, and maternal and paternal depression screening.
- All newborns should be put on their back to sleep.
- Additional anticipatory guidance for newborns includes car safety, water safety, avoidance of exposing infants to smoking and vaping, pacifier use, and nutrition.
- Exclusive breastfeeding is recommended for the first year of life.

## REFERENCES

American Academy of Family Physicians. (2021). *Breastfeeding, family physicians supporting (position paper).* https://www.aafp.org/about/policies/all/breastfeeding-position-paper.html

American Academy of Pediatrics, Committee on Fetus and Newborn. (2010, reaffirmed 2015). Hospital stay for healthy term newborns. *Pediatrics, 125*(2), 405–409. https://doi.org/10.1542/peds.2009-3119

American Academy of Pediatrics, Section on Breastfeeding. (2012). Breastfeeding and the use of human milk—Policy Statement. *Pediatrics, 129*(3), e827–e841. https://doi.org/10.1542/peds.2011-3552

American College of Nurse Midwives. (2018). *Statement in support of breastfeeding.* https://www.midwife.org/ACNM-Releases-Statement-in-Support-of-Breastfeeding

American College of Obstetrics and Gynecologists. (2018a). *Optimizing support for breastfeeding as part of obstetric practice.* https://www.acog.org/clinical/clinical-guidance/committee-opinion/articles/2018/10/optimizing-support-for-breastfeeding-as-part-of-obstetric-practice

American College of Obstetrics and Gynecologists. (2018b). *Screening for perinatal depression.* https://www.acog

.org/clinical/clinical-guidance/committee-opinion/articles/2018/11/screening-for-perinatal-depression

American Nurses Association. (2019). *Expanded historical review of nursing and the ANA*. https://www.nursingworld.org/~4ab5e0/globalassets/docs/ana/ana-expandedhistoricalreview.pdf

Association of Women's Health, Obstetric, and Neonatal Nurses. (2015a). AWHONN position statement: Mood and anxiety disorders in pregnant and postpartum women. *Journal of Obstetric, Gynecologic, and Neonatal Nursing, 44*(1), 158–160. https://doi.org/10.1111/1552-6909.12734

Association of Women's Health, Obstetric, and Neonatal Nurses. (2015b). *Breastfeeding support: Preconception care through the first year* (3rd ed.). Author.

Ballard, J. L., Khoury, J. C., Wedig, K., Wang, L., Eilers-Wlasman, B. L., & Lippo, R. (1991). New Ballard score, expanded to include extremely premature infants. *Journal of Pediatrics, 119*(3), 417–423. https://doi.org/10.1016/S0022-3476(05)82056-6

Carley, A., & Duderstadt, K. (2019). Newborn assessment. In K. Duderstadt (Ed.), *Pediatric physical exam: An illustrated edition* (3rd ed., pp. 67–88). Elsevier.

Centers for Disease Control and Prevention. (2020). *Birth–18 years immunization schedule*. https://www.cdc.gov/vaccines/schedules/hcp/imz/child-adolescent.html

Chantry, C. J., Eglash, A., & Labbok, M. (2015). Position on breastfeeding—Revised 2015. *Breastfeeding Medicine, 10*(9), 94–104. https://doi.org/10.1089/bfm.2015.29012.cha

Cox, J., Holden, J., & Henshaw, C. (2014). *Perinatal mental health: The Edinburgh postpartum depression scale (EPDS)* (2nd ed.). RCPsych Publications.

Di Florio, A., Putnam, K., Altemus, M., Apter, G., Bergink, V., Bilszta, J., Brock, R., Buist, A., Deligiannidis, K. M., Devouche, E., Epperson, C. N., Guille, C., Kim, D., Lichtenstein, P., Magnusson, P. K. E., Martinez, P., Munk-Olsen, T., Newport, J., Payne, J., & the Postpartum Depression: Action Towards Causes and Treatment (PACT) Consortium. (2017). The impact of education, country, race, ethnicity on the self-report of postpartum depression using the Edinburgh Postnatal Depression Scale. *Psychological Medicine, 47*(5), 787–798. https://doi.org/10.1017/S0033291716002087

Farrow, A. (2015). Lactation support and the LGBTQI community. *Journal of Human Lactation, 31*(1), 26–28. https://doi.org/10.1177%2F0890334414554928

Flaherman, V. J., Schaefer, E. W., Kuzniewicz, M. W., Li, S. X., Walsh, E. M., & Paul, I. M. (2015). Early weight loss nomograms for exclusively breastfed newborns. *Pediatrics, 135*(1), e16–e23. https://doi.org/10.1542/peds.2014-1532

Foronda, C., Baptiste, D.-L., Reinholdt, M. M., & Ousman, K.(2016). Cultural humility. *Journal of Transcultural Nursing,27*(3), 210–217. https://doi.org/10.1177%2F1043659615592677

Gooding, J. R., & McClead, R. E., Jr. (2015). Initial assessment and management of the newborn. *Pediatric Clinics of North America, 62*(2), 345–365. https://doi.org/10.1016/j.pcl.2014.12.001

Hagan, J. F., Shaw, J. S., & Duncan, P. M. (Eds.). (2017). *Bright futures* (4th ed.). American Academy of Pediatrics.

Isley, M. M. (2021). Postpartum care and long-term health considerations. In M. B. Landon, H. L. Galan, E. L. M. Jauniaux, D. A. Driscoll, V. Berghella, W. A. Grobman, S. J. Kilpatrick, & A. G. Cahill (Eds.), *Gabbe's obstetrics: Normal and problem pregnancies* (8th ed., pp. 459–474). Elsevier.

National Association of Pediatric Nurse Practitioners. (2019). NAPNAP position statement on breastfeeding. *Journal of Pediatric Health Care, 33*(1), A11–A15. https://doi.org/10.1016/j.pedhc.2018.08.011

Pineles, B. L., Hsu, S., Park, E., & Samet, J. M. (2016). Systematic review and meta-analyses of perinatal death and maternal exposure to tobacco smoke during pregnancy. *American Journal of Epidemiology, 184*(2), 87–97. https://doi.org/10.1093/aje/kwv301

Salandy, S., Rai, R., Gutierrez, S., Ishak, B., & Tubbs, R. S. (2019). Neurological examination of the infant: A comprehensive review. *Clinical Anatomy, 32*(6), 770–777. https://doi.org/10.1002/ca.23352

Scharf, R. J., Scharf, G. J., & Stroustrup, A. (2016). Developmental milestones. *Pediatrics in Review, 37*(1), 25–47. https://doi.org/10.1542/pir.2014-0103

Schillie, S., Vellozzi, C., Reingold, A., Harris, A., Haber, P., Ward, J. W., & Nelson, N. P. (2018). Prevention of hepatitis B virus infection in the United States: Recommendations of the advisory committee on immunization practices. *MMWR Recommendations and Reports, 67*(No. RR-1), 1–31. http://doi.org/10.15585/mmwr.rr6701a1

Siu, A. L., & U.S. Preventive Services Task Force. (2016). Screening for depression in adults: US Preventive Services Task Force recommendation statement. *Journal of American Medical Association, 31*(4), 380–387. https://doi.org/10.1001/jama.2015.18392

Snodgrass, A. M., Tan, P. T., Soh, S. E., Goh, A., Shek, L. P., van Bever, H. P., Gluckman, P. D., Godfrey, K. M., Chong, Y. S., Saw, S. M., Kwek, K., Teoh, O. H., & GUSTO Study Group. (2016). Tobacco smoke exposure and respiratory morbidity in young children. *Tobacco Control, 25*(e2), e75–e82. http://doi.org/10.1136/tobaccocontrol-2015-052383

Sriraman, N. K., Pham, D. Q., & Kumar, R. (2017). Postpartum depression: What do pediatricians need to know? *Pediatrics in Review, 38*(12), 541–551. https://doi.org/10.1542/pir.2015-0133

Tervalon, M., & Murray-Garcia, J. (1998). Cultural humility versus cultural competence: A critical distinction in defining physician training outcomes in multicultural education. *Journal of Health Care for the Poor and Underserved, 9*(2), 117–125. https://doi.org/10.1353/hpu.2010.0233

Warren, J. B., & Phillipi, C. A. (2012). Care of the well newborn. *Pediatrics in Review, 33*(1), 4–18. https://doi.org/10.1542/pir.33-1-4

Webber, E., & Serowoky, M. (2017). Breastfeeding curriculum content of family nurse practitioner programs. *Journal of Pediatric Health Care, 31*(2), 189–195. https://doi.org/10.1016/j.pedhc.2016.07.006

Wielek, T., Del Giudice, R., Lang, A., Wislowska, M., Ott, P., & Schabus, M. (2019). On the development of sleep states in the first weeks of life. *PLoS ONE, 14*(10), e0224521. https://doi.org/10.1371/journal.pone.0224521

Wolfe-Roubatis, E., & Spatz, D. L. (2015). Transgender men and lactation. *Maternal-Child Nursing Journal, 40*(1), 32–38. https://doi.org/10.1097/NMC.0000000000000097

World Health Organization. (2019). *Exclusive breastfeeding for optimal growth, development and health of infants*. https://www.who.int/elena/titles/exclusive_breastfeeding/en

Zickler, C. F. (2020). Making newborn rounds. In B. Richardson (Ed.), *Pediatric primary care: Practice guidelines for nurses* (4th ed., pp. 27–38). Jones & Bartlett Learning.

# Well-Child Visits During Infancy

Theresa Kyle

## Student Learning Outcomes

**Upon completion of this chapter the reader should be able to:**

1. Determine adequacy of growth of infants.
2. Evaluate developmental milestones of infants.
3. Choose appropriate screening tests based on current recommendations for child's age and risk status.
4. Select immunizations based on current recommendations for child's age and risk status.
5. Determine applicable anticipatory guidance for each scheduled visit during infancy.

## INTRODUCTION

The period of infancy provides an opportunity for the family and the healthcare provider to work collaboratively to support the infant's health. Parents become more attuned to their baby, are increasingly able to interpret their baby's cues, and improve their own behavioral responses based on the infant's behavior. As they learn more about their infant, they grow to understand the infant's ability to self-regulate. They also are able to adapt to respond best to the infant's emerging personality. The focus in early infancy is most frequently related to feeding, elimination, sleep and wake patterns, and increasing integration into the family. Later in infancy, emotional attachment is secured and mutual reciprocity is prominent. As the infant demonstrates increasing mobility, it becomes necessary for parents to choose and set limits. Because infants don't really understand the word "no," redirection away from an undesired behavior is very helpful. Parents should decide when saying "no" is important, such as when the infant is in possible danger. Infancy yields a large shift in development for both the infant and the parents.

During this period, Bright Futures recommends six standard outpatient well-child visits. Health supervision should occur at 1, 2, 4, 6, 9, and 12 months of age in the otherwise healthy infant (Hagan et al., 2017). Infants born prematurely, or who demonstrate other health concerns, may need more frequent visits.

The content in this chapter maps to the following areas on the Pediatric Nursing Certification Board (PNCB) Pediatric Nurse Practitioner—Primary Care certification examination:

### CONTENT AREAS:

#### I. Health Maintenance and Promotion

- **A. Partner with patients/caregivers to support growth and development from infancy to young adulthood**
- **B. Provide patients/caregivers with age/developmentally appropriate anticipatory guidance**
- **C. Recommend and prescribe immunizations according to current CDC guidelines**
- **D. Educate about illness prevention and early warning signs of pediatric illness and emergencies**
- **E. Advise patients/caregivers about age appropriate injury prevention and safety (environmental exposure, risk taking behaviors, social situations, sports and recreation, and vehicle safety)**
- **F. Counsel about age-appropriate social, behavioral, and mental health concerns (e.g., substance abuse, social media use, grief and loss, and sexual orientation/LGBTQ)**

## II. Assessment and Diagnosis

**A. Growth and Development**

1. Evaluate and interpret growth parameters
2. Perform developmental surveillance

**B. History and Physical Examination**

1. Obtain history of present illness
2. Obtain a comprehensive health history for new patients
3. Complete an interval history for established patients
4. Perform a review of systems
5. Perform a complete physical examination

**C. Diagnostic Testing and Screening**

1. Order and interpret office/clinic based screening tests
4. Select, utilize, and interpret developmental, behavioral and mental health screening and assessment tools

**D. Analyzing Information**

1. Integrate health history and physical examination findings into the plan of care
2. Assimilate findings from screening and diagnostic testing into plan of care

## IV. Professional Role and Responsibilities

**B. Practice Management**

1. Document patient encounters in a manner which supports applicable diagnostic and procedure codes
2. Utilize appropriate billing and coding to facilitate reimbursement

# PARENT-CHILD INTERACTION

The parent-infant relationship is vital to the infant's growth and development. Secure attachment is fundamental to the infant's confidence in their world, and when experiencing secure attachment the infant feels assured the parent will be there for them when needed (Cassidy & Shaver, 2016). Observe the parents' interaction with the child and the infant's responses. Table 14.1 provides examples of behavior for each type of attachment. Support the parent in interactions that promote secure attachment.

▶ ALERT: Warning signs of poor emotional attachment include:

- Demonstrates poor eye contact
- Does not brighten or smile upon seeing parent
- Lacks vocalization
- Does not turn to sound of parent's voice, nor quiet with it
- Difficulty with calming or is excessively irritable
- At 3 months of age, facial expression is somber or sad
- At 4 months of age infant appears wary
- At 9 months of age infant demonstrates fear

# DEVELOPMENTAL SURVEILLANCE

At each well-child visit, assess the infant's achievement of developmental milestones. At the 9-month infant visit, use a validated screening tool. Parent-completed developmental screening questionnaires recognize the parent as expert on their infant, provide assessment information valuable for developmental surveillance, and are recommended for use by the American Academy of Pediatrics (AAP; Aites & Schonwald, 2020; Hagan et al., 2017). Tools with demonstrated reliability and validity appropriate for use in infancy include:

- Ages and Stages Questionnaires (ASQ-3; Paul H. Brookes Publishing, 2020)—may begin use at 1 month of age
- Parent's Evaluation of Developmental Status (PEDS test; Pedstest.com, 2016)—use throughout infancy

**TABLE 14.1 Patterns of Attachment**

| Attachment Pattern | Parent Behavior | Infant Behavior |
|---|---|---|
| **Secure** | Is responsive and available, demonstrates sensitivity to infant's cues | Will interact with provider, but seeks reassurance from parent |
| **Insecure, Ambivalent/ Resistant** | Inconsistent in care, unpredictable in responses to infant's cues | Appears anxious, is dependent or clingy |
| **Insecure, Avoidant** | Avoids contact, may reject, is insensitive to infant's cues | May be fearful, sad, or angry; seeks parental reassurance but pulls away |

*Source*: Data from Cassidy, J., & Shaver, P. R. (2016). *Handbook of attachment: Theory, research, and clinical applications* (3rd ed.). Guilford Press.

- PEDS: Developmental Milestones (PEDS: DM)—use throughout infancy
- Survey of Well-being of Young Children (SWYC; Tufts Children's Hospital, 2020)—may begin use at 2 months of age

Periodic evaluation at each well-child visit during infancy will allow for early identification of infants who may be at risk for developmental delay (Lipkin et al., 2020; Treitz et al., 2020). In addition to the screening questionnaire, begin the health history at each well-infant visit by asking, "Since the last visit, what changes have you seen in your baby's development?" Or start the conversation with, "What's your baby doing that's new since the last visit?" Concerning findings include extremely low activity level or low muscle tone, as well as lack of mouthing of objects. Expected developmental milestones for each age in infancy may be found in chapter 7.

## HEALTH ASSESSMENT

Each infant well-child visit will include a comprehensive health assessment. The assessment includes developmental surveillance, as noted earlier, as well as health history and physical examination data. Each visit also includes prevention (immunization or screening as appropriate) and anticipatory guidance appropriate for age, always including but not limited to nutrition, sleep, and safety (Hagan et al., 2017).

### SUBJECTIVE DATA

Along with developmental surveillance, obtain information from the caregiver in relation to past medical history (since last health supervision visit), diet, sleep, dental care, changes in family or social history, and results of prior screenings. Always address any concerns the parents may have.

### OBJECTIVE DATA

In addition to observation of the parent-infant interaction, perform a comprehensive physical examination, beginning with observation of the infant's general appearance (happy, calm, well-appearing, active, neatly/cleanly clothed). Note body build and nutritional status. The infant's weight, recumbent length, occipitofrontal head circumference, and weight-for-length should be plotted on the gender-appropriate World Health Organization (WHO) growth chart, as these charts provide a better representation of growth of infancy (Centers for Disease Control and Prevention [CDC], 2010). The young infant may be examined on the parent's lap or the examination table. By 9 months of age the infant is more wary of strangers. Approach the older infant slowly and begin the examination while the child is in the parent's arms. Distract the infant with a toy as needed to gain cooperation.

> ALERT: If the infant lacks animation or makes no eye contact, or after 4 months of age has no social smile, consider the possibility of child maltreatment (abuse or neglect; Drutz, 2020).

On examination of the skin, note any birthmarks, bruises, or other skin changes. Palpate the skull, fontanel(s), and sutures, noting any skull deformities (expect posterior fontanel closing by 2 months, anterior fontanel closing between 9 and 18 months). Examine the eyelids and eyes, looking for opacification (not desired) and presence of a bilateral red reflex. Screen visual acuity by determining the ability to fix and follow. When teeth emerge, observe for hygiene, caries, plaque, staining, or white spots (demineralization). Respirations should be unlabored, although they are often irregular, particularly in the younger infant. Auscultate the heart for murmur and palpate the femoral pulses for equality. Note healing of the umbilicus in younger infants and palpate the abdomen for masses (none should be found).

Observe the extremities for equality of size, tone, and movement. Healthy infants should be normotonic. Through 6 months of age, perform the Ortolani and Barlow maneuvers (see chapter 34) to screen for developmental dysplasia of the hip. Assess the infant's resting posture. Evaluate the quality and integration of the primitive reflexes (through 6 months) and emergence of the protective reflexes (postural responses) after 6 months. Assess deep tendon reflexes, noting that they may be brisk until 4 months of age, after which time they should be average. Observe the infant's level of consciousness and interaction with the environment. Note the infant's response to auditory and visual stimuli. In boys, determine whether testes are fully descended, and in girls whether the labia are open. Any alterations noted on the physical examination may warrant further screening or other investigation.

> **PRO TIP** Talk through the examination while performing it, commenting on normal findings and reinforcing developmentally appropriate actions and reactions of the infant. Role-model attentiveness to the infant's cues.

## PREVENTION

Prevention during the infant health supervision visits includes routine recommended immunizations and targeted health screenings. The AAP recommendations for preventive pediatric health care may be found at https://downloads.aap.org/AAP/PDF/periodicity_schedule.pdf (AAP/Bright Futures, 2020).

## IMMUNIZATIONS

The Advisory Committee on Immunization Practices (ACIP) recommends immunizations for infants at 2, 4, 6, 9, and 12 months of age. The CDC, AAP, and American Academy of Family Physicians, among others, agree with these recommendations. The current immunization schedule is available at www.cdc.gov/vaccines/schedules/hcp/child-adolescent.html. Refer to Table 14.2 for quick access to immunizations recommended at particular ages.

## SCREENINGS

Well-child visits during infancy also provide an opportunity for other screenings, including for physical issues and postpartum depression.

### Anemia

Screen all 12-month-old infants for anemia by obtaining a serum hemoglobin. By risk assessment at 4 months of age, other infants needing a screening at 4 months include those born prematurely, those with low birth weight, and non-breastfeeding infants drinking non-iron-fortified or low-iron formula or cow's milk.

### Blood Pressure

Blood pressure (BP) screening is not ordinarily performed at health supervision visits during infancy. Perform a risk assessment to determine risk status and obtain BP measurement at each infant well child visit if the infant has:

- History of premature birth, low birth weight, or other neonatal condition requiring a neonatal intensive care stay
- History of congenital heart disease
- History of urinary tract infection, hematuria, proteinuria, known renal disease, urological malformation, or family history of congenital kidney disease
- History of malignancy, or bone marrow/stem cell/solid organ transplant
- Use of medications known to raise BP
- Systemic illness associated with hypertension such as tuberous sclerosis or neurofibromatosis
- Increased intracranial pressure (Treitz et al., 2020)

### Hearing

- Determine results of the hearing screen obtained at birth. At each visit, note the infant's response to sound as well as language development. If concerns exist related to the infant's hearing, obtain a formal audiologic evaluation (Hagan et al., 2017)

**TABLE 14.2 Recommended Immunizations by Infant Age**

| Immunization | 2 months | 4 months | 6 months | 9 months | 12 months |
|---|---|---|---|---|---|
| **Hepatitis B (Hep B)** | 2nd dose | | 3rd dose | | |
| **Diphtheria, tetanus, acellular pertussis (DTaP)** | 1st dose | 2nd dose | 3rd dose | | 4th dose may be given |
| **Haemophilus influenzae type b (Hib)** | 1st dose | 2nd dose | * | | 3rd or 4th dose* |
| **Inactivated poliovirus (IPV)** | 1st dose | 2nd dose | 3rd dose | | |
| **Influenza (IIV)** | | | Annually (1 to 2 doses) | | |
| **Rotavirus (RV)** | 1st dose | 2nd dose | ^ | | |
| **Measles, mumps, rubella (MMR)** | | | | | 1st dose may be given |
| **Varicella** | | | | | 1st dose may be given |
| **Hepatitis A** | | | | | 1st dose may be given |

*PedvaxHIb is a 3-dose series, the other brands are a 4-dose series

^RV1 is a 2-dose series. RV5 is a 3-dose series

*Source*: Data from Centers for Disease Control and Prevention. (2020). *Immunization schedules: Recommended child and adolescent immunization schedule for ages 18 years or younger, United States, 2020.* https://www.cdc.gov/vaccines/schedules/hcp/child-adolescent.html

### Lead Exposure

Infants 6 months and older should be screened for risk of lead exposure. Increased risk is associated with:

- Living in or visiting a home built before the 1970s (in poor repair or recently renovated) or with an identified lead hazard
- Lower socioeconomic status
- Use of folk remedies, ceramics, or pewter
- Exposure in countries still utilizing lead in gasoline, cookware, jewelry, toys, candy wrappers, and paint
- Parental occupation of smelting, soldering, or auto body repair
- Child abuse or neglect (Kelly, 2020)

Obtain a blood lead level if the infant has been determined to be at high risk based on the screenings at 6 and 9 months of age. At 12 months of age, obtain a blood lead level if the infant lives in a high prevalence area for lead poisoning or is on Medicaid.

### Postpartum Depression

Continue screening for maternal postpartum depression at the 1-month, 2-month, 4-month, and 6-month infant health supervision visits (see Chapter 13).

### Vision

Screen the infant's vision by determining the ability to fix and follow. If concerns exist, refer to pediatric ophthalmology for a full visual assessment (Hagan et al., 2017).

# ANTICIPATORY GUIDANCE

Provide anticipatory guidance related to nutrition, commonly occurring development concerns, dental health, screen time, sleep, and safety.

## NUTRITION

Exclusive breastfeeding is recommended until 6 months of age (see chapter 13). After 6 months of age, in addition to their breast milk or formula, infants usually require the nutrients available in solid foods. Successful solid food consumption best occurs when the tongue extrusion reflex is disappearing or has disappeared. In the newborn and young infant, the tongue automatically protrudes when a nipple is placed in the mouth, triggering sucking. With disappearance of this reflex around 4 to 6 months of age, the spoon may be successfully introduced (Duryea & Fleisher, 2020). The infant should also be capable of sitting up (even if supported). Additionally, ability to swallow solid food does not become completely functional until 4 to 6 months of age, at which time the enzymes necessary for digestion and absorption of food other than breast milk and formula become available.

Begin solid food introduction by mixing iron-fortified infant cereal with a small amount of breast milk or formula. The cereal's taste is generally well accepted and additionally it is easily digested. Mix the cereal quite thin at first, mixing it to a thicker consistency as the infant gets older. Once successful feeding of cereal with a spoon is achieved, other single foods puréed to a smooth consistency may be introduced. These foods may be purchased as prepackaged baby food or puréed at home. Instruct parents not to add sugar, salt, or other seasoning to these first foods. Introducing one new food every 3 to 5 days is recommended (Buchanan & Marquez, 2019). Offer the older infant soft foods such as sliced bananas, Cheerios, or cooked green bean pieces to encourage self-feeding and development of the pincer grasp. Teach the parent to avoid hard foods that the infant may choke on, such as peanuts, popcorn, and raw carrots, and to cut grapes and hot dog slices into smaller pieces to avoid blocking the airway. All foods except honey may be introduced throughout later infancy, including nut-containing foods. Strained, puréed, or mashed meats are more likely to be accepted if introduced at 10 to 12 months of age.

At 6 to 8 months of age, the cup may be introduced. Tell the parent to place one ounce of breast milk or formula in the cup while the infant is learning (to decrease the amount of mess should the cup be spilled). Avoid the use of newer no-spill sippy cups, as they require sucking (similar to the bottle), do not encourage learning of cup-drinking, and permit milk or other sugar-containing fluids to be in contact with the infant's teeth for long periods of time, increasing the risk for dental caries (American Academy of Pediatric Dentistry [AAPD], 2016). Older infants quickly learn to drink from an ordinary cup with assistance when they are thirsty, and are also able to drink from a straw. The AAP recommends against the introduction of fruit juice in infancy (Abrams, 2017).

▶ ALERT: Ordinary cow's milk is not recommended for the first year of life, as it is lacking in iron and does not provide the carbohydrate/fat/protein balance required by infants for optimal growth.

### Promoting Healthy Eating Habits

Learning about food occurs within a social context, with infants learning about eating through watching others. Therefore, it is important for the family to model appropriate eating behaviors for healthy eating habits to be created. Emphasizing healthy eating practices begins in infancy and both the permissive feeding style and authoritarian feeding style should be avoided. Allowing the infant to eat whatever they want (permissive) may lead to fights about eating in the future. Coercing the infant into eating all that is provided (authoritarian) not only sets the child up for overeating in the future but may also lead to power struggles (Duryea & Fleisher, 2020). A balance between the styles needs to be found for the establishment of lifelong healthy eating patterns in children.

## COMMON CONCERNS

Commonly occurring developmental issues may raise concern among parents and caregivers of infants. These include spitting up, colic, and the use of pacifiers, thumb sucking, and security items.

### Spitting Up

Spitting up occurs nearly universally in infants and can be concerning for parents. Strategies to decrease spitting-up episodes include:

- Feeding smaller amounts on a more frequent basis
- Always burp the infant at least two or three times per feeding
- Keep the infant in an upright position for 30 minutes after feeding
- Do not:
    - Bounce or provide excess activity immediately after feeding
    - Lay the infant prone after feeding
    - Position in an infant seat after feeding, as the stomach is compressed (AAP, 2019)

**PRO TIP** Instruct parents to notify the primary care provider if the infant chokes when vomiting, vomits one-third or more of most feedings, or experiences forceful emesis.

### Colic

Prolonged infant crying causes increased caregiver stress among parents, and failure to stop the crying leads to frustration. When crying prevents the caregivers from sleeping, the exhaustion they are already experiencing is exacerbated. For the colicky infant, parents should utilize a stepwise approach to check that all of the infant's basic needs are met. When all needs are met, attempts at soothing the infant may be used, one intervention at a time to avoid overstimulation. Strategies to manage colic include:

- Reduce stimulation to decrease the length of crying
- Carry the infant more often
- Incorporate motion or vibration (infant swing or a car ride)
- Provide white noise
- Swaddle younger infants
- A pacifier may be useful in the infant who needs additional nonnutritive sucking (Goldson et al., 2020).

### Pacifiers, Thumb Sucking, and Security Items

Cultural preferences and individual family values regarding sucking habits and security items should be explored with the family. Physical removal of pacifiers and security items may occur at some point, but the infant's thumb is attached, so this habit may be more difficult to break. Parents may observe that when the infant is intensely trying to master a new skill, such as sitting or walking, an increased need for self-soothing occurs. A stressful time for the infant is not the right time to break the sucking habit, nor to remove the security item. Parents should not try to break the habit during a stressful time for the infant. An optimal time for pacifier weaning is when the infant approaches 1 year of age, as this is the time when the need for additional sucking naturally decreases. Additional attention should not be drawn to the infant who sucks a thumb, as it may prolong thumb sucking. Weaning the child from a security blanket or toy should probably be reserved for after infancy.

## DENTAL HEALTH

Prior to the first tooth erupting, wipe the infant's mouth after feeding with a moistened cloth. After first tooth eruption in later infancy, in order to facilitate the best oral health, teach the family to:

- Never permit the infant to have a bottle in bed (if absolutely necessary, ensure that the bottle contains only water)
- Wean to the cup by 12 months of age
- Avoid juices in infants less than 12 months of age
- Avoid using foods with added sugars, such as "fruit"-flavored candy, or yogurt snacks (Hagan et al., 2017; Turner, 2018)

Once the first tooth has erupted, it is recommended to utilize fluoride, as it inhibits tooth demineralization while enhancing remineralization (Turner, 2018). Fluoride varnish should be applied to teeth of all infants at least once every 6 months, and every 3 months if at increased risk for dental caries. Establish a dental home at first tooth eruption and no later than 12 months of age (Hagan et al., 2017). Brush the infant's teeth with a very small smear of fluoridated toothpaste (size no more than a grain of rice) twice daily using a soft toothbrush or washcloth.

### Teething

Later in infancy, teething begins. As the tooth breaks through the periodontal membrane, inflammation occurs and infant discomfort is common. Drooling, biting on hard objects, or increased finger sucking may occur in teething infants. Increased irritability, refusal to eat, and poor sleep may also occur. Fever, vomiting, and diarrhea are generally not considered a sign of teething but rather of illness. Strategies to manage teething pain include:

- Apply cold to the gums:
  - Provide a cold (not frozen) teething ring for chewing on
  - Rub an ice cube wrapped in a washcloth on the gums
- Numerous over-the-counter natural teething remedies are available; review their ingredient lists prior to recommending to avoid potentially dangerous substances
- On occasion, oral acetaminophen or ibuprofen may be needed for pain relief (Gandhi et al., 2020)

▶ ALERT: Avoid use of topical numbing ointments containing benzocaine, as its use in infants has been linked to the development of methemoglobinemia.

## SCREEN TIME

Children under 2 years of age should be encouraged to participate in hands-on exploration of their environment. Digital media should be a avoided except in the case of video chatting (Turner, 2018).

## SLEEP

To decrease the risk of sudden infant death syndrome (SIDS), the AAP recommends that all infants sleep on their backs on a firm mattress for the first year of life. There should be no blankets, soft toys, or other objects in the crib with the infant. Breastfeeding, pacifier use, and sleeping in the same room with the parents (not the same bed) also seem to have protective effects against SIDS (Turner, 2018).

## SAFETY

Provide safety guidance in relation to the home, car, water, and environment.

### Car Safety

The infant should be fastened securely in a car safety seat, in the middle of the back seat, in the rear-facing position. Instruct parents not to allow the car seat to be placed in the front seat if the vehicle is equipped with air bags.

▶ ALERT: Never leave the infant unattended in the car. Heat levels rise very quickly within a closed vehicle, placing the infant at risk for injury or death (AAP, 2020).

### Environmental Exposures

With higher respiratory rates, developing organs, breathing areas closer to the floor or ground, and the repeated putting of substances into their mouths, infants are at increased risk for harmful exposures inside and outside of the home (Galvez & Balk, 2017). To prevent environmental exposures:

- Do not permit infants to be exposed to tobacco smoke or nicotine. Counsel the parent or caregiver to stop smoking (Treitz et al., 2020).
- Encourage better indoor air quality by frequently changing heat, air, and air conditioning (HVAC) filters.
- Avoid using pesticides and harsh cleaning agents in the home.
- Increased ventilation is important when using cleaning products or art supplies such as paint and glue.
- If the home was built before 1978, lead paint maybe present. Avoid home renovations when the child is in the home. Ascertain that water piping in the home is of a material other than lead.
- Advise parents to explore radon testing for in homes lower than a third floor and install a radon reduction system if needed.
- Repair any visible mold or water damage as soon as it is noted to avoid mold exposure of the infant. If the home is serviced by well water, rather than municipal water, ensure that the water is tested for contaminants and bacteria.
- Avoid exposure to neuroendocrine disrupters (phthalate and bisphenol A [BPA]) by advising

families to choose unprocessed foods, avoid heating foods in plastic containers, choose glass containers when possible, purchase products labeled phthalate and BPA free, and use wet methods to dust and mop to avoid phthalates in dust (Galvez & Balk, 2017).

### Sun Exposure

Protect the infant's skin from sun exposure by:

- Dressing the infant in protective clothing and a wide-brimmed hat
- Avoiding being outside between the hours of 10:00 a.m. and 4:00 p.m. in the warmer months
- Using sunscreen, with an SPF of at least 15, in the infant 6 months of age and older

### Water Safety

Infants can drown in a very small amount of water. Never leave an infant unattended in any body of water, including a draining bathtub. Infant swimming lessons have not been demonstrated to protect the infant from drowning; adult supervision is required at all times while the infant is in or around water.

## KEY POINTS

- Provide developmental surveillance of the infant by direct observation, questioning the parent in relation to milestones recently met, and the use of valid and reliable questionnaires.
- Update the infant's health history and perform a comprehensive physical examination at each health supervision visit.
- Plot the infant's weight, length, head circumference, and weight-for-length on the appropriate WHO growth charts.
- Provide immunizations to the infant as recommended by the ACIP.
- At 12 months of age, screen for anemia with a serum hemoglobin level.
- It is not necessary to check the infant's BP unless certain risk factors are present.
- Beginning at 6 months of age, screen infants for the risk of lead exposure.
- While breastfeeding is the preferred method for infant feeding, both breastfed and bottle-fed infants should be fed on cue rather than on a parent-designed schedule.
- The spoon may be used to introduce solid foods at the age of 4 to 6 months; the cup may be introduced at 6 months of age.
- Spitting up, colic, and teething occur as a part of normal development in the otherwise thriving infant and do not require medical intervention.
- Provide anticipatory guidance to parents in relation to dental health, car/home/water safety, and environmental exposures.

## REFERENCES

Abrams, S. J. (2017). *Weighing in on fruit juice: AAP now says no juice before age 1*. https://www.aappublications.org/news/2017/05/22/FruitJuice052217

Aites, J., & Schonwald, A. (2020). Developmental-behavioral surveillance and screening in primary care. In M. Augustyn (Ed.), *UpToDate*. Retrieved November 11, 2020, from https://www.uptodate.com/contents/developmental-behavioral-surveillance-and-screening-in-primary-care

American Academy of Pediatric Dentistry. (2016). *Perinatal and infant oral health care*. http://www.aapd.org/media/Policies_Guidelines/BP_PerinatalOralHealthCare.pdf

American Academy of Pediatrics. (2019). *Why babies spit up*. https://www.healthychildren.org/English/ages-stages/baby/feeding-nutrition/Pages/Why-Babies-Spit-Up.aspx

American Academy of Pediatrics. (2020). *Prevent child car deaths in hot cars*. https://www.healthychildren.org/English/safety-prevention/on-the-go/Pages/Prevent-Child-Deaths-in-Hot-Cars.aspx

American Academy of Pediatrics/Bright Futures. (2020). *Recommendations for preventive pediatric health care*. https://downloads.aap.org/AAP/PDF/periodicity_schedule.pdf

Buchanan, A. O., & Marquez, M. L. (2019). Pediatric nutrition and nutritional disorders. In K. J. Marcdante & R. M. Kliegman (Eds.), *Nelson's essentials of pediatrics* (8th ed., Section 6). Elsevier.

Cassidy, J., & Shaver, P. R. (2016). *Handbook of attachment: Theory, research, and clinical applications* (3rd ed.). Guilford Press.

Centers for Disease Control and Prevention. (2010). *WHO growth standards are recommended for use in the U.S. for infants and children 0 to 2 years of age*. https://www.cdc.gov/growthcharts/who_charts.htm#The%20WHO%20Growth%20Charts

Drutz, J. E. (2020). The pediatric physical examination: General principles and standard measurements. In T. K. Duryea (Ed.), *UpToDate*. Retrieved November 11, 2020, from https://www.uptodate.com/contents/the-pediatric-physical-examination-general-principles-and-standard-measurements

Duryea, T. K., & Fleisher, D. M. (2020). Patient education: Starting solid foods during infancy (Beyond the basics). In K. J. Motil & J. E. Drutz (Eds.), *UpToDate*. Retrieved November 18, 2020, from https://www.uptodate.com/contents/starting-solid-foods-during-infancy-beyond-the-basics#H3

Galvez, M. P., & Balk, S. J. (2017). Environmental risks to children: Prioritizing health messages in pediatric practice. *Pediatrics in Review, 38*(6), 263–279. http://dx.doi.org/10.1542/pir.2015-0165

Gandhi, R. P., Puranik, C. P., Wilson, A., & Chin, K. L. (2020). Oral medicine and dentistry. In W. W. Hay, M. J. Levin, M. J. Abzug, & M. Bunik (Eds.), *Current diagnosis & treatment: Pediatrics* (25th ed., Chapter 17). McGraw-Hill Education.

Goldson, E., Angulo, A. S., Raz, D. M., & Reynolds, A. (2020). Child development and behavior. In W. W. Hay, M. J. Levin, M. J. Abzug, & M. Bunik (Eds.), *Current diagnosis & treatment: Pediatrics* (25th ed., Chapter 3). McGraw-Hill Education.

Hagan, J. F., Shaw, J. S., & Duncan, P. M. (Eds.). (2017). *Bright Futures: Guidelines for health supervision of infants, children, and adolescents* (4th ed.). Bright Futures/American Academy of Pediatrics.

Kelly, N. R. (2020). Screening tests in children and adolescents. In J. E. Drutz (Ed.), *UpToDate*. Retrieved November 11, 2020, from https://www.uptodate.com/contents/screening-tests-in-children-and-adolescents

Lipkin, P. H., Macias, M. M., & the Council on Children with Disabilities, Section on Developmental and Behavioral Pediatrics. (2020). Promoting optimal development: Identifying infants and young children with developmental disorders through developmental surveillance and screening. *Pediatrics, 145*(1), e20193449. https://doi.org/10.1542/peds.2019-3449

Paul H. Brookes Publishing. (2020). *ASQ: Ages and Stages Questionnaires*. https://agesandstages.com

Pedstest.com. (2016). *PEDS test*. https://pedstest.com/index.html

Treitz, M., Nicklas, D., & Fox, D. (2020). Ambulatory & office pediatrics. In W. W. Hay, M. J. Levin, M. J. Abzug, & M. Bunik (Eds.), *Current diagnosis & treatment: Pediatrics* (25th ed., Chapter 9). McGraw-Hill Education.

Tufts Children's Hospital. (2020). *The survey of well-being of young children*. https://www.tuftschildrenshospital.org/The-Survey-of-Wellbeing-of-Young-Children/Age-Specific-Forms

Turner, K. (2018). Well-child visits for infants and young children. *American Family Physician, 98*(6), 347–353. https://www.aafp.org/afp/2018/0915/p347.html

# Well-Child Visits During Toddlerhood

Theresa Kyle

## Student Learning Outcomes

**Upon completion of this chapter the reader should be able to:**

1. Determine expected and healthy growth of toddlers.
2. Evaluate developmental milestones of toddlers.
3. Choose appropriate screening tests based on current recommendations for child's age and risk status.
4. Select immunizations based on current recommendations for child's age and risk status.
5. Determine applicable anticipatory guidance for each scheduled visit during toddlerhood.

The content in this chapter maps to the following areas on the Pediatric Nursing Certification Board (PNCB) Pediatric Nurse Practitioner—Primary Care certification examination:

CONTENT AREAS:

**I. Health Maintenance and Promotion**

**A. Partner with patients/caregivers to support growth and development from infancy to young adulthood**

**B. Provide patients/caregivers with age/developmentally appropriate anticipatory guidance**

**C. Recommend and prescribe immunizations according to current CDC guidelines**

**D. Educate about illness prevention and early warning signs of pediatric illness and emergencies**

**E. Advise patients/caregivers about age appropriate injury prevention and safety (environmental exposure, risk taking behaviors, social situations, sports and recreation, and vehicle safety)**

**F. Counsel about age-appropriate social, behavioral, and mental health concerns (e.g., substance abuse, social media use, grief and loss, and sexual orientation/LGBTQ)**

**II. Assessment and Diagnosis**

**A. Growth and Development**

1. Evaluate and interpret growth parameters
2. Perform developmental surveillance

## INTRODUCTION

The toddler period is a time of activity, curiosity, and lack of internal limits, which are all important and wonderful parts of toddler development. However, this crucial learning period can be a source of ongoing stress for parents, as constant supervision and guidance are required around the clock. The normal developmental milestones of toddlerhood can also cause frustration in the toddler. During this time of critical learning for the child and the parents, the parent can best help their child by remaining patient and consistent, and this comes more easily when the parent knows what to expect as well as what behaviors are considered to be typical.

Regarding this period, Bright Futures recommends five standard outpatient well-child visits. Health supervision should occur at 15 months, 18 months, 2 years, 30 months, and 3 years of age in the otherwise healthy toddler (Hagan et al., 2017). Toddlers born prematurely or who demonstrate other health concerns may need more frequent visits.

**B. History and Physical Examination**

1. Obtain history of present illness
2. Obtain a comprehensive health history for new patients
3. Complete an interval history for established patients
4. Perform a review of systems
5. Perform a complete physical examination

**C. Diagnostic Testing and Screening**

1. Order and interpret office/clinic based screening tests
4. Select, utilize, and interpret developmental, behavioral and mental health screening and assessment tools

**D. Analyzing Information**

1. Integrate health history and physical examination findings into the plan of care
2. Assimilate findings from screening and diagnostic testing into plan of care

### IV. Professional Role and Responsibilities

**B. Practice Management**

1. Document patient encounters in a manner which supports applicable diagnostic and procedure codes
2. Utilize appropriate billing and coding to facilitate reimbursement

## PARENT-CHILD INTERACTION

The parent-toddler relationship is vital to the toddler's growth and development. Secure attachment is fundamental to the toddler's confidence in their world, and when experiencing secure attachment the toddler feels assured that the parent will be there for them when needed (Cassidy & Shaver, 2016). Observe the parents' interaction with the child and the toddler's responses. Refer to Table 14.1 in chapter 14 for information about secure and insecure attachment. Support the parent in interactions that promote secure attachment.

▶ ALERT: Warning signs of poor emotional attachment include:

- Demonstrates poor eye contact
- Excessive fearfulness
- Clingy behaviors
- Frequent crying
- Is not consoled by parent
- Frequent nightmares or other sleep problems

## DEVELOPMENTAL SURVEILLANCE

Parent-completed developmental screening questionnaires recognize the parent as expert on their toddler, provide assessment information valuable for developmental surveillance, and are recommended for use by the American Academy of Pediatrics (AAP; Aites & Schonwald, 2020; Hagan et al., 2017). These questionnaires can be completed prior to the visit, saving time during the visit. Tools with demonstrated reliability and validity appropriate for use in toddlerhood include:

- Ages and Stages Questionnaires (ASQ-3; Paul H. Brookes Publishing, 2020)
- Parent's Evaluation of Developmental Status (PEDS test; Pedstest.com, 2016)
- PEDS: Developmental Milestones (PEDS: DM)
- Survey of Well-being of Young Children (SWYC; Tufts Children's Hospital, 2020)

Periodic evaluation at each well-child visit during this period will allow for early identification of toddlers who may be at risk for developmental delay (Lipkin et al., 2020; Treitz et al., 2020). In addition to the screening questionnaire, begin the health history at each well-toddler visit by asking, "Since the last visit, what changes have you seen in your child's development?" Or start the conversation with, "What's your toddler doing that's new since the last visit?" Expected developmental milestones for each age in toddlerhood may be found in chapter 8.

## HEALTH ASSESSMENT

Each toddler well-child visit will include a comprehensive health assessment. The assessment includes developmental surveillance, as noted earlier, as well as health history and physical examination data. Each visit also includes prevention (immunization or screening as appropriate) and anticipatory guidance appropriate for age, always including but not limited to nutrition, sleep, and safety (Hagan et al., 2017).

### SUBJECTIVE DATA

Along with development surveillance, obtain information from the caregiver in relation to past medical history (since last health supervision visit), diet, sleep, dental care, changes in family or social history, and results of prior screenings. Always address any concerns the parents may have (Turner, 2018). Toddlerhood is a pivotal time for social and emotional development and expected toddler behavior can be quite trying for parents.

While obtaining the health history, permit the toddler to safely explore the examination room, returning to the parent as needed for comfort. As the toddler exhibits a particular behavior, point out the typical nature of it, although it may be a frustrating behavior. Throughout the interview speak with both the toddler and the parent, allowing time for the toddler to become a bit more at ease.

## OBJECTIVE DATA

In addition to observation of the parent-toddler interaction, perform a comprehensive physical examination, beginning with observation of the toddler's general appearance (happy, calm, well-appearing, active, neatly/cleanly clothed). Note body habitus and nutritional status. The toddler's weight, recumbent length, occipitofrontal head circumference, and weight-for-length should be plotted on the gender-appropriate World Health Organization (WHO) growth chart until age 2 years (Centers for Disease Control and Prevention [CDC], 2010). After age 2 years, begin measuring standing height instead of recumbent length and plot weight, height, and body mass index (BMI) for age on the gender-appropriate charts (CDC, 2016).

Begin the examination with the young toddler on the parent's lap. Approach the toddler slowly, as most toddlers experience stranger anxiety. Always begin with the least intrusive portions of the assessment first, saving the most intrusive for last. Some toddlers respond well to seeing the equipment first being used on the parent or on a doll or stuffed animal. Talking to the toddler and/or singing throughout the examination may assist the provider with gaining the toddler's cooperation.

On examination of the skin, note nevi, café-au-lait spots, bruises, or other skin changes. Palpate the young toddler's anterior fontanel to determine it has closed by 18 months of age. Assess for strabismus or an unequal Hirschberg reflex. Evaluate the pupils' presence of a bilateral red reflex and for opacification (not desired). Screen visual acuity by determining the ability to fix and follow (15 months). Assess the teeth for hygiene, caries, plaque, staining, injury, or white spots (demineralization). The gums should be healthy and pink. Respirations should be unlabored and more regular than in infancy. Auscultate the heart for murmur and palpate the femoral pulses for equality. Palpate the abdomen for masses (none should be found).

Observe the extremities for equality of size, tone, and movement. Observe the toddler walking or running. Evaluate hand control, arm and spine movement. Assess deep tendon reflexes, which should be average. Observe the toddler's level of consciousness and interaction with the environment. In the 2- to 3-year-old, observe for socialization and note language acquisition and clarity. Additional neurologic assessments by age include:

- 2 years: Scribbling, ability to follow commands
- 30 months and 3 years: Coordination

Note the toddler's response to auditory and visual stimuli. In boys, determine whether testes are fully descended, and in girls whether the labia are open. Any alterations noted on the physical examination may warrant further screening or other investigation (Drutz, 2020).

**PRO TIP** To assess gross motor development, make it a game. Have the toddler copy the examiner's movements (lift hands over head, touch toes, crouch down like a frog, jump with both feet). To assess fine motor development, bring a crayon into the examination room and ask the toddler to draw a particular picture or item on the examination table paper.

# PREVENTION

Prevention during the toddler health supervision visits includes routine recommended immunization and targeted health screenings. The AAP recommendations for preventive pediatric health care may be found at https://downloads.aap.org/AAP/PDF/periodicity_schedule.pdf (AAP/Bright Futures, 2020).

## IMMUNIZATIONS

The Advisory Committee on Immunization Practices (ACIP) recommends immunizations for toddlers at 12 to 18 months, and influenza vaccination annually. The CDC, AAP, and American Academy of Family Physicians, among others, agree with these recommendations. The current immunization schedule is available at www.cdc.gov/vaccines/schedules/hcp/child-adolescent.html. Refer to Table 15.1 for quick access to immunizations recommended at particular ages.

## SCREENINGS

Well-child visits during infancy also provide an opportunity for other screenings, including for particular health conditions, hearing, vision, and lead exposure.

**TABLE 15.1 Recommended Immunizations by Toddler Age**

| Immunization | 12–15 months | 18 months | 2 years | 3 years |
|---|---|---|---|---|
| **Hepatitis B (Hep B)** | 3rd dose may be given between 6 and 18 months | | | |
| **Diphtheria, tetanus, acellular pertussis (DTaP)** | 4th dose may be given between 12 and 18 months | | | |
| ***Haemophilus influenzae* type b (Hib)** | *3rd dose or 4th dose between 12 and 15 months | | | |
| **Inactivated poliovirus (IPV)** | 3rd dose may be given between 6 and 18 months | 2nd dose | | |
| **Measles, mumps, rubella (MMR)** | 1st dose between 12 and 15 months | | | |
| **Varicella** | 1st dose between 12 and 15 months | | | |
| **Hepatitis A** | 2-dose series (minimum age 12 months, minimum 6-month interval between doses) | | | |

*PedvaxHIb is a 3-dose series, the other brands are a 4-dose series.

*Source*: Data from Centers for Disease Control and Prevention. (2020). *Immunization schedules: Recommended child and adolescent immunization schedule for ages 18 years or younger, United States, 2020.* https://www.cdc.gov/vaccines/schedules/hcp/child-adolescent.html

## Anemia

Ask parents if the toddler's diet includes iron-rich foods (meat, beans, iron-fortified cereals). Determine if the family is experiencing food insecurity. Screen all 12-month-old toddlers for anemia by determining hemoglobin level, either by point-of-care testing (if available) or serum sent out to the lab. According to risk assessment, other toddlers needing a screening at that time include those born prematurely, those with low birth weight, and non-breastfeeding toddlers drinking large quantities of cow's milk.

## Autism

Screen for early signs of autism. These signs are often noted by parents prior to 18 months of age and include:

- 6 to 12 months:
  - Decreased response to name, gaze to faces, shared smiles
  - Decreased vocalizations to others
  - Tendency to fixate on particular objects in the environment
- 12 months: Lack of orientation to name
- 14 months: Lack of pointing to object of interest
- 12 to 24 months:
  - Decreased frequency of sharing experiences, interests, or attention with other
  - Repetitive or perseverative behavior
  - Delayed receptive and expressive language
  - Lack of pretend play by 18 months
- Other red flags parents report include:
  - Intolerance to change
  - Eye contact avoidance
  - Prefers being alone

Regardless of the presence or absence of these parentally reported signs, all children should be screened for autism at 18 and 24 months of age with a valid, reliable tool such as the Modified Checklist for Autism in Toddlers, Revised with Follow-up (M-CHAT-R/F) or the Screening Tool for Autism in Toddlers and Young Children (SCAT). If the toddler screens positive with the initial tool, follow-up and further screening are warranted.

## Blood Pressure

Blood pressure (BP) screening begins at age 3 years in the healthy child. Perform a risk assessment to determine risk status and obtain BP measurement at each toddler well child visit if the toddler has:

- History of premature birth, low birth weight, or other neonatal condition requiring a neonatal intensive care stay
- History of congenital heart disease
- History of urinary tract infection, hematuria, proteinuria, known renal disease, urological malformation, or family history of congenital kidney disease
- History of malignancy, or bone marrow/stem cell/solid organ transplant
- Use of medications known to raise BP
- Systemic illness associated with hypertension, such as tuberous sclerosis or neurofibromatosis
- Increased intracranial pressure (Treitz et al., 2020)

### Hearing

Review the results of the hearing screen obtained at birth. At each visit, note the toddler's response to sound as well as language development. Ask the parents if they have any concerns about how the toddler hears or speaks. If concerns exist related to the toddler's hearing, obtain a formal audiologic evaluation (Hagan et al., 2017).

### Lead Exposure

Perform a risk assessment at 18 and 24 months of age. If the toddler lives in a high-prevalence area for lead poisoning or is on Medicaid, obtain a blood lead level (Kelly, 2020).

### Vision

Screen the toddler's vision by determining the ability to fix and follow. If available, screen vision using photo screening (special camera measuring light reflexes in the eye determining visual acuity and risk for amblyopia) (American Academy of Pediatric Ophthalmology and Strabismus, 2020). The average 3-year-old is usually developmentally capable of completing visual acuity screening with an age-appropriate chart such as the Tumbling E chart or the Allen chart (or similar picture-type chart). If concerns exist, refer to pediatric ophthalmology for a full visual assessment (Hagan et al., 2017).

## ANTICIPATORY GUIDANCE

Teach parents about the importance of physical activity. Toddlers need at least 3 hours per day of physical activity with at least 30 minutes of the activity being planned and directed by an adult. Limit screen time (television, computer, any digital media) to no more than 1 hour per day. Additionally, provide anticipatory guidance related to nutrition, discipline, commonly occurring developmental concerns, dental health, sleep, and safety.

## NUTRITION

Extending breastfeeding into toddlerhood is believed to be beneficial to the child, as it provides nutritional, immunologic, and emotional benefits. Cultural beliefs, local and regional ethnic beliefs, societal feelings about the nature of the mother–infant relationship, desired child spacing, and/or the mother's work schedule may influence the timing of weaning from breastfeeding. The AAP recommends breastfeeding for at least 12 months, then for as long as is mutually agreeable to mother and child (2020a).

By toddlerhood, the child should be adept at drinking from the cup, is developmentally capable of consuming adequate fluid volume using a cup, and should be weaned from the bottle by 12 to 15 months of age. Prolonged bottle-feeding and the use of no-spill sippy cups (the type with a valve requiring sucking) are associated with the development of dental caries. The use of no-spill sippy cups is not recommended (American Academy of Pediatric Dentistry [AAPD], 2016). Use of a cup with a spout that does not contain a valve is acceptable. Encourage the toddler to drink water and limit fruit juice intake to 4 to 6 ounces per day. Serve juice or milk in a cup with meals and snacks, and offer water from the cup for between-meal drinking.

**PRO TIP** When weaning from breastfeeding or infant formula occurs, breast milk is often replaced with cow's milk, which is iron-poor. Limit milk intake to 16 to 24 ounces per day to encourage the intake of other foods, including those rich in iron and vitamin C, in order to prevent iron deficiency.

Although the toddler continues to grow rapidly, toddler growth is not as fast-paced as that of the infant. Thus, the toddler may demonstrate periods of physiologic anorexia and food jags, preferring to eat only one type of food for a period of time. Self-regulation of food intake occurs in the toddler who, although not eating well every day, tends to consume the amounts and types of food needed for further growth and development (Satter, 2019). Large portion size may intimidate the toddler. Recommended serving sizes for toddlers are:

- Dairy—½ cup milk, ½ ounce cheese, or ⅓ cup yogurt
- Fruits—½ of a fresh fruit; ½ cup cooked, frozen, or canned fruit; or 2 ounces 100% fruit juice
- Grains—⅓ cup dry cereal, 2 to 3 crackers, ½ slice bread, or ¼ cup cooked cereal, rice, or pasta
- Meats (and other proteins)—½ egg, ¼ cup cooked beans, or 1 ounce chicken, fish, meat, or tofu
- Vegetables—¼ cup cooked vegetables (AAP, 2015)

Teach parents to offer three full meals and two snacks daily. Toddlers can be picky eaters. A new food on the plate may result in reluctance of the toddler to try new things. Encourage parents to be flexible about the toddler's potential rejection of a new food. Some parents perceive the developmentally normal behaviors of mouthing, handling, tasting,

**BOX 15.1 Guidance for Feeding Toddlers**

- Cut food into bite-size pieces
- Make sure some of the food on the plate is moist and soft
- Serve food near room temperature
- At each meal, include foods the toddler is known to like, and at some meals introduce a new food as well
- Offer praise for trying a new food and do not punish if a new food is refused
- Permit toddlers to eat with their fingers
- Provide child-sized spoon and fork (with dull tines)
- Limit fruit juice to 4 to 6 ounces per day
- Ensure adequate fiber intake
- Have the toddler sit in a secure highchair or booster chair with feet supported
- Serve the toddler with the rest of the family and do not leave unattended while eating
- Minimize distractions during meals (television, etc.)
- Provide a calm and pleasant eating environment

*Sources*: Data from Haemer, M. A., Diab, L. K., Primak, L. E., & Krebs, N. F. (2020). Normal childhood nutrition & its disorders. In W. W. Hay, M. J. Levin, M. J. Abzug, & M. Bunik (Eds.), *Current diagnosis & treatment: Pediatrics* (25th ed., Chapter 11). McGraw-Hill Education; Satter, E. (2019). *Child feeding ages and stages.* https://www.ellynsatterinstitute.org/how-to-feed/child-feeding-ages-and-stages

extruding the food from the mouth, and then resampling the food to be distasteful. Educate parents to tolerate these behaviors rather than scolding the toddler when they occur (Lieberman, 2018). When the toddler refuses the healthy food choice provided, instruct the parents not to provide high-sugar, high-fat, or processed food just to make sure the toddler eats something (Parks et al., 2020). To avoid power struggles, the parent should decide which foods are offered, while the toddler decides how much will be eaten. Refer to Box 15.1 for additional guidance on feeding toddlers.

▶ **ALERT:** Provide young children with only pasteurized juice. Unpasteurized juice consumption places the toddler at increased risk of *Escherichia coli*, *Salmonella*, and *Cryptosporidium* infection.

To avoid choking in toddlers, always cut foods into bite-sized pieces. Grate raw carrots rather than cutting them. Always cut grapes and hotdog slices into quarters. Do not give the toddler gumdrops or other chewy candies, nuts, peanut butter by itself, or popcorn. If the toddler will not drink milk, ensure adequate calcium intake with cheese, regular or frozen yogurt, pudding, or warm cocoa. When meat intake is poor, cook with an iron skillet. The toddler may also obtain iron through unsweetened iron-fortified cereals or breakfast bars, or raisins. If the toddler loves processed white bread, encourage adequate fiber intake with fresh fruits and vegetables, bran muffins, beans, or peas (can be in soup). When a toddler refuses vegetables, adequate vitamin A intake may be achieved with apricots, sweet potatoes, and vegetable juices.

## Healthy Eating

The foundation for health eating habits throughout life is laid in early childhood, with lifelong diet having a significant influence on overall health and the prevention of obesity (Haemer et al., 2020). Early overweight and obesity may result in metabolic programming and is associated with subsequent obesity and metabolic syndrome as early as in childhood (Klish & Skelton, 2020). Childhood obesity has also been linked to the future development of hypertension (Flynn et al., 2017). The greatest risk factor for the development of overweight or obesity in children is having a parent with a high BMI (Klish & Skelton, 2020), with juice intake also being a contributing factor (Parks et al., 2020).

Prevention of overweight and obesity during early childhood is best achieved via family role modeling of appropriate eating, and family mealtime results in better nutritional status for children, including age-appropriate BMI (Dallacker et al., 2018). Learning about food occurs within a social context, with toddlers learning about eating through watching others; therefore, it is important for the family to model appropriate eating behaviors for healthy eating habits to be created. Emphasizing healthy eating practices begins in infancy, continues through early childhood, and should not utilize either the permissive feeding style or the authoritarian feeding style. Allowing the toddler to eat whatever they want (permissive) may lead to fights about eating in the future. Coercing the toddler into eating all that is provided (authoritarian) not only sets the child up for overeating in the future but may also lead to power struggles. A balance between the styles needs to be found for the establishment of lifelong healthy eating patterns in children.

**PRO TIP** Toddlers consuming a strictly vegan diet with no food from animal sources are at risk for deficiencies in iron, vitamin $B_{12}$, and vitamin D. Provide supplementation with these nutrients to promote adequate nutrition and growth (Parks et al., 2020).

## DISCIPLINE

Toddlers experience a great deal of frustration as they learn about their lives in this world. They have temper tantrums, exhibit difficulty with impulse control, and experience extremes of emotions and intense feelings, all without having the maturity to effectively deal with them. They need assistance with learning self-regulation, controlling impulses, and dealing with emotions and feelings. With appropriate guidance and discipline (rather than punishment), a toddler can learn those things as well as learn to recognize others' feelings and develop empathy (Brazelton & Sparrow, 2015).

Toddlers' intense personalities and extreme emotions are difficult for some parents to understand and learn to cope with. Gentle, firm guidance is needed about expectations and how to meet them. Affection and respect are important guidance aspects of discipline. Yet toddlers naturally tend to push the limits imposed upon them, and many parents resort to spanking. Although historically commonly accepted, the AAP (2018) and the American Academy of Child and Adolescent Psychiatry (2018) recommend against corporal or physical punishment. The toddler younger than 18 months of age is at increased risk for physical injury from spanking and is not able to make the correct connection between the undesired behavior and the spanking (Global Initiative to End All Corporal Punishment of Children, 2018). Spanking is less effective than other discipline techniques at decreasing unwanted toddler behaviors. Physical punishment is not a good model for learning effective problem solving, may create resentment and lead to a pro-violence attitude, and may weaken the parent-child relationship when used frequently. Later effects of physical punishment include increased aggression as older children and adults, increased risk for substance abuse and depression in adulthood, criminal and antisocial behavior, and more frequent incidence of hitting their own children or spouse (Global Initiative to End All Corporal Punishment of Children, 2018).

It is recommended to provide a childproof environment to allow the toddler to participate in safe exploration, meeting his or her developmental needs and decreasing the frequency of intervention needed on the part of the parents. One of the most important aspects of toddler discipline is providing consistency and committing to the limits set. Offer the toddler realistic choices to promote their sense of mastery. Choose a limited number of rules and keep them simple. Toddlers do not understand the concept of sharing and should not be forced to do so. Encourage simple activities that each child enjoys to avoid confrontation over toys or other items. Parents should maintain the toddler's routine as much as possible (including meals, naps, and sleep) in an attempt to prevent conflicts occurring as a result of fatigue or hunger. When a choice exists, offer the toddler a choice to help them develop autonomy.

Focus toddler discipline on limit setting, negotiation, and techniques to assist the toddler to learn problem solving. Use positive reinforcement as much as possible. Reinforce desirable behaviors by catching the toddler being good. When an appropriate behavior is displayed, the parent should reward the child consistently with physical affection and praise. At around 2.5 to 3 years of age, time-out can be used effectively (refer to chapter 15 for details). For the 2- to 3-year-old, extinction should be used (systematic ignoring of the undesired behavior). While an annoying behavior can be difficult for the parent to ignore, the results of doing so are well worth the effort.

## COMMON CONCERNS

Commonly occurring developmental issues may raise concern among parents and caregivers of toddlers. These include temper tantrums, aggressive behavior, and the approach to discipline.

### Temper Tantrums and Aggressive Behavior

Although the toddler is progressing quickly in the ability to communicate, they still experience a great deal of frustration with expressing themselves. Instruct parents to pay attention to how the toddler communicates their wants and interests. Remember that as the toddler struggles with individuation and separation, life may be a bit like an emotional roller coaster. Temper tantrums typically occur in toddlerhood as a result of the toddler's quest for independence. When parents pay attention to the toddler's behavioral cues, they are able to identify when to limit an activity that is frustrating to the toddler. The parent may use a friendly warning initially when the beginnings of frustration are noted, as intervening early with an activity change may prevent a tantrum. Educate the parent to use refocusing, distraction, or removal from the situation (Sears & Sears, 2020).

When the frustration actually progresses to a temper tantrum, the parent needs to ensure the toddler's safety and ignore the behavior. Tantrums are often prolonged and result in more intense negative behavior when physical punishment is used. Immobilizing the toddler with a big bear hug and using a calm, soothing voice may also be effective. Parents are role models for their children and modeling self-control is a very important activity. This role-modeling teaches toddlers to control their temper when they cannot get what they want (O'Donnell, 2018). Otherwise, aggressive behaviors may also occur and are typical during the toddler years. Educate parents to guide the toddler toward socially acceptable actions in order to foster development of appropriate social judgment. Promote empathy-building in the toddler by pointing out when someone is hurt and explaining what happened. To help the toddler come to have control over their environment and establish a sense of mastery, the parent should offer limited choices (rather than the opportunity to respond with "no").

## DENTAL HEALTH

If not completed in infancy, establish a dental home at 12 months of age and ensure annual visits (Hagan et al., 2017). Twice daily, brush the toddler's teeth with a very small amount of fluoridated toothpaste (a smear; the size of a grain of rice). To prevent dental caries:

- To avoid continual contact of the teeth with milk sugars, do not permit the toddler to have a bottle in bed or utilize a no-spill sippy cup.
- Do not feed the toddler foods with added sugars, such as fruit-flavored candy or yogurt snacks.
- Limit eating to meal and snack times rather than permitting grazing throughout the day.
- Supplement with fluoride as appropriate and have fluoride varnishes applied to primary teeth (Hagan et al., 2017; Nowak & Warren, 2020)

To ensure that most children receive adequate fluoride intake to prevent dental caries, many municipal water sources are fluoridated. If the water supply contains less than 0.3 parts per million (ppm) of fluoride, prescribe fluoride supplement 0.25 mg daily (AAPD, 2018). Teach parents to avoid the development of fluorosis (mottling of the enamel) by avoiding excess fluoride ingestion. Fluoride varnish should be applied to teeth of all toddlers at least once every 6 months, and every 3 months if at increased risk for dental caries.

## SLEEP

The toddler needs consistent rituals in order to achieve adequate sleep. Teach parents to choose a bedtime routine and remain consistent with it. An evening bedtime is very helpful in preparing toddlers for sleep. A warm bath followed by reading a story or quietly singing a song is a good idea. Minimize outside distractions during the bedtime routine. Toddlers often need security items to help them fall asleep. The toddler should not take a bottle to bed. A nightlight may also be helpful, as older toddlers are sometimes afraid of the dark. Night waking may occur in some toddlers, either as a result of change in routine or as a desire for nighttime attention. It is important to minimize attention during night waking, so the toddler is not rewarded for being awake at night. Sometime the night waking occurs a result of nightmares, which occur as the toddler's imagination capacity for make-believe expands. Teach parents to limit television viewing shortly before bedtime and to hold and comfort the toddler after a nightmare.

## SAFETY

Provide safety guidance in relation to the home, car, water, and environment.

### Preventing Poisoning

Innate curiosity and an expanding ability to explore the environment, along with the toddler's increasing mobility, allow the toddler to more efficiently gain access to materials that may be unsafe for them to handle. Additionally, poor taste discrimination in toddlers allows for ingestion of chemicals or other materials that older children would find too unpleasant to swallow. Discuss poisoning prevention with the parents at each well-child visit. Potentially poisonous substances (e.g., medications, cleaners, hair care products, car care products) must be stored out of the toddler's reach, out of the toddler's sight, and in a childproof, locked cabinet (AAP, 2019). Teach the parents to post the poison control center phone number [(800) 222-1222] in an easily accessible area in the home and to program it into their mobile phones. If the toddler ingests anything they should not, the parent should call the poison control center immediately. Inform parents that syrup of ipecac is no longer recommended to be kept in the home for use in the event of accidental ingestion.

Educate families to follow these safety measures:

- Store all substances in original containers only and never store any other liquid in a soda pop bottle other than the soda that came in it.
- Confirm that all medications have child-safety caps.
- Keep out of reach of the toddler:
  - Lozenges
  - Transdermal patch medications (prior to and following use)
  - Sample medications not packaged in safety containers
  - Baby powder, lotions, creams, and other hygiene products
  - Button batteries
  - House plants
- Never refer to medicine as candy, as the toddler may mistake pills for candy and ingest them.
- Avoid exposing toddlers to hazardous vapors such as paints, cleaners, tobacco smoke, marijuana, crack (cocaine), or heroin (AAP, 2019; American Association of Poison Control Centers, n.d.).

## Car Safety

The toddler should be fastened securely in an appropriately sized car safety seat, in the middle of the back seat in the rear-facing position, until they reach 2 years of age. Car seats should have harness straps and a clip for securing the child, and tethers for anchoring the seat in the vehicle. After 2 years of age, an appropriately sized forward-facing seat may be used. Instruct parents not to allow the car seat to be placed in the front seat if the vehicle is equipped with air bags. Teach parents not to permit children to ride in the cargo bed of a truck (Durbin et al., 2018).

▶ **ALERT:** The level of heat in a closed vehicle rises quickly, so the toddler should *never* be left unattended in the car, to avoid risk for injury or death (AAP, 2020b).

## Environmental Exposures

Similar to infants, toddlers are at increased risk for harmful exposures inside and outside of the home (Galvez & Balk, 2017). Refer to chapter 14 for information related to preventing environmental exposures in toddlers.

### Sun Exposure

Protect the toddler's skin from sun exposure by:

- Dressing the toddler in protective clothing and a wide-brimmed hat
- Avoiding being outside between the hours of 10:00 a.m. and 4:00 p.m. in the warmer months
- Using sunscreen with an SPF of at least 15 with UVA and UVB (broad spectrum) protection.

## Water Safety

Toddlers can drown in a very small amount of water, such as a bucket, toilet, bathtub, or puddle. The top-heavy toddler is at increased risk for drowning due to body proportions. Never leave a toddler unattended in any body of water, including a draining bathtub. Toddler swimming lessons have not been demonstrated to protect the toddler from drowning, although water safety classes may be helpful. Adult supervision is required at all times while the toddler is in or around water.

## KEY POINTS

- Provide developmental surveillance of the toddler by direct observation, questioning the parent in relation to milestones recently met, and using valid and reliable questionnaires.
- Update the toddler's health history and perform a comprehensive physical examination at each health supervision visit.
- Plot the toddler's weight, length, head circumference, and weight-for-length on the appropriate WHO growth charts, until age 2 years. After age 2 years, plot the toddler's weight, height, and BMI on the gender-appropriate CDC growth charts.
- Provide immunizations to the toddler as recommended by ACIP.
- At 12 months of age, screen for anemia by determining hemoglobin level.
- It is not necessary to check the toddler's BP until age 3 years, unless certain risk factors are present.
- Screen toddlers for the risk of lead exposure.
- Toddlers may demonstrate physiologic anorexia and go on food jags, yet they should still be provided with nutritious, healthy food options rather than high-sugar, high-fat, processed snacks.
- Respond to temper tantrums calmly; ignore them while keeping the toddler safe, rather than punishing the toddler.
- Toddler discipline should focus on clear limits and consistency, not spanking. Limits should be balanced with a caring and nurturing environment along with frequent praise for appropriate behavior.

- A prime safety focus of the toddler years is the prevention of accidental ingestion.
- Provide anticipatory guidance to parents in relation to dental health, car/home/water safety, and environmental exposure avoidance.

## REFERENCES


Aites, J., & Schonwald, A. (2020). Developmental-behavioral surveillance and screening in primary care. *UpToDate*. https://www.uptodate.com/contents/developmental-behavioral-surveillance-and-screening-in-primary-care

American Academy of Child and Adolescent Psychiatry. (2018). *Physical punishment*. https://www.aacap.org/aacap/families_and_youth/facts_for_families/fff-guide/Physical-Punishment-105.aspx

American Academy of Pediatric Dentistry. (2016). *Perinatal and toddler oral health care*. http://www.aapd.org/media/Policies_Guidelines/BP_PerinatalOralHealthCare.pdf

American Academy of Pediatric Dentistry. (2018). *Fluoride therapy*. http://www.aapd.org/media/Policies_Guidelines/BP_FluorideTherapy.pdf

American Academy of Pediatric Ophthalmology and Strabismus. (2020). *Photoscreening*. https://aapos.org/glossary/photoscreening

American Academy of Pediatrics. (2015). *Portions and serving sizes*. https://www.healthychildren.org/English/healthy-living/nutrition/Pages/Portions-and-Serving-Sizes.aspx

American Academy of Pediatrics. (2018). *Where we stand: Spanking*. https://www.healthychildren.org/English/family-life/family-dynamics/communication-discipline/Pages/Where-We-Stand-Spanking.aspx

American Academy of Pediatrics. (2019). *Poison prevention and treatment tips*. https://www.healthychildren.org/English/safety-prevention/all-around/Pages/Poison-Prevention.aspx

American Academy of Pediatrics. (2020a). *Breastfeeding*. https://www.healthychildren.org/English/ages-stages/baby/breastfeeding/Pages/default.aspx

American Academy of Pediatrics. (2020b). *Prevent child car deaths in hot cars*. https://www.healthychildren.org/English/safety-prevention/on-the-go/Pages/Prevent-Child-Deaths-in-Hot-Cars.aspx

American Academy of Pediatrics/Bright Futures. (2020). *Recommendations for preventive pediatric health care*. https://downloads.aap.org/AAP/PDF/periodicity_schedule.pdf

American Association of Poison Control Centers. (n.d.). *Prevention*. https://aapcc.org/prevention/home

Brazelton, T. B., & Sparrow, J. (2015). *Discipline: The Brazelton way* (2nd ed.). Capo Press.

Cassidy, J., & Shaver, P. R. (2016). *Handbook of attachment: Theory, research, and clinical applications* (3rd ed.). Guilford Press.

Centers for Disease Control and Prevention. (2010). *WHO growth standards are recommended for use in the U.S. for infants and children 0 to 2 years of age*. https://www.cdc.gov/growthcharts/who_charts.htm#The%20WHO%20Growth%20Charts

Centers for Disease Control and Prevention. (2016). CDC growth charts. https://www.cdc.gov/growthcharts/cdc_charts.htm

Dallacker, M., Hertwig, R., & Mata, J. (2018). The frequency of family meals and nutritional health in children: A meta-analysis. *Obesity Reviews, 19*(5), 638–653. https://doi.org/10.1111/obr.12659

Drutz, J. E. (2020). The pediatric physical examination: General principles and standard measurements. *UpToDate*. https://www.uptodate.com/contents/the-pediatric-physical-examination-general-principles-and-standard-measurements

Durbin, D. R., Hoffman, B., & Council on Injury, Violence, and Poison Prevention. (2018). Child passenger safety. *Pediatrics, 142*(5), e20182460. https://doi.org/10.1542/peds.2018-2460

Flynn, J. T., Kaelber, D. C., Baker-Smith, C. M., Blowey, D., Carroll, A. E., Daniels, S. R., de Ferranti, S. D., Dionne, J. M., Falkner, B., Flinn, S. K., Gidding, S. S., Goodwin, C., Leu, M. G., Powers, M. E., Rea, C., Samuels, J., Simasek, M., Thaker, V. V., Urbina, E. M., & the Subcommittee on Screening and Management of High Blood Pressure in Children. (2017). Clinical practice guideline for screening and management of high blood pressure in children and adolescents. *Pediatrics, 140*(3), e20171904. https://doi.org/10.1542/peds.2017-1904

Galvez, M. P., & Balk, S. J. (2017). Environmental risks to children: Prioritizing health messages in pediatric practice. *Pediatrics in Review, 38*(6), 263–279. http://dx.doi.org/10.1542/pir.2015-0165

Global Initiative to End All Corporal Punishment of Children. (2018). *Global initiative to end corporal punishment*. www.endcorporalpunishment.org

Haemer, M. A., Diab, L. K., Primak, L. E., & Krebs, N. F. (2020). Normal childhood nutrition & its disorders. In W. W. Hay, M. J. Levin, M. J. Abzug, & M. Bunik (Eds.), *Current diagnosis & treatment: Pediatrics* (25th ed., Chapter 11). McGraw-Hill Education.

Hagan, J. F., Shaw, J. S., & Duncan, P. M. (Eds.). (2017). *Bright Futures: Guidelines for health supervision of toddlers, children, and adolescents* (4th ed.). Bright Futures & American Academy of Pediatrics.

Kelly, N. R. (2020). Screening tests in children and adolescents. *UpToDate*. https://www.uptodate.com/contents/screening-tests-in-children-and-adolescents

Klish, W. J., & Skelton, J. A. (2020). Definition, epidemiology, and etiology of obesity in children and adolescents. *UpToDate*. https://www.uptodate.com/contents/definition-epidemiology-and-etiology-of-obesity-in-children-and-adolescents

Lieberman, A. (2018). *The emotional life of a toddler*. Simon & Schuster.

Lipkin, P. H., Macias, M. M., & the Council on Children with Disabilities, Section on Developmental and Behavioral Pediatrics. (2020). Promoting optimal development: Identifying toddlers and young children with developmental disorders through developmental surveillance and screening. *Pediatrics, 145*(1), e20193449. https://doi.org/10.1542/peds.2019-3449

Nowak, A. J., & Warren, J. J. (2020). Preventive dental care and counseling for infants and young children. *UpToDate*. https://www.uptodate.com/contents/preventive-dental-care-and-counseling-for-infants-and-young-children

O'Donnell, L. M. (2018). *Disciplining your toddler*. https://kidshealth.org/en/parents/toddler-tantrums.html#

Parks, E. P., Shaikhkhalil, A., Sainath, N. N., Mitchell, J. A., Brownell, J. N., & Stallings, V. A. (2020). Feeding healthy infants, children, and adolescents. In R. M. Kliegman, J. W. St. Geme III, N. J. Blum, S. S. Shah, R. C. Tasker, K. M. Wilson, & R. E. Behrman (Eds.), *Nelson textbook of pediatrics* (21st ed., Chapter 56). Elsevier.

Paul H. Brookes Publishing. (2020). *ASQ: Ages and stages questionnaires.* https://agesandstages.com

Pedstest.com. (2016). *PEDS test.* https://pedstest.com/index.html

Satter, E. (2019). *Child feeding ages and stages.* https://www.ellynsatterinstitute.org/how-to-feed/child-feeding-ages-and-stages

Sears, W., & Sears, M. (2020). *8 tools for toddler discipline.* http://www.askdrsears.com/topics/parenting/discipline-behavior/8-tools-toddler-discipline

Treitz, M., Nicklas, D., & Fox, D. (2020). Ambulatory & office pediatrics. In W. W. Hay, M. J. Levin, M. J. Abzug, & M. Bunik (Eds.), *Current diagnosis & treatment: Pediatrics* (25th ed., Chapter 9). McGraw-Hill Education.

Tufts Children's Hospital. (2020). *The survey of well-being of young children.* https://www.tuftschildrenshospital.org/The-Survey-of-Wellbeing-of-Young-Children/Age-Specific-Forms

Turner, K. (2018). Well-child visits for infants and young children. *American Family Physician, 98*(6), 347–353. https://www.aafp.org/afp/2018/0915/p347.html

# Well-Child Visits During Preschool Years

Theresa Kyle

## Student Learning Outcomes

**Upon completion of this chapter the reader should be able to:**

1. Determine adequacy of growth of preschool-age children.
2. Evaluate developmental milestones of preschoolers.
3. Choose appropriate screening tests based on current recommendations for a child's age and risk status.
4. Select immunizations based on current recommendations for a child's age and risk status.
5. Determine applicable anticipatory guidance for each scheduled visit during the preschool years.

## INTRODUCTION

The preschool period, from ages 3 to 5 years, is a time of slower growth but with substantial gains in cognitive, language, and psychosocial development. With a longer attention span and the ability to tolerate separation from parents, preschool children are preparing for school entry. Parents can best help their children prepare for this transition by continuing to support these gains in development while maintaining appropriate discipline in preparation for success in school. During this period, Bright Futures recommends annual outpatient well-child visits (American Academy of Pediatrics [AAP]/Bright Futures, 2020). Health supervision should occur at 4 years and 5 years of age in the otherwise healthy preschooler (Hagan et al., 2017). Children with chronic illness may need more frequent visits.

The content in this chapter maps to the following areas on the Pediatric Nursing Certification Board (PNCB) Pediatric Nurse Practitioner—Primary Care certification examination:

### CONTENT AREAS:

#### I. Health Maintenance and Promotion

**A. Partner with patients/caregivers to support growth and development from infancy to young adulthood**

**B. Provide patients/caregivers with age/developmentally appropriate anticipatory guidance**

**C. Recommend and prescribe immunizations according to current CDC guidelines**

**D. Educate about illness prevention and early warning signs of pediatric illness and emergencies**

**E. Advise patients/caregivers about age appropriate injury prevention and safety (environmental exposure, risk taking behaviors, social situations, sports and recreation, and vehicle safety)**

**F. Counsel about age-appropriate social, behavioral, and mental health concerns (e.g., substance abuse, social media use, grief and loss, and sexual orientation/LGBTQ)**

#### II. Assessment and Diagnosis

**A. Growth and Development**

1. Evaluate and interpret growth parameters
2. Perform developmental surveillance

**B. History and Physical Examination**

1. Obtain history of present illness
2. Obtain a comprehensive health history for new patients
3. Complete an interval history for established patients
4. Perform a review of systems
5. Perform a complete physical examination

**C. Diagnostic Testing and Screening**

1. Order and interpret office/clinic based screening tests
4. Select, utilize, and interpret developmental, behavioral and mental health screening and assessment tools

**D. Analyzing Information**

1. Integrate health history and physical examination findings into the plan of care
2. Assimilate findings from screening and diagnostic testing into plan of care

### IV. Professional Role and Responsibilities

**B. Practice Management**

1. Document patient encounters in a manner which supports applicable diagnostic and procedure codes
2. Utilize appropriate billing and coding to facilitate reimbursement

## PARENT-CHILD INTERACTION

The parent-child relationship continues to be vital to the child's growth and development throughout the preschool years. The preschool well-child visit presents the nurse practitioner (NP) with the opportunity to observe the parent-child interaction during a time when the child is more mature in their communication abilities and is learning to demonstrate initiative. The NP has the opportunity to offer positive reinforcement for parental behaviors that may foster initiative in the child, as well as time to role model positive interactions. During the visit, observe the manner in which the parent/caregiver communicates with and about the child. Note the body language between parent and child:

- Does the parent-child relationship occur with ease, or is it strained?
- When communicating with the child, does the parent acknowledge and support the child?
- Is the child able to undress themself?
- Does the child separate easily from the parent for weighing and measuring?
- For incorrect behavior, is the parent paying attention and offering appropriate verbal correction?

## DEVELOPMENTAL SURVEILLANCE

Begin the health history at each well-child visit by asking, "Since the last visit, what changes have you seen in your child's development?" or start the conversation with, "What's your child doing that's new since the last visit?" Expected developmental milestones for each age during the preschool years may be found in chapter 9. Parent-completed developmental screening questionnaires recognize the parent as expert on their preschooler, provide assessment information valuable for developmental surveillance, and are recommended for use by the AAP (Aites & Schonwald, 2020; Hagan et al., 2017). Tools with demonstrated reliability and validity appropriate for use in during the preschool years include:

- Ages and Stages Questionnaires (ASQ-3)
- Parent's Evaluation of Developmental Status (PEDS test)
- PEDS: Developmental Milestones (PEDS: DM)
- Survey of Well-being of Young Children (SWYC)

TABLE 16.1 **Signs of Developmental Delay**

| Age | Concern |
|---|---|
| 4 years | Cannot stack four blocks<br>Has difficulty with scribbling<br>Cannot copy a circle<br>Does not grasp crayon with thumb and fingers<br>Cannot throw ball overhand<br>Cannot jump in place or ride a tricycle<br>Does not use sentences with three or more words<br>Cannot use the words "me" and "you" appropriately<br>Ignores other children or does not show interest in interactive games<br>Will not respond to people outside the family<br>Still clings or cries if parents leave<br>Resists using toilet, dressing, sleeping<br>Does not engage in fantasy play |
| By 5 years | Cannot build tower of six to eight blocks<br>Cannot brush teeth, wash and dry hands, or undress efficiently<br>Cannot use plurals or past tense<br>Is unhappy or sad often<br>Has little interest in playing with other children<br>Is unable to separate from parent without major protest<br>Is extremely aggressive<br>Is extremely fearful or timid, or unusually passive<br>Is easily distracted; cannot concentrate on single activity for 5 minutes<br>Rarely engages in fantasy play<br>Has trouble with eating, sleeping, or using the toilet |

Question the parent about language development and social skills, while observing the child. Periodic evaluation at each well-child visit during this time will allow for early identification of preschool-age children who may be at risk for developmental delay and who may not be demonstrating school readiness (Lipkin et al., 2020; Treitz et al., 2020). Refer to Table 16.1 for signs of developmental delay.

## HEALTH ASSESSMENT

Each preschool well-child visit will include a comprehensive health assessment. The assessment includes developmental surveillance, as noted earlier, as well as health history and physical examination. Each visit also includes prevention (immunization or screening as appropriate) and anticipatory guidance appropriate for age, always including but not limited to nutrition, sleep, and safety (Hagan et al., 2017).

### SUBJECTIVE DATA

Along with development surveillance, obtain information from the caregiver in relation to past medical history (since the last health supervision visit), diet, sleep, dental care, changes in family or social history, and results of prior screenings (Turner, 2018). Always address any concerns the parents may have. Direct questions to the child as appropriate and engage them in conversation about their life.

### OBJECTIVE DATA

In addition to observation of the parent-child interaction, perform a comprehensive physical examination, beginning with observation of the child's general appearance (happy, interactive, well-appearing, active, neatly/cleanly clothed). Note body habitus and nutritional status (Drutz, 2020). The child's weight, height, and body mass index (BMI) for age should be plotted on the gender-appropriate charts (Centers for Disease Control and Prevention [CDC], 2016). The preschooler will likely be willing to sit independently on the examination table. Save the genitalia examination for last. Preschool-age children respond well to trying out the equipment first on the parent or examiner. Talk with the child throughout the examination, explaining in simple terms what you are doing.

On examination of the skin, note any rashes or bruises. Assess for strabismus or an unequal Hirschberg reflex. Evaluate the pupils for presence of a bilateral red reflex and for opacification (not desired). Assess ocular motility. Assess the teeth for hygiene, caries, plaque, staining, or malocclusion. The gums should be healthy and pink. Respirations should be unlabored and regular. Auscultate the heart for murmur and palpate the pulses throughout for strength and equality. Palpate the abdomen for masses (none should be found).

Observe the extremities for equality of size, tone, and movement. Observe the child walking, running, and climbing onto the examination table. Evaluate hand control, and arm and spine movement. Assess deep tendon reflexes, which should be average. The 4-year-old should be able to draw a picture. While talking with the child, note the level of language acquisition, thought content, and abstraction. Is the speech fluent and clear? Are there articulation difficulties? Note the child's affect, effort to make eye contact, and responses, assessing for signs of anxiety or depression.

## PREVENTION

The physical examination should include measurements with comparison to norms for age and sex, including BMI, and blood pressure (BP) readings. Neurodevelopmental status should be assessed with observation of gait and coordination, and dental health should be assessed (Hagan et al., 2017). Hearing and visual acuity with ocular movement assessment should also be evaluated (CDC, Bright Futures, 2020). As more than 1.25 million children are victims of maltreatment, it is critical to assess for signs of abuse at each health encounter (Riley et al., 2019). The NP should ask health screening questions during this portion of the examination and address concerns presented by the child or caregiver. The AAP recommendations for preventive pediatric health care can be accessed at https://downloads.aap.org/AAP/PDF/periodicity_schedule.pdf).

### IMMUNIZATIONS

Prevention during the preschool health supervision visits includes routine recommended immunization and targeted health screenings. The AAP recommendations for preventive pediatric health care may be found at https://downloads.aap.org/AAP/PDF/periodicity_schedule.pdf).

The Advisory Committee on Immunization Practices (ACIP) recommends immunizations for preschool children at 4 to 5 years, and influenza vaccination annually. The CDC, AAP, and American Academy of Family Physicians, among others, agree with these recommendations. At 4 to 6 years of age the following vaccinations are recommended:

- Diphtheria, tetanus, acellular pertussis (DTaP)—5th dose
- Inactivated poliovirus (IPV)—4th dose
- Measles, mumps, rubella (MMR)—2nd dose
- Varicella—2nd dose

The current immunization schedule is available at www.cdc.gov/vaccines/schedules/hcp/child-adolescent.html.

## SCREENINGS

Well-child visits during the preschool years also provide an opportunity for other screenings, including school readiness, screening for specific health issues, vision and hearing screenings, and screening for exposure to lead.

### Anemia

Ask parents if the child's diet includes iron-rich foods (meat, beans, iron-fortified cereals). Determine if the family is experiencing food insecurity. If the child is determined to be at risk for anemia, obtain serum hemoglobin.

### Blood Pressure Screening

Measure BP annually in the healthy preschool-age child (Flynn et al., 2017).

### Dyslipidemia

During the preschool years the AAP recommends select screening for dyslipidemia. Twice between the ages of 2 years and 8 years, the child should be screened with a fasting lipid profile as determined by risk assessment. The risk assessment includes:

- Child has diabetes, hypertension, BMI greater than or equal to 95%, or a moderate to high risk condition
- Family history:
  - Parent, grandparent, aunt, uncle, or sibling with myocardial infarction, angina, stroke, or coronary artery bypass graft before age 55 in males and before age 65 in females
  - Parent with known dyslipidemia or total cholesterol greater than or equal to 240 mg/dL (Kelly, 2020; U.S. Preventive Services Task Force [USPSTF], 2016)

### Hearing Screening

Screen hearing annually in the preschool years with audiometry.

### Vision Screening

Screen the child's vision with the HOTV or Lea chart. Visual acuity should be equal in both eyes. If concerns exist, refer to pediatric ophthalmology for a full visual assessment (Hagan et al., 2017; USPSTF, 2017a).

### Lead Exposure

Perform a risk assessment at 4 and 5 years of age. If positive risk is determined, obtain a blood lead level.

## ANTICIPATORY GUIDANCE

Teach parents about the importance of physical activity. Preschoolers need at least 2 hours per day of physical activity (preferably some of it outdoors), with at least 60 minutes of the activity being moderate to vigorous in intensity (AAP, 2020c). Limit screen time (television, computer, tablet, any digital media) to no more than 2 hours per day, avoiding commercials and advertisements. The AAP recommends not having a television, tablet, or other device in the child's bedroom. Additionally, provide anticipatory guidance related to nutrition, discipline, commonly occurring developmental concerns, dental health, sleep, and safety.

## NUTRITION

With a full set of primary teeth, the preschooler is able to chew and swallow competently and has learned to use utensils fairly well, thus should be able to feed themselves. Younger preschoolers may be inconsistent, eating very little one day, then eating well the next day. During this time period, similar to toddlerhood, the child is continuing to learn and build upon healthy eating habits; these will develop into lifelong habits. The preschooler should consume a nutrient-rich diet including whole grains, lean meats, vegetables, fruits, and appropriate dairy foods. Providing a diet high in fiber is important as it is associated with decreased risk for obesity (Haemer et al., 2020). As with the toddler, nutrient-poor, high-calorie foods such as typical fast foods and sweets should be limited.

▶ ALERT: Preschoolers who drink excess amounts of milk are at risk for iron deficiency, as the calcium in milk blocks iron absorption. Limit milk intake to 16 ounces per day.

### Healthy Eating

As it is with the toddler, family mealtime is important for role modeling healthy eating habits and preventing obesity (Dallacker et al., 2018). Although preschool children may be picky eaters and want to eat only certain foods over several days, as they get older this pickiness lessens. The parent should continue to maintain a patient and positive demeanor at mealtime, choose and provide healthy foods for meals and snacks, then permit the child to choose how much they will eat. By 5 years of age the child is less picky, may help with food preparation and clean-up as appropriate, and demonstrates more focus on the social context of meals such as manners and table conversation. The United States Department of Agriculture's website provides parents with planning a healthy diet for their child with foods from all groups provided over the course of the day (U.S. Department of Agriculture, n.d.). For the overweight or obese preschooler, weight management goals based on BMI for age/gender include:

- Overweight (BMI 85%–94%)—maintain weight
- Obese (BMI 95%–58%), without complications—maintain weight
- Obese (BMI 95%–58%), with complications—lose 1 pound per month
- Obese with BMI 99% or greater—lose 1 pound per month (Haemer et al., 2020).

## DENTAL HEALTH

During the preschool years, it is important to continue daily brushing and flossing to prevent dental caries. To prevent excess fluoride consumption (and avoid fluorosis), use only a pea-sized amount of toothpaste (Nowak & Warren, 2020). The parent must continue to supervise the preschooler while brushing to ensure adequate brushing. The preschool child cannot perform flossing adequately, so the parent will need to do so. Continue to avoid cariogenic foods, but if they are consumed have the child rinse the mouth with water if it is not possible to immediately brush the teeth (Nowak & Warren, 2020). Continue fluoride varnish application for high-risk children throughout the preschool years (see chapter 12 for additional information). Remind parents that dental visits should occur every 6 months. Prescribe fluoride supplementation depending upon the fluoride level in drinking water (in parts per million [ppm]):

<0.3 ppm—0.5 mg daily
0.3–0.6 ppm—0.25 mg daily (American Academy of Pediatric Dentistry, 2018)

> **PRO TIP** Take care to prevent dental caries prevention in the primary teeth. If these teeth are lost due to caries, the proper formation of permanent teeth as well as the width of the dental arch may be affected.

## SLEEP

Each day the preschool child should sleep 10 to 13 hours, including naps (AAP, 2020b). Occasionally, the preschool child resists going to bed unless very tired, thus bedtime rituals continue to be important and reassuring to children during this time. The child will fall asleep more easily if a period of relaxation and decreased stimulation occurs near bedtime. Some children this age will continue to need a security item at naptime or bedtime. Being afraid of the dark is common at this age, so a nightlight in the bedroom may help.

With their increased imagination and continued struggle to distinguish reality from fantasy, preschool children often have nightmares. Rather than discounting the nightmare, parents should validate the child's fear (e.g., agree that monsters are scary but remind the child that monsters are not real; Goldson et al., 2020). Sleep terrors may also occur. They can be frightening to parents as the child does not seem respond but eventually goes back to sleep, whereas with a nightmare the child may be screaming and crying but will converse with the parent. If sleep terrors recur, it may be helpful to awaken the child 15 to 20 minutes prior to the usual time of occurrence in order to abort them (Kotagal, 2019). For a comparison of sleep terrors and nightmares, refer to Table 16.2.

## DISCIPLINE

Choosing limits well, enforcing them consistently, and providing a loving and nurturing environment in which the preschooler's self-esteem is fostered sets the stage for successful discipline. Children this age are becoming capable of understanding the concept of right and wrong, understanding another's feelings, and are cognitively capable of remembering basic rules. Parents need to encourage the preschooler's normal growth and development of imagination and make-believe, yet be consistent with discipline so the child will learn to accept that certain things are not allowed. When rules are clear and enforced consistently, guilt in the child can be avoided and the

**TABLE 16.2 Nightmares Versus Sleep Terrors**

| | Nightmare | Sleep Terror |
|---|---|---|
| **Definition** | Scary or bad dream followed by awakening | Partial arousal from deep sleep |
| **Timing** | Usually in the second half of the night | Usually in the first 1/3 of the night, often about an hour after falling asleep |
| **Parental awareness** | After the episode is over, the child awakens the parent | Screaming and thrashing during the episode is heard by the parent |
| **Child's behavior** | Crying, may be scared after awakening | Thrashes and sits up, while crying and/or screaming, may talk. May look wild-eyed, and/or have racing heartbeat |
| **Responsiveness** | Responsive to parent's reassurances and soothing | Child is unaware of parent's presence, does not respond to attempts at soothing, may thrash and scream more if restrained |
| **Return to sleep** | May have difficulty going back to sleep if continues to be afraid | Rapidly returns to sleep without full awakening, usually abruptly |
| **Memory of occurrence** | May remember the dream and talk about it later | No memory of event |

*Source*: Data from Kotagal, S. (2019). Sleepwalking and other parasomnias in children. *UpToDate.* https://www.uptodate.com/contents/sleepwalking-and-other-parasomnias-in-children#H27172832

child's sense of initiative can be preserved (Brazelton & Sparrow, 2015).

Parents should learn to anticipate conditions likely to lead to the undesired or risky action in order to minimize the occurrence of the misbehavior. Distraction may be used to change the child's focus. To preserve the preschooler's self-esteem, educate parents to be certain to label the behavior and not the child when discussing the misbehavior. Parents should not only teach the child about the undesired behavior, but also ensure that the child understands the reason why it is wrong or unacceptable to do it. This understanding will help the child to use internal controls over behavior. Additionally, parents should serve as role models for self-control, including tone of voice, choice of words, and the actions accompanying them. Encourage parents to always reward positive behaviors, as the child will work harder to obtain praise than to avoid punishment.

Time-out can be very effective in preschool-age children. With an intentional misbehavior (knowing something is forbidden but doing it anyway), use time-out for the punishment. Provide a warning that time-out will occur if the behavior does not stop. When the behavior does not stop, remove the child from the situation and place the child in time-out for a specified period of time. It is helpful to have a particular area used specifically for time-out (such as a boring corner of the room without distractions). The time-out should last 1 minute per year of age (a 4-year-old would be in time-out for 4 minutes). Setting a timer helps the child know when the time-out is over. The child must sit in time-out for the entire prescribed length of time, and if they get up before the timer alarms, they are replaced in time-out and the timer is restarted. This technique works best if used consistently (every time the undesirable behavior occurs). The child should also be praised when they follow the rules and behave appropriately. Provide the child with a simple and clear explanation of the misbehavior and talk about acceptable alternative strategies that the child can use. Removing a privilege or a favorite toy can be as effective as time-out, and must be used similarly with consistency.

Corporal punishment is discouraged by the American Academy of Child and Adolescent Psychiatry [AACAP] (2018) and the AAP (2018). Spanking is the least effective discipline practice. Striking with the open hand, a belt, switch, paddle, or other items should never be done. Refer to chapter 4 for information on negative outcomes associated with physical punishment.

▶ ALERT: In addition to the resultant physical and emotional pain, learning capacity is decreased with the use of corporal punishment (AACAP, 2018).

## School Readiness

The early years (toddler and preschool years) set the stage for the child to be able to have a successful school journey. For the child to succeed in school, the home environment needs to be safe and responsive, allowing the child to learn and explore within a structure and with limits, allowing the child to learn the socially acceptable behaviors needed in school. Encourage language development through books and reading, as language is critical to the ability to succeed in school. All of these are important in readying the child for education in a more formal setting (Nierengarten, 2018).

### Promoting Language Development

Parent-child interactions in relation to books and other play activities model the types of interactions that the child will later have in school; thus, the parent serves as the child's first teacher. To stimulate the development of thinking and language, the parent should ask the child open-ended questions. As the preschooler is a great imitator, the parent should role model appropriate language, and also avoid swearing, as the child is sure to repeat those words. Encourage the parent to allow the child to pursue interests at their own pace, helping them to develop the literacy and numeric skills that will enable them to later focus on academic skills. Reading story books with pictures helps the child to develop early literacy skills.

▶ ALERT: Risk factors for lack of school readiness include maternal depression, insecure attachment in the early years, parental substance abuse, and low socioeconomic status.

### Choosing a Preschool

Preschool serves as a foundation for later education, allowing the child the opportunity to build self-esteem and the skills needed for the more formal setting of elementary school. Preschool attendance fosters the development of the child's social skills and accustoms the child to the group environment. When selecting a preschool, the parent may want to consider:

- Recommendations from other parents
- The focus of the school environment (daily schedule, very structured or with a looser approach)
- How focused a curriculum the parent would prefer
- Teachers' qualifications
- School accreditation
- Type of discipline used (corporal punishment is unacceptable)

Parents may want to observe the classroom, evaluating the environment, noise level, sanitary practices, child-to-child interaction, and teacher-child interaction. Touring the school with the child or attending an open house may help the child transition to the preschool. This is helpful with kindergarten transition as well.

## SAFETY

Provide safety guidance in relation to the home, car, water, and environment.

### Preventing Poisoning

Although continuing to develop, preschool-age children continue have unrefined taste discrimination, placing them at risk for accidental ingestion. To prevent poisoning, advise parents as follows:

- Never try to coax a child to take a vitamin supplement, tablet, or pill by calling it "candy."
- Store dangerous fluids in their original containers; never pour into containers looking like ordinary drinking glasses or cups.
- Keep all potentially dangerous substances out of reach of preschoolers (preferably in a locked cabinet).
- Always have childproof caps on medication containers and keep medicines in a locked cabinet. Post the Poison Control Center telephone number in a prominent place in the home and program into mobile phones (1-800-222-1222; American Association of Poison Control Centers, 2017).

### Car Safety

Up until 4 years of age, the child whose height meets the car seat size requirement should be fastened securely in an appropriately sized forward-facing car safety seat. Car seats should have harness straps and a clip for securing the child, and tethers for anchoring in the vehicle. After reaching the car seat height restriction, the child should ride in a booster seat that uses both the lap and shoulder belts (Durbin et al., 2018). The AAP recommends that the booster seat continue to be used until a height of 145 cm (4 feet 9 inches) and age of 8 to 12 years are reached (2020a). The safest place for a child to ride is always the back seat of the car. Instruct parents not to allow the car seat to be placed in the front seat if the vehicle is equipped with air bags.

▶ ALERT: Never allow a young child to ride in the cargo area of a pickup truck. Their risk for dying in the event of an accident is increased ten-fold as compared with riding inside the vehicle, appropriately restrained (Stanford Children's Health, 2020).

### Sports Safety

It is important to establish the habit of daily physical activity in the early years to reach the long-term goal of avoiding obesity. Many preschool-age children become involved in sports, and while fun and enjoyable safety must remain a priority. Teach families the importance of having their child always wear protective equipment appropriate for the activity (CDC, 2019). The child this age may also learn to ride a tricycle or big wheel, or a bicycle (with or without training wheels). Any time the child is riding a wheeled vehicle, the child must wear an approved bicycle helmet, even if it is just in the driveway (CDC, 2020). Helmet requirement in the early years not only promotes child safety, but also helps lead to the habit of helmet use as the child gets older. If parents allow the preschooler to choose the helmet, it may encourage the child to use it. To promote bicycle safety, the parent must ensure that the size is correct; while sitting on the seat with both hands on the handlebars, the balls of the child's feet should reach both pedals. Traditional pedal-back brakes are recommended for preschool-age children, as children under 5 years of age have difficulty learning to use hand-operated brakes. Preschoolers should always ride on the sidewalk, as they are not mature enough to ride a bicycle in the street even if they are riding with an adult (AAP, 2015).

## Environmental Exposures

Similar to infants and toddlers, preschool-age children are at increased risk for harmful exposures inside and outside of the home (Galvez & Balk, 2017). Refer to chapter 14 for information related to preventing environmental exposures in toddlers.

### Sun Exposure

Protect the child's skin from sun exposure by:

- Dressing the child in protective clothing and a wide-brimmed hat
- Avoiding being outside between the hours of 10:00 a.m. and 4:00 p.m. in the warmer months
- Using sunscreen with an SPF of at least 15

## Water Safety

An appropriate time for a child to learn to swim is at 4 years of age, as they are able to voluntarily hold their breath by then (AAP, 2019). They also demonstrate physical capability and cognitive maturity for swimming and basic water safety. In addition to appropriate swim techniques, the swimming lesson should also focus on safety measures. Additional safeguards related to water safety include:

- Never leave a preschool-age child unattended around any body of water, even if they know how to swim.
- Parents and caregivers should be trained in infant/child cardiopulmonary resuscitation (CPR). Teach preschoolers to never dive into water until an adult has verified its depth.
- Never allow a preschool-age child to swim in a canal or any fast-moving water.
- If the home has a swimming pool, life-saving devices should be readily accessible.
- When riding in boats or fishing off riverbanks, the child should wear a personal flotation device.
- Caution parents about close supervision of young children walking, skating, or riding near thin or weak ice.

## KEY POINTS

- Provide developmental surveillance of the child by direct observation, questioning the parent in relation to milestones recently met, and using valid and reliable questionnaires.
- Update the child's health history and perform a comprehensive physical examination at each health supervision visit.
- Plot the child's weight, height, and BMI on the gender-appropriate CDC growth charts.
- Provide immunizations to the preschool-age child as recommended by ACIP.
- Complete risk assessments for anemia, dyslipidemia, and lead exposure at annual well child visits, obtaining screening if the risk assessment is positive.
- The child's BP should be checked at the annual well child visit beginning at 3 years of age.
- The promotion of healthy eating habits in the preschool years sets a foundation for lifelong healthy eating.
- Provide nutritious healthy food options to the preschooler rather than high-sugar, high-fat, processed snacks.
- Nurturing, appropriate limits, and consistency are necessary for preschool discipline.
- Time-out with 1 minute of time per age in years works well as a punishment for inappropriate behavior in the preschool-age child.
- The prevention of accidental ingestion continues to be a prime safety focus during the preschool years.
- Ensure that the preschooler always uses the appropriate sports protective equipment, and always wears a helmet when riding a wheeled vehicle.
- Provide anticipatory guidance to parents in relation to dental health, car/home/water safety, and environmental exposure avoidance.

## REFERENCES


Aites, J., & Schonwald, A. (2020). Developmental-behavioral surveillance and screening in primary care. *UpToDate.* https://www.uptodate.com/contents/developmental-behavioral-surveillance-and-screening-in-primary-care

American Academy of Child and Adolescent Psychiatry. (2018). *Physical punishment.* https://www.aacap.org/aacap/families_and_youth/facts_for_families/fff-guide/Physical-Punishment-105.aspx

American Academy of Pediatric Dentistry. (2018). *Fluoride therapy.* http://www.aapd.org/media/Policies_Guidelines/BP_FluorideTherapy.pdf

American Academy of Pediatrics. (2015). *Safety for your child: 5 years.* http://www.healthychildren.org/english/tips-tools/Pages/Safety-for-Your-Child-5-Years.aspx

American Academy of Pediatrics. (2018). *Where we stand: Spanking.* https://www.healthychildren.org/English/family-life/family-dynamics/communication-discipline/Pages/Where-We-Stand-Spanking.aspx

American Academy of Pediatrics. (2019). *Swim lessons: When to start & what parents should know.* https://www.healthychildren.org/English/safety-prevention/at-play/Pages/Swim-Lessons.aspx

American Academy of Pediatrics. (2020a). *Car seats: Information for families.* http://www.healthychildren.org/English/safety-prevention/on-the-go/Pages/Car-Safety-Seats-Information-for-Families.aspx

American Academy of Pediatrics. (2020b). *Healthy sleep habits: How many hours does your child need?* https://www.healthychildren.org/English/healthy-living/sleep/Pages/Healthy-Sleep-Habits-How-Many-Hours-Does-Your-Child-Need.aspx

American Academy of Pediatrics. (2020c). *Preschooler—Physical activity.* https://www.aap.org/en-us/advocacy-and-policy/aap-health-initiatives/HALF-Implementation-Guide/Age-Specific-Content/Pages/Preschooler-Physical-Activity.aspx

American Academy of Pediatrics/Bright Futures. (2020). *Recommendations for preventive pediatric health care.* https://downloads.aap.org/AAP/PDF/periodicity_schedule.pdf

American Association of Poison Control Centers. (2017). *Prevention.* https://aapcc.org/Prevention

Brazelton, T. B., & Sparrow, J. (2015). *Discipline: The Brazelton way* (2nd ed.). Capo Press.

Centers for Disease Control and Prevention. (2016). *CDC growth charts.* https://www.cdc.gov/growthcharts/cdc_charts.htm

Centers for Disease Control and Prevention. (2019). *Protect the ones you love: Child injuries are preventable.* https://www.cdc.gov/safechild/sports_injuries/

Centers for Disease Control and Prevention. (2020). *Helmet safety.* https://www.cdc.gov/headsup/helmets/index.html

American Academy of Pediatrics, Bright Futures. (2020). *Recommendations for preventive pediatric health care.* https://downloads.aap.org/AAP/PDF/periodicity_schedule.pdf

Dallacker, M., Hertwig, R., & Mata, J. (2018). The frequency of family meals and nutritional health in children: A meta-analysis. *Obesity Reviews, 19*(5), 638–653. https://doi.org/10.1111/obr.12659

Drutz, J. E. (2020). The pediatric physical examination: General principles and standard measurements. *UpToDate.* https://www.uptodate.com/contents/the-pediatric-physical-examination-general-principles-and-standard-measurements

Durbin, D. R., Hoffman, B., & Council on Injury, Violence, and Poison Prevention. (2018). Child passenger safety. *Pediatrics, 142*(5), e20182460. https://doi.org/10.1542/peds.2018-2460

Flynn, J. T., Kaelber, D. C., Baker-Smith, C. M., Blowey, D., Carroll, A. E., Daniels, S. R., de Ferranti, S. D., Dionne, J. M., Falkner, B., Flinn, S. K., Gidding, S. S., Goodwin, C., Leu, M. G., Powers, M. E., Rea, C., Samuels, J., Simasek, M., Thaker, V. V., Urbina, E. M., & the Subcommittee on Screening and Management of High Blood Pressure in Children. (2017). Clinical practice guideline for screening and management of high blood pressure in children and adolescent. *Pediatrics, 140*(3), e20171904. https://doi.org/10.1542/peds.2017-1904

Galvez, M. P., & Balk, S. J. (2017). Environmental risks to children: Prioritizing health messages in pediatric practice. *Pediatrics in Review, 38*(6), 263–279. http://dx.doi.org/10.1542/pir.2015-0165

Goldson, E., Angulo, A. S., Raz, D. M., & Reynolds, A. (2020). Child development and behavior. In W. W. Hay, M. J. Levin, M. J. Abzug, & M. Bunik (Eds.), *Current diagnosis & treatment: Pediatrics* (25th ed., Chapter 3). McGraw-Hill Education.

Haemer, M. A., Diab, L. K., Primak, L. E., & Krebs, N. F. (2020). Normal childhood nutrition & its disorders. In W. W. Hay, M. J. Levin, M. J. Abzug, & M. Bunik (Eds.), *Current diagnosis & treatment: Pediatrics* (25th ed., Chapter 11). McGraw-Hill Education.

Hagan, J. F., Shaw, J. S., & Duncan, P. M. (2017). *Bright futures: Guidelines for health supervision of infants, children, and adolescents.* American Academy of Pediatrics.

Kelly, N. R. (2020). Screening tests in children and adolescents. *UpToDate.* https://www.uptodate.com/contents/screening-tests-in-children-and-adolescents

Kotagal, S. (2019). Sleepwalking and other parasomnias in children. *UpToDate.* https://www.uptodate.com/contents/sleepwalking-and-other-parasomnias-in-children#H27172832

Lipkin, P. H., Macias, M. M., & the Council on Children with Disabilities, Section on Developmental and Behavioral Pediatrics. (2020). Promoting optimal development: Identifying infants and young children with developmental disorders through developmental surveillance and screening. *Pediatrics, 145*(1), e20193449. https://doi.org/10.1542/peds.2019-3449

Nierengarten, M. B. (2018). School readiness: Why early intervention is key. *Contemporary Pediatrics, 35*(8), 24–26, 28–29.

Nowak, A. J., & Warren, J. J. (2020). Preventive dental care and counseling for infants and young children. *UpToDate.* https://www.uptodate.com/contents/preventive-dental-care-and-counseling-for-infants-and-young-children

Riley, M., Morrison, L., & McEvoy, A. (2019). Health maintenance in school-aged children: Part I. History, physical examination, screening, and immunizations. *American Family Physician, 100*(4), 213–218.

Stanford Children's Health. (2020). *Motor vehicle safety for children.* https://www.stanfordchildrens.org/en/topic/default?id=motor-vehicle-safety-for-children-85-P01038

Treitz, M., Nicklas, D., & Fox, D. (2020). Ambulatory & office pediatrics. In W. W. Hay, M. J. Levin, M. J. Abzug, & M. Bunik (Eds.), *Current diagnosis & treatment: Pediatrics* (25th ed., Chapter 9). McGraw-Hill Education.

Turner, K. (2018). Well-child visits for infants and young children. *American Family Physician, 98*(6), 347–353. https://www.aafp.org/afp/2018/0915/p347.html

U.S. Department of Agriculture. (n.d.). *MyPlate tips for preschoolers.* https://www.choosemyplate.gov/browse-by-audience/view-all-audiences/children/health-and-nutrition-information/preschoolers-food-groups

U.S. Preventive Services Task Force. (2016). *Final recommendations summary: Lipid disorders in children and adolescents: Screening*. https://www.uspreventiveservicestaskforce.org/Page/Document/UpdateSummaryFinal/lipid-disorders-in-children-screening1

U.S. Preventive Services Task Force. (2017a). *Final recommendations summary: Vision in children ages 6 months to 5 years: Screening*. https://www.uspreventiveservicestaskforce.org/Page/Document/UpdateSummaryFinal/vision-in-children-ages-6-months-to-5-years-screening

# Well-Child Visits During School-Age Years

Keeley A. Harding, Jennifer Ridgway, and Terry Witherington

## Student Learning Outcomes

Upon completion of this chapter the reader should be able to:

1. Determine adequacy of growth of school-age children.
2. Evaluate developmental milestones of school-age children.
3. Choose appropriate screening tests based on current recommendations for child's age and risk status.
4. Select immunizations based on current recommendations for child's age and risk status.
5. Determine applicable anticipatory guidance for each scheduled visit during school-age years.

The content in this chapter maps to the following areas on the Pediatric Nursing Certification Board (PNCB) Pediatric Nurse Practitioner—Primary Care certification examination:

### CONTENT AREAS:

### I. Health Maintenance and Promotion

**A. Partner with patients/caregivers to support growth and development from infancy to young adulthood**

**B. Provide patients/caregivers with age/developmentally appropriate anticipatory guidance**

**C. Recommend and prescribe immunizations according to current CDC guidelines**

**D. Educate about illness prevention and early warning signs of pediatric illness and emergencies**

**E. Advise patients/caregivers about age appropriate injury prevention and safety (environmental exposure, risk taking behaviors, social situations, sports and recreation, and vehicle safety)**

**F. Counsel about age-appropriate social, behavioral, and mental health concerns (e.g., substance abuse, social media use, grief and loss, and sexual orientation/LGBTQ)**

### II. Assessment and Diagnosis

**A. Growth and Development**

1. Evaluate and interpret growth parameters
2. Perform developmental surveillance

**B. History and Physical Examination**

1. Obtain history of present illness
2. Obtain a comprehensive health history for new patients
3. Complete an interval history for established patients
4. Perform a review of systems
5. Perform a complete physical examination

**C. Diagnostic Testing and Screening**

1. Order and interpret office/clinic based screening tests
4. Select, utilize, and interpret developmental, behavioral and mental health screening and assessment tools

**D. Analyzing Information**

1. Integrate health history and physical examination findings into the plan of care
2. Assimilate findings from screening and diagnostic testing into plan of care

**IV. Professional Role and Responsibilities**

**B. Practice Management**

1. Document patient encounters in a manner which supports applicable diagnostic and procedure codes
2. Utilize appropriate billing and coding to facilitate reimbursement

## INTRODUCTION

Middle childhood is a dynamic time of industry and change, marking the transition between the tremendous development in early childhood and the tumultuous development in puberty. The clinical objectives of the health supervision visits for the school-age child include health facilitation and disease identification along with illness and injury prevention (Riley et al., 2019). During this period of development, school-age children are seen less frequently by healthcare providers than in early childhood; therefore, it is critical for nurse practitioners (NPs) to seize all opportunities for prevention and intervention in this vulnerable population. The health supervision visits in school-age children should provide evidence-based health screenings, immunizations, and counseling to children and their caregivers.

Involving the child and family in the decision-making process and plan of care is crucial when developing healthcare goals to facilitate positive change and healthcare behaviors. Collaboration with other healthcare professionals is also necessary to meet the needs of the patient. Incorporating cultural awareness and inclusiveness into all aspects of care is essential when caring for children. Referrals to specialists, as indicated, may be necessary for evaluation, counseling, and treatment.

## PARENT-CHILD INTERACTION

Positive family support is of great importance during visits with the healthcare provider. The first step in offering family support is for the provider to know who constitutes the family for the child (Hagan et al., 2017). The well-child examination for the school-age child presents the NP with the opportunity to observe the parent-child interaction and to offer guidance on how these interactions between the child and caregiver can have an impact on child wellness and overall health. Parent-child interactions are integral to growth and development as children learn social skills, cooperation, communication, and respect of others via this relationship.

**PRO TIP** Model eye contact with the school-age child as a positive reinforcement for parents to also engage in this behavior with their child.

During the well-child visit, the provider should engage in observing the manner in which the caregiver communicates with and about the child. Body language between parent and child may be a nonverbal indicator of the nature of the relationship.

- Is communication positive or negative?
- Does the relationship appear supportive or strained?
- Does the caregiver speak about behavior difficulties?
- Are stressors evident in the family?
- With cultural considerations in mind, do the parent and child make eye contact when speaking with each other?

**PRO TIP** The electronic health record (EHR) has led to convenient accessibility of patient data. However, the use of desktop and laptop computers as well as other mobile devices during assessment of the child can be a distraction. Be aware of this distraction, as it is critical during the well-child visit to be engaged in observation of the parent-child interaction and development of a trusting relationship.

## DEVELOPMENTAL SURVEILLANCE

Developmental surveillance is the process of ongoing, periodic evaluation of the child's development in an effort to identify children who may be at risk for developmental delays (Lipkin et al., 2020). Developmental surveillance is more defined for infants and young children than for school-age children. However, developmental surveillance and psychosocial/behavioral assessment should occur at each well-child visit during middle childhood (American Academy of Pediatrics [AAP], 2019). Currently, collecting comprehensive health surveillance data on children with intellectual and developmental disabilities is challenging, even with the advancement of today's technology and availability of EHRs (Wagner et al., 2019).

The NP evaluates the child's development through information obtained in the initial and ongoing history and physical examinations. In addition, routine questions and conversations about the child's development, behavior, and learning will help elicit concerns from the patient or family. Letting the parents' concerns or questions guide the discussion is sometimes helpful. Involving the parent or caregiver as well as school and after-school program professionals is important when a child is at risk for suspected developmental delay (Lipkin et al., 2020). Screening tools are also used to help identify the child who is at-risk or delayed. Regardless of whether a screening tool is used or referral is made, the NP evaluates the plan of care and modifies the plan based on the child's response or outcomes. Establishing a plan for follow-up care is part of this process.

**PRO TIP** Promote development through education. Provide anticipatory guidance by offering the parent something they "could" do instead of "should" do.

## SUBJECTIVE DATA

### Screening Tools to Identify At-Risk Children

Screening tools are a standardized way to identify children at risk. The goal is to determine if the child is achieving or progressing in their development. Currently, there is no *comprehensive* developmental screening tool for this age group. There are numerous screening tools available in a variety of languages depending on the age of the child and the intended measurement. The AAP offers *Screening Time*, an online resource of screening tools available at: https://screeningtime.org/star-center/#/screening-tools#top. In addition, there are a variety of mental health screening tools available, along with their psychometric properties, at: https://www.aap.org/en-us/advocacy-and-policy/aap-health-initiatives/mental-health/documents/mh_screeningchart.pdf.

Common age-appropriate psychosocial and behavioral assessment tools with translations include the Pediatric Symptom Checklist (PSC; https://www.brightfutures.org/mentalhealth/pdf/professionals/ped_sympton_chklst.pdf), and Safe Environment for Every Kid (SEEK) Parent Questionnaire (Q-R; https://seekwellbeing.org/wp-content/uploads/2019/09/English_PQ-R.pdf).

### Depression

Mental disorders in childhood, such as depression, can have a negative impact on a child's learning and behavior, resulting in impaired functioning at home or school. The prevalence of major depressive disorder in children 8 to 15 years of age is 2% for boys and 4% for girls (Forman-Hoffman et al., 2016). It is essential to be diligent in assessing for depression in school-age children, as 10% of children 5 to 13 years of age with major depressive disorder have a suicide attempt.

Children with major depressive symptoms may have functional impairment in multiple arenas, including family, social, school, and work (Mullen, 2018). The AAP (2019) recommends depression screening starting at 12 years of age, while the United States Preventive Services Task Force (USPSTF, 2016a) did not find sufficient evidence for routine depression screening in children younger than 12 years. Although these younger children may not present with classic symptoms of depression, NPs should consider depression in children presenting with unexplained somatic symptoms, restlessness, separation anxiety, academic problems, or issues with behavior at school (Mullen, 2018).

## OBJECTIVE DATA

The school-age years come with an increasing growth of independence. Strong parent-child interactions build the foundation for independence with strong self-esteem and model appropriate peer interactions. The NP may provide anticipatory guidance to help build resilience. Assisting with realistic expectations for this stage of childhood may prevent unneeded negative interactions between parent and child. During the school-age years, children are developing peer relationships in addition to increasing academic challenges. Success and failure are both anticipated during this stage. Caregivers should offer support in both of these experiences. Development of a strong and positive self-esteem is cultivated not only in success but also in how the parent responds to failures that the child experiences. Positive parent-child interactions provide a protective factor that has also been credited with decreasing the likelihood of risk-taking behaviors (Hagan et al., 2017).

A detailed history and physical examination should be performed on the child who has an actual or suspected developmental delay (Lipkin et al., 2020). In addition to annual evaluations, more frequent or periodic assessments are needed to help establish a diagnosis as the child's development progresses. There is increasing evidence of the impact of social determinants of health on a child's development, which support the continuous monitoring at visits (Lipkin et al., 2020). Maintenance of a standardized surveillance schedule at each visit is important, even for the school-age child. This is especially important if the child is identified as being at risk or delayed (Lipkin et al., 2020). An important task of the medical home provider is to utilize a developmental surveillance and referral tracking system that monitors the child's development and documentation of referrals with outcomes. Specialty referral is important to ensure early treatment and access to educational and community resources (Lipkin et al., 2020).

In the child with increased muscle tone, neuroimaging may be indicated, whereas in a child with normal or low muscle tone, serum creatine kinase and a thyroid function test should be obtained. Genetic testing and referral to a developmental specialist is recommended for the child suspected of having autism spectrum disorder, intellectual disability, or global developmental delay (Lipkin et al., 2020).

The AAP Task Force on Mental Health identified indicators of mental health problems in school-age children: depression (low mood), anxious and avoidant behaviors, impulsivity and/or inattention with or without hyperactivity, disruptive behavior, aggression, substance use, and learning difficulty (Foy et al., 2019, p. 9).

**PRO TIP** Identify and reinforce strengths in the child's development to promote engagement, optimism, and alliance (Foy et al., 2019).

School-age children are becoming more independent from their parents, interested in learning about their bodies, and are developing a body image of themselves. Perform the physical examination, respect modesty, and use a talk-through approach. Allow the child to participate in the examination by listening to their heart with the stethoscope while teaching them the importance of good hygiene practice by wiping off the earpieces and other components with an alcohol swab.

## PREVENTION

The health supervision visit for school-age children should allow for appropriate time to evaluate the child's physical and developmental status while effectively addressing all concerns from the child and family. This visit should include comprehensive health history, review of systems, and complete physical examination with appropriate screening tests and counseling about health risks, as well as a discussion regarding preventive health strategies. Developmental surveillance is critical in pediatrics with every clinical encounter, as these evaluations are central to health supervision for children. For children 7 or 8 years of age, it is appropriate to offer a portion of the examination without parents present. By age 12, the parents should be excused for a part of the examination to give opportunities for children to confide in the NP about pertinent health issues or risk-taking behaviors (Hagan et al., 2017).

A comprehensive history is obtained to assess physical and developmental strengths and areas of concern while fostering the NP's understanding of the child and their unique health qualities. A comprehensive history should include past medical history, family history, and social history. The social history should include lifestyle patterns, living situations, school performance, and safety issues. The NP needs to be aware of the total context of the child's environment and how these elements affect overall health status and developmental milieu. A standard review of systems is obtained in the health supervision examination and is an effective means to ensure that significant issues are highlighted (Hagan et al., 2017).

Although the focus of the well-child visit is the child, parental well-being should be addressed. Does the parent have a support system? Employment status or military deployment of the parent may lead to discussion of parent schedule, sources of stress, and economic stability (Hagan et al., 2017). What is the housing situation? Is there food insecurity? These factors affect the child on a daily basis and may lead to the need for additional resources or specialty referral.

The physical examination should include measurements with comparison to norms for age and sex, including body mass index (BMI), and blood pressure readings. Neurodevelopmental status should be assessed with observation of gait and coordination, and dental health should be assessed (Hagan et al., 2017). Hearing and visual acuity with ocular movement assessment should also be evaluated. As more than 1.25 million children are victims of maltreatment, it is critical to assess for signs of abuse at each health encounter (Riley et al., 2019). The NP should ask health screening questions during this portion of the examination and address concerns presented by the child or caregiver. The AAP recommendations for preventive pediatric health care can be accessed at https://downloads.aap.org/AAP/PDF/periodicity_schedule.pdf.

**PRO TIP** Education aimed at prevention should be ongoing and pertinent to the geographic location or season. Educational handouts or dedicated pages on websites and social media pages allow for the timely dissemination of important health-related information regarding safety promotion and illness or injury prevention. Educational content should be available in various forms, including printed materials and multimedia formats, and sensitive to diverse backgrounds and various cultural or religious beliefs. Materials can be created or reprinted with permission from authoritative or professional organization websites.

## IMMUNIZATIONS

School-age children should receive appropriate immunizations and catch-up immunizations as needed. Immunizations are a pivotal component of pediatric health maintenance and have been shown consistently to reduce the incidence of disease and complications. The recommended immunizations are approved annually by the AAP, the Advisory Committee on Immunization Practices (ACIP) of the Centers for Disease Control and Prevention (CDC), the American Academy of Family Physicians (AAFP), and the American College of Obstetricians and Gynecologists (ACOG). The recommended immunization schedule can be accessed at https://www.cdc.gov/vaccines/schedules/hcp/child-adolescent.html.

Strategies should be implemented in pediatric offices to encourage adherence to recommended vaccine schedules and increased rates of immunizations across the pediatric population. Pediatric providers should give clear and strong recommendations for immunizations, as this strategy has been shown to increase adherence to immunizations (Dempsey & Zimet, 2015). Immunization status should be reviewed at each health visit to ensure that catch-up immunizations are given if indicated. The rates of immunizations vary across the United States and are related to many factors, including school entry requirements and inaccurate information about immunizations.

**PRO TIP** Teach children and families how to prevent the flu and other illnesses by using proper handwashing technique and that the optimal length of time is 20 seconds of scrubbing. Encourage patients to hum or sing a song, such as the ABCs or "Happy Birthday," twice. Children and parents can time themselves singing or humming their favorite song to ensure they scrubbed their hands adequately. Inform them of proper handwashing and the CDC national Handwashing Campaign website: www.cdc.gov/handwashing

It is recommended that school-age children between 4 and 6 years old receive immunizations that include diphtheria, tetanus, and acellular pertussis (DTaP); inactivated poliovirus (IPV); measles, mumps, and rubella (MMR); and varicella (chickenpox). Completion rates in the United States for the 4- to 6-year-old vaccine series is 93% for DTaP, MMR, and varicella (Seither et al., 2017). It is recommended that school-age children between 11 to 12 years of age receive tetanus toxoid, diphtheria toxoid, and acellular pertussis (Tdap); the human papillomavirus vaccine (HPV), and the meningococcal vaccine. The influenza vaccine is also recommended annually (CDC, 2021). Although the rate for Tdap completion is 88%, the rates fall dramatically for the HPV at 49% and meningococcal vaccine at 44% (CDC, 2021; Walker et al., 2019).

## SCREENINGS

Well-child visits during the school-age years also provide an opportunity for other screenings, including school readiness, screening for specific health issues, vision and hearing screening, dental status, scoliosis screening, and adequacy of sleep.

### School Readiness

Although formal developmental screenings are not routinely performed after toddlerhood, the pediatric healthcare provider should assess developmental issues in this age group with questions related to school performance and social interactions. Children may have adjustment issues, special health needs, developmental disorders, or learning disabilities that negatively affect school readiness and success. The NP will be key in identifying at-risk school-age children and in developing strategies to assist the child in reaching their academic, social, and emotional potential. School-age children may also begin displaying signs of attention-deficit hyperactivity disorder (ADHD) due to academic demands (Riley et al., 2019). It is also important to screen for school absenteeism, which is linked to poor school performance and poor health outcomes. Chronic absenteeism varies between states, but approximately 13% of all students miss more than 15 days a year (Allison & Attisha, 2019).

### Screening for Specific Health Issues

Screening for health issues in the school-age child is a critical portion of the health supervision examination. The AAP has developed recommendations for screenings for specific conditions in this pediatric population.

#### Hypertension

Elevated blood pressure is defined as blood pressure at or above the 90th percentile. Hypertension should be diagnosed in children and adolescents who have auscultatory-confirmed blood pressure readings greater than or equal to the 95th percentile, based on sex, age, and height tables, at three different visits (Flynn et al.,

2017). Beginning at age 3, the AAP recommends blood pressure screening annually or at a healthcare encounter that identifies risks for hypertension with published recommendations for the management of hypertension in children (AAP, 2021). The USPSTF (2013) found insufficient evidence to recommend universal blood pressure screening in asymptomatic children and adolescents.

## Overweight and Obesity

The prevalence of obesity in children remains high. Approximately 1 in 5 children have obesity despite decades of intense efforts to reduce the childhood obesity epidemic in the United States (Skinner et al., 2018). The AAP recommends annual BMI measurements starting at age 2, while the USPSTF recommends measuring BMI beginning at age 6 (Grossman et al., 2017). Obesity in children is diagnosed with a BMI at or above the 95th percentile for age and sex, while overweight is defined as a BMI at or above the 85th percentile.

> **PRO TIP** EHRs may automatically calculate and classify BMI, making that information easily accessible to the NP.

An important strategy for preventing overweight and obesity is the concept of family mealtime. Studies have shown that greater frequency of meals eaten together as a family results in better nutritional status for children, including BMI (Dallacker et al., 2018). Children who meet the diagnostic criteria of overweight or obesity should receive counseling about lifestyle changes and dietary changes. Referral to an intensive behavioral program may be warranted, as that type of program has been demonstrated to lead to improvement in weight parameters (Grossman et al., 2017).

## Dyslipidemia

Pediatric patients with lipids disorders are at risk for cardiovascular disease in adulthood. Due to the serious health outcome of childhood dyslipidemia, the AAP recommends universal screening with a lipid profile once between 9 and 11 years of age (AAP/Bright Futures, 2021). The USPSTF (2016b) did not find significant evidence to obtain routine dyslipidemia screening in children.

## Vision and Hearing

Vision screening is an important part of the well child visit and the AAP (2021) recommends routine vision testing at 5, 6, 8, 10, and 12 years of age using an age-appropriate visual acuity test, such as a Snellen chart. The USPSTF (2017a) recommends starting vision screening between the ages of 3 and 5 to identify amblyopia. When visual acuity is assessed less than 20/40 for children 3 to 5 years of age or less than 20/30 for children older than 5 years, and in all children if there are more than two lines of difference between the eyes, the child should receive a referral to a pediatric ophthalmologist. Although the USPSTF does not have a recommendation for hearing screenings in school-age children, the AAP advises assessing audiometry at 5, 6, 8, and 10 years of age, and once between 11 and 14 years of age (Hagan et al., 2017). A referral is required for a hearing evaluation that reveals conduction thresholds greater than 20 dB to determine hearing impairment (Harlor et al., 2009).

## Dental Care

The NP should screen for dental care in school-age children, including identifying at-risk children who have an inadequate intake of fluoride (0.6 ppm or less). As fluoride in drinking water has been shown to decrease caries, children with low fluoride levels in their water supply should be given daily supplemental fluoride to promote dental health (Clark et al., 2014). Another component of screening for dental health is to promote dental sealants on back teeth to decrease the incident of caries. Although dental sealants are recommended to maintain dental health, less than half of children 6 to 11 have this effective intervention utilized. A definite health disparity is seen with decreased use of dental sealants and the treatment of caries in children within lower socioeconomic settings (CDC, 2020b).

## Scoliosis Screening

*Scoliosis* is defined as a three-dimensional spine deformity with lateral and rotational curvature of the spine. Idiopathic scoliosis is the most common form and is usually found in early adolescence, with a prevalence of approximately 3% of children under 16 years of age. Although the majority of children do not have progressive spinal curvature, a small subset may develop rapid progression with possibly devastating results if undetected early enough for effective interventions. Although the USPSTF (2018) concluded that the current evidence is insufficient to assess the benefit of screening for scoliosis in children and adolescents age 10 to 18 years, a joint statement from multiple entities, including the AAP, agrees that scoliosis screening should be performed on females twice at 10 and 12 years of age and on boys once, at age 13 or 14 (Hresko et al., 2015).

### Sleep

Sleep is increasingly highlighted as an element of health in children, with an adequate amount of sleep preventing obesity, type 2 diabetes, behavior problems, poor mental health, and injuries. Children age 6 to 12 years need 9 to 12 hours of sleep a night for optimal health outcomes. The NP should work to increase the family's awareness of the importance of sleep in their children, encourage parents to model good sleep patterns, and promote methods that foster quality sleep behavior (CDC, 2020).

## ANTICIPATORY GUIDANCE

Anticipatory guidance in pediatrics is a process in which pediatric providers anticipate the developmental challenges of infancy, childhood, and adolescence by providing guidance to the caregivers and the child. This guidance should be developmentally relevant and timely to foster the emergence of developmental tasks. Attention should be given to developing interventions that will promote wellness and identify physical, mental, and developmental diversion from normative standards. The NP should enhance anticipatory guidance with questions and information to aid the families in navigating expected developmental tasks. Anticipatory guidance is essential at all ages to promote positive healthcare outcomes, but it is particularly critical in school-age children because they are establishing health patterns that will extend into adulthood.

School-age children should be encouraged to lead a healthy lifestyle with a diet rich in fruits and vegetables, whole grains, fish, lean meats, adequate fluid intake, daily physical activity, limited screen time, adequate sleep, and dental hygiene. High-risk behaviors may begin in early adolescence; therefore, NPs should give preventive strategies related to tobacco, alcohol, and drug use starting at 11 years of age. Safety issues are also a critical element in anticipatory guidance, as unintentional injury is the leading cause of death in this age group in the United States (Locke et al., 2019).

After addressing the concerns of the parents, Bright Futures Middle Childhood Expert Panel has set five priority areas to be addressed during the anticipatory guidance for health supervision visits (Hagan et al., 2017), as follows:

1. The first of these outline priorities for this age group is social determinants of health and involves evaluating risks for environmental and family violence, food security, family substance use and protective elements of self-esteem, and family support and involvement.
2. The second priority is focused on developmental and mental health with the assessment of discipline patterns, conflict resolution, and family structure.
3. School readiness and academics is critical third priority for this age group.
4. Physical growth and developmental tasks of the school-age child is a priority in anticipatory guidance and include lifestyle and healthy choices related to activity and diet, while ensuring the developmental milestones are being successfully mastered.
5. Safety issues is the fifth priority and will be discussed in detail below (Hagan et al., 2017).

## SAFETY

The well-child examination for the school-age child focuses on health promotion and injury prevention; safety guidance is a key responsibility of the NP. Some guidance on safety and injury prevention may be tailored to various geographic regions and urban versus rural areas of habitation. Increased independence, steady growth and development, and curiosity put this age group at risk for a multitude of accidental and nonaccidental injuries.

### Environmental Exposures

Children are at risk for harmful and unhealthy exposures inside and outside of the home. Younger children are at higher risk for exposures due to factors such as higher respiratory rates, breathing areas closer to the ground or floor, likelihood of putting substances in their mouths, and developing internal organs (Galvez & Balk, 2017). During the well-child visit the NP will assess and educate caregivers and children on how to prevent and minimize unhealthy environmental exposures.

### Home Exposures

Poor indoor air quality can lead to an increased number of respiratory illnesses and asthma exacerbations. Air quality can be improved by frequently changing heat, air, and air conditioning (HVAC) filters. Pollutants such as pesticides and harsh cleaning agents should be reduced or eliminated in the home. Increasing ventilation is important when using cleaning products or art supplies such as paint and glue (Galvez & Balk, 2017).

#### *Smoke and Nicotine Exposure*

Children should never be exposed to tobacco smoke or nicotine. If the parent or caregiver does smoke, the NP should strongly advise the adult to quit smoking. If the parent does express interest, then counsel them on available resources for smoking cessation. In the case that the parent is not motivated to quit smoking, education should be given on how to keep the home and car smoke-free. Children should also be advised to avoid the use of tobacco- or nicotine-containing products, including vaping pens, as these substances can lead to multiple adverse health outcomes (Galvez & Balk, 2017).

#### *Lead and Radon Exposure*

Lead and radon exposure should be assessed based on the type and age of housing the family inhabits. Homes lower than the third floor should be tested for radon. Radon reduction systems are available for installation. Radon exposure can be reduced by not using basements for sleep or play. School-age children are less likely to be exposed to lead, as the typical exposure to lead occurs when children ingest lead-based paint chips. Lead is not present in paints manufactured after 1978, though home renovations may pose a risk. Children with developmental delays living in homes built before 1978 should be tested for lead exposure. Routine follow-up is recommended for blood lead levels between 5 to 45 mcg/dL and treatment is warranted for lead levels greater than 45 mcg/dL (Galvez & Balk, 2017).

#### *Mold Exposure*

Water damage and visible mold in the home should be repaired and removed, as even the smallest amount of mold can cause allergic and respiratory illnesses. When assessing the child with asthma or chronic respiratory disorders, the NP should address this potential trigger at well-child and acute illness visits. If water or mold damage is present in the home, a contractor trained in mold removal may be hired to repair the damage (Galvez & Balk, 2017).

#### *Well-Water Exposure*

The NP should determine if the family's home has municipal water or well water. If the family or child drinks water from a well, specific guidance should be offered to ensure safe drinking water. Well water requires annual testing because it may contain pesticides, heavy metals, coliform bacteria, arsenic, radon, lead, fuel additives, and uranium. As children drink a higher ratio of water to their body weight than do adults, they are at increased risk for *Cryptosporidium*. In the case where well water safety is questioned, bottled water should be advised as a safer drinking option (Galvez & Balk, 2017).

#### *Phthalates and BPA Exposure*

Exposure to endocrine-disrupting molecules, such as phthalates and bisphenol A (BPA), can lead to disorders such as hyperactive behavior, wheezing, obesity, insulin insensitivity, heart disease, and type 2 diabetes. The NP can educate on decreasing exposure to these substances by advising families to choose unprocessed foods, avoid heating foods in plastic containers, choose glass containers when possible, purchase products labeled phthalate and BPA free, and use wet methods to dust and mop to avoid phthalates in dust (Galvez & Balk, 2017).

### Outdoor and Community Exposures

#### *Sun Exposure*

The sun is the most common cause of ultraviolet (UV) exposure for the school-age child. Skin cancer is the most frequently diagnosed cancer among Americans (Galvez & Balk, 2017). Sun exposure at younger ages is a large contributor to the development of melanoma; therefore, avoidance and reduction of sun exposure should be addressed yearly at the annual well-child visit. NPs should advise caregivers and patients on avoidance of deliberate tanning; wearing sun protective clothing, wide brimmed hats, and sunblock; minimizing sun exposure between 10:00 a.m. and 4:00 p.m.; and wearing sunglasses while participating in activities in the sun (Galvez & Balk, 2017).

#### *Noise Exposure*

Excessive exposure to loud noises can have an adverse impact on health by causing increased stress levels, sleep deprivation, headache, and fatigue (Galvez & Balk, 2017). Noisy environments can also lead to adverse outcomes for children, including learning difficulties, speech and language delay, and reading and writing problems. During the well-child visit, the healthcare provider should assess the child's exposure to noise. Toys such as cap guns and exposure to firecrackers may cause long-term hearing damage. If children are exposed to loud music, such as from a radio or while playing a musical instrument, they should wear earplugs or use a noise muffling device (Galvez & Balk, 2017).

## Risk-Taking Behavior

Risk-taking behavior in the middle childhood years can be part of healthy psychosocial development that provides confidence and increases self-esteem. Peers become a more influential and important part of the child's life, which also leads to exposures to new experiences. Unfortunately, seeking out new experiences may also lead to situations where danger or injury may occur (Bottomley, 2013). At each well-child visit, the NP will offer anticipatory guidance to encourage positive risk taking while discouraging dangerous or unhealthy risk-taking behavior.

Healthy risks that encourage industry and increased self-esteem include trying out for a sports team, indoor supervised rock climbing, engaging in an organized extracurricular activity, trying new foods, kayaking, or going to a theme or amusement park. These activities allow for the excitement of trying new things with the possibility of success or challenges, but do not pose a dangerous risk (Bottomley, 2013).

Interventions discouraging substance use in middle childhood can decrease the use of tobacco, alcohol, and drugs into adolescence (Castellanos-Ryan et al., 2013). Peers or older siblings may introduce school-age children to tobacco, alcohol, and drugs. Parents and healthcare providers should take an active stance on discouraging experimentation with these substances and know how to monitor for use from childhood through adolescence.

### Broadcast and Social Media Use

Exposure to broadcast media and social media has increased dramatically with the school-age population. While media use may offer the ability to quickly gain information, it also provides opportunities for unhealthy risk-taking situations. Media use may increase exposure to alcohol, drugs, and sexual behaviors, as the display of these activities may be presented as attractive to children and adolescents (AAP, Council on Communications and Media, 2016).

The NP should counsel the parent on closely monitoring media use and content. Social media and internet use provide access to child predators by way of chat rooms, gaming, and email which the child may access via a mobile phone, tablet, or computer. Unmonitored access to the internet puts children in danger of exploitation by child sex offenders (AAP, Council on Communications and Media, 2016). Guidance for parental modeling of appropriate internet and media use should be provided at well-child visits, as children and adolescents emulate the actions of parents and caregivers. If attention is given to a mobile device such as a cell phone or tablet while spending time with a child, the parent is less likely to engage in conversation with the child. Parental engagement is critical in social and emotional well-being of the child. Lack of parental engagement has negative short- and long-term results in child development (AAP, Council on Communications and Media, 2016).

## Social Situations

Social development is of great importance for the school-age child because social environments, such as school, play a predominant part in the child's life. While providers and parents hope that the social environment is positive, children may find themselves in scenarios that are very negative and potentially dangerous, physically and mentally. Awareness of bullying should be addressed during the well-child visit. There are three important questions to ask about bullying:

- Do you ever see kids picking on other kids?
- Do kids ever pick on you?
- Do you ever pick on kids? (And tell the truth; you are not in trouble) (Korioth, 2016).

*Bullying* is defined as "unwanted, aggressive behavior among school-aged children that involves a real or perceived difference in power" (Korioth, 2016, para. 2). These unwanted behaviors can be perpetrated physically, verbally, through cyber-harassment, by social media, and socially; often the bully attempts to destroy the victim's reputation. These types of situations and behaviors should be addressed immediately, as victims of bullying often present with many types of physical complaints/illnesses, depression, anxiety, and suicidal thoughts, and may also become bullies themselves (Korioth, 2016).

Adults and peers may offer support for victims. Parents and providers should encourage all children to form strong friendships and to not join others in bullying behaviors. Counseling should be provided to bullies and victims. Children who engage in bullying activities often learn the behavior at home and may have been victims of bullying. A strong sense of belonging and engagement is more effective than punishment (Korioth, 2016).

## Vehicle Safety

Education on vehicle safety should be communicated with each caregiver who transports a child in a vehicle. Motor vehicle accidents are the leading cause of death in children in the United States (National Center for Health Statistics, 2018). All passengers should be properly restrained before the vehicle is put into motion. Each passenger should be restrained with their own individual seat belt; seat belts should not be shared (AAP, 2020).

All children ages 13 and younger should be restrained in the back seat while in transit. An adult seat belt will properly fit a child when they reach the height of 4 feet and 9 inches. However, most children will not reach this height until 10 or 11 years old. A seat belt that fits correctly will fit snugly across the lap, not the abdomen. The shoulder strap should restrain across the middle of the chest, not the neck or throat. If the child has not yet reached the height of 4 feet and 9 inches, the caregiver should be instructed that the child should use a booster seat until the minimum height requirement is met. Children under age 13, and less than 4 feet 9 inches in height, should always ride in the back seat of the car to avoid risk of air bag injury. An indication that the child may still require a booster seat is that he or she is unable to sit comfortably against the back of the seat with legs bent over the seat (AAP, 2020).

Children should never be left alone in a vehicle for *any* length of time. Educating caregivers on not leaving young children alone in a vehicle has become more critical than ever. Child death by heat stroke is the primary cause of non-crash, vehicle-related deaths under the age of 15. The interior of a vehicle increases 20 degrees Fahrenheit every 10 minutes. Heat stroke is possible even when environmental temperature is as low as 57 degrees Fahrenheit (AAP, 2019).

### Sports and Recreation

Participation in sports and recreation positively affects overall physical health by promoting an active lifestyle and the development of cooperative peer relationships. The NP, when offering guidance in injury prevention, should reinforce involvement in sports and recreation. Depending on the sport or activity, appropriate safety gear should be used for both practice and competitive games or matches. Safety gear may include helmets, mouth or wrist guards, kneepads, elbow pads, or reflective clothing. Gear should fit properly and not be damaged, as this may lead to discomfort and suboptimal protection (CDC, 2019c).

When sports or recreation take place outdoors, environmental temperature should be addressed. In seasons and regions where heat and humidity pose a health threat, adequate physical breaks and hydration are preventative against dehydration and heat stroke. Uniforms or practice gear should be worn based on temperature in order to prevent injuries caused by overheating or hypothermia (CDC, 2019c).

The use of helmets should be addressed at each well-child visit, as the appropriate use of this piece of protective equipment can decrease occurrence of devastating head/brain injury and death. Helmets should be worn for specific sports such as football, baseball, lacrosse, and rugby. Helmets should also be worn for riding a bicycle, inline skating, and skateboarding. For optimal protection helmets should be properly fitting, undamaged, and worn every time the child participates in the activity. To increase the likelihood of the child forming a habit of wearing a helmet, encourage parents and caregivers to model this behavior by also wearing a helmet during recreation (CDC, 2019).

In the event that a head injury results from sports or recreation, the child should follow up with a healthcare provider to rule out concussion or a more severe brain injury. The CDC (2020a) has developed the HEADS UP campaign in order to standardize concussion assessment and provide guidance for return to school and sports. The healthcare provider concussion assessment tool can be accessed by visiting www.cdc.gov/headsup/pdfs/providers/ace_v2-a.pdf.

## KEY POINTS

- Adhere to best practices by creating, disseminating, and actively engaging patients and families at all visits and address issues.
- Direct families to appropriate resources.
- Assist families in identifying and implementing patient safety best practices.
- Engage families by creating safety materials and participating in safety committees or safety events in the community.

## REFERENCES

Allison, M. A., & Attisha, E. (2019). The link between school attendance and good health. *Pediatrics, 143*(2), e20183648. https://doi.org/10.1542/peds.2018-3648

American Academy of Pediatrics. (2019). *Prevent child car deaths in hot cars.* https://www.healthychildren.org/English/safety-prevention/on-the-go/Pages/Prevent-Child-Deaths-in-Hot-Cars.aspx

American Academy of Pediatrics. (2020). *Seatbelts for older children.* https://www.healthychildren.org/English/safety-prevention/on-the-go/Pages/Seat-Belts-for-Older-Children-Adults.aspx

American Academy of Pediatrics/Bright Futures. (2021). *Recommendations for preventive pediatric health care.* https://downloads.aap.org/AAP/PDF/periodicity_schedule.pdf

American Academy of Pediatrics, Council on Communications and Media. (2016). Media use in school-aged children and adolescents. *Pediatrics, 138*(5), e20162592. http://dx.doi.org/10.1542/peds.2016-2592

Bottomley, L. (2013). *Healthy risk-taking.* https://www.canr.msu.edu/news/healthy_risk_taking

Castellanos-Ryan, N., O'Leary-Barrett, M., & Conrod, P. J. (2013). Substance-use in childhood and adolescence:

A brief overview of developmental processes and their clinical implications. *Journal of the Canadian Academy of Child and Adolescent Psychiatry, 22*(1), 41–46. https://www.ncbi.nlm.nih.gov/pmc/articles/PMC3565714/

Centers for Disease Control and Prevention. (2019). *Protect the ones you love: Child injuries are preventable*. https://www.cdc.gov/safechild/sports_injuries

Centers for Disease Control and Prevention. (2020a). *HEADS UP to youth sports*. https://www.cdc.gov/headsup/youthsports/index.html

Centers for Disease Control and Prevention. (2020b). *Promoting health for children and adolescents*. https://www.cdc.gov/chronicdisease/resources/publications/factsheets/children-health.htm

Centers for Disease Control and Prevention. (2021). *Immunization schedules. For health care providers*. https://www.cdc.gov/vaccines/schedules/index.html

Clark, M. B., Slayton, R. L., & Section on Oral Health. (2014). Fluoride use in caries prevention in the primary care setting. *Pediatrics, 134*(3), 626–633. https://doi.org/10.1542/peds.2014-1699

Dallacker, M., Hertwig, R., & Mata, J. (2018). The frequency of family meals and nutritional health in children: A meta-analysis. *Obesity Reviews, 19*(5), 638–653. https://doi.org/10.1111/obr.12659

Dempsey, A. F., & Zimet, G. D. (2015). Interventions to improve adolescent vaccination: What may work and what still needs to be tested. *American Journal of Preventative Medicine, 49*(6), S445–S454. https://doi.org/10.1016/j.amepre.2015.04.013

Flynn, J. T., Kaelber, D. C., Baker-Smith, C. M., Blowey, D., Carroll, A. E., Daniels, S. R., de Ferranti, S. D., Dionne, J. M., Falkner, B., Flinn, S. K., Gidding, S. S., Goodwin, C., Leu, M. G., Powers, M. E., Rea, C., Samuels, J., Simasek, M., Thaker, V. V., Urbina, E. M., & the Subcommittee on Screening and Management of High Blood Pressure in Children. (2017). Clinical practice guideline for screening and management of high blood pressure in children and adolescent. *Pediatrics, 140*(3), e20171904. https://doi.org/10.1542/peds.2017-1904

Forman-Hoffman, V., McClure, E., McKeeman, J., Wood, C. T., Middleton, J. C., Skinner, A. C., Perrin, E. M., & Viswanathan, M. (2016). Screening for major depressive disorder among children and adolescents: A systematic review for the U.S. Preventive Services Task Force [Publication No. 13-05192-EF-1]. *Annals of Internal Medicine, 164*(5), 342–349. https://doi.org/ 10.7326/M15-2259

Foy, J. M., Green, C. M., Earls, M. F., & Members of the Committee on Psychosocial Aspects of Child and Family Health, Mental Health Leadership Work Group. (2019). Mental health competencies for pediatric practice [Policy statement]. *Pediatrics, 144*(5), e20192757. https://pediatrics.aappublications.org/content/144/5/e20192757

Galvez, M. P., & Balk, S. J. (2017). Environmental risks to children: Prioritizing health messages in pediatric practice. *Pediatrics in Review, 38*(6), 263–279. http://dx.doi.org/10.1542/pir.2015-0165

Grossman, D. C., Bibbins-Domingo, K., Curry, S. J., Barry, M. J., Davidson, K. W., Doubeni, C. A., Epling, J. W., Kemper, A. R., Krist, A. H., Kurth, A. E., Landefeld, C. S., Mangione, C. M., Phipps, M. G., Silverstein, M., Simon, M. A., Tseng, C., & the members of U.S. Preventive Services Task Force. (2017). Screening for obesity in children and adolescents: U.S. Preventive Services Task Force recommendation statement. *JAMA: The Journal of the American Medical Association, 317*(23), 2417–2426. https://doi.org/10.1001/jama.2017.6803

Hagan, J. F., Shaw, J. S., & Duncan, P. M. (Eds.). (2017). *Bright Futures: Guidelines for health supervision of infants, children, and adolescents* (4th ed.). Bright Futures/American Academy of Pediatrics.

Harlor, A. D. B., Bower, C., & the Committee on Practice and Ambulatory Medicine, the Section on Otolaryngology-Head and Neck Surgery. (2009). Hearing assessment in infants and children: Recommendations beyond neonatal screening. *Pediatrics, 124*(4), 1252–1263. https://doi.org/10.1542/peds.2009-1997

Hresko, M. T., Talwalkar, V. R., & Schwend, R. M. (2015). *Position statement—Screening for the early detection for idiopathic scoliosis in adolescents*. https://bit.ly/2HkZvht

Korioth, T. (2016). *Signs of bullying: Important questions for parents to ask*. https://www.healthychildren.org/English/safety-prevention/at-play/Pages/Bullies-Beat-Down-Self-Esteem.aspx

Lipkin, P. H., Macias, M. M., & the Council on Children with Disabilities, Section on Developmental and Behavioral Pediatrics. (2020). Promoting optimal development: Identifying infants and young children with developmental disorders through developmental surveillance and screening. *Pediatrics, 145*(1), e20193449. https://doi.org/10.1542/peds.2019-3449

Locke, A., Stoesser, K., & Pippitt, K. (2019). Health maintenance in school-aged children: Part II. Counseling recommendations. *American Family Physician, 100*(4), 219–226.

Mullen, S. (2018). Major depressive disorder in children and adolescents. *The Mental Health Clinician, 8*(6), 275–283. https://doi.org/10.9740/mhc.2018.11.275

National Center for Health Statistics, National Vital Statistics System. (2018). *10 leading causes of injury deaths by age group highlighting unintentional injury deaths, United States—2017*. National Center for Injury Prevention and Control, Centers for Disease Control and Prevention. https://www.cdc.gov/injury/wisqars/pdf/leading_causes_of_injury_deaths_highlighting_unintentional_2017-508.pdf

Riley, M., Morrison, L., & McEvoy, A. (2019). Health maintenance in school-aged children: Part I. History, physical examination, screening, and immunizations. *American Family Physician, 100*(4), 213–218. https://www.aafp.org/afp/2019/0815/p213.html

Seither, R., Calhoun, K., Street, E. J., Mellerson, J., Knighton, C. L., Tippins, A., & Underwood, M. (2017). Vaccine coverage for selected vaccines, exemption rates, and provisional enrollment among children in kindergarten—United States, 2016-17 school year. *Morbidity and Mortality Weekly Report, 66*(40), 1073–1080. http://dx.doi.org/10.15585/mmwr.mm6640a3

Skinner, A. C., Ravanbakht, S. N., Skelton, J. A., Perrin, E. M., & Armstrong, S. C. (2018). Prevalence of obesity and severe obesity in U.S. children, 1999–2016. *Pediatrics, 141*(3), Article e20173459. https://doi.org/10.1542/peds.2017-3459

U.S. Preventive Services Task Force. (2013). *Final recommendation statement: Blood pressure in children and adolescents (hypertension): Screening*. https://www.uspreventiveservicestaskforce.org/Page/Document/RecommendationStatementFinal/blood-pressure-in-children-and-adolescents-hypertension-screening

U.S. Preventive Services Task Force. (2016a). *Final recommendations summary: Depression in children and adolescents: Screening*. https://www.uspreventiveservicestaskforce

.org/Page/Document/UpdateSummaryFinal/depression-in-children-and-adolescents-screening

U.S. Preventive Services Task Force. (2016b). *Final recommendations summary: Lipid disorders in children and adolescents: Screening*. https://www.uspreventiveservicestaskforce.org/Page/Document/UpdateSummaryFinal/lipid-disorders-in-children-screening

U.S. Preventive Services Task Force. (2017a). *Final recommendations summary: Vision in children ages 6 months to 5 years: Screening*. https://www.uspreventiveservicestaskforce.org/Page/Document/UpdateSummaryFinal/vision-in-children-ages-6-months-to-5-years-screening

U.S. Preventive Services Task Force. (2018). *Final recommendation statement: Adolescent idiopathic scoliosis: Screening*. https://www.uspreventiveservicestaskforce.org/Page/Document/RecommendationStatementFinal/adolescent-idiopathic-scoliosis-screening

Wagner, J. B., Kim, M., & Tassé, M. J. (2019). Technology tools: Increasing our reach in national surveillance of intellectual and developmental disabilities. *Intellectual and Developmental Disabilities, 57*(5), 463–475. https://doi.org/10.1352/1934-9556-57.5.463

Walker, T. Y., Elam-Evans, L. D., Yankey, D., Markowitz, L. E., Williams, C. L., Fredua, B., & Singleton, J. A. (2019). National, regional, state, and selected local area vaccination coverage among adolescents aged 13–17 years—United States, 2018. *Morbidity and Mortality Weekly Report, 68*(33), 718–723. http://dx.doi.org/10.15585/mmwr.mm6833a2external icon

# Well-Child Visits During Adolescence

Tedra S. Smith and Imelda Reyes

## Student Learning Outcomes

**Upon completion of this chapter the reader should be able to:**

1. Determine the adequacy of adolescent growth.
2. Evaluate developmental milestones of adolescents.
3. Choose appropriate screening tests based on current recommendations for an adolescent's age and risk status.
4. Select immunizations based on current recommendations for an adolescent's age and risk status.
5. Determine applicable anticipatory guidance for each scheduled visit during adolescence.

## INTRODUCTION

Remarkable changes occur during the adolescent period. The adolescent experiences dramatic physical, developmental, and emotional maturation between the ages of 11 and 21 years. During this time, it is important to recognize that the adolescent is not a small adult or a large child. As the adolescent is changing, the family dynamic is shifting. The nurse practitioner (NP) is in a unique position as primary care provider to assist the child and family with this challenging transition. This may be achieved through a trusting and respectful relationship.

Adolescents demonstrate particular vulnerabilities related to their developmental stage. The adolescent period may be divided into three substages: early, middle, and late. The changes adolescents experience can vary widely. During each of the substages, it is critical to focus care specifically to the adolescent's needs on an individualized basis. Well-child visits provide the perfect opportunity for screening and educating the adolescent and the family. Developmental surveillance, primary prevention (immunizations, safety education), secondary prevention (screenings), and anticipatory guidance are individualized based on the adolescent's needs.

The content in this chapter maps to the following areas on the Pediatric Nursing Certification Board (PNCB) Pediatric Nurse Practitioner—Primary Care certification examination:

CONTENT AREAS:

### I. Health Maintenance and Promotion

**A. Partner with patients/caregivers to support growth and development from infancy to young adulthood**

**B. Provide patients/caregivers with age/developmentally appropriate anticipatory guidance**

**C. Recommend and prescribe immunizations according to current CDC guidelines**

**D. Educate about illness prevention and early warning signs of pediatric illness and emergencies**

**E. Advise patients/caregivers about age appropriate injury prevention and safety (environmental exposure, risk taking behaviors, social situations, sports and recreation, and vehicle safety)**

**F. Counsel about age-appropriate social, behavioral, and mental health concerns (e.g., substance abuse, social media use, grief and loss, and sexual orientation/LGBTQ)**

## II. Assessment and Diagnosis

**A. Growth and Development**

1. Evaluate and interpret growth parameters
2. Perform developmental surveillance

**B. History and Physical Examination**

1. Obtain history of present illness
2. Obtain a comprehensive health history for new patients
3. Complete an interval history for established patients
4. Perform a review of systems
5. Perform a complete physical examination

**C. Diagnostic Testing and Screening**

1. Order and interpret office/clinic based screening tests
4. Select, utilize, and interpret developmental, behavioral and mental health screening and assessment tools

**D. Analyzing Information**

1. Integrate health history and physical examination findings into the plan of care
2. Assimilate findings from screening and diagnostic testing into plan of care

## IV. Professional Role and Responsibilities

**B. Practice Management**

1. Document patient encounters in a manner which supports applicable diagnostic and procedure codes
2. Utilize appropriate billing and coding to facilitate reimbursement

## SETTING THE STAGE

Respect for the adolescent is of the upmost importance while you gain the trust of the patient and family. The adolescent gains trust in the provider as confidentiality is maintained and when the adolescent feels listened to. Rephrasing what the adolescent tells the provider may help clarify issues and result in the adolescent's voice or opinion being valued. Adolescents want and need a trusted healthcare provider. They want a friendly provider who listens, but do not desire the provider to be their friend. Health promotion for the adolescent begins with a sensitive approach to both the patient and the family member present with the adolescent. Always start by introducing yourself and your role as the provider to the adolescent. At this age, it is also recommended that you ask for preferred pronouns; do not assume gender based on the chart or electronic medical record. For privacy, the parent can be asked about any concerns and then escorted out of the room to wait either in another room or the waiting room. This will ensure that the adolescent is given privacy either to review the paperwork the adolescent has completed or to ask sensitive questions, and places the responsibility for having the private conversation with the provider. With this approach, the provider takes the lead and is able to negotiate with the parent regarding the privacy issues.

Privacy and confidentiality for the adolescent are important, but you must clearly state what can be kept confidential and what must be shared. During the assessment, it is important to allow for time with only the adolescent in the room in order to ask sensitive questions. These might include questions about drug and alcohol use, sexuality and reproductive health, pregnancy, or contraception. Videos demonstrating confidential care are available for viewing on the American Academy of Pediatrics' (AAP) website (www.aap.org/en-us/about-the-aap/aap-press-room/campaigns/adolescent-health-care/Pages/default.aspx).

Privacy laws vary by state and becoming aware of nuances regarding confidentiality of testing or treatment of the adolescent is essential. For example, in some states, the minor does not have the right to confidentiality regarding certain testing or treatment (AAP, 2020b). The Guttmacher Institute can be very helpful in providing guidance as to what a teen is entitled to and what can be kept confidential.

## DEVELOPMENTAL SURVEILLANCE

Developmental surveillance is completed at each substage of adolescence, beginning with early adolescence. In the early adolescent years (11–14 years old), the patient may experience a change from having their parents answer questions to having the focus be on them taking charge of their own health. It is important to help in this transition. As you ask questions, be sensitive and responsive to the patient. If the adolescent is not forthcoming, e.g., regarding sexual health, take the time to use motivational interviewing to find out what is known and how to engage the adolescent with anticipatory guidance. Resources for conducting motivational interviewing may be found in the resource "Behavioral Health: An Adolescent Provider Toolkit" (https://ahwg.org).

In the middle adolescent years (15–17 years old), the patient is generally more independent, and approaching adult physical size. But the adolescent is still in a stage of flux, with great variability in emotional development. The patient should take the lead in answering questions. Reviewing confidentiality becomes more important and ensuring privacy with the adolescent is of utmost importance.

In late adolescent years (18–21 years old), the adolescent is usually transitioning to becoming an independent adult. This is a time of finishing high school or the equivalent and considering college, including technical schools, or joining the workforce. The transition can feel daunting to the young adult.

## SUBJECTIVE DATA

During the review of systems, ask about these items if they have not been covered within any screening tool used:

- **Constitutional**:
  - *Nutrition*: food insecurity
  - *Sleep:* fatigue, What is bedtime? Is there a television in the bedroom? Are electronic devices used before going to bed?
- **HEENT**: Vision (ensure the adolescent is being screened per the AAP Periodicity Schedule every 2 years)
- **Gastrointestinal**: stomach pains
- **Genitourinary:** If the adolescent is sexually active, ask what type of contraception or protection is in use. Is the adolescent interested in learning about or gaining access to birth control or protection? For girls: Has she started her period? How regular, heavy, and frequent is the period?

### Risk Screening Tools

As a starting point for assessing key aspects of the adolescent's home and school life, use of illicit substances or alcohol, sex, and risk for depression and suicide, it can be useful to utilize a questionnaire. Completing a screening tool either on paper or digitally can help to eliminate or reduce the burden on the teen of disclosing confidential information to a relative stranger (Ho et al., 2019). These screening questionnaires can be used in the office to help expedite the process, but following up with clarifying questions or comments and incorporating anticipatory guidance improves individualized care for the adolescent. Suggestions for questionnaires:

- Develop a questionnaire for use in the office or clinic based on the **HEEADSSS** (Home, Education/Employment, Eating, Activities, Drugs, Sexuality, Suicide/Depression, Safety) assessment (Exhibit 18.1). The questionnaire could be delivered on paper or digitally depending upon the office resources.
- Use the cloud-based **RAAPS** (Rapid Assessment for Adolescent Preventive Services©), available from https://possibilitiesforchange.org/raaps/. A preview of the standardized 21-question RAAPS is shown in Exhibit 18.2.

When reviewing the results of the screening tools, tailor further questioning to the age of the adolescent. By questioning the adolescent, the adolescent's relationship with the parents or caregivers may also be determined. Screening may reveal protective behaviors, which the provider can encourage, as well as risk factors, which need to be addressed through either gaining additional resources, referring to a specialist, creating a detailed management plan, or a combination of these things. These questions should be routinely addressed at every adolescent visit, whether it is a sick- or well-child examination (AAP, 2020a).

Suggested questions for following up on the screening tool include:

- *Home:* Do you have someone you can talk to at home? How is your home life?
- *Education/Environment*: How is school going? Are you bullied at school? What is a favorite subject at school?
- *Eating:* Tell me what you eat in a typical day. Do you ever go hungry because of lack of food?
- *Activities:* Tell me about clubs, sports, or other extracurricular activities you are involved in. Do you work?
- *Drugs:* Have you ever tried recreational drugs including tobacco, vaping, or alcohol? Do you use marijuana? Have you taken any drug that was not prescribed for you?
- *Sex:* What gender do you identify with? When was the last time you engaged in sex? May specify by asking: Have you had oral, anal, or vaginal sex with a boy or girl? Ask about safety, consent for sex, birth control, and infection prevention (Simmonds et al., 2017).
- *Suicide/depression (emotions):* Have you ever had thoughts of hurting yourself?
- *Safety:* Do you ever feel sad or anxious? Which one? (expand on this depending upon the adolescent's answers) Do you feel safe at home or at school?

## OBJECTIVE DATA

Perform a complete physical examination at each scheduled well child visit.

### Parental or Caregiver Interaction

While interviewing the parent and adolescent together, carefully observe the interactions between the parent/

ADDRESSING *Mental Health* CONCERNS IN PRIMARY CARE
A CLINICIAN'S TOOLKIT

## HEADSSS ASSESSMENT: RISK AND PROTECTIVE FACTORS

**FOR PROVIDERS:** SCREENING, ASSESSMENT AND REFERRAL

# HEADSSS Assessment: Risk and Protective Factors

*Risk factors increase the likelihood that an adolescent will engage in risky behaviors. Protective factors, on the other hand, build an adolescent's resiliency and contribute to his/her ability to cope with stress and thrive. Identify the adolescent's risk and protective factors during each visit. Encourage all of your patients to build upon their assets and reach out for help.*

**Biological Risk Factors:**

- Genetics: family history of mood, anxiety, and/or eating disorders, schizophrenia, substance addiction.
- In-utero and childhood risks: fetal alcohol exposure, toxin exposure, brain injury, infections, nutritional deficits.

| PSYCHOSOCIAL REALMS | PROTECTIVE FACTORS | RISK FACTORS |
|---|---|---|
| **HOME** | • Positive relationship with parent(s)<br>• Parent(s)/family seen as resource<br>• Good communication with parent(s)/family<br>• Caring adults involved in his/her life | • Conflicted/negative relationship with parent(s)<br>• Absent or excessive rules, structure, or supervision<br>• Uncomfortable asking parent(s)/family for help<br>• Poor communication with parent(s)/family<br>• Caring adults cannot be identified |
| **EDUCATION/ EMPLOYMENT** | • Positive attitude about school<br>• Involvement in school and school activities<br>• Belief that teachers and school are caring and fair<br>• High academic expectations communicated by parent(s)<br>• Good academic achievement<br>• Future educational attainment goals | • Belief that school is boring, useless, and/or unsafe<br>• Isolated, disengaged, or discriminated in school<br>• Belief that teachers and school mistreat him/her<br>• Low or extremely high academic expectations from parent(s)<br>• Grade(s) repeated, ↓ school performance/attendance<br>• Education not seen as part of her/his future life<br>• 20 hours or more per week of work |
| **ACTIVITIES** | • Involvement in supervised group activities such as after-school, community-based, sports, arts and/or faith-based programs<br>• Religious and/or spiritual practice<br>• Involvement in social justice, advocacy, and/or community work<br>• At least one meal per day eaten with family | • Lack of supervision in school or after school<br>• Engaged in risky and/or harmful behaviors<br>• Isolated or disconnected from peers, community, and family<br>• Overscheduled and without down time<br>• Inadequate nutrition or sleep<br>• Excessive preoccupation with diet and/or exercise |
| **DRUGS** | • Not associated w/ substance-involved peers<br>• Parent(s)/family members do not use substances<br>• Negative attitude towards substances<br>• Past substance use but now abstinent | • Substance use by peers<br>• Substance use by parent(s)/family members<br>• Early, intense, and/or consistent substance involvement |
| **SEXUALITY** | • Intention to abstain from sexual intercourse until late adolescence/young adulthood<br>• Not currently sexually active or using reliable methods to reduce pregnancy and STI/HIV risk<br>• Sexual debut after 15 years of age<br>• Trusted adult to talk to about sexual issues | • Engaged in unprotected sex<br>• Pregnancy or STI in the past<br>• Sexual debut before 14 years of age<br>• Peers are only source of sexual information<br>• History of sexual assault or abuse |
| **SUICIDE/ DEPRESSION/ SELF-IMAGE** | • Caring adult to talk to when stressed<br>• Peer support network<br>• Healthy coping skills<br>• Positive self-esteem/ self-image<br>• Acceptance of appearance and weight | • Current depression/isolation/disengagement<br>• Current suicidal ideation<br>• History of suicide attempt and/or major trauma<br>• Family member/friend who committed suicide<br>• Unreasonable expectations from self or others<br>• Extreme dissatisfaction with appearance or weight |
| **SAFETY** | • Seat belt and protective gear usage<br>• Good problem solving skills when faced with dangerous situations<br>• Non-violent conflict resolution skills | • No or inconsistent seat belt & protective gear usage<br>• Easy access to weapons or carrying weapons<br>• Victimization through family, intimate partner, gang, or school violence/bullying |

Sources:
1) Simmons M, Shalwitz J, Pollock S, Young A. *Adolescent Health Care 101: The Basics.* Adolescent Health Working Group. 2003: B-9. http://www.ahwg.net/resources/toolkit.htm Annotated HEADSSS assessment can be found in *Adolescent Health Care 101.*
2) Erica Monasterio, RN, MN, FNP. University of California San Francisco, Division of Adolescent Medicine. 2006.

Adolescent Provider Toolkit D-9 

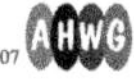




American Academy of Pediatrics
DEDICATED TO THE HEALTH OF ALL CHILDREN™

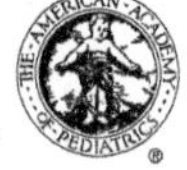

**EXHIBIT 18.1 HEEADSSS Assessment Tool**

*Sources*: From Adolescent Health Working Group. (2007). www.ahwg.net. Data from Simmons, M., Shalwitz, J., Pollock, S., & Young, A. (2003). *Adolescent Health Care 101: The basics*. Adolescent Health Working Group, B-9. http://www.ahwg.net/resources/toolkit.htm; Erica Monasterio, RN, MN, FNP. University of California San Francisco, Division of Adolescent Medicine. 2006.

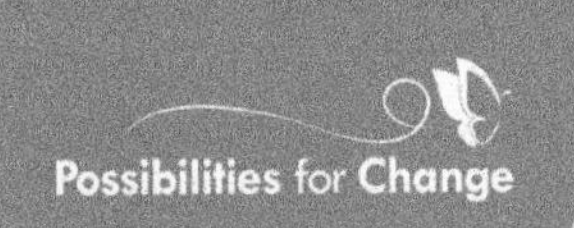


# Standard RAAPS Assessment Preview

The RAAPS assessments are comprised of 21 evidence-based questions proven to elicit honest responses from teens. The standardized, validated comprehensive assessments are available to license in a cloud-based or paper format, with three age-specific assessments available: **older child** (9-12yrs), **standard** (13-18yrs), and **young adult** (18-24yrs).

*A sample question for each risk category in the **RAAPS standard assessment** is below.*

Nutrition/Physical Activity:
Are you active after school or on weekends (walking, running, dancing, swimming, biking, playing sports) for **at least 1 hour, on at least 3 or more days each week?**
Substance Use:
**In the past 3 months**, have you drunk more than a few sips of alcohol (beer, wine coolers, liquor, other)?
Sexual Health:
If you have had sex, do you **always** use a condom and/or another method of birth control to prevent sexually transmitted infections and pregnancy?
Violence:
**During the past month**, have you been threatened, teased, or hurt by someone (on the internet, by text, or in person) causing you to feel sad, unsafe, or afraid?
Protective:
Do you have at least one adult in your life that you can talk to about any problems or worries?
Mental Health:
**During the past month**, did you **often** feel sad or down as though you had nothing to look forward to?
Safety:
**In the past 12 months**, have you driven a car while texting, drunk or high, or ridden in a car with a driver who was?

*When an adolescent responds positively to any of the questions, a pre-populated health message appears upon completion of the assessment. The health messages can be used by professionals as talking points to help guide the adolescent toward positive behavior change. In the example below, the adolescent responded positively for **safety risks.***

HEALTH MESSAGE
Driving drunk, high, or while texting is risky and you're much more likely to be in a car crash. All of these things slow down your reaction time and makes it harder to focus while driving. You can lower your chance of an accident by following a few simple tips.

**To limit the temptation to text while driving:**
- Put your phone in your glove box or back seat while driving.
- Turn your phone off while driving.
- Wait until you are parked to use your phone.
- Ask a friend riding with you to text for you.

**Never drive a car after using even a small amount of drugs or alcohol and avoid riding with someone who has.**
- Before you go out for the night, decide who is going to be the designated driver and stick to it.
- Identify someone you can call for a ride if you find yourself in a situation that is unsafe.
- Offer to drive if you are sober.
- Find a ride from someone else.
- Call a taxicab.
- Make plans to stay the night wherever you are going.

**You can make a difference in your life and the lives of your friends by making safe driving choices.**

http://www.drivingsober.net/Teen-page.html
www.takethewheel.net

National Alcohol/Drug Abuse Hotline:1-800-662-HELP(4357)

RAPID ASSESSMENT FOR ADOLESCENT PREVENTIVE SERVICES RAAPS
Youth don't always share. But they will RAAP.

**Email info@Pos4Chg.org for details on how to use RAAPS to empower youth to make healthy lifelong decisions.**

**EXHIBIT 18.2 Rapid Assessment for Adolescent Preventive Services (RAAPS)**

*Source*: From Possibilities for Change, LLC. (2020). https://possibilitiesforchange.org.

caregiver and the adolescent. Examine and review the relationship of the parent/caregiver with the adolescent:

- Does the child seem comfortable with the accompanying adult?
- Who takes the lead in answering questions?

### Physical Examination

Generally, with adolescents it is best to leave them with their clothes on as you ask probing questions. When complete, give the teen some time to change into a patient gown. Take a head-to-toe approach, leaving the genitourinary part of the exam until the end with a chaperone, either the parent or another clinical team member. Perform a comprehensive physical exam with particular attention to:

- Measuring and plotting height, weight, and body mass index (BMI) on the appropriate growth chart, for patient's age
- Measure blood pressure and use appropriate charts to interpret, based on gender, age, and height
- Skin: Check for nevi, acne, piercings or tattoos, signs of self-harm or abuse
- Breasts:
  - Female: Sexual maturity rating using visual inspection and palpation (Table 11.1 in Chapter 11)
  - Male: Observe for abnormal changes
- Spine: Check for deformities, including scoliosis
- Genitalia:
  - Female: Sexual maturity rating using visual inspection. (Table 11.1 in Chapter 11) (Simmonds et al., 2017).
  - Pelvic examination is recommended to start at age 21 years.
  - Male: Sexual maturity rating using visual inspection and palpation of testicles (Table 11.1 in Chapter 11) (Simmonds et al., 2017).

## PREVENTION

Primary prevention is achieved via health teaching and the provision of immunizations. Refer to the section on anticipatory guidance for information about health teaching. Secondary prevention is achieved via health screenings, discussed later.

## IMMUNIZATIONS

Discussions regarding vaccines should happen at every visit and the importance of illness prevention should be stressed. The adolescent visits are a time to ensure that the patient is up to date on essential vaccines. The conversation regarding which vaccines are appropriate should happen with the adolescent and the parent/caregiver. All questions should be answered and if there is any hesitation on the part of the adolescent or the caregiver, using motivational interviewing can help the discussion. Adolescent immunization recommendations from the Centers for Disease Prevention and Control follow:

- Influenza, given annually
- Tetanus, diphtheria, and acellular pertussis (Tdap), routinely given at 11 years old
- Meningococcal, routinely given at 11 years (second dose at 16 years old)
- Meningococcal B (MenB), first dose routinely given at 16 years, with second dose given a month later
- Human papillomavirus vaccination (HPV), recommended to start at ages 11 or 12 years (may start as early as 9 years); two-dose series (2nd dose 6–12 months following 1st dose). If series starts at age 15 years or older, three-dose series (initial, 1–2 months following first dose, 6 months following first dose) (Centers for Disease Control and Prevention, 2020)

### Health Screenings

During the adolescent well child visits, perform universal screenings as recommended by the AAP, as follows:

- *Tobacco, alcohol, and drug use (including **vaping**)*: Beginning at 12-year visit, use the CRAFFT 2.1+N self-administered questionnaire, on paper or digitally (see Exhibit 18.3). If positive, consider using Screening, Brief Intervention, and Referral to Treatment (SBIRT) in the office (www.samhsa.gov/sbirt) (Substance Abuse and Mental Health Administration, 2017 & Breuner, 2020).
- *Depression*: Begin at 12-year visit. A useful tool to screen for depression is the Patient Health Questionnaire 9, modified for adolescents (PHQA; Siu, 2016; available at hrsa.gov/behavioral-health/phg-9-modified-teens).
- *Dyslipidemia*: Once between 9 and 11 years, then once again between 17 and 21 years.
- *Hearing*: Once between 11 and 14 years, once between 15 and 17 years, and once between 18 and 21 years.
- *Vision*: 12-year and 15-year visits.
- *Human immunodeficiency virus* (HIV): Once between 15 and 18 years).

Selective screenings (based on individual situation) include:

- Oral health (make sure a dental home established)
- Sexually transmitted infections (STIs) including HIV
- Tuberculosis
- Anemia

# The CRAFFT+N Questionnaire

**To be completed by patient**

Please answer all questions **honestly**; your answers will be kept **confidential**.

## During the PAST 12 MONTHS, on how many days did you:

| | | |
|---|---|---|
| **1.** | Drink more than a few sips of beer, wine, or any drink containing **alcohol**? Put "0" if none. | ☐ # of days |
| **2.** | Use any **marijuana** (cannabis, weed, oil, wax, or hash by smoking, vaping, dabbing, or in edibles) or "**synthetic marijuana**" (like "K2," "Spice")? Put "0" if none. | ☐ # of days |
| **3.** | Use **anything else to get high** (like other illegal drugs, pills, prescription or over-the-counter medications, and things that you sniff, huff, vape, or inject)? Put "0" if none. | ☐ # of days |
| **4.** | Use a **vaping device* containing nicotine and/or flavors**, or use any **tobacco products**[†]? Put "0" if none.<br>**Such as e-cigs, mods, pod devices like JUUL, disposable vapes like Puff Bar, vape pens, or e-hookahs. †Cigarettes, cigars, cigarillos, hookahs, chewing tobacco, snuff, snus, dissolvables, or nicotine pouches.* | ☐ # of days |

**READ THESE INSTRUCTIONS BEFORE CONTINUING:**

- **If you put "0" in ALL of the boxes above, ANSWER QUESTION 5 BELOW, THEN STOP.**
- **If you put "1" or more for Questions 1, 2, or 3 above, ANSWER QUESTIONS 5-10 BELOW.**
- **If you put "1" or more for Question 4 above, ANSWER ALL QUESTIONS ON BACK PAGE.**

| | | **Circle one** | |
|---|---|---|---|
| **5.** | Have you ever ridden in a CAR driven by someone (including yourself) who was "high" or had been using alcohol or drugs? | **No** | **Yes** |
| **6.** | Do you ever use alcohol or drugs to RELAX, feel better about yourself, or fit in? | **No** | **Yes** |
| **7.** | Do you ever use alcohol or drugs while you are by yourself, or ALONE? | **No** | **Yes** |
| **8.** | Do you ever FORGET things you did while using alcohol or drugs? | **No** | **Yes** |
| **9.** | Do your FAMILY or FRIENDS ever tell you that you should cut down on your drinking or drug use? | **No** | **Yes** |
| **10.** | Have you ever gotten into TROUBLE while you were using alcohol or drugs? | **No** | **Yes** |

**NOTICE TO CLINIC STAFF AND MEDICAL RECORDS:**
The information on this page is protected by special federal confidentiality rules (42 CFR Part 2), which prohibit disclosure of this information unless authorized by specific written consent.

EXHIBIT 18.3 **The CRAFFT+N Questionnaire.** © John Rogers Knight, MD, Boston Children's Hospital, 2020

*Source*: Reproduced with permission from the Center for Adolescent Substance Use and Addiction Research (CeASAR), Boston Children's Hospital. For more information and versions in other languages, see www.crafft.org

(*continued*)

The following questions ask about your use of any **vaping devices containing nicotine and/or flavors**, or use of any **tobacco products***. Circle your answer for each question.

| | Circle one | |
|---|---|---|
| **1.** Have you ever tried to QUIT using, but couldn't? | **Yes** | **No** |
| **2.** Do you vape or use tobacco NOW because it is really hard to quit? | **Yes** | **No** |
| **3.** Have you ever felt like you were ADDICTED to vaping or tobacco? | **Yes** | **No** |
| **4.** Do you ever have strong CRAVINGS to vape or use tobacco? | **Yes** | **No** |
| **5.** Have you ever felt like you really NEEDED to vape or use tobacco? | **Yes** | **No** |
| **6.** Is it hard to keep from vaping or using tobacco in PLACES where you are not supposed to, like school? | **Yes** | **No** |
| **7.** When you HAVEN'T vaped or used tobacco in a while (or when you tried to stop using)... | | |
| **a.** did you find it hard to CONCENTRATE because you couldn't vape or use tobacco? | **Yes** | **No** |
| **b.** did you feel more IRRITABLE because you couldn't vape or use tobacco? | **Yes** | **No** |
| **c.** did you feel a strong NEED or urge to vape or use tobacco? | **Yes** | **No** |
| **d.** did you feel NERVOUS, restless, or anxious because you couldn't vape or use tobacco? | **Yes** | **No** |

**References:*

Wheeler, K. C., Fletcher, K. E., Wellman, R. J., & DiFranza, J. R. (2004). Screening adolescents for nicotine dependence: the Hooked On Nicotine Checklist. *J Adolesc Health*, *35*(3), 225–230;

McKelvey, K., Baiocchi, M., & Halpern-Felsher, B. (2018). Adolescents' and Young Adults' Use and Perceptions of Pod-Based Electronic Cigarettes. *JAMA Network Open*, *1*(6), e183535.

**NOTICE TO CLINIC STAFF AND MEDICAL RECORDS:**
The information on this page is protected by special federal confidentiality rules (42 CFR Part 2), which prohibit disclosure of this information unless authorized by specific written consent.

EXHIBIT 18.3 **The CRAFFT+N Questionnaire.** (*continued*)

**BOX 18.1 Anticipatory Guidance for Adolescents**

*Growth and Development*

- School work and attendance
- Brush teeth twice daily, establish dental home (need dental cleaning every 6 months)
- Eat a well-balanced diet (overview of nutritional needs—variety of fruits, vegetables, nuts, low-fat dairy, healthy snacks, and foods rich in calcium and iron) (Kumar et al., 2018).
- Drink water, avoid sugary beverages
- Encourage exercise *at least* 3 days a week for at least 60 minutes
- Use bike helmets and other sports equipment for protection
- Recommend *at least* 8 hours of sleep each day
- Discuss pubertal development and associated changes
- Provide information on anticipated body changes.
- Teach self breast and testicular examinations (Figures 18.1 and 18.2)
- Provide a list of red flags (refer to Table 11.2 in chapter 11)

*Risk Reduction*

- Use motivational interviewing to ascertain level of knowledge regarding risky behavior
- Avoid drug use, including tobacco (vaping) and alcohol
- Discuss safe sex, including abstinence, but ensure that teen is aware of all forms of protection including condoms and birth control
- Continuously emphasize responsible sexual behavior

*Social and Emotional Well-being*

- Have someone that you can talk to
- Limit social media and screen time
- Discuss safe use of the internet and avoidance of exploitation
- Talk about handling bullying and peer pressure
- Discuss coping strategies related to emotional and psychological changes (for LGBTQ youths, refer to chapter 44 for additional information)
- Offer stress reduction strategies
- Plans for a future career beyond high school (begin in middle adolescence)

*Safety*

- Always use seatbelt
- Discuss firearm safety. Encourage caregivers to remove guns from the home. If guns are in the home, store ammunition separate from the guns and keep guns in locked safe
- Avoid riding in cars with others who might be impaired (may be captured by CRAFFT screener)
- No texting and driving: follow safety rules (beginning with middle adolescence)
- Wear sunscreen

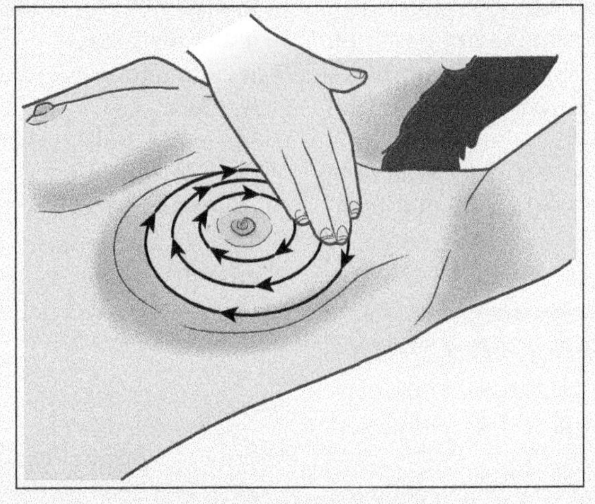

FIGURE 18.1 Breast self-examination.

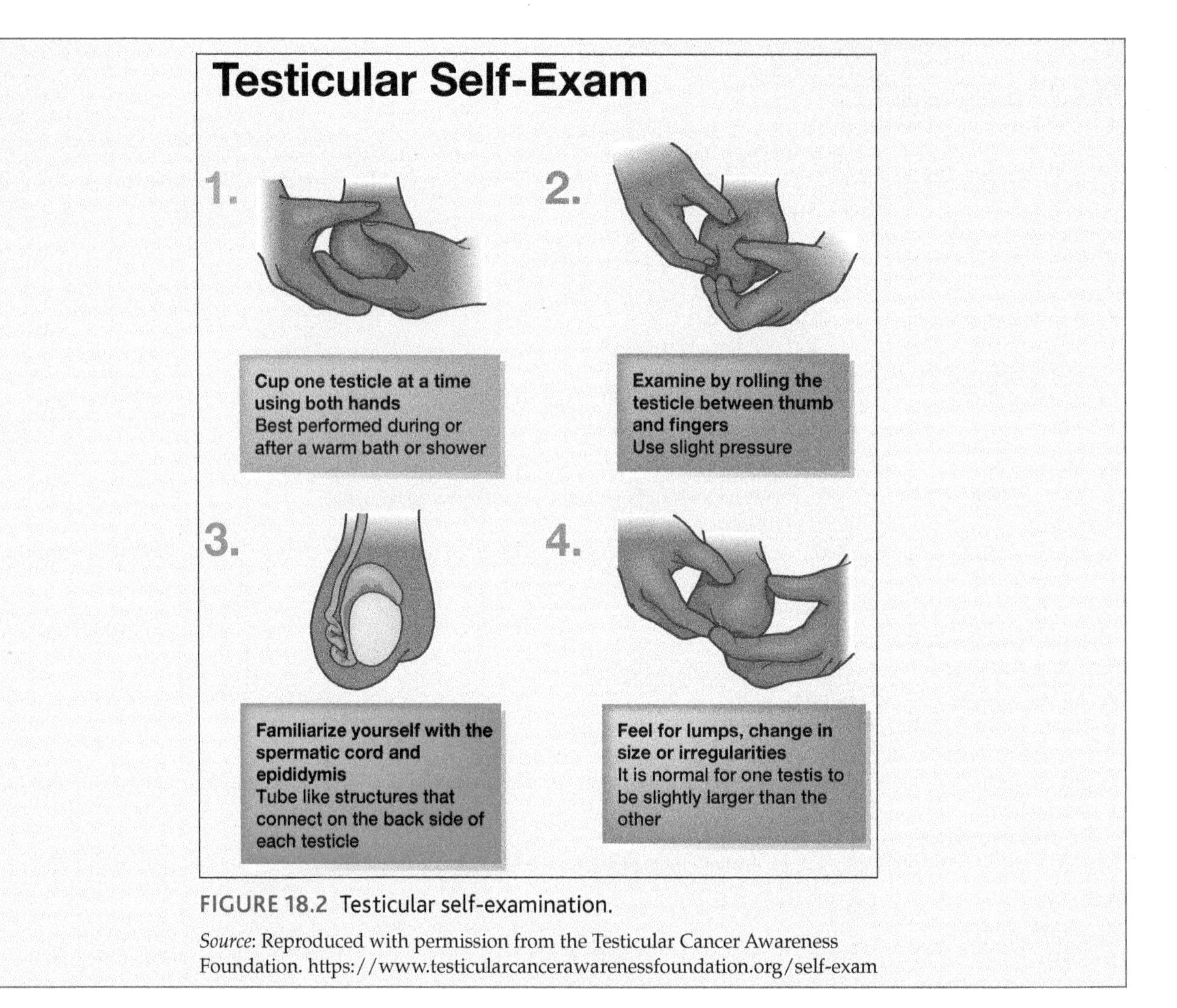


FIGURE 18.2 Testicular self-examination.

*Source*: Reproduced with permission from the Testicular Cancer Awareness Foundation. https://www.testicularcancerawarenessfoundation.org/self-exam

## ANTICIPATORY GUIDANCE

Provide anticipatory guidance at each well child visit. (Hagan et al., 2017). The guidance may vary based on the developmental stage of the adolescent or individual circumstances. Include the parent/caregiver and the adolescent.

Box 18.1 provides information on risk reduction, growth and development, social and emotional well-being, and safety for adolescents in every age range.

## KEY POINTS

- Adolescents experience dramatic changes while transitioning from childhood to adulthood (physiological growth and maturation).
- Provide frequent reassurance and maintain confidentiality during each health visit.
- Conduct the patient interview by being culturally sensitive, nonjudgmental, and nonthreatening.
- Interview the adolescent with and without the parent at each visit. The adolescent is more likely to disclose more information when the parent is not in the room.
- Seek to understand the adolescent's concerns and feelings.
- Screening tools provide helpful information to the provider; consider using them with each visit before entering the room.
- Take the opportunity at each visit to assess physical growth and development, emotional well-being, social issues, risk behaviors, and safety.

## REFERENCES

American Academy of Pediatrics. (2020a). *Assessing the adolescent patient*. https://www.aap.org/en-us/advocacy-and-policy/aap-health-initiatives/adolescent-sexual-health/Pages/Assessing-the-Adolescent-Patient.aspx

American Academy of Pediatrics. (2020b). *Confidential health care services*. https://www.aap.org/en-us/advocacy

-and-policy/aap-health-initiatives/adolescent-sexual-health/Pages/Confidential-Health-Care-Services.aspx

Breuner, C. C. (2020). Substance abuse. In R. M. Kliegman, J. St. Geme III, N. J. Blum, S. S. Shah, R. C. Tasker, K. M. Wilson, & R. E. Behrman (Eds.), *Nelson textbook of pediatrics* (21st ed., Chapter 140). Elsevier.

Centers for Disease Control and Prevention. (2020). *Recommended child and adolescent immunization schedule for age 18 years or younger, United States, 2020.* https://www.cdc.gov/vaccines/schedules/hcp/imz/child-adolescent.html

Hagan, J. F., Shaw, J. S., & Duncan, P. M. (2017). *Bright futures: Guidelines for health supervision of infants, children, and adolescents* (4th ed.). American Academy of Pediatrics.

Ho, J., Fong, C. K., Iskander, A., Towns, S., & Steinbeck, K. (2019). Digital psychosocial assessment: An efficient and effective screening tool. *Journal of Paediatrics and Child Health, 56*, 521–531. https://doi.org/10.1111/jpc.14675

Kumar, M. M., AlBuhairan, F., Galagali, P., Docter, A. D., Weiss, A., & Keough, L. (2018). Addressing nutritional disorders in adolescents. *Journal of Adolescent Health, 63*(1), 120–123. https://doi.org/10.1016/j.jadohealth.2018.05.010

Possibilities for Change. (2020). *RAAPS.* https://possibilitiesforchange.org/raaps/

Simmonds, K., Hewitt, C. M., Aztlan, E. A., & Skinner, E. (2017). Pathways to competence in sexual and reproductive health care for advanced practice nurses. *Journal of Obstetric, Gynecologic and Neonatal Nursing, 46*(5), e168–e179. https://doi.org/10.1016/j.jogn.2017.02.007

Siu, A. L. (2016). Screening for depression in children and adolescents: U.S. Preventive Services Task Force recommendation statement. *Pediatrics, 137*(3), e20154467. https://doi.org/10.1542/peds.2015-4467

Substance Abuse and Mental Health Services Administration. (2017). *Screening, Brief Intervention, and Referral to Treatment (SBIRT).* https://www.samhsa.gov/sbirt

# UNIT IV

# Disease Management in Pediatric Patients

# Management of Integumentary Disorders

Jacquelyn Sink, Lacey L. Kruse, Allison Sindle, and Kari Lyn Martin

## Student Learning Outcomes

**Upon completion of this chapter the reader should be able to:**

1. Discuss pathophysiology and epidemiology of selected integumentary disorders in children.
2. Differentiate subjective and objective findings of selected integumentary disorders in children.
3. Choose appropriate laboratory or diagnostic tests for particular integumentary disorders in children.
4. Utilize the differential diagnosis process to determine integumentary diagnosis in children.
5. Determine treatment plan, child/family education, and need for referral in children with an integumentary diagnosis.

The content in this chapter maps to the following areas on the Pediatric Nursing Certification Board (PNCB) Pediatric Nurse Practitioner—Primary Care certification examination:

### CLINICAL PROBLEMS: DERMATOLOGY

CONTENT AREAS:

#### II. Assessment and Diagnosis

**B. History and Physical Examination**

1. Obtain history of present illness
2. Obtain a comprehensive health history for new patients
3. Complete an interval history for established patients
4. Perform a review of systems
5. Perform a complete physical examination

**C. Diagnostic Testing and Screening**

1. Order and interpret office/clinic based screening tests
2. Order and interpret diagnostic laboratory tests
3. Order and interpret the results of diagnostic imaging tests

**D. Analyzing Information**

1. Integrate health history and physical examination findings into the plan of care
2. Assimilate findings from screening and diagnostic testing into plan of care

**E. Diagnosis**

1. Develop and prioritize differential diagnoses
2. Establish a diagnosis based on evaluation of patient data

#### III. Management

**A. Child and Caregiver Counseling and Education**

1. Provide condition-specific counseling and education, including treatment options
2. Educate about benefits and potential adverse reactions of pharmacological interventions
3. Discuss non-pharmacological interventions
4. Counsel regarding the threshold for seeking follow-up care
5. Review the risks of non-adherence to recommended treatment

**B. Therapeutic Interventions**

1. Prescribe pharmacologic agents
2. Recommend the use of over-the-counter pharmacologic agents
3. Order or recommend non-pharmacologic treatments for the management of symptoms
4. Discuss use of complementary and alternative therapies as appropriate

**C. Procedures**

1. Perform procedures in accordance with diagnostic guidelines and plan of care (rapid tests)
2. Initiate life-saving techniques in response to urgent or emergent situations

**D. Collaboration and Referral**

2. Refer to specialists as indicated for evaluation, counseling, and/or treatment

**E. Care Coordination**

1. Facilitate patient and family-centered care for children of all ages with acute and chronic conditions

**F. Evaluation and Follow-up**

2. Establish a plan for follow-up care

### IV. Professional Role Responsibilities

**A. Leadership and Evidence-based Practice**

4. Develop, implement, and/or modify clinical practice guidelines

## INTRODUCTION

Skin changes are very common in children and are a frequent cause for visits to primary care clinics and urgent care. At times, diagnoses are straightforward and easily managed. Other times, the differential diagnosis may be complex, and may require a more thorough history, physical examination, and diagnostic tests such as laboratory evaluations or skin biopsies. Additionally, caring for children with chronic and complex skin disease poses its own set of challenges. There are not as many rigorous trials or Food and Drug Administration (FDA)-approved medications for pediatric as there are for adult skin disease. Yet, the burden of pediatric skin disease can take a toll on the entire family unit.

## ANATOMY AND PHYSIOLOGY

The overall anatomy of the skin is similar between adults and children, but there are some subtle differences (Figure 19.1). A child's skin, especially early in infancy, is thinner overall and may be more sensitive to irritants and friction. Some of the glands of the skin are also not as well-developed or prominent early in childhood. For example, sebaceous glands, stimulated by adrenal androgens, demonstrate an increase in sebum production occurring about 2 years before the onset of puberty (Zouboulis, 2019).

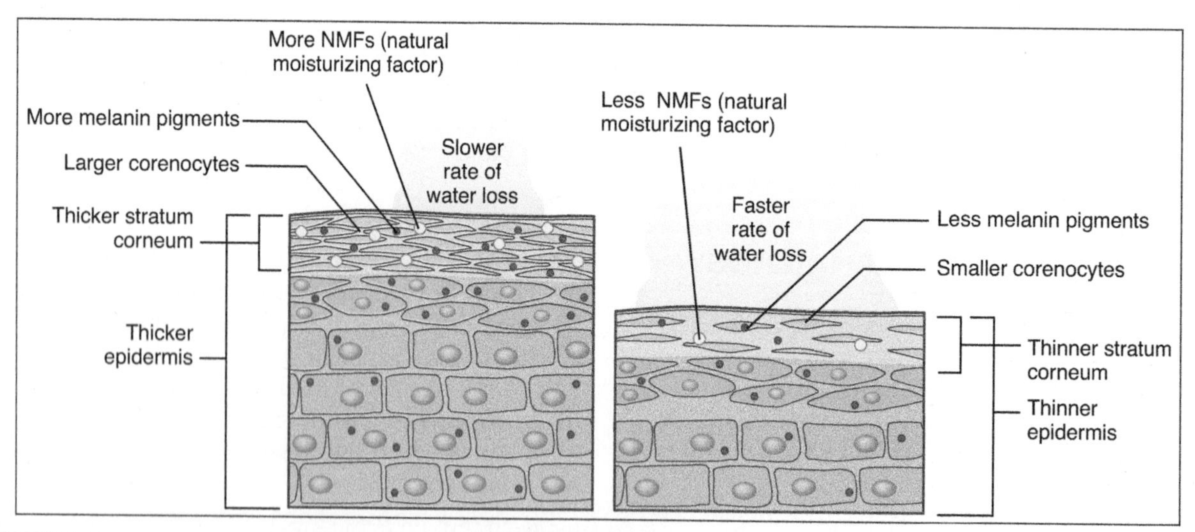


FIGURE 19.1 Comparison of skin between an adult and an infant.

## GENERAL APPROACH TO THE CHILD WITH AN INTEGUMENTARY DISORDER

### Subjective Findings

The health history may reveal:

- Color changes: red, brown, purplish, white
- Texture changes: dryness, scaling
- Pruritus
- Pain
- New growths
- Hair loss or texture changes
- Nail changes
- Mucosal sores or lesions: oral and genital

### Risk Factors

The most common risk factors for integumentary disorders are:

- Family history: helpful in atopic disorders, evaluation of nevi or possible skin cancer, psoriasis, and additional autoimmune or genetic skin disease
- Sun exposure: important to ask when evaluating rashes for photosensitivity, and also helpful when evaluating risk for skin cancer and educating on sun protection
- Cutaneous exposures: important when evaluating atopic disorders, contact dermatitis, and injuries
- Personal contacts with similar symptoms: for assessing infectious exposures

### Review of Systems

The most common manifestations revealed during the review of systems include:

- **Constitutional:** fever, fatigue, irritability, difficulty sleeping
- **Integumentary:** rash, itching, pain, blisters
- **HEENT:** hair loss, itchy/watery eyes, vision changes, rhinorrhea, sore throat, oral sores
- **Respiratory:** cough, shortness of breath, wheezing
- **Cardiovascular:** high blood pressure
- **Gastrointestinal:** poor feeding, nausea, vomiting, diarrhea, constipation, abdominal pain
- **Genitourinary:** dysuria
- **Reproductive:** irregular menses, dysmenorrhea
- **Musculoskeletal:** arthralgias, joint swelling, myalgias, weakness
- **Neurologic:** seizures, headache
- **Lymphatic:** lymphadenopathy, limb swelling
- **Psychiatric:** mood changes

### Objective Findings

When performing the physical examination of the child with an integumentary disorder, it is important to note the morphology of individual skin lesions as well as their shapes, arrangement, and distribution. The physical examination of the child with an integumentary disorder may reveal:

Lesion morphology:

- *Macule*: flat area of differing skin color or texture, <1 cm
- *Patch*: flat area of differing skin color or texture, >1 cm
- *Papule*: raised, solid elevation of skin, <1 cm
- *Plaque*: raised, solid (mesa-like) elevation of skin, >1 cm
- *Nodule:* solid skin lesion, with >1 cm palpable depth or height
- *Vesicle*: fluid-filled elevation of skin, <1 cm
- *Bulla*: fluid-filled elevation of skin, <1 cm
- *Pustule*: pus-filled elevation of skin

Lesion shape/configuration/distribution:

- *Guttate*: drop-shaped
- *Nummular*: coin-shaped
- *Polygonal:* multiple sides
- *Serpiginous:* snake-like, wavy
- *Annular:* ring-shaped
- *Targetoid*: target-shaped; concentric rings
- *Linear*: straight, follows a line
- *Disseminated:* scattered
- *Grouped*: clustered together
- *Herpetiform*: tightly grouped, may be partially confluent

Secondary characteristics:

- *Scale*
- *Erosions*
- *Excoriations*
- *Crust*
- *Fissures*

# BACTERIAL INFECTIONS

## IMPETIGO

Impetigo is a contagious, superficial infection of the skin that is common in children (Mancini & Krowchuk, 2016). The principal causative pathogen is *Staphylococcus aureus*. Carriage of staphylococci commonly occurs in the upper respiratory tract of asymptomatic individuals. Spread occurs via close contact with carriers. A minority of cases are caused by β-hemolytic streptococci (usually group A *Streptococccus*). Streptococci appear to be spread mainly via the infected skin of other affected individuals.

Impetigo is subclassified into two types: bullous and nonbullous. Bullous impetigo occurs when strains of *S. aureus* produce exfoliative toxin A, which leads to cleavage and blistering of the superficial epidermis. Nonbullous impetigo is the most common form of impetigo (Baddour, 2020). The infection is easily spread by autoinoculation to other areas of the body.

## Subjective Findings

The health history may reveal:

- Superficial blisters occurring in an infant or young child (older children and adolescents are less commonly affected) located on the diaper region, face, or extremities

### Risk Factors

The most common risk factors for impetigo are:

- Skin breakdown, such as that caused by atopic dermatitis, trauma, scabies infestations, and insect bites, contributes to a higher risk of infection
- Any condition that places individuals in close contact with carriers, including warm or humid conditions, poverty, overcrowding, and poor hygiene.

### Review of Systems

Impetigo may be asymptomatic, but the most common manifestations revealed during the review of systems include:

- **Constitutional:** pain
- **Integumentary:** pruritus

Systemic symptoms are rare.

## Objective Findings

The physical examination of the child with nonbullous impetigo may reveal:

- Pinpoint papules that progress to form vesicles with a rim of erythema
- Eventual development of pustules that easily rupture and dry to form thick, adherent plaques with characteristic honey-colored crust (Figure 19.2a)

The physical examination of the child with bullous impetigo may reveal:

- Vesicles that enlarge to form large, flaccid bullae filled with clear or purulent fluid
- Initial blisters eventually rupture and leave round, erythematous plaques with overlying scale-crust (Figure 19.2b)

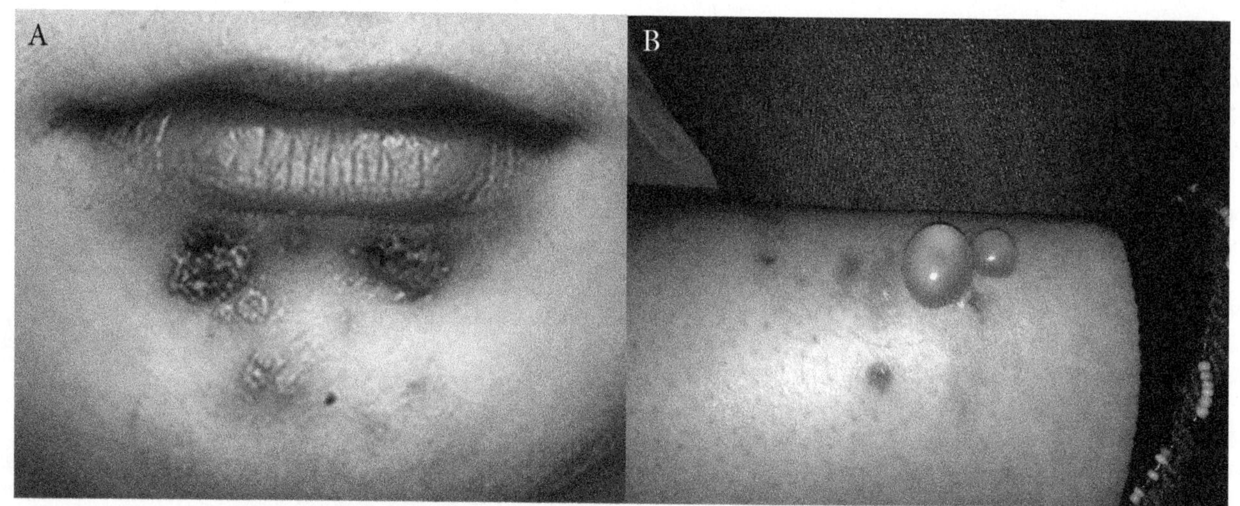


FIGURE 19.2 **(A)** Impetigo. **(B)** bullous impetigo.

*Sources:* **(A)** From Gawlik, K., Melnyk, B. M., & Teall, A. M. (Eds.). (2021). *Evidence-based physical examination: Best practices for health and well-being assessment*. Springer Publishing Company; **(B)** From Lyons, F., & Ousley, L. E. (2015). *Dermatology for the advanced practice nurse*. Springer Publishing Company.

### Laboratory/Diagnostic Testing

The diagnosis of impetigo can usually be made clinically, but it can be confirmed by swabbing an active skin lesion for Gram stain and bacterial culture. Cultures are helpful in order to identify the specific etiologic bacteria and associated antibiotic sensitivities.

### Differential Diagnosis

The differential diagnosis for impetigo includes:

- Autoimmune blistering diseases
- Bullous insect bite reactions
- Contact dermatitis
- Dermatophyte infections
- Folliculitis
- Herpes simplex infection
- Varicella zoster infection

### Treatment/Management Plan

For children with mild disease or localized skin involvement, topical treatment is usually sufficient. First-line therapy is a topical antibiotic ointment such as mupirocin applied three times daily for seven to 10 days. In the setting of recurrent impetigo or multiple affected family members, intranasal mupirocin may be used to reduce nasal carriage of *S. aureus*.

When skin disease is widespread, oral antibiotic therapy may be necessary. A 7-day course of an antibiotic with appropriate coverage for both streptococcus and staphylococcus, such as oral cephalexin or dicloxacillin, is recommended. Amoxicillin can be considered if only β-hemolytic streptococci are detected on bacterial culture. Switching to an antibiotic with coverage for methicillin-resistant *S. aureus* (MRSA) should be considered if the child does not respond to therapy within 48 hours, as expected, or if MRSA is confirmed with a bacterial culture (Table 19.1).

### Family Education

Teach the following:

- Wash affected skin gently with water or aluminum acetate compresses to facilitate crust removal.
- Handwashing is critical for reducing spread.

### Referral

The prognosis is very good with appropriate therapy. Consider referral to a pediatric dermatologist if child has severe or extensive disease or is not responding to standard therapy.

**TABLE 19.1 Medication for Impetigo**

| Generic Drug (Brand Name) | Dosage | Comments |
|---|---|---|
| **Amoxicillin (Amoxil)** | 40–45 mg/kg/day divided in 3 doses<br>>12 years of age: 775 mg once daily extended release (ER) | |
| **Cephalexin (Keflex)** | 25–50 mg/kg/day divided in 2 doses | |
| **Clindamycin (Cleocin)** | 10–25 mg/kg/day divided in 3 doses | Active against MRSA |
| **Dicloxacillin** | 12–25 mg/kg/day divided in 4 doses, maximum 1 g per day | For severe or widespread *S. aureus* infection |
| **Doxycycline (Vibramycin)** | 2.2–4.4 mg/kg/day divided in 2 doses, maximum 200 mg per day | Active against MRSA; avoid in children <8 years old |
| **Trimethoprim-sulfamethoxazole (TMP-SMX; Bactrim, Septra)** | 8–10 mg/kg/day divided in 2 doses | Active against MRSA |

*Source*: Data from Kimberlin, D. W., Brady, M. T., Jackson, M. A., Long, S. S., & the Committee on Infectious Diseases. (2018). *American Academy of Pediatrics red book: 2018–2021 Report of the Committee on Infectious Diseases* (31st ed.). American Academy of Pediatrics.

## METHICILLIN-RESISTANT STAPHYLOCOCCUS AUREUS

*Staphylococcus aureus* normally colonizes human skin. Methicillin-resistant *Staphylococcus aureus* (MRSA) is resistant to certain commonly prescribed antibiotics (oxacillin, methicillin, and beta-lactam agents such as most cephalosporins). This resistance can lead to major complications in severely ill or immunocompromised children, including sepsis and death. The clinical presentation of MRSA can range from asymptomatic colonization to skin and soft tissue infection to invasive disease. Community spread is generally via direct, skin-to-skin contact or fomites (Paller & Mancini, 2016).

### Subjective Findings

The health history may reveal:

- Fever
- Sore or red skin at a wound site
- Enlarged, tender lymph node proximal to a wound site
- Past history of MRSA colonization or infection

### Risk Factors

The high-risk factors for MRSA infection are:

- history of eczema, MRSA infection or colonization
- close contact with someone who has MRSA infection or colonization
- exposure to crowded living conditions (community living conditions such as shelters)
- Attend school or daycare
- implanted medical device(s) or nasogastric/endotracheal/tracheostomy tubes, and/or parenteral/enteral tubes in place
- recently hospitalized longer than 14 days or recently had surgery
- on dialysis (Kaplan, 2019)

Neonates (less than 28 days old) are at high risk for developing systemic disease.

### Review of Systems

The most common manifestations revealed during the review of systems include:

- **Constitutional:** fever, malaise
- **Integumentary:** swelling, redness, warmth, pain, purulent drainage

### Objective Findings

The physical examination of the child with MRSA may reveal:

- Pustules
- Furuncle or carbuncle (abscess)
- Erythema, induration, warmth, and tenderness of a localized area of skin (cellulitis)
- Erythematous papules and plaques with crusting (impetigo)
- Lymphadenopathy
- Hypotension or tachycardia (suggestive of systemic disease)

### Laboratory/Diagnostic Testing

Culture and sensitivity testing are necessary to confirm infection and determine the appropriate antimicrobial therapy (Kaplan, 2021).

### Differential Diagnosis

The differential diagnosis for MRSA includes:

- bacterial skin and soft tissue infections of other causes, including:
  - Impetigo
  - Folliculitis
  - Skin abscess
  - Furuncle
  - Carbuncle
  - Cellulitis

### Treatment/Management Plan

Treatment depends on the age of the child at diagnosis, presence of systemic indications, and size, extent, and location of infection. If appropriate, incision and drainage of a purulent or fluctuant lesion must be performed initially; otherwise, moist heat may be applied. Targeted antibiotic therapy is determined through culture, susceptibility testing, and knowledge of local resistance patterns. Common antibiotic choices with coverage for MRSA include clindamycin, trimethoprim-sulfamethoxazole (TMP-SMX), and doxycycline for children 8 years of age or older. Dosing is noted in Table 19.1 In individuals with frequent or recurrent MRSA infections, screening for intranasal colonization, followed by decolonization with intranasal mupirocin or antibacterial washes (chlorhexidine), may be considered and include other household members.

### Family Education

Teach the following:

- Monitor the child's response to therapy.
- A decrease in erythema, size of wound, and pain is an indication that the therapy is effective.
- Notify a healthcare provider if fever occurs or local symptoms worsen (redness, swelling, or pain increase).

### Referral

Consider referral to a pediatric infectious disease specialist or hospitalization for any child who:

- Has fever, hypotension, tachycardia, rapidly progressing erythema, inability to tolerate oral medications, infection near an implantable device, or multiple sites of infection
- Shows no improvement within 48 hours of initiating treatment
- Is less than 1 year of age or immunocompromised

## CELLULITIS

Cellulitis is an acute bacterial infection of the skin and subcutaneous tissues. Cellulitis generally refers to an infection of the deeper dermis and subcutaneous fat, whereas erysipelas (a form of cellulitis) involves the superficial dermis and lymphatics and is typified by sharply defined borders.

The most common etiologic agents in cellulitis are *S. aureus* and group A β-hemolytic streptococcus (GABHS). In young children, *Haemophilus influenzae* and *Streptococcus pneumoniae* have been implicated in the development of facial cellulitis; however, since the introduction of the conjugated Hib and heptavalent-conjugated pneumococcal vaccines, this type of infection is much less common (Paller & Mancini, 2016). Perianal streptococcal dermatitis is a notable subtype of cellulitis frequently seen in the pediatric population and caused by GABHS. Although more commonly associated with streptococcal pharyngitis, guttate psoriasis has been associated with perianal streptococcal dermatitis. Finally, a more severe type of cellulitis caused by group B streptococci (GBS) has been described in young infants under 3 months old and can lead to invasive disease, including bacteremia and meningitis.

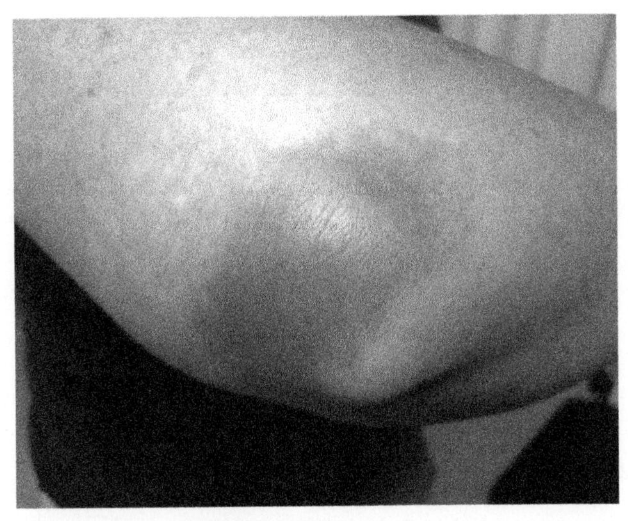

**FIGURE 19.3** Cellulitis.

*Source*: Lyons, F., & Ousley, L. E. (2015). *Dermatology for the advanced practice nurse*. Springer Publishing Company.

## Subjective Findings

The health history may reveal:

- Acute onset of redness, warmth, pain, and swelling of a localized area of skin

### Risk Factors

The most common risk factors for cellulitis are:

- Trauma
- Underlying inflammatory skin disease
- Fungal infections of the skin

All of the preceding can lead to skin breakdown.

### Review of Systems

The most common manifestations revealed during the review of systems include:

- **Constitutional:** fever, malaise

Symptoms associated with perianal cellulitis may include:

- **Constitutional:** pain with defecation
- **Gastrointestinal:** constipation, blood-streaked stools
- **Neurologic:** irritability

## Objective Findings

The physical examination of the child with cellulitis may reveal:

- Localized skin erythema, pain, edema, and warmth (Figure 19.3)
- Purulence or superficial bullae

Erysipelas is characterized by a well-defined, erythematous, indurated plaque with a raised border. Perianal cellulitis manifests as sharply demarcated, intense perianal erythema. The skin surface is sometimes macerated with fissuring.

### Laboratory/Diagnostic Testing

The diagnosis of cellulitis is usually made clinically. Laboratory findings are not generally required in uncomplicated cases, but may include leukocytosis and elevated inflammatory markers such as erythrocyte sedimentation rate (ESR) and C-reactive protein (CRP). Blood and/or bacterial cultures of intact skin are unlikely to be high yield, with the notable exception of perianal swabs for GABHS in perianal cellulitis. In rare cases in which the diagnosis is uncertain, a skin biopsy with tissue cultures may be helpful (Spelman & Baddour, 2020).

## Differential Diagnosis

The differential diagnosis for cellulitis includes:

- Candidiasis
- Contact dermatitis
- Drug eruption
- Erythema migrans
- Staph scalded skin syndrome
- Toxic shock syndrome

## Treatment/Management

Management of cellulitis and erysipelas requires systemic therapy with an antibiotic that covers for

**TABLE 19.2 Antibiotic Dosing for Cellulitis**

| Medication | Dose |
|---|---|
| Amoxicillin (Amoxil) | 40–45 mg/kg/day divided in 3 doses; >12 years of age: 775 mg ER once daily |
| Azithromycin (Zithromax) | 5–10 mg/kg/day daily (immediate release), maximum 500 mg/dose |
| Cephalexin (Keflex) | 25–50 mg/kg/day divided in 2 doses |
| Erythromycin ethylsuccinate | 40–50 mg/kg/day divided in 3 doses, maximum 4 g/day |

*Source*: Kimberlin, D. W., Brady, M. T., Jackson, M. A., Long, S. S., & the Committee on Infectious Diseases. (2018). *American Academy of Pediatrics red book: 2018–2021 Report of the Committee on Infectious Diseases* (31st ed.). American Academy of Pediatrics.

GABHS and *S. aureus*, such as penicillin, amoxicillin, a first-generation cephalosporin, or a macrolide in the case of penicillin allergy. Recommended dosing is provided in Table 19.2.

### Family Education

Teach the following:

- Monitor closely for any systemic signs of worsening infection.
- Seek medical care immediately if the child does not improve as expected.

### Referral

Outpatient treatment is generally sufficient for uncomplicated cases. If GBS is suspected in an infant under 3 months of age, workup for sepsis and meningitis should be performed. Hospitalization for parenteral therapy should be considered for children with periorbital or orbital cellulitis and any child who appears toxic.

## FOLLICULITIS

Folliculitis refers to superficial inflammation of the skin surrounding hair follicles. The most common cause of bacterial folliculitis is *S. aureus*; less commonly etiologic agents include MRSA and Gram-negative organisms. Other, nonbacterial folliculitis causes include *Pityrosporum* (a yeast) and fungal organisms. "Hot tub folliculitis" is caused by *Pseudomonas aeruginosa*, which may be found in whirlpools, hot tubs, or swimming pools in the setting of inadequate chlorine levels (Jackson, 2020). Folliculitis can also be "sterile," triggered by exposure to oils or occlusive products, or as a result of irritation from shaving. The most common locations affected in folliculitis are the upper back, buttocks, and thighs (Paller & Mancini, 2016).

### Subjective Findings

The health history may reveal:

- Red, mildly itchy bumps or pimples occurring in skin folds or on the buttocks or thighs
- Recent exposure to a long course of antibiotic therapy (e.g., for the treatment of acne)
- Frequent application of thick, topical emollients or oils
- History of shaving or waxing the affected area
- Participation in sports or activities associated with tight-fitting, nonbreathable clothing or sweating

### Risk Factors

Gram-negative folliculitis, in particular, can occur after prolonged exposure to oral antibiotic therapy in children with acne.

### Review of Systems

The most common manifestations revealed during the review of systems include:

- **Integumentary:** itching, burning, mild tenderness

### Objective Findings

The physical examination of the child with folliculitis may reveal:

- Grouped erythematous papules and pustules associated with individual hair follicles (Figure 19.4)

### Laboratory/Diagnostic Testing

Folliculitis is a clinical diagnosis. However, a bacterial culture will usually confirm the causative organism.

### Differential Diagnosis

The differential diagnosis for folliculitis includes:

- Acne vulgaris
- Drug eruption
- Keratosis pilaris
- Periorificial dermatitis
- Scabies
- Viral exanthem

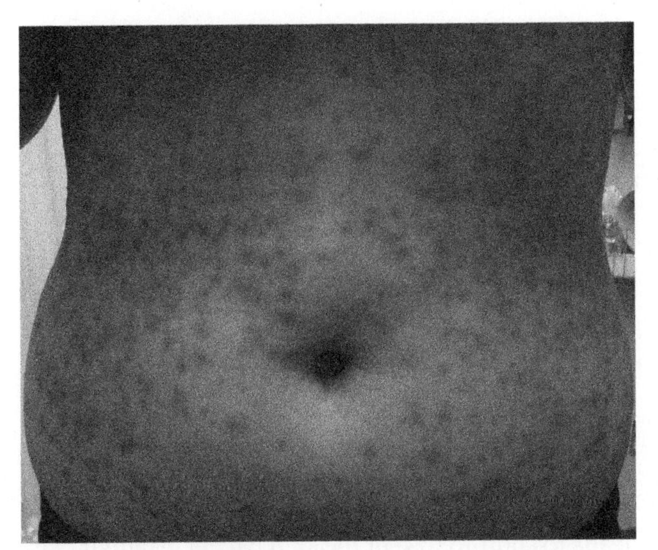

FIGURE 19.4 Folliculitis.

*Source*: Gawlik, K., Melnyk, B. M., & Teall, A. M. (Eds.). (2021). *Evidence-based physical examination: Best practices for health and well-being assessment*. Springer Publishing Company.

### Treatment/Management Plan

Mild cases of bacterial folliculitis can be treated empirically with antibacterial soaps (containing benzoyl peroxide, chlorhexidine, or triclosan) or topical antibiotics such as clindamycin, erythromycin, or mupirocin. If MRSA is suspected or cultured, antibiotic options include TMP-SMX, doxycycline, or clindamycin. Long-term, continuous oral antibiotic therapy for acne should be avoided whenever possible to prevent Gram-negative folliculitis. For severe or widespread cases, an oral antistaphylococcal antibiotic such as cephalexin or dicloxacillin for 7 days should be considered. Refer to Table 19.1 for systemic antibiotic dosing.

For those children who are found to be nasal carriers of *S. aureus* or who suffer from recurrent episodes of bacterial folliculitis, decolonization with intranasal mupirocin ointment or sodium hypochlorite (bleach) bath soaks (one-eighth of a cup of household liquid bleach added to a half bathtub of water, or one-fourth of a cup added to a full tub) can be recommended for 10 minutes two to three times weekly for prevention. Any underlying hyperhidrosis should be addressed.

#### Family Education

Teach the following:

- Avoid tight-fitting clothing.
- Weight loss (if applicable) may be helpful.

#### Referral

Consider referral to a pediatric dermatologist if the diagnosis is in doubt, in cases of severe or widespread disease, or if children are not responding to therapy as expected.

## ABSCESS

An abscess is a localized collection of pus within the skin. It usually begins as a superficial folliculitis that progresses to involve the deep portion of a hair follicle, referred to as a furuncle or "boil." A collection of several contiguous furuncles coalescing together is known as a carbuncle. As in folliculitis, the most common cause of a skin abscess is *S. aureus* (including MRSA), although sometimes multiple bacterial pathogens are responsible. Common locations of involvement include frequently occluded, hair-bearing areas such as the back, thighs, buttocks, groin, and axillae.

### Subjective Findings

The health history may reveal:

- Acute onset of a painful, enlarging pimple that may have drained pus
- History of participation in contact sports

#### Risk Factors

The most common risk factors for abscess are:

- Local skin trauma
- Immunodeficiency
- Obesity
- Diabetes

#### Review of Systems

The most common manifestations revealed during the review of systems include:

- **Constitutional:** pain, fever, chills, malaise
- **Lymphatic:** lymph node swelling

### Objective Findings

The physical examination of the child with an abscess may reveal:

- A fluctuant, tender, erythematous nodule with or without a central punctum
- Purulent drainage

### Laboratory/Diagnostic Testing

The diagnosis of a skin abscess is based on the clinical findings. However, if the abscess is incised and drained, a swab should be sent for bacterial culture and antibiotic sensitivities. Blood cultures are rarely positive.

### Differential Diagnosis

The differential diagnosis for abscess includes:

- Acne vulgaris
- Epidermal inclusion cyst
- Hidradenitis suppurativa
- Insect bites

### Treatment/Management Plan

When possible, incision and drainage of the skin abscess should be performed. Warm compresses can help to facilitate drainage. In otherwise healthy children with mild disease and without evidence of systemic infection or risk factors, incision and drainage alone may be sufficient. In most other situations, particularly in recurrent or complicated cases, an oral antistaphylococcal antibiotic such as cephalexin or dicloxacillin should be considered. If MRSA is confirmed or suspected, TMP-SMX, doxycycline, or clindamycin should be used, depending on local resistance patterns. Refer to Table 19.1 for dosing. Caregivers should also be asked about other affected family members or close contacts. Recurrences are common if underlying risk factors are not addressed.

### Family Education

Teach the following:

- Avoid tight-fitting clothing.
- Weight loss (if applicable) may be helpful.

### Referral

Referral to a pediatric dermatologist should be considered for children who are not responding to therapy as expected.

# FUNGAL INFECTIONS

## CANDIDIASIS

*Candida* species, particularly *C. albicans*, are yeast-like fungi that are found as part of the normal microbiota of the oral cavity, gastrointestinal tract, and vagina of humans. Disruption of the body's natural defenses predisposes to overgrowth and infection. Clinical manifestations of *Candida* infection in infants and children include oral candidiasis (thrush, discussed in chapter), diaper candidiasis, intertrigo, vulvovaginitis, angular cheilitis, and paronychia. Oropharyngeal candidiasis or thrush is commonly seen in young infants, although it may also be seen in older children with immunodeficiency disorders or who have been treated with antibiotics, inhaled or systemic glucocorticoids, or chemotherapy.

*Candida* infection of the skin folds (neck folds, axillae, inguinal folds, diaper area, intergluteal folds) is known as intertrigo. Candidal diaper dermatitis is usually precipitated by an irritant contact dermatitis (exposure to urine, feces, exacerbated by friction) that leads to compromise of the skin barrier. Angular cheilitis (perlèche) is a form of candidal infection involving the corners of the mouth due to moisture accumulation. Underlying precipitants include excessive salivation, drooling, lip-licking, or dental malalignment. Superinfection with *C. albicans* is often present.

Whereas acute inflammation of the nail apparatus is often due to bacterial infection, chronic paronychia is usually associated with *Candida* infection. It is often present in children who are thumb suckers or nail biters/pickers and presents with mild inflammation of the proximal and lateral nail folds. In severely ill, immunocompromised, or hospitalized individuals, *Candida* species can cause serious, invasive infections including candidemia, endocarditis, and meningitis.

### Subjective Findings

The health history may reveal:

- Beefy red diaper rash
- Painful cracking or fissuring of the corners of the mouth
- Excessive thumb-sucking or repeated exposure of the hands to wetness
- Pain, redness, and swelling of the nail folds, which may be associated with nail changes

### Risk Factors

The most common risk factors for candidiasis include:

- moist and humid environments
- immunodeficiency
- moist or macerated skin
- exposure to inhaled or oral corticosteroids, chemotherapy or antibiotics.

## Review of Systems

The most common manifestations revealed during the review of systems include:

- **Integumentary:** pruritus
- **Neurologic:** irritability

## Objective Findings

The physical examination of the child with intertrigo may reveal:

- Moist, macerated, beefy red patches in skin folds
- Presence of satellite papulo-pustules at the border of the rash (helpful to differentiate intertrigo from other causes of intertriginous rashes, in particular, GABHS)

The physical examination of the child with diaper candidiasis may reveal:

- Moist erythema of both the inguinal creases and convexities of the diaper area (unlike in contact dermatitis, where the rash usually only involves the convex surfaces)
- Presence of satellite papulo-pustules

The physical examination of the child with angular cheilitis may reveal:

- Erythema, fissuring, and maceration of the corners of the mouth

The physical examination of the child with chronic paronychia may reveal:

- Erythema and swelling of the proximal nail fold
- Loss of the cuticle
- Dystrophy of the nail plate

## Laboratory/Diagnostic Testing

In the vast majority of cases, uncomplicated cases of candidiasis can be diagnosed clinically. When the diagnosis is uncertain, a fungal culture or a potassium hydroxide wet-mount preparation demonstrating budding yeast or pseudohyphae can be used to confirm the diagnosis (Campell & Palazzi, 2019). A bacterial culture should be obtained if there is suspicion for a secondary bacterial infection. A fungal culture of the dystrophic nail plate can help to exclude the diagnosis of tinea unguium.

## Differential Diagnosis

The differential diagnosis for intertrigo includes:

- Irritant dermatitis
- Nutritional deficiency
- Psoriasis
- Seborrheic dermatitis

The differential diagnosis for angular cheilitis includes:

- Contact dermatitis
- Lip-licker's dermatitis

The differential diagnosis for chronic paronychia includes:

- Acute paronychia
- Blistering dactylitis
- Herpetic whitlow
- Tinea unguium

## Treatment/Management Plan

The recommended treatment for intertrigo is a topical azole antifungal (such as clotrimazole, econazole, or ketoconazole cream) applied two to three times daily. A low-potency topical corticosteroid may be temporarily added to reduce symptoms including pruritus. In the case of bacterial superinfection, addition of an oral antibiotic with antistaphylococcal and antistreptococcal activity is recommended.

Treat diaper candidiasis with a topical antifungal cream (such as nystatin or an azole) applied with diaper changes. For persistent redness, use only a low-potency corticosteroid cream sparingly, as occlusion with a diaper may increase systemic absorption.

Treatment of angular cheilitis consists of a low-strength topical corticosteroid ointment applied two to three times daily. Addition of a topical antifungal agent such as nystatin or clotrimazole is often recommended to address any underlying infection with *C. albicans*.

Topical antifungal therapy applied twice a day usually leads to improvement in chronic paronychia. Oral fluconazole may be needed in severe or refractory cases. Even with successful treatment, the nail plate can take many months to grow out normally.

▶ ALERT: Families should avoid the use of diaper dermatitis products containing benzocaine, boric acid, camphor, salicylates, or phenol, as they pose a risk for systemic toxicity and/or methemoglobinemia.

## Family Education

Teach the following:

- *Intertrigo, diaper candidiasis*: Consider measures to minimize moisture and friction in the affected areas.

(frequent diaper changes, superabsorbent diapers, treat hyperhidrosis), allow child to go diaper-free several times daily.

- *Angular cheilitis*: Avoid lip-licking behavior.
- *Chronic paronychia:* Minimize nail biting and thumb sucking.

### Referral

Referral to a pediatric dermatologist is indicated in children with severe or recalcitrant disease, or when the diagnosis is in question. Special consideration should be given to children with multiple, recurrent mucocutaneous infections and should raise suspicion for cellular immune deficiency. In the child with angular cheilitis, referral for corrective orthodontia should be considered if malocclusion is suspected.

## DERMATOPHYTE INFECTIONS

The dermatophytes are a group of fungi that are responsible for a variety of infections involving the skin, hair, and nails. Dermatologic diseases caused by dermatophytes are named depending on the location affected. They include tinea capitis (scalp), tinea faciei (face), tinea corporis (body), tinea manuum (hands), tinea pedis or "athlete's foot" (feet), tinea cruris or "jock itch" (groin), and tinea unguium (nails).

Each subtype of dermatophyte infection is associated with a different set of dermatophyte species. The most common examples include tinea capitis (*Trichophyton tonsurans, Microsporum canis*), tinea corporis (*Trichophyton tonsurans, Microsporum canis, Trichophyton mentagrophytes, Trichophyton rubrum*), tinea cruris (*Trichophyton mentagrophytes, Epidermophyton floccosum*), and tinea pedis (*Trichophyton rubrum, Trichophyton mentagrophytes, Epidermophyton floccosum*; Goldstein, A. & Goldstein, B., 2020a).

### Subjective Findings

The health history may reveal:

- Localized itching and scaling of the scalp associated with hair loss
- Red, itchy rash of the inner thighs and groin folds in an adolescent male
- Dry scaling and itching of the bottoms of the feet, along with maceration between the toes
- Itchy, red, scaly rash on the body in the shape of rings
- Recent use of a topical steroid without resolution or improvement

### Risk Factors

The most common risk factors for dermatophyte infection are:

- African American and prepubertal children are more likely to acquire tinea capitis.
- Sports associated with close contact (e.g., wrestling), and household pets, especially puppies and kittens, predispose to infection with dermatophytes.
- Additional risk factors for infection include obesity, diabetes, immunodeficiency, hot and humid climates, friction, sweating, nonbreathable footwear, tight-fitting clothing, pre-existing tinea pedis, and onychomycosis.
- Tinea cruris most commonly affects male adolescents.
- Tinea pedis is most common in adolescents.

### Review of Systems

The most common manifestations revealed during the review of systems include:

- **Constitutional:** localized pain (severe, inflammatory cases of tinea capitis)
- **Integumentary:** pruritus
- **HEENT:** scalp swelling (severe, inflammatory cases of tinea capitis)

### Objective Findings

The physical examination of the child with *tinea capitis* may reveal:

- Diffuse, dry scaling on the scalp (similar to seborrheic dermatitis)
- Patches of complete or partial alopecia with scaling (in a pattern analogous to alopecia areata)
- Broken-off hair shafts
- Pustules
- Crusting
- Painful, boggy, inflammatory nodule(s) or plaque(s) with purulent discharge (known as kerion)
- Posterior cervical or suboccipital lymphadenopathy

The physical examination of the child with *tinea corporis* may reveal:

- Singular or multiple, annular to polycyclic, well-demarcated, thin erythematous plaques with an advancing, scaly border and central clearing (Figure 19.5)
- Inflammatory papules and pustules
- Scale may be less noticeable or absent if the infection was previously treated with topical corticosteroids, which can delay diagnosis

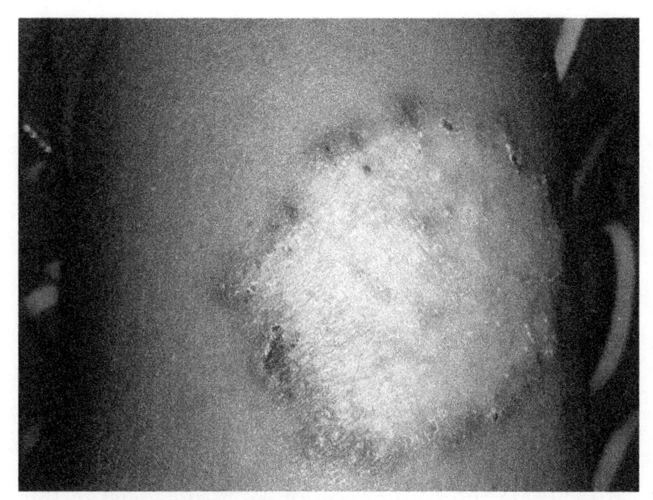

FIGURE 19.5 Tinea corporis.

*Source*: Lyons, F., & Ousley, L. E. (2015). *Dermatology for the advanced practice nurse*. Springer Publishing Company.

The physical examination of the child with *tinea cruris* may reveal:

- Symmetric, sharply defined, erythematous to hyperpigmented plaques with a leading edge of scale located on the bilateral inguinal folds and upper thighs

The physical examination of the child with *tinea pedis* may reveal:

- Scaling and erythema on the plantar surfaces and sides of the feet (so-called "moccasin distribution"), less commonly on the dorsal feet and toes
- Maceration, desquamation, or fissuring in the interdigital spaces
- Inflammatory vesicles or bullae on the insteps of the feet

Rarely, an autosensitization reaction known as an "id reaction" can occur as a result of a dermatophyte infection. It is characterized by a widespread, eczematous eruption.

**PRO TIP** The presence of satellite papulo-pustules or involvement of the scrotum should raise suspicion for candidiasis rather than a dermatophyte infection.

## Laboratory/Diagnostic Testing

The diagnosis of a dermatophyte infection is usually made clinically. However, testing can be very helpful in confirming the diagnosis. Fungal culture using dermatophyte test medium (DTM) is the gold standard for diagnosis and may be obtained using a cytobrush or premoistened cotton-tipped applicator. In tinea capitis, examination of infected hair shafts under a light microscope with potassium hydroxide will show spores either in or around the hair shaft. In other forms of dermatophyte infections, a potassium hydroxide preparation performed using scale scraped from the border of the lesion should demonstrate branching hyphae.

## Differential Diagnosis

The differential diagnosis for *tinea capitis* includes:

- Alopecia areata
- Atopic dermatitis
- Bacterial folliculitis or abscess
- Psoriasis
- Seborrheic dermatitis
- Traction alopecia
- Trichotillomania

The differential diagnosis for *tinea corporis* includes:

- Nummular eczema
- Tinea (pityriasis) versicolor
- Pityriasis rosea (PR)
- Psoriasis
- Seborrheic dermatitis

The differential diagnosis for *tinea cruris* includes:

- Erythrasma
- Intertrigo (candidiasis)
- Psoriasis

The differential diagnosis for *tinea pedis* includes:

- Contact dermatitis
- Dyshidrotic eczema
- Juvenile plantar dermatosis
- Pitted keratolysis

## Treatment/Management Plan

Tinea capitis must be treated with systemic therapy for at least 4 to 6 weeks. Options include griseofulvin and terbinafine (Table 19.3). Terbinafine has been demonstrated to be more effective for *T. tonsurans* infection, whereas griseofulvin has been shown to be superior to terbinafine for treatment of *M. canis*. An antifungal shampoo such as selenium sulfide 1% or 2.5% or ketoconazole 2% twice weekly is usually used as adjuvant therapy and may reduce spread. Treatment of a kerion may require the addition of a short course of oral corticosteroids to address the underlying inflammation. Evaluation and treatment of any suspected secondary bacterial infection should be addressed, particularly in the case of a kerion.

**TABLE 19.3 Medication for Dermatophyte Infections**

| Drug (Trade Name) | Dosage | Comments |
|---|---|---|
| **Griseofulvin** | Ultramicrosize: 10–15 mg/kg/day daily dose<br>Microsize: 20–25 mg/kg/day divided in 2 doses | Administer with a fatty meal |
| **Terbinafine** | <25 kg: 125 mg daily dose<br>25–35 kg: 187.5 mg daily dose<br>>35 kg: 250 mg daily dose | Consider baseline and lab monitoring for liver enzyme abnormalities |

*Source*: Data from Kimberlin, D. W., Brady, M. T., Jackson, M. A., Long, S. S., & the Committee on Infectious Diseases. (2018). *American Academy of Pediatrics red book: 2018–2021 Report of the Committee on Infectious Diseases* (31st ed.). American Academy of Pediatrics.

Topical antifungal therapy is usually sufficient for localized tinea corporis, tinea cruris, and tinea pedis. Topical options include ciclopirox, clotrimazole, econazole, miconazole, ketoconazole, terbinafine, and tolnaftate applied twice daily until resolution. Clinical improvement is expected within a few weeks. Combination products containing topical steroids should generally be avoided. Occasionally, systemic therapy may be needed in the case of severe, recalcitrant, or widespread infection. Reinfection is common. Siblings and close contacts should also be screened for infection and treated appropriately.

### Family Education

Teach the following:

- Avoid sharing potential fomites (hats, combs, brushes).
- Avoid tight-fitting clothing.
- Affected areas of the skin should be dried thoroughly after bathing or exercising.
- Avoid bare feet in communal spaces (such as locker rooms, gyms, and pool decks).
- Occlusive footwear should be avoided when possible.
- Weight loss should be advised for obese children.
- Antifungal, absorbent powders can be used for prevention in the intertriginous folds and for the feet.
- Hyperhidrosis should be managed with antiperspirants.

### Referral

Referral to a pediatric dermatologist should be considered if the child fails to respond to standard therapies as expected, or if the diagnosis is uncertain.

## TINEA VERSICOLOR

Tinea versicolor, also known as pityriasis versicolor, is a common superficial fungal infection caused by the lipid-dependent, dimorphic fungus *Malassezia furfur* (*Pityrosporum ovale*, *Pityrosporum orbiculare*). *M. furfur* is a normal part of the skin flora and is not contagious. In tinea versicolor, external conditions such as heat and humidity, hyperhidrosis, and oil facilitate the conversion of *M. furfur* yeast to the pathogenic mycelial form. It most commonly affects adolescents and young adults (Goldstein, B. & Goldstein, A., 2020).

### Subjective Findings

Most patients are asymptomatic, but the health history may reveal:

- Hyper- or hypopigmented spots on the upper trunk, arms, neck, or face in a young adult or teenager
- Recent exposure to high humidity and temperatures

### Risk Factors

The most common risk factors for tinea versicolor are hot, humid environments and sweating.

### Review of Systems

During the review of systems, some individuals may report

- **Integumentary:** mild pruritus

### Objective Findings

The physical examination of the child with tinea versicolor may reveal:

- Hypo- or hyperpigmented round to oval macules coalescing into patches with or without fine scale located predominantly on the chest, upper back, neck, and proximal extremities (Figure 19.6)

Hypopigmented skin lesions are most prominent in individuals with fair skin during the summer months, during which time exposure to the sun exacerbates the color difference between normal and affected skin.

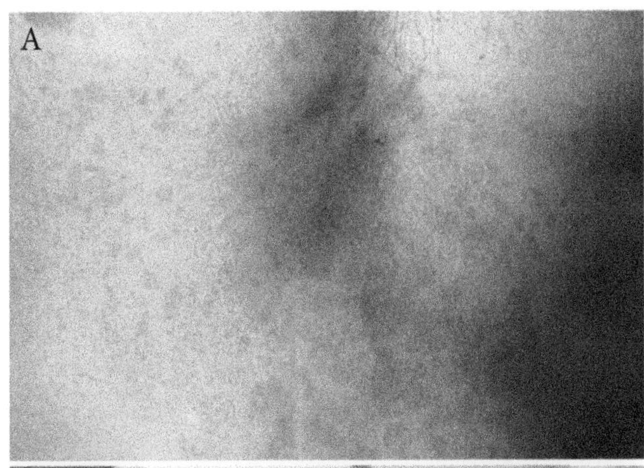


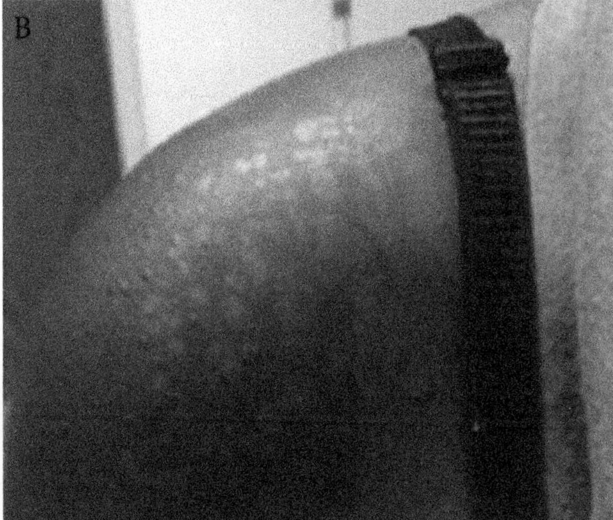


FIGURE 19.6 **(A)** Tinea versicolor on light skin. **(B)** Tinea versicolor on dark skin.

*Sources*: (**A**) From Gawlik, K., Melnyk, B. M., & Teall, A. M. (Eds.). (2021). *Evidence-based physical examination: Best practices for health and well-being assessment*. Springer Publishing Company; (**B**) From Lyons, F., & Ousley, L. E. (2015). *Dermatology for the advanced practice nurse*. Springer Publishing Company.

### Laboratory/Diagnostic Testing

Although the diagnosis is usually made based on its characteristic clinical appearance, tinea versicolor may be confirmed with a potassium hydroxide preparation of skin scrapings, which will demonstrate many clusters of short hyphae and yeast spores (often described as resembling "spaghetti and meatballs"). Examination with a Wood's lamp typically reveals yellow-green fluorescence of the affected areas of the skin.

### Differential Diagnosis

The differential diagnosis for tinea versicolor includes:

- Confluent and reticulated papillomatosis
- Idiopathic guttate hypomelanosis
- Postinflammatory pigmentary alteration
- Pityriasis alba
- PR
- Psoriasis
- Seborrheic dermatitis
- Secondary syphilis
- Vitiligo

### Treatment/Management Plan

Most cases of tinea versicolor are too widespread for topical antifungal creams to be convenient or effective. Therefore, the preferred treatment is typically an antifungal shampoo (selenium sulfide 1% shampoo or 2.5% lotion, or ketoconazole 2% shampoo), which should be lathered and applied to the affected areas as a shampoo and body wash daily. It should be left on for at least 5 to 10 minutes prior to rinsing. The treatment course is usually 1 to 2 weeks, followed by once or twice monthly as needed for maintenance. An alternative option is terbinafine 1% spray applied once or twice daily for 1 to 2 weeks.

Systemic therapy is typically reserved for patients who have frequent recurrences or who have failed topical therapy. Oral options include a single dose of fluconazole 400 mg. An alternative treatment is itraconazole 200 mg daily for 5 to 7 days. Oral ketoconazole is no longer recommended by the FDA for treatment of fungal infections of the skin or nails due to concerns regarding liver toxicity, adrenal insufficiency, and potential for drug-drug interactions. Even with successful treatment, recurrences are common.

### Family Education

Teach the following:

- It may take months to years for the pigmentary change to return to normal.

# VIRAL INFECTIONS

## HERPES SIMPLEX VIRUS INFECTION

Herpes simplex virus (HSV) is a double-stranded DNA virus that belongs to the herpesvirus family. Infections are common in both adults and children. HSV is categorized into two immunologic types:

HSV-1 and HSV-2. HSV-1 predominantly causes oral and mucosal lesions in children and is transmitted via contact with active skin lesions or infectious mucosal secretions. HSV-2 is primarily spread through sexual transmission or via vertical transmission to the neonate. Genital herpes is discussed in chapter 31.

Infection may be primary or recurrent. Symptomatic infection is not necessary to spread the disease to others. When symptomatic, primary HSV infection is typically more severe, initially presenting with constitutional symptoms (primary herpes gingivostomatitis—see chapter 22). However, acquisition of infection is most commonly asymptomatic. Once an individual is infected, HSV remains latent in the nerve ganglia. Recurrences of localized cutaneous disease are possible with reactivation of the latent virus. Triggers may include sunlight, fever, physical trauma, stress, or immunodeficiency. Recurrent HSV is usually self-limited; however, certain populations are at increased risk for complications or severe disease from HSV.

HSV-1 infections are further characterized based on clinical subtype. Herpetic gingivostomatitis is the most common manifestation of herpes virus in children, occurring most often in children between the ages of 6 months and 5 years old (Keels & Clements, 2019). Mild constitutional symptoms may arise 1 to 2 days prior to the appearance of lesions. The duration of the infection ranges from 5 to 14 days. Herpes labialis refers to a cold sore on the lips. Herpetic whitlow is an infection of the digit that results from autoinoculation in children with orofacial herpes and is commonly seen in children who are thumb suckers. Herpes gladiatorum is an infection usually located on the face, neck, and arms of children who engage in certain contact sports or activities such as wrestling or rugby. Ocular herpes refers to infection of the eye. It may have serious complications, including permanent vision loss. Eczema herpeticum refers to a severe, rapidly progressive, widespread HSV infection of the skin in a child with atopic dermatitis.

## Subjective Findings

The health history may reveal:

- Fever
- Painful perioral or mucosal blister(s)
- Localized blistering on the face, neck, arm, or digit

## Risk Factors

The most common risk factors for HSV-1 infection are:

- Are 6 months to 5 years old (herpes labialis)
- Attend day care (herpes labialis)
- Participate in wrestling or rugby (herpes gladiatorum)
- Are immunocompromised or malnourished (more severe disease; Johnston & Wald, 2019)

## Review of Systems

The most common manifestations revealed during the review of systems include:

- **Constitutional:** fever, anorexia, malaise, pain
  - On the lip (herpes labialis)
  - On the face, neck, or arms (herpes gladiatorum)
  - On the digit (herpetic whitlow)
  - Around the eye (ocular herpes)
- **Neurologic:** irritability, headache

## Objective Findings

The physical examination of the child with HSV-1 infection may reveal:

- Early stage: 2–3 mm clusters of vesicles on an erythematous base
- Later stage (after rupture of vesicle): healing erosion with crusting
- Individual lesions with a "punched-out" appearance (eczema herpeticum)

## Laboratory/Diagnostic Testing

HSV is usually diagnosed based on its characteristic clinical presentation. Viral culture, direct immunofluorescence, or polymerase chain reaction can be used if the diagnosis is unclear.

## Differential Diagnosis

The differential diagnosis for *herpes labialis/herpes gladiatorum* includes:

- Aphthous ulcers
- Bullous impetigo
- Contact dermatitis
- Hand, foot, and mouth disease
- Stevens-Johnson syndrome

The differential diagnosis of herpetic whitlow includes:

- Bacterial paronychia
- Blistering dactylitis

The differential diagnosis of ocular herpes includes:

- Conjunctivitis

## Treatment/Management Plan

Supportive care is the predominant focus for treatment. Oral analgesics may be prescribed for pain. Topical antiviral therapies are of modest benefit. Severe or frequent recurrences may warrant oral antiviral therapy, either as needed for outbreaks or for daily suppressive therapy (depending on the frequency of recurrences). Oral acyclovir, valacyclovir, or famciclovir are most frequently used.

Dehydration accounts for most complications of HSV infection. Secondary infection should be considered if a child's symptoms worsen or fail to resolve as expected.

### Family Education

Teach the following:

- Good oral hygiene practices may prevent secondary infection.
- Contact precautions may decrease the risk of transmission to others.
- Manage pain with age-appropriate acetaminophen or nonsteroidal anti-inflammatory drugs (NSAIDs, e.g., ibuprofen).
- Local skin care includes a barrier cream, such as petroleum jelly.
- Follow up with a healthcare provider if symptoms do not improve within 72 hours after starting treatment.

### Referral

Herpetic lesions near the eyes warrant prompt referral to a pediatric ophthalmologist for evaluation and management of herpetic keratitis. Newborn age, dehydration, immunocompromise, and eczema herpeticum all warrant hospitalization.

## PITYRIASIS ROSEA

PR is a benign, self-limited, papulosquamous eruption. The etiology is not well understood, although an infectious etiology has been proposed. PR is most commonly seen in older children and adolescents. There are data supporting the causative role of reactivation of human herpesvirus 7 (HHV-7). However, other studies have failed to validate this association (Goldstein, A. & Goldstein, B., 2020b).

### Subjective Findings

PR is typically asymptomatic. The health history may reveal:

- Report of a ring-shaped or oval red patch on the skin, followed days to weeks later by a rash on the trunk and upper extremities in an adolescent
- Rarely, affected individuals will describe a viral-like prodrome (headache, malaise, pharyngitis)

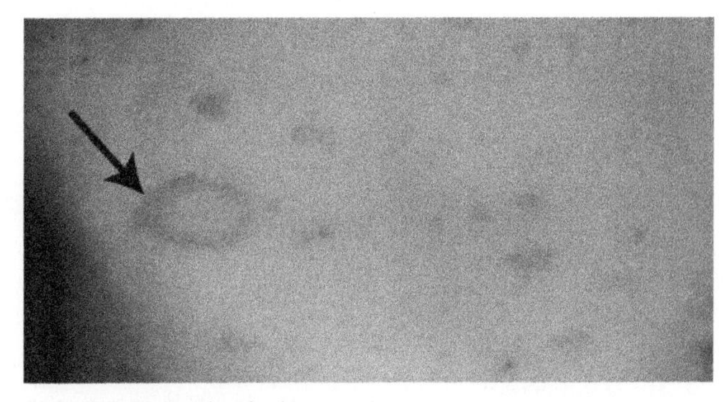

FIGURE 19.7 Pityriasis rosea.

*Source*: Lyons, F., & Ousley, L. E. (2015). *Dermatology for the advanced practice nurse*. Springer Publishing Company.

### Risk Factors

There are no risk factors for PR.

### Review of Systems

During the review of systems, some children may report

- **Integumentary:** mild pruritus

### Objective Findings

The physical examination of the child with PR may reveal (Figure 19.7):

- Initial lesion is a "herald patch," characterized by a single, round to oval, pink- to salmon-colored patch with a border ("collarette") of scale and central clearing
- Within about 2 weeks of the initial herald patch, the eruption becomes generalized, consisting of numerous scaly papules and small, oval plaques appearing in crops
- Lesions tend to be distributed parallel to the skin cleavage lines of the trunk and proximal extremities, following a "Christmas tree" or "fir tree" distribution
- Less commonly, PR presents in an atypical or inverse pattern, primarily affecting the face and skin folds with relative sparing of the trunk
- The eruption normally resolves in 4 to 8 weeks, leaving postinflammatory pigment changes

### Laboratory/Diagnostic Testing

The diagnosis of PR is based on the characteristic clinical morphology and distribution of skin lesions. A potassium hydroxide preparation of skin scrapings can help to differentiate PR from tinea versicolor and tinea corporis.

### Differential Diagnosis

The differential diagnosis for PR includes:

- Guttate psoriasis
- Nummular eczema
- Pityriasis lichenoides chronica
- Tinea corporis
- Tinea versicolor
- Secondary syphilis

### Treatment/Management Plan

PR is a self-limited eruption, and treatment is not required. However, low- to medium-strength topical corticosteroids may be prescribed one to two times daily as needed for pruritus. Oral antihistamines and lotions containing pramoxine or menthol may also be helpful for reducing symptoms of itch. Exposure to ultraviolet light has been reported to hasten resolution of lesions.

#### Family Education

Teach the following:

- The expected clinical course is up to 8 weeks, sometimes longer; provide reassurance.
- PR does not leave permanent skin changes or scarring.
- PR is not thought to be contagious and in most cases does not recur.

#### Referral

Refer to a pediatric dermatologist if the eruption is atypical or lasts longer than 2 to 3 months. A workup for syphilis should be considered if risk factors are present and the clinical history is suggestive.

## MOLLUSCUM CONTAGIOSUM

Molluscum contagiosum is a common, benign, self-limited viral infection of the skin caused by a poxvirus. It has no associated systemic complications. In children, cutaneous spread occurs via direct skin-to-skin contact, scratching, shaving, or via fomites (Isaacs, 2020). Autoinoculation frequently occurs in affected patients, especially those with atopic dermatitis. In adolescents and adults, molluscum may be spread by sexual contact. In children, however, involvement of the skin folds, including the genital area, is common and does not necessarily indicate sexual transmission.

### Subjective Findings

The health history may reveal:

- Random appearance of persistent, small, pink bumps on the trunk and extremities
- Siblings with similar bumps

#### Risk Factors

Children with immune deficiency syndromes and atopic dermatitis tend to have more widespread disease.

#### Review of Systems

The most common manifestations revealed during the review of systems include:

- **Constitutional:** lesion pain
- **Integumentary:** erythema, and inflammation of individual lesions (usually indicative of a host response to the molluscum virus), pruritus due to a localized, eczematous dermatitis ("molluscum dermatitis")

### Objective Findings

The physical examination of the child with molluscum contagiosum may reveal:

- Variable number of discrete, 1- to 5-mm, flesh-colored to erythematous, dome-shaped papules with or without central umbilication (Figure 19.8)
- Distribution of molluscum may be localized or generalized.

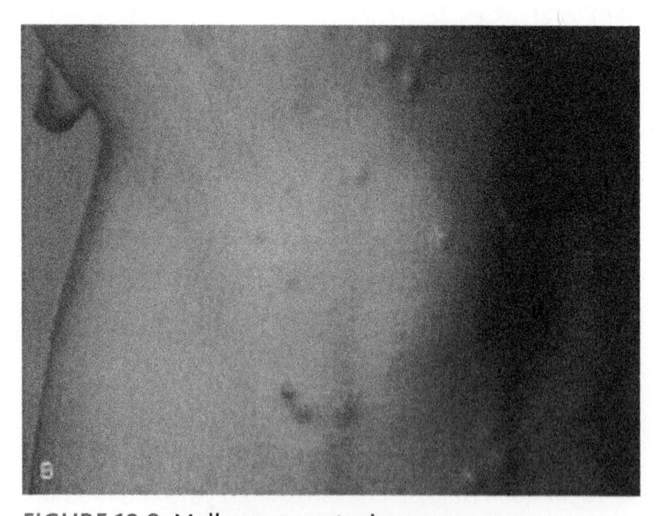

FIGURE 19.8 Molluscum contagiosum.

*Source*: Singleton, J. K., DiGregorio, R. V., Green-Hernandez, C., Holzemer, S. P., Faber, E. S., Ferrara, L. R., & Slyer, J. T. (2014). *Primary care: An interprofessional perspective*. Springer Publishing Company.

### Laboratory/Diagnostic Testing

The diagnosis of molluscum is usually made clinically based on its characteristic appearance. If the diagnosis is in doubt, Wright or Giemsa staining can be obtained from a scraping of the central core of a papule and will demonstrate characteristic intracytoplasmic inclusions (known as Henderson-Patterson bodies). A skin biopsy is rarely indicated.

### Differential Diagnosis

The differential diagnosis for molluscum includes:

- Cryptococcus
- Genital warts
- Histoplasmosis
- Milia
- Verruca plana (flat warts)

### Treatment/Management Plan

Molluscum is a self-limited infection. Reassurance and observation are frequently all that is needed. However, the total course may span months to years. Despite its tendency to spontaneously involute, concerns regarding contagiousness and psychosocial distress over the appearance of lesions often prompt parents and children to request treatment.

Painful procedures such as cryotherapy and curettage are generally discouraged because they are not well tolerated in the pediatric population and may result in scarring. A frequently used, relatively painless option for in-office treatment is topical cantharidin, an extract derived from the blister beetle. A small drop of cantharidin 0.7% or 0.9% liquid is applied to individual papules of molluscum using a wooden applicator. Sensitive areas (skin folds and face) are generally avoided. The treated areas are allowed to dry over several minutes. Parents are instructed to gently wash the treated areas at home approximately four hours after cantharidin application. Treated areas are expected to blister over the next 1 to 2 days, followed by healing and resolution over the next week. Cantharidin treatments can be repeated at 3- to 4-week intervals as needed.

At-home treatment options include topical imiquimod and tretinoin creams applied nightly to the affected areas. Irritant contact dermatitis is common and may limit tolerability. Treatment of molluscum dermatitis (e.g., with a topical corticosteroid ointment) is important to prevent scratching and further autoinoculation of the virus. Secondary bacterial superinfection occasionally occurs and should be treated appropriately.

### Family Education

Teach the following:

- Reassure regarding the benign and self-limited nature of the condition.
- Educate about the expected clinical course, which may last months to years.
- Risks and benefits of treatment versus observation should be discussed before considering any intervention.

### Referral

In-office application of cantharidin is considered off-label and should be performed by an experienced clinician. Referral to a pediatric dermatologist may be indicated depending on cantharidin availability and provider comfort level. Referral should also be considered for severe or widespread cases or for children with coexistent severe atopic dermatitis.

## WARTS

Warts (verrucae) are a common viral infection of the skin and mucous membranes caused by human papillomavirus (HPV). There are many different clinical forms corresponding to distinct HPV subtypes. Terminology related to warts includes:

- *Verruca vulgaris*—common wart
- *Verruca plana*—flat warts
- *Verruca plantaris*—plantar warts affecting the soles of the feet
- *Condyloma acuminatum*—anogenital warts (Tong et al., 2019)

Infection occurs via spread from direct skin-to-skin contact, fomites, or autoinoculation. The incubation period is relatively long (up to 6 months or more; Goldstein et al., 2019).

### Subjective Findings

The health history may reveal:

- Appearance of rough bumps on sites prone to frequent trauma such as the fingers, hands, knees, and elbows
- Warts may appear in a linear array after scratching

### Risk factors

The most common risk factors for warts are:

- Exposure to family members or classmates with warts
- Localized skin trauma or maceration

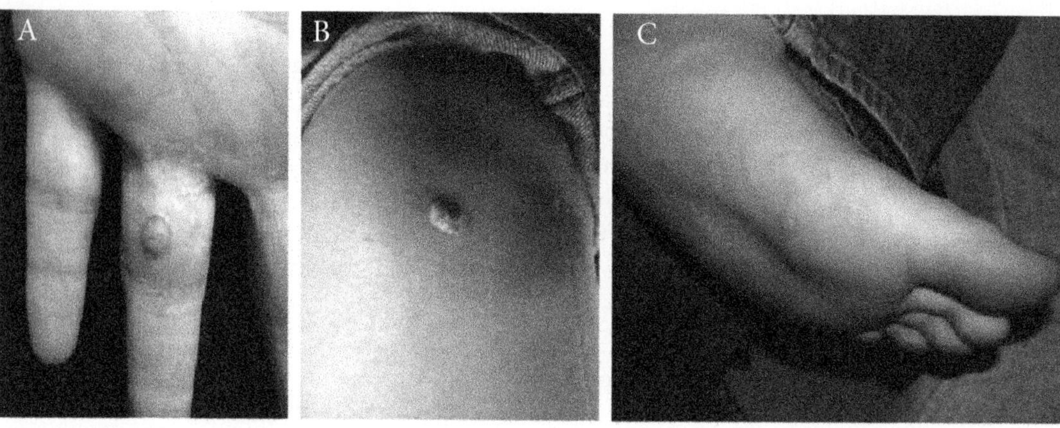


FIGURE 19.9 **(A–C)** Warts.

*Source*: From Lyons, F., & Ousley, L. E. (2015). *Dermatology for the advanced practice nurse*. Springer Publishing Company, LLC.

- Decreased cell-mediated immunity
- Any underlying inflammatory skin disease associated with impaired skin barrier function, such as atopic dermatitis

## Review of Systems

Most children with warts are asymptomatic. However, during the review of systems children may report:

- **Constitutional:** pain on weight-bearing areas of the foot (large plantar warts)

## Objective Findings

The physical examination of the child with warts may reveal (Figure 19.9):

- Verruca vulgaris (common warts):
    - Discrete, flesh-colored, rough papules that are dome-shaped, exophytic, or filiform
    - Common locations include the hands, fingers (particularly peri- or subungual), elbows, and knees
    - May also be found on the oral mucosa
- Verruca plana (flat warts):
    - Multiple, small, smooth, pink-to-brown, flat-topped papules
    - Common locations include the face and distal extremities
- Verruca plantaris (plantar warts):
    - Large, endophytic rough papules on the soles of the feet
- Condyloma acuminata (anogenital warts):
    - Soft, flesh-colored verrucous papules
    - May resemble skin tags
    - Most commonly found in the perianal area
    - May also affect the genitalia or other mucosal surfaces

## Laboratory/Diagnostic Testing

The diagnosis of warts is made clinically. A helpful diagnostic feature is the presence of punctate black dots on the surface of the wart, which represent thrombosed capillaries. Gentle paring of the wart and a magnifying tool may allow for better visualization of these structures.

## Differential Diagnosis

The differential diagnosis for warts includes:

- Hyperkeratosis (corn or callus)
- Skin tag
- Epidermal nevus
- Knuckle pads
- Lichen niditus
- Molluscum contagiosum
- Perianal pyramidal protrusion
- Condyloma lata (syphilis)

## Treatment/Management Plan

Observation is an appropriate management strategy given the tendency of warts to spontaneously resolve over time. However, resolution is slow and may take several years or longer. Recurrences are common. If treatment is desired by the family and child, options include local destructive therapies (paring/filing, cryotherapy) and/or topical formulations (salicylic acid, imiquimod 3.75% or 5% cream, 5-flurouracil 5% cream). Painful procedures such as cryotherapy should generally be avoided in young children and should only be considered after a discussion of the risks and benefits of therapy.

One of the most frequently utilized options for initial therapy is an over-the-counter 17% salicylic acid liquid applied nightly to the wart(s), followed by occlusion with duct tape. The tape is removed in the morning, after which the wart can be gently pared with an emery board or a pumice stone. This process is repeated nightly until wart resolution, which can take weeks to months. Prescription-strength topical options include 2% 5-fluorouracil + 17% salicylic acid solution and 1% cidofovir cream, which can be compounded by certain specialty pharmacies upon request.

Tretinoin cream or adapalene gel are often used for sensitive areas, such as for treatment of flat warts on the face. For all topical therapies, treatment should be held for 1 to 3 days in the case of significant inflammation or irritation. Oral cimetidine 30 to 40 mg/kg per day divided into two or three doses for at least 2 months has also been effective for certain children. The exact mechanism of action of cimetidine in wart clearance is unknown.

### Family Education

Teach the following:

- Warts can be a frustrating problem for children and families.
- Treatments do not always work for every patient, and therapy may take weeks to months to be effective.
- Effective treatment requires consistency and adherence.
- Make routine HPV vaccination recommendations for age-appropriate children.

### Referral

Referral to a pediatric dermatologist should be considered for children with warts not responding to standard therapies or severe cases in children who are immunocompromised. Anogenital warts may be a sign of sexual abuse, although autoinoculation and vertical transmission also frequently occur. If there is any concern for potential abuse based on a thorough history and physical examination, referral to child protective services is indicated.

# INFLAMMATORY DISORDERS

## ACNE VULGARIS

Acne is extremely common and will at some point affect the vast majority of all adolescents and young adults (Zaenglein et al., 2016). Although it is considered a benign skin condition, it has the ability to cause a significant degree of psychosocial distress and have an impact on quality of life. Pediatric acne is divided into categories based on age of the child:

- Neonatal acne (less than 1 month of age)
- Infantile acne (between 1 and 12 months of age)
- Mid-childhood acne (between 1 to 6 years of age)
- Prepubertal acne (between 7 and 11 years of age)
- Adolescent acne (12 years of age and older)

Neonatal acne is believed to occur as a result of exposure to maternal or internally produced androgens. Neonatal cephalic pustulosis is a papulopustular eruption in the neonatal acne spectrum that is thought to represent an inflammatory response to the resident yeast species *Malassezia furfur*. Infantile acne occurs slightly later in life, but is also believed to be associated with androgen and sebaceous gland activity. Mid-childhood acne is considered atypical and should immediately raise suspicion for an underlying endocrinologic disorder (Zaenglein et al., 2016).

Adolescent acne tends to occur at puberty, mirroring the rise in androgen and sebum production. Acne begins with plugging of the pilosebaceous unit (formation of a microcomedone), leading to overgrowth of the resident bacterium *Propionibacterium acnes* and eventual development of a pro-inflammatory state (Thiboutot & Zaenglein, 2021).

### Subjective Findings

The health history may reveal:

- Pimples, blackheads, and/or whiteheads on the face, back, and upper chest

### Risk Factors

Triggers for adolescent acne include stress, mechanical occlusion or friction (e.g., sports gear), and use of comedogenic skin care or hair products. Common medications that can trigger or worsen acne include anabolic steroids, progestins, lithium, antiepileptics, and isoniazid. Androgen excess leading to severe acne may be due to an underlying endocrinologic abnormality, such as polycystic ovarian syndrome. The effect of diet on acne is controversial, although it seems that diets with high glycemic loads and skim milk may worsen acne.

## Review of Systems

Acne is usually asymptomatic, although during the review of systems, some individuals may report:

- **Constitutional:** pain with larger, inflammatory lesions

## Objective Findings

The physical examination of the baby with neonatal acne may reveal:

- Erythematous papules and pustules affecting the face and scalp
- Comedones are usually not seen

The physical examination of the child with infantile or mid-childhood acne may reveal:

- Open comedones (blackheads)
- Closed comedones (whiteheads)
- Inflammatory papules, pustules, and occasionally nodules
- Scarring may be present

The physical examination of the child with adolescent acne may reveal:

- Open and closed comedones (Figure 19.10)
- Inflammatory lesions become more prominent with worsening severity and may include erythematous papules, pustules, cysts, and nodules
- Permanent scarring from cysts and nodules
- Hyperpigmentation and erythema (common sequelae following the resolution of acne lesions and can last up to several months, especially in individuals with darker skin tones)
- Acne is most common in areas with the highest density of sebaceous glands, namely the face, chest, back, and shoulders

## Laboratory/Diagnostic Testing

Acne is a clinical diagnosis. A biopsy is rarely indicated to differentiate acne from other skin disorders.

## Differential Diagnosis

The differential diagnosis for acne includes:

- Adenoma sebaceum
- Candidiasis
- Eosinophilic folliculitis
- Erythema toxicum neonatorum
- Keratosis pilaris
- Milia
- Miliaria

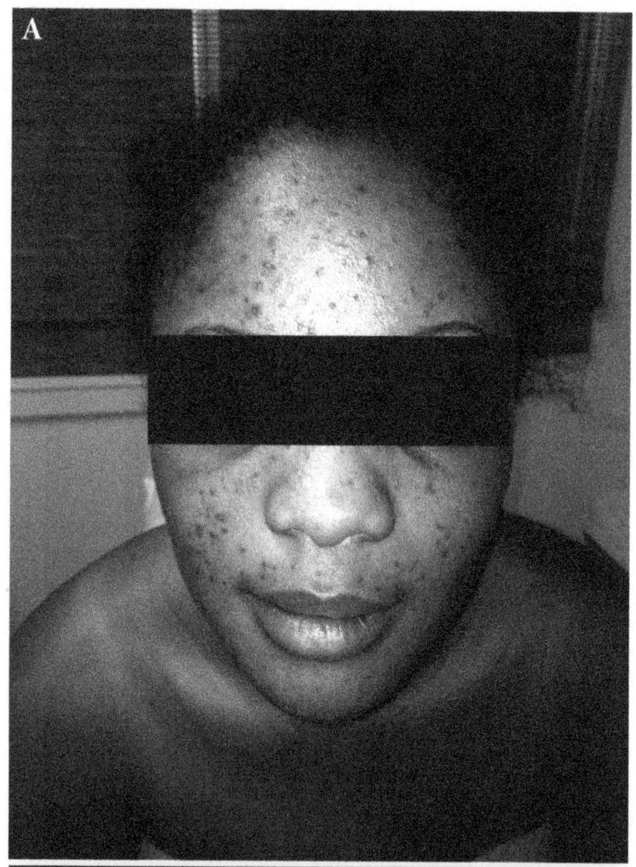


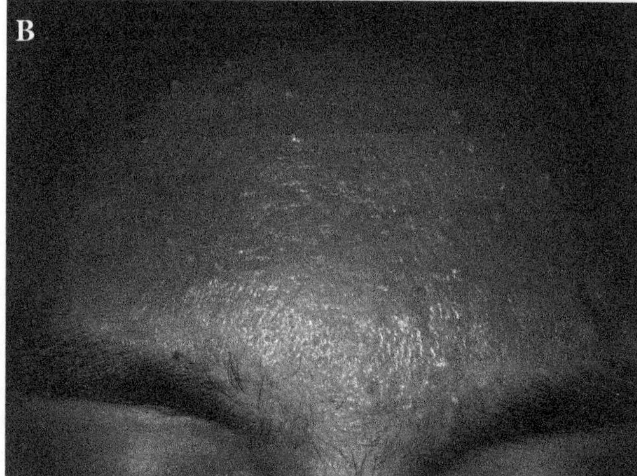


FIGURE 19.10 Acne vulgaris—note open and closed comedomes.

*Source*: From Lyons, F., & Ousley, L. E. (2015). *Dermatology for the advanced practice nurse*. Springer Publishing Company; Gawlik, K., Melnyk, B. M., & Teall, A. M. (Eds.). (2021). *Evidence-based physical examination: Best practices for health and well-being assessment*. Springer Publishing Company.

- Pityrosporum folliculitis
- Rosacea
- Sebaceous hyperplasia

## Treatment/Management Plan

Neonatal acne tends to self-resolve over several months. In the majority of cases, mild daily cleansing with soap and water is sufficient. Topical creams, oils, and emollients should generally be avoided on the affected areas. If treatment is needed, benzoyl peroxide 2.5% gel or erythromycin 2% solution or gel may be used. In the case of neonatal cephalic pustulosis, topical ketoconazole 2% cream is the preferred treatment.

Early treatment of infantile acne is important to prevent scarring. Options for therapy for mild to moderate inflammatory disease include topical benzoyl peroxide 2.5% gel and erythromycin 2% gel or solution. Topical retinoids (adapalene 0.1 or 0.3% gel or tretinoin 0.025% cream) should be used when comedones are present. Oral erythromycin ethylsuccinate is most commonly prescribed for moderate to severe, inflammatory cases, especially if scarring is present (Table 19.4).

For adolescents with mild acne, topical therapy options include benzoyl peroxide, a topical retinoid, or a combination product containing a retinoid + benzoyl peroxide or benzoyl peroxide + antibiotic. Topical retinoids should be applied to a dry face. A pea-sized amount (two pea-sized amounts for the chest and back) is applied in a thin layer to all acne-prone areas. Topical acne treatments should not be used as spot therapy, as they also function to prevent acne. If significant irritation occurs, they may be stopped for several days and restarted every other day, increasing the frequency as tolerated.

In the case of moderate acne with inflammatory lesions, an oral antibiotic such as doxycycline or minocycline should be added (see Table 19.4). Benzoyl peroxide should always be employed if a topical or oral antibiotic is prescribed in order to minimize the risk of bacterial resistance. Ideally, the duration of oral antibiotic treatment should be limited to 3 months of continuous therapy to avoid the development of resistance. Multiple courses of oral antibiotic therapy may be needed.

Severe, nodulocystic acne requires aggressive treatment with oral treatment, including early referral to a dermatologist for consideration of isotretinoin therapy. Hormonal therapies such as spironolactone and combined oral contraceptive pills containing a low- or anti-androgen progesterone should be considered as adjuvant treatment in females with moderate to severe acne (Graber, 2021).

## Family Education

Teach the following:

- Neonatal acne is self-limited and does not usually carry any risk of scarring; provide reassurance.
- Infantile acne should be treated to avoid long-term scarring.

**TABLE 19.4 Medications for Acne**

| Drug (Brand Name) | Dosage | Comments |
|---|---|---|
| **Doxycycline** | 50 to 100 mg twice a day or 100 mg once daily | Delayed-release formulations available. Side effects include photosensitivity and gastrointestinal distress<br>Calcium and iron-containing products decrease absorption<br>Should not be given to children <8 years old or pregnant women |
| **Minocycline** | 50 to 100 mg twice a day | Extended-release formulation available. Side effects include dizziness, drug-induced lupus, skin discoloration. Calcium and iron-containing products decrease absorption. Should not be given to children <8 years old or pregnant women |
| **Erythromycin ethylsuccinate** | 250 to 500 mg once or twice a day<br>Maximum daily dose 50 mg/kg/day | Typically reserved for children <8 years old who cannot receive tetracycline antibiotics |
| **Azithromycin** | Dosing regimens vary | Typically reserved for children <8 years old who cannot receive tetracycline antibiotics |
| **Combination oral contraceptives** | Once daily | Side effects include nausea, breast tenderness, thromboembolic events, weight gain |
| **Spironolactone** | 50 to 200 mg/day in 1 or 2 divided doses | Side effects include menstrual irregularity, breast tenderness, dizziness, hyperkalemia |

*Source*: Data from Graber, E. (2021). Acne vulgaris: Overview of management. *UpToDate*. https://www.uptodate.com/contents/acne-vulgaris-overview-of-management; Lexicomp. (2020). *Lexicomp clinical drug information* (version 5.7.1) [Mobile app]. App store. https://apps.apple.com/us/app/lexicomp/id313401238

- Noticeable improvement can take up to 4 to 6 weeks with any therapy.
- Prescription acne medications should generally not be combined with over-the-counter medicated acne treatments (containing salicylic acid or benzoyl peroxide), as this may lead to unnecessary drying and irritation of the skin.
- Everyday use of a noncomedogenic gentle cleanser, noncomedogenic moisturizer with sun protection, and noncomedogenic makeup should be encouraged.
- Acne products must be used regularly and applied appropriately in order to work.

### Referral

Referral to a pediatric dermatologist is indicated for patients with severe or refractory disease. As mentioned previously, a referral to a pediatric endocrinologist is necessary for those with mid-childhood acne or other signs of precocious puberty. Also refer to a pediatric endocrinologist adolescent girls with severe or recalcitrant acne, menstrual irregularity, hirsutism, androgenetic alopecia, and/or signs of metabolic syndrome.

## SEBORRHEIC DERMATITIS

Seborrheic dermatitis is a chronic, relapsing skin condition that commonly affects infants (referred to as "cradle cap") and adolescents. The etiology is not well known, although a relationship to sebum production and the resident yeast *Pityrosporum ovale* (*Malassezia ovalis*) has been suggested.

In infants, seborrheic dermatitis occurs most commonly within the first several months of life and may overlap with atopic dermatitis (Sasseville, 2021a). In adolescents, it occurs after puberty and is commonly referred to as dandruff (Sasseville, 2021b).

### Subjective Findings

The health history may reveal:

- Red, scaly rash on the scalp or diaper area of a young child or infant
- Greasy scaling of the scalp, eyebrows, ears, nose, and/or the chest in an adolescent
- Light patches with or without scaling on the face of children with darker skin phenotypes

### Risk Factors

Immunodeficiency results in more severe disease.

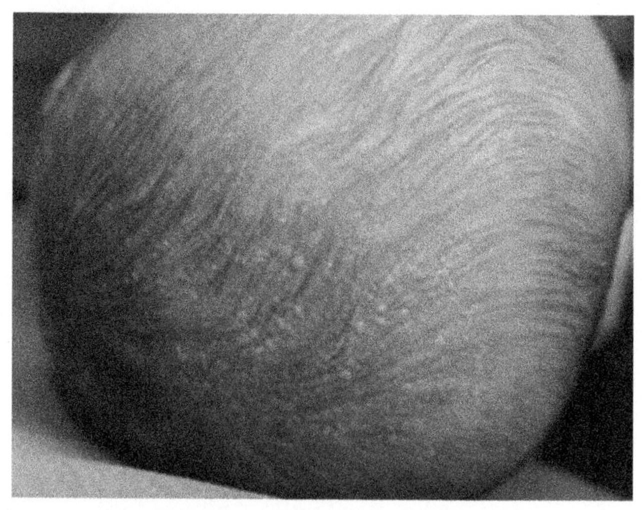

FIGURE 19.11 Infantile seborrheic dermatitis.

*Source*: From Gawlik, K., Melnyk, B. M., & Teall, A. M. (Eds.). (2021). *Evidence-based physical examination: Best practices for health and well-being assessment*. Springer Publishing Company.

### Review of Systems

The most common manifestation revealed during the review of systems includes:

- **Integumentary:** mild pruritus

### Objective Findings

The physical examination of the child with seborrheic dermatitis may reveal (Figure 19.11):

In infants:

- Erythematous, scaly, round to ovoid plaques
- Thick, yellow-brown, and greasy scale
- Most commonly seen on the scalp and the diaper area
- Less frequently, it affects the face, skin folds, trunk, and umbilicus

In adolescents:

- Dry, flaky, fine scaling on the scalp with or without erythema
- The face may also demonstrate ill-defined, erythematous thin plaques with greasy scale, particularly between the eyebrows and around the nose and ears
- Pustules are occasionally seen

### Laboratory/Diagnostic Testing

Seborrheic dermatitis is a clinical diagnosis. However, when the diagnosis is in doubt (particularly in atypical, severe, or recalcitrant cases), a skin biopsy may differentiate seborrheic dermatitis from a potentially serious condition such as Langerhans cell histiocytosis.

## Differential Diagnosis

The differential diagnosis for seborrheic dermatitis includes:

- Atopic dermatitis
- Candidiasis
- Congenital ichthyoses
- Dermatophyte infection
- Immunodeficiency syndromes
- Langerhans cell histiocytosis
- Nutritional deficiency
- Psoriasis

## Treatment/Management Plan

Most cases of infantile seborrheic dermatitis will self-resolve over several months, even without treatment. Reassurance may be sufficient. Daily use of a gentle, "no-tears" shampoo can be recommended. Mineral or baby oil may be applied to the scalp followed by a gentle scalp massage prior to shampooing. Anti-dandruff shampoos (containing ketoconazole, pyrithione zinc, or selenium sulfide) can also be tried. For seborrheic dermatitis affecting the face or body in infants, a low-potency topical corticosteroid such as hydrocortisone 1% or 2.5% can be prescribed.

The first-line therapy for adolescent dandruff is an anti-seborrheic shampoo. Examples include over-the-counter or prescription shampoos containing tar, salicylic acid, ketoconazole, tea tree oil, selenium sulfide, or zinc pyrithione. Shampoos should be lathered and left in place on the scalp for 5 to 10 minutes prior to rinsing. As with infants, mineral oil can be massaged gently onto the scalp prior to shampooing to facilitate removal of scale. To treat any associated erythema or pruritus, a mid-potency topical corticosteroid, preferably in a lotion, oil, gel, or foam formulation, can be given. Affected areas on the face or body should be treated with a mild topical corticosteroid, calcineurin inhibitor, and/or ketoconazole cream.

## Family Education

Teach the following:

- Provide reassurance that cradle cap is expected to self-resolve over a few months.
- In the case of adolescents, seborrheic dermatitis is usually a chronic condition that requires ongoing maintenance therapy.
- For most individuals, daily or every other day shampooing is appropriate.

## Referral

Referral to a pediatric dermatologist should be considered for cases of severe, generalized, seborrheic-like dermatitis, as well as for any children with unexplained constitutional symptoms or who are nonresponsive to therapy.

# PSORIASIS

Psoriasis is a chronic, immune-mediated, inflammatory disorder of the skin. It is characterized by a chronic, relapsing, and remitting course. Up to one-third of adult patients with psoriasis report onset in childhood or adolescence (Paller & Broun Lund, 2020b). The incidence of psoriasis has been steadily increasing, perhaps due to increased awareness, along with an increasing prevalence of known risk factors. Genetics also likely play a role (Paller & Broun Lund, 2020b).

A recent history of throat pain or fever should prompt evaluation for a GABHS infection given its potential association with the guttate subtype of psoriasis. All patients with psoriasis should be screened for symptoms of psoriatic arthritis, which usually manifests as pain and swelling of several joints, inflammation of the digits (dactylitis), stiffness after rest or sleep that improves with activity, heel pain (enthesitis), or back pain (ankylosing spondylitis; Menter et al., 2020).

## Subjective Findings

The health history may reveal:

- Scaly rash
- History of obesity, hyperlipidemia, diabetes, inflammatory bowel disease, arthritis, depression, or anxiety (Menter et al., 2020)

## Risk Factors

Psoriasis may be elicited or exacerbated by psychosocial stress, certain medications, increased body mass index, second-hand cigarette smoke, pharyngeal or perianal GABHS infections, and withdrawal of systemic corticosteroids. Paradoxically, anti-tumor necrosis factor α agents used for psoriasis and other inflammatory or autoimmune diseases can also induce psoriasis or make it worse (Eickstaedt et al., 2017). A common characteristic of psoriasis is the Koebner phenomenon, in which psoriasis develops in areas of prior trauma, for example, due to mechanical irritation or secondary candidal or streptococcal colonization or infection in the diaper area (Menter et al., 2020).

### Review of Systems

Although some children with psoriasis are asymptomatic except for the rash, during the review of systems the following manifestations may be revealed:

- **Integumentary:** mild pruritis associated with the rash, nail changes
- **Musculoskeletal:** tender, swollen joints

## Objective Findings

The physical examination of the child with psoriasis may reveal:

- Plaque psoriasis (most common variant in children):
  - Well-demarcated, erythematous plaques with adherent, silvery-white scale
  - Typical sites of involvement are the scalp, posterior auricular region, extensor elbows and knees, groin, and trunk (including the umbilicus)
- Guttate psoriasis:
  - Few to numerous, drop-like, erythematous, scaly papules and small plaques
- Scalp psoriasis:
  - Well-demarcated erythematous plaques with thick, adherent scale
  - Scale may also be greasy and diffuse, closely resembling seborrheic dermatitis (referred to as "sebopsoriasis")
- Nail psoriasis:
  - Irregularly spaced depressions of the nail plate (known as pitting)
  - Oil spots
  - Discoloration, thickening, lifting, or separation of the nail plate

In infants, scaling may be obscured in the diaper area due to moisture, which may make it difficult to differentiate from other common diaper rashes. Involvement of the umbilicus may be helpful in diagnosing such ambiguous cases.

### Laboratory/Diagnostic Testing

The diagnosis of psoriasis is largely clinical based on the characteristic morphology and distribution of lesions. Rarely, a skin biopsy may be indicated to differentiate psoriasis from other skin disorders. In the case of guttate psoriasis, a pharyngeal or perianal culture for *S. pyogenes* should be considered if the history is suggestive of it.

## Differential Diagnosis

The differential diagnosis for psoriasis includes:

- Lichen planus
- Nummular eczema
- Pityriasis lichenoides
- PR
- Pityriasis rubra pilaris
- Seborrheic dermatitis

## Treatment/Management Plan

Topical corticosteroids are the mainstay of therapy in psoriasis. Topical calcineurin inhibitors (tacrolimus, pimecrolimus) are the preferred option for off-label use as monotherapy for pediatric psoriasis of the face, body folds, and genital region. Alternative topical options include topical vitamin D3 analogs (calcipotriol, calcipotriene), anthralin, tar, topical retinoids, and keratolytic agents such as salicylic acid. Keratolytic agents can be used as single agents or compounded into preparations with topical corticosteroids for thicker, recalcitrant plaques. Rotational therapy with vitamin D analogues, topical calcineurin inhibitors, emollients, tar-based therapies, and topical corticosteroids is often used to reduce potential adverse effects from long-term corticosteroid monotherapy.

A popular topical treatment regimen is combination therapy with a high- or ultra-high potency topical steroid and a topical vitamin D analogue twice daily for 2 weeks, followed by a maintenance regimen of weekend application of a high-potency topical steroid twice daily paired with weekday application of a vitamin D analogue twice daily.

Narrowband-ultraviolet B phototherapy (311–313 nm wavelength) performed two to three times per week is considered a safe and effective treatment for moderate-to-severe pediatric plaque-type and guttate psoriasis (Paller & Broun Lund, 2020a). Referral to a health center with phototherapy equipment is required. At-home phototherapy units of various sizes are also commercially available with a prescription.

Systemic therapy may be needed for children with moderate-to-severe psoriasis who do not respond to skin-directed therapies, especially in the case of impaired function or quality of life. Referral to a pediatric dermatologist is warranted for children who require systemic therapy.

### Family Education

Teach the following:

- Risk and clinical manifestations of psoriatic arthritis.
- Children with psoriasis require routine screening for metabolic syndrome.
- A healthy lifestyle should be encouraged.

### Referral

Referral to a pediatric dermatologist should be considered for severe cases of psoriasis or children who are refractory to standard therapies. Children with metabolic comorbidities or symptoms of arthritis should be referred to the appropriate specialist for further evaluation and management.

## CONTACT DERMATITIS

Contact dermatitis is an eczematous dermatitis that is either a direct response to an irritating substance (irritant contact dermatitis) or the result of a delayed type IV allergic reaction (allergic contact dermatitis). Frequent causes of irritant contact dermatitis in the pediatric population may include antiseptics, saliva, acid, urine, feces, sweat, soaps, and detergents. The most common forms of irritant dermatitis in children include lip-licker's dermatitis and diaper dermatitis. In contrast, true allergic contact dermatitis of the diaper area is rare. In young children, irritation around the mouth is frequently seen from drool, saliva, and certain foods (such as citrus). In older children, excessive handwashing commonly leads to hand dermatitis, especially in individuals who also have atopic dermatitis.

Relevant sources of allergic contact dermatitis in children include poison ivy (also sumac, oak), metals (nickel, cobalt), topical antibiotics (neomycin), fragrances, preservatives, dyes, surfactants, rubber, and adhesives. Unlike in irritant contact dermatitis, sensitization is required for an allergic contact dermatitis to occur and only develops after repeated exposures to the offending substance.

Identification of the offending allergen or irritant is critical and requires a thoughtful review of all potential exposures on the part of the family. The particular area of involvement is helpful in determining the cause. For example, involvement of the earlobes (jewelry), wrist (watch), or umbilicus (buckle or snap) may be indicative of an allergic contact dermatitis due to nickel. An acute-onset rash with a linear or streaky distribution affecting an exposed area of the body such as an extremity, along with a clinical history of outdoor exposure, is highly suggestive of a plant dermatitis.

### Subjective Findings

The health history may reveal:

- Red diaper rash in an infant affecting the areas of the skin in greatest contact with the diaper
- Red, itchy rash localized to one area of the body following exposure of the skin to an irritating substance or potential allergen

### Risk Factors

The most common risk factors for contact dermatitis are:

- Impairment of the skin barrier. Examples include individuals with atopic dermatitis or areas of the body that are predisposed to sweat, friction, occlusion, and skin breakdown (such as the diaper area).
- In addition, areas of the body with thin or delicate skin, such as the eyelids, are more likely to be affected.
- Environmental conditions with low humidity contribute to the development of irritant dermatitis, particularly hand dermatitis.
- Caregivers of infants affected by irritant diaper dermatitis may report a history of increased stooling.

### Review of Systems

The most common manifestations revealed during the review of systems include:

- **Integumentary:** pruritus, burning sensation

### Objective Findings

The physical examination of the child with contact dermatitis may reveal (Figure 19.12):

- Localized, well-demarcated erythematous patches and plaques (may be geometric or linear)
- Secondary changes including excoriation
- Vesicles or blisters (especially in cases of allergic contact dermatitis due to poison ivy, oak, or sumac)
- Lip-licker's dermatitis and hand dermatitis: significant xerosis and scaling, with or without cracking and fissuring
- Irritant diaper dermatitis: erythematous papules, patches, or plaques affecting the convex surfaces of the diaper area with sparing of the skin folds (in contrast to intertrigo and candidiasis)

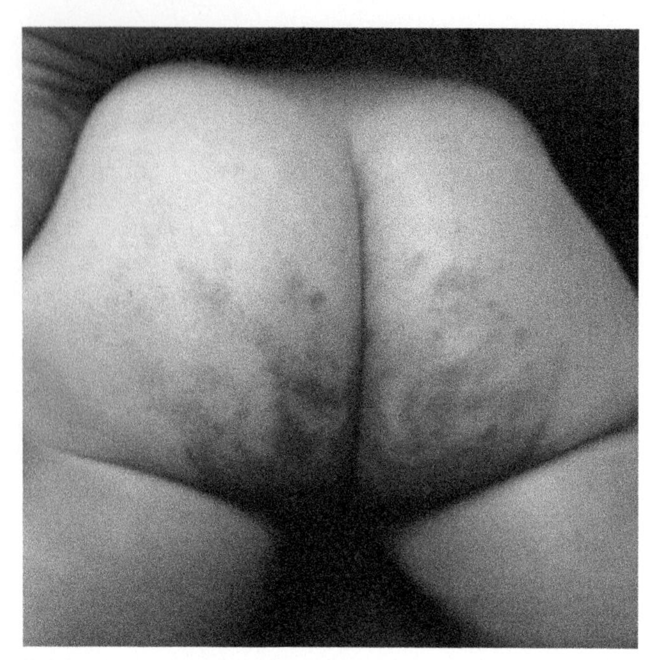

FIGURE 19.12 Diaper dermatitis.

*Source*: Lyons, F., & Ousley, L. E. (2015). *Dermatology for the advanced practice nurse*. Springer Publishing Company.

- Jacquet's erosive diaper dermatitis (severe variant of irritant diaper dermatitis): shallow erosions and inflamed papulonodules in the diaper area

### Laboratory/Diagnostic Testing

Contact dermatitis is a clinical diagnosis.

### Differential Diagnosis

The differential diagnosis for contact dermatitis includes:

- Atopic dermatitis
- Bullous impetigo
- Candidiasis
- Intertrigo
- Langerhans cell histiocytosis
- Nutritional deficiency
- Psoriasis
- Seborrheic dermatitis
- Streptococcal perianal dermatitis

### Treatment/Management Plan

The mainstay of therapy in contact dermatitis is topical corticosteroids. Topical calcineurin inhibitors may also be used for sensitive areas such as the face and skin folds, especially if a prolonged treatment course is anticipated. A common regimen for diaper dermatitis includes a combination of a low-potency topical corticosteroid (such as hydrocortisone 1% or 2.5% ointment) and an antifungal ointment such as nystatin as needed for areas of active inflammation. Occasionally, severe or widespread cases of allergic contact dermatitis (for example, due to poison ivy) may require a course of systemic corticosteroids. Oral steroids should be slowly tapered over 2 to 3 weeks to avoid rebound.

### Family Education

Teach the following:

- Avoid potential irritants; this is key for improvement and prevention.
- Gentle skin care should be encouraged: daily baths (<10 minutes duration) with a non-soap cleanser, followed by moisturization with a fragrance-free cream or emollient.
- Diapers should be fragrance-free, super-absorbent, and changed frequently.
- Cleanse the diaper area with tap water only (avoid harsh soaps and fragranced wipes).
- An emollient or barrier cream containing zinc oxide should be applied with every diaper change and after application of any prescription ointments.
- Individuals with hand dermatitis should be instructed to use gentle cleansers followed by an emollient after every episode of handwashing.

### Referral

Individuals with evidence of a severe, recurrent, or chronic allergic contact dermatitis to an unknown substance should be referred to a pediatric dermatologist or allergist who specializes in patch testing.

# INJURIES

Injuries are common in children of all ages and may be accidental or a sign of abuse. For many of these conditions, the management is similar to that for adults. This section will cover burns, cuts and abrasions, and cutaneous signs of abuse.

## BURNS

Burns encompass a variety of thermal injuries to the skin including scald injury, fire injury, and sunburn. Scald injuries are most common for children under the age of five, while flame injuries are the most common in older children and adolescents (Antoon, 2020).

Burns also may be accidental or a component of child abuse. They are classified by body surface area involved and depth. Localized burn injuries can be managed in an outpatient setting, but more severe burns can cause multisystem organ failure due to massive loss of the skin barrier, and should be managed by a multidisciplinary team in a specialized setting.

Thermal burns are classified by depth and need for specialty referral or surgical intervention. Only minor thermal burns will be discussed here. Minor burns (previously referred to as first-degree burns) are defined as partial-thickness burns affecting less than 10% of the total body surface area (TBSA) in adolescents and less than 5% TBSA in children under 10 years of age. Minor burns are isolated, noncircumferential, and do not involve sensitive areas. The primary sources of burn injury in children are scalding, flames, and electrical sources. Minor thermal burns are characterized by isolated epidermal involvement and heal without scarring.

Sunburns are common, acute inflammatory reactions due to prolonged exposure to ultraviolet radiation. Ultraviolet B light is primarily responsible for the sunburn response (Young & Tewari, 2020).

## Subjective Findings

The health history may reveal:

- Pain; lack of pain, especially at the center of burned areas of skin, is a sign of nerves having been destroyed by the thermal injury and is indicative of deeper burns
- Localized redness and pain of the skin following exposure to hot water, open flame, or a hot surface
- Redness and tenderness of exposed skin between 12 to 24 hours after ultraviolet exposure

During the health history, also determine:

- Type of burn (scald vs. fire vs. sun)
- Duration of exposure
- Clothing or other protective factors in place at the time of injury
- Any immediate care provided prior to the visit

Providers must always have a high degree of suspicion in all types of fire or scald burns for child abuse, regardless of the history given.

## Risk Factors

The most common risk factors for burns are:

- The most common risk factor for complications due to burns is comorbid illness, such as diabetes or immunosuppression.
- Severe, widespread, or frequent burns may be a sign of abuse or neglect.

The most common risk factors for sunburn are:

- Fair skin and lighter skin phenotypes
- Photosensitizing medications or supplements
- Exposure to midday sun
- Lack of sun protective clothing or sunscreen

Risk of sunburn is highest near the equator and during midday.

Additional predisposing factors include indoor tanning, higher altitude, and reflection from snow, sand, and water.

Certain commonly prescribed medications may cause photosensitization, such as doxycycline.

## Review of Systems

The most common manifestations revealed during the review of systems include:

- **Constitutional:** fever, chills, malaise (in the case of severe or widespread burns)
- **Integumentary:** Pain, tenderness, redness and swelling of the affected area, blistering, drainage from longer-standing burns (may be a sign of secondary infection)
- **Respiratory:** shortness of breath or cough (signs of inhalational injury for burns caused by fire)
- **Gastrointestinal:** nausea/vomiting (in the case of severe or widespread burns)
- **Neurologic:** headache (severe or widespread burns), changes in orientation or alertness (may be a sign of hemodynamic or respiratory compromise and should prompt emergent transfer)

## Objective Findings

The physical examination of the child with burns may reveal (Figure 19.13):

- Char around the mouth and nose may be signs of possible inhalational injury
- Scalding burns in a "stocking" distribution or of the buttocks, especially without splash injuries, should raise suspicion of child abuse
- Minor thermal burns:
  - Initial: tender, erythematous patches
  - Subsequent: superficial desquamation, hyper- or hypopigmentation
- Sunburns:
  - Initial: erythematous patches within several hours of sun exposure
  - Intensity peaks by about 24 to 48 hours

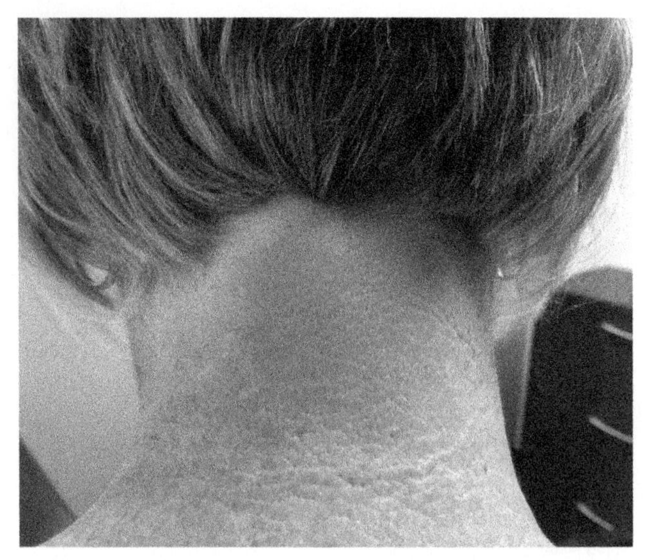

FIGURE 19.13 Sunburn.

*Source*: From Lyons, F., & Ousley, L. E. (2015). *Dermatology for the advanced practice nurse*. Springer Publishing Company.

- Blistering may occur in severe cases
- Subsequent: scaling, desquamation, and hyperpigmentation occur over the course of several days to a week

Skin findings for burns vary based on the thickness of the thermal injury (Rice & Orgill, 2021); only superficial and superficial partial-thickness burns will be discussed here:

- Superficial: affects epidermis only and presents with erythema and pain
- Superficial partial-thickness: affects epidermis and superficial dermis and presents with erythema, pain, and blistering

ALERT: Refer all children with burns suspicious for physical abuse to Child Protective Services. Types of burns include:

- Looks like a distinct shape of object
- Small circular burns matching the size of a cigarette or cigar tip
- Scald burns with a sharply demarcated edge, possibly in a sock or glove pattern, on the perineal area from being dipped into hot fluid (Wiktor & Richards, 2019)

## Laboratory/Diagnostic Testing

A swab for culture should be performed if there is suspicion for a secondary bacterial infection.

## Differential Diagnosis

The differential diagnosis for burns includes:

- Cellulitis
- Polymorphous light eruption
- Systemic lupus erythematosus
- Allergic contact dermatitis
- Irritant contact dermatitis
- Vasculitis or other autoinflammatory disease

## Treatment/Management Plan

Minor thermal burns and sunburns can be managed as an outpatient. Management consists of cool compresses, gentle cleansing with mild soap and tap water, bland emollients, and pain management. Topical antibiotic medications, such as silver sulfadiazine, are frequently prescribed to prevent infection but are usually not needed for superficial burns. If dressings are needed, they should be nonadherent.

Pain management is important for all types of burns. Most pain can be successfully controlled with alternating acetaminophen and ibuprofen. Timing doses 30 minutes prior to bathing and dressing changes can also be helpful.

## Family Education

Teach the following:

- Monitor for signs and symptoms of infection (fevers/chills, increasing redness, drainage, swelling, pain).
- Follow up to ensure proper healing of a thermal burn.
- Sunburns:
  - Sunburns are generally expected to self-resolve within 1 week.
  - Sunburns are an important marker of susceptibility to skin cancer and are associated with an increased risk of melanoma.
  - Daily sun protection with broad-spectrum sunscreen SPF 30 or higher should be advised for all children and adolescents for sunburn prevention.
  - Sunscreens should be reapplied at least every two hours and after swimming.
  - Protective clothing including long sleeves, dark colors, tightly woven fabrics, and hats should be worn while outdoors.
  - Complete avoidance of sun exposure is recommended for infants less than 6 months old.
  - Indoor tanning should be discouraged.
- Wound care: cleanse any areas of open skin daily with gentle cleanser and water. Apply emollient or

topical antibiotic ointment if prescribed. Cover with bandaging as directed.

- Pain control: alternate ibuprofen and acetaminophen as tolerated for pain control. It may be helpful to give a dose of one of these medications 30 minutes prior to bathing or dressing changes. Provider should be contacted if the child is continuing to have breakthrough pain.

### Referral

Localized superficial and superficial partial-thickness burns can be managed well in an outpatient setting. Any burns that are suspicious for child abuse or neglect (in the shape of an object or scald burns) should be reported to Child Protective Services. For any patients with more extensive body surface area involvement, or involvement of high-risk areas (face, ears, neck, hands, feet, genitals), referral to a clinic specializing in burn care is recommended. Children with extensive blistering sunburns associated with severe pain, systemic symptoms, and signs of dehydration may require hospitalization. For children who may have suspected inhalation injury, are unstable hemodynamically, or have signs of deep partial-thickness or beyond-depth burns, emergent referral is indicated.

## CUTS/ABRASIONS

Cuts and abrasions of varying extent are common in children of all ages. In general, they can be easily cared for with appropriate cleansing and wound care, although it is important to note when certain cuts will benefit from skin closure or referral.

### Subjective Findings

The health history may reveal:

- Timing and details around incident leading to the cut/abrasion
- Underlying health history that may be pertinent, such as bleeding disorders or genetic disorders leading to poor wound healing

### Risk Factors

The most common risk factors for cuts and abrasions are physical activities or hobbies that increase chances of being cut. Additionally, intentional cutting may occur either by the child themselves or in instances of child abuse.

### Review of Systems

The most common manifestations revealed during the review of systems include:

- **Constitutional:** pain, fever, or chills (indicating secondary infection)
- **Integumentary:** wound bleeding, drainage from older lesions indicating secondary infection

### Objective Findings

The physical examination of the child with cuts/abrasions may reveal:

- Linear cut or laceration
- Broader, superficial erosions
- Bleeding or hemorrhagic crust

The depth of the wound and involvement of underlying structures should be assessed

### Laboratory/Diagnostic Testing

The diagnosis of cuts/abrasions is based upon the clinical findings. No laboratory or diagnostic testing is needed.

### Differential Diagnosis

There is no differential diagnosis for cuts/abrasions.

### Treatment/Management Plan

The first goal in the management of cuts and abrasions is to stop bleeding. This is usually easily done by applying direct, firm pressure to the site for 15 to 30 minutes with a clean cloth/gauze without lifting. Wounds should be gently cleansed with soap and water and then covered with an emollient and bandage. For clean wounds, topical antibiotics are not generally needed. If an antibiotic is needed, it is best to use mupirocin, polysporin, or bacitracin, because topical neomycin can frequently cause allergic contact dermatitis.

### Family Education

Teach the following:

- Wound care as noted earlier

### Referral

Cuts and lacerations with arterial bleeding, or for bleeding persists that despite 30 minutes of firm pressure, should be referred to the emergency department for further evaluation and care. The depth of lacerations should also be carefully evaluated for involvement of underlying structures (e.g., tendons or ligaments on hands). Additionally, cuts extending to the mid-dermis or deeper may require skin closure with suture and/or skin glue, so may require referral depending on the provider's comfort and expertise. Any cuts or abrasions due to suspected child abuse (see later) or self-harm should be referred to Child Protective Services.

## CUTANEOUS SIGNS OF ABUSE

In 2018, of the 2.4 million reports of potential child maltreatment recorded by all 50 states in the United States, close to 700,000 children were determined to have been maltreated, and nearly 2,000 of them died from the abuse (Children's Bureau, 2020). As many as 3 million children are at risk for child abuse (Boos, 2020). As healthcare professionals, we are uniquely positioned to advocate for these children and it is our responsibility to be aware of the signs of neglect and abuse so these children can be identified and protected from further harm. Child abuse refers to nonaccidental trauma. In as many as 90% of cases of child abuse, cutaneous signs are noted (Christian & Oranje, 2015). Therefore, it is critical for providers to remain knowledgeable and alert for signs of abuse during every encounter. Here we review cutaneous signs of abuse which are often noted during the examination of a child presenting to a clinic, often for an unrelated reason.

### Subjective Findings

When possible, older children and adolescents should be interviewed alone to evaluate for abuse. Parents may be hostile or uncooperative during the interview. The health history may reveal:

- Stories of how the signs of trauma (bruises, cuts, burns, etc.) occurred may be incongruent with findings on examination
- Stories may change over time or be inconsistent between family members, implausible, or vague
- Delay in seeking care
- History of multiple injuries, multiple emergency department visits, or domestic violence in the home
- Behavioral problems or mental health disorders including depression, suicidal ideation, low self-esteem, and social withdrawal, among others

### Risk Factors

The most common risk factors for child abuse are:

- Young age
- History of abuse
- Comorbid disorders (learning disabilities, conduct disorders, chronic illnesses, cognitive impairment)
- Family disorganization, lack of support, stressors (parental substance abuse, unemployment and poverty), and community violence (Boos, 2020)

Younger children and infants, particularly those with disabilities and intellectual delay, tend to be the most vulnerable to abuse. Risk factors for abuse perpetrated by a caregiver include lack of familial support, financial stressors including unemployment, intimate partner violence, personal history of abuse, substance abuse, and mental illness. Children who have been abused are at high risk for future episodes of abuse.

### Review of Systems

During the review of systems, the description of the injuries may be incompatible with the presentation. The most common manifestations revealed during the review of systems include:

- **Constitutional:** lethargy
- **Neurologic:** irritability
- **Psychiatric:** withdrawal or anxiety

### Objective Findings

The physical examination of the child with cutaneous signs of child abuse may reveal (Figures 19.14–19.18):

- Bruising, particularly if located on the head and neck, clustered, occurring in characteristic shapes (handprints, cords, belt buckles, ropes, sticks or rods), or in various stages of healing; especially in unusual locations or patterns or in the shape of a household object, occurring in a nonmobile child, or in varying ages of healing
- Injuries of any kind in a nonambulatory infant (in contrast, normal bruising, as is seen in ambulatory children, occurs most commonly on bony surfaces such as the shins, knees, and forehead)
- Adult-sized bite marks
- Abrasions, lacerations, or burns (from scalding liquid, hot irons, chemical burns, electrical burns, cigarettes, or immersion burns)
  - Burns: may appear older than expected based on history; symmetric; scald injuries suggestive of immersion (no splash, clear tide levels, stocking or glove pattern); buttocks; sparing of flexure creases
- Patterned hyperpigmentation or scars

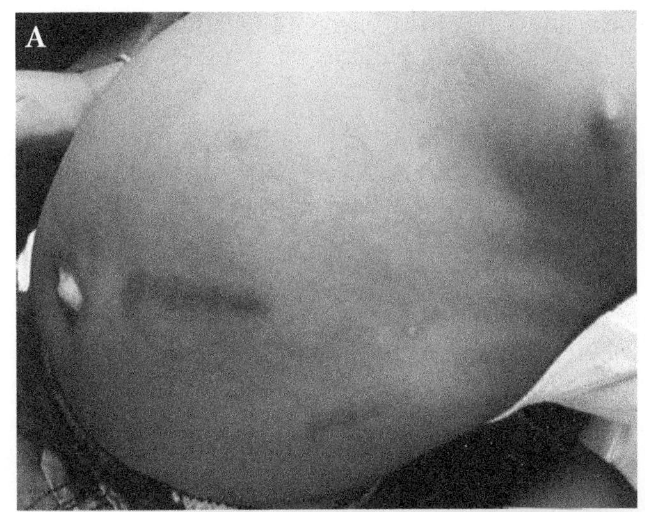


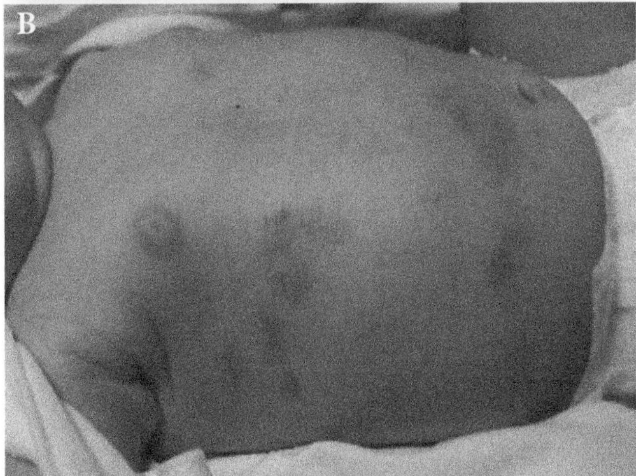


FIGURE 19.14 **(A)** Torso bruising in older child. **(B)** Torso ecchymosis in infant.

*Source*: From Gawlik, K., Melnyk, B. M., & Teall, A. M. (Eds.). (2021). *Evidence-based physical examination: Best practices for health and well-being assessment*. Springer Publishing Company.

- Oral and genital lesions including abrasions, tearing, ecchymoses, hematomas, lacerations, and scarring
- Signs of physical neglect such as poor growth, evidence of nutritional deficiencies, poor hygiene, and severe periodontal disease

Thorough medical documentation of all physical examination findings is critical.

## Laboratory/Diagnostic Testing

Radiographic imaging may be used to evaluate for new or healing fractures. Laboratory testing for

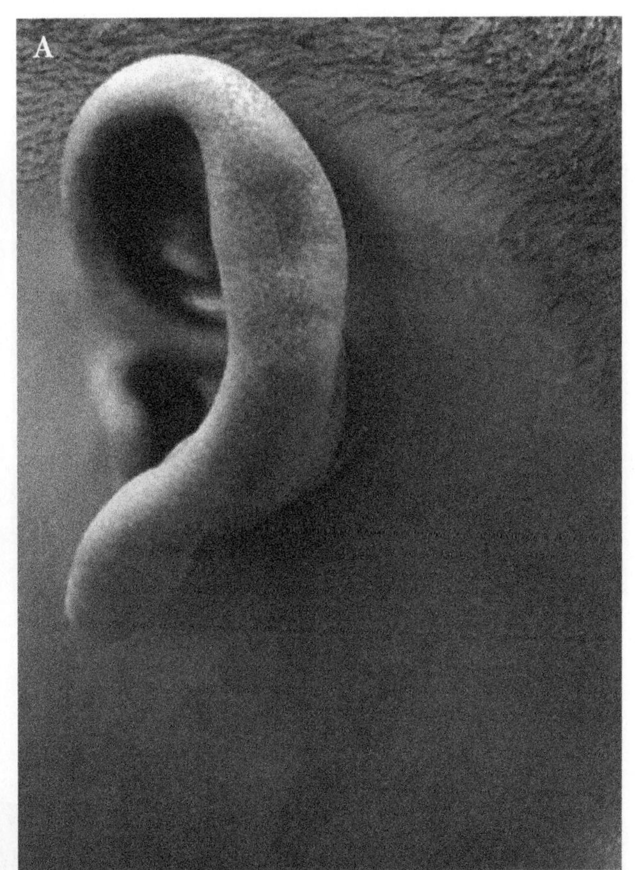


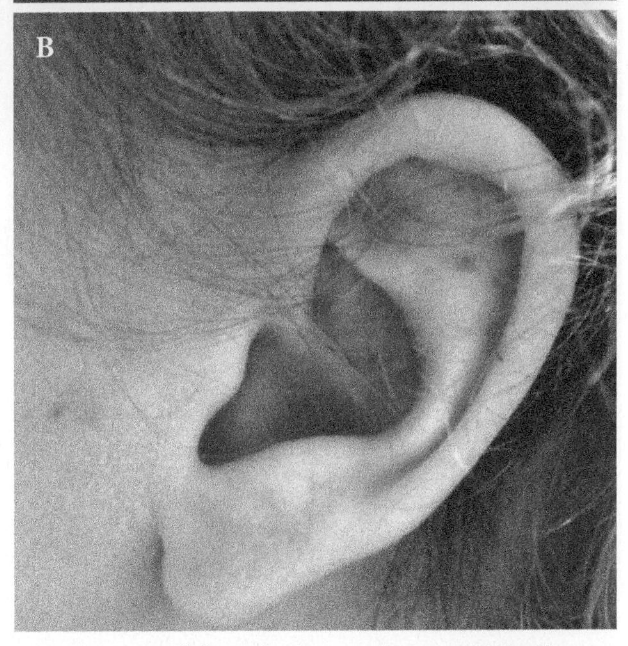


FIGURE 19.15 **(A)** Battle sign, consistent with basilar skull fracture. **(B)** Pinpoint ecchymoses on pinna.

*Source*: From Gawlik, K., Melnyk, B. M., & Teall, A. M. (Eds.). (2021). *Evidence-based physical examination: Best practices for health and well-being assessment*. Springer Publishing Company.

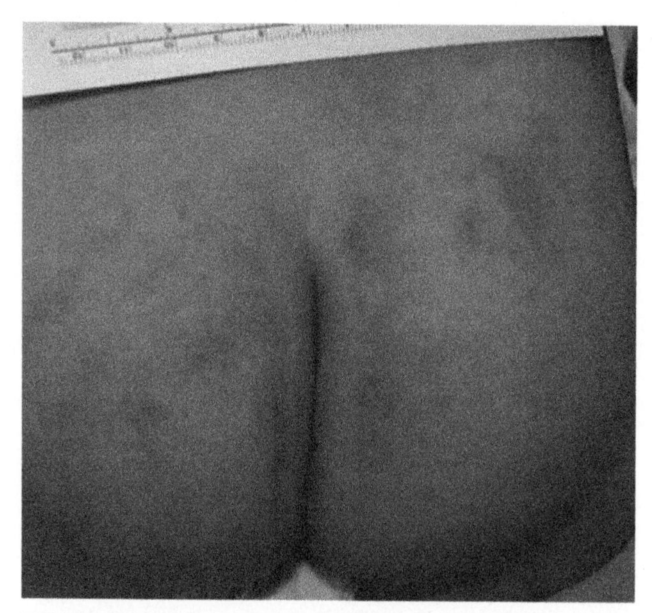

FIGURE 19.16 **Bruising on buttocks.**

*Source*: From Gawlik, K., Melnyk, B. M., & Teall, A. M. (Eds.). (2021). *Evidence-based physical examination: Best practices for health and well-being assessment*. Springer Publishing Company.

sexually transmitted infections is indicated if sexual abuse is disclosed or highly suspected.

## Differential Diagnosis

The differential diagnosis for cutaneous signs of child abuse includes:

- Findings attributable to accidental injury: bruises, abrasions, cuts, burns
- Benign skin conditions that may mimic abuse: dermal melanocytosis and café-au-lait macule may mimic bruising.
- Pathologic conditions that may mimic abuse: Ehlers-Danlos syndrome, bleeding disorder, erythema nodosum, purpura, vasculitis may mimic bruising. Impetigo, dermatitis herpetiformis, hemangiomas, varicella, herpes, ecthyma, and contact dermatitis may mimic burns.
- Cultural practices: Coining and cupping may mimic bruises
- Dermal melanocytosis (historically referred to as Mongolian spots)
- Factitial disorders (self-inflicted)

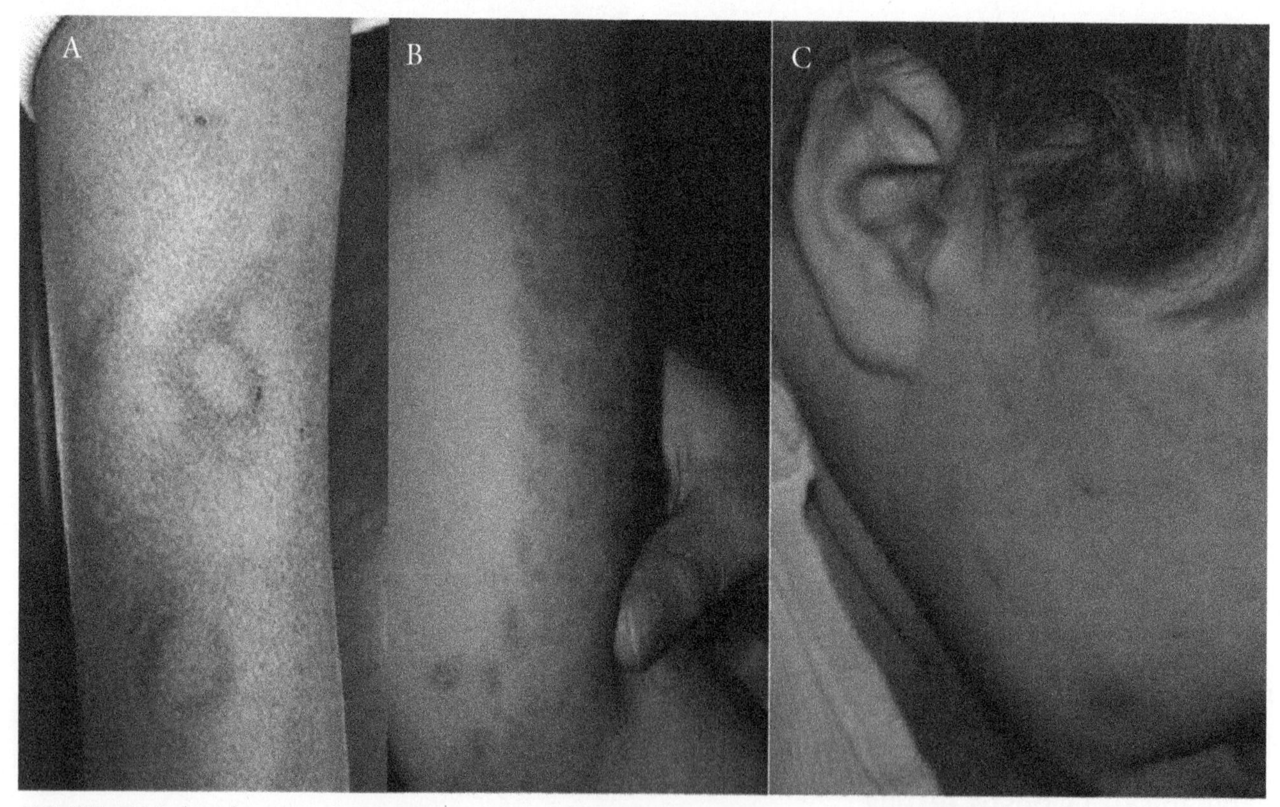


FIGURE 19.17 **(A, B) Pattern bruising from a belt. (C) Healing bruise from slap.**

*Source*: From Gawlik, K., Melnyk, B. M., & Teall, A. M. (Eds.). (2021). *Evidence-based physical examination: Best practices for health and well-being assessment*. Springer Publishing Company.

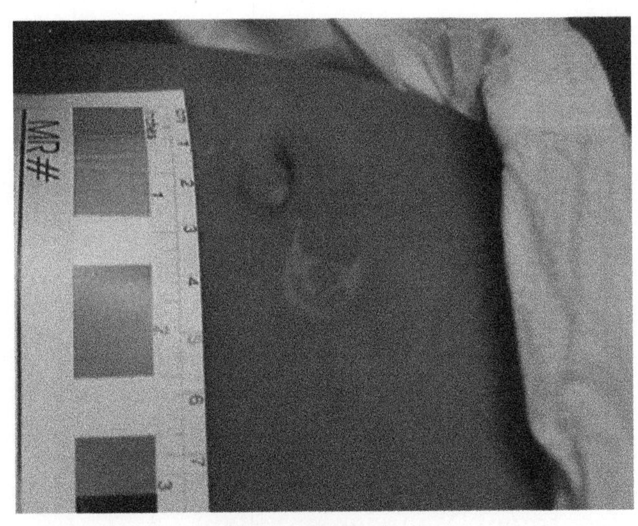


FIGURE 19.18 Scar from a lighter burn.

*Source*: From Gawlik, K., Melnyk, B. M., & Teall, A. M. (Eds.). (2021). *Evidence-based physical examination: Best practices for health and well-being assessment*. Springer Publishing Company.

### Treatment/Management Plan

If a healthcare provider has reasonable suspicion that child abuse is taking place or has taken place, a report to Child Protective Services is mandated by law. For children with serious or life-threatening injuries, or for those at risk for imminent harm, hospitalization may be indicated. Any child who shares a household with the affected child should also be screened for abuse.

### Family Education

Teach the following:

- Once the decision has been made to report a concern to Child Support Services, the provider will need to disclose the report to the parent(s) or caregiver(s).
- It is important not to place blame on the caregiver; rather, it is more helpful to focus on the provider's concern for a particular injury, and to inform the caregiver that reporting is mandated by law.
- Child Support Services may be able to provide the family with helpful resources and support.

### Referral

Consultation with a multidisciplinary team is always recommended. Many medical centers have specialized child abuse teams that serve as an excellent resource. If available, these teams should be involved as early as possible.

# BITES AND INFESTATIONS

## INSECT BITES

Arthropod bites and stings are a common nuisance throughout the world. Cutaneous reactions can occur as a response to the bites of mosquitos, ticks, flies, fleas, mites, bees, wasps, ants, caterpillars, and beetles. Common fleas of significance in the United States include *Pulex irritans* (human flea), *Ctenocephalides felis* (cat flea), and *Ctenocephalides canis* (dog flea). Notable mites include the harvest mite (chiggers), grain mite, house mouse mite, wheat mite, avian mite, dust mites, scrub mites, mold mites, and rat/fowl mites. Bedbugs (*Cimex lenticularis*) are obligate blood-feeders, nocturnal, and reside in homes on mattresses and furniture. Bedbug infestations can be very difficult to eradicate. Several insects are known to be vectors for infectious diseases; therefore, bite prevention is important. Reactions to arthropod bites and stings range from mild irritation to life-threatening anaphylaxis (Goddard & Stewart, 2020).

### Subjective Findings

The health history may reveal:

- Rapid appearance of localized swelling, redness, burning, and itching of the skin
- Recent travel, exposure to pets or outdoor activities
- Other family members or close contacts with similar skin lesions

### Risk Factors

The most common risk factors for infestations and insect bites are:

- Fleas may be carried by pets, but can also be found in carpets, floors, sandboxes, beaches, and in grassy areas.
- *Cheyletiella* mites can also be carried by household pets (known as "walking dandruff") and are known to bite humans.
- Bedbug infestations are more common in areas with crowded housing such as economically disadvantaged areas, urban cities, and refugee camps.
- Individuals who travel frequently are also at higher risk for acquiring bedbugs.
- Children and adolescents at higher risk for tick bites include those living in endemic regions and those with occupational or recreational exposure to wooded areas, such as forestry, hunting, camping, hiking, and gardening.

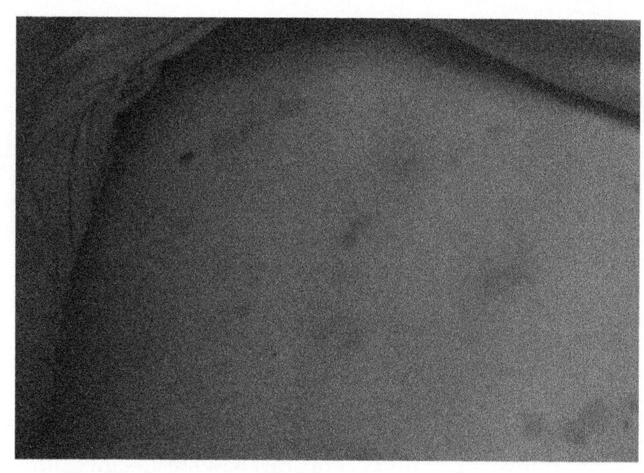

FIGURE 19.19 Bed bug bites.

*Source*: From Lyons, F., & Ousley, L. E. (2015). *Dermatology for the advanced practice nurse*. Springer Publishing Company.

## Review of Systems

The most common manifestations revealed during the review of systems include:

- **Integumentary:** localized pruritus, redness, mild tenderness and swelling.

Rarely, patients may present with symptoms of anaphylaxis, including dizziness, airway swelling, nausea and vomiting.

## Objective Findings

The physical examination of the child with insect bites may reveal:

- Erythematous, edematous, pruritic papules or wheals that appear with a few minutes of the bite (Figure 19.19)
- A central punctum may be seen
- Vesicle or bullae
- Linear clustering of bites (especially in the case of fleas and bedbugs; "breakfast, lunch, and dinner" sign; see Figure 19.19)

Most bite reactions resolve within a few hours to days. Papular urticaria, common in younger children, refers to a localized wheal and flare hypersensitivity reaction that becomes recurrent and chronic, sometimes lasting months to years. It may be localized or generalized. Younger children are also more likely to have exaggerated insect bite reactions. Patients with allergies (most commonly to stings of the Hymenoptera order) or mast cell disorders may experience severe reactions that present with systemic signs including flushing and hypotension.

## Laboratory/Diagnostic Testing

The diagnosis is made clinically based on history and physical examination. Skin biopsy is rarely needed to differentiate from other conditions.

## Differential Diagnosis

The differential diagnosis for insect bites includes:

- Bullous impetigo
- Cellulitis
- Folliculitis
- Lymphomatoid papulosis
- Pityriasis lichenoides
- Urticaria

## Treatment/Management Plan

Treatment of insect bites is based on symptoms. Oral antihistamines, cool compresses, mid-potency topical corticosteroids, and reassurance are usually sufficient until the bite has self-resolved. Anaphylaxis due to insect bites should be treated emergently with epinephrine. Patients with severe allergies to insect bites or stings should be given an epinephrine autoinjector to carry with them, and every caregiver should be instructed in how to use it.

## Family Education

Teach the following:

- Infected household pets should be identified and treated.
- Carpets, floors, and furniture should be disinfected (when appropriate).
- Bedbug infestations usually require evaluation and treatment by a licensed professional in order to achieve successful eradication.
- Prevention of insect bites involves diligent use of protective clothing and insect repellents, especially during high-risk outdoor activities.
- Repellents with N,N-Diethyl-meta-toluamide (DEET, 10%–30%) are the most effective, provide broad-spectrum protection against most insects, and should be applied to all exposed skin.
  - DEET should not be used in infants younger than 2 months of age.
  - Application of DEET near the eyes, mouth, and hands should be avoided (Breisch, 2020).
- Avoid combination insect repellent-sunscreen preparations, as these may be less effective.
- Other options for insect repellents include picaridin and oil of lemon eucalyptus (efficacy is variable).

### Referral

Refer to a pediatric allergist for formal testing and possible immunotherapy in the child with severe or life-threatening bite reactions. Referral should also be considered when the diagnosis is in doubt or when an insect bite reaction does not self-resolve as expected.

## PEDICULOSIS

Lice are small, wingless insects that have infected humans for centuries and feed on their blood to survive. *Pediculosis humanus capitis* (the head louse) most commonly affects children (Coates et al., 2020). Two additional species of lice are known to infest humans: *Pediculus humanus corporis* (the body louse) and *Phthirus pubis* (the pubic or "crab" louse; Goldstein, A. & Goldstein, B., 2021). Each louse type has six legs and a slightly different body shape. Adult female lice lay nits (eggs), which hatch after about 1 week. While head lice and pubic lice live directly on affected persons or attached to hairs, body lice live on clothing and bedding.

### Subjective Findings

The health history may reveal:

- Severe itching of the scalp (head lice) or body (body lice)
- Nits or live lice identified on the scalp (head lice)
- Recent exposure to an affected child (head lice)
- Poor hygiene, poverty, or homelessness (body lice)

### Risk Factors

The most common rick factors for lice are:

- Head lice are transmitted via close person-to-person contact with an affected individual or by sharing fomites (hats, headgear, combs, brushes, hooded clothing).
- Infestations of head lice are more common in girls and less common in African Americans.
- Head lice are not associated with low socioeconomic status or poor hygiene.
- Body lice are most common in individuals living in crowded conditions, such as the homeless and refugee populations.
- Pubic lice are almost always transmitted via sexual contact.

### Review of Systems

The most common manifestations revealed during the review of systems include:

- **Integumentary:** pruritus

### Objective Findings

The physical examination of the child with lice may reveal:

- Live head lice on the scalp
- Viable nits (usually firmly secured to hair shafts within a few centimeters of the scalp)
- Cervical and suboccipital lymphadenopathy

Body lice may be suspected on the basis of severe excoriation or the presence of urticarial papules from individual bites in areas of the body, usually in contact with the seams of clothing. A characteristic finding indicative of pubic lice is *maculae ceruleae*, or gray-blue macules usually seen on the lower abdomen and thighs that are thought to occur from bites.

### Laboratory/Diagnostic Testing

The diagnosis is confirmed by identifying live lice or viable nits on the hair, eyelashes, scalp, or body, or on the inner seams of clothing or bedding in the case of body lice. To confirm the presence of a viable nit, a hair mount preparation can be performed and viewed under a light microscope, which may demonstrate an intact nit cemented to the hair shaft with a developing louse inside it.

### Differential Diagnosis

The differential diagnosis for lice includes:

- Bedbug infestation
- Hair casts
- Piedra
- Seborrheic dermatitis

### Treatment/Management Plan

Head lice are usually treated with permethrin 1% cream rinse, which is available over the counter and should be applied to damp hair and rinsed after 10 minutes. A repeat treatment is recommended after 1 week.

Body lice are usually treated with permethrin 5% cream or lindane 1% lotion. Permethrin can be used for children as young as 2 months of age. There have been reports of increasing resistance to permethrin. Other options for topical therapy include lindane 1% shampoo, benzyl alcohol 5% lotion, malathion 0.5% lotion, spinosad 0.9% suspension, and ivermectin 0.5% lotion.

Manual removal of lice and nits is very difficult to achieve and is not recommended as a singular therapy. Infestation of eyelashes with pubic lice may be treated with petroleum jelly, which functions by suffocating live lice. Any secondary bacterial infection should be treated appropriately. Prophylactic treatment of close contacts and other household members should be considered. The American Academy of Pediatrics (AAP) recommends against no-nit policies, which require children to remain home from school despite the fact that nonviable nits may remain on hair shafts for several months after successful treatment (AAP, 2020).

### Family Education

Teach the following:

- All clothing and bed linens should be machine-washed in hot water and dried using high heat.
- Minimize direct contact with others to avoid sharing potential fomites.

### Referral

Referral to a pediatric dermatologist or lice clinic is indicated for children who are refractory to treatment.

## SCABIES

Scabies is an infestation of the skin caused by the human scabies mite, *Sarcoptes scabiei*. It is a relatively common infestation and can occur in any age group, including children and infants. Female mites burrow into the skin and lay eggs that hatch after several days (Thomas et al., 2020). Scabies is contagious and is spread via prolonged, direct skin-to-skin contact or, less commonly, from fomites such as clothing or bedding (Goldstein, B. & Goldstein, A., 2019). Under normal circumstances, the overall mite burden is low and an affected individual may only carry up to 15 mites at a time. However, in crusted ("Norwegian") scabies, individuals can harbor thousands or even millions of mites and are extremely contagious (Thomas et al., 2020).

Symptoms begin several weeks after infestation, owing to a delayed-type hypersensitivity reaction. Individuals who have been previously sensitized may experience symptoms more quickly. Other household members may report similar symptoms.

### Subjective Findings

The health history may reveal:

- Severe itching associated with redness, bumps, or scaling of the skin
- Recent exposure to an affected individual
- Crowded living conditions, poverty, poor hygiene, or homelessness

### Risk Factors

Crowded conditions predispose to scabies infestation. Epidemics may occur in institutional settings.

### Review of Systems

The most common manifestations revealed during the review of systems include:

- **Integumentary:** severe pruritus that may be worse at night

### Objective Findings

The physical examination of the child with scabies may reveal:

- Scattered, erythematous papules, nodules (Figure 19.20a)
- Vesicles or pustules
- Excoriations
- Nodules (more likely to occur in the groin and buttocks)
- Burrows, which appear as thread-like white lines on the skin up to a few millimeters in size, are a characteristic feature but may be difficult to appreciate (Figure 19.20b)

The most common locations affected include the webs and sides of the fingers, the palms, soles, wrists, ankles, axillae, waist, periumbilical skin, areola, male genitalia, and buttocks. Although rare in adults, scalp involvement is possible in infants.

- Crusted scabies presents as erythematous, thick, scaly plaques that may mimic common inflammatory skin diseases such as psoriasis.
- Nails may appear thickened and dystrophic.

### Laboratory/Diagnostic Testing

The best test for confirming a scabies infestation is a scabies preparation. A small amount of mineral oil is applied to an affected area on the skin and scraped with a number 15 blade or disposable curette. The best sites for obtaining specimens are the distal extremities; in particular, burrows and new lesions. Magnification (dermoscopy) can be helpful for identification of burrows. The scabies preparation is viewed using a light microscope and examined for scabies mites, eggs, and feces, all of which are diagnostic of infection.

### Differential Diagnosis

The differential diagnosis for scabies includes:

- Acropustulosis of infancy
- Eosinophilic folliculitis

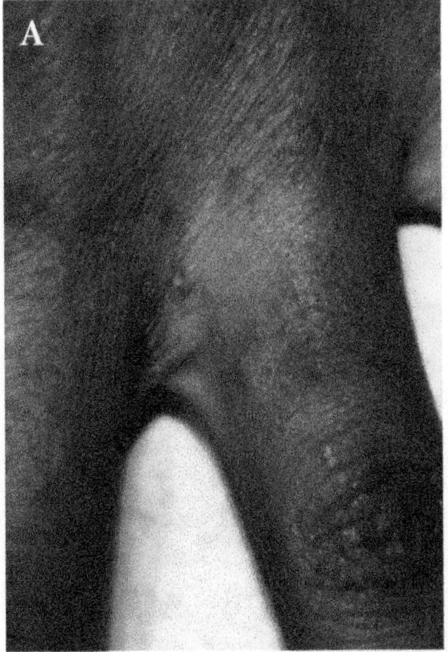

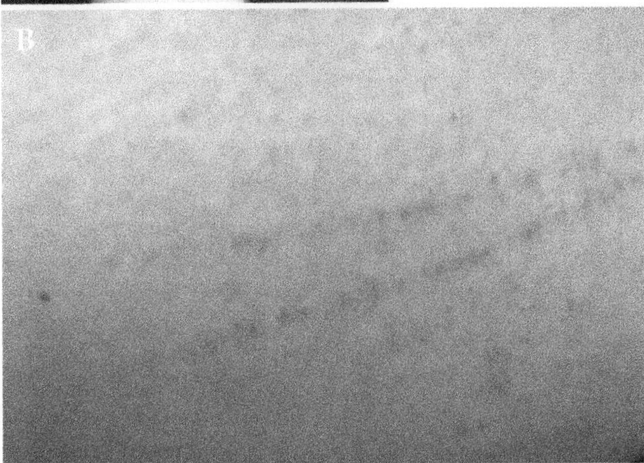

FIGURE 19.20 **(A) Appearance of scabies on dark skin. (B) Note burrow with scabies.**

*Source*: From Lyons, F., & Ousley, L. E. (2015). *Dermatology for the advanced practice nurse*. Springer Publishing Company.

- Impetigo
- Insect bites
- Langerhans cell histiocytosis
- Psoriasis
- Seborrheic dermatitis
- Viral exanthem (Gianotti-Crosti)

### Treatment/Management Plan

The gold stand therapy for scabies is permethrin 5% cream, applied evenly to the entire body from the neck down and left in place for at least 8 hours prior to rinsing (usually overnight). The scalp should also be treated in infants. The treatment is repeated in 1 week. Treatment of all household members and close contacts is recommended at the same time to prevent recurrence.

Permethrin is not recommended for infants under 2 months of age. Alternative treatment options include sulfur 6% ointment, crotamiton cream, and benzyl benzoate. Oral ivermectin 200 ug/kg per dose given in two doses, 2 weeks apart, has also been shown to be very effective in children weighing over 15 kg (Goldstein, B. & Goldstein, A., 2018). Crusted scabies is usually always treated with oral ivermectin in three- to seven-dose regimens, in combination with topical therapies. Topical corticosteroids and oral antihistamines can be used for symptomatic management of pruritus.

### Family Education

Teach the following:

- Recurrences are possible.
- All clothing, linens, and towels in the household should be machine-washed and dried with high heat.
- Items that cannot be washed can be dry cleaned or stored in airtight bags for up to 1 week to kill the mites.
- The body's hypersensitivity reaction to the mite, including pruritus, often continues for weeks to months even after successful treatment and does not necessarily indicate treatment failure.

### Referral

Referral to pediatric dermatology should be considered for severe cases and those not responding to standard therapy as expected.

## VASCULAR AND PIGMENTARY ANOMALIES

Many vascular and pigmentary anomalies are present at birth or shortly thereafter such as capillary malformations (CMs; port wine stains). Others present later in childhood, including nevi and pyogenic granulomas. Here we discuss common vascular and pigmentary anomalies. Many do not require therapy, but can be associated with underlying systemic disease, so it is important to know when to refer children needing further evaluation.

## VASCULAR ANOMALIES

Vascular anomalies are divided into two groups: vascular tumors and vascular malformations. Vascular tumors have active growth phases and include pyogenic granulomas and infantile hemangiomas (IH). Vascular malformations are present from birth and grow with the patient slowly over time, but do not actively have growth of their own; this includes CMs and nevus simplex.

## Subjective Findings

During the health history, determine the timing of onset; any associated bleeding, ulceration or pain,;whether the lesion is more pronounced when the child is crying or upset; and change of appearance over time. IH have a unique life cycle in which they proliferate early in infancy (from about 4 weeks up to 6 months of age), then reach a plateau in growth, and then slowly involute over the following several years. CMs may slowly darken and develop firm papules (blebs) within them over years, but do not have this same characteristic growth pattern in early infancy.

### Risk Factors

Most of the vascular anomalies do not have clearly associated risk factors other than IHs, which are more likely in low-weight birth, Caucasian, and female infants.

### Review of Systems

The most important manifestations revealed during the review of systems include:

- **Constitutional:** difficulty feeding
- **Integumentary:** lesion bleeding
- **HEENT:** poor visual tracking
- **Respiratory:** wheezing, stridor, or labored respirations
- **Neurologic:** seizure

## Objective Findings

The physical examination of the child with vascular anomalies may reveal:

- Infantile hemangioma (three presentations):
  - Superficial hemangiomas—brightly erythematous velvety plaque
  - Deep hemangiomas—a blue-hued subcutaneous nodule
  - Mixed hemangiomas have both superficial and deep components
- CMs present as a light pink-to-red patch without epidermal or surface change. In teens and young adults, the color may become more dusky red or purple and firm red papules may form within the patch.
- Both CMs and IH may be localized or segmental (requiring further evaluation and referral)
- Pyogenic granulomas present as a domed red papule that is usually friable and bleeds easily; may have hemorrhagic crust present
- Nevus simplex presents as a faint pink patch commonly on bilateral upper eyelids, mid forehead and glabella, and/or on the occipital scalp/posterior neck
- Erosion, ulceration, or hemorrhagic crust

### Laboratory/Diagnostic Testing

The diagnosis of most vascular anomalies is based upon the clinical findings. No laboratory or diagnostic testing is needed unless indicated to screen for associated underlying diseases (see Referral section).

## Differential Diagnosis

The differential diagnosis for vascular anomalies includes:

- Other types of vascular tumors or malformations
- Other tumors of childhood: pilomatricoma, lipoma, juvenile xanthogranuloma, Spitz nevus, dermoid cyst, fibrosarcoma, rhabdomyosarcoma

## Treatment/Management Plan

For small, focal IH in low-risk areas of the body, observation without active therapy is appropriate. Superficial IH can be treated effectively with timolol ophthalmic gel or solution, applied twice daily. Higher-risk and deep tumors often require oral propranolol after appropriate referral and evaluation. Ulcerated IH can be initially treated with topical metronidazole gel or petroleum jelly covered with a thin hydrocolloid dressing while waiting on referral.

Pyogenic granulomas are small enough to be removed in the office with simple shave removal and curettage and electrodessication of the base of the lesion.

CMs themselves do not require urgent treatment, but may be lightened over time with laser therapy by a specialist. Segmental CM or CM of the head and neck should undergo further evaluation (see Referral section).

Nevus simplex is a benign, common finding and does not require therapy.

### Family Education

Teach the following:

- Educate families on what to expect with the growth and resolution of IH, as well as the risk of ulceration.

- CMs are generally stable over time but may darken and develop blebs. Laser treatment is available by specialists if desired to lighten the malformation.
- Families of infants with nevus simplex should be reassured of its benign nature and that lesion on facial skin will fade with time. Occipital scalp/posterior neck patches are usually persistent.
- Pyogenic granuloma papules may recur after removal, so families should be encouraged to reach back out to their healthcare provider if that happens.

### Referral

IH that are segmental and expand to cover larger areas of the face, neck, lower back/buttocks, or genital regions should be further evaluated for underlying associated syndromes and malformations. Infants with >5 hemangiomas (multifocal cutaneous IH) should also be referred to a pediatric dermatologist to receive evaluation for internal organ involvement. IHs that occur in high-risk areas for cosmetic deformity or ulceration should also be referred early in infancy; these include involvement of the eyelids, nose, lips, ears, neck creases, axillae, palms/fingers, genitals and buttocks, or perianal skin.

CMs occurring on the head and neck, as well as segmental lesions, should be referred to a pediatric dermatologist for further evaluation, as they may be associated with underlying syndromes.

## PIGMENTARY ANOMALIES

Pigmentary anomalies encompass a wide variety of disorders and can include both increased or decreased pigmentation and can be localized or generalized. Here we will cover the most common pigmentary anomalies including café-au-lait macules (CALMs), melanocytic nevi, and hypomelanotic macules.

### Subjective Findings

Determine the age of onset. CALMs may not be present at birth, but may increase in number and pigmentation over time. Melanocytic nevi may be congenital in nature or may be acquired and increase in number throughout childhood. The health history may reveal:

- Family history of similar lesions
- Changes in color, size, or shape

### Risk Factors

Pigmentary abnormalities also do not have unified, overarching risk factors, although specific associations are seen for some of the individual conditions. Acquired melanocytic nevi are more commonly seen in children with fair skin, family history of numerous nevi, and those with increased intermittent sun exposure (Kinsler, 2019). CALMs are often hereditary in an autosomal dominant manner, whether or not they are a component of neurofibromatosis 1. Hypopigmented macules may be associated with tuberous sclerosis, which is also inherited in an autosomal dominant manner.

### Review of Systems

The most common manifestations revealed during the review of systems include:

- **Constitutional:** pain (irritated nevi)
- **Integumentary:** itch (irritated nevi)
- **Cardiovascular:** any cardiac symptoms (with hypopigmented macules [tuberous sclerosis])
- **Neurologic:** includes seizures, developmental delay, or skin nodules (with CALMs); seizures, developmental delay, behavioral problems (with hypopigmented macules [tuberous sclerosis])

### Objective Findings

The physical examination of the child with pigmentary anomalies may reveal:

- CALMs present as well-defined light to medium brown macules or patches.
- Melanocytic nevi are varying shades of brown and may be macules, papules, or plaques. Terminal hairs may be present, especially in adolescents. It is important to note varying colors, symmetry, and the sharpness and regularity of the borders of the lesion. Congenital melanocytic nevi may be quite large and children may also have scattered smaller "satellite" nevi.
- Hypopigmented macules are light tan to white (although not completely depigmented) and often oval shaped, but may also be round.

### Laboratory/Diagnostic Testing

The diagnosis of most pigmentary anomalies is based upon the clinical findings. No laboratory or diagnostic testing is typically needed. Clinically atypical nevi may require biopsy to rule out malignancy.

### Differential Diagnosis

The differential diagnosis for pigmentary anomalies includes other pigmentary disorders:

- Vitiligo
- Post-inflammatory pigmentary alteration

- Acanthosis nigricans
- Pigmentary moisaicism

### Treatment/Management Plan

Treatment for most isolated pigmentary anomalies consists of observation for change or development of any new associated symptoms or clinical findings.

### Family Education

Teach the following:

- For children with melanocytic nevi, families should be educated on home self-skin checks and how to monitor for the ABCDEs of melanoma: **A**symmetry, irregular **B**orders, multiple or worrisome **C**olors, **D**iameter >6 mm, **E**volving/changing.

### Referral

Refer the following children accordingly:

- Children with CALMs should be referred to a geneticist if they have >5 CALMs measuring more than 5 mm before puberty, neurofibromas, axillary or inguinal freckling, iris hamartomas, or a family history of neurofibromatosis.
- Children with changing or symptomatic nevi, or nevi with concerning features, may require excision, and should be referred to a pediatric dermatologist depending on the comfort of the primary care provider.
- Infants with large congenital melanocytic nevi (estimated to be >20 cm when the child reaches adult size) or with satellite nevi should be referred to a pediatric neurologist for close follow-up, and in some cases evaluation of meningeal involvement.
- Children with more than three hypopigmented macules (or with other cutaneous stigmata including angiofibromas) should be referred to a pediatric neurologist for further workup of tuberous sclerosis.

## URTICARIA

Urticaria (hives) is a hypersensitivity reaction to antigens such as medications, infections, or other stimuli which cause degranulation of mast cells (Perez & Dyer, 2020). Classically, urticarial lesions are transient, lasting less than 24 hours. The eruption can be categorized as acute or chronic depending on how long a child is affected. If the eruption is less than 6 weeks in duration, it is considered acute. If the eruption is greater than 6 weeks, it is considered chronic. Oral antihistamines are the mainstay of management in both acute and chronic forms of urticaria.

### Subjective Findings

The health history may reveal:

- Transient pruritic rash
- In some children, there may be a preceding viral infection, bacterial infection, introduction of a new medication, or new food
- In many children, there may be no clear identifiable factor

### Risk Factors

The most common risk factors for urticaria are:

- Viral infection. It is estimated that acute urticaria is secondary to preceding viral infections in 80% of children (Paller & Mancini, 2016).
- Bacterial infections (i.e., streptococcal)
- Medications (i.e., penicillins, sulfonamides, NSAIDs)
- Introduction of new foods (i.e., dairy, seafood, nuts; Paller & Mancini, 2016).

### Review of Systems

There is usually a lack of systemic symptoms. The most common manifestations revealed during the review of systems include:

- **Integumentary:** Transient rash (each lesion lasting for less than 24 hours), pruritus

▶ ALERT: If systemic symptoms of anaphylaxis occur after urticarial lesions (i.e., weakness, difficulty breathing, abdominal pain, diarrhea, vomiting, loss of consciousness), the child should receive emergency care.

### Objective Findings

The physical examination of the child with urticaria may reveal:

- Widespread pink pruritic edematous patches and plaques
- Lesions may become violaceous as they fade
- Transient lesions lasting less than 24 hours

### Laboratory/Diagnostic Testing

The diagnosis of urticaria is based upon the clinical findings. No laboratory or diagnostic testing is needed.

### Differential Diagnosis

The differential diagnosis for urticaria includes:

- Serum sickness/serum sickness-like reaction
- Urticarial vasculitis
- Erythema multiforme

### Treatment/Management Plan

The mainstay of urticarial treatment is to remove the causative factor (if identifiable) and initiate oral nonsedating antihistamines (i.e., cetirizine, levocetirizine; Paller & Mancini, 2016). If pruritus is leading to difficulty sleeping, consider addition of a sedating antihistamine at bedtime. Antihistamines should be continued at least until clearance of the eruption and for several weeks after resolution before slowly tapering to achieve best control (Paller & Mancini, 2016).

### Family Education

Teach the following:

- Pediatric urticaria is most often secondary to a viral infection.
- Most urticarial eruptions will resolve within 6 weeks.
- The mainstay of treatment is oral antihistamines to reduce pruritus.

### Referral

If urticarial eruptions are not responding to antihistamine therapy, consider referral to a pediatric dermatologist for further workup and consideration of other systemic treatments.

# NAIL DISORDERS

Nail disorders are frequently encountered in both urgent care and primary care clinics. In the pediatric population, common nail disorders include paronychia and ingrown toenails. Onychomycosis is also seen, although it is less common in young children and more prevalent with increasing age (Solis-Arias & Garcia-Romero, 2016). In this section, we will expand upon these diagnoses to ensure accurate diagnosis and management.

## ONYCHOMYCOSIS

Onychomycosis, also known as tinea unguium, is defined as fungal infection of the nails. The most common etiologic organisms are dermatophytes (i.e., tinea rubrum, tinea mentagrophytes, tinea tonsurans, and microsporum canis; Solis-Arias & Garcia-Romero, 2016). It is uncommon in the pediatric population, only estimated to occur in up to 2.6% of children (Solis-Arias & Garcia-Romero, 2016). When present, it is common to see concurrent tinea pedis or tinea manuum or an affected family member (Solis-Arias & Garcia-Romero, 2016).

### Subjective Findings

The health history may reveal:

- Discoloration and/or thickening of nails
- History of red/scaly rash on hands or feet
- Family members with similar findings

### Risk Factors

The most common risk factors for onychomycosis are concurrent dermatophyte infections of hands/feet or affected family members. Common risk factors for tinea pedis (dermatophyte infection of the feet) are increased heat/moisture, use of shared pools/gyms, etc.

### Review of Systems

The most common manifestations revealed during the review of systems include:

- **Integumentary:** Discoloration and/or thickening of nails; red, itchy, scaly rash on hands or feet

### Objective Findings

The physical examination of the child with onychomycosis may reveal:

- Thickened nail plate leading to a yellow/brown discoloration
- Onycholysis (detachment of the nail plate from the nailbed)
- Powdery subungual debris
- If tinea manuum/pedis is present, erythematous macules, patches, and papules in an annular configuration with leading scaly border on hands or feet

### Laboratory/Diagnostic Testing

The diagnosis of onychomycosis is achieved via nail clipping, which is sent for fungal culture or histopathologic evaluation (Solis-Arias & Garcia-Romero, 2016).

### Differential Diagnosis

The differential diagnosis for onychomycosis includes:

- Onychodystrophy secondary to trauma
- Psoriasis
- Lichen planus
- Chronic paronychia
- Congenital disorder of the nails

### Treatment/Management Plan

Antifungal medications are the mainstay of treatment for onychomycosis. Topical treatments are safest, yet have decreased efficacy given their poor penetration through the nail plate (Paller & Mancini, 2016). Because pediatric nail plates are thinner than those of adults, it is reasonable to try topical antifungal therapies initially. Ciclopirox 8% nail lacquer has shown effectiveness in a study conducted over 32 weeks of treatment, with 77% of children achieving clearance (Solis-Arias & Garcia-Romero, 2016). Topical therapy with antifungal creams (i.e., terbinafine 1% cream) is an important consideration if concurrent tinea pedis or tinea manuum is present.

Oral antifungal therapy is considered a definitive treatment; however, careful consideration should be given to the risks and benefits of treatment, severity of infection, age of the child, and response to topical therapies. Systemic therapy is typically considered when topical therapies have failed, or when multiple nails are affected. Antifungals discussed in the literature include itraconazole and terbinafine (Solis-Arias & Garcia-Romero, 2016).

### Family Education

Teach the following:

- Onychomycosis is uncommon in the pediatric population.
- If onychomycosis is suspected, a nail clipping should be obtained by a healthcare provider and evaluated for the presence of fungal infection.
- If onychomycosis is diagnosed, both the child and family members should be evaluated for the presence of other fungal infections of the skin.

### Referral

If there is extensive disease and consideration is given to oral antifungal therapy, referral to a dermatologist is recommended.

## PARONYCHIA

Paronychia is defined as inflammation involving the nailfolds surrounding the nail. It can be further categorized as acute or chronic. Acute paronychia is most commonly seen with concurrent bacterial infection (typically *Staphylococcus aureus*); however, it is often polymicrobial (Leggit, 2017). Chronic paronychia is related to repeated exposure to moisture (i.e., thumb sucking, wet environments) and can be seen with subsequent candidal infection (Leggit, 2017).

### Subjective Findings

The health history may reveal:

- Painful, swollen nailfolds with or without purulent drainage and nail dystrophy
- Possible history of thumb sucking or frequent exposures to wet environments

### Risk Factors

The most common risk factors for paronychia are:

- Manipulation of the nail cuticle
- Trauma of the nail/cuticle
- Thumb sucking
- Repeated exposure to wet environments

### Review of Systems

There is usually a lack of systemic symptoms. The most common manifestations revealed during the review of systems include:

- **Integumentary:** pain and redness of affected nail folds, purulent drainage at edge of nail bed, nail dystrophy if chronic in nature

### Objective Findings

The physical examination of the child with paronychia may reveal:

- Erythematous, indurated proximal or lateral nailfolds that are tender to palpation
- If acute in nature, purulent drainage may be present
- If chronic in nature, dystrophy of the nail may be present

### Laboratory/Diagnostic Testing

The diagnosis of paronychia is based upon the clinical findings. No laboratory or diagnostic testing is needed. If purulent drainage is present, consider obtaining a bacterial culture for directed therapy.

### Differential Diagnosis

The differential diagnosis for paronychia includes:

- Trauma
- Ingrown toenail
- Herpetic whitlow
- Digital mucous cyst
- Onychomycosis

### Treatment/Management Plan

In acute paronychia, antibacterial dilute vinegar soaks along with topical antibiotics (e.g., mupirocin) may be used on a trial basis. If more extensive involvement or an abscess is present, antibiotic treatment with staphylococcal coverage should be administered, along with local wound care. In chronic paronychia, efforts should be made to remove irritating factors (e.g., frequent exposure to a wet environment) and inflammation may be treated with a low to mid potency topical corticosteroid (Leggit, 2017).

### Family Education

Teach the following:

- Paronychia is inflammation of the skin around the nail that may be related to bacterial infection or repeated exposure to wet environments.
- Dilute vinegar soaks have antibacterial properties and may be used on a trial basis; however, treatment with an antibiotic may be required.

### Referral

If paronychia is not resolving despite the use of appropriate therapies as discussed earlier, consider referral to a dermatologist for further evaluation and management.

## INGROWN TOENAIL

Ingrown toenail, also known as onychocryptosis, is defined as curvature of the lateral edge of the nail leading to penetration of the underlying tissue and subsequent pain and erythema. The great toenail is most commonly affected and is typically secondary to compression from poor-fitting footwear or inappropriate nail trimming. As a whole, ingrown toenails represent approximately 20% of nail complaints in primary care clinics (Mayeaux et al., 2019).

### Subjective Findings

The health history may reveal:

- Pain and redness of the skin surrounding the great toenail
- Recurring symptoms

### Risk Factors

The most common risk factors for ingrown toenails are:

- Improperly fitted footwear
- Inappropriate nail trimming

### Review of Systems

Usually lacking systemic symptoms, the most common manifestations revealed during the review of systems include:

- **Integumentary:** pain and redness of the skin surrounding the great toenail

### Objective Findings

The physical examination of the child with an ingrown toenail may reveal:

- Erythematous edematous lateral nailfold with inward curvature of the nail plate
- Most often involvement of the great toenail
- Granulation tissue and serosanguinous drainage may be present

### Laboratory/Diagnostic Testing

The diagnosis of ingrown toenails is based upon the clinical findings. No laboratory or diagnostic testing is needed.

### Differential Diagnosis

The differential diagnosis for ingrown toenails includes:

- Trauma
- Paronychia
- Pincer nail

## Treatment/Management Plan

The management of an ingrown toenail involves preventative measures, including wearing footwear that fits appropriately and avoiding trimming nails too frequently (allowing nail to grow past the free edge; Mayeaux et al., 2019). If secondary bacterial infection is present, topical or systemic antibiotics should be employed as appropriate.

## Family Education

Teach the following:

- Ingrown toenails are most commonly caused by ill-fitting footwear or inappropriate nail trimming.
- Ensure proper fit of footwear and avoid trimming nails too short to reduce the risk of ingrown toenails.

## Referral

If a child has recurrent ingrown nails and/or they do not respond to the management previously described, referral should be made to a podiatrist or pediatric dermatologist for consideration of surgical treatment (i.e., lateral avulsion of the nail plate; Mayeaux et al., 2019).

# KEY POINTS

- Impetigo may present in both bullous and nonbullous forms, with the most common pathogen being *Staphylococcus aureus and* nonbullous impetigo also caused by group A *Streptococccus.*
- Treatment of impetigo consists of topical and oral antibiotics with coverage for both streptococcus and staphylococcus.
- MRSA causes a variety of skin and soft tissue infections and its incidence has increased over the last decade.
- Obtain bacterial cultures when treating skin and soft tissue infections whenever possible to appropriately direct antibiotic therapy.
- Cellulitis is an acute bacterial infection of the skin and subcutaneous fat commonly caused by *S. aureus* and GABHS.
- Antibiotic therapy for cellulitis should cover both staphylococcus and streptococcus.
- Bacterial folliculitis presents as a pustular eruption and is most commonly caused by *S. aureus.*
- Consider pseudomonal "hot tub folliculitis" in children with a history of hot tub use.
- The mainstay of therapy for an abscess is incision and drainage; antibiotic therapy may be considered on a case-by-case basis as adjunctive therapy.
- Clinical presentations of *Candida* infection in infants and children include oral candidiasis (thrush), diaper candidiasis, intertrigo, vulvovaginitis, angular cheilitis, and paronychia.
- Treatment for *Candida* infection is typically with a topical antifungal formulation and preventative measures, especially related to the control of moisture, which are important to reduce the chance of recurrence.
- Dermatophyte infections are common in children and have various clinical presentations, including tinea capitis (scalp), tinea faciei (face), tinea corporis (body), tinea manuum (hands), tinea pedis or "athlete's foot" (feet), tinea cruris or "jock itch" (groin), and tinea unguium (nails).
- Although most localized dermatophyte infections can usually be treated successfully with a topical antifungal medication, treatment of tinea capitis requires oral therapy.
- Tinea versicolor is a common, noncontagious superficial fungal infection caused by *Malassezia furfur*, usually presenting with asymptomatic pigmentary changes of the skin in highly sebaceous areas such as the chest and back.
- Treatment options for tinea versicolor include topical and systemic antifungal agents, but recurrence is common.
- Herpes simplex virus type 1 and type 2 (HSV-1 and HSV-2) are common recurrent infections of the skin that present with pain, vesicle formation, erosions, and crusting.
- Treatment of HSV infection is largely supportive, although systemic antiviral therapy may be necessary for recurrent or severe disease.
- PR is a self-limited cutaneous eruption that classically begins with a single, larger patch or plaque with a fine collarette of scale ("herald patch"), followed days to weeks later by an asymptomatic eruption on the trunk.
- Treatment of PR is not necessary, as the condition typically self-resolves within 4 to 8 weeks.
- Molluscum is a benign viral infection of the skin that is characterized by pink or flesh-colored, dome-shaped, umbilicated papules and spread by contact with other children or by autoinoculation due to scratching.
- Infection is self-limited, but if treatment is requested, in-office topical cantharidin may be used.

- Warts (verrucae) are a common viral infection of the skin and mucous membranes caused by HPV.
- Treatment options include observation, topical therapies, and cryotherapy (limit use to older, cooperative children), but successful clearance of warts requires patience, consistency, and adherence to recommended therapy.
- Acne is an extremely common inflammatory condition of the pilosebaceous unit.
- Use of a topical or oral antibiotic for acne should always be paired with use of benzoyl peroxide to minimize the risk of bacterial resistance.
- Seborrheic dermatitis most commonly presents as cradle cap in infants and dandruff in adolescents, although other areas of the body may also be affected.
- Treatment of seborrheic dermatitis is typically with topical antifungal preparations in combination with a topical steroid to use as needed for any associated inflammation and itching.
- Psoriasis is a chronic, inflammatory disorder of the skin that is characterized by multiple different clinical patterns.
- Treatment options for psoriasis include various anti-inflammatory topical formulations, narrow band ultraviolet light therapy, and systemic medications.
- Contact dermatitis is either a response to an irritating substance (irritant contact dermatitis) or the result of an allergic reaction (allergic contact dermatitis).
- Treatment of contact dermatitis is typically with topical steroids, in addition to identification of the offending substance.
- Minor burns (first-degree burns) are partial-thickness burns affecting a limited body surface area.
- Treatment for minor burns is largely supportive and includes monitoring for secondary bacterial infection in the case of thermal burns.
- Healthcare providers must be alert for signs of child abuse during every encounter with a child.
- Abuse should be considered in a child presenting with an inconsistent, implausible, or vague history related to the cutaneous injury, or atypical bruising, abrasions, lacerations, or burns (especially if the child is nonambulatory), or evidence of neglect (poor growth).
- Treatment of insect bites is supportive and should be paired with education regarding eradication of infestations and counseling on preventative measures (e.g., protective clothing and insect repellent).
- Head lice are a common nuisance among the pediatric population, confirmed by identifying live lice on the hair or scalp or viable nits on hair shafts, and are usually treated with permethrin 1% cream rinse, with a repeat treatment in 1 week.
- Scabies is a relatively common cutaneous infestation that can occur in any age group.
- The mainstay of therapy for scabies is permethrin 5% cream, which should also be given to all household members at the same time to prevent recurrence.

## REFERENCES


American Academy of Pediatrics. (2020). *Head lice: What parents need to know.* https://healthychildren.org/English/health-issues/conditions/from-insects-animals/Pages/Signs-of-Lice.aspx

Antoon, A. (2020). Burn injuries. In R. M. Kliegman, J. St. Geme, N. J. Blum, S. S. Shah, R. C. Tasker, K. M. Wilson, & R. E. Behrman (Eds.), *Nelson textbook of pediatrics* (21st ed., Chapter 92). Elsevier.

Baddour, L. M. (2020). Impetigo. *UpToDate.* https://www.uptodate.com/contents/impetigo

Boos, S. C. (2020). Physical child abuse: Recognition. *UpToDate.* https://www.uptodate.com/contents/physical-child-abuse-recognition

Breisch, N. L. (2020). Prevention of arthropod and insect bites: Repellents and other measures. *UpToDate.* https://www.uptodate.com/contents/prevention-of-arthropod-and-insect-bites-repellents-and-other-measures

Campbell, J. R., & Palazzi, D. L. (2019). Candida infections in children. *UpToDate.* https://www.uptodate.com/contents/candida-infections-in-children

Children's Bureau. (2020). *Child maltreatment 2018.* https://www.acf.hhs.gov/cb/research-data-technology/statistics-research/child-maltreatment

Christian, C., & Oranje, A. (2015). Cutaneous clues of child abuse. *Contemporary Pediatrics.* https://www.contemporarypediatrics.com/view/cutaneous-clues-child-abuse

Coates, S. J., Thomas, C., Chosidow, O., Engelman, D., & Chang, A. Y. (2020). Ectoparasites: Pediculosis and tungiasis. *Journal of the American Academy of Dermatology, 82*(3), 551–569. https://doi.org/10.1016/j.jaad.2019.05.110

Eickstaedt, J. B., Killpack, L., Tung, J., Davis, D., Hand, J. L., & Tollefson, M. M. (2017). Psoriasis and psoriasiform eruptions in pediatric patients with inflammatory bowel disease treated with anti-tumor necrosis factor alpha agents. *Pediatric Dermatology, 34*(3), 253–260. https://doi-org.resource.ahu.edu/10.1111/pde.13081

Gawlik, K., Melnyk, B. M., & Teall, A. M. (Eds.). (2021). *Evidence-based physical examination: Best practices for health and well-being assessment.* Springer Publishing Company.

Goddard, J., & Stewart, P. H. (2020). Insect and other arthropod bites. *UpToDate.* https://www.uptodate.com/contents/insect-and-other-arthropod-bites/

Goldstein, A. O., & Goldstein, B. G. (2020a). Dermatophyte (tinea) infections. *UpToDate.* https://www.uptodate.com/contents/dermatophyte-tinea-infections

Goldstein, A. O., & Goldstein, B. G. (2020b). Pityriasis rosea. *UpToDate.* https://www.uptodate.com/contents/pityriasis-rosea

Goldstein, A. O., & Goldstein B. G. (2021). Pediculosis capitis. *UpToDate*. https://www.uptodate.com/contents/pediculosis-capitis

Goldstein, B. G., & Goldstein, A. O. (2019). Scabies: Epidemiology, clinical features, and diagnosis. *UpToDate*. https://www.uptodate.com/contents/scabies-epidemiology-clinical-features-and-diagnosis

Goldstein, B. G., & Goldstein, A. O. (2020). Tinea versicolor (pityriasis versicolor). *UpToDate*. https://www.uptodate.com/contents/tinea-versicolor-pityriasis-versicolor

Goldstein, B. G., & Goldstein, A. O. (2021). Scabies: Management. *UpToDate*. https://www.uptodate.com/contents/scabies-management

Goldstein, B. G., Goldstein, A. O., & Morris-Jones, R. (2019). Cutaneous warts (common, plantar, and flat warts). *UpToDate*. https://www.uptodate.com/contents/cutaneous-warts-common-plantar-and-flat-warts

Graber, E. (2021). Acne vulgaris: Overview of management. *UpToDate*. https://www.uptodate.com/contents/acne-vulgaris-overview-of-management

Isaacs, S. N. (2020). Molluscum contagiosum. *UpToDate*. https://www.uptodate.com/contents/molluscum-contagiosum

Jackson, J. D. (2020). Infectious folliculitis. *UpToDate*. https://www.uptodate.com/contents/infectious-folliculitis

Johnston, C., & Wald, A. (2019). Epidemiology, clinical manifestations, and diagnosis of herpes simplex virus type 1. *UpToDate*. https://www.uptodate.com/contents/epidemiology-clinical-manifestations-and-diagnosis-of-herpes-simplex-virus-type-1-infection

Kaplan, S. L. (2019). Methicillin-resistant *Staphylococcus aureus* infections in children: Epidemiology and clinical spectrum. *UpToDate*. https://www.uptodate.com/contents/methicillin-resistant-staphylococcus-aureus-infections-in-children-epidemiology-and-clinical-spectrum

Kaplan, S. L. (2021). Suspected *Staphylococcus aureus* and streptococcal skin and soft tissue infections in children >28 days: Evaluation and management. *UpToDate*. https://www.uptodate.com/contents/suspected-staphylococcus-aureus-and-streptococcal-skin-and-soft-tissue-infections-in-children-greater-than28-days-evaluation-and-management

Keels, M. A., & Clements, D. A. (2019). Herpetic gingivostomatitis in young children. *UpToDate*. https://www.uptodate.com/contents/herpetic-gingivostomatitis-in-young-children

Kimberlin, D. W., Brady, M. T., Jackson, M. A., Long, S. S., & the Committee on Infectious Diseases. (2018). *American Academy of Pediatrics red book: 2018–2021 Report of the Committee on Infectious Diseases* (31st ed.). American Academy of Pediatrics.

Kinsler, V. A. (2019). Chapter 105: Melanocytic naevi. In P. H. Hoeger, D. Purvis, V. Kinsler, & A. C. Yan (Eds.), *Harper's textbook of pediatric dermatology* (4th ed.). John Wiley & Sons.

Leggit, J. (2017). Acute and chronic paronychia. *American Family Physician, 96*(1), 44–51.

Lexicomp. (2020). *Lexicomp clinical drug information* (version 5.7.1) [Mobile app]. App store. https://apps.apple.com/us/app/lexicomp/id313401238

Lyons, F., & Ousley, L. E. (2015). *Dermatology for the advanced practice nurse*. Springer Publishing Company.

Mancini, A. J., & Krowchuk, D. P. (Eds.). (2016). *Pediatric dermatology: A quick reference guide*. American Academy of Pediatrics.

Mayeaux, E. J., Carter, C., & Murphy, T. (2019). Ingrown toenail management. *American Family Physician, 100*(3), 158–164.

Menter, A., Cordoro, K. M., Davis, D. M. R., Kroshinsky, D., Paller, A. S., Armstrong, A. W., Connor, C., Elewski, B. E., Gelfand, J. M., Gordon, K. B., Gottlieb, A. B., Kaplan, D. H., Kavanaugh, A., Kiselica, M., Kivelevitch, D., Korman, N. J., Lebwohl, M., Leonardi, C. L., Lichten, J., ... Elmets, C. A. (2020). Joint American Academy of Dermatology–National Psoriasis Foundation guidelines of care for the management and treatment of psoriasis in pediatric patients. *Journal of the American Academy of Dermatology, 82*(1), 161–201. https://doi.org/10.1016/j.jaad.2019.08.049

Paller, A. S., & Broun Lund, E. (2020a). Management of chronic plaque psoriasis. *UpToDate*. https://www.uptodate.com/contents/psoriasis-in-children-management-of-chronic-plaque-psoriasis

Paller, A. S., & Broun Lund, E. (2020b). Psoriasis in children: Epidemiology, clinical manifestations, and diagnosis. *UpToDate*. https://www.uptodate.com/contents/psoriasis-in-children-epidemiology-clinical-manifestations-and-diagnosis

Paller, A. S., & Mancini, A. J. (2016). *Hurwitz clinical pediatric dermatology: A textbook of skin disorders of childhood and adolescence* (5th ed.). Elsevier.

Perez, C. E., & Dyer, J. A. (2020). Cutaneous drug eruptions in pediatrics: A primer. *Pediatric Annals, 49*(3), e132–e139. https://doi.org/10.3928/19382359-20200224-01

Rice, P. L., & Orgill, D. P. (2021). Assessment and classification of burn injury. *UpToDate*. https://www.uptodate.com/contents/assessment-and-classification-of-burn-injury

Sasseville, D. (2021a). Cradle cap and seborrheic dermatitis in infants. *UpToDate*. https://www.uptodate.com/contents/cradle-cap-and-seborrheic-dermatitis-in-infants

Sasseville, D. (2021b). Seborrheic dermatitis in adolescents and adults. *UpToDate*. https://www.uptodate.com/contents/seborrheic-dermatitis-in-adolescents-and-adults

Singleton, J. K., DiGregorio, R. V., Green-Hernandez, C., Holzemer, S. P., Faber, E. S., Ferrara, L. R., & Slyer, J. T. (2014). *Primary care: An interprofessional perspective*. Springer Publishing Company.

Solis-Arias, M. P., & Garcia-Romero, M. T. (2016). Onychomycosis in children: A review. *International Journal of Dermatology, 56*(2), 123–130. https://doi.org/10.1111/ijd.13392

Spelman, D., & Baddour, L. M. (2020). Cellulitis and skin abscess: Clinical manifestations and diagnosis. *UpToDate*. https://www.uptodate.com/contents/cellulitis-and-skin-abscess-clinical-manifestations-and-diagnosis

Thiboutot, D., & Zaenglein, A. (2021). Pathogenesis, clinical manifestations, and diagnosis of acne vulgaris. *UpToDate*. https://www.uptodate.com/contents/pathogenesis-clinical-manifestations-and-diagnosis-of-acne-vulgaris

Thomas, C., Coates, S. J., Engelman, D., Chosidow, O., & Chang, A. Y. (2020). Ectoparasites: Scabies. *Journal of the American Academy of Dermatology, 82*(3), 533–548. https://doi.org/10.1016/j.jaad.2019.05.109

Tong, Y., Tyring, S. K., & Szalai, Z. Z. (2019). Chapter 49: Human papillomavirus infection. In P. H. Hoeger, D. Purvis, V. Kinsler, & A. C. Yan (Eds.), *Harper's textbook of pediatric dermatology* (4th ed.). John Wiley & Sons.

Weston, W. L. (2020). Contact dermatitis in children. *UpToDate*. https://www.uptodate.com/contents/contact-dermatitis-in-children

Wiktor, A., & Richards, D. (2019). Treatment of minor thermal burns. *UpToDate*. https://www.uptodate.com/contents/treatment-of-minor-thermal-burns

Young, A. Y., & Tewari A. (2020). Sunburn. *UpToDate*. https://www.uptodate.com/contents/sunburn

Zaenglein, A. L., Pathy, A. L., Schlosser, B. S., Alikhan, A., Baldwin, H. E., Berson, D. S., Bowe, W. P., Graber, E. M., Harper, J. C., Kang, S., Keri, J. E., Leyden, J. J., Reynolds, R. B., Silverberg, N. B., Stein Gold, L. F., Tollefson, M. M., Weiss, J. W., Dolan, N. C., Sagan, A. A., ... Bhushan, R. (2016). Guidelines of care for the management of acne vulgaris. *Journal of the American Academy of Dermatology, 74*(5), 945–973.e33.

Zouboulis, C. C. (2019). Skin glands: Sebaceous, eccrine, and apocrine glands. In S. Kang, M. Amagai, A. L. Bruckner, A. H. Enk, D. J. Margolis, A. J. McMichael, & J. S Orringer (Eds.), *Fitzpatrick's dermatology* (9th ed.) McGraw-Hill Education.

# Management of Eye Disorders

Jamie H. Andre and Morgan Rockwell

## Student Learning Outcomes

**Upon completion of this chapter the reader should be able to:**

1. Discuss pathophysiology and epidemiology of selected eye disorders in children.
2. Differentiate subjective and objective findings of selected eye disorders in children.
3. Choose appropriate laboratory or diagnostic tests for particular eye disorders in children.
4. Utilize the differential diagnosis process to determine the diagnosis of eye disorders in children.
5. Determine treatment plan, child/family education, and need for referral in children with an eye disorder.

## INTRODUCTION

Eye disorders are common complaints seen in the primary care setting. It is important to evaluate each child and identify disorders that require urgent referral and intervention. Other disorders are benign and can be treated in an outpatient setting. It might be difficult for young children to verbalize changes in vision or eye pain. Practitioners rely heavily on the parent's history of present illness, on thorough physical examination, and on evaluation of visual acuity.

The content in this chapter maps to the following areas on the Pediatric Nursing Certification Board (PNCB) Pediatric Nurse Practitioner—Primary Care certification examination:

**CLINICAL PROBLEMS: HEAD, EYE, EAR, NOSE, AND THROAT**

CONTENT AREAS:

**II. Assessment and Diagnosis**

**B. History and Physical Examination**

1. Obtain history of present illness
2. Obtain a comprehensive health history for new patients
3. Complete an interval history for established patients
4. Perform a review of systems
5. Perform a complete physical examination

**C. Diagnostic Testing and Screening**

1. Order and interpret office/clinic based screening tests

**D. Analyzing Information**

1. Integrate health history and physical examination findings into the plan of care
2. Assimilate findings from screening and diagnostic testing into plan of care

**E. Diagnosis**

1. Develop and prioritize differential diagnoses
2. Establish a diagnosis based on evaluation of patient data

## III. Management

**A. Child and Caregiver Counseling and Education**

1. Provide condition-specific counseling and education, including treatment options
2. Educate about benefits and potential adverse reactions of pharmacological interventions
3. Discuss non-pharmacological interventions
4. Counsel regarding the threshold for seeking follow-up care
5. Review the risks of non-adherence to recommended treatment

**B. Therapeutic Interventions**

1. Prescribe pharmacologic agents
2. Recommend the use of over-the-counter pharmacologic agents
3. Order or recommend non-pharmacologic treatments for the management of symptoms

**C. Procedures**

1. Perform procedures in accordance with diagnostic guidelines and plan of care (rapid tests)

**D. Collaboration and Referral**

2. Refer to specialists as indicated for evaluation, counseling, and/or treatment

**E. Care Coordination**

1. Facilitate patient and family-centered care for children of all ages with acute and chronic conditions

**F. Evaluation and Follow-up**

2. Establish a plan for follow-up care

## IV. Professional Role Responsibilities

**A. Leadership and Evidence-based Practice**

4. Develop, implement, and/or modify clinical practice guidelines

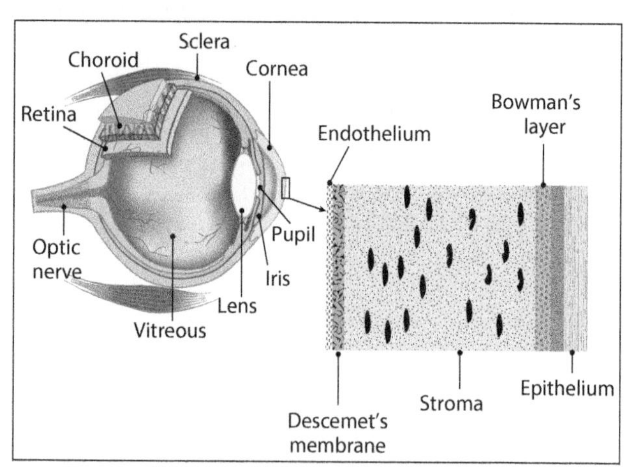


FIGURE 20.1 Internal structure of the eye.

*Source*: Gawlik, K., Mazurek Melnyk, B., & Teall, A. M. (Eds.). (2021). *Evidence-based physical examination: Best practices for health & well-being assessment: Comprehensive book for teaching physical and health assessment techniques*. Springer Publishing Company.

## ANATOMY AND PHYSIOLOGY

The anatomy of a child's eye and visual pathway is very similar to that of an adult (Figure 20.1). However, during the first few months of life, there are some conditions that are normal but would be abnormal if they persisted as the child ages or are present in an adult. An understanding of the anatomy and physiology is important to guide diagnosis and determine need for referral.

The visual pathway extends from the occipital lobe to the cornea. Posterior to the globe, the pathway includes the occipital lobe, the optic tract, the optic chiasm, and the optic nerve. The optic chiasm is the point along the visual pathway where the optic tracks from the left and right brain each divide and provide part of the optic nerve to each eye. The globe itself consists of the optic disc, macula, choroid, retina, ciliary body, sclera, conjunctiva, lens, iris, pupil, and cornea. The lens divides the eye into the posterior chamber (vitreous body) and anterior chamber. There are six extraocular muscles controlled by three different cranial nerves. The abducens nerve (CN VI) innervates the lateral rectus muscle, the trochlear nerve (CN IV) innervates the superior obliques muscle, and the oculomotor nerve (CN III) innervates the superior, medial, and inferior rectus as well as the inferior oblique (Figure 20.2).

## GENERAL APPROACH TO CHILD WITH EYE DISORDERS

Many eye conditions occurring in children also occur in adults. Although the newborn has poor visual acuity at birth, with visual acuity progressing to that of the adult by school age. Certain eye conditions may be normal in the newborn, yet resolve as the child ages. It is necessary to approach the assessment of eye conditions in infants and children, keeping in mind that earlier treatment of conditions may preserve visual acuity development. For instance, although present in adults as well, the presence of a bilateral red reflex is critical to note in the

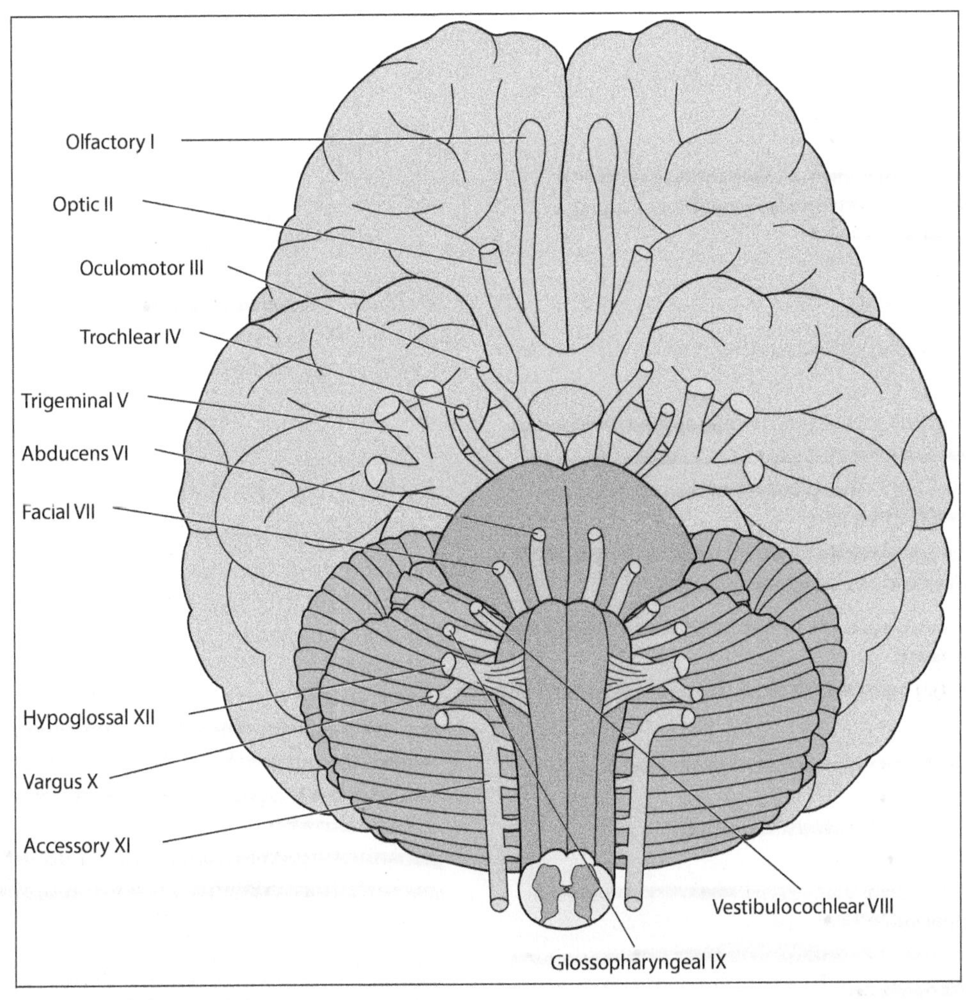


FIGURE 20.2 Location of the cranial nerves.

*Source*: Myrick, K., Karosas, L., & Smeltzer, S. (Eds.). (2020). *Advanced health assessment and differential diagnosis: Essentials for clinical practice*. Springer Publishing Company.

newborn, as its absence may indicate congenital cataract (needing early treatment). An abnormal red reflex can be a sign of serious conditions. Without high visual acuity, newborns are unable to focus well on objects. Because of this, it is not abnormal for the infant to have strabismus (malalignment) during the first few months of life. This should resolve by 6 months of age as binocularity develops and visual acuity improves. Children also do not develop full depth perception until around 5 years of age, which can account for apparent clumsiness that parents may be concerned about.

## Subjective Findings

Explore the health history for recent trauma or infectious contacts. The health history may reveal:

- Eye pain
- Changes in vision
- Noticeable changes to the eye, eyelid, or surrounding structures
- Watery or mucopurulent discharge
- Foreign body sensation (Donahue et al., 2016)

## Risk Factors

The most common risk factors for eye disorders are:

- Prematurity
- Congenital disorders
- Trauma or sports injury
- Upper respiratory tract infection

### Review of Systems

- The most common manifestations revealed during the review of systems include
- **Constitutional:** pain
- **HEENT:** eye redness, eye discharge or increased lacrimation, visual acuity changes, blurred vision, diplopia, photophobia

### Objective Findings

The physical examination of the child with an eye disorder may reveal:

- Orbit and conjunctivae may reveal edema, erythema or other discoloration, icterus hematoma, drainage
- Eyelids may show drooping, laceration, erythema, edema, or foreign body
- Pupils may reveal inequality of size and shape, reactivity to light, and/or accommodation

Use tracking of an object for assessment of extraocular muscle function.
An ophthalmoscope will show fundus and retinal vessels.

- Evaluate the eyelids for foreign body, laceration, edema, erythema
- Evaluate the pupils, reactivity to light, accommodation
- Evaluate the extraocular muscle function by asking the patient to track an object
- Evaluate the interior of the eye using a funduscope for ruptured vessels (Donahue et al., 2016)

Eyelids, following palpation, may reveal masses. Evaluate visual acuity using a Snellen chart, tumbling Es, or other developmentally appropriate vision chart.

## EYE PROCEDURES

There are procedures that can be done safely in the outpatient setting that can help with both diagnosis and treatment. In this section, fluorescein staining and eyelid eversion are discussed. Fluorescein staining is helpful in identifying corneal abrasion and eyelid eversion can be used to remove a foreign body.

### FLUORESCEIN STAINING

Fluorescein staining can be used when the history and physical examination are concerning for corneal abrasion. This should be done after all other eye examinations and visual acuity testing are complete, as it can affect the results.

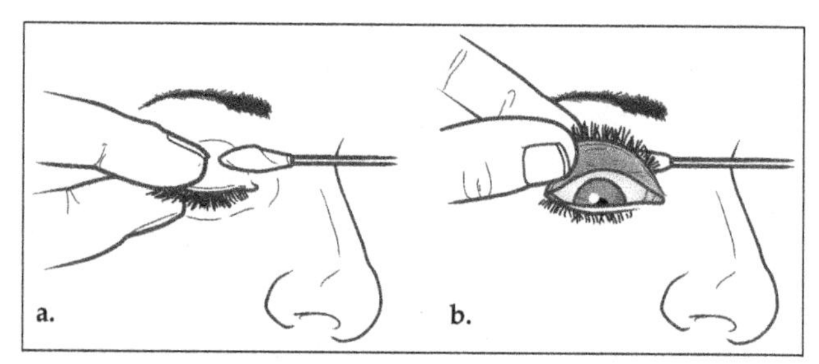


FIGURE 20.3 Eyelid eversion

*Source*: Chiocca, E. M. (2019). *Advanced pediatric assessment* (3rd ed.). Springer Publishing Company.

Perform the examination as follows:

1. Pull the lower eyelid down.
2. Allow a drop from a moistened fluorescein strip to drip into this area or gently wipe the strip against the cornea. Ensure maintainance of sterile technique.
3. The dye will distribute when the child blinks.
4. An abrasion may be visible upon examination without tools but will be enhanced with the use of a slit lamp, the filter on an ophthalmoscope, or a Wood's lamp.
5. Flush the eye with saline following the examination to remove the fluorescein.

### REMOVAL OF FOREIGN BODY

Performing eyelid eversion to remove a foreign body:

1. Gently pull the upper eyelid away from the eye.
2. Place a cotton-tipped applicator against the outside of the eyelid (Figure 20.3a).
3. While gently moving the swab downward, pull the eyelid up and around the swab so the inside of the eyelid is exposed (Figure 20.3b).
4. A foreign body can then be removed with sterile irrigation or gently with another sterile cotton-tipped applicator.
5. It is important to examine the inside of the eyelid, sclera, and cornea thoroughly. Similarly, a cotton-tipped swab can be used to gently pull down the lower eyelid to expose the inside of the eyelid.

## VISION IMPAIRMENT

Although vision impairment can be caused by a broad spectrum of conditions, it is important to identify a decrease in visual acuity or a condition that can lead to a decrease in visual acuity or blindness. In addition to vision impairment, amblyopia and strabismus are also discussed, as they may contribute to vision impairment if left untreated.

## LOSS IN VISUAL ACUITY

Vision screening should be performed in children regularly to assess for loss in visual acuity in one or both eyes. Decreased visual acuity or blurred vision may be caused by a lesion along the visual pathway anywhere from the occipital lobe to the cornea. The history of the vision loss as well as the physical examination can help determine where the lesion is. This can be a result of a congenital or neurological disorder, abnormal development along the visual pathway, or trauma. A lesion posterior to the chiasm or at the optic chiasm will affect both eyes, whereas a lesion anterior to the chiasm along the optic nerve will affect only one eye.

### Subjective Findings

The vision loss may be of acute or gradual onset. The health history may reveal:

- Poor tracking of objects
- Crossed eyes, or wandering eye

### Risk Factors

The most common risk factors for visual impairment are:

- Prematurity
- Family history of vision impairment
- Trauma
- Cataracts
- Retinoblastoma
- Neurodevelopmental delay
- Genetic disorders

### Review of Systems

The most common manifestations revealed during the review of systems include:

- **HEENT:** visual acuity changes, blurred vision, diplopia, foreign body in eye

### Objective Findings

The physical examination of the child with visual impairment may reveal:

- Esotropia or exotropia
- Abnormal red reflex, abnormal cover/uncover test
- Cataract
- Decreased visual acuity in one or both eyes
- Foreign body in the eye, retinal detachment, or hyphema
- Torticollis

### Laboratory/Diagnostic Testing

Depending on the history and physical examination findings, no further diagnostic or laboratory testing may be necessary.

### Differential Diagnosis

The differential diagnosis for visual impairment includes:

- Strabismus
- Amblyopia
- Trauma to the globe or optic nerve
- Cataracts
- Central nervous system process or disorder of the visual pathway
- Hyphema
- Foreign body
- Corneal abrasion

### Treatment/Management Plan

Treatment and management will depend on what is causing the vision impairment.

### Family Education

Teach the following:

- It is important to follow up with the ophthalmologist for evaluation and treatment of visual impairment, as delay in treatment initiation can result in permanent blindness

### Referral

Refer the child to a pediatric ophthalmologist for further evaluation and treatment of the visual impairment. If there is concern for damage to the globe or surrounding structures, urgent referral should be made, as delay in evaluation and treatment may lead to permanent blindness.

## STRABISMUS

Strabismus is a misalignment of the eyes resulting in the inability of the eyes to focus on an object simultaneously. Although each eye can focus on an object individually, if strabismus is uncorrected, amblyopia (see definition later) may develop. Strabismus can be caused by weakness or paralysis of any of the six extraocular muscles, increase in intraocular pressure, or damage to cranial nerves. Strabismus may be horizontal (esotropia or exotropia), vertical (hypertropia or hypotropia), or torsional depending on which extraocular muscles and nerves are involved (Gunton, 2015).

## Subjective Findings

Ask if the strabismus has been present since birth or if it developed later. The child or parent may report that one eye deviates from the other. There may be a family history of strabismus. The health history may reveal:

- Genetic or neuromuscular problems
- History of head or eye trauma

### Risk Factors

The most common risk factors for strabismus are:

- Positive family history of strabismus
- Prematurity
- Associated ocular conditions
- Genetic syndromes
- Neuromuscular conditions such as cerebral palsy

### Review of Systems

The most common manifestations revealed during the review of systems include:

- **HEENT:** diplopia, visual acuity changes
- **Neurologic:** headache

## Objective Findings

The physical examination of the child with strabismus may reveal (Figure 20.4):

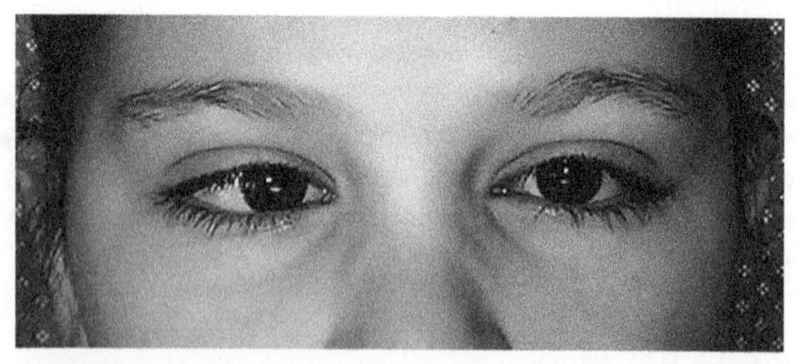

FIGURE 20.4 A toddler with strabismus. Also note the asymmetric Hirschberg reflex.

*Source*: Myrick, K., Karosas, L., & Smeltzer, S. (Eds.). (2020). *Advanced health assessment and differential diagnosis: Essentials for clinical practice*. Springer Publishing Company.

- Visible misalignment of eyes
- Asymmetric Hirschberg test
- Asymmetric Bruckner test
- Strabismus manifested during the cover test
- Latent strabismus noted on cover/uncover test
- Abnormal eye movement upon examination
- Poor vision—inability to focus with both eyes simultaneously but able to focus with either eye individually
- Torticollis

### Laboratory/Diagnostic Testing

The diagnosis of strabismus is based on the clinical findings. Blood tests and neuroimaging are only indicated when craniofacial malformations, neurologic disorders, trauma, or acute onset of strabismus is present.

## Differential Diagnosis

The differential diagnosis for strabismus includes:

- **Pseudostrabismus:** ocular alignment is normal but appears abnormal
- **Retinoblastoma**
- **Congenital esotropia:** requires surgical repair
- **Accommodative esotropia:** occurs with farsighted refractive errors, will require surgery if referral for glasses is too delayed

## Treatment/Management Plan

The goal of therapy is to improve muscular alignment. Treatment may include any or all of the following: occlusion therapy with patching, visual training exercises, glasses or prism therapy, or miotic drops. Surgical repair may be required if training exercises and glasses are ineffective. Some types of strabismus will require surgery regardless.

### Family Education

Teach the following:

- Regular follow-up with a pediatric ophthalmologist is recommended to evaluate the need for surgery if nonsurgical therapy is ineffective.
- It is normal for children to have misalignment of their eyes for the first few months of life. This is generally brief and resolves as the oculomotor system develops.

### Referral

Refer to a pediatric ophthalmologist infants older than 4 months of age with continued intermittent strabismus, children with constant strabismus at any age, and any child with diplopia or an abnormality in the corneal light reflex test, cover test, or Bruckner test.

## AMBLYOPIA

Amblyopia is a result of abnormal visual development that causes a disconnect between the brain and the eye, leading to unilateral blindness. It is important to detect amblyopia early on because treatment may improve the long-term visual outcome. Amblyopia is generally unilateral but can be bilateral in rare cases. Classifications of amblyopia include:

- Strabismic amblyopia caused by misalignment of the eyes
- Refractive amblyopia caused by differing visual acuity between the eyes
- Deprivational amblyopia caused by obstruction of the visual axis (Taylor et al., 2016)

Amblyopia can recur, so it is important to have continued surveillance after successful treatment.

### Subjective Findings

The health history may reveal:

- Unequal vision between the two eyes
- Crossed eyes or wandering eye
- Cataracts
- Squinting

**PRO TIP** Parents may note that their child is reading slower compared with other children but is comprehending the material (Birch & Kelly, 2017).

### Risk Factors

The most common risk factors for amblyopia are:

- Prematurity
- Small size for gestational age
- Cataract or glaucoma
- Neurodevelopmental delay
- Eyelid ptosis
- First-degree relative with amblyopia

### Review of Systems

The most common manifestations revealed during the review of systems include:

- **HEENT:** visual acuity changes—generally unilateral, blurred vision, nystagmus
- **Musculoskeletal:** torticollis

### Objective Findings

The physical examination of the child with amblyopia may reveal:

- Ptosis
- Cataract or corneal opacity
- Asymmetric Hirschberg (see Figure 20.4) and Bruckner tests
- Fixation reflex test or cover/uncover testing: while occluding one eye, move a visual target from side to side; it will reveal different points of fixation for each eye. In younger children with strabismus and amblyopia, the eye with amblyopia will have a hard time fixating on the object when both eyes are uncovered.
- Unlike children with equal vision, children with amblyopia will be more irritated when their eye with better visual acuity is occluded compared to their eye with worse visual acuity.
- Red reflex test may reveal a unilateral abnormality.
- Visual chart testing in children 3 years or older will reveal difference in visual acuity between the two eyes
- Torticollis
- Strabismus (McConaghy & McGuirk, 2019)

### Laboratory/Diagnostic Testing

The diagnosis of amblyopia is made based on the presence of differences in visual acuity between the eyes; this is the only diagnostic test needed. No additional testing is required.

### Differential Diagnosis

The differential diagnosis for amblyopia includes:

- Strabismus
- Central nervous system process or disorder/injury affecting the visual pathway including optic nerve and retina
- Refractive error such as myopia or astigmatism

### Treatment/Management Plan

The goal of therapy is to promote equal visual acuity development for both eyes. Treatment may include any or all of the following: occlusion therapy with patching (better eye is patched), atropine eye drops, exercises, glasses, or optical penalization of the nonamblyopic eye. The underlying condition must also be addressed.

### Family Education

Teach the following:

- After successful treatment of amblyopia, it is possible for it to recur, so it is important to monitor for any signs of different acuity between the eyes

### Referral

In children in whom amblyopia is a concern, referral to a pediatric ophthalmologist should be made for further evaluation and initiation of treatment.

# DISORDERS OF THE EYELID AND ADNEXA

The eyelids and adnexa are structures that surround and protect the eye. Disorders of these structures can affect the eyelids, eyelashes, eyebrows, medial canthus, and lateral canthus. Hordeolum, chalazion, and blepharitis are disorders of the eyelids. Dacryostenosis affects lacrimation somewhere between the nasal canal and the medial canthus.

## HORDEOLUM

A hordeolum, commonly known as a stye, is a small, painful, inflamed nodule on the eyelid. It can be external or internal to the eyelid. Hordeola develop acutely due to obstruction of eyelid glands and secondary infection, usually with *Staphylococcus aureus* (Schabowski & McGruk, 2018).

### Subjective Findings

The health history may reveal:

- Painful bump on the eyelid
- Sensation of foreign body under eyelid
- Sudden appearance

### Risk Factors

The most common risk factor for hordeolum is a history of hordeolum or blepharitis.

### Review of Systems

The most common manifestations revealed during the review of systems include:

- **Constitutional:** pain

### Objective Findings

The physical examination of the child with hordeolum may reveal (Figure 20.5):

- External hordeolum: Palpable painful mass on the eyelid, pointing anteriorly
- Internal hordeolum: Palpable painful mass through the eyelid, pointing internally
- Surrounding edema and erythema

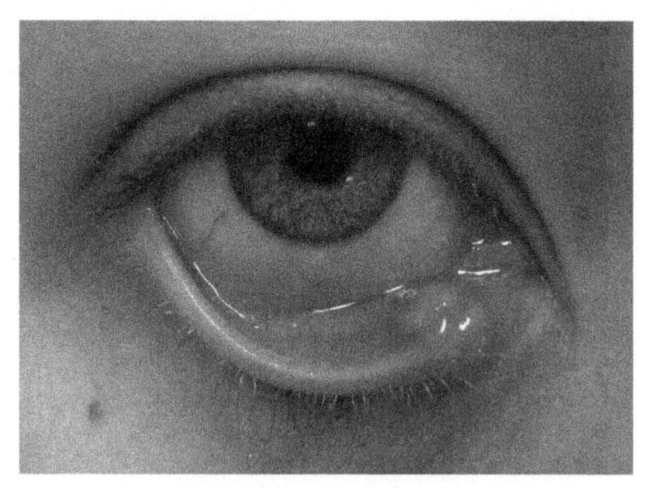

FIGURE 20.5 Hordeolum.

*Source*: Chiocca, E. M. (2019). *Advanced pediatric assessment* (3rd ed.). Springer Publishing Company.

### Laboratory/Diagnostic Testing

The diagnosis of hordeolum is based upon the clinical findings. Slit-lamp examination and corneal evaluation should be performed to rule out other causes of pain and inflammation.

### Differential Diagnosis

The differential diagnosis for hordeolum includes:

- Chalazion
- Blepharitis
- Nasolacrimal obstruction
- Foreign body

### Treatment/Management Plan

Treatment of hordeolum includes supportive care with warm compresses. If there is concern for associated conjunctivitis, topical antibiotic drops or ointment should be considered. Symptoms typically resolve in 1 to 2 weeks.

### Family Education

Teach the following:

- Seek medical attention if changes in vision develop.
- Hordeola are not considered contagious.

### Referral

In severe cases of internal hordeolum, referral to a pediatric ophthalmologist might be necessary for incision and drainage.

## CHALAZION

A chalazion is a firm, nontender nodule on the eyelid. It develops over time due to long-standing glandular obstruction and chronic glandular inflammation.

### Subjective Findings

The health history may reveal:

- Formation of an eyelid nodule over time
- Feeling of pressure on the eye
- History of internal hordeolum

### Risk Factors

The most common risk factor for chalazion is history of internal hordeolum.

### Review of Systems

The most common manifestations revealed during the review of systems include:

- **Constitutional:** absence of pain

### Objective Findings

The physical examination of the child with chalazion may reveal:

- Well-circumscribed nodule on eyelid
- Nontender to palpation
- Possible surrounding erythema
- Lesion might be white or grayish in appearance

### Laboratory/Diagnostic Testing

The diagnosis of chalazion is based upon the clinical findings. Special attention should be made to ensure the nodule is not causing corneal injury.

### Differential Diagnosis

The differential diagnosis for chalazion includes:

- Hordeolum
- Blepharitis
- Nasolacrimal obstruction
- Foreign body

### Treatment/Management Plan

Treatment of chalazion includes warm compresses and nonemergent referral to a pediatric ophthalmologist for elective excision.

### Family Education

Teach the following:

- Counsel that the chalazion might require elective excision by a pediatric ophthalmologist if it does not resolve with supportive measures.
- Advise seeking medical attention if acute pain or changes in vision develop.

### Referral

Treatment of chalazion includes nonemergent referral to a pediatric ophthalmologist for elective excision.

## BLEPHARITIS

Blepharitis is inflammation of the eyelid. Inflammation can occur on the anterior portion of the eyelid due to dermatitis or bacterial infection, or on the posterior portion of the eyelid due to chronic dysfunction of the Meibomian glands. Blepharitis is commonly a chronic condition with periods of exacerbations and remissions.

### Subjective Findings

The health history may reveal:

- Red rims of the eyelids
- Eyelashes adhere together
- Mucopurulent discharge might be present in posterior blepharitis

### Risk Factors

The most common risk factors for blepharitis are:

- Seborrheic dermatitis
- Systemic inflammatory conditions
- Environmental factors

### Review of Systems

The most common manifestations revealed during the review of systems include:

- **HEENT:** redness, discharge or increased lacrimation

### Objective Findings

The physical examination of the child with blepharitis may reveal:

- Fibrous scales known as collarettes
- Dandruff-like debris known as scurf

- Matted and oily eyelashes, stuck together
- Erythema and edema at the eyelid margin
- Possible mucopurulent discharge associated with posterior blepharitis

### Laboratory/Diagnostic Testing

The diagnosis of blepharitis is based upon the clinical findings.

### Differential Diagnosis

The differential diagnosis for blepharitis includes:

- Eyelid carcinoma
- Eyelid lice

### Treatment/Management Plan

There is no definitive treatment for blepharitis. Good eye hygiene, warm compresses, and gentle scrubs with a mild shampoo can be helpful. Topical antibiotics can be prescribed if there is suspicion of *Staphylococcus* or *Streptococcus* infection. In cases refractory to conservative treatment, oral antibiotics can be prescribed (Duncan & Jeng, 2015).

### Family Education

Teach the following:

- Good eye hygiene

## DACRYOSTENOSIS

Dacryostenosis, also known as nasolacrimal duct obstruction, is a common finding in the newborn. The most common etiology is failure of the nasolacrimal duct to open completely. In some cases, known as dacryocystitis, obstruction might be caused by a bacterial pathogen. Infants with dacryostenosis typically present at several weeks or months of life with symptoms of excessive tear production and possible erythema or irritation of the eye.

### Subjective Findings

The health history may reveal:

- Excessive tear production
- Purulent drainage
- Ocular and eyelid erythema

### Risk Factors

The most common risk factors for dacryostenosis are accompanying facial anomalies including cleft lip and palate and children with trisomy 21 or CHARGE (**C**oloboma of the eye, **H**eart defects, **A**tresia of the choanae, **R**etardation of growth and development, and **E**ar abnormalities and deafness) syndrome.

### Review of Systems

The most common manifestations revealed during the review of systems include:

- **Constitutional:** ocular and eyelid pain or tenderness
- **HEENT:** discharge or increased lacrimation, eyelid and periorbital redness

### Objective Findings

The physical examination of the child with dacryostenosis may reveal:

- Excessive tearing
- Eyelid debris
- Edema and/or erythema of the lacrimal sac
- Expression of fluid with palpation of the lacrimal sac
- Prominent tear meniscus

### Laboratory/Diagnostic Testing

The diagnosis of dacryostenosis is typically based upon the clinical findings. Fluorescein-stained saline can be applied to the inferior portion of the infant's eye. If there is no nasolacrimal duct obstruction, saline should drain completely into the nose within 5 minutes of application (Perez et al., 2021).

### Differential Diagnosis

The differential diagnosis for dacryostenosis includes:

- Conjunctivitis
- Dacryocystitis
- Allergic rhinitis
- Corneal abrasion
- Congenital glaucoma

### Treatment/Management Plan

Dacryostenosis typically resolves by 6 to 9 months of age with conservative management. Warm compresses and lacrimal massages are recommended two to three times per day. Topical antibiotics can be prescribed if there is concern for infectious obstruction (Perez et al., 2021).

### Family Education

Teach the following:

- How to provide warm compresses and nasolacrimal duct massage at home (Figure 20.6).

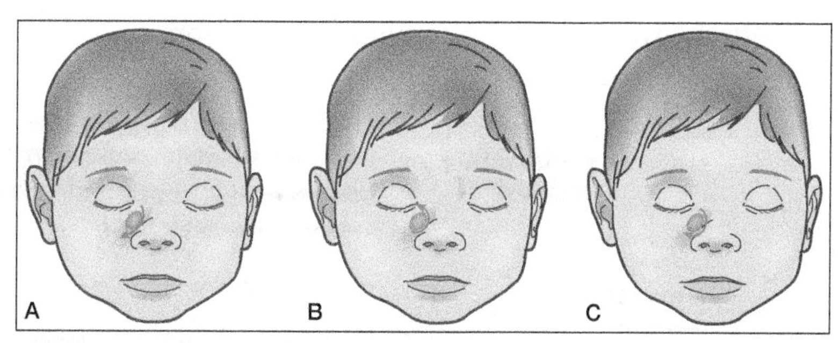


FIGURE 20.6 Nasolacrimal duct massage. (A) Using the forefinger or little finger, push on top of the bone (the puncta must be blocked). (B) Gently push in and up. (C) Gently push downward along the side of the nose.

- Signs/symptoms to look out for in the event of an infected lacrimal gland and surrounding structures.

## Referral

Referral to a pediatric ophthalmologist is recommended in the event of abscess formation for possible incision and drainage, or for possible surgical intervention if nasolacrimal obstruction continues past 12 months of age.

# INFECTIOUS DISORDERS

Infectious disorders that affect the eye and surrounding structures can be related to contagious contacts or due to local trauma to the area that makes it prone to infection. Special attention should be paid by the clinician to recognize infectious eye disorders in order to properly treat them and, when necessary, prescribe topical or systemic antibiotics. This section describes conjunctivitis and periorbital cellulitis.

## CONJUNCTIVITIS

Conjunctivitis, or pink eye, is one of the most common eye complaints seen in a primary care setting. The etiology is viral infection, bacterial pathogen, or allergic reaction. Viral conjunctivitis is the most common etiology, followed by bacterial conjunctivitis. Infectious causes of conjunctivitis are highly contagious. Although these infections usually originate in one eye, they often eventually affect both eyes due to spread from the primarily infected eye.

Viral conjunctivitis is usually caused by adenovirus, and in some rare cases can be caused by herpes simplex virus. Bacterial conjunctivitis is usually caused by *Streptococcus pneumoniae*, *Haemophilus influenza*, and *Moraxella catarrhalis*. Less common but more serious causes of bacterial conjunctivitis include *Chlamydia trachomatis* and *Neisseria gonorrhoeae* (Yeu & Hauswirth, 2020). Allergic conjunctivitis is typically due to seasonal allergies. The key in the treatment of conjunctivitis is identifying the etiology.

### Subjective Findings

The health history may reveal:

- Red eye (unilateral or bilateral)
- Pain or itching (unilateral or bilateral)
- Tearing or discharge (unilateral or bilateral)
- Waking in the morning with eyes glued shut due to discharge

### Risk Factors

The most common risk factors for conjunctivitis are sick contacts and seasonal allergies.

### Review of Systems

The most common manifestations revealed during the review of systems include:

- **Constitutional:** eye pain
- **HEENT:** eye redness, discharge or increased lacrimation, upper respiratory infection symptoms
- **Neurologic:** irritability

### Objective Findings

The physical examination of the child with conjunctivitis may reveal (unilateral or bilateral):

- Conjunctival erythema
- Ocular pruritus
- Tearing or purulent discharge
- Preauricular lymphadenopathy
- Signs of acute otitis media

Refer to Table 20.1.

**TABLE 20.1 Conjunctivitis Signs and Symptoms**

| Etiology | Involvement | Pruritus | Discharge | Lymphadenopathy |
|---|---|---|---|---|
| Viral | Unilateral or bilateral | Rare | Watery | Yes—preauricular |
| Bacterial | Unilateral or bilateral | Rare | Mucopurulent, stuck to eyelids | No |
| Allergic | Bilateral | Yes | Rare | No |

▶ ALERT: Signs of hyperacute conjunctivitis concerning for *Chlamydia trachomatis* or *Neisseria gonorrhoeae* include those listed here in addition to decreased visual acuity, eye tenderness, and copious amount of discharge.

### Laboratory/Diagnostic Testing

The diagnosis of conjunctivitis is primarily based upon the clinical findings. In-office rapid adenovirus testing or polymerase chain reaction may be collected to identify viral etiology. Eye culture may be sent if there is a concern for a possible bacterial etiology.

### Differential Diagnosis

The differential diagnosis for conjunctivitis includes:

- Ocular trauma
- Corneal abrasion
- Foreign body
- Keratitis
- Acute angle-closure glaucoma

### Treatment/Management Plan

Treatment for viral conjunctivitis includes supportive measures with normal saline eye lavage two times per day for 1 to 2 weeks. Warm or cool compresses can help relieve discomfort. Prescribe topical antibiotics for bacterial conjunctivitis. Common antibiotic choices include sulfonamides, fluoroquinolones, and aminoglycosides. If there is concern for infection with *Chlamydia trachomatis* or *Neisseria gonorrhoeae*, systemic antibiotics should be prescribed. Infection with these two pathogens is serious and in some cases might lead to permanent visual impairment. Treatment for allergic conjunctivitis includes supportive measures in addition to topical or systemic antihistamines.

### Family Education

Teach the following:

- The importance of hand and eye hygiene, as infectious conjunctivitis is highly contagious.
- Child may return to school or day care after 24 hours on antibiotic treatment.

### Referral

Children presenting with pain, photophobia, blurred vision, or severe purulent discharge should be referred to a pediatric ophthalmologist for further investigation and treatment.

## PERIORBITAL CELLULITIS

Periorbital cellulitis is an infection of the anterior portion of the eyelid in front of the septum. This infection does not involve the orbit. This is generally mild and does not lead to more serious conditions such as vision loss. This condition is more common in children than orbital cellulitis; however, it is important to eliminate orbital cellulitis during the examination due to its possible severe complications (Williams & Allen, 2019).

### Subjective Findings

The health history may reveal:

- Local trauma or insect bite
- Dacryocystitis (more likely with orbital cellulitis)
- Sinusitis (more likely with orbital cellulitis)

### Risk Factors

The most common risk factors for periorbital cellulitis are:

- Recent local trauma
- Bug bite
- Upper respiratory infection (Baiu & Melendez, 2020)

### Review of Systems

The most common manifestations revealed during the review of systems include:

- **Constitutional:** unilateral ocular pain
- **HEENT:** redness around the eye

### Objective Findings

The physical examination of the child with periorbital cellulitis may reveal:

- Pain/tenderness
- Redness

- Eyelid swelling
- No increase in pain with eye movements
- No proptosis
- Normal pupillary reflex
- Normal vision

▶ ALERT: Signs of orbital cellulitis include eyelid edema and discoloration, bulging of the eyeball, pain, decreased vision, and decreased eyeball movement.

### Laboratory/Diagnostic Testing

The diagnosis of periorbital cellulitis is generally based on the clinical findings. Computed tomography may be used if unable to rule out orbital cellulitis with clinical examination.

### Differential Diagnosis

The differential diagnosis for periorbital cellulitis includes:

- Orbital cellulitis
- Allergic reaction/allergies
- Hordeolum
- Chalazion
- Conjunctivitis

### Treatment/Management Plan

Prescribe oral antibiotics that cover *Staphylococcus aureus* and *Streptococcus pyogens* for a 7 to 10 day course.

### Family Education

Teach the following:

- It is important to complete the entire antibiotic course.

### Referral

Referral to a pediatric ophthalmologist is recommended when orbital cellulitis is suspected (for further examination and computed tomography imaging). Surgical intervention is only indicated if there is a possible foreign body or eyelid abscess.

## EYE TRAUMA

Eye trauma severity depends on the location and the degree of injury to the eye. Open-globe trauma, orbital fractures, hyphemas, or other injuries that cannot be addressed in an outpatient setting should be referred immediately to an emergency center or pediatric ophthalmologist. Minor injuries, such as corneal abrasions and subconjunctival hemorrhages, can typically be treated by a primary care provider.

## SUBCONJUNCTIVAL HEMORRHAGE

Subconjunctival hemorrhage is the rupture of blood vessels between the conjunctiva and sclera leading to blood spots or blood pooling on the conjunctiva. This is a benign condition usually caused by bearing down, straining, coughing, vomiting, or any activity that acutely raises blood pressure. It can also be caused by minor injuries or irritation to the eye. Subconjunctival hemorrhages should not cause vision changes. They typically resolve over several days to weeks.

### Subjective Findings

The health history may reveal:

- Blood spot(s) noted on the white surface of the eye
- History of straining or bearing down (Boyd, 2020)

### Risk Factors

The most common risk factors for subconjunctival hemorrhage are:

- Acute changes in blood pressure

Other risk factors can include

- Diabetes
- Hypertension
- Anticoagulation

### Review of Systems

The most common manifestations revealed during the review of systems include:

- **HEENT:** Redness/blood spots

### Objective Findings

The physical examination of the child with subconjunctival hemorrhage may reveal:

- Blood spot(s) limited to the conjunctiva
- No involvement of the cornea
- No change in vision

### Laboratory/Diagnostic Testing

The diagnosis of subconjunctival hemorrhage is based upon the clinical findings. If the child is taking blood thinners, consider checking coagulation levels.

### Differential Diagnosis

The differential diagnosis for subconjunctival hemorrhage includes:

- Anterior uveitis
- Globe rupture
- Corneal abrasion
- Hyphemia

### Treatment/Management Plan

Subconjunctival hemorrhages typically heal on their own over time. Artificial tears can be recommended to help relieve irritation (Boyd, 2020).

### Family Education

Teach the following:

- Avoid bearing down or straining if the child is able.
- Seek medical attention if vision becomes affected or if severe pain develops.

### Referral

Consider referral to a pediatric ophthalmologist if the child has a history of frequent subconjunctival hemorrhages.

## CORNEAL ABRASION

Corneal abrasions are minor injuries to the corneal surface due to tearing or scratching. Trauma or contact with foreign body causes a defect of the corneal epithelium.

### Subjective Findings

The health history may reveal:

- Scratchy pain and discomfort
- Foreign body sensation
- Excessive tearing
- Blurred vision

### Risk Factors

The most common risk factors for corneal abrasions are:

- Contact lens use
- Eye trauma
- Contact with a foreign body

### Review of Systems

The most common manifestations revealed during the review of systems include:

- **Constitutional:** pain
- **HEENT:** eye redness, visual acuity changes, photophobia, eye discharge or increased lacrimation

### Objective Findings

The physical examination of the child with corneal abrasion may reveal:

- Conjunctival and scleral injection
- Tearing
- Decreased visual acuity
- Epithelial defect seen on slit-lamp exam or fluorescein staining
- Rule out presence of foreign body under the eyelid (Lawe, 2018)

### Laboratory/Diagnostic Testing

The diagnosis of corneal abrasion is based upon the clinical findings in addition to epithelial defect seen on slit-lamp examination or fluorescein staining.

### Differential Diagnosis

The differential diagnosis for corneal abrasion includes:

- Conjunctivitis
- Hordeolum or chalazion
- Corneal ulcer
- Glaucoma

### Treatment/Management Plan

If a foreign body is visualized and is penetrating the globe, it should be removed urgently in an emergency room or pediatric ophthalmology setting. For simple corneal abrasions, saline irrigation can be used in the office to remove debris. Topical antibiotic should be prescribed if concerned for secondary infection; antipseudomonal coverage should be considered if the child wears contact lenses. Pain control can be achieved with over-the-counter analgesic agents.

### Family Education

Teach the following:

- Avoid contact lens use until the abrasion is healed.

### Referral

Foreign body trauma to the globe or penetrating injury warrants urgent referral to a pediatric ophthalmologist. Referral should also be made in the event that the corneal abrasion fails to heal with standard treatment.

## HYPHEMA

Hyphema is blood in the anterior chamber of the eye, usually caused by trauma to the eye or head. However, a hyphema can be the result of a stressful birth or juvenile xanthogranuloma. Spontaneous hyphema are rare in children. It is important to identify orbital and ocular injuries that can be associated with traumatic hyphema and need to be addressed more emergently. If hyphemas are not appropriately treated or cared for, they can lead to unilateral blindness.

### Subjective Findings

The health history may reveal:

- A blunt trauma injury to the eye or head
- Associated injuries to the head, orbital area, or posterior eye
- Intraocular surgery

### Risk Factors

The most common risk factors for hyphema are:

- Blunt trauma to the ocular area
- Bleeding disorders such as sickle cell disease or Von Willebrand
- Retinoblastoma
- Metastatic tumors
- Leukemia
- Clotting disorder
- Child abuse
- Juvenile xanthogranuloma
- Increase in intraocular pressure which leads to rupture of fragile vasculature
- Intraocular surgery

### Review of Systems

The most common manifestations revealed during the review of systems include:

- **Constitutional:** pain
- **HEENT:** redness/blood, visual acuity changes, photophobia

### Objective Findings

The physical examination of the child with hyphema may reveal:

- Blood in the anterior chamber of the eye
- Orbital fracture—restriction in ocular motility
- Open-globe or closed-globe injuries
- Detached retina or retinal tear, which requires emergent intervention
- Corneal abrasion
- Light sensitivity
- Increased intraocular pressure
- Foreign body
- Visual acuity may be affected depending on grade of hyphema
- The grading scale to use when evaluating a hyphema:
  - Grade 1 is <1/3 of the anterior chamber
  - Grade 2 is 1/3 to 1/2 of the anterior chamber
  - Grade 3 is >1/2 but not total filling of the anterior chamber
  - Grade 4 is total filling of the anterior chamber (Gharaibeh et al., 2019)

### Laboratory/Diagnostic Testing

Use the slit lamp to diagnose a small hyphema. X-ray can be performed to evaluate for foreign body. More advanced imaging may be required if suspected or foreign body is not detected by x-ray.

### Differential Diagnosis

The differential diagnosis for hyphema includes:

- Orbital compartment syndrome
- Open globe

### Treatment/Management Plan

An eye shield over the affected eye should be worn until hyphema resolves, to prevent further eye injury. Strict avoidance of activity is required until full evaluation has been completed. Dim light and refraining from reading are sometimes recommended so as not to further stress the eye. Elevation of the head helps reduce obstruction of the visual field and prevent clots in the pupillary axis. Intraocular pressure should be monitored daily. Anticoagulant and antiplatelets (such as nonsteroidal anti-inflammatory drugs [NSAIDs]) are contraindicated due to risk for rebleeding. Topical corticosteroids may prevent rebleeding. Cycloplegia eye drops are prescribed for comfort (Bansal et al., 2016).

### Family Education

Teach the following:

- Limit use of the eye while hyphema is still present and until further consultation with ophthalmologist (must be within 24 hours).
- If emergent, consult an ophthalmologist immediately.

## Referral

If there is concern for a grade 4 hyphema, orbital compartment syndrome, retinal tear/detachment, or orbital fracture, emergent referral to a pediatric ophthalmologist for further evaluation is needed. If this is not an immediate concern, follow-up with the pediatric ophthalmologist is still recommended within the following 24 hours for complete evaluation. The ophthalmologist will also provide ongoing evaluation of ocular pressure.

## KEY POINTS

- Visual impairment can be caused by a broad spectrum of things. It is important to identify what requires emergency referral and what requires routine referral to a pediatric ophthalmologist.
- Strabismus is an anomaly of ocular alignment that may affect visual development. Referral to a pediatric ophthalmologist is recommended to initiate therapies and evaluate need for surgical repair.
- Amblyopia is a decrease or loss of visual acuity (unilaterally) caused by abnormal development and should be suspected if there is a discrepancy in visual acuity between the eyes. Early recognition and prompt treatment are necessary for the promotion of optimal visual acuity development.
- A hordeolum, commonly known as a stye, is a painful glandular obstruction on the eyelid, typically caused by *Staphylococcus aureus* and treated with warm compresses.
- A chalazion is a firm, nontender nodule on the eyelid caused by chronic glandular obstruction; children should be referred to a pediatric ophthalmologist for elective excision of the nodule.
- Blepharitis is chronic inflammation of the eyelid characterized by periods of exacerbations and remissions; treatment should emphasize good eye hygiene.
- Nasolacrimal duct obstruction is commonly observed in the newborn period and is usually spontaneously resolved before 12 months of life; management includes warm compresses and lacrimal massage.
- Careful attention to history and physical examination will help differentiate between conjunctivitis etiologies, and treatment should be aimed at the suspected source of conjunctivitis.
- It is important to differentiate between periorbital cellulitis (which may be treated with a course of oral antibiotics) and orbital cellulitis, due to the serious complications associated with orbital cellulitis.
- Assess for emergent injuries associated with hyphema that require immediate care from a specialist; provide eye rest with a patch until hyphema is resolved or further treatment plan is made by a pediatric ophthalmologist.
- Subconjunctival hemorrhage is a benign rupture of the conjunctival vessels due to straining or trauma, which spontaneously resolves in days to weeks without treatment.
- Corneal abrasions are defects of corneal epithelium due to trauma or contact with a foreign body.

## REFERENCES

Baiu, I., & Melendez, E. (2020). Periorbital and orbital cellulitis. *JAMA, 323*(2), 196. https://jamanetwork.com/journals/jama/fullarticle/2758601

Bansal, S., Gunasekeran, D. V., Ang, B., Lee, J., Khandelwal, R., Sullivan, P., & Agrawal, R. (2016). Controversies in the pathophysiology of management of hyphema. *Survey of Ophthalmology, 61*(3), 297–308. https://doi.org/10.1016/j.survophthal.2015.11.005

Birch, E. E., & Kelly, K. R. (2017). Pediatric ophthalmology and childhood reading difficulties: Amblyopia and slow reading. *Journal of AAPOS, 21*(6), 442–444. https://doi.org/10.1016/j.jaapos.2017.06.013

Boyd, K. (2020). *What is a subconjunctival hemorrhage?* http://www.aao.org/eye-health/diseases/what-is-subconjunctival-hemorrhage

Donahue, S., Nixon, C., Section on Ophthalmology, American Academy of Pediatrics; Committee on Practice and Ambulatory Medicine, American Academy of Pediatrics; American Academy of Ophthalmology; American Association for Pediatric Ophthalmology and Strabismus; & American Association of Certified Orthoptists. (2016). Visual system assessment in infants, children, and young adults by pediatricians. *Pediatrics, 137*(1), 28–30. https://doi.org/10.1542/peds.2015-3596

Duncan, K., & Jeng, B. H. (2015). Medical management of blepharitis. *Current Opinion in Ophthalmology, 26*(4), 289–294. https://doi.org/10.1097/icu.0000000000000164

Gharaibeh, A., Savage, H. I., Scherer, R. W., Goldberg, M. F., & Lindsley, K. (2019). Medical interventions for traumatic hyphema. *Cochrane Database of Systematic Reviews.* https://www.cochranelibrary.com/cdsr/doi/10.1002/14651858.CD005431.pub4/abstract

Gunton, K. B., Wasserman, B. N., & DeBenedictis, C. (2015). Strabismus. *Primary Care: Clinics in Office Practice, 42*(3), 393–407. https://doi.org/10.1016/j.pop.2015.05.006

Lawe, D. S. (2018). Corneal abrasion. In J. J. Schaider, R. M. Barkin, S. R. Hayden, R. E. Wolfe, A. Z. Barkin, & P. Shayne (Eds.), *Rosen & Barkin's 5-minute emergency medicine consult* (5th ed., pp. 266–267). Wolters Kluwer Health.

McConaghy, J. R., & McGuirk, R. (2019). Amblyopia: Detection and treatment. *American Family Physician, 100*(12), 745–750. https://www.aafp.org/afp/2019/1215/p745.html

Perez, Y., Patel, B. C., & Mendez, M. D. (2021). Nasolacrimal duct obstruction. *StatPearls.* http://www.ncbi.nlm.nih.gov/books/NBK532873/

Schabowski, S., & McGruk, K. J. (2018). Hordeolum and chalazion. In J. J. Schaider, R. M. Barkin, S. R. Hayden, R. E. Wolfe, A. Z. Barkin, P. Shayne, & Rosen, P. (Eds.), *Rosen & Barkin's 5-minute emergency medicine consult* (5th ed., pp. 542–543). Wolters Kluwer Health.

Taylor, V., Bossi, M., Greenwood, J. A., & Dahlmann-Noor, A. (2016). Childhood amblyopia: Current management and new trends. *British Medical Bulletin, 119*, 75–86. https://doi.org/10.1093/bmb/ldw030

Williams, K. J., & Allen, R. C. (2019). Paediatric orbital and periorbital infections. *Current Opinion in Ophthalmology, 30*(5), 349–355. https://doi.org/10.1097/ICU.0000000000000589

Yeu, E., & Hauswirth, S. (2020). A review of the differential diagnosis of acute infectious conjunctivitis: Implications for treatment and management. *Clinical Ophthalmology, 14*, 805–813. https://doi.org/10.2147/opth.s236571

# Management of Ear Disorders

Theresa Kyle

## Student Learning Outcomes

**Upon completion of this chapter the reader should be able to:**

1. Discuss the pathophysiology and epidemiology of selected ear disorders in children.
2. Differentiate subjective and objective findings of selected ear disorders in children.
3. Choose appropriate laboratory or diagnostic tests for particular ear disorders in children.
4. Utilize the differential diagnosis process to determine the diagnosis of ear disorders in children.
5. Determine treatment plan, child/family education, and need for referral for children with an ear disorder.

## INTRODUCTION

Ear disorders in children may lead to alterations in sensory perception, specifically hearing, negatively affecting the young child's language development and the older child's academic achievement. Children commonly suffer from ear disorders (Conover, 2013). Otitis media and otitis externa (OE) are two very common infectious and inflammatory disorders that affect a child's ears. Some children may be born with ear anomalies or deficits in hearing. Alternatively, chronic or recurrent ear disorders may cause hearing impairment. The nurse practitioner must become astute in the assessment of children's ears in order to make accurate diagnoses and promote adequate hearing in the child.

The content in this chapter maps to the following areas on the Pediatric Nursing Certification Board (PNCB) Pediatric Nurse Practitioner—Primary Care certification examination:

**CLINICAL PROBLEMS: HEAD, EYE, EAR, NOSE, AND THROAT**

CONTENT AREAS:

**II. Assessment and Diagnosis**

**B. History and Physical Examination**

1. Obtain history of present illness
2. Obtain a comprehensive health history for new patients
3. Complete an interval history for established patients
4. Perform a review of systems
5. Perform a complete physical examination

**C. Diagnostic Testing and Screening**

1. Order and interpret office/clinic based screening tests
2. Order and interpret diagnostic laboratory tests
3. Order and interpret the results of diagnostic imaging tests

**D. Analyzing Information**

1. Integrate health history and physical examination findings into the plan of care
2. Assimilate findings from screening and diagnostic testing into plan of care

**E. Diagnosis**

1. Develop and prioritize differential diagnoses
2. Establish a diagnosis based on evaluation of patient data

## III. Management

### A. Child and Caregiver Counseling and Education

1. Provide condition-specific counseling and education, including treatment options
2. Educate about benefits and potential adverse reactions of pharmacological interventions
3. Discuss non-pharmacological interventions
4. Counsel regarding the threshold for seeking follow-up care
5. Review the risks of non-adherence to recommended treatment

### B. Therapeutic Interventions

1. Prescribe pharmacologic agents
2. Recommend the use of over-the-counter pharmacologic agents
3. Order or recommend non-pharmacologic treatments for the management of symptoms
4. Discuss use of complementary and alternative therapies as appropriate

### C. Procedures

1. Perform procedures in accordance with diagnostic guidelines and plan of care (rapid tests)
2. Initiate life-saving techniques in response to urgent or emergent situations

### D. Collaboration and Referral

2. Refer to specialists as indicated for evaluation, counseling, and/or treatment

### E. Care Coordination

1. Facilitate patient and family-centered care for children of all ages with acute and chronic conditions

### F. Evaluation and Follow-up

2. Establish a plan for follow-up care

## IV. Professional Role Responsibilities

### A. Leadership and Evidence-based Practice

4. Develop, implement, and/or modify clinical practice guidelines

# ANATOMY AND PHYSIOLOGY

The anatomy of children's ears differs from that of adults, but hearing is intact at birth. The infant's eustachian tubes are relatively short, wide, and horizontally placed, allowing viruses and bacteria to gain access to the middle ear. Thus, children experience a higher incidence of middle ear effusion and ear infections than do adults (Pagano et al., 2017). With growth and maturation, the eustachian tubes assume a more downward, slanted position. Children may also experience enlargement of the adenoids, causing obstruction of the eustachian tubes and leading to infection. Children produce cerumen in the ear canal. The acidic pH of this waxy substance acts as a hydrophobic protective barrier to the underlying skin of the ear canal by inhibiting bacterial and fungal growth. If a child has a congenital ear anomaly, other congenital anomalies or syndromes may also be present (Table 21.1).

**TABLE 21.1 Congenital Malformations of the Ear**

| Malformation | Significance |
|---|---|
| **Atresia:** failure of the ear canal to form<br>Often associated with microtia and anotia | Resultant conductive hearing loss; pediatric audiology and otolaryngology should evaluate within first 3 months of life |
| **Microtia:** small, collapsed outer ear, or only an ear lobe present (usually deficiency of cartilage and tissue)<br>**Anotia:** absent external ear | Auricle reconstruction around 6 to 8 years of age with introduction of tissue or implants |
| **Prominotia:** ears protrude from the skull<br>**Folded ears:** due to lack of cartilage stiffness or in utero positioning | Taping of ears into correct anatomic position within first 72 to 96 hours of life, continuing until 2 weeks of age<br>If unsuccessful, otoplasty may be performed at school age |
| **Low-set ears:** upper pole is below the eyebrow | Associated with other congenital anomalies; refer to genetics |
| Preauricular tags or pits, ectopic cartilage, fistulas, and cysts | Surgical correction primarily for cosmetic reasons, though pits may become infected |
| *** During embryogenesis, ear formation occurs at the same time as renal development. Test hearing and consider a renal ultrasound *** | |

*Source*: Data from Yoon, P. J., Scholes, M. A., & Herrmann, B. W. (2020). Ear, nose, & throat. In W. W. Hay, M. J. Levin, M. J. Abzug, & M. Bunik (Eds.), *Current diagnosis & treatment: Pediatrics* (25th ed., Chapter 18). McGraw-Hill Education.

# INFECTIOUS DISORDERS

Infectious and inflammatory disorders related to the ears include OE, types of otitis media, and mastoiditis. Inflammation of the external ear canal is termed OE. Inflammation of the middle ear with the presence of fluid is called otitis media. Otitis media is further divided into two categories: acute otitis media (AOM) and otitis media with effusion (OME). *Mastoiditis* refers to an infection involving the mastoid process.

## ACUTE OTITIS MEDIA

AOM is an acute infectious process of the middle ear that may produce fever with a rapid onset of ear pain. Young children contract multiple viral upper respiratory infections annually. These infections permit fluid backup from the nasopharynx into the eustachian tubes. This stagnant fluid provides a prime opportunity for infectious invasion. Infants and young children also have limited response to antigens and lack of previous exposure to common pathogens, placing them at further risk. AOM is most frequently diagnosed in the fall and winter months, associated with the timing of increased respiratory viral activity in temperate climates (Stockmann et al., 2013).

Frequently, an upper respiratory infection precedes AOM. Traveling upward from the nasopharyngeal area along short eustachian tubes, fluid and pathogens invade the middle ear space. With the horizontal positioning of the eustachian tubes, fluid behind the tympanic membrane (TM) has difficulty draining back outward. As these pathogens gain access to the eustachian tube, they proliferate, invading the mucosa. In AOM, ear pain and fever begin acutely. Pain is caused by the increased pressure behind the TM (which may also lead to TM perforation). When the TM perforates, pain is usually decreased because the pressure is relieved and the fluid may drain into the ear canal. Most perforations are completely benign, healing spontaneously (Conover, 2013).

Most commonly, AOM is caused by viral pathogens, but may also be caused by bacteria, specifically *Streptococcus pneumoniae, Haemophilus influenzae,* or *Moraxella catarrhalis*. Viral causes of AOM resolve spontaneously. After the infection clears, fluid may remain in the middle ear space behind the TM, sometimes for several months. The most common complications of AOM are hearing loss, expressive speech delay, TM perforation (acute with resolution or chronic), chronic suppurative otitis media (chronic drainage via perforation or tympanostomy tubes), and less frequently acute mastoiditis, bacterial meningitis, and intracranial abscess.

### Subjective Findings

The health history may reveal:

- Concurrent upper respiratory infection
- Acute onset of pain and fever

#### Risk Factors

The most common risk factors for AOM are:

- Age 1 to 3 years
- Eustachian tube dysfunction (at any age)
- Previous history of AOM or OME
- Passive smoke exposure
- Nasopharyngeal colonization with *Streptococcus pneumoniae, Haemophilus influenzae, or Moraxella catarrhalis*
- Bottle feeding
- Day care attendance
- Immunocompromise
- Native American, Inuit, or Australian aborigine ethnicity
- Genetic susceptibility (family history of AOM; Kaur et al., 2017)

#### Review of Systems

The most common manifestations revealed during the review of systems include:

- **Constitutional:** ear pain, fever, poor feeding, anorexia, difficulty sleeping
- **HEENT:** runny nose, holding or rubbing ear, shaking or banging head (infant), hearing loss
- **Neurologic:** dizziness or vertigo, lethargy, irritability or fussing, inconsolable crying when lying down (infant)

### Objective Findings

The physical examination of the child with AOM may reveal:

- Otoscopic findings specific for AOM (Figure 21.1):
  - Bulging TM
  - Impaired visibility of bony landmarks
  - White or yellow effusion (pus)
  - Opacified/inflamed TM
  - Squamous exudate or bullae on the TM (occasionally)
- Drainage in the ear canal if TM is perforated (Figure 21.2)

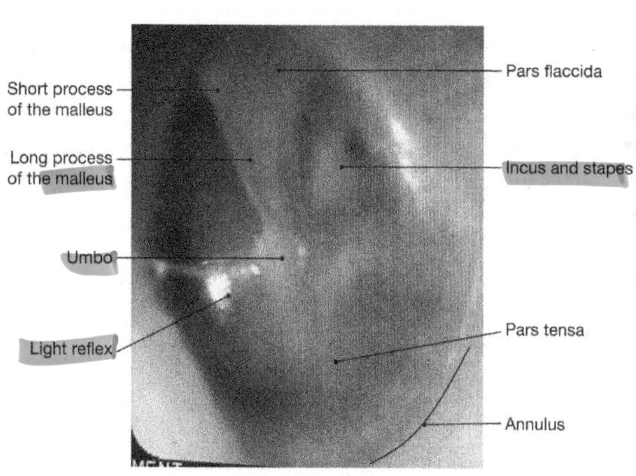


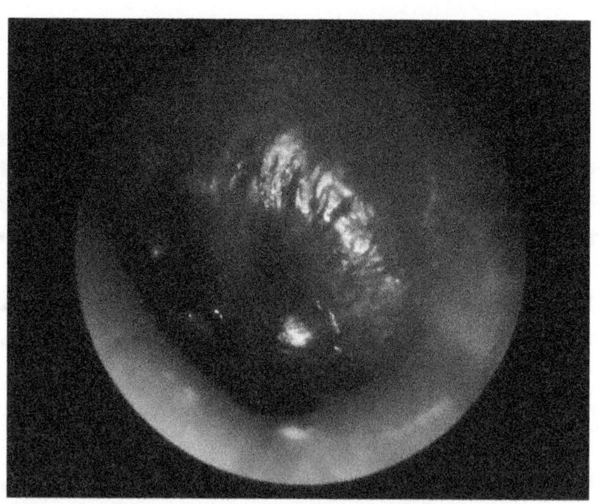

FIGURE 21.1 (A) Normal tympanic membrane (pearly gray with cone of light and bony landmarks visible). (B) Acute otitis media—note bulging of tympanic membrane with obscured bony landmarks.

*Source*: From Gawlik, K. S., Mazurek Melnyk, B., & Teall, A. M. (Eds.). (2021). *Evidence-based physical examination*. Springer Publishing Company.

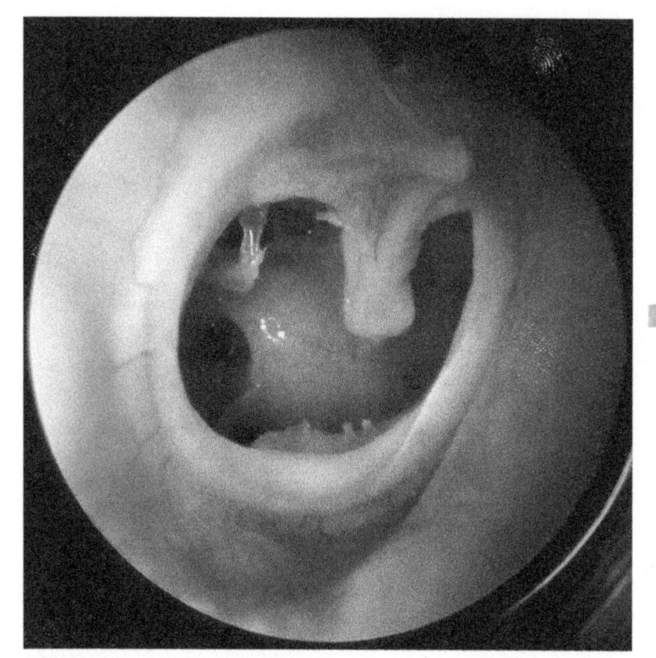

FIGURE 21.2 Note perforation in tympanic membrane.

*Source*: From Gawlik, K. S., Mazurek Melnyk, B., & Teall, A. M. (Eds.). (2021). *Evidence-based physical examination*. Springer Publishing Company.

- Conjunctivitis (same side—termed otitis-conjunctivitis syndrome)
- Ipsilateral anterior cervical lymphadenopathy
- Immobility (Wald, 2020)

**PRO TIP** Redness of the TM is NOT diagnostic of AOM. TM erythema is often a vascular flush caused by fever or crying.

## Laboratory/Diagnostic Testing

The diagnosis of AOM is based upon the clinical findings. No laboratory or diagnostic testing is needed. If diagnosis is uncertain, tympanometry may be utilized to determine presences of effusion.

## Differential Diagnosis

The differential diagnosis for AOM includes:

- OME
- Acute mastoiditis
- Bullous myringitis
- Middle ear mass

## Treatment/Management Plan

Fever and pain may be treated with acetaminophen or ibuprofen. Some children may allow a cool or warm compress to the ear for pain relief, others may not accept it. Over-the-counter numbing ear drops (containing ingredients such as benzocaine) are not advised for use in children as they are not approved by the U.S. Food and Drug Administration (FDA) to be safe and effective (FDA, 2015). Additionally,

TABLE 21.2 **Antibiotic Therapy for Acute Otitis Media**

| Child characteristics | Standard choice | Received a beta-lactam in past 30 days or nonresponsive after 48–72 hours initial antibiotic | Mild or remote allergy to penicillins | Severe reaction to beta-lactams |
|---|---|---|---|---|
| **Under 2 years of age OR with tympanic membrane perforation OR history of recurrent AOM** | Amoxicillin (oral) 90 mg/kg/day in 2 divided doses, max 4 g daily—for 10 days | Amoxicillin/clavulanate [600 mg amoxicillin/5 ml] (oral) 90 mg amoxicillin/kg/day in 2 divided doses, max 4 g amoxicillin daily—for 10 days **OR**<br>Ceftriaxone (intramuscular or intravenous) 50 mg/kg/dose once daily. Max 1 g daily—for 1–3 doses depending on persistence of illness | Cefdinir (oral) 14 mg/kg/day once daily or in 2 divided doses, max 600 mg daily—for 10 days **OR**<br>Cefpodoxime (oral) 10 mg/kg/day in 2 divided doses, max 400 mg daily—for 10 days **OR** | Over 6 months of age: Clindamycin (oral) 20 to 30 mg/kg/day in 3 divided doses, max 1.8 g/day, for 5 to 7 days |
| | | | Cefuroxime (oral) 30 mg/kg/day in 2 divided doses, max 1 g daily—for 10 days | |
| **2 years of age or older with intact tympanic membrane and no history of recurrent AOM** | Amoxicillin (oral) 90 mg/kg/day in 2 divided doses, max 3 g daily—for 5 to 7 days | Amoxicillin/clavulanate (oral) 90 mg amoxicillin/kg/day in 2 divided doses, max 3 g daily—for 5 to 7 days **OR**<br>Ceftriaxone (intramuscular or intravenous) 50 mg/kg/dose once daily. Max 1 g daily—for 1–3 doses depending on persistence of illness | Cefdinir (oral) 14 mg/kg/day once daily or in 2 divided doses, max 600 mg daily—for 5 to 7 days **OR**<br>Cefpodoxime (oral) 10 mg/kg/day in 2 divided doses, max 500 mg daily—for 5 to 7 days | Clindamycin (oral) 20 to 30 mg/kg/day in 3 divided doses, max 1g/day, for 5 to 7 days |
| | | Cefuroxime (oral) 30 mg/kg/day in 2 divided doses, max 1 g daily [children >17 kg, can swallow tablet, 250 mg twice daily]—for 5 to 7 days | | |
| **Otitis-conjunctivitis syndrome** | Amoxicillin/clavulanate (oral) 90 mg amoxicillin/kg/day in 2 divided doses, max 3 g daily—for 10 days in child less than 2 years of age, for 5–7 days age 2 years and older | | | |
| **Uncomplicated acute otorrhea, child 6 months or older** | Ofloxacin (ear drops), 5 drops in affected ear once daily, for 7 days (adolescent 10 drops)<br>**OR** ciprofloxacin 0.25 mL in affected ear, twice daily for 7 days | | | |

*(continued)*

TABLE 21.2 **Antibiotic Therapy for Acute Otitis Media *(continued)***

| Child characteristics | Standard choice | Received a beta-lactam in past 30 days or nonresponsive after 48–72 hours initial antibiotic | Mild or remote allergy to penicillins | Severe reaction to beta-lactams |
|---|---|---|---|---|
| **TM perforation with otorrhea, child 6 months or older** | Ofloxacin (ear drops), 5 drops in affected ear once daily, for 7 days (adolescent 10 drops)<br>**OR** ciprofloxacin 0.25 mL in affected ear, twice daily for 7 days (may use either, with or with steroids) | | | |

*Sources*: Data from Lexicomp. (2020). *Lexicomp clinical drug information* (version 5.7.1) [Mobile app]. App store. https://apps.apple.com/us/app/lexicomp/id313401238; Lieberthal, A. S., Carroll, A. E., Chonmaitree, T., Ganiats, T. G., Hoberman, A., Jackson, M. A., Joffe, M. D., Miller, D. T., Rosenfeld, R. M., Sevilla, X. D., Schwartz, R. H., Thomas. P. A., & Tunkel, D. E. (2013). The diagnosis and management of acute otitis media. *Pediatrics, 131*(3), e964–e999. https://doi.org/10.1542/peds.2012-3488; Pelton, S. (2019). Acute otitis media in children: Treatment. *UpToDate*. https://www.uptodate.com/contents/acute-otitis-media-in-children-treatment; Yoon, P. J., Scholes, M. A., & Herrmann, B. W. (2020). Ear, nose, & throat. In W. W. Hay, M. J. Levin, M. J. Abzug, & M. Bunik (Eds.), *Current diagnosis & treatment: Pediatrics* (25th ed., Chapter 18). McGraw-Hill Education.

the numbing action is of quite short duration. Immediate antibiotic therapy (Table 21.2) is recommended for:

- All infants less than 6 months of age, with unilateral or bilateral AOM
- Those with severe signs or symptoms (moderate to severe ear pain, ear pain for at least 48 hours, temperature ≥39 °C [102.2 °F])
- Children less than 24 months of age with bilateral AOM (Lieberthal et al., 2013)

The choice of either immediate antibiotic therapy or watchful waiting (with pain management) may be used in children:

- 6 to 24 months of age with unilateral nonsevere AOM
- Greater than or equal to 24 months of age with unilateral or bilateral nonsevere AOM (Lieberthal et al., 2013)

With watchful waiting, if the child is improved within 48 to 72 hours, antibiotics are not necessary. Bring the child back into the office for an ear recheck in 3 to 4 weeks' time to determine resolution of effusion.

## Family Education

Teach the following:

- Complete entire course of antibiotics even if the child seems to have improved significantly
- Importance of follow-up, as OME has a potential negative impact on hearing and speech
- Return to or call the office if not improving
- Prevention:
  - Avoid passive smoke exposure for the child
  - Breastfeed for at least 6 to 12 months
  - Do not prop the bottle nor use the pacifier past 6 months of age
  - Avoid excess exposure to individuals with upper respiratory infections
  - Ensure the child is immunized against pneumococcus and influenza

## Referral

Children who fail to demonstrate improvement after several appropriate antibiotic courses may benefit from organism identification (culture) by tympanocentesis performed by pediatric otolaryngology (Lieberthal et al., 2013). Also, refer to pediatric otolaryngology the child with a TM perforation persisting for 3 months (with or without drainage) or with persistent treatment failure.

# OTITIS MEDIA WITH EFFUSION

OME is a collection of fluid in the middle ear space that does not result in any signs and symptoms of infection. It results from the backup of fluid from the nasopharyngeal area. Frequent upper respiratory infections and eustachian tube positioning contribute to the development of OME. OME is a common occurrence, with up to 90% of children having at least one episode of OME by age 5 years (Rosenfeld et al., 2016). OME may occur independent of bouts of AOM or effusion may persist after the infection of AOM has resolved. When OME lasts longer than 3 months, it is termed chronic OME. Complications of OME include AOM, hearing loss, language delay, and deafness.

## Subjective Findings

The health history may reveal complaint of feeling of fullness in the ear.

### Risk Factors

The most common risk factors for OME are:

- Exposure to tobacco smoke
- Absence of breastfeeding (Rosenfeld et al., 2016)
- Otitis-prone parents
- Male gender
- Daycare center attendance
- Hypertrophied adenoids
- Cleft palate
- Low socioeconomic status (Pelton & Marom, 2020)

### Review of Systems

The most common manifestations revealed during the review of systems include:

- **HEENT:** hearing loss (most often noted by parent, not child), tinnitus
- **Neurologic:** balance issues (stumbling, falling, clumsiness)

## Objective Findings

The physical examination of the child with OME may reveal:

- Neutral or retracted TM (not bulging)
- TM light amber to gray-white in color, possibly with air fluid level (Figure 21.3)
- TM is immobile with pneumatic otoscopy

## Procedure 21.1 Performing Pneumatic Otoscopy

**Materials:**

- Insufflator
- Otoscope
- Speculum

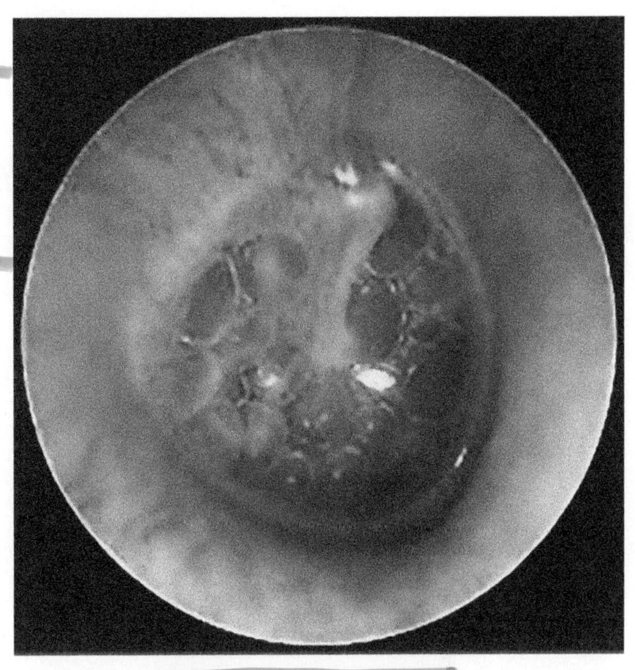

FIGURE 21.3 Otitis media with effusion.

*Source*: From Gawlik, K. S., Mazurek Melnyk, B., & Teall, A. M. (Eds.). (2021). *Evidence-based physical examination*. Springer Publishing Company.

**Steps in the Procedure:**

1. Connect the insufflator to the otoscope (Figure 21.4).
2. Ensure a good seal between the ear canal and the speculum.
3. Gently squeeze the bulb to provide a small puff of air.
4. Observe lack of movement of the TM in response to the negative pressure created.

**PRO TIP** A pearly white or greasy-looking mass seen in a retraction pocket or perforation behind the TM is suggestive of a cholesteatoma (Figure 21.5). Refer the child to pediatric otolaryngology for further evaluation.

### Laboratory/Diagnostic Testing

The diagnosis of OME is based upon the clinical findings. Tympanometry is useful in verifying the presence of fluid behind the TM. The tympanometer measures TM compliance and displays it in a graphical form. Accuracy of the reading is depending upon the child holding still and a good seal in the ear canal. Normal movement of the TM results

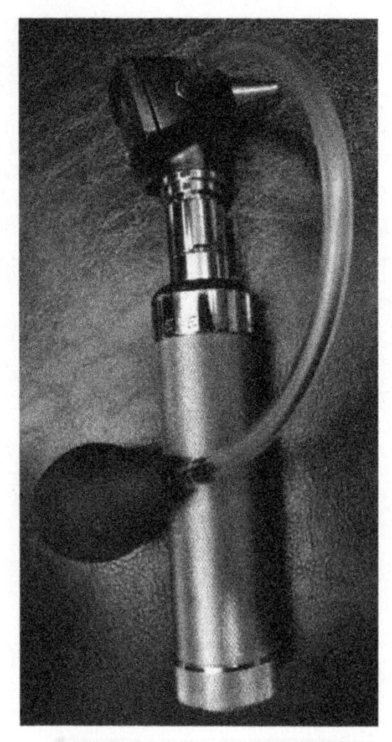

FIGURE 21.4 Insufflator attached to otoscope for pneumatic otoscopy.

*Source*: From Gawlik, K. S., Mazurek Melnyk, B., & Teall, A. M. (Eds.). (2021). *Evidence-based physical examination*. Springer Publishing Company.

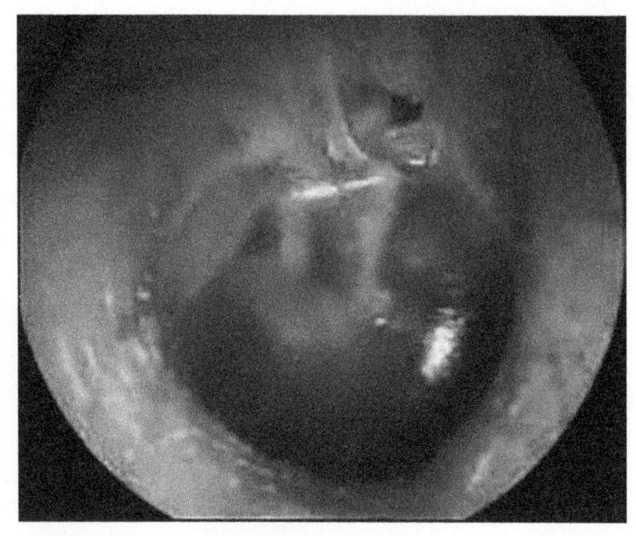

FIGURE 21.5 Cholesteatoma.

*Source*: From Gawlik, K. S., Mazurek Melnyk, B., & Teall, A. M. (Eds.). (2021). *Evidence-based physical examination*. Springer Publishing Company.

in in a bell-shaped curve on the graph (Figure 21.6). When the TM becomes immobile (with OME or AOM), the graph is flattened.

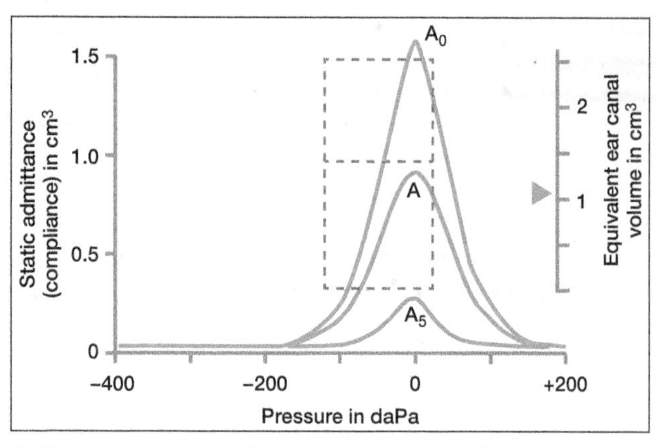


FIGURE 21.6 Normal tympanometry result.

*Source*: Reproduced with permission from Dr. David Klemm.

## Differential Diagnosis

The differential diagnosis for OME includes AOM.

## Treatment/Management Plan

Management of uncomplicated OME includes observation for up to 3 months. In children with no or minimal hearing changes, no risk factors for language delay, and a structurally normal TM, observation may last for a longer period.

ALERT: Do not treat OME with antibiotics, as there is no infection present (Rosenfeld et al., 2016). The use of antibiotics in the absence of infection contributes to antibiotic resistance (World Health Organization, 2020). Additionally, treatment with antihistamines or corticosteroids is also inappropriate, as they have not been shown to alter the course of OME.

## Family Education

Teach the following:

- The natural history of OME
- Observe for worsening hearing loss or lack of speech development
- Comply with follow-up appointment to determine resolution of OME
- For the child experiencing mild hearing loss with OME, communicate more effectively with the child by doing the following:
  - Turn off music or the television, position yourself within 3 feet of the child before speaking, and face the child while speaking

- Only increase the volume of speech slightly, speaking clearly
- Use visual cues as needed
- Request preferential classroom seating

### Referral

In the young child with hearing loss and possible delay in development, the placement of tympanostomy tubes may be helpful. Referal to pediatric otolaryngology is indicated for:

- TM retraction pockets or adhesive atelectasis
- Hearing loss greater than 40 dB
- Ossicular erosion
- Cholesteatoma

## OTITIS EXTERNA

OE refers to an infection with inflammation (cellulitis) of the skin of the external ear canal, with *Pseudomonas aeruginosa* and *Staphylococcus aureus* being typical causative agents. Other bacteria, and fungi such as *Aspergillus* may also cause OE. Pathogens grow in the ear canal particularly when it is moist, as the altered pH created by the moisture contributes to the inflammatory process. OE is commonly called swimmer's ear, as the often-wet ear canals of swimmers contribute to the development of OE (Yoon et al., 2020).

### Subjective Findings

The health history may reveal ear pain and drainage, worsening over a 3-day period.

### Risk Factors

The most common risk factors for OE:

- Frequently wet ears
- Summer season
- Swimming in a pool, ocean, or lake
- Humid climate
- Trauma to the ear canal skin (use of cotton swabs, earbuds, ear plugs, or by scratching)
- Atopic dermatitis

### Review of Systems

The most common manifestations revealed during the review of systems include:

- **Constitutional:** pain
- **HEENT:** ear itching, feeling of ear canal fullness, decreased hearing

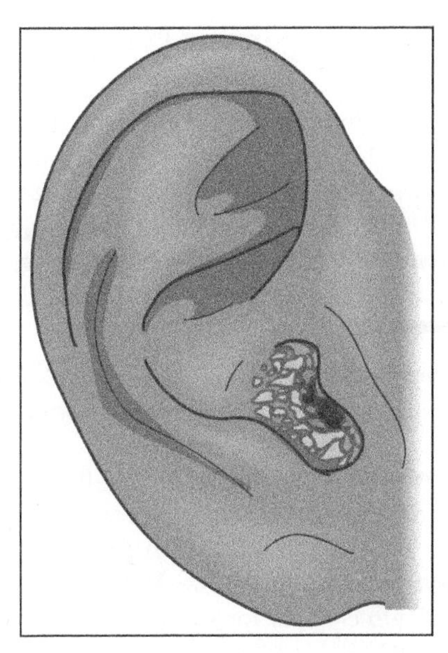

FIGURE 21.7 Note the edematous canal and drainage occurring with OE.

### Objective Findings

The physical examination of the child with OE may reveal:

- Clear, white, or purulent drainage
- Swollen, narrow, erythematous external ear canal (Figure 21.7)
- Child resistance to otoscopy
- Normal TM (though it may be difficult to see due to ear canal debris and edema)

**PRO TIP** Pressure on the tragus results in significant pain.

### Laboratory/Diagnostic Testing

The diagnosis of OE is based upon the clinical findings. Laboratory or diagnostic testing is not needed, unless the condition is resistant to treatment, in which case a fungal culture of ear drainage may be warranted.

### Differential Diagnosis

The differential diagnosis for OE includes:

- Acute or chronic otitis media with TM rupture
- Mastoiditis
- Furunculosis of the ear canal
- Chronic OE
- *Herpes zoster oticus*

### Treatment/Management Plan

The primary goals of treatment of OE are clearance of the infection, pain relief, and prevention of recurrence. Analgesics and a warm compress or heating pad to the affected ear are helpful in some children. Gently remove debris from the canal as able. Prescribe an otic fluoroquinolone with or without otic corticosteroid (to decrease ear canal inflammation) in children over 6 months of age:

- Ciprofloxacin otic solution 0.2%—0.25 mL twice daily in each affected ear for 7 days (doses about 12 hours apart)
- Ciprofloxacin otic suspension 0.6%—0.2 mL in each affected ear once (by healthcare provider; liquid becomes a gel upon contact with ear canal)
- Ofloxacin otic solution 0.3%—5 drops once daily in each affected ear for 7 days (10 drops for adolescents)

An ear wick may have to be placed if the ear canal is too edematous to allow passage of the ear drops. Insertion of the ear wick can be quite painful; ensure that the child is restrained in an atraumatic fashion during the insertion to maintain safety.

### Family Education

Teach the following:

- Keep the ear dry until the infection has cleared.
- It is important to keep the ear canals dry to prevent future episodes. After showering or swimming:
  - Avoid the use of cotton swabs, headphones, and earbuds
  - Wear earplugs when swimming
  - To promote ear canal dryness and alternate pH, use one of the following:
    - After showering or swimming, dry the ear canals using a hair dryer set on a lower setting.
    - Administer a drying solution such as a mixture of half rubbing alcohol and half vinegar (gently squirt into the canal and allow to run out), Domeboro solution (place a few drops in canal and allow to run out), or other available over-the-counter drying solution (Cook, 2016)

▶ ALERT: Use the alcohol solution ONLY when the canals are healthy, as it may cause a significant stinging and burning sensation if used when the child has OE.

### Referral

Refer the child whose OE is nonresponsive to treatment to pediatric otolaryngology for further evaluation.

## MASTOIDITIS

A suppurative complication of AOM, acute mastoiditis occurs when purulent material accumulates within the mastoid cavities, although some children with mastoiditis do not have a history of AOM. It may range in severity from inflammation of the mastoid periosteum to bony destruction of the mastoid air cells and abscess development. The primary bacteria most common in acute mastoiditis are *Streptococcus pneumoniae, Streptococcus pyogenes*, and *Staphylococcus aureus* (Wald, 2018). More than 60% of cases of mastoiditis occur in children younger than 2 years of age (Yoon et al., 2020). Complications of mastoiditis include subperiosteal, neck, or intracranial abscess; hearing loss; labyrinthitis; facial nerve paralysis; osteomyelitis; and meningitis.

### Subjective Findings

Some children may be asymptomatic, and in others the health history may reveal fever and ear pain.

### Risk Factors

The most common risk factor for mastoiditis is AOM.

### Review of Systems

The most common manifestations revealed during the review of systems include:

- **Constitutional:** lethargy, malaise, poor feeding, pain
- **Gastrointestinal:** diarrhea
- **Neurologic:** irritability (young children)

### Objective Findings

The physical examination of the child with mastoiditis may reveal:

- Erythema and induration of the mastoid area
- Edema and fluctuance of the mastoid area as the disease progresses
- Narrowing of the external ear canal
- Otorrhea
- Evidence of AOM
- Ear protrusion (late finding)
  - Outwardly displaced pinna (children)
  - Downwardly displaced pinna (infants)

### Laboratory/Diagnostic Testing

The diagnosis of mastoiditis is based upon the clinical findings. If obtained, the white blood cell count may be elevated and demonstrate a left shift, while C-reactive protein and erythrocyte sedimentation rates may also be elevated. Early mastoiditis may be difficult to distinguish from AOM on computed tomography (CT) scan, but as it progresses the CT scan may show coalescence of mastoid air cells characteristic of bone destruction.

### Differential Diagnosis

The differential diagnosis for mastoiditis includes:

- Lymphadenitis
- OE
- Parotitis
- Furuncle
- Trauma
- Tumor
- Histiocytosis

### Treatment/Management Plan

Mastoiditis is treated with intravenous (IV) antibiotic therapy.

### Family Education

Teach the following:

- The prognosis for full recovery is good

### Referral

Refer the child with mastoiditis for hospitalization for IV antibiotic therapy. The child who is not demonstrating improvement within 24 to 48 hours of IV antibiotics should be referred to pediatric otolaryngology for possible surgical intervention.

## FOREIGN BODY IN THE EAR CANAL

Foreign bodies may enter the ear canal intentionally (the child places something in) or accidentally (such as an insect or playground mulch). Additionally, cerumen may impact the ear canal, effectively acting as a foreign body.

### Subjective Findings

The health history may reveal the child reporting there is something in the ear.

### Risk Factors

The most common risk factors for a foreign body in the ear canal are:

- Young age (intentional foreign body insertion)
- Use of cotton swabs (cerumen impaction)

### Review of Systems

The most common manifestations revealed during the review of systems include:

- **Constitutional:** possibly pain
- **HEENT:** difficulty hearing (cerumen impaction)

### Objective Findings

The physical examination of the child with ear canal foreign body may reveal the foreign body or impacted cerumen.

▶ ALERT: If the foreign object is a disk-type battery, an electric current can be generated in the moist canal, resulting in a burn. Immediate referral to pediatric otolaryngology or the emergency department is warranted.

### Laboratory/Diagnostic Testing

The diagnosis of foreign body in the ear canal or cerumen impaction is based upon the clinical findings.

### Differential Diagnosis

The differential diagnosis for foreign body in the ear canal includes trauma.

### Treatment/Management Plan

Small objects not close to the TM may be gently irrigated out of the canal, avoiding aggressive irritation to prevent canal trauma. Vegetative objects may be retrieved with a curette in some instances. If the object is close to the orifice, straight alligator forceps may be used to grip and remove it. Never irrigate the canal if a vegetative object is noted or suspected, as the water causes the object to swell, making removal more difficult. Also do not irrigate the canal if the TM cannot be visualized, as a perforation could be present. To encourage live insects to exit the ear canal independently, turn off the light in the room, straighten the ear canal, and shine a penlight directly toward the canal (Alfaifi et al., 2019).

## Procedure 21.2 Cerumen Removal

**Materials:**

Metal or plastic cerumen curette (loop on end)
Cerumenolytic, e.g., hydrogen peroxide

**Steps in the Procedure:**

1. Utilize a metal or plastic cerumen curette (loop on end) to gently remove cerumen from the canal.
2. Use of a cerumenolytic such as hydrogen peroxide helps to soften the cerumen, facilitating removal.
3. Irrigation should only be used for cerumen removal if the TM is visualized and intact, which is rare with cerumen impaction.

### Family Education

Teach the following:

- The child should not put anything in the ears
- Cerumen is normal and helps to protect the ear canal
- Do not use cotton swabs to clean the ears

### Referral

Do not attempt to remove the foreign body if it is large enough to obscure the TM, or is so deep in the ear canal as to be adjacent to the TM. Refer these children to pediatric otolaryngology for safe removal of the foreign body.

## EAR TRAUMA

Traumatic perforation of the TM, hearing loss, hematoma of the middle ear, facial nerve injury, vertigo, or ossicular chain disruption may occur as a result of head or blast injury, an ear canal blow, sudden impact with water, or by insertion of pointed objects into the ear canal. Of note is that serious penetrating wounds of the TM may occur with parental use of cotton swabs (Yoon et al., 2020). When middle ear trauma occurs, sensorineural hearing loss may result from a perilymphatic fistula and can be prevented/reversed with emergency surgery.

### Subjective Findings

The health history may reveal the mechanism of injury.

### Risk Factors

The most common risk factors for ear trauma are:

- Parental use of cotton swabs for ear cleaning
- Lack of helmet use with recommended sports
- Water or snow skiing
- Firearm/explosive use

### Review of Systems

The most common manifestations revealed during the review of systems include:

- **Constitutional:** pain
- **HEENT:** hearing loss, ear drainage or bleeding, tinnitus
- **Gastrointestinal:** nausea, vomiting
- **Neurologic:** imbalance

### Objective Findings

The physical examination of the child with ear trauma may reveal:

- Bruising in and around the ear
- Ear drainage or bleeding
- Perforation of or hematoma on the TM
- Hearing deficit by audiometric testing, or by Weber or Rinne testing in cooperative child over 5 years old (Evans & Handler, 2019)

### Laboratory/Diagnostic Testing

The diagnosis of ear trauma is based upon the clinical findings. Ear drainage should be evaluated for the presence of cerebrospinal fluid, which if present could indicate basilar skull fracture warranting a head CT scan.

### Treatment/Management Plan

Most cases of ear trauma warrant referral to a specialist. The child with TM perforation and minimal hearing loss (<40 dB on formal audiometry), and without nausea, vomiting, ataxia, or nystagmus, may be observed by the primary care provider. If the wound is contaminated, ofloxacin or ciprofloxacin ear drops may be administered. Repeat audiometry and check TM healing in 4 weeks (as both should be restored by then) (Evans & Handler, 2019).

### Family Education

Teach the following:

- Do not put anything in the ears, including cotton swabs
- Use helmet and ear protection as appropriate to the situation

### Referral

Urgently refer to pediatric otolaryngology any child who experiences subjective hearing loss, facial paralysis, or severe vertigo after ear trauma, as emergent surgery may be needed. If child maltreatment is suspected, refer to child protective services.

## HEARING IMPAIRMENT

Hearing loss may be congenital or acquired. Ordinarily, infants are born with the sense of hearing fully developed. In the United States, congenital hearing loss occurs at the rate of 1.33 per 1,000 live births, with most being inherited through a single gene or associated with a syndrome, although it may also occur as a result of prenatal infection (Korver et al., 2017). Newborn universal hearing screening mandates have been passed by legislation in 43 states, allowing for earlier identification of infants with congenital hearing loss (National Center for Hearing Assessment and Management, 2020).

Language development in infancy and early childhood is dependent upon adequate hearing; thus, it is imperative to identify congenital hearing loss so it can be treated early. Intermittent episodes of AOM and chronic or intermittent OME may result in fluctuating hearing loss which can delay language development (Searight et al., 2020). Hearing loss may be unilateral or bilateral. Measuring the softest intensity of sound that is perceived in decibels (dB) determines the extent of hearing loss. Levels of hearing loss are:

- 0 to 20 dB: normal
- 20 to 40 dB: mild loss
- 40 to 60 dB: moderate loss
- 60 to 80 dB: severe loss
- Greater than 80 dB: profound loss (American Speech-Language-Hearing Association [ASHA], n.d.-b)

Acquired hearing loss may be conductive, sensorineural, or mixed:

- **Conductive hearing loss:** transmission of sound through the middle ear is disrupted (OME)
- **Sensorineural hearing loss:** damage to the hair cells in the cochlea or along the auditory pathway
- **Mixed hearing loss:** cause is attributed to both sensorineural and conductive problems

Whether conductive, sensorineural, or mixed hearing loss, early identification allows for intervention with hearing aids, cochlear implants, communication devices, and/or speech education. These interventions may enable children with hearing loss to communicate verbally, and enhanced communication beginning in infancy and early childhood also has the potential to improve the child's school achievement.

### Subjective Findings

The health history may reveal:

- Parental perception that infant or child does not seem to hear well
- Child speaks loudly
- Sits close to television or radio, or turns volume up loud

### Risk Factors

The most common risk factors for hearing impairment are:

- Premature birth
- History of persistent pulmonary hypertension of the newborn
- Genetic syndrome
- Conductive hearing loss:
  - OME
- Sensorineural hearing loss:
  - Severe neonatal respiratory depression
  - Intrauterine infection with cytomegalovirus or rubella
  - Kernicterus
  - Neonatal or postnatal infection (e.g., meningitis)
  - Use of ototoxic medication
  - Exposure to excess noise

### Review of Systems

The most common manifestations revealed during the review of systems include:

- **Behavioral/Developmental:**
  - *Infant:*
    - Only wakes to touch, not environmental noises
    - Loud noises do not result in startle
    - Does not turn to sound by 4 months of age, babble at 6 months of age, or progress with speech development
  - *Young child:*
    - Communicates needs through gestures, does not speak by 2 years of age, or does not speak distinctly, as appropriate for age
    - Cognitive delay
    - Immature emotional behavior, prefers solitary play
    - When communicating, focuses on facial expressions
  - *Older child:*
    - Monotone or other abnormal speech
    - Often asks for statements to be repeated or inappropriate answers to questions except when able to view face of speaker
    - Inattentive, daydreams, performs poorly at school

### Objective Findings

Determine the child's level of interaction with the environment. The physical examination of the child with hearing impairment may reveal:

- Abnormal external or internal ear development
- Potential hearing loss with whisper, Weber, or Rinne tests (preschoolers and older children)
- Actual hearing loss with brainstem evoked-response, otoacoustic emission, or audiometry tests

### Laboratory/Diagnostic Testing

The diagnosis of hearing impairment is based upon objective documentation of hearing loss as noted earlier. Several methods of audiometry exist:

- Conventional audiometry: child indicates when they hear a sound (5 years and over)
- Conditioned play audiometry: child responds to sound stimulus by performing activity (e.g., putting a peg into a board; 2.5 to 5 years)
- Visual reinforcement audiometry: auditory stimulus paired with positive reinforcement. (Child reacts appropriately by turning toward a sound source, behavior rewarded by activation of a toy that lights up. After a brief conditioning period, the child localizes toward the tone (if audible) in anticipation of the lighted toy (6 months to 2.5 years)
- Behavioral observational audiometry: performed by audiologist watching closely for a reaction to sound presented (birth to 6 months)

### Differential Diagnosis

The differential diagnosis for hearing impairment involves determining the type of hearing loss—either conductive, sensorineural, or mixed type—in order to best guide further evaluation and treatment.

### Treatment/Management Plan

A multidisciplinary approach is recommended for optimal management of hearing loss. Specialists may prescribe hearing aids, or recommend and train the child in augmentative communication devices (American Speech Language Association, n.d. -a). Alternatively, cochlear implants may be recommended (National Institute of Deafness and Other Communication Disorders, 2021).

### Family Education

Teach the following:

- If hearing aids are prescribed, how to use, change batteries, and otherwise care for them and reinforce the specialist's instructions
- Follow through with augmentative communication devices to best support the child's communication skills
- Use lights rather than bells or alarms to alert the child; use text telephone service and closed-caption television
- Educate children with disabilities, have an individualized family service plan, and advocate for their child with the school
- Reinforce family education of American Sign Language if being used

▶ ALERT: Hearing aid batteries are a serious aspiration risk. Keep them out of the reach of young children.

### Referral

Refer the child with hearing impairment to early intervention (if less than 3 years of age), audiologist experienced with infants and children, pediatric otolaryngology, speech-language pathology, and educational specialists (when ready to attend school).

## KEY POINTS

- AOM is identified by acute onset of fever and pain, with a bulging, dull TM.
- Treatment of AOM is dependent upon the child's history and age.
- OME may last for weeks at a time. Refer children in whom hearing loss from OME is affecting their language development.
- Maintain dry ears to prevent OE.
- Mastoiditis requires IV antibiotics.
- Carefully evaluate foreign bodies in the ear canal to determine method for removal or if the problem should be referred to an ear, nose, and throat specialist.
- Most cases of ear trauma require referral to pediatric otolaryngology, although a small TM perforation with mild hearing loss should clear by 4 weeks and can be followed by the primary care provider.
- Hearing loss, whether congenital or acquired, conductive or sensorineural, requires early intervention to best develop the child's communication skills.

## REFERENCES

Alfaifi, A. J., Khan, L. A., & Mokarbesh, H. M. (2019). Light-assisted removal of ear canal live insect—A noninvasive approach for first level responders. *Journal of Family Medicine and Primary Care, 8*(9), 3042–3044. https://doi.org/10.4103/jfmpc.jfmpc_443_19

American Speech-Language-Hearing Association. (n.d.-a). *Augmentative and alternative communication (AAC).* https://www.asha.org/practice-portal/professional-issues/augmentative-and-alternative-communication/

American Speech-Language-Hearing Association. (n.d.-b). *Degree of hearing loss.* https://www.asha.org/public/hearing/degree-of-hearing-loss/

Conover, K. (2013). Earache. *Emergency Medicine Clinics of North America, 31*(2), 413–442. https://doi.org/10.1016/j.emc.2013.02.001

Cook, S. P. (2016). *Swimmer's ear.* http://kidshealth.org/kid/ill_injure/aches/swimmers_ear.html

Evans, A. K., & Handler, S. D. (2019). Evaluation and management of middle ear trauma. *UpToDate.* https://www.uptodate.com/contents/evaluation-and-management-of-middle-ear-trauma

Food and Drug Administration. (2015). *FDA: Use only approved prescription ear drops.* https://www.fda.gov/consumers/consumer-updates/fda-use-only-approved-prescription-ear-drops

Kaur, R., Morris, M., & Pichichero, M. E. (2017). Epidemiology of acute otitis media in the postpneumococcal conjugate vaccine era. *Pediatrics, 140*(3), e20170181. https://doi.org/10.1542/peds.2017-0181

Korver, A., Smith, R., Van Camp, G., Schleiss, M., Bitner-Glindzicz, M., Lustig, L., Usami, S., & Boudewyns, A. (2017). Congenital hearing loss. *Nature Reviews Disease Primers, 3*, 16094. https://doi.org/10.1038/nrdp.2016.94

Lexicomp. (2020). *Lexicomp clinical drug information* (version 5.7.1) [Mobile app]. App store. https://apps.apple.com/us/app/lexicomp/id313401238

Lieberthal, A. S., Carroll, A. E., Chonmaitree, T., Ganiats, T. G., Hoberman, A., Jackson, M. A., Joffe, M. D., Miller, D. T., Rosenfeld, R. M., Sevilla, X. D., Schwartz, R. H., Thomas, P. A., & Tunkel, D. E. (2013). The diagnosis and management of acute otitis media. *Pediatrics, 131*(3), e964–e999. https://doi.org/10.1542/peds.2012-3488

National Center for Hearing Assessment and Management. (2020). *EDHI legislation: Overview.* http://www.infanthearing.org/legislation/

National Institute on Deafness and Other Communication Disorders. (2021). *Cochlear implants.* http://www.nidcd.nih.gov/health/hearing/pages/coch.aspx

Pagano, A., Wang, E., Yuan, D., Fischer, D., Bluestone, C. D., Marquez, S., & Laitman, J. T. (2017). Cranial indicators identified for peak incidence of otitis media. *Anatomical Record: Advances in Integrative Anatomy and Evolutionary Biology, 300*, 1721–1740. https://doi.org/10.1002/ar.23625

Pelton, S. (2019). Acute otitis media in children: Treatment. *UpToDate.* https://www.uptodate.com/contents/acute-otitis-media-in-children-treatment

Pelton, S., & Marom, T. (2020). Otitis media with effusion (serous otitis media) in children: Management. *UpToDate.* http://www.uptodate.com/contents/otitis-media-with-effusion-serous-otitis-media-in-children-management

Rosenfeld, R. M., Shin, J. J., Schwartz, S. R., Coggins, R., Gagnon, L., Hackell, J. M., Hoelting, D., Hunter, L. L., Kummer, A. W., Payne, S. C., Poe, D. S., Veling, M., Vila, P. M., Walsh, S. A., & Corrigan, M. D. (2016). Clinical practice guideline: Otitis media with effusion (update). *Otolaryngology—Head and Neck Surgery, 154*(1 Suppl.), S1–S41. https://doi.org/10.1177/0194599815623467

Searight, F. T., Singh, R., & Peterson, D. C. (2020). *Otitis media with effusion.* https://www.ncbi.nlm.nih.gov/books/NBK538293/

Stockmann, C., Ampofo, K., Hersh, A. L., Carleton, S. T., Korgenski, K., Sheng, X., Pavia, A. T., & Byington, C. L. (2013). Seasonality of acute otitis media and the role of respiratory viral activity in children. *The Pediatric Infectious Disease Journal, 32*(4), 314–319. https://doi.org/10.1097/INF.0b013e31827d104e

Wald, E. R. (2018). Acute mastoiditis in children: Clinical features and diagnosis. *UpToDate.* https://www.uptodate.com/contents/acute-mastoiditis-in-children-clinical-features-and-diagnosis

Wald, E. R. (2020). Acute otitis media in children: Clinical manifestations and diagnosis. *UpToDate.* https://www.uptodate.com/contents/acute-otitis-media-in-children-clinical-manifestations-and-diagnosis

World Health Organization. (2020). *Antibiotic resistance.* https://www.who.int/news-room/fact-sheets/detail/antibiotic-resistance

Yoon, P. J., Scholes, M. A., & Herrmann, B. W. (2020). Ear, nose, & throat. In W. W. Hay, M. J. Levin, M. J. Abzug, & M. Bunik (Eds.), *Current diagnosis & treatment: Pediatrics* (25th ed., Chapter 18). McGraw-Hill Education.

# Management of Mouth Disorders

Theresa Kyle

## Student Learning Outcomes

**Upon completion of this chapter the reader should be able to:**

1. Discuss pathophysiology and epidemiology of selected mouth disorders in children.
2. Differentiate subjective and objective findings of selected mouth disorders in children.
3. Choose appropriate laboratory or diagnostic tests for selected mouth disorders in children.
4. Utilize the differential diagnosis process to determine the diagnosis of mouth and tooth disorders in children.
5. Determine treatment plan, child/family education, and need for referral for children with a mouth or tooth disorder.

## INTRODUCTION

Nutrition is critical during childhood to appropriately support growth and development, and having a healthy mouth is key to being able to eat and drink properly. Younger children are susceptible to infectious disorders of the mouth owing to their developmental stage (always putting thing in their mouths). Younger children are also developing their primary teeth, then later their permanent teeth. Ensuring that the teeth remain healthy is important not only to the ability to eat properly, but also to avoid other morbidities.

The content in this chapter maps to the following areas on the Pediatric Nursing Certification Board (PNCB) Pediatric Nurse Practitioner—Primary Care certification examination:

**CLINICAL PROBLEMS: HEAD, EYE, EAR, NOSE, AND THROAT**

CONTENT AREAS:

### II. Assessment and Diagnosis

**B. History and Physical Examination**

1. Obtain history of present illness
2. Obtain a comprehensive health history for new patients
3. Complete an interval history for established patients
4. Perform a review of systems
5. Perform a complete physical examination

**C. Diagnostic Testing and Screening**

1. Order and interpret office/clinic based screening tests
2. Order and interpret diagnostic laboratory tests

**D. Analyzing Information**

1. Integrate health history and physical examination findings into the plan of care
2. Assimilate findings from screening and diagnostic testing into plan of care

**E. Diagnosis**

1. Develop and prioritize differential diagnoses
2. Establish a diagnosis based on evaluation of patient data

### III. Management

**A. Child and Caregiver Counseling and Education**

1. Provide condition-specific counseling and education, including treatment options
2. Educate about benefits and potential adverse reactions of pharmacological interventions
3. Discuss non-pharmacological interventions
4. Counsel regarding the threshold for seeking follow-up care
5. Review the risks of non-adherence to recommended treatment

**B. Therapeutic Interventions**

1. Prescribe pharmacologic agents
2. Recommend the use of over-the-counter pharmacologic agents
3. Order or recommend non-pharmacologic treatments for the management of symptoms
4. Discuss use of complementary and alternative therapies as appropriate

**D. Collaboration and Referral**

2. Refer to specialists as indicated for evaluation, counseling, and/or treatment

**E. Care Coordination**

1. Facilitate patient and family-centered care for children of all ages with acute and chronic conditions

**F. Evaluation and Follow-up**

2. Establish a plan for follow-up care

### IV. Professional Role Responsibilities

**A. Leadership and Evidence-based Practice**

4. Develop, implement, and/or modify clinical practice guidelines

## ANATOMY AND PHYSIOLOGY

The mouth is a highly vascular area of the body that allows for easy absorption of medications or microorganisms. Additionally, the cells of the oral mucosa experience rapid cell turnover. Normal development in infants and younger children involves exploration of objects with the mouth, placing them at increased risk for invading infectious organisms. Newborns are usually born without teeth, with initial tooth eruption occurring by the second half of infancy. Refer to chapter 7 for additional information on tooth eruption. The primary teeth are usually all established by 33 months of age. They then begin shedding at around 6 to 7 years of age, when the permanent teeth begin erupting. Children have a full set of 28 permanent teeth by about 13 years of age. The third molars (wisdom teeth) may begin erupting between 17 and 21 years of age. Adolescents may demonstrate intraoral piercings or tattoos, and they may chew tobacco or betel (areca) nuts, which place them at increased risk for infection and mouth cancer.

# ORAL LESIONS

A number of oral lesions may affect infants and children, resulting in stomatitis. *Stomatitis* is an inflammation of the oral cavity and may present with particular lesions or as more generalized erythema and inflammation. A few commonly occurring oral lesions are aphthous ulcers, herpetic gingivostomatitis, and herpangina. Aphthous ulcers may occur without a identifiable cause or may result from trauma, vitamin deficiency, or celiac or Crohn disease. Herpes simplex virus type 1 (HSV-1) is the causative agent for gingivostomatitis. Herpangina results from infection with an enterovirus (typically Coxsackie virus). Regardless of type, oral lesions are often painful and can interfere with the child's ability to eat.

## APHTHOUS ULCERS

Aphthous ulcers are commonly called canker sores. Most children with will experience at least one episode of aphthous ulcer eruption. Sometimes the ulcers recur and in this situation it is termed recurrent aphthous stomatitis.

### Subjective Findings

Note the onset of the lesion(s) and progression over time. Determine the history of present illness from the parent and child (as age allows); the health history is generally otherwise negative.

#### Risk Factors

The most common risk factors for aphthous ulcers are:

- Stress
- Exposure to infectious agents
- Trauma
- Immune deficiency, cancer chemotherapy, or radiation treatment
- Celiac or Crohn disease

## Review of Systems

The most common manifestations revealed during the review of systems include:

- **Constitutional:** pain, difficulty eating or drinking (refusal in the young child or infant), absence of fever
- **Lymphatic:** absence cervical lymphadenopathy

## Objective Findings

Inspect the oral cavity, including the tongue, buccal mucosa, palate, and hypoglossal area. Note the presence of lesions and their distribution. Typically, the minor variety occurs and small round craters (<5 mm in diameter) may occur on any of the surfaces of the oral cavity. They most commonly occur on nonkeratonized oral surfaces such as the lips, cheeks, ventral surface of the tongue, or floor of the mouth. Refer to Table 22.1 for descriptions and illustrations of various oral lesions, including aphthous ulcers.

**PRO TIP** Lesions >5 mm may also occur and are considered the major variety. They may last as long as 6 weeks, and leave a scar (Nield, 2017).

## Laboratory/Diagnostic Testing

Generally, the diagnosis of aphthous ulcer is based on the history and clinical presentation, but occasionally oral lesions are cultured for HSV.

## Differential Diagnosis

The differential diagnosis for aphthous ulcer includes:

- Irritant or allergic contact stomatitis
- Herpetic gingivostomatitis

**TABLE 22.1 Comparison Chart: Oral Lesions**

| | Aphthous Ulcers | Gingivostomatitis | Herpangina |
|---|---|---|---|
| **Appearance** | Erythematous border, often yellow appearance to the ulcer, anywhere on oral mucosa or lips | Vesicular lesions on erythematous base, anywhere in oral cavity, including lips | Bright-red ulcers, generally in posterior oral cavity |
| **Fever** | Generally absent | May have high fever with initial outbreak | Abrupt onset of high fever (up to 39.4–40.6 °C), lasting 1–4 days |
| **Length of illness** | Generally heal within 7–14 days; may recur | 10–12 days initially; may recur with stress, febrile illness, or intense sunlight exposure (as virus lies dormant in system) | Generally resolves within 5–7 days |
| **Therapeutic management** | Topical corticosteroid in dental paste may help | Acyclovir | Supportive treatment only |

*Sources*: Data from Keels, M. A., & Clements, D. A. (2019). Herpetic gingivostomatitis in young children. *UpToDate*. Retrieved October 14, 2020, from http://www.uptodate.com/contents/herpetic-gingivostomatitis-in-young-children; Solo-Josephson, P. (2017). *Canker sores*. Retrieved October 14, 2020, from http://kidshealth.org/parent/general/aches/canker.html#; Romero, J. R. (2020). Hand, foot, and mouth disease and herpangina. *UpToDate*. Retrieved October 14, 2020, from http://www.uptodate.com/contents/hand-foot-and-mouth-disease-and-herpangina

Aphthous ulcer photograh courtesy of Centers for Disease Control and Prevention, ID 12620, 1967.

Herpangina photograph from Gawlik, K. S., Mazurek Melnyk, B., & Teall, A. M. (Eds.). (2021). *Evidence-based physical examination*. Springer Publishing Company.

- Herpangina
- Acute cutaneous lupus erythematosus
- Behçet disease

### Treatment/Management Plan

Pain management and hydration maintenance are the focus of care. A corticosteroid-containing dental paste may hasten resolution of the ulcers. Prescribe triamcinolone dental paste, thin film over the lesion(s) to to three times per day. Common over-the-counter medications such as Anbesol, Oragel, or Kank-A may be helpful for topical pain relief, though oral analgesics are often necessary.

### Family Education

Teach the following:

- Encourage oral liquids or frozen ice pops to maintain hydration.
- Avoid carbonated beverages and citrus juices in the presence of oral lesions, as they may result in increased burning or stinging.
- Children may not like having the dental paste applied. The area should be as dry as possible prior to application. The most important dosage time is at bedtime, as this allows the medication to be in contact with the lesion longer.
- The dental paste forms a sticky film that should be permitted to stay on.

## HERPETIC GINGIVOSTOMATITIS

HSV is usually contracted via direct contact with infected secretions or lesions. Herpetic gingivostomatitis occurs most frequently in children between 6 months and 5 years of age, without a particular seasonal distribution (Keels & Clements, 2019). The virus is usually shed for at least 1 week, and up to several weeks, with asymptomatic reactivation and shedding occurring throughout life. After primary infection, HSV-1 remains latent unless reactivated. Reactivation may occur as a result of sunlight or cold exposure, immunosuppression, stress, or trauma. Recurrent episodes tend to be less severe than the initial infection and are not usually associated with other systemic symptoms (Nield, 2017). Secondary bacterial infection may occur as a complication of herpetic gingivostomatitis.

### Subjective Findings

Note the onset of the lesion(s) and progression over time. The health history may reveal:

- An initial lesion(s) following by merging with other lesions

### Risk Factors

The most common risk factors for herpetic gingivostomatitis are:

- Exposure to the oral secretions or lesions of an infection individual
- Immunodeficiency
- Cancer chemotherapy or radiation treatment

### Review of Systems

The most common manifestations revealed during the review of systems include:

- **Constitutional:** fever, malaise, anorexia, refusal to drink, oral pain, headache
- **HEENT:** sore throat
- **Musculoskeletal:** joint discomfort

### Objective Findings

The physical examination of the child with herpetic gingivostomatitis (see Table 22.1) may reveal:

- Erythematous, edematous gingival margin lesions with clusters of small vesicles (usually anterior oropharynx: lips, tongue, buccal mucosa)
- Erupted lesions will be yellow with an erythematous halo
- Vesicles that have bled (happens easily) will have black crust
- Swollen, erythematous gingivae
- Halitosis
- Submandibular and/or cervical lymphadenopathy

### Laboratory/Diagnostic Testing

The diagnosis of herpetic stomatitis is based upon the clinical findings. If the etiologic diagnosis must be confirmed, viral culture, immunofluorescence, or polymerase chain reaction can identify HSV-1.

### Differential Diagnosis

The differential diagnosis for herpetic stomatitis includes:

- Aphthous ulcer
- Oral candidiasis
- Irritant or allergic contact stomatitis
- Gingivostomatitis
- Herpangina
- Acute cutaneous lupus erythematosus

- Behçet disease
- Stevens-Johnson syndrome

### Treatment/Management Plan

Of primary concern with herpetic gingivostomatitis is pain management and hydration maintenance. Oral analgesics such as acetaminophen or ibuprofen are usually necessary. Older children may "swish and spit" varied formulations of "magic mouthwash" to achieve some pain relief. Magic mouthwash formulations typically contain a combination of liquid diphenhydramine, kaolin or sucralfate, and milk of magnesia. There is not a standard recipe and the evidence for its use has not yet been proven.

If the immunocompetent child presents within 96 hours of disease onset with severe pain and the inability to eat, oral acyclovir may be helpful for reducing length of symptoms and possibly the duration of viral shedding. Dose acyclovir at 15 to 20 mg/kg/dose orally, five times daily, for 5 to 7 days (Keels & Clements, 2019; Lexicomp, 2020). As the fever subsides, and the lesions begin to heal, frequency of dosing may be decreased to three times daily.

#### Family Education

Teach the following:

- Encourage oral liquids or frozen ice pops to maintain hydration.
- Avoid carbonated beverages and citrus juices in the presence of oral lesions, as they may result in increased burning or stinging.
- Acyclovir's adverse effects include headaches, nausea, vomiting, and diarrhea.
- Notify provider if unable to maintain oral hydration while taking acyclovir, as there is a risk of renal tubule crystal formation in the presence of dehydration.

#### Referral

Refer for hospitalization those children who are unable to maintain hydration, who are immunocompromised, and those who also have eczema herpitcum or herpes keratitis.

## HERPANGINA

Infection with enterovirus, particularly coxsackievirus Type A serotypes, may result in the febrile illness of herpangina. The infection is self-limiting, yet fever can be high and the oral lesions are very painful. Outbreaks occur most often in the summer and early autumn, most frequently in children younger than 5 to 7 years of age (Romero, 2020). The lesions usually resolve spontaneously within 3 to 5 days (Nield, 2017). Complications are rare.

### Subjective Findings

Note the onset of the lesion(s) and progression over time. The health history may reveal:

- Fever
- Oral lesions in the back of the mouth

#### Risk Factors

The most common risk factors for herpangina are young age, daycare, school, or summer camp attendance, and exposure to an infected individual.

#### Review of Systems

The most common manifestations revealed during the review of systems include:

- **Constitutional:** high fever, refusal to drink, anorexia, mouth pain, malaise
- **HEENT:** mouth sores, drooling, difficulty swallowing
- **Neurologic:** fussiness, irritability

### Objective Findings

The physical examination of the child with herpangina may reveal (see Table 22.1):

- Irritable child
- Pharyngeal erythema
- Posterior oral cavity (soft palate, tonsils, uvula, faucial pillars) papulovesicular lesions (yellow-grey to white

> **PRO TIP** Infection with Coxsackie virus A16 may result in hand, foot, and mouth disease (HFMD). HFMD results in not only posterior oral cavity lesions, but also blanching macules (typically football-shaped) with an erythematous halo or vesicles on the palms, soles, or buttocks. HFMD spontaneously resolves within a week and treatment is consistent with that of herpangina (Nield, 2017).

### Laboratory/Diagnostic Testing

The diagnosis of herpangina is based upon the clinical findings. No laboratory or diagnostic testing is needed.

### Differential Diagnosis

The differential diagnosis for herpangina includes:

- Aphthous ulcers
- Herpetic gingivostomatitis

### Treatment/Management Plan

No antiviral therapy is indicated. The focus of care is on hydration maintenance and fever management. Ibuprofen or acetaminophen may be used. Older children may benefit from swishing and spitting magic mouthwash or viscous lidocaine, although care must be taken to avoid swallowing it.

Common over-the-counter medications such as Anbesol, Oragel, and Kank-A may be helpful for topical pain relief, though oral analgesics are often necessary.

▶ ALERT: It is not advised to utilize viscous lidocaine, nor preparations containing in it, in young children. They may swallow it, resulting in serious toxic effects or fatality.

### Family Education

Teach the following:

- Encourage oral liquids or frozen ice pops to maintain hydration. Playing games to encourage hydration may be helpful with a young child.
- Avoid carbonated beverages and citrus juices in the presence of oral lesions, as they may result in increased burning or stinging.
- Notify the provider if altered mental status or apparent muscle weakness occurs.

### Referral

Refer for hospitalization those children unable to maintain hydration orally, or if they are exhibiting neurologic or musculoskeletal signs (rare).

PRO TIP A small callus in the mid, upper lip in the young infant is termed a *labial sucking tubercle*. It may result from strong sucking in utero and after birth, usually disappearing once cup feeding is started.

# TONGUE DISORDERS

## ANKYLOGLOSSIA

When the lingual frenulum is shortened or tight, the resulting condition is termed ankyloglossia, or tongue-tie. The tongue cannot elevate or protrude properly. Ankyloglossia restricts proper tongue movement and extension, thereby hindering breastfeeding in infants and resulting in articulation difficulties and dental problems in children. Poor latch and maternal pain may lead to early cessation of breastfeeding. The incidence of ankyloglossia ranges between 1% and 10% (Isaacson, 2019).

### Subjective Findings

The health history may reveal:

- Poor latch (newborn, infant)
- Maternal nipple pain (newborn, infant)
- Speech difficulties

### Risk Factors

The most common risk factor for ankyloglossia is male gender (Isaacson, 2019).

### Review of Systems

The most common manifestations revealed during the review of systems include:

- **HEENT:** cannot protrude the tongue past 1 to 2 millimeters (children)

### Objective Findings

The physical examination of the child with ankyloglossia may reveal:

- Abnormally short frenulum
- Notched or heart-shaped tongue end when protruded
- In the child: difficulty lifting or protruding the tongue

### Laboratory/Diagnostic Testing

The diagnosis of ankyloglossia is based upon the clinical findings.

### Differential Diagnosis

The differential diagnosis for ankyloglossia includes:

- Posterior ankyloglossia
- Lip tie

### Treatment/Management Plan

Definitive treatment is surgical correction.

### Family Education

Teach the following:

- Follow through with lactation consultant or speech pathologist recommendations.

### Referral

Newborns with difficulty establishing adequate breastfeeding should be referred to a pediatric otolaryngologist for surgical release (frenotomy). Pending frenotomy, a lactation consultant may be able to assist with breastfeeding establishment. Refer the child with persisting ankyloglossia and who has speech/articulation issues to a pediatric speech pathologist.

## BENIGN MIGRATORY GLOSSITIS

Benign migratory glossitis, also termed geographic tongue, occurs in about 1% to 2% of the population (Yoon et al., 2020). The pattern on the tongue changes over time as desquamation and regeneration occur. It is a painless condition. The etiology of geographic tongue is unknown.

### Subjective Findings

The health history may reveal:

- Red/pink/white patches on the tongue, changing over time

### Risk Factors

There are no known risk factors for benign migratory glossitis.

### Review of Systems

The review of systems is negative in the child with benign migratory glossitis.

### Objective Findings

The physical examination of the child with benign migratory glossitis will reveal:

- Smooth areas on the tongue with reddish, minimally raised borders

### Laboratory/Diagnostic Testing

The diagnosis of benign migratory glossitis is based upon the clinical findings.

### Differential Diagnosis

The differential diagnosis for benign migratory glossitis includes:

- Oral candidiasis
- Stomatitis

### Treatment/Management Plan

No treatment is needed.

### Family Education

Teach the following:

- This is a benign condition, changing in appearance over time.

## ORAL CANDIDIASIS

Oral candidiasis (also known as thrush) is infection of the mouth with *Candida albicans*. It may be acquired from the birth canal or through skin colonization or the environment. Persistent infection may occur in breastfed infants when the mother's nipples are also infected (Bishop & Ebach, 2020).

### Subjective Findings

The health history may reveal:

- White patches on the tongue and inside the cheeks

### Risk Factors

The most common risk factors for oral candidiasis are:

- Broad spectrum antibiotic use
- Immunodeficiency
- Corticosteroid use
- Diabetes mellitus

### Review of Systems

The most common manifestations revealed during the review of systems include:

- **Constitutional:** poor feeding, mouth pain
- **Neurologic:** irritability

### Objective Findings

The physical examination of the child with oral candidiasis may reveal:

- Whitish, friable plaques on an erythematous base involving the buccal mucosa, palate, or tongue
- Unlike milk or formula residue, oral candidiasis cannot be easily removed or scraped with a tongue depressor and may bleed when rubbed or scraped

### Laboratory/Diagnostic Testing

The diagnosis of oral candidiasis is based upon the clinical findings. No laboratory or diagnostic testing is needed. Fungal culture or potassium hydroxide smear may be obtained if the diagnosis is uncertain.

### Differential Diagnosis

The differential diagnosis for oral candidiasis includes:

- Milk or formula residue
- Benign migratory glossitis

### Treatment/Management Plan

Oral candidiasis can be treated with nystatin oral suspension (100,000 units/mL), 1 mL to each cheek administered 4 times daily for at least 7 days. Evaluate the breastfed infant's mother for infection. Severe or refractory cases can be treated with oral fluconazole.

### Family Education

Teach the following:

- Pacifiers and bottle nipples should be properly sterilized.
- Avoid feeding for 5 to 10 minutes after administration of nystatin.
- Older children should swish nystatin for several minutes before swallowing.

**PRO TIP** *Cheilitis*—scaling of the lips with dryness and cracking—may be caused by sun or wind exposure, contact with musical instruments, or excessive licking (which exacerbates it). When the cracking is only in the corners it is termed angular cheilitis. Recommend lip balm and licking avoidance.

# TOOTH DISORDERS

Several disorders of the teeth are discussed here, including dental caries, avulsed tooth, bruxism, and malocclusion.

## DENTAL CARIES

Dental caries or cavities result from a tooth exposure to cariogenic microorganisms, most commonly *Streptococcus mutans* or *Streptococcus sobrinus*. *S. mutans* is commonly passed from mother or primary caregiver to child, as early as 3 months through usually around 19 to 30 months of age. Dental plaque harbors acidogenic bacteria close to the tooth enamel. The acidogenic bacteria cause enamel demineralization, which is followed by bacterial penetration of the enamel and advancement through the dentin. Early childhood caries (ECC; baby bottle caries) begin on the smooth surfaces of the primary teeth soon after eruption, then spreading rapidly.

### Subjective Findings

The health history may reveal:

- Discoloration of the teeth

### Risk Factors

The most common risk factors for dental caries are:

- Ingestion of sugary foods
- Maternal low socioeconomic status or low educational level (Gandhi et al., 2020)
- Infants permitted to have a bottle in the mouth for prolonged periods (e.g., during sleep) are also at high risk (Bishop & Ebach, 2020)

### Review of Systems

The most common manifestations revealed during the review of systems include:

- **HEENT:** tooth sensitivity, particularly to sweets or temperature change (especially cold)

### Objective Findings

The physical examination of the child with dental caries may reveal:

- White-spot lesion on the tooth (initial defect)
- Light to dark brown spots of cavities on the tooth (frank carious lesions)

### Laboratory/Diagnostic Testing

The diagnosis of dental caries is based upon visualization of a cavitated tooth. X-ray confirmation is usually performed by a dentist. ECC is noted in children under age 6 with one or more decayed, missing, or filled tooth surfaces (American Academy of Pediatric Dentistry, 2016).

### Differential Diagnosis

The differential diagnosis for dental caries includes:

- Dental fluorosis
- Developmental tooth anomaly

### Treatment/Management Plan

Prevention of dental caries is the focus. The American Academy of Pediatric Dentistry (2016) advocates the following:

- Dietary and oral hygiene recommendations (see Family Education).
- Apply fluoride varnish during well-child visits in high-risk children (see chapter 12).
- Establish dental home within 6 months of first tooth eruption (no later than 12 months of age).

Once caries are present, treatment is managed by the pediatric dentist (preferably pediatric, if available in the child's local area).

### Family Education

Teach the following:

- Avoid frequent consumption of sugar-sweetened beverages or sugary foods, as well as ad lib (on demand) breastfeeding after the first tooth erupts.
- Provide only water in the bottle, if the infant is taking a bottle to bed, as soon as teeth erupt.
- Wean from the baby bottle at 12 to 18 months.
- Use only regular cups (avoid no-spill sippy cups).
- Milk and cheese are considered to be protective.
- Begin oral hygiene with first tooth eruption (clean with soft cloth or soft toothbrush).
- Brush toddler and preschool children's teeth at least twice daily using a rice-sized amount of fluoridated toothpaste from ages 1 to 3 years, and a pea-sized amount in ages 3 to 6 years.
- School-age children should brush their teeth with fluoridated toothpaste for 2 to 3 minutes, two to three times per day. Parents should brush the teeth until age 8 years.
- Replace toothbrush every 3 to 4 months.
- Teach older children how to floss their teeth.
- Xylitol-containing products have limited evidence for caries reduction, but they have not been shown to be harmful (Gandhi et al., 2020).

**PRO TIP** Children do not have the manual dexterity to properly brush their teeth until they are about 8 years of age. The ability to tie the shoes demonstrates appropriate manual dexterity (Nowak & Warren, 2020).

### Referral

Refer infants to the dentist (preferably pediatric if available in the local area) after first tooth eruption for establishment of dental home. Also refer any child with suspected caries to the dentist.

## AVULSED TOOTH

Children of all ages may accidentally experience a dislodged tooth, with the highest incidence being between 2 and 3 years of age (Gandhi et al., 2020). When primary teeth are accidentally dislodged, complications to the permanent teeth may include hypocalcification of the enamel, angular distortions of the root or crown, impaction, and ectopic eruption. Older children typically experience an avulsed tooth from a fall or as a result of injury from sports or other activity.

### Subjective Findings

The health history may reveal:

- Fall, hit, or other accident resulting in dislodgement of the tooth

### Risk Factors

The most common risk factors for avulsed tooth are toddler age and sports participation.

### Review of Systems

The most common manifestations revealed during the review of systems include:

- **Constitutional:** pain at the site of the avulsion
- **HEENT:** possible split lip or mild bleeding from the gum

### Objective Findings

The physical examination of the child with an avulsed tooth may reveal:

- Missing tooth, empty socket

### Laboratory/Diagnostic Testing

The diagnosis of avulsed tooth is based upon the clinical findings. No laboratory or diagnostic testing is needed.

### Differential Diagnosis

The differential diagnosis for avulsed tooth includes:

- Displaced tooth
- Fractured tooth
- Swallowed tooth

### Treatment/Management Plan

Rarely are avulsed primary teeth reimplanted, due to the risk of further complications to the forthcoming permanent tooth. A permanent tooth that has been dislodged should be placed in cold milk or saline for transport. The tooth should be reimplanted as quickly as possible.

### Family Education

Teach the following:

- Provide adequate supervision to young children
- Encourage all children participating in contact sports and/or bicycle riding to wear mouth guards for tooth protection.

### Referral

Promptly refer the child with an avulsed tooth to the pediatric dentist.

## BRUXISM

Bruxism is the act of grinding the teeth, occurring while the child is awake or asleep (most often). It may begin within the first 5 years and occur in as many as 30% of children (Ryan et al., 2020). Bruxism may occur as a result of anxiety. It can wear away tooth enamel and may contribute to malocclusion and tooth malalignment.

### Subjective Findings

The health history may reveal:

- Teeth grinding observed by another person

### Risk Factors

The most common risk factors for bruxism are anxiety, other parasomnias, or family history of bruxism.

### Review of Systems

The most common manifestations revealed during the review of systems include:

- **Constitutional:** temporomandibular joint pain, temporal headache
- **HEENT:** snoring

### Objective Findings

The physical examination of the child with bruxism may reveal:

- Maloccluded teeth
- Alterations in tooth enamel or abnormal wear on biting surfaces of the teeth
- Pain with palpation of the temporomandibular joint

### Laboratory/Diagnostic Testing

The diagnosis of bruxism is based upon the clinical findings. No laboratory or diagnostic testing is needed.

### Differential Diagnosis

The differential diagnosis for bruxism includes:

- Facial myoclonus
- Chewing movements, swallowing, or sleep talking
- Expiratory groaning
- Nocturnal seizure (rare; Gerstner, 2020)

### Treatment/Management Plan

Treatment for bruxism is not always necessary but may include behavior interventions or dental appliances.

### Family Education

Teach the following:

- Use a calming bedtime routine to help the child relax.
- If prescribed, use dental appliance as instructed.
- Follow through with behavioral interventions if recommended.

### Referral

Refer children with troublesome bruxism to the pediatric dentist for evaluation and treatment.

## MALOCCLUSION

Tooth formation, speech development, and physical appearance are reliant upon proper alignment of teeth. *Malocclusion* refers to misalignment of the top teeth with the bottom teeth. It results from altered facial and mandibular bone growth.

### Subjective Findings

The health history may reveal:

- Crooked teeth
- Difficulty biting or chewing

### Risk Factors

The most common risk factors for malocclusion are:

- Thumb sucking after permanent teeth eruption
- History of dental caries
- Persistent bruxism

### Review of Systems

The most common manifestations revealed during the review of systems include:

- **HEENT:** digit sucking, chewing only on one side

### Objective Findings

The physical examination of the child with malocclusion may reveal:

- Crowded, crooked, or misaligned teeth
- Overbite or crossbite

### Laboratory/Diagnostic Testing

The diagnosis of malocclusion is based upon the clinical findings. The dental provider may perform X-rays once the child is referred by the primary care provider.

### Differential Diagnosis

The differential diagnosis for malocclusion includes:

- Facial structural anomaly

### Treatment/Management Plan

Treatment for dental malocclusion includes orthodontic braces or other dental devices.

### Family Education

Teach the following:

- With braces or other dental devices, more frequent toothbrushing with fluoridated toothpaste is required to prevent the development of dental caries and gingivitis.
- Limit high-sugar, high-carbohydrate, sticky foods when the child has braces.

### Referral

Refer children with malocclusion to a pediatric dentist or orthodontist.

## KEY POINTS

- Pain management and hydration maintenance are the mainstays of the management of oral lesions.
- Oral candidiasis appears as nonremovable white patches on the surfaces in the mouth. It should be treated with an antifungal mediation.
- Ankyloglossia may contribute to difficulty with breastfeeding.
- Geographic tongue is a benign condition requiring no treatment.
- Counsel parents to avoid baby bottles in bed or constant use of baby bottles by toddlers, as well as sippy cups, to avoid the development of dental caries.
- Keep an avulsed tooth in milk or saline and refer the child to the pediatric dentist immediately.
- Children with persistent bruxism or dental malocclusion should be referred to the pediatric dentist.

## REFERENCES

American Academy of Pediatric Dentistry. (2016). *Policy on early childhood caries (ECC): Classifications, consequences, and preventive strategies.* https://www.aapd.org/media/Policies_Guidelines/P_ECCClassifications.pdf

Bishop, W. B., & Ebach, D. R. (2020). Oral cavity. In R. M. Kliegman, J. St. Geme, N. J., Blum, S. S. Shah, R. C. Tasker, K. M. Wilson, & R. E. Behrman (Eds.), *Nelson textbook of pediatrics* (21st ed., Chapter 127). Elsevier.

Gandhi, R. P., Puranik, C. P., Wilson, A., & Chin, K. L. (2020). Oral medicine & dentistry. In W. W. Hay, M. J. Levin, M. J. Abzug, & M. Bunik (Eds.), *Current diagnosis & treatment: Pediatrics* (25th ed., Chapter 17). McGraw-Hill Education.

Gerstner, G. E. (2020). Sleep-related bruxism (tooth grinding). *UpToDate.* https://www.uptodate.com/contents/sleep-related-bruxism-tooth-grinding

Isaacson, G. C. (2019). Ankyloglossia (tongue-tie) in infants and children. *UpToDate.* https://www.uptodate.com/contents/ankyloglossia-tongue-tie-in-infants-and-children

Keels, M. A., & Clements, D. A. (2019). Herpetic gingivostomatitis in young children. *UpToDate.* http://www.uptodate.com/contents/herpetic-gingivostomatitis-in-young-children

Lexicomp. (2020). *Lexicomp clinical drug information* (version 5.7.1) [Mobile app]. App store. https://apps.apple.com/us/app/lexicomp/id313401238

Nield, L. S. (2017). Stomatitis. In In T. K. McInerny, H. M. Adam, D. E. Campbell, T. G. DeWitt, J. M. Foy, & D. M. Kamat (Eds.), *American Academy of Pediatrics textbook of pediatric care* (2nd ed., Chapter 335). American Academy of Pediatrics.

Nowak, A. J., & Warren, J. J. (2020). Preventive dental care and counseling for infants and young children. *UpToDate.* Retrieved October 14, 2020, from https://www.uptodate.com/contents/preventive-dental-care-and-counseling-for-infants-and-young-children

Romero, J. R. (2020). Hand, foot, and mouth disease and herpangina. *UpToDate.* Retrieved October 14, 2020, from https://www.uptodate.com/contents/hand-foot-and-mouth-disease-and-herpangina

Ryan, C. A., Walter, H. J., & DeMaso, D. R. (2020). Motor disorders and habits. In R. M. Kliegman, J. St. Geme, N. J. Blum, S. S. Shah, R. C. Tasker, K. M. Wilson, & R. E. Behrman (Eds.), *Nelson textbook of pediatrics* (21st ed., Chapter 37). Elsevier.

Solo-Josephson, P. (2017). *Canker sores.* http://kidshealth.org/parent/general/aches/canker.html#

Yoon, P. J., Scholes, M. A., & Herrmann, B. W. (2020). Ear, nose, & throat. In W. W. Hay, M. J. Levin, M. J. Abzug, & M. Bunik (Eds.), *Current diagnosis & treatment: Pediatrics* (25th ed., Chapter 18). McGraw-Hill Education.

# Management of Upper Respiratory Disorders

Theresa Kyle

## Student Learning Outcomes

**Upon completion of this chapter the reader should be able to:**

1. Discuss pathophysiology and epidemiology of selected upper respiratory disorders in children.
2. Differentiate subjective and objective findings of selected upper respiratory disorders in children.
3. Choose appropriate laboratory or diagnostic tests for particular upper respiratory disorders in children.
4. Utilize the differential diagnosis process to determine upper respiratory diagnosis in children.
5. Determine treatment plan, child/family education, and need for referral in children with an upper respiratory diagnosis.

## INTRODUCTION

Respiratory illness (upper and lower) accounts for a significant percentage of infant and child morbidity. Increased secretions and mucosal congestion may quickly contribute to respiratory distress in infants and young children, as their nasal passages are anatomically smaller (Allen, 2019). Foreign bodies in the nose may also occlude a nasal passage; yet the most commonly occurring upper respiratory disorders result from infection.

Typical healthy children may have six to eight upper respiratory infections annually, although some may have as many as 15. Infants and young children have relatively immature immunologic responses and are frequently exposed to respiratory pathogens (Goldman, 2017). Day care attendance and second-hand smoke exposure play important roles in the occurrence of infection. Most of these illnesses are self-limited, and children experience a healthy period between infections. To practice antibiotic stewardship as promoted by the American Academy of Pediatrics (AAP, 2020) and the Centers for Disease Control and Prevention (CDC, 2019b), the provider must become adept at distinguishing viral from bacterial infection to avoid unnecessary antibiotic prescription.

The content in this chapter maps to the following areas on the Pediatric Nursing Certification Board (PNCB) Pediatric Nurse Practitioner—Primary Care certification examination:

**CLINICAL PROBLEMS: HEAD, EYE, EAR, NOSE, AND THROAT**

CONTENT AREAS:

**II. Assessment and Diagnosis**

**B. History and Physical Examination**

1. Obtain history of present illness
2. Obtain a comprehensive health history for new patients
3. Complete an interval history for established patients
4. Perform a review of systems
5. Perform a complete physical examination

**C. Diagnostic Testing and Screening**

1. Order and interpret office/clinic based screening tests
2. Order and interpret diagnostic laboratory tests
3. Order and interpret the results of diagnostic imaging tests

**D. Analyzing Information**

1. Integrate health history and physical examination findings into the plan of care
2. Assimilate findings from screening and diagnostic testing into plan of care

**E. Diagnosis**

1. Develop and prioritize differential diagnoses
2. Establish a diagnosis based on evaluation of patient data

## III. Management

**A. Child and Caregiver Counseling and Education**

1. Provide condition-specific counseling and education, including treatment options
2. Educate about benefits and potential adverse reactions of pharmacological interventions
3. Discuss non-pharmacological interventions
4. Counsel regarding the threshold for seeking follow-up care
5. Review the risks of non-adherence to recommended treatment

**B. Therapeutic Interventions**

1. Prescribe pharmacologic agents
2. Recommend the use of over-the-counter pharmacologic agents
3. Order or recommend non-pharmacologic treatments for the management of symptoms
4. Discuss use of complementary and alternative therapies as appropriate

**C. Procedures**

1. Perform procedures in accordance with diagnostic guidelines and plan of care (rapid tests)
2. Initiate life-saving techniques in response to urgent or emergent situations

**D. Collaboration and Referral**

2. Refer to specialists as indicated for evaluation, counseling, and/or treatment

**E. Care Coordination**

1. Facilitate patient and family-centered care for children of all ages with acute and chronic conditions

**F. Evaluation and Follow-up**

2. Establish a plan for follow-up care

## IV. Professional Role Responsibilities

**A. Leadership and Evidence-based Practice**

4. Develop, implement, and/or modify clinical practice guidelines

## ANATOMY AND PHYSIOLOGY

The upper respiratory tract consists of the nose and sinuses, oropharynx, larynx, and upper trachea (Figure 23.1). The nose is divided into two passages, separated by a midline and nearly straight septum. The nasal passages are covered with a vascular epithelium and serve to warm, humidify, and filter inspired air. Air passing over the nasal superior, middle, and inferior turbinates experiences turbulence, which warms it to near body temperature (Scanlon & Sanders, 2019). The turbinates mature to resemble an adult's by 12 years of age (Allen, 2019). The goblet cells in the nasal mucosa produce mucus, which traps inhaled pathogens and air pollutants. Cilia in the nasal epithelium sweep the mucus to the oropharynx where it is swallowed (Scanlon & Sanders, 2019).

Newborns are preferential nose breathers, which facilitates their ability to suckle for nourishment. They generally open their mouths to breathe only when the nares are occluded or when they are crying (Tolomeo, 2019). Additionally, newborns produce very little upper respiratory mucus (a cleansing agent), thus they are more susceptible to infection. Naturally, the younger the child is, the smaller the airways are, making newborns and younger infants increasingly susceptible to airway obstruction in the presence of excess mucus. This may result in difficulty sucking or feeding in the young infant. The nose also drains the nasolacrimal duct, resulting in increased nasal drainage in young children, especially while crying or if the eyes are irritated (Allen, 2019).

The paranasal sinuses consist of paired cavities: the maxillary, ethmoid, frontal, and sphenoid sinuses (Figure 23.2). The sinuses are lined with ciliated epithelium, and mucus produced within them drains into the nasal cavity (Scanlon & Sanders, 2019). Goblet cells and submucosal glands are responsible for the production of mucus and immune mediators. The maxillary and ethmoid sinuses are present at birth but are small and less functional. The frontal sinuses begin to develop around 6 to 8 years of age, and the sphenoid sinuses develop in early adolescence. By 12 to 14 years of age, the sinuses are mature (Allen, 2019).

Posterior to the nasal cavity lies a muscular tube known as the pharynx (Figure 23.1). The uppermost portion, the nasopharynx, is surrounded by bone, which helps to maintain its patency (Allen, 2019). The adenoids (pharyngeal tonsils) are lymph nodes containing macrophages and are housed in the nasopharynx (Scanlon & Sanders, 2019). The eustachian tubes drain middle ear secretions into the nasopharynx. In the bony portion of the eustachian tubes,

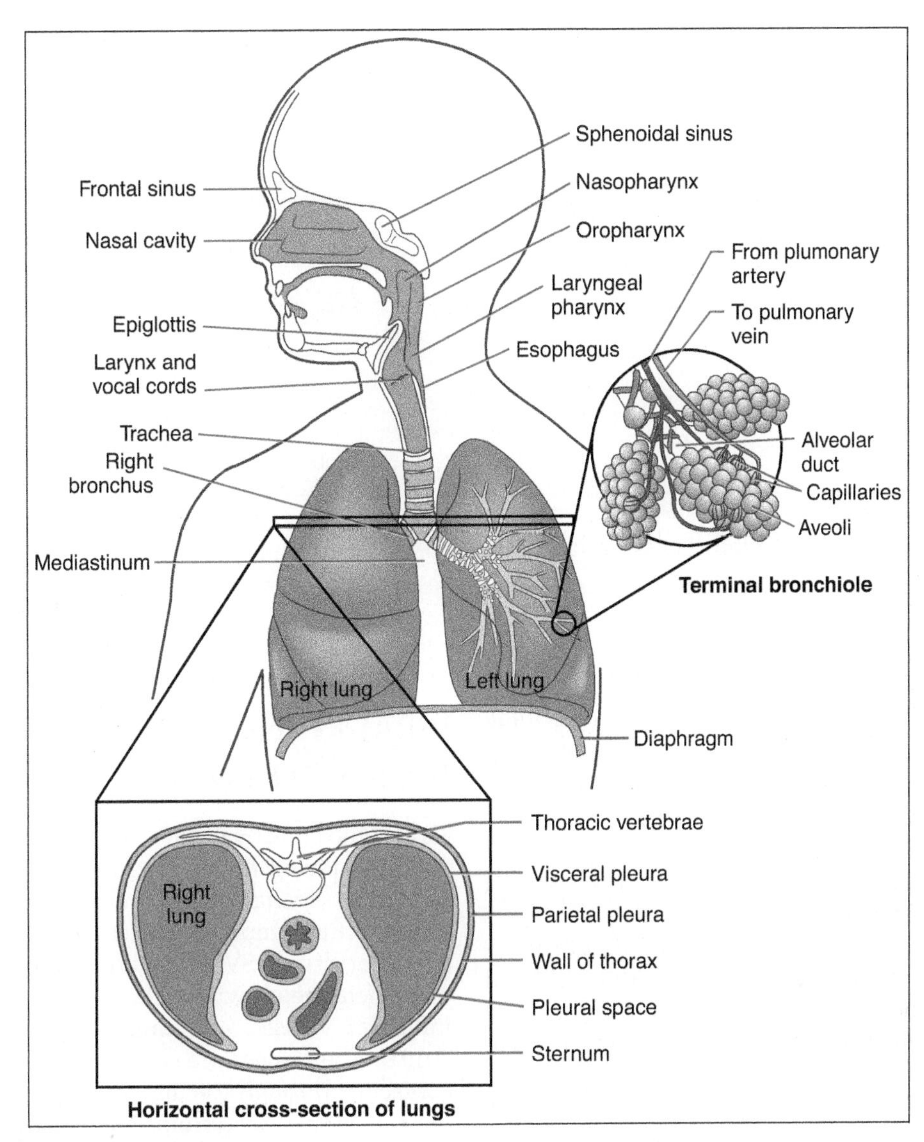


FIGURE 23.1 The respiratory system.

*Source*: Chiocca, E. M. (2020). *Advanced pediatric assessment* (3rd ed.). Springer Publishing Company.

the respiratory epithelium blends with the middle ear mucosa. The adenoids are often enlarged in early childhood, contributing to middle ear issues during that time period (Tewfik & Singh, 2018). On the lateral edges of the oropharynx (posterior to the mouth) lie the palatine tonsils, which are frequently significantly enlarged (4+, tonsils are touching each other, also termed kissing) throughout early childhood. Both the adenoids and the tonsils decrease to the average adult size of 1+ or 2+ in middle childhood (Allen, 2019).

▶ ALERT: A congenital anomaly termed **choanal atresia** occurs when either a membranous or bony abnormality blocks the space between the posterior wall of the nasopharynx and the posterior nasal turbinates on either one or both sides, resulting in respiratory distress in the newborn (Allen, 2019).

Similar to the remainder of the upper respiratory tract, the larynx is lined with ciliated epithelium, except for the vocal cords, which have squamous epithelium. The larynx is comprised of nine rings of cartilage that assist with keeping the airway open. In adolescents and adults, the shape of the larynx is that of a fairly uniform cylinder. Up until about 10 years of age, the cricoid cartilage (ring of cartilage around the trachea) is underdeveloped, resulting in laryngeal narrowing and more of a funnel shape (Nagler, 2020). Audible

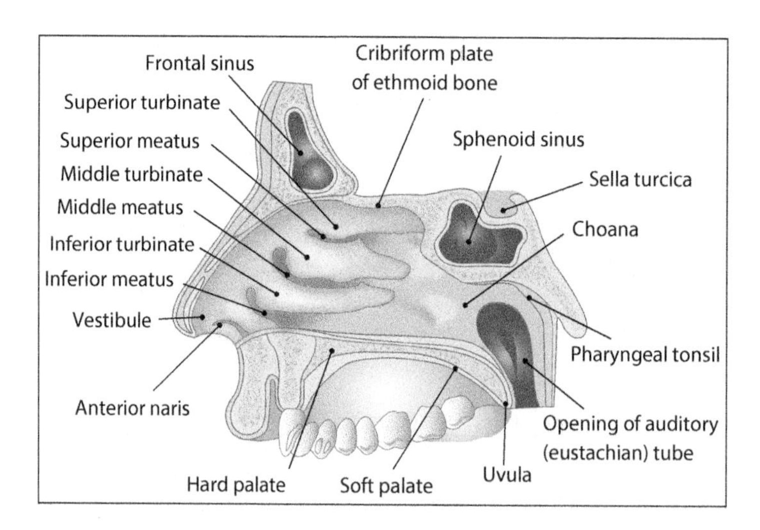


FIGURE 23.2 Anatomy of the internal nasal cavity.

*Source*: Gawlik, K. M., Melnyk, B. M., & Teall, A. M. (2020). *Evidence-based physical examination: Best practices for health and well-being assessment*. Springer Publishing Company.

adventitious sounds such as crowing, snoring, stridor, and upper airway noises transmitted into the chest often occur in infants and younger children because of these anatomical differences.

Additional differences in young children make the airway susceptible to dynamic collapse when airway obstruction is present. The young child's airway is highly compliant, its supporting musculature functioning less efficiently than that of the older child and adult. The mucous membranes lining the airway and the large amount of soft tissue surrounding the trachea are less firmly affixed as compared with adults, increasing the risk for obstruction and edema (Nagler, 2020). Upper airway obstruction caused by croup, epiglottitis, or a foreign body may lead to tracheal collapse with inspiration.

## INFECTIOUS DISORDERS

Common upper airway infections occurring in children include viral rhinosinusitis, acute and chronic bacterial rhinosinusitis, and croup. Because of immunizations, less commonly occurring infections include epiglottitis, diphtheria, and pertussis. When an upper respiratory tract infection is suspected, always ask about recent foreign travel or recent immigration, exposure to ill contacts, immunization status, and any hospitalizations (Allen, 2019; Striegel et al., 2019; Tolomeo, 2019).

## VIRAL RHINOSINUSITIS (COMMON COLD)

Viral rhinosinusitis occurs frequently in children, particularly during the cooler months. Over 100 viruses have been identified as causing the common cold. These include rhinoviruses, parainfluenza, respiratory syncytial virus (RSV), enteroviruses, adenoviruses, human metapneumovirus (Fischer, 2017), human parainfluenza viruses, and human coronaviruses (CDC, 2019a). The viruses are spread from person-to-person contact or through the air, with direct inoculation via the eye or nose. Symptoms are usually worse near the beginning of the illness, and the cold spontaneously resolves without treatment after about 7 to 10 days (Wald, 2019). Occasionally, cilia function in the nasal and sinus cavities may take up to 3 weeks for full recovery; mild rhinorrhea and dry cough may persist during that time frame. Potential complications include acute otitis media, asthma exacerbation, epistaxis, bacterial pharyngitis, bacterial rhinosinusitis, and pneumonia.

### Subjective Findings

The health history may reveal:

- Sneezing
- Runny nose or nasal congestion
- Cough (see Table 23.1 for further descriptive questions related to cough)

**TABLE 23.1 Cough Descriptors**

| Characteristics | Associated Questions |
|---|---|
| Timing and duration | Occurs during the day, night, or both? Continuous or intermittent?<br>Acute (less than 2 weeks), subacute (2–4 weeks), recurrent, or chronic (longer than 4 weeks)? |
| Quality | Wet, dry, tight, or hacking? Is it barking or staccato-like? Paroxysmal with an inspiratory whoop? |
| Productivity | Produces mucus or not? (Infants often have a nonproductive cough.) |
| Effect on child and family | Child or parent sleep disrupted? Child missing school? Parents missing work? Parents frustrated? |

*Source*: Data from Chiocca, E. M. (2020). *Advanced pediatric assessment* (3rd ed.). Springer Publishing Company; Marcus, M. G. (2017). Cough. In T. K. McInerny, H. M. Adam, D. E. Campbell, J. M. Foy, & D. M. Kamat (Eds.), *American Academy of Pediatrics textbook of pediatric care* (2nd ed., Chapter 135). American Academy of Pediatrics

- Fever (near the beginning of the illness, occurring more frequently in younger children)
- Contact with ill family, friends, or classmates

### Risk Factors

The most common risk factors for viral rhinosinusitis are day care attendance and exposure to second-hand smoke.

### Review of Systems

The most common risk factors for viral rhinosinusitis are:

- **Constitutional:** fatigue, irritability (infants), poor feeding (infants), possible malaise
- **HEENT:** headache, fullness in the ears, scratchy or sore throat
- **Gastrointestinal:** mild diarrhea (infants)

### Objective Findings

The physical examination of the child with viral rhinosinusitis may reveal:

- Mild conjunctival injection (often occurs with adenovirus)
- Full, immobile tympanic membrane (especially infants and younger children)
- Erythema or flaking around the nares (from nose blowing)
- Nasal discharge (usually watery near the beginning of the cold and may become thicker and discolored later in the illness)
- Edematous, erythematous nasal turbinates
- Mild pharyngeal erythema
- Cough (may be productive depending upon volume of nasal discharge)
- Mildly elevated respiratory rate (infants)
- Clear breath sounds throughout lung fields, although upper airway congestion noises may be transmitted into the chest in infants and younger children

### Laboratory/Diagnostic Testing

The diagnosis of a common cold is based upon the clinical findings. No laboratory or diagnostic testing is needed.

### Differential Diagnosis

The differential diagnosis for viral rhinosinusitis includes:

- Allergic rhinitis
- Streptococcal pharyngitis (not usually accompanied by rhinorrhea or cough)
- Acute bacterial rhinosinusitis
- Nasal foreign body
- Cocaine or medicated nasal spray use
- *Bordetella pertussis* infection

### Treatment/Management Plan

Supportive care for the common cold may yield some symptomatic relief. Cough and cold preparations have not been demonstrated to be effective in children younger than 6 years of age (Lopez & Williams, 2019). The older child or adolescent may experience some symptom relief with the use of an antihistamine or decongestant, which should be avoided altogether in children under age 2 (due to critical side effects). Saline nose drops and a bulb syringe help liquefy and mobilize secretions in young children. Older children may utilize normal saline nose spray. Utilizing a cool mist humidifier may also be useful. Avoid aspirin use because of the risk of Reye syndrome; acetaminophen or ibuprofen may be used for fever or malaise. Discourage the use of vasoconstricting nasal sprays such as oxymetazoline hydrochloride because of the risk of rebound nasal congestion associated with its use. The use of complementary therapies such as zinc, vitamin C, and echinacea has demonstrated mixed results. While not likely harmful, they have not consistently demonstrated improvement in or shortening of symptom duration (Fischer, 2017).

▶ ALERT: Do not give children under 4 years of age decongestants or antihistamines for the common cold, because of the increased risk of serious side effects in this age group (U.S. Food and Drug Administration, 2018).

## Family Education

Teach the following:

- Avoid forceful nose blowing.
- Nasal wash solution may be made with 8 ounces of distilled water, 1/2 teaspoon table salt, and 1/4 teaspoon baking soda. Instill in the nares with a bulb syringe or Neti pot.
- Teach parents that neither dextromethorphan nor codeine have been demonstrated to effectively suppress cough in children, and may have serious side effects, including respiratory depression.

# BACTERIAL RHINOSINUSITIS

Bacterial rhinosinusitis is a bacterial infection of the paranasal sinuses, usually following a course of viral rhinosinusitis. As many as 9% of colds are complicated by bacterial infection (Wald, 2019). Most colds improve or resolve completely within 7 to 10 days. In bacterial sinusitis, the cold symptoms worsen nearer the predicted natural history end of illness, and the child becomes sicker. The main sites of infection in young children are the maxillary and ethmoid sinuses, whereas the frontal sinuses are more commonly involved in children over 10 years of age (Yoon et al., 2018).

Typically, bacteria are removed from the paranasal sinuses by mucociliary clearance. During viral rhinosinusitis and other conditions, the ciliary epithelium is damaged and/or the cilia function is altered. The production of mucus, increase in mucus viscosity, or altered ostia patency also decrease mucociliary clearance. This allows for microbial invasion and bacterial overgrowth (Wald, 2019). Commonly, *Streptococcus pneumoniae, Haemophilus influenza* (nontypeable), or *Moraxella catarrhalis* are the responsible pathogens. The classification of bacterial sinusitis is presented in Table 23.2. Complications from bacterial sinusitis include orbital cellulitis and intracranial infection (i.e., subdural empyema).

TABLE 23.2 **Classification of Sinusitis**

| Classification | Duration and Recurrence |
|---|---|
| Acute | Completely resolved in less than 30 days |
| Subacute | Completed resolved between 30 and 90 days |
| Recurrent acute | Within a 6-month period: At least 3 episodes less than 30 days in length, quickly responding to antibiotic therapy, with at least 10 days symptom-free in between<br>Within a 12-month period: At least 4 episodes as described above |
| Chronic | Paranasal sinus inflammation lasting longer than 90 days (child has persistent symptoms of cough, rhinorrhea, nasal obstruction) |

*Source*: Data from Wald, E. R. (2019). Acute bacterial rhinosinusitis in children: Clinical features and diagnosis. *UpToDate*. Retrieved March 11, 2020, from https://www.uptodate.com/contents/acute-bacterial-rhinosinusitis-in-children-clinical-features-and-diagnosis

## Subjective Findings

When obtaining the history of the present illness, note if the cold persists longer than 10 days or the worsening of cold symptoms rather than the natural history of improvement over time. The health history may reveal:

- Cough (must be present during day but is often worse at night)
- Nasal discharge, often thick
- Malaise, or feeling more ill than earlier in the course of illness

## Risk Factors

The most common risk factors for bacterial rhinosinusitis are:

- History of common cold or allergic rhinitis
- Anatomic obstruction (such as nasal polyps)
- Mucosal irritants (smoke, dry air, chlorinated water)
- Descent in an airplane

## Review of Systems

The most common manifestations revealed during the review of systems include:

- **Constitutional:** fever, fatigue, poor appetite, facial pain may or may not be present
- **HEENT:** eyelid edema (ethmoid sinus involvement), decrease in or inability to smell (anosmia), toothache, sore throat
- **Respiratory:** snoring, mouth breathing
- **Gastrointestinal:** vomiting (due to postnasal discharge)
- **Neurological:** irritability, headache

## Objective Findings

The physical examination of the child with bacterial rhinosinusitis may reveal:

- Periorbital edema
- Sinus pain upon palpation
- Clear, mucoid, or purulent nasal discharge
- Halitosis
- Erythematous oropharynx with postnasal drainage
- Nasal quality of speech
- Cough (wet or dry)

### Laboratory/Diagnostic Testing

Uncomplicated acute bacterial sinusitis may be diagnosed by clinical presentation (see below); thus, imaging is not recommended. Complicated bacterial sinusitis may require contrast-enhanced computed tomography or magnetic resonance imaging. Microbiological studies are not needed (Wald, 2019).

## Differential Diagnosis

To distinguish acute bacterial rhinosinusitis from the common cold, it is recommended that two of the following criteria be met:

- Daytime cough, nasal symptoms, or both
  and one of the following:
  - Duration of symptoms without improvement longer than 10 days, up to 30 days
  - Severe symptoms (ill appearance, temperature greater than or equal to 39 °C (102.2 °F), and purulent nasal discharge for 3 or more consecutive days)
  - Worsening of symptoms (new-onset severe headache or fever, increased respiratory symptoms, or recurring fever after initial resolution)

The clinical guidelines for bacterial rhinosinusitis may be found at https://pediatrics.aappublications.org/content/pediatrics/132/1/e262.full.pdf.

The differential diagnosis for acute bacterial rhinosinusitis includes:

- Viral rhinosinusitis
- Allergic rhinitis
- Infected/enlarged adenoids
- Nasal foreign body
- Catarrhal (initial) stage of pertussis
- Structural abnormality

## Treatment/Management Plan

The child with acute bacterial sinusitis of severe presentation or worsening symptoms is treated with antibiotics. Children with persistent illness may be prescribed antibiotic treatment or may be observed for up to 3 days before prescription. Refer to Table 23.3 for recommended medications.

**TABLE 23.3 Antibiotic Treatment for Acute Bacterial Rhinosinusitis**

| Criteria | Medication |
|---|---|
| Mild to moderate illness, no day care attendance, no antibiotic treatment in past 4 weeks | Amoxicillin (oral)—45 mg/kg/day, in two divided doses for a minimum of 10 days |
| Community with high prevalence of nonsusceptible *S. pneumoniae* | Amoxicillin (oral)—80–90 mg/kg/day, in two divided doses for a minimum of 10 days |
| Moderate to severe illness, age younger than 2 years, day care attendance, antibiotic treatment in past 4 weeks | Amoxicillin with clavulanate (oral)—80–90 mg/kg/day of amoxicillin component, in two divided doses for a minimum of 10 days |
| Vomiting, unable to tolerate oral medication, unlikely oral medication adherence | Ceftriaxone (intravenous or intramuscular)—50 mg/kg/dose times 1; if improving at 24 hours, switch to oral medication; if not improving may redose parenterally |
| Penicillin-allergic | Usually safe to prescribe cefdinir, cefuroxime, or cefpodoxime. If serious type 1 allergy, may use cefixime in combination with clindamycin or linezolid; or use a quinolone such as levofloxacin |

*Source*: Data from Wald, E. R., Applegate, K. E., Bordley, C., Darrow, D. H., Glode, M. P., Marcy, S. M., Nelson, C. E., Rosenfeld, R. M., Shaikh, N., Smith, M. J., Williams, P. V., & Weinberg, S. T. (2013). Clinical practice guideline for the diagnosis and management of acute bacterial sinusitis in children aged 1 to 18 Years. *Pediatrics, 132*(1), e262–e280. https://doi.org/10.1542/peds.2013-1071

## Family Education

Teach the following:

- Teach families to complete the full course of antibiotics in order to eradicate the infection.
- Decongestants, antihistamines, and intranasal steroids have not been demonstrated to be effective in the treatment of bacterial rhinosinusitis.
- Normal saline nose spray or nasal washes may promote drainage in some children, resulting in increased comfort.

- Advise the child and family that clinical improvement should occur within 48 hours (Yoon et al., 2018).

### Referral

Children with complicated cases of bacterial rhinosinusitis should be referred to the physician to evaluate for chronic sinusitis, recalcitrant recurrent sinusitis, orbital cellulitis, or intracranial infection.

## VIRAL CROUP

Croup (also called acute laryngotracheobronchitis) is an upper airway inflammatory condition resulting in laryngeal and subglottic swelling. It occurs most commonly in younger children who have narrow cricoid and thyroid cartilage (Hall & Hall, 2017). Significant airway obstruction may occur where the airway is narrowest. Viral croup results most often from parainfluenza infection, though other viruses are also implicated (Striegel et al., 2019). Outbreaks occur most often in the fall. The natural history of viral croup is resolution without intervention within 4 to 5 days.

### Subjective Findings

The health history may reveal:

- Nasal congestion and cough for 1 to 2 days
- Night awakening with spasmodic cough (barking or brassy)
- Inspiratory crowing sound (stridor)
- Fast breathing or difficulty breathing

The symptoms are often absent upon arising from bed in the morning, only to return with a subsequent coughing spell. The child may act quite well between coughing fits.

### Risk Factors

The most common risk factors for croup are:

- Age 3 months to 3 years
- Male gender

### Review of Systems

The most common manifestations revealed during the review of systems include:

- **Constitutional:** fever as high as 39.4 °C (102.9 °C)
- **HEENT:** hoarseness or laryngitis
- **Respiratory:** possible antecedent upper respiratory tract symptoms

### Objective Findings

The physical examination of the child with croup may reveal:

- Hoarseness
- Inspiratory stridor
- Distinctive barking or brassy cough
- Suprasternal, supraclavicular, and substernal retractions particularly on inspiration
- Tachypnea (usually not higher than 50 breaths/minute)
- Prolonged inspiratory phase with coarse crackles
- Wheeze or rhonchi on expiration

In worsening obstruction, cyanosis may occur.

▶ ALERT: The child with a toxic appearance may have **bacterial tracheitis** rather than viral croup.

### Laboratory/Diagnostic Testing

Although not necessary for diagnosis of croup, laboratory and diagnostic testing may reveal:

- Neck anteroposterior radiograph may show the "steeple sign" (subglottic narrowing)
- Lack of leukocytosis with complete blood count (CBC)

### Differential Diagnosis

The differential diagnosis for croup includes:

- Epiglottitis
- Bacterial tracheitis
- Retropharyngeal or parapharyngeal abscess
- Foreign body aspiration
- Laryngomalacia
- Subglottic stenosis
- Hemangioma
- Vascular ring
- Vocal cord paralysis

Refer to Table 23.4 for a comparison of the clinical manifestations of croup and epiglottis.

Determine the level of croup severity based on the Westley Croup Score (for children less than or equal to 6 years of age). See Table 23.5.

### Treatment/Management Plan

Cough suppressants, decongestants, and antibiotics are not recommended for the treatment of croup. Cool mist humidification or 10 minutes in a steamy bathroom has not been proven to be beneficial, but if children with mild croup or their parents perceive

**TABLE 23.4 Croup Compared with Epiglottis**

| Manifestation | Croup | Epiglottitis |
|---|---|---|
| Stridor | Loud | Quiet |
| Cough | Barking | None |
| Voice | Hoarse | Muffled |
| Drooling | No | Yes |
| Dysphagia | No | Yes |
| Tripod position | No | Yes |
| Trismus | No | Yes |
| Toxic appearance | No | Yes |

*Source*: Data from Conrad, C., & Cornfield, D. N. (2017). Airway obstruction. In T. K. McInerny, H. M. Adam, D. E. Campbell, J. M. Foy, & D. M. Kamat (Eds.), *American Academy of Pediatrics textbook of pediatric care* (2nd ed., Chapter 348). American Academy of Pediatrics.

**TABLE 23.5 Level of Croup Severity Based on the Westley Croup Score**

| Assessment | Points |
|---|---|
| **Level of consciousness:**<br>normal (including sleep)—0 points<br>disoriented—5 points | |
| **Cyanosis:**<br>none—0 points<br>with agitation—4 points<br>at rest—5 points | |
| **Stridor:**<br>none—0 points<br>with agitation—1 point<br>at rest—2 points | |
| **Air entry:**<br>normal—0 points<br>decreased—1 point<br>markedly decreased—2 points | |
| **Retractions:**<br>none—0 points<br>mild—1 point<br>moderate—2 points<br>severe—3 points | |
| **Total** | |

**Scoring:**
Mild croup: 0–2 points
Moderate croup: 3–7 points
Severe croup: 8–11 points
Impending respiratory failure: 12–17 points

*Source*: Reproduced with permission from Woods, C. R. (2018). Croup: Clinical features, evaluation, and diagnosis. *UpToDate*. Retrieved from https://www.uptodate.com/contents/croup-clinical-features-evaluation-and-diagnosis

**TABLE 23.6 Treatment of Croup With Medications**

| Medication | Mild Croup | Moderate Croup | Severe Croup |
|---|---|---|---|
| Dexamethasone (0.6 mg/kg, one dose orally or intramuscularly) | Consider an oral dose | Recommended | Recommended |
| Racemic epinephrine (2.25%, 0.5 mL in 2.5 mL saline, nebulized) | Not recommended | Recommended | Recommended—may repeat after 20 minutes |

*Note*: Nebulized racemic epinephrine has an effect duration of 2 to 3 hours; children should be observed for rapid recurrence of symptoms.

*Source*: Data from Hall, C. B., & Hall, W. J. (2017). Croup (acute laryngotracheobronchitis). In T. K. McInerny, H. M. Adam, D. E. Campbell, J. M. Foy, & D. M. Kamat (Eds.), *American Academy of Pediatrics textbook of pediatric care* (2nd ed., Chapter 352). American Academy of Pediatrics

it to be helpful, it is not harmful (Woods, 2019). Humidification is not recommended for moderate or severe croup. Medications for croup are presented in Table 23.6.

The child with mild croup may be observed at home. Following observation after treatment with racemic epinephrine (one dose for moderate croup, two doses for severe croup), the child with moderate or severe croup may be discharged home in the absence of stridor and retractions. If the child does not improve with nebulization treatment, hospitalization may be necessary (Hall & Hall, 2017). Consult the physician for a child who appears toxic, who is lethargic or dehydrated, or who has significant respiratory distress. Refer the child with recurrent croup to the otolaryngologist (ENT).

## Family Education

Teach the following:

- Do not expect improvement with the use of humidity.
- The cough is usually worse at night. Maintain a calm demeanor and soothe the child.
- Return if not improved in 3 days.
- If cyanosis occurs, call 911.

## EPIGLOTTITIS

**Epiglottitis** is a life-threatening bacterial infection of the epiglottis. Swelling of the epiglottis may result in complete airway obstruction. Prior to implementation of the *Haemophilus influenzae* type B (Hib) vaccine, epiglottitis occurred at a rate of 5 per 100,000 children less than or equal to age 5 years. Since the Hib vaccine, that rate has dropped to 0.6 to 0.8 (Woods, 2019). *Staphylococcus aureus, Moraxella catarrhalis, Neisseria* species, *Pseudomonas* species, and others may also cause epiglottitis (although less frequently). Epiglottitis more commonly occurs from December to May (Conrad & Cornfield, 2017). Airway obstruction may occur within hours of illness onset (Woods, 2019).

### Subjective Findings

The health history may reveal:

- Abrupt onset of symptoms (a defining feature)
- Choking sensation
- Sore throat (older children)
- Difficulty breathing (as reported by the parent)

### Risk Factors

The most common risk factors for epiglottitis are:

- Lack of immunization or underimmunization for Hib
- Immune deficiency

### Review of Systems

The most common manifestations revealed during the review of systems include:

- **Constitutional:** high fever
- **Neurologic:** anxiety, restlessness, irritability

### Objective Findings

Allow the child to maintain a position of comfort, such as in the parent's lap. Care should be taken to keep the child calm and not to incite crying in order to avoid abrupt airway obstruction. The physical examination of the child with epiglottitis may reveal:

- Tripod sitting (leaning forward with neck hyperextended, chin stretching forward)
- Muffled voice or cry
- Trismus (difficulty opening mouth)
- Toxic appearance
- Dysphagia, drooling
- Cyanosis
- Distress with inspiration
- Inspiratory retractions
- Soft stridor (late finding)

▶ ALERT: Do not attempt to inspect the oropharynx, utilize a tongue depressor, or elicit a gag reflex in the child suspected of having epiglottitis.

### Laboratory/Diagnostic Testing

A lateral neck radiograph demonstrates the characteristic "thumb sign" (thickened bulging epiglottis), although airway visualization should not be delayed in order to obtain the x-ray. Ideally, the x-ray should be obtained in the emergency room or intensive care unit, rather than the radiology department, and only if the child is stable and without stridor. CBC will reveal an elevated white blood cell count, and a blood culture may confirm the type of bacteria causing the infection.

### Differential Diagnosis

Definitive diagnosis is made by direct visualization by an experienced airway specialist during intubation. The epiglottis is cherry red, and the aryepiglottic folds are edematous. Emergency tracheostomy may be required if complete airway obstruction occurs. The differential diagnosis for epiglottitis includes:

- Croup
- Bacterial tracheitis
- Peritonsillar or retropharyngeal abscess
- Uvulitis
- Upper airway foreign body
- Angioedema
- Diphtheria
- Congenital anomaly
- Trauma or thermal injury to the upper airway

Refer to Table 23.4 for a comparison of the clinical manifestations of croup and epiglottitis.

### Treatment/Management Plan

Avoid agitation of the child until an airway is secured. Provide 100% oxygen by blow-by (Conrad & Cornfield, 2017). The parent can hold the oxygen if it keeps the child calm. Intubation should occur in the operating room, and the child will be hospitalized. Ceftriaxone or amoxicillin/clavulanate are the antibiotics of choice.

# DIPHTHERIA

Respiratory-tract diphtheria is a rare infection in the developed world caused by toxigenic strains of *Corynebacterium diphtheriae*, spread only through humans via droplet transmission or contact with skin lesions (AAP, 2018). With infection, the toxin is absorbed into the mucous membranes, destroying the epithelium and causing inflammation. A gray, tenacious pseudomembrane forms and adheres to the pharynx and trachea, resulting in bleeding when disrupted (Gaensbauer et al., 2018). Complications of diphtheria are life-threatening: airway obstruction, circulatory collapse, or myocarditis with heart block. Reversible cranial or peripheral neuropathies may also occur (AAP, 2018).

## Subjective Findings

The health history may reveal a gradual onset of symptoms, including:

- Sore throat
- Malaise

### Risk Factors

The most common risk factors for diphtheria are:

- Lack of immunization
- Living in unsanitary or crowded conditions
- Homelessness
- Travel to areas where diphtheria is common

### Review of Systems

The most common manifestations revealed during the review of systems include:

- **Constitutional:** low-grade to moderate fever
- **HEENT:** nasal speech, bloody nasal discharge
- **Lymphatic:** swollen cervical lymph nodes

## Objective Findings

The physical examination of the child with diphtheria may reveal:

- Significant cervical lymphadenitis
- Serosanguinous nasal discharge
- Gray pharyngeal membrane with erythema and edema
- Stridor
- Tachycardia unjustified by height of fever
- Edema of the neck ("bull neck" appearance)

### Laboratory/Diagnostic Testing

Polymerase chain reaction (PCR) and enzyme-linked immunoassay (ELISA) tests for diphtheria are now available. A culture must be obtained when diphtheria is suspected. The CBC may reveal a normal white blood cell count and decreased hemoglobin, hematocrit, and platelets.

## Differential Diagnosis

Diphtheria diagnosis should be considered in the presence of the aforementioned clinical manifestations, particularly an oropharyngeal membrane resulting in bleeding when disrupted. Definitive diagnosis is based on a positive culture. The differential diagnosis for diphtheria includes:

- Group A strep pharyngitis
- Epstein-Barr virus (EBV) infection
- Purulent sinusitis
- Nasal foreign body
- Epiglottitis
- Croup

## Treatment/Management Plan

When clinical suspicion for diphtheria is high, a single dose of equine diphtheria antitoxin (DAT) should be administered intravenously prior to culture or other laboratory results, as the risk of rapid respiratory deterioration is very high. Information related to administration of the antitoxin may be found on the Centers for Disease Control and Prevention website (www.cdc.gov/diphtheria/dat.html), and the emergency phone number as of this publication is (770) 488-7100. Following antitoxin administration, eradication of the bacteria may be achieved with a 14-day course of either oral or parenteral erythromycin, or intravenous or intramuscular penicillin G benzathine. Carriers must also be treated. Culture-confirmed cases of diphtheria must be immediately reported to the local health department.

# PERTUSSIS (WHOOPING COUGH)

Pertussis infection occurs with human-to-human transmission via droplets of the bacteria *Bordetella pertussis*. Immunity to pertussis via both immunization and natural infection wanes over time. The catarrhal stage (mild respiratory symptoms) lasts 1 to 2 weeks, followed by the paroxysmal phase lasting 2 to 4 weeks. Paroxysms of coughing occur, causing loss of breath in infants and young children. The coughing dislodges mucous plugs and necrotic epithelial tissue. Inhalation forced against a narrow glottis produces the characteristic whooping sound in infants (Kronman et al., 2019). Emesis often occurs post-tussively.

Younger infants are more severely affected, tend to require hospitalization, and may present first with apnea. One percent of cases in infants younger than 2 months of age results in death (AAP, 2018). Maternal immunization during pregnancy provides a protective effect. The convalescent phase lasts 1–2 weeks, with the cough waning over time. Cough may continue for several months, especially in adolescents. Complications in infants include pneumonia, pulmonary hypertension, hernia, conjunctival bleeding, and hypoxia resulting in seizures, encephalopathy, or apnea. Among adolescents, complications may include pneumonia, weight loss, sleep disturbance, and syncope.

### Subjective Findings

Determine the child's immunization status. Parents may report the coughing fits to be worse at night. The health history may reveal:

- Early
  - Rhinitis
  - Sneezing
  - Irritating cough
- Later
  - Forceful coughing followed by whooping (especially older infants and young children)
  - Persistent nonproductive cough (adolescents)

#### Risk Factors

The most common risk factor for pertussis is lack of immunization or underimmunization (in the child or in the mother if the infant is less than 2 months of age).

#### Review of Systems

The most common manifestations revealed during the review of systems include:

- **Constitutional:** low-grade fever earlier in the illness, sweating with coughing fits, exhaustion
- **Respiratory:** worsened coughing at night, cyanosis, and/or difficulty catching the breath with coughing fit
- **Gastrointestinal:** vomiting after a coughing fit

### Objective Findings

The physical examination of the child with pertussis may reveal:

- Watery rhinorrhea
- Staccato-like cough, possibly with whoop following

#### Laboratory/Diagnostic Testing

The PCR assay demonstrates optimal sensitivity during the first 3 weeks of the cough, in the absence of antibiotic treatment. For accuracy, the specimen for PCR testing must be collected appropriately. It must be obtained via a Dacron swab or nasopharyngeal wash and aspirate. Refer to the CDC resources for best practice related to pertussis PCR testing (www.cdc.gov/pertussis/clinical/diagnostic-testing/diagnosis-pcr-bestpractices.html). Leukocytosis with absolute lymphocytosis is noted on CBC.

### Differential Diagnosis

The CDC case definition for pertussis allows for clinical diagnosis without laboratory testing in children with a cough lasting 2 weeks or more and having at least one of the following: cough paroxysm, inspiratory whooping, post-tussive vomiting, or apnea in infants. The differential diagnosis for pertussis includes:

- Pneumonia (particularly *Mycoplasma pneumoniae*)
- Bronchiolitis (RSV or adenovirus)
- Cystic fibrosis
- Upper airway foreign body

### Treatment/Management Plan

The first-line treatment for pertussis infection is a 5-day course of azithromycin, ideally begun earlier in the illness. If not begun until the paroxysmal stage, the purpose is to prevent spread to others. Hospitalized infants and children should be isolated with droplet precautions, continuing for 5 days after the start of effective antibiotic treatment. Treatment of contacts should also occur. Underimmunized children younger than 7 years of age should receive a DTaP booster vaccine if one has not been received in the past 3 years. Children 7 to 10 years of age who are underimmunized should receive a Tdap booster vaccine. All close contacts should receive a 5-day course of azithromycin.

## PHARYNGITIS AND TONSILLITIS

Pharyngitis refers to inflammation of the pharynx, whereas tonsillitis refers to inflammation of the tonsils. The term tonsillopharyngitis may also be used. The approach to treatment is the same for both. Acute pharyngitis is a common occurrence in childhood. It may be caused by a number of viruses or bacteria, which varies based on season and geographic location. An important bacterial cause of pharyngitis is group A β-hemolytic streptococcus (GABSH) and is the most common problem for which antibiotics are prescribed in school-age children. GABHS pharyngitis usually results about 2 to 5 days after exposure to an infected individual. In children under 3 years of age, GABHS only accounts for about 3% of cases, yet in children over 3 years of age, the incidence increases to an estimated 15% to 20% of cases (Steele, 2017). Untreated GABHS may lead to acute rheumatic fever or glomerulonephritis, so when present must be treated with antibiotics.

## Subjective Findings

The health history may reveal:

- Fever
- Headache
- Malaise
- Sore or scratchy throat

### Risk Factors

Risk factors for the development of pharyngitis/tonsillitis include day care attendance and school attendance.

### Review of Systems

The most common manifestations revealed during the review of systems include:

- **Constitutional:** anorexia, fatigue, fever
- **HEENT:** sore throat, pain with swallowing, snoring, red tongue
- **Gastrointestinal:** abdominal pain, nausea, vomiting
- **Musculoskeletal:** achiness
- **Integumentary:** rash, particularly on abdomen or trunk
- **Neurologic:** headache
- **Hematologic/Lymphatic:** painful or swollen cervical lymph nodes

## Objective Findings

The physical examination of the child with pharyngitis/tonsillitis may reveal:

- Erythema of the mouth, tongue, pharynx, or tonsils
- Petechiae on the palate or gums
- Enlarged tonsils, with or without exudate
- Anterior cervical lymphadenopathy with tenderness
- Scarletinaform rash on abdomen or trunk, with possible coalescing in skin folds (with GABHS)
- Redness around the anus in infants

▶ ALERT: Palpate for organomegaly and percuss the liver and spleen (they should not be enlarged). As GABHS may lead to the sequela of acute rheumatic fever, and certain strains of *Streptococcus pyogenes* may cause glomerulonephritis, it is important to examine the heart, lungs, and kidneys. Signs of renal or cardiovascular involvement include coarse breath sounds (fluid retention), murmur (flow, related to anemia), elevated heart rate or blood pressure, costovertebral angle tenderness, and inadequate urine output.

▶ ALERT: If the child has a toxic appearance, a muffled voice ("hot potato"), and/or trismus, suspect peritonsillar abscess and carefully palpate the peritonsillar area with a gloved finger.

### Laboratory/Diagnostic Testing

A positive rapid antigen detection test (RADT) for Group A *Streptococcus* confirms the diagnosis of GABHS pharyngitis within about 10 minutes. The RADT is 95% specific, and 70% to 90% sensitive, so a throat culture should be sent if the RADT is negative (Wald, 2020).

## Differential Diagnosis

Diagnosis is made based upon the history and physical examination, as well as rapid strep test and/or throat culture. The differential diagnosis for pharyngitis/tonsillitis includes:

- Mononucleosis
- Peritonsillar abscess
- Epiglottitis

When assessing a child with pharyngitis, it is important to distinguish the pharyngitis from mononucleosis, as the treatment plan differs. Refer to Table 23.7 for a comparison of pharyngitis/tonsillitis with mononucleosis.

## Treatment/Management Plan

Supportive care is recommended for all children with pharyngitis/tonsillitis (see "Family Education" following). If RADT or throat culture is positive for GABHS, prescribe antibiotic treatment, with penicillin being the first-line treatment. Antibiotic options include:

- Penicillin V potassium (PenVK) 500 mg twice daily for both adolescents and adults for 10 days
- PenVK 250 mg two to three times daily (children) for 10 days
- Amoxicillin 50 mg/kg once daily (children) for 10 days

TABLE 23.7 **Pharyngitis/Tonsillitis Compared with Mononucleosis**

| Clinical Manifestation | Pharyngitis/ Tonsillitis | Infectious Mononucleosis |
|---|---|---|
| Fatigue | Present | Pronounced |
| Malaise | Present | Pronounced |
| Sore throat | Present | Present |
| Pharyngeal or tonsillar exudate | May be present | May be present |
| Cervical lymphadenopathy | Usually anterior | May be posterior |
| Scarletinaform rash | With scarlet fever | Not present |
| Hepatosplenomegaly | Not present | May be present |

*Source*: Data from Krilov, L. R. (2017). Infectious mononucleosis and other Epstein-Barr infections. In T. K. McInerny, H. M. Adam, D. E. Campbell, J. M. Foy, & D. M. Kamat (Eds.), *American Academy of Pediatrics textbook of pediatric care* (2nd ed., Chapter 275). American Academy of Pediatrics; Steele, R. W. (2017). Pharyngitis and tonsillitis. In T. K. McInerny, H. M. Adam, D. E. Campbell, J. M. Foy, & D. M. Kamat (Eds.), *American Academy of Pediatrics textbook of pediatric care* (2nd ed., Chapter 311). American Academy of Pediatrics; Wald, E. R. (2020). Group A streptococcal tonsillopharyngitis in children and adolescents: Clinical features and diagnosis. *UpToDate*. Retrieved March 11, 2020, from https://www.uptodate.com/contents/group-a-streptococcal-tonsillopharyngitis-in-children-and-adolescents-clinical-features-and-diagnosis

- Penicillin G benzathine 600,000 units (patients less than 27 kg) or 1,200,000 units (patients greater than 27 kg) intramuscularly times one (1) dose
- A 5-day course of azithromycin, or 10-day course of cephalosporin may be used in the penicillin-allergic client (Steele, 2017; Wolters Kluwer Clinical Drug Information, 2020).

### Family Education

Teach the following:

- Provide warm or cool fluids to soothe the throat; increase fluid intake.
- Lozenges (in the child age 6 years and older) and avoidance of salty or spicy foods may be helpful.
- Give acetaminophen 10 to 15 mg/kg/dose every 4 hours as needed to ease the fever and pain.
- If antibiotics are prescribed, complete the entire course of medication.
- Notify the nurse practitioner if swallowing or breathing becomes difficult due to the sore throat (Schmitt, 2019).

### Referral

If peritonsillar abscess or retropharyngeal abscess is suspected, refer the child to the ENT for possible incision and drainage. If epiglottitis is suspected, refer to the hospital emergency department for immediate airway management. Refer the child with recurrent GABHS-documented tonsillitis to the ENT for possible tonsillectomy based on the following;

- >7 per year, in the past year
- >5 per year, in the past 2 years
- >3 per year, in the past 3 years (Mitchell et al., 2019)

## MONONUCLEOSIS

Infectious mononucleosis is caused by infection with the EBV. It may result in a subclinical infection or as disease. Infectious mononucleosis is a systemic viral infection and can affect every organ system. The acute clinical manifestations usually last 2 to 3 weeks. Large percentages of children are infected in the early years, but historically infectious mononucleosis has occurred most often in teenagers and young adults. Among Caucasian high school and college students the incidence is one in 2500 (Krilov, 2017). EBV establishes latency in the oropharynx and may be spread throughout the lifetime. It is spread via saliva; thus the reason for its nickname, the “kissing disease.” After exposure the incubation period is 2 to 6 weeks, most often 20 to 30 days (Krilov, 2017).

### Subjective Findings

The health history may reveal:

- Fever
- Malaise
- Sore throat (can be excruciating)

### Risk Factors

The most common risk factors for Epstein-Barr infection are:

- High school or college attendance
- Drink or glass sharing, toothbrush sharing, sexual contact, and blood transfusion

### Review of Systems

The most common manifestations revealed during the review of systems include:

- **Constitutional:** fever, malaise (may be significant)
- **HEENT:** sore throat

- **Respiratory:** rhinitis, cough (less frequent)
- **Gastrointestinal:** abdominal pain
- **Integumentary:** rash
- **Hematologic/Lymphatic:** painful or swollen cervical lymph nodes

### Objective Findings

The physical examination of the child with infectious mononucleosis may reveal:

- Eyelid edema
- Injected pharynx and tonsils (with or without exudate)
- Posterior cervical lymphadenopathy (tender)
- Hepatomegaly
- Splenomegaly

### Laboratory/Diagnostic Testing

Positive rapid mononuclear heterophile testing (completed within 2 minutes in the office), is 96% to 99% specific in children over 4 years of age, although it may also be negative very early in the infection (Krilov, 2017). If the rapid test is negative and infectious mononucleosis is strongly suspected in the child who is under 4 years of age, EBV infection can be confirmed with EBV antibody testing. A CBC with differential will reveal lymphocytosis greater than 50%, as well as atypical lymphocytosis (Krilov, 2017). Ultrasound may be used to verify and monitor splenomegaly.

### Differential Diagnosis

The differential diagnosis for infectious mononucleosis includes:

- Influenza
- Upper respiratory infection
- Pharyngitis or tonsillitis
- Lymphadenopathy
- Chronic fatigue

### Treatment/Management Plan

Supportive care is recommended for all children with infectious mononucleosis (see "Family Education" section following). Children and adolescents should rest as they feel necessary. If the child is continuing to experience fatigue during convalescence, then completing schoolwork at home is an option, or the provider may write a note for half-day school attendance until the child's energy level returns. If significant tonsillar hypertrophy occurs and there is a concern about airway obstruction, a short course of corticosteroids may be helpful (dexamethasone 0.25 mg/kg, methylprednisolone 1 mg/kg every 6 hours, or oral prednisone 40 mg per day; Krilov, 2017).

### Family Education

Teach the following:

- Follow the same instructions for pharyngitis/tonsillitis for palliation of sore throat.
- Rest in bed, gradually returning to the normal activity level.
- Fatigue may last for several weeks.
- Avoid strenuous physical activity (especially contact sports) until cleared by the nurse practitioner—minimum of 3 weeks for noncontact sports, 4 weeks for contact sports (and resolution of splenomegaly).
- If severe pain in the upper left abdomen occurs (splenic rupture), seek medical attention immediately.
- If antibiotics are prescribed for a concomitant bacterial infection, a rash may follow their use.

### Referral

Referral to a sub-specialist and/or hospitalization may be needed for children and adolescents with airway compromise, splenic rupture, thrombocytopenia, or if neurologic complications occur.

## INFLUENZA

Infection with the influenza virus occurs primarily during the winter and early spring and affects as many as 10% to 40% of children annually (Munoz, 2020). Influenza is spread through droplet inhalation or fine-particle aerosol contact. In children, shedding of the virus starts 1 to 2 days before symptoms begin and may continue for as long as 2 weeks. Primarily, the upper respiratory epithelium is affected, but systemic effects may also occur.

Complications of influenza include secondary bacterial infection resulting in severe pneumococcal pneumonia, acute otitis media, and acute myositis (unique to children—bilateral calves with severe pain resulting in refusal to walk). Prolonged fever, or return of fever during convalescence, should be investigated, due to the risk for these complications.

**PRO TIP** Current immunization recommendations include annual influenza vaccine for all children older than 6 months of age (CDC, 2020).

## Subjective Data

The health history may reveal:

- Fever
- Achiness
- Headache
- Cough
- Congestion

## Risk Factors

Unimmunized children are at highest risk for contracting influenza infection. Day care and school attendance also increase risk of infection. Risk factors for more severe influenza infection include:

- Chronic heart or lung conditions
- Diabetes
- Chronic renal disease
- Immune deficiency or treatment with chemotherapy

## Review of Systems

The review of systems may yield the following:

- **Constitutional:** abrupt onset of fever (often greater than 39.5 °C [103.1 °F] in infants and younger children), chills, malaise
- **Integumentary:** facial flushing
- **HEENT:** photophobia, tearing, burning, eye pain, sore or dry throat, nasal discharge, pain with swallowing
- **Respiratory:** cough
- **Gastrointestinal:** possibly diarrhea
- **Musculoskeletal:** myalgia
- **Neurologic:** headache, irritability (infants)

## Objective Findings

Upon physical examination, the following clinical manifestations may be noted:

- Mildly toxic appearance (infants)
- Reddened conjunctivae
- Injected pharynx
- Possible wheezing (especially infants and younger children)
- Erythematous rash

## Laboratory/Diagnostic Testing

The diagnosis of influenza infection may be made based on the history and physical examination, particularly during the influenza season. Reverse transcription-polymerase chain reaction (RT-PCR) testing is highly sensitive and highly specific. Another test for influenza is the rapid molecular assay (66%–100% sensitive; CDC, 2019c).

▶ ALERT: Do not withhold influenza treatment based on laboratory results if the clinical picture suggests influenza.

## Differential Diagnosis

The differential diagnosis for influenza includes:

- Other viral respiratory illness (RSV, parainfluenza viruses, adenovirus, rhinovirus, enteroviruses)
- Pneumonia
- Tonsillopharyngitis
- Rhinosinusitis

## Treatment/Management Plan

Supportive care includes treatment of cough and fever, and maintenance of hydration (see "Family Education" section following). If the clinical picture demonstrates influenza infection or laboratory testing confirms it, begin anti-flu medication and prescribe a 5-day course. Options (with doses) include:

- Oseltamivir
  - Term infant 0 to 8 months—3 mg/kg per dose, twice daily
  - Infant 9 to 11 months—3.5 mg/kg per dose, twice daily
  - Child 12 months or older:
    - ≤15 kg (≤33 lb)—30 mg, twice daily
    - >15 to 23 kg (33–51 lb)—45 mg, twice daily
    - >23 to 40 kg (>51–88 lb)—60 mg, twice daily
    - >40 kg (>88 lb)—75 mg, twice daily
- Zanamivir
  - Children 7 years or older—10 mg (two 5-mg inhalations), twice daily (Committee on Infectious Diseases, 2019)

## Family Education

Teach the following:

- Provide warm or cool fluids to soothe the throat; increase fluid intake.
- Lozenges or hard candies (in the child 6 years or older) may soothe throat.
- Give acetaminophen 10 to 15 mg/kg/dose every 4 hours or ibuprofen 4 to 10 mg/kg/dose every 6 hours as needed to ease the fever and pain.

- Avoid use of aspirin (to prevent development of Reye syndrome).
- If antiviral medication is prescribed, complete the entire course of medication (Schmitt, 2019).
- Notify the nurse practitioner if breathing becomes difficult, fever lasts more than 3 days, fever goes away for 24 hours then returns, or cough lasts for more than 3 weeks (Schmitt, 2019).

### Referral

Refer to a pediatric infectious disease specialist if the child does not improve with appropriate antiviral treatment.

# NONINFECTIOUS DISORDERS

## CONGENITAL LARYNGOMALACIA

Congenital laryngomalacia is a condition in which the newborn's laryngeal structure is weaker than normal, yielding dynamic collapse on inspiration. The problem is compounded by the newborn's increased respiratory rate, smaller airways, and more compliant chest wall and soft tissues. Stridor generally begins by 2 weeks of age and is worse when the infant is supine, improving when the infant is in an upright or prone position (Conrad & Cornfield, 2017). In infants with mild laryngomalacia, the stridor may worsen with respiratory infections, yet weight gain is adequate. Stridor is most pronounced at 4 to 8 months of age and resolves by 12 to 18 months of age. Infants with moderate to severe laryngomalacia should be referred a pediatric otolaryngologist for possible treatment (Isaacson, 2018).

## NASAL FOREIGN BODY

Nasal foreign bodies may be of soft material such as clay, eraser material, or paper; or of hard composition such as candy pieces, popcorn kernels, pebbles, or most commonly jewelry beads. There is danger of electrical burns or tissue necrosis when a small alkaline battery ("button" battery) is placed in the nose. Paired disc magnets may migrate upward and create erosion over time. A foreign body in the nose may lead to complications of infection, inflammation, epistaxis, or nasal septum perforation; thus the foreign body should be promptly and skillfully removed (Skae & Parikh, 2017).

### Subjective Findings

The health history may reveal unilateral nasal drainage that has become foul-smelling. Keep in mind that children will not usually admit to having put something in their nose.

### Risk Factors

The most common risk factors for a nasal foreign body are:

- Young age
- Developmental delay

### Review of Systems

The most common manifestations revealed during the review of systems include:

- **HEENT:**
  - May reveal epistaxis
  - Complaint of "clogged nose"
  - Mouth breathing

### Objective Findings

The physical examination of the anterior nose of a child with a nasal foreign body requires adequate illumination and a nasal speculum. The foreign body may be visualized, although nasal secretions may first have to be suctioned in order to increase visibility.

### Laboratory/Diagnostic Testing

In most instances, radiographs are not needed, although they may be helpful to identify disc batteries or paired disc magnets.

### Differential Diagnosis

Diagnosis is made based upon the history and direct visualization. Differential diagnosis for nasal foreign body includes:

- Epistaxis
- Adenoiditis
- Suppurative rhinitis
- Sinusitis
- Nasal polyp
- Tumor

### Treatment/Management Plan

Soft or smooth foreign bodies in the anterior nasal cavity may often be successfully expelled in the child older than 3 years of age by occluding the opposite naris and having the child blow the nose. Positive pressure from parent's mouth to child's mouth has also been successfully utilized. The opposite naris must be occluded; with the child in a sitting or standing position, the parent creates a firm seal over the child's mouth and provides a short, sharp puff of air (Isaacson & Ojo, 2020). Both of these techniques have an increased success rate when the foreign body has been in the nose a shorter period of time. With appropriate restraint, local anesthesia, and the use of a curette or alligator forceps, the practitioner may manually remove the foreign object. Local anesthesia is achieved with one part oxymetazoline and one part lidocaine (do NOT use with lodged button batteries; Isaacson & Ojo, 2020).

### Family Education

Teach the following:

- Teach the child not to place foreign objects in the nose.
- Educate parents to ensure that children under 3 years of age do not have access to any small items that would fit in the nose.

## EPISTAXIS (NOSEBLEED)

Epistaxis (nosebleed) in childhood is relatively common and self-limited. It is more common in dry climates and during the winter months. Peak occurrence is between the ages of 3 and 8 years, with about 90% of nose bleeds occurring in the anterior region where the thin mucosa overlies a rich vasculature (Schechter & Stevens, 2017). Exposure to trauma and/or dry air makes the nose susceptible to bleeding. Allergic rhinitis and viral upper respiratory infection may also result in epistaxis.

### Subjective Findings

The health history may reveal:

- When the bleeding started
- What has been attempted to control the bleeding

### Risk Factors

The most common risk factors for epistaxis are:

- Male gender
- Age 3 to 8 years
- Picking the nose
- Blunt trauma to the nose
- Nasal foreign body
- Nasal septum deviation
- Use of intranasal drugs such as corticosteroids and cocaine

### Review of Systems

The review of systems for the hematologic system may reveal bleeding from other sites (not commonly occurring in children without hematologic disorders).

### Objective Findings

The physical examination of the child with epistaxis may reveal:

- Nasal erythema or edema
- Active nasal bleeding
- Scabbing
- Determine blood pressure and pulse, noting age appropriateness of both. Check the skin for an unusual presence or number of petechiae or bruises.

▶ ALERT: Further evaluation for child abuse should be considered in the child under 2 years of age with epistaxis.

### Laboratory/Diagnostic Testing

Laboratory and diagnostic testing is generally not needed for simple anterior epistaxis. Obtain a CBC if petechiae or unusual ecchymosis are present or in the ill-appearing child. In the child who has experienced blunt force trauma (in intentional or nonintentional injury), plain radiographs may reveal facial fracture as the cause of the bleeding.

### Differential Diagnosis

The differential diagnosis for epistaxis includes:

- Nasal polyps
- Neoplasm (benign and malignant)

### Treatment/Management Plan

Ensure that the child's head is elevated to avoid aspiration. In the child older than 3 years of age, have the child gently blow the nose to expel clots. Apply pressure by pinching the nostrils without interruption for 5 to 10 minutes. If the bleeding stops, provide child and family education for epistaxis prevention.

If the bleeding does not stop, have the child gently blow the nose again to expel clots. Apply a topical decongestant (such as oxymetazoline or phenylephrine) and hold pressure as before, then examine the nose (Tunkel et al., 2020). If anterior bleed is identified, cauterize carefully with silver nitrate stick.

### Family Education

Teach the following:

- Avoid forceful nose blowing and nose picking, to prevent epistaxis.
- Use a cool mist humidifier in the home.
- Apply a water-based lubricant gently inside the nares.
- If bleeding recurs, have the child sit up, and pinch the nares closed without interruption for 5 to 15 minutes.
- If cauterized, lubricate nose 1 to 3 times daily. Avoid nose blowing, strenuous activity, or placing anything in the nose (including cotton swabs and tissues) for 1 week.

### Referral

If a posterior bleed is suspected, refer to the ENT specialist immediately. Children with recurrent episodes of epistaxis should also be referred to the ENT and to the hematologist for further evaluation of a possible bleeding disorder or leukemia.

## UPPER AIRWAY FOREIGN BODY

Foreign bodies may find their way into a child's larynx or trachea as a result of curiosity, boredom, or inadequate dentition or chewing required for the size of a food piece. Lodging of foreign bodies in the larynx carries a high risk of mortality and anoxic encephalopathy. The most frequently inhaled items are shelled nuts and seeds. In one study, 40% of deaths from foreign body aspiration were attributed to grapes (Conrad & Cornfield, 2017).

### Subjective Findings

The health history may reveal a parental report of a choking, gagging, or coughing episode often followed by an asymptomatic period.

### Risk Factors

The highest risk factors for upper airway foreign body are:

- Young age
- Developmental or behavioral delay

Adolescents who play blow darts are also at increased risk.

### Review of Systems

The most common manifestations revealed during the review of systems include:

- **Constitutional:** pain or discomfort
- **HEENT:** dysphonia, stridor
- **Respiratory:** hemoptysis (with sharp item inhalation)

### Objective Findings

The physical examination of the child with an upper airway foreign body may reveal:

- Hoarseness
- Cyanosis
- Stridor
- Cough
- Wheeze

### Laboratory/Diagnostic Testing

If the child's condition permits, plain-film upper airway radiograph may reveal the foreign body's location.

### Treatment/Management Plan

The recently inhaled foreign body may be expelled by use of the Heimlich maneuver in children and chest thrusts/back blows in the infant. Refer children with a suspected or confirmed upper airway foreign body to the ENT for removal.

### Family Education

Teach the following:

- Avoid toys with small removable parts for children under 3 years of age.
- Keep beaded jewelry with small parts away from young children.
- Cut toddlers' food into tiny pieces (hotdogs, grapes, berries).
- Do not provide children under 5 years of age with small, round, or hard food such as hard candy, nuts, grapes, cheese chunks or sticks, hot dogs, popcorn, or marshmallows.
- Keep button batteries, disc magnets, broken crayons, and other items away from small children.
- Encourage children not to put crayons, pencils, or pens in their mouth.
- Do not allow children to run, ride in the car, or play sports with gum, candy, or lollipops in their mouths (Pitone, 2020; Safe Kids Worldwide, 2020).

## KEY POINTS

- A careful history and thorough physical examination is important for diagnosis and treatment of upper respiratory disorders in children.
- Many upper respiratory disorders in infants and children are viral in nature and self-limited, requiring only supportive management.
- Antiviral medications are prescribed for influenza, though not for other viral upper respiratory illnesses.
- For pharyngitis/tonsillitis, infectious mononucleosis, and influenza, supportive care related to hydration and throat pain palliation is important.
- Prescribe antibiotics for pharyngitis only in documented cases of bacterial infection.
- Perform skillful abdominal assessment in the patient with mononucleosis to determine extent of hepatosplenomegaly.

## REFERENCES


Allen, P. J. (2019). Nose, mouth, and throat. In K. G. Duderstadt (Ed.), *Pediatric physical examination: An illustrated handbook* (3rd ed., Chapter 14). Elsevier.

American Academy of Pediatrics. (2018). *Red book: 2018–2021 report of the Committee on Infectious Diseases* (31st ed.).

American Academy of Pediatrics. (2020). *Pediatric ASP toolkit for outpatient settings*. http://www.pids.org/asp-toolkit/tools/outpatient.html

Centers for Disease Control and Prevention. (2019a). *Common cold: Protect yourself and others*. https://www.cdc.gov/features/rhinoviruses/index.html

Centers for Disease Control and Prevention. (2019b). *Core elements of outpatient antibiotic stewardship for healthcare professionals*. https://www.cdc.gov/antibiotic-use/core-elements/outpatient.html

Centers for Disease Control and Prevention. (2019c). *Information on rapid molecular assays, RT-PCR, and other molecular assays for diagnosis of influenza virus infection*. https://www.cdc.gov/flu/professionals/diagnosis/molecular-assays.htm

Centers for Disease Control and Prevention. (2020). *Seasonal influenza vaccination resources for health professionals*. https://www.cdc.gov/flu/professionals/vaccination/index.htm

Committee on Infectious Diseases. (2019). Recommendations for prevention and control of influenza in children, 2019–2020. *Pediatrics, 144*(4), e20192478. https://doi.org/10.1542/peds.2019-2478

Conrad, C., & Cornfield, D. N. (2017). Airway obstruction. In T. K. McInerny, H. M. Adam, D. E. Campbell, J. M. Foy, & D. M. Kamat (Eds.), *American Academy of Pediatrics textbook of pediatric care* (2nd ed., Chapter 348). American Academy of Pediatrics.

Fischer, H. (2017). Common cold. In T. K. McInerny, H. M. Adam, D. E. Campbell, J. M. Foy, & D. M. Kamat (Eds.), *American Academy of Pediatrics textbook of pediatric care* (2nd ed., Chapter 233). American Academy of Pediatrics.

Gaensbauer, J., Nomura, Y., Ogle, J. W., & Anderson, M. S. (2018). Infections: Bacterial & spirochetal. In W. W. Hay, M. J. Levin, R. R. Deterding, M. J. Abzug, & J. M. Sondheimer (Eds.), *Current diagnosis and treatment: Pediatrics* (24th ed., Chapter 42). McGraw-Hill Education.

Goldman, D. L. (2017). Recurrent infections. In T. K. McInerny, H. M. Adam, D. E. Campbell, J. M. Foy, & D. M. Kamat (Eds.), *American Academy of Pediatrics textbook of pediatric care* (2nd ed., Chapter 187). American Academy of Pediatrics.

Hall, C. B., & Hall, W. J. (2017). Croup (acute laryngotracheobronchitis). In T. K. McInerny, H. M. Adam, D. E. Campbell, J. M. Foy, & D. M. Kamat (Eds.), *American Academy of Pediatrics textbook of pediatric care* (2nd ed., Chapter 352). American Academy of Pediatrics.

Isaacson, G. C. (2018). Congenital anomalies of the larynx. *UpToDate*. Retrieved March 11, 2020, from https://www.uptodate.com/contents/congenital-anomalies-of-the-larynx

Isaacson, G. C., & Ojo, A. (2020). Diagnosis and management of intranasal foreign bodies. *UpToDate*. https://www.uptodate.com/contents/diagnosis-and-management-of-intranasal-foreign-bodies

Krilov, L. R. (2017). Infectious mononucleosis and other Epstein-Barr infections. In T. K. McInerny, H. M. Adam, D. E. Campbell, J. M. Foy, & D. M. Kamat (Eds.), *American Academy of Pediatrics textbook of pediatric care* (2nd ed., Chapter 275). American Academy of Pediatrics.

Kronman, M. P., Crowell, C. S., & Vora, S. B. (2019). Infectious diseases. In K. J. Marcdante & R. M. Kliegman (Eds.), *Nelson's essentials of pediatrics* (8th ed., Section 16). Elsevier.

Lopez, S. M. C., & Williams, J. V. (2019). The common cold. In K. J. Marcdante & R. M. Kliegman (Eds.), *Nelson's essentials of pediatrics* (8th ed., Chapter 407). Elsevier.

Mitchell, R. B., Archer, S. M., Ishman, S. L., Rosenfeld, F. M., Coles, S., Finestone, S. A., Friedman, N. R., Giordano, T., Hildrew, D. M., Kim, T. W., Lloyd, R. M., Parikh, S. R., Shulman, S. T., Walner, D. L., Walsh, S. A., & Nnacheta, L. C. (2019). Clinical practice guideline: Tonsillectomy in children (update)—Executive summary. *Otolaryngology—Head and Neck Surgery, 160*(2), 187–205. https://doi.org/10.1177/0194599818807917

Munoz, F. M. (2020). Seasonal influenza in children: Clinical features and diagnosis. *UpToDate*. https://www.uptodate.com/contents/seasonal-influenza-in-children-clinical-features-and-diagnosis

Nagler, J. (2020). Emergency airway management in children: Unique pediatric considerations. *UpToDate*. https://www.uptodate.com/contents/emergency-airway-management-in-children-unique-pediatric-considerations

Pitone, M. L. (2020). *Household safety: Preventing choking*. Retrieved March 11, 2020, from http://kidshealth.org/parent/firstaid_safe/home/safety_choking.html

Safe Kids Worldwide. (2020). *Choking and strangulation*. https://www.safekids.org/choking

Scanlon, V., & Sanders, T. (2019). *Essentials of anatomy and physiology* (8th ed.). F. A. Davis.

Schechter, M., & Stevens, D. M. (2017). Epistaxis. In T. K. McInerny, H. M. Adam, D. E. Campbell, J. M. Foy, & D. M. Kamat (Eds.), *American Academy of Pediatrics textbook of pediatric care* (2nd ed., Chapter 146). American Academy of Pediatrics.

Schmitt, B. D. (2019). *Pediatric telephone protocols: Office version* (16th ed.). American Academy of Pediatrics.

Skae, C. C., & Parikh, S. R. (2017). Foreign bodies of the ear, nose, airway, and esophagus. In T. K. McInerny, H. M. Adam, D. E. Campbell, J. M. Foy, & D. M. Kamat (Eds.), *American Academy of Pediatrics textbook of pediatric care* (2nd ed., Chapter 251). American Academy of Pediatrics.

Steele, R. W. (2017). Chapter 311: Pharyngitis and tonsillitis. In T. K. McInerny, H. M. Adam, D. E. Campbell, J. M. Foy, & D. M. Kamat (Eds.), *American Academy of Pediatrics textbook of pediatric care* (2nd ed.). American Academy of Pediatrics.

Striegel, A., Ong, T., & Marshall, S. G. (2019). Section 18: Respiratory system. In K. J. Marcdante & R. M. Kliegman (Eds.), *Nelson's essentials of pediatrics* (8th ed.). Elsevier.

Tewfik, T. L., & Singh, H. (2018). Eustachian tube function. *eMedicine*. https://emedicine.medscape.com/article/874348-overview

Tolomeo, C. (2019). Chapter 9: Respiratory assessment. In K. G. Duderstadt (Ed.), *Pediatric physical examination: An illustrated handbook* (3rd ed.). Elsevier.

Tunkel, D. E., Anne, S., Payne, S. C., Ishman, S. L., Rosenfled, R. M., Abramson, P. J., Alikhaani, J. D., Benoit, M. M., Bercovitz, R. S., Brown, M. D., Chernobilsky, B., Feldstein, D. A., Hackell, J. M., Holbrook, E. H., Holdsworth, S. M., Lin, K. W., Lind, M. M., Poetker, D. M., Riley, C. A., … Monjur, T. M. (2020). Clinical practice guideline: Nosebleed (epistaxis). *Otolaryngology—Head and Neck Surgery, 162* (Suppl. 1), S1–S38. https://journals.sagepub.com/doi/full/10.1177/0194599819890327

U.S. Food and Drug Administration. (2018). *Use caution when giving cough and cold products to kids*. https://www.fda.gov/drugs/special-features/use-caution-when-giving-cough-and-cold-products-kids

Wald, E. R. (2019). Acute bacterial rhinosinusitis in children: Clinical features and diagnosis. *UpToDate*. Retrieved March 11, 2020, from https://www.uptodate.com/contents/acute-bacterial-rhinosinusitis-in-children-clinical-features-and-diagnosis

Wald, E. R. (2020). Group A streptococcal tonsillopharyngitis in children and adolescents: Clinical features and diagnosis. *UpToDate*. https://www.uptodate.com/contents/group-a-streptococcal-tonsillopharyngitis-in-children-and-adolescents-clinical-features-and-diagnosis

Wald, E. R., Applegate, K. E., Bordley, C., Darrow, D. H., Glode, M. P., Marcy, S. M., Nelson, C. E., Rosenfeld, R. M., Shaikh, N., Smith, M. J., Williams, P. V., & Weinberg, S. T. (2013). Clinical practice guideline for the diagnosis and management of acute bacterial sinusitis in children aged 1 to 18 Years. *Pediatrics, 132*(1), e262–e280. https://doi.org/10.1542/peds.2013-1071

Wolters Kluwer Clinical Drug Information. (2020). *Lexi-comp online*. https://online.lexi.com/lco/action/home

Woods, C. R. (2018). Croup: Clinical features, evaluation, and diagnosis. *UpToDate*. https://www.uptodate.com/contents/croup-clinical-features-evaluation-and-diagnosis

Woods, C. R. (2019). Epiglottitis (supraglottitis): Clinical features and diagnosis. *UpToDate*. https://www.uptodate.com/contents/epiglottitis-supraglottitis-clinical-features-and-diagnosis

Yoon, P. J., Scholes, M. A., & Friedman, N. R. (2018). Chapter 18: Ear, nose, & throat. In W. W. Hay, M. J. Levin, R. R. Deterding, & M. J. Abzug (Eds.), *Current diagnosis & treatment: Pediatrics* (24th ed.). McGraw-Hill Education.

# Management of Lower Respiratory Disorders

Sonia A. Smith

## Student Learning Outcomes

**Upon completion of this chapter the reader should be able to:**

1. Discuss pathophysiology and epidemiology of selected respiratory disorders.
2. Differentiate subjective and objective assessment findings of selected respiratory disorders.
3. Choose appropriate laboratory or diagnostic tests for selected respiratory disorders.
4. Utilize the differential diagnosis process to determine respiratory diagnoses.
5. Determine treatment plan, child/family education, and need for referral for children with respiratory disorder diagnoses.

## INTRODUCTION

Lower respiratory problems, including viral and bacterial respiratory infections (i.e., bronchiolitis, pneumonia) as well as chronic disease (i.e., asthma) commonly occur in children. For infections, it is important for the primary care provider to correctly distinguish viral from bacterial infection in order to demonstrate antibiotic stewardship as promoted by the American Academy of Pediatrics (Gerber et al., 2021) and the Centers for Disease Control and Prevention (CDC, 2019). To arrive at a correct diagnosis, the primary care provider carefully obtains a thorough health history, performs a systematic physical examination of the respiratory system, and orders and interprets laboratory and diagnostic tests if indicated. A successful treatment and management plan begins with accurate diagnosis. Additionally, the comprehensive and systematic approach to assessment of respiratory status allows for identification of potentially life-threatening situations.

Respiratory disorders are the most common causes of illness in children and range from acute infections to serious chronic conditions (Federico et al., 2018). Chronic diseases such as cystic fibrosis (CF) can affect quality of life and the child's development, but frequent infections can also alter the child's well-being.

The child's age, general health status, and socioeconomic status can influence the course of the illness. Due to differences in their anatomy and physiology, healthy infants and younger children are more likely to worsen quickly when ill with a respiratory infection. When experiencing a respiratory infection, children with other chronic conditions experience a more severe illness. The season of the year also influences the development of respiratory infections (e.g., certain viruses are more prevalent in the fall or winter). It is important for the advanced practice provider to be aware of illness patterns in the local area at any given time.

The content in this chapter maps to the following areas on the Pediatric Nursing Certification Board (PNCB) Pediatric Nurse Practitioner—Primary Care certification examination:

## CLINICAL PROBLEMS: PULMONOLOGY

CONTENT AREAS:

### II. Assessment and Diagnosis

**B. History and Physical Examination**

1. Obtain history of present illness
2. Obtain a comprehensive health history for new patients
3. Complete an interval history for established patients
4. Perform a review of systems
5. Perform a complete physical examination

**C. Diagnostic Testing and Screening**

1. Order and interpret office/clinic based screening tests
2. Order and interpret diagnostic laboratory tests
3. Order and interpret the results of diagnostic imaging tests

**D. Analyzing Information**

1. Integrate health history and physical examination findings into the plan of care
2. Assimilate findings from screening and diagnostic testing into plan of care

**E. Diagnosis**

1. Develop and prioritize differential diagnoses
2. Establish a diagnosis based on evaluation of patient data

### III. Management

**A. Child and Caregiver Counseling and Education**

1. Provide condition-specific counseling and education, including treatment options
2. Educate about benefits and potential adverse reactions of pharmacological interventions
3. Discuss non-pharmacological interventions
4. Counsel regarding the threshold for seeking follow-up care
5. Review the risks of non-adherence to recommended treatment

**B. Therapeutic Interventions**

1. Prescribe pharmacologic agents
2. Recommend the use of over-the-counter pharmacologic agents
3. Order or recommend non-pharmacologic treatments for the management of symptoms
4. Discuss use of complementary and alternative therapies as appropriate

**C. Procedures**

1. Perform procedures in accordance with diagnostic guidelines and plan of care (rapid tests)
2. Initiate life-saving techniques in response to urgent or emergent situations

**D. Collaboration and Referral**

2. Refer to specialists as indicated for evaluation, counseling, and/or treatment

**E. Care Coordination**

1. Facilitate patient and family-centered care for children of all ages with acute and chronic conditions

**F. Evaluation and Follow-up**

2. Establish a plan for follow-up care

### IV. Professional Role Responsibilities

**A. Leadership and Evidence-based Practice**

4. Develop, implement, and/or modify clinical practice guidelines

## ANATOMY AND PHYSIOLOGY

The lower airway is comprised of the thorax and lungs (Figure 24.1). The trachea, bronchi, bronchioles, and aveoli are structures all below the sternal notch; air exchange occurs at the aveolar level. The chest wall is comprised of cartilage, bone, and muscle, which provides a protective enclosure for the heart and the lungs. Primitive lungs begin to form at approximately 4 weeks of gestation. By week 28, the lungs are capable of producing the phospholipid surfactant. Alveolar ducts and air sacs form starting at 24 weeks' gestation. Alveoli separate toward the end of gestation and continue to increase in number until 8 years of age (Hill, 2020). The right and left lungs differ in their number of lobes, with the right lobe containing three and the left containing two. The chest wall continues to mature and change throughout childhood. In an infant, the ribcage is more cartilaginous and the ribs are more horizontal. With time, the ribcage becomes more ossified and more vertical.

Infants have a greater rate of oxygen consumption than adults and have a lower functional residual capacity (the amount of air left in the lungs following a

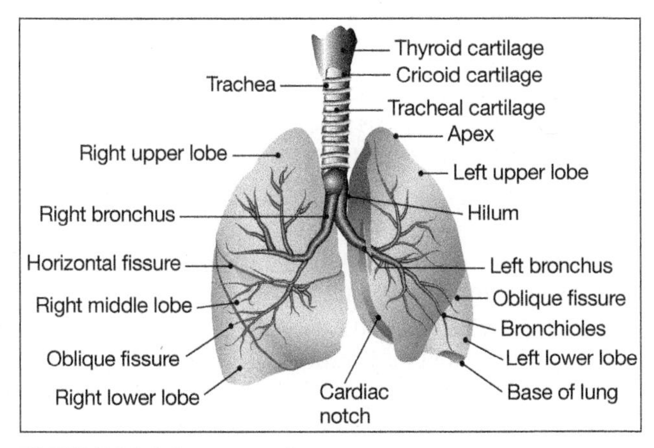


FIGURE 24.1 Lower respiratory tract.

normal respiration). Therefore, they are at increased risk for rapid desaturation during periods of apnea. In addition, because airways are smaller in young children, there is an increase in airway resistance. Infants and young children can develop significant respiratory distress with disease processes that cause narrowing of airway structures due to edema or compression (Harless et al., 2014). Infants and young children have a higher respiratory rate than older children and adults, increased chest compliance due to the cartilaginous ribcage, and less supporting muscle and adipose tissue (Harris & Homnick, 2011).

Developmental considerations must be employed when examining the respiratory system of the infant and young child. Younger children may be examined comfortably in the arms or the lap of the parent or caretaker (Harris & Homnick, 2011). The order of the examination may vary; however, inspection and auscultation should precede palpation and percussion in younger children.

Common variations in the pediatric physical examination may include congenital anomalies such as pectus excavatum or pectus carinatum (Harris & Homnick, 2011). Infants have increased chest wall compliance. Chest wall compliance becomes more pronounced during periods of respiratory distress when intercostal retractions are present. Practitioners should be alert for common signs of respiratory distress in children, such as increased respiratory rate, retractions, grunting, cyanosis, abnormal body positions at rest, use of accessory muscles, and the presence of adventitious breath sounds (University of Rochester Medical Center, 2020). See Table 24.1.

TABLE 24.1 **Adventitious Breath Sounds**

| Breath Sounds | Definition/Description |
|---|---|
| Crackles (rales) | High- or low-pitched sound caused by secretions in the airways; high-pitched, cracking, popping sound is termed *fine crackles*; low-pitched gurgling sound is termed *coarse crackles*; does not clear with coughing |
| Rhonchi | Low-pitched sound caused by large airway narrowing or the presence of secretions; may sound like bubbling, gurgling, or rattling; often will clear with coughing |
| Stridor | Audible (without a stethoscope) high-pitched sound caused by upper airway narrowing; sounds loud and coarse |
| Wheezes | High-pitched sound caused by lower airway narrowing; sound squeaky, like whistling or musical |

*Source*: Adapted from Chiocca, E. M. (2020). *Advanced pediatric assessment* (3rd ed.). Springer Publishing Company.

# INFECTIOUS DISORDERS

## BRONCHIOLITIS

Bronchiolitis is an acute lower respiratory condition found in children under the age of 2 years. It is most commonly caused by viral infections. The infection results in inflammation and edema of the airways along with necrosis of the epithelial airway lining and increased mucus production. Initially occurring in the upper airways, the infection travels to the lower airways in a few days. Symptoms are manifested by rhinorrhea, coughing, tachypnea, and respiratory distress. Wheezing is common as the airway becomes impaired due to bronchiolar changes that result in air trapping and hyperinflation (Mozun et al., 2019; Ralston et al., 2015). The most common pathogen causing bronchiolitis, respiratory syncytial virus (RSV), infects up to 90% of all children by 2 years of age and is most common during the months of November through April. Bronchiolitis is the most common cause of hospitalization in infants and young children and can be a significant cause of morbidity and mortality for children with compromised immune function or cardiorespiratory disease (Ralston et al., 2015).

### Subjective Findings

The health history may reveal:

- Symptoms of a common cold
- Irritability
- Difficulty breathing
- Decreased feeding behavior (Piedra & Stark, 2020)

### Risk Factors

The most common risk factors for bronchiolitis are:

- Prematurity or low birth weight
- Lack of breastfeeding
- Passive smoking
- Household crowding
- Day care attendance
- Presence of siblings in the home
- Indoor air pollution
- Presence of atopy
- Underlying cardiovascular disease
- Immunodeficiency (AAP, 2014; Shi et al., 2015)

### Review of Systems

The most common manifestations revealed during the review of systems include:

- **Constitutional:** Fever, decreased activity
- **Respiratory:** Coryza, rhinorrhea, frequent coughing, apnea
- **Genitourinary:** Possible poor urine output (due to dehydration)
- **Neurologic:** Lethargy (Piedra & Stark, 2020; Ralston et al., 2015)

### Objective Findings

The physical examination of the child with bronchiolitis may reveal:

- Respiratory distress manifested by retractions and nasal flaring
- Adventitious breath sounds to include wheezing and crackles
- Nasal congestion
- Tachypnea
- Hypoxia
- Apnea
- Signs of dehydration (Piedra & Stark, 2020; Ralston et al., 2015)

### Laboratory/Diagnostic Testing

The diagnosis of bronchiolitis can be made on the basis of the history and physical examination. Routine laboratory or imaging studies are not recommended (Breakell et al., 2017; Ralston et al., 2015). However, if the diagnosis is in question, or for children in whom severe or secondary disease is suspected, the following labs and diagnostic tests may be ordered:

- Respiratory viral panels may be positive for RSV or other pathogens such as human metapneumovirus, adenovirus, coronavirus, and influenza, among others
- Complete blood count (CBC) may indicate the probability of a viral infection
- Chemistry panel may indicate signs of dehydration
- Blood gas analysis may indicate respiratory acidosis
- Chest x-rays may be consistent with a viral infection (Piedra & Stark, 2020)

### Differential Diagnosis

The differential diagnosis for bronchiolitis includes:

- Pneumonia
- Reactive, asthma-like wheezing
- Upper respiratory tract infection
- Congenital cardiopulmonary disease
- CF
- Gastroesophageal reflux

### Treatment/Management Plan

Outpatient treatment of bronchiolitis is indicated in patients who are not severely affected. Antibiotics, bronchodilators, chest physiotherapy, and steroids are not recommended (Ralston et al., 2015). Suctioning of nasal secretions, maintenance of hydration, and careful monitoring are the mainstays of treatment (Piedra & Stark, 2020; Figure 24.2). There are no supportive studies advocating for the use of over-the-counter cough and cold medications.

> **PRO TIP** There are many effective nasal aspirators on the market; however, 2-ounce bulb syringes continue to be cost-effective and adequate for suctioning. Adding two to three drops of sterile saline to each nare prior to suctioning can help loosen secretions.

Patients presenting with hypoxia, severe tachypnea, or dehydration require hospitalization. Inpatient treatment includes nebulized hypertonic normal saline, intravenous (IV) hydration, nasal suctioning, and supplemental oxygen (Piedra & Stark, 2020). Severely affected patients may require high-flow nasal cannula oxygen therapy or mechanical ventilation and intensive care unit monitoring (Franklin et al., 2018).

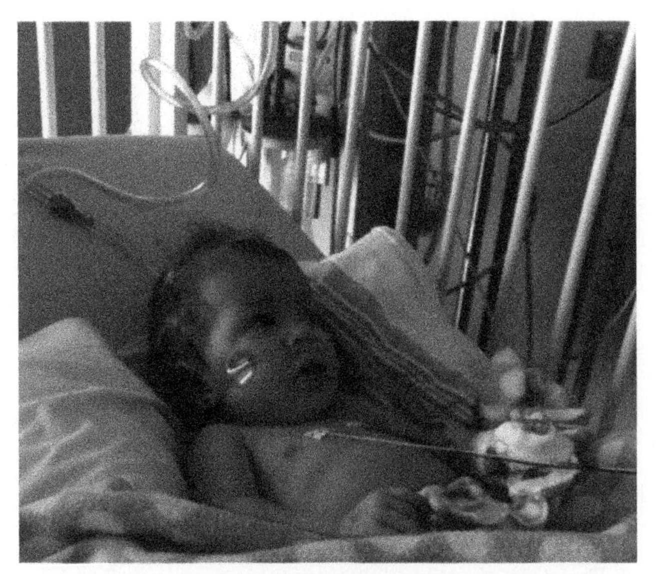

FIGURE 24.2 Infant with history of prematurity hospitalized with bronchiolitis caused by respiratory syncytial virus. Note intercostal retractions.

All patients should be closely observed for development of secondary pulmonary infections.

For infants who meet criteria as outlined by the AAP, monthly injections throughout the RSV season with palivizumab for RSV prophylaxis may prevent the development of bronchiolitis (AAP, 2014 [reaffirmed 2019]; Ralston et al., 2015).

▶ ALERT: Patients with tachypnea can have insensible losses that contribute to dehydration. In addition, prolonged fevers, respiratory distress, and failure to progress may indicate development of a secondary bacterial infection, such as pneumonia.

## Family Education

Teach the following:

- Monitor for signs of respiratory distress and dehydration.
- Perform nasal suctioning.
- Maintain hydration.
- Perform infection control with handwashing and use of alcohol-based products.
- Risk factors include attendance at day care and passive smoking.
- For qualifying infants and young children, ensure monthly receipt of palivizumab for RSV prevention (during the RSV season).

## Referral

The majority of patients can be safely managed by primary care providers throughout the course of their illness. However, hospitalized patients with severe disease and patients with risk factors for more severe outcomes, including those with underlying cardiorespiratory disease, should be referred to a pulmonologist for co-management.

### COVID-19 Impact on Children

The family of Coronaviridae have long been known to be implicated in viral upper respiratory infection in children. Coronaviruses are single-strand RNA viruses that mutate easily. Over the years a few different coronaviruses have resulted in severe respiratory disease, particularly in locations outside of the United States.

In early 2020, an increase in coronavirus disease 19 (COVID-19) was noted and a worldwide pandemic declared. The virus was mutating and spreading rapidly, resulting in increasing numbers of deaths along the way. Thus, the United States implemented country-wide quarantine recommendations to contain spread of the virus. Populations most at risk for severe disease and death included those under age 1 year, the elderly, and immunosuppressed populations.

After many months, as new cases of COVID-19 and deaths began decreasing, quarantines were lifted and recommendations for limiting large public gatherings and requiring face coverings in public places were enacted. During the quarantine, many businesses closed (leaving parents out of work) and children were not permitted to attend day care or school. The long-term psychosocial effects of these restrictions remain to be seen, yet increased stress in all populations has been noted.

Coronavirus 19 infection affects children slightly differently than it does adults. Some children may be mildly affected (mainly presenting with fever and cough), though severe disease may result in pediatric intensive care stays for some children. CT scans revealed a preference for subpleural areas in children rather than lung consolidation. The majority of children testing positive for COIVD-19 had a history of family cluster of disease (Bal et al., 2020; Ma et al., 2020).

The CDC currently recommends administration of the COVID-19 vaccine to all eligible patients age 16 years and older (CDC, 2021). With the expectation of vaccinating young population groups, researchers are currently gathering data about vaccine efficacy in children and in infants as young as six months of age. Despite impending vaccine recommendations for young children, parental vaccine hesitancy will remain a potential challenge for healthcare providers (Goldman et al., 2020). Pediatric nurses will be instrumental in the attempt to educate families with evidence-based information in an ongoing effort to improve vaccination rates and achieve herd immunity against the COVID-19 pandemic (Goldschmidt, 2021).

The World Health Organization (WHO) maintains a "Mythbusters" website useful for accurately educating children and families about COVID-19 infection (WHO, 2020).

# BRONCHITIS

Bronchitis can be acute or chronic and can be caused by viruses or bacteria. Bronchitis in children is frequently characterized by the presence of a wet cough. Protracted bacterial bronchitis (PBB) is the leading cause of wet cough in young children and is one of the primary reasons for referral for subspecialist care (Gilchrist, 2019). The diagnostic criteria for PBB include the presence of a wet cough for 4 weeks or longer, resolution of the cough following a regimen of antibiotics, and identification of bacteria in the lower airways through bronchoscopy (Wang et al., 2019).

## Subjective Findings

The health history may reveal:

- The presence of a wet cough for at least 4 weeks
- Lack of other systemic symptoms (Kantar, 2017; Marchant & Chang, 2019)

### Risk Factors

The most common risk factor for PBB in young children is day care attendance (Kantar, 2017).

### Review of Systems

The most common manifestations revealed during the review of systems include:

- **Constitutional:** lack of fever or malaise
- **Respiratory:** rattling chest, wet cough (Kantar, 2017; Marchang & Chang, 2019)

## Objective Findings

The physical examination of the child with PBB may reveal:

- Loose cough
- Crackles, wheezes, or rhonchi on auscultation
- Mucopurulent secretions if the child is able to expectorate (Marchant & Chang, 2019)

### Laboratory/Diagnostic Testing

The diagnosis of PBB is usually derived from the history and physical examination. There is an absence of symptoms of other etiologies for the cough. If obtained from sputum culture or bronchoalveolar lavage, *Streptococcus pneumoniae* and *Haemophilus influenzae* are the organisms most commonly found. Chest x-rays, if obtained, are typically unremarkable (Kantar, 2017, p. 908).

## Differential Diagnosis

The differential diagnosis for PBB includes:

- Pneumonia
- Bronchiectasis
- Airway malacia
- Asthma
- Residual post-infection cough

## Treatment/Management Plan

- Antibiotics (amoxicillin-clavulanate and second- or third-generation cephalosporins are most commonly prescribed)
- Duration of antibiotic treatment ranges from 2 to 4 weeks
- There are no indications for the use of bronchodilators or inhaled steroids in the treatment of PBB (Gilchrist, 2019; Marchant & Chang, 2019)

### Family Education

Teach the following:

- Supportive care in the form of maintenance of hydration and good handwashing.
- Adherence to the prolonged course of antibiotics.

### Referral

Refer as follows:

- Children unresponsive to an appropriate regimen of antibiotics
- Children with low pulse oximetry readings
- Children with atypical features of PBB

# PNEUMONIA

Pneumonia is a disease characterized by infection and inflammation of the lung parenchyma and alveoli (Mohakud et al., 2018). It typically follows an upper respiratory tract infection that travels to the lungs, which then triggers an immune response leading to inflammation and cytokine production, which leads to tissue edema and capillary leakage. Pneumonia can be community-acquired, hospital-acquired, ventilator-assisted, atypical, or the result of aspiration. Both bacterial and viral pneumonias can induce significant morbidity. In children under the age of

5 years, 15% to 18.3% of all deaths can be attributed to pneumonia, making it the single largest cause of death by infection in children worldwide (Falup-Pecurariu et al., 2018; Mathur et al., 2018). The most vulnerable are very young children who are immunocopromised. *Streptococcus pneumonia* and *Haemophilus influenzae* type b (Hib) were previously the most common bacterial causes of pneumonia prior to immunization. Due to the Hib vaccine, *H. influenzae* type b has been mostly eradicated, with now non-typable *H. influenzae* becoming the most prominent pathogen in pediatric pneumonia. Outside the neonatal period, *S. pneumoniae* is the most common bacterial cause of pneumonia.

## Subjective Findings

The health history may reveal symptoms similar to other infectious lung diseases (see bronchiolitis). Patients with pneumonia may also complain of:

- Chest pain
- Cough
- Difficulty breathing (Barson, 2019a)

## Risk Factors

The most common risk factors for pneumonia are:

- Immunocompromised host
- Lack of immunization against *Haemophilus influenzae*, influenza, and pneumococcus
- Low socioeconomic status
- Crowding
- Exposure to secondhand smoke
- Smoking and vaping
- Underlying cardiorespiratory disease
- Neuromuscular disease
- Respiratory disease such as asthma and CF
- Sickle cell disease
- Any disease process that predisposes a child to aspiration (Barson, 2020; Mathur et al., 2018)

## Review of Systems

The most common manifestations revealed during the review of systems include:

- **Constitutional:** lethargy, abdominal pain (due to mesenteric adenitis; Barson, 2019a)
- **Respiratory:** coryza, rhinorrhea, frequent coughing
- **Gastrointestinal:** vomiting
- **Genitourinary:** poor urine output due to decreased oral intake (Barson, 2019a)

▶ ALERT: Symptoms of pneumonia can be atypical and subtle in children. Coughing may not be an initial presenting symptom. Young children may present with fussiness and poor feeding. Older children may complain of abdominal pain. Chest x-rays are not always definitive, as they can lag behind the patient's clinical presentation.

## Objective Findings

Upon physical examination, the following clinical manifestations may be noted:

- Irritability
- Fever
- Tachypnea
- Respiratory distress
- Hypoxia/cyanosis
- Grunting, nasal flaring (young infants)
- Wheezing, crackles, diminished lung sounds
- Dullness on percussion
- Positive findings on performing egophony, bronchophony, whispered pectoriloquy, and tactile fremitus (Barson, 2019a)

**PRO TIP** A two-view chest with a lateral view may be recommended to illuminate areas of consolidation that may be hidden behind the heart shadow.

## Laboratory/Diagnostic Testing

- Chest x-ray (two view) may be obtained if the child is severely affected, unresponsive to treatment, or if the diagnosis is in doubt. X-rays may reveal areas of focal airspace consolidation or interstitial infiltrates (Figure 24.3).
- CBC findings may depend on the severity and etiology of the disease.
- Acute phase reactants (C-reactive protein and erythrocyte sedimentation rate) are not routinely performed, but may be helpful to document the course of the disease.
- Chemistry panels may be helpful to determine the degree of dehydration in children with poor oral intake.
- Sputum cultures or viral respiratory panels may be helpful to identify pathogens to help guide treatment or antibiotic selection.
- Blood cultures may be obtained when bacteremia is suspected or from those who are not fully immunized (Barson, 2019b; Bradley et al., 2011; Falup-Pecurariu et al., 2018).

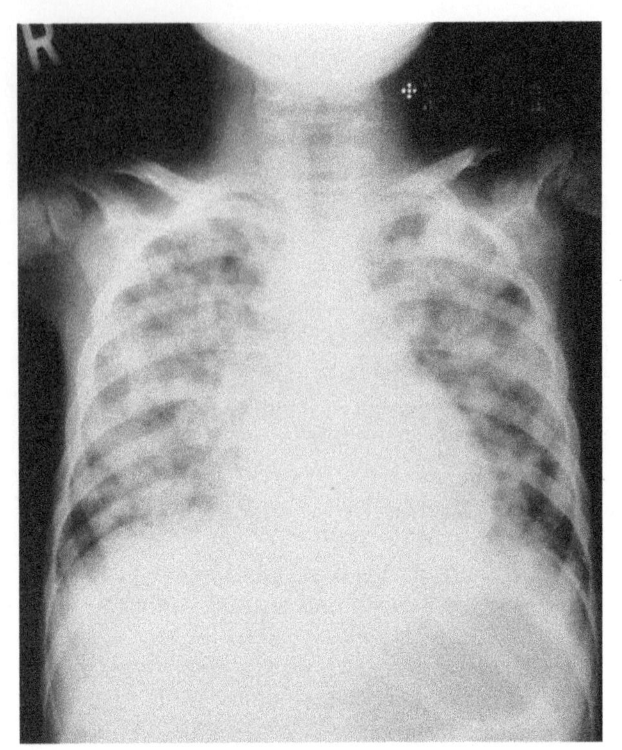


FIGURE 24.3 Chickenpox pneumonia. This anteroposterior radiograph revealed bilateral pulmonary infiltrates throughout the entirety of each lung field in the case of a child with leukemia, as well as chickenpox pneumonia. The fact that this child had leukemia made him that much more susceptible to contracting a pneumonic infection.

*Source*: Image courtesy of Joel D. Meyers, MD/Centers for Disease Control and Prevention.

**PRO TIP** The thymus "sail sign" in young children is a normal finding that can be mistaken for pneumonia on x-ray (Figure 24.4).

## Differential Diagnosis

The diagnosis of pneumonia is usually based on the clinical findings. The differential diagnosis for pneumonia includes:

- Bronchiolitis
- Bronchitis
- Asthma
- Hemoglobinopathy
- Foreign body aspiration (FBA)
- Metastatic malignancy
- Pleural effusion

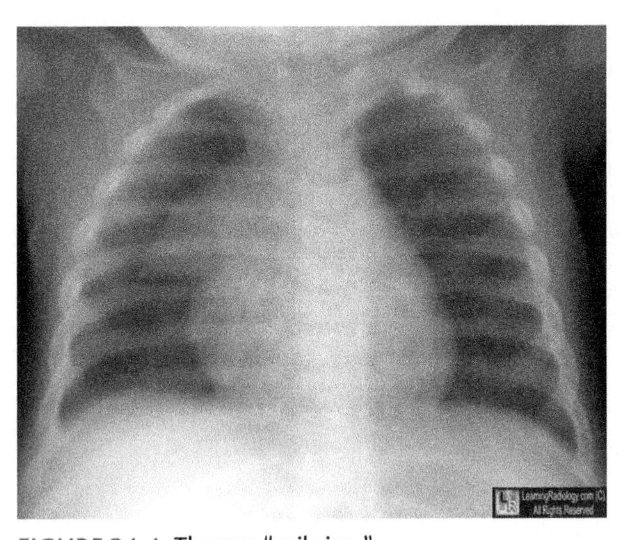

FIGURE 24.4 Thymus "sail sign."

*Source*: Reproduced with permission from LearningRadiology. http://learningradiology.com/notes/chestnotes/thymicsailsigns.htm

## Treatment/Management Plan

The treatment of pneumonia is dependent upon several factors, including the etiology of the disease, the baseline condition of the patient, and the severity of the disease. The aims of treatment for all patients are to eradicate the infection, correct hypoxia, maintain hydration, and prevent complications. Many children can be successfully treated on an outpatient basis. *Streptococcus pneumoniae* is the most common community-acquired pathogen. Amoxicillin is the first-line treatment for healthy, immunized children with community-acquired pneumonia. Macrolides are recommended for treatment of atypical pneumonia caused by *M. pneumoniae* or for other causes in children who have a penicillin allergy (Bradley et al., 2011).

The decision to hospitalize is based on the age of the child, underlying illnesses, and patient response to the infection (Barson, 2019b). Hospitalization should be considered for all infants age 3 to 6 months (Bradley et al., 2011). In moderately ill patients, laboratory studies, such as a CBC or blood culture, can be somewhat useful. Parenteral antibiotic choices depend upon the level of bacterial resistance in the community, the etiology of the infection, and the condition of the child. Outpatient antibiotic therapy should be between 7 and 10 days with an evaluation in 48 hours if fever and symptoms continue.

Because viral infections cannot be treated with antibiotics, supportive care and close observation for signs of a secondary bacterial infection are indicated. In cases of pneumonia caused by influenza, viral therapy is recommended if given within the designated period of time (Bradley et al., 2011).

## Family Education

Teach the following:

- Monitor for signs of respiratory distress and dehydration.
- Perform nasal suctioning for young infants and children.
- Maintain hydration.
- Maintain infection control with the use of handwashing and alcohol-based products.
- Reduce risk factors, including obtaining required immunizations.
- Administer antibiotics or antiviral medication.
- Monitor for signs of worsening condition, which may necessitate hospitalization.

## Referral

Practitioners should consider referral to a pulmonologist in the following groups of patients:

- Immunocompromised
- Underlying cardiorespiratory disease
- Recurrent pneumonia
- Development of complications of pneumonia such as empyema or lung abscess
- Unusual pathogens such as *Staphylococcus aureus*
- Suspected aspiration pneumonia
- Patients requiring bronchoscopy

ALERT: A new phenomenon leading to significant morbidity and growing mortality is e-cigarette vaping associated lung injury (EVALI). Guidance for the care of these patients can be found in the October 2019 *Morbidity and Mortality Weekly Report* (Siegel et al., 2019). Providers should be aware of this potential diagnosis in older children and adolescents who present with respiratory and gastrointestinal symptoms. Patients may complain of coughing, difficulty breathing, abdominal pain, nausea, and diarrhea (Siegel et al., 2019). There is no specific test to evaluate for the presence of EVALI; however, products containing nicotine with and without tetrahydrocannabinol (THC) have been implicated as possible causative agents (Siegel et al., 2019). Treatment considerations for patients with EVALI include the use of antibiotics, steroids, and antivirals with supplemental oxygen and respiratory support, as needed (Siegel et al., 2019; Figure 24.5).

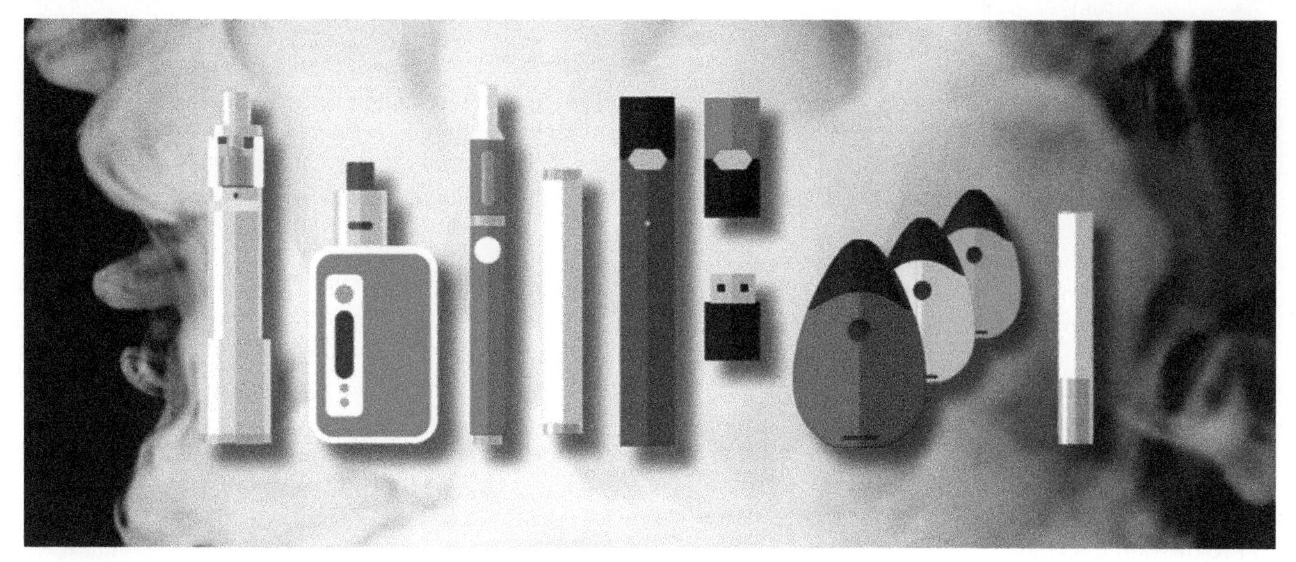

FIGURE 24.5 E-cigarette types.

*Source*: Centers for Disease Control and Prevention. (n.d.). *E-cigarette, or vaping, products visual dictionary*. https://www.cdc.gov/tobacco/basic_information/e-cigarettes/pdfs/ecigarette-or-vaping-products-visual-dictionary-508.pdf

# TUBERCULOSIS

Tuberculosis (TB) is an infectious disease caused by *Mycobacterium tuberculosis* or *Mycobacterium bovis*, an acid-fast bacillus, and is transmitted by aerosolized particles (Adams & Starke, 2019a). The World Health Organization estimated 10 million cases of TB worldwide in 2018 with approximately 1 million children affected (Adams & Starke, 2019b). The disease can be characterized as either latent or active. A diagnosis of latent TB is given to those individuals who demonstrate prior infection without clinical evidence of active disease (Adams & Starke, 2019a).

The majority of children who test positive for TB are infected due to exposure to an affected adult. The diagnosis of TB in children is hampered by challenges in laboratory testing as well as the often nonspecific nature of physical manifestations of the disease (Cowger et al., 2019). Although pulmonary TB is the most common, extrapulmonary disease can be found in the lymph nodes, central nervous system (CNS), and other organs (Adams & Starke, 2019b).

## Subjective Findings

The health history may reveal:

- Fever
- Chronic cough for longer than 3 weeks
- Weight loss/failure to thrive
- Decreased energy/playfulness (Adams & Starke, 2019b)

## Risk Factors

The most common risk factors for TB are:

- Being born outside of the United States
- Having lived in a foreign country for at least 2 months
- Having at least one parent who is foreign born
- Spending time in a shelter, with someone in prison, or with someone who is HIV positive or who uses illegal drugs
- Immunodeficiency
- Consuming unpasteurized dairy products
- Older children are more likely to test positive than younger children
- Younger children are at higher risk for disease progression than older children (Adams & Starke, 2019b; Cowger et al., 2019; AAP Pediatric Tuberculosis Collaborative Group, 2004; Whittaker et al., 2019)

## Review of Systems

Children with latent TB are asymptomatic. The most common manifestations revealed during the review of systems for children with active TB include:

- **Constitutional:** fever for at least 2 weeks in the absence of other diseases, weight loss
- **Respiratory:** lower respiratory tract symptoms with an unremitting cough, hemoptysis
- **Lymphatic:** Swollen lymph nodes (Adams & Starke, 2019b).

## Objective Findings

The physical examination of the child with TB may reveal:

- Failure to gain weight/falling off growth curve
- Adventitious breath sounds or decreased breath sounds
- Lymphadenopathy (Adams & Starke, 2019b)

## Laboratory/Diagnostic Testing

*The Official American Thoracic Society/Infectious Diseases Society of America/Centers for Disease Control and Prevention Clinical Practice Guidelines* for the diagnosis of tuberculosis in adults and children (Lewinsohn et al., 2016) provide a detailed overview of laboratory and diagnostic testing for patients with latent and active TB. The guidelines have been endorsed by the AAP. Practitioners screening and caring for children with active or latent TB should be aware of the following:

- The TB skin test using purified protein derivative by Mantoux technique is the preferred method of testing for children under the age of 5 years. The TB skin test cannot distinguish between latent and active disease.

▶ ALERT: A negative skin test does not rule out TB disease. Testing must be interpreted in the context of the patient's history and clinical presentation (Adams & Starke, 2019b).

- The interferon gamma release assay (IGRA) blood test may be used for children over the age of 5 years and for any child who received the bacille Calmette-Guerin (BCG) vaccine for TB prevention.
- Acid-fast bacilli smear microscopy should be performed for all patients suspected of having pulmonary TB.

- Mycobacterial cultures with drug susceptibility testing should be performed for all patients suspected of having pulmonary TB.
- Specimens from other sites of potential TB infection may be obtained for culture.
- Chest x-rays may show areas of opacification and hilar adenopathy.
- Chest computed tomography (CT) may be indicated if the pathology on x-ray requires further clarity.
- Routine CBCs and chemistry panels may be obtained (Adams & Starke, 2019b; Ishikawa et al., 2018; Lewinsohn et al., 2016).

**PRO TIP** Sputum induction should be used as the initial respiratory sampling method for all patients unable to expectorate a sufficient sample.

- Flexible bronchoscopy sampling should be used for patients for whom sputum induction was not successful.
- An early morning gastric aspiration is the preferred method for obtaining a sputum sample in very young children.

▶ ALERT: TB is transmitted via airborne droplets (Lewinsohn et al., 2016). Therefore, appropriate personal protective equipment (N95, gown, and gloves) must be utilized during specimen collection and care of persons suspected of having TB.

### Differential Diagnosis

The differential diagnosis for TB includes:

- Pneumonia caused by other organisms
- Malignancy
- Lymphadenopathy caused by other organisms, including cat scratch fever
- Other systemic febrile illnesses

### Treatment/Management Plan

*The Official American Thoracic Society/Infectious Diseases Society of America/Centers for Disease Control and Prevention Clinical Practice Guidelines* for the diagnosis of TB in adults and children (Lewinsohn et al., 2016) provides a detailed overview of treatment for patients with latent and active TB. The guidelines have been endorsed by the AAP. Multidrug treatment regimens include a combination of rifampin, isoniazid, and rifapentine. For complete eradication of the bacillus, treatment regimens can last up to 9 months. All patients should be closely monitored for clinical progression or resolution of the disease and medication adherence (Adams & Starke, 2019a).

### Family Education

Teach the following:

- Avoid consuming unpasteurized dairy products.
- Adherence to the prescribed medical regimen is necessary for complete eradication of the bacillus.
- All persons to whom the child was exposed should be screened for latent or active TB.

### Referral

Refer as follows:

- Tuberculosis is a reportable disease to local departments of health.
- Practitioners should consider referrals to infectious disease specialists, pulmonologists, and other subspecialists, as appropriate.

## COCCIDIOIDOMYCOSIS

Coccidioidomycosis, also known as Valley Fever, is a fungal respiratory disease caused by soil-bearing fungi *Coccidioides immitis* or *Coccidioides posadasii*. The disease is endemic to the southwestern United States. The airborne spores are especially prevalent in Arizona and California but can also be found in Mexico and South America (Matlock et al., 2019). Approximately 150,000 cases of coccidioidomycosis are documented in the United States each year (Blair & Ampel, 2020).

Transmission is via inhalation of fungal spores found in environmental dust. Once the spores are inhaled into the lung, small spore-producing spheres are released into the lung tissue and cellular immunity is activated. The disease is not transmitted person-to-person.

### Subjective Findings

The health history may reveal:

- Exposure, however brief, to endemic areas within the past 21 days
- Flu-like symptoms (malaise, fever, cough, myalgia, joint pains, difficulty breathing, night sweats; Blair & Ampel, 2020; Matlock et al., 2019)

### Risk Factors

The most common risk factors for coccidioidomycosis are:

- Exposure to dust in areas endemic to coccidioidomycosis
- Immunocompromised individuals are particularly susceptible (Blair & Ampel, 2020; Matlock et al., 2019)

### Review of Systems

The most common manifestations revealed during the review of systems include:

- **Constitutional:** fever, night sweats, weight loss, fatigue, chest pain
- **Integumentary:** rashes
- **Respiratory:** difficulty breathing, cough
- **Musculoskeletal:** Muscle aches, joint pain
- **Neurologic:** headache (Blair & Ampel, 2020)

### Objective Findings

The physical examination of the child with coccidioidomycosis may reveal:

- Pulmonary symptoms similar to those found in patients with bronchitis or community-acquired pneumonia
- Erythema nodosum or, less commonly, erythema multiforme (Blair & Ampel, 2020)

### Laboratory/Diagnostic Testing

- Routine lab tests may be normal, with the exception of an elevated erythrocyte sedimentation rate
- Coccidioidal IgG and IgM
- Direct examination of cultures using potassium hydroxide preparation
- Polymerase chain reaction (PCR) testing may also be available
- Chest x-ray findings may demonstrate findings consistent with pneumonia and may show hilar adenopathy (Blair & Ampel, 2020)

### Differential Diagnosis

The differential diagnosis for coccidioidomycosis includes:

- Bacterial community-acquired pneumonia or bronchitis
- Viral respiratory infections
- Atypical mycobacterial infection
- Tuberculosis
- Other fungal infections
- Erythema nodosum and erythema multiforme from other sources
- Histiocytosis
- Sarcoidosis
- Leukemias
- Lymphoproliferative disorders (Alexander et al., 2017)

▶ ALERT: Basic laboratory testing and chest x-rays may be normal. Consideration of a diagnosis of Valley Fever should be given to all individuals with the potential for exposure with accompanying signs and symptoms of the disease.

### Treatment/Management Plan

- Many infections in healthy individuals resolve without intervention.
- Although there is no cure for coccidioidomycosis, treatment with antifungal medications (including fluconazole and itraconazole) is indicated for more seriously affected individuals as well as for those who are at risk for dissemination of the infection.
- Amphotericin B may be used for treatment of the most serious cases.
- Close examination and serologic monitoring every few weeks until significantly improved, then every 6 months for up to 1 to 2 years following the initial infection (Alexander et al., 2017; Blair & Ampel, 2020).

### Family Education

Teach the following:

- Signs of dissemination of the disease and pulmonary complications.
- Prolonged fatigue, night sweats, fever, joint pain, muscle aches, and weight loss can persist for weeks or months.

### Referral

Refer as follows:

- Valley Fever is a reportable disease in certain states, including Arizona.
- Patients with dissemination of the disease, or complications of coccidioidomycosis, should have appropriate referrals to subspecialists, including pediatric pulmonology and infectious disease

## CONGENITAL DISORDERS

Congenital disorders affecting the lower respiratory tract in children include CF, congenital central hypoventilation (CCH) syndrome, congenital diaphragmatic hernia (CDH), and congenital pulmonary airway malformation (CPAM).

## CYSTIC FIBROSIS

Cystic fibrosis (CF) is an autosomal recessive disorder producing a multitude of systemic manifestations, including chronic pulmonary and sinus infections, pancreatic insufficiency, and nutritional deficiencies. The underlying mechanism of the disease is a mutation in the CF transmembrane conductance regulator (CFTR) gene involved in the transport of chloride and water to the cell membrane (Katkin, 2019). The defect in water and chloride transport results in the formation of thick, tenacious mucus which obstructs the airways and the ducts in the pancreas, liver, and other organs. The thickened mucus serves as a breeding ground for bacteria and produces inflammatory responses, most often affecting the lungs and sinuses (Bono-Neri et al., 2019). Involvement of the pancreas often leads to development of insulin-dependent diabetes.

The severity of CF depends upon the type of mutation involved (Cystic Fibrosis Foundation, n.d.). In 2016, the median life expectancy of adults with CF was 47.7 years (Bono-Neri et al., 2019). Treatment of patients with CF involves a multidisciplinary team consisting of pulmonologists, gastroenterologists, endocrinologists, respiratory therapists, nutritionists, and primary care providers.

### Subjective Findings

The health history may reveal:

- Meconium ileus in the neonatal period
- Prolonged neonatal jaundice
- Recurrent or persistent cough
- Recurrent mucopurulent mucus production
- Inability to gain weight
- Infection with bacteria to include *P. aeruginosa* and *s. aureus* (Jancelewicz et al., 2019; Katkin, 2019)

▶ ALERT: Consider CF in patients with recurrent pulmonary or sinus infections as well as children with poor growth.

### Risk Factors

In patients with non-Hispanic White or Ashkenazi Jewish heritage, the carrier rate for CF at 1:29 is higher than for other ethnic groups. Because the disease is autosomal recessive, the risk of having CF, if both parents are carriers of the CFTR mutation, is 25% (Bono-Neri et al., 2019).

### Review of Systems

The most common manifestations revealed during the review of systems include:

- **Constitutional:** malnutrition, delayed growth
- **HEENT:** recurrent or persistent ear or sinus infections
- **Respiratory:** recurrent or persistent respiratory infections, episodes of wheezing and cough
- **Gastrointestinal:** constipation, abnormal stools (fatty, floating, loose, foul-smelling)
- **Reproductive:** reduced fertility (Bono-Neri et al., 2019)

### Objective Findings

The physical examination of the child with CF may reveal:

- Adventitious lung sounds including wheezing, rhonchi, and crackles
- Frequent, productive cough
- Signs of respiratory distress
- Hypoxia
- Barrell chest
- Digital clubbing
- Hemoptysis
- Nasal polyps
- Delayed development of secondary sex characteristics
- Abdominal distension
- Signs of pancreatitis or cholelithiasis
- Rectal prolapse
- Intussusception (Katkin, 2019)

### Laboratory/Diagnostic Testing

The following diagnostic tests are common in the diagnosis and management of CF:

- Prenatal testing for the CFTR gene mutation via chorionic villus sampling or amniocentesis
- Newborn screening
- Sweat chloride test: considered positive for CF with a concentration of 60 mmol/L or greater
- Post-neonatal CFTR gene mutation testing

- CBC may reveal signs of infection or anemia
- Chemistry panels may reveal hyponatremia and hypochloremia. Patients may also suffer from hypokalemia and hyperglycemia
- Sputum samples may grow bacteria not commonly found in healthy individuals
- Stool samples often show a high content of fecal fat
- Hypovitaminosis of fat-soluble vitamins is common
- Chest x-rays and CTs may reveal hyperinflation and findings consistent with pneumonia or bronchiectasis
- Pulmonary function testing often reveals obstructive lung disease
- Sinus x-rays and CTs are often positive for acute or chronic sinus disease
- Echocardiogram may show evidence of pulmonary hypertension (Sabharwal & Schwarzenberg, 2019; Simon, 2020)

## Differential Diagnosis

The differential diagnosis for CF includes:

- Asthma
- Sinusitis
- Congenital lung malformations
- Primary ciliary dyskinesia
- Bronchiectasis
- Bronchitis

## Treatment/Management Plan

The treatment of patients with CF is focused on management of acute exacerbations, prevention and treatment of sequelae of the disease, and promotion of growth and development.

- Management of acute exacerbations
  - Aggressive bacteria-specific IV and inhaled antibiotic therapy
  - Inhaled bronchodilators and airway clearance agents and techniques
  - Treatment of hypoxia and hypercapnia
  - Correction of dehydration and nutritional deficiencies (Sabharwal & Schwarzenberg, 2019; Simon, 2020)
- Prevention and treatment of sequelae of disease
  - Treatment with CFTR modulators
  - Promotion of a nutritionally balanced, calorie-dense diet
  - Administration of fat-soluble vitamins and formula supplements
  - Administration of pancreatic enzyme supplements
  - Maintenance bronchodilator and anti-inflammatory medications
  - Airway clearance techniques (chest physiotherapy, cough assist devices, exercise)
  - Inhaled airway clearance agents (recombinant human deoxyribonuclease and hypertonic normal saline)
  - Administration of azithromycin for anti-inflammatory effects
  - Treatment of gastroesophageal reflux, if present
  - Treatment of CF-related diabetes
  - Immunizations including yearly influenza vaccines
  - Employing isolation principles, when appropriate
  - Use of positive airway pressure during sleep, if needed (Bono-Neri et al., 2019; Sabharwal & Schwarzenberg, 2019; Simon, 2020)
- Promotion of growth and development
  - Education about respiratory triggers including cigarette smoking and vaping
  - Reproductive health education regarding infertility, pregnancy prevention, and disease prevention
  - Promotion of normal school activities based on the patient's ability to participate
  - Assessment of symptoms of anxiety or depression
  - Promotion of compliance in order to maximize growth and developmental potential (Bono-Neri et al., 2019; Sabharwal & Schwarzenberg, 2019; Simon, 2020)

Patients with advanced lung disease with impending respiratory failure may be candidates for bilateral lung transplant. Pediatric patients undergoing the procedure have a 50% survival rate of 5.2 years (Simon, 2020). End-of-life discussions should be initiated, when appropriate, with advance care directives agreed upon by the patient and family.

## Family Education

Teach the following:

- Know respiratory care and airway clearance techniques.
- Be able to administer oral and IV medication.
- Care for central line catheters (if applicable).
- Care for gastrostomy tubes (if applicable).
- Promote healthy living including nutrition, exercise, and sleep.
- Know signs of respiratory distress and when to contact medical providers.
- Promote normal growth and developmental milestones.

### Referral

Patients and families should be referred to an accredited CF care center for primary management of the disease. At the center, patients will have the benefit of a multidisciplinary team of care providers and will be able to take advantage of the latest research and advances in the care of patients with CF. Another advantage of center-based care is the ability to network with other similarly affected families for support.

## CONGENITAL CENTRAL HYPOVENTILATION SYNDROME

Congenital central hypoventilation (CCH), also known as "Ondine's curse," is a rare, autosomal dominant genetic syndrome that affects the autonomic nervous system and in which neonates present with periods of apnea, hypoventilation, and hypoxia in the absence of signs of respiratory distress. Children with this condition do not response to the usual stimulus of elevated carbon dioxide or decreased oxygen levels. Apneic periods are most commonly seen during non-rapid eye movement (REM) sleep. If the condition is mild, older children may first present following respiratory tract infections or induction of anesthesia (Kasi et al., 2016).

### Subjective Findings

The health history may reveal:

- Inability to breathe independently at birth
- Chronic cyanosis
- Episodes of apnea, particularly during sleep (Kasi et al., 2016)

### Risk Factors

The most common risk factors for CCH are:

- The presence of the paired-like homeobox 2B (PHOX2B) gene in one or both parents
- The presence of Hirschsprung disease and neural crest tumors that also arise from expression of the PHOX2B gene (Kasi et al., 2016)

### Review of Systems

The most common manifestations revealed during the review of systems include:

- **Respiratory:** apnea in the absence of respiratory distress, cyanosis during sleep
- **Gastrointestinal:** history of Hirschsprung disease
- **Neurologic:** other neurologic abnormalities (Brouillette, 2019; Kasi et al., 2016)

### Objective Findings

The physical examination of the child with CCH may reveal:

- Ocular abnormalities
- Persistent or recurrent central cyanosis
- Witnessed apnea or shallow breathing during sleep
- Respiratory arrest
- Bradycardia and other problems regulating the heart rate
- Cognitive deficits in older child (Brouillette, 2019; Kasi et al., 2016)

▶ ALERT: Clinicians should be aware of CCH in older children who present with apnea or cyanosis following anesthesia, respiratory infections, or with administration of other CNS depressants.

### Laboratory/Diagnostic Testing

- Polysomnography may reveal central apnea, hypoxia, and hypoventilation
- PHOX2B mutation testing
- Screen for inborn errors of metabolism
- Brain magnetic resonance imaging (MRI) to exclude other possible etiologies for central apnea (e.g., Chiari malformation)
- Chest x-ray
- Cardiac evaluation to evaluate for other possible etiologies of cyanosis
- Barium enema and rectal biopsy for evaluation of Hirschsprung disease
- Imaging and biopsy for evaluation of neural crest tumors (Brouillette, 2019; Kasi et al., 2016)

### Differential Diagnosis

The differential diagnosis for CCH includes:

- Central apnea of other etiologies
- Cardiac disease
- Inborn errors of metabolism

### Treatment/Management Plan

The primary treatment for CCH is management of the patient's oxygenation ventilatory status. This can be accomplished via:

- Home ventilatory support

- Tracheostomy placement
- Bilevel positive pressure support
- Diaphragmatic pacing (Brouillette, 2019; Kasi et al., 2016)

### Family Education

Teach the following:

- Home ventilatory care.
- Tracheostomy care.
- Foster growth and developmental milestones.

### Referral

All children with CCH should be referred to a center with pulmonologists experienced in caring for children with atypical pulmonary diseases and who have the capacity to provide family education regarding home ventilator management (Brouillette, 2019).

## CONGENITAL DIAPHRAGMATIC HERNIA AND CONGENITAL PULMONARY AIRWAY MALFORMATION

Congenital diaphragmatic hernia (CDH) is an in utero defect manifested by herniation of abdominal contents into the chest cavity resulting in varying degrees of pulmonary hypoplasia in one or both lungs. Many infants with CDH are diagnosed antenatally, resulting in improved rates of survival. Some infants, however, are not diagnosed until after birth, when they may present with signs of respiratory distress within the first minutes or hours of life (Hedrick & Adzick, 2019). Despite technological advances, mortality is still approximately 30% (Jancelewicz et al., 2019).

Congenital pulmonary airway malformation (CPAM) is the most common congenital pulmonary lesion. Most cases are found in the neonatal period or during infancy (Amraoui et al., 2017). Cysts vary in size and number and compress normal lung tissue, resulting in respiratory distress. CPAM is often misdiagnosed on radiological exam. Despite the presence of abnormal lungs, approximately 25% of newborns with CPAM are asymptomatic at birth (Oermann, 2019). Management of infants with CDH and CPAM is complex and requires the services of a multidisciplinary team.

### Subjective Findings

The health history may reveal:

- Identification of CDH or CPAM on antenatal ultrasound
- Respiratory distress at birth (Hedrick & Adzick, 2019)

### Risk Factors

CDH is often associated with other anomalous conditions including cardiac defects, chromosomal abnormalities, and neural tube defects. Adrenal insufficiency is another condition commonly found in infants with CDH. Identification of any of these comorbid conditions should alert the practitioner to the possibility of CDH (Hedrick & Adzick, 2019). Risk factors and etiology of CPAM are unknown.

### Review of Systems

The most common manifestations revealed during the review of systems include:

- **Constitutional:** poor feeding behavior (CDH), failure to thrive (CDH)
- **Respiratory:** respiratory distress (severe in CDH and in CPAM associated with significant compression of lung tissue), recurrent pulmonary infections (CPAM), spontaneous pneumothorax (CPAM; Hedrick & Adzick, 2019; Oermann, 2019)

### Objective Findings

The physical examination of the infant with CDH may reveal:

- Decreased or absent breath sounds over the affected lung(s)
- Severe respiratory distress on examination
- Barrel-shaped chest
- Scaphoid-appearing abdomen
- Pulmonary hypertension
- Cardiac anomalies (found in 50% of infants with CDH)
- Cardiac sounds more prominent over the right side of the chest (Hedrick & Adzick, 2019)

The physical examination of the infant or child with CPAM may reveal:

- Varying degrees of respiratory distress or respiratory failure
- Recurrent cough and dyspnea in older children

- Pneumothorax
- Abnormal lung sounds
- Mediastinal shift (in severe cases; Oermann, 2019)

### Laboratory/Diagnostic Testing

The diagnostic tests for CDH include:

- The primary diagnostic tool is radiographic evidence from chest and abdominal x-rays that reveal intrusion of the abdominal contents into the hemithorax.
- Blood gas analysis findings include acidosis and hypoxia.
- Low cortisol levels may be found in infants with concomitant adrenal insufficiency.
- Echocardiogram is necessary for evaluation of cardiac defects and functioning.
- MRI is helpful to provide a detailed evaluation of the defect (Hedrick & Adzick, 2019).

Diagnostic tests for CPAM include:

- Chest x-rays; useful in the initial evaluation of pulmonary disease
- CT scans and MRI of the thorax; help to distinguish CPAM from other pulmonary diseases
- Histopathological evaluation of surgical specimens
- Blood gas analysis; may reveal impaired gas exchange (Amraoui et al., 2017, p. 3; Oermann, 2019)

### Differential Diagnosis

The differential diagnosis for CDH should include other possible etiologies of respiratory distress:

- Oligohydramnios
- Meconium aspiration
- Cardiac defects.

The differential diagnosis for CPAM should include:

- Bronchopulmonary sequestration
- CDH
- Congenital lobar emphysema
- Bronchogenic cysts
- Pneumatoceles

### Treatment/Management Plan

Treatment for CDH includes immediate attention to stabilization of breathing with intubation and the use of mechanical ventilation and extracorporeal membranous oxygenation (ECMO). Central IV lines are placed, and a nasogastric tube is used to decompress the stomach and decrease pressure on the lungs. Once the infant is stable, surgical repair of the defect is planned (Jancelewicz et al., 2019).

Once the respiratory status has stabilized, surgical wedge resection or lobectomy is the curative option for symptomatic infants and children with CPAM. Asymptomatic patients may be observed with caution, as they are at increased risk for recurrent infections, malignancy, pneumothorax, increased lung tissue compression, and repeated radiation exposure (Hedrick & Adzick, 2019; Jancelewicz et al., 2019).

### Family Education

Teach the following:

- Educate family members about the diagnosis, etiology (if known), course of treatment, and prognosis.
- Anticipatory guidance about potential complications following the acute phase of treatment is especially important for severely affected infants, particularly if ECMO was used in the initial treatment phase:
  - Ongoing respiratory vulnerability to infection
  - Cognitive and developmental delays
  - Poor growth
  - Feeding problems
- Need for prophylaxis against RSV.
- Potential for development of malignancy in patients with CPAM who do not undergo surgical resection or lobectomy.

### Referral

One of the primary responsibilities of the primary care advanced practice nurse (APN) is development of clinical suspicion for congenital pulmonary defects in infants presenting with respiratory distress. The APN should initiate early referrals to, and collaborate with, appropriate subspecialists while caring for the child in the acute and post-hospitalization phases of treatment.

## OTHER LOWER RESPIRATORY DISORDERS

Other disorders affecting the lower respiratory system in children include FBA, spontaneous pneumothorax, obstructive sleep apnea syndrome (OSAS), and brief, resolved, unexplained event (BRUE).

## FOREIGN BODY ASPIRATION

Tracheobronchial FBA occurs at a rate of approximately 2,000 cases annually in the United States. Most cases occur in children under the age of 3 years. FBA is more common in young children due to their small airway diameters, immature dentition necessary for thorough chewing, and a tendency to explore their environment with introduction of objects into their mouths (Vivisenco et al., 2019; Figure 24.6).

Fifty-two percent of aspirated items travel to the right mainstem bronchus (Ruiz, 2020). Food items are most commonly aspirated by infants and toddlers. Round objects may cause a complete airway obstruction resulting in asphyxiation if not quickly removed. Medications containing iron or potassium may cause airway inflammation and stenosis if not removed urgently (Ruiz, 2020). Due to the electrochemical properties of the object, aspirated button batteries can also cause extensive damage if not removed promptly (Swain et al., 2017). A retained foreign body in the airway may result in treatment-resistant pneumonia, bronchiectasis, pulmonary atelectasis, pulmonary abscess, subcutaneous emphysema, pneumomediastinum, or airway stenosis (Bourrous et al., 2019; Mehta et al., 2019; Ruiz, 2020; Vivisenco et al., 2019).

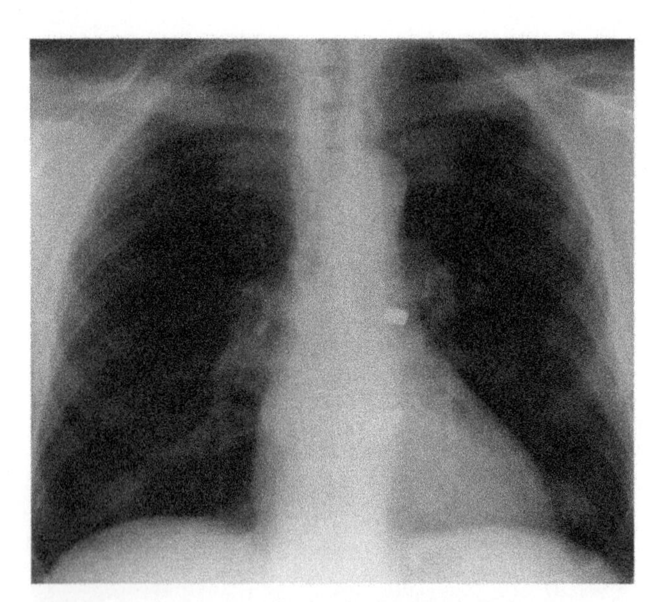

FIGURE 24.6 Chest radiograph showing a radiopaque foreign body in the left main stem bronchus.

*Source*: Swanson, K. L., Prakash, U. B. S., McDougall, J. C., Midthun, D. E., Edell, E. S., Brutinel, M. W., & Utz, J. P. M (2003). Airway foreign bodies in adults. *Journal of Bronchology & Interventional Pulmonology, 10*(2), 107–111. https://journals.lww.com/bronchology/Fulltext/2003/04000/Airway_Foreign_Bodies_in_Adults.4.aspx

### Subjective Findings

The health history may reveal:

- Sudden-onset or persistent coughing
- Noisy or rapid breathing
- Witnessed episode of choking
- Recurrent pneumonia (Ruiz, 2020; Vivisenco et al., 2019)

▶ ALERT: The American Academy of Pediatrics recommends screening all children for OSAS during routine well-child visits (Marcus et al., 2012).

### Risk Factors

The most common risk factors for FBA are:

- Young age of the child
- Difficulty swallowing or chewing
- Putting nonfood items in the mouth (Vivisenco et al., 2019)

### Review of Systems

The most common manifestations revealed during the review of systems include:

- **Respiratory:** presence of lower respiratory symptoms in the absence of signs of upper respiratory infection (Ruiz, 2020)

### Objective Findings

The physical examination of the child with FBA may reveal:

- Fever
- The triad of coughing, wheezing, and diminished breath sounds (particularly on one side)
- Audible stridor
- Tachypnea
- Hypoxia
- Mediastinal shift
- Dyspnea
- Hoarseness
- Hemoptysis
- Cyanosis (Ruiz, 2020)

### Laboratory/Diagnostic Testing

- Chest x-ray findings may be normal or may include:
  - Opacities or atelectasis in the affected region
  - Radio opaque foreign body
  - Unilateral lung hyperinflation (Ruiz, 2020).
- Chest CT may be ordered if the plain x-rays are inconclusive. A CT scan can be a valuable tool to detect radiolucent objects not visible on x-ray (Ruiz, 2020).

ALERT: The cough, wheeze, diminished breath sound triad may not be present in all children. Symptoms may be very nonspecific (Ruiz, 2020). Therefore, FBA should be included in the differential for any child with sudden onset of pulmonary symptoms or respiratory distress. In children with occult FBA, a careful history should be obtained, as parents may ignore a recent episode of brief of choking and gagging that resolved without intervention.

### Differential Diagnosis

The differential diagnosis for FBA includes:

- Pneumonia
- Airway mass
- Congenital, traumatic, or infectious etiologies for airway stenosis

### Treatment/Management Plan

- Rigid bronchoscopy for foreign body removal is the treatment of choice (Ruiz, 2020)

### Family Education

Teach the following:

- Be aware of appropriate food choices based on the age and developmental level of the child.
- Babyproof the home for choking hazards.
- Monitor signs of respiratory distress.
- Know infant/child cardiopulmonary resuscitation.

### Referral

Patients with suspected or confirmed FBA should be referred to an ear, nose, and throat specialist for rigid bronchoscopy and foreign body removal.

## SPONTANEOUS PNEUMOTHORAX

Spontaneous pneumothorax occurs in approximately 3.4 per 100,000 children under the age of 18. The areas that are most often affected are the lung apices. The ruptured alveola and emphysematous changes in the impacted areas are referred to as *blebs* (Williams et al., 2018). Primary spontaneous pneumothorax (PSP) occurs in the absence of an identifiable cause. Secondary causes for pneumothorax can be the result of trauma or underlying lung disease (Janahi, 2019). A tension pneumothorax occurs when air becomes trapped in the pleural space, causing lung restriction and, in some instances, hemodynamic instability (Janahi, 2019). There are no evidence-based, standardized guidelines for the treatment of PSP in children (Williams et al., 2018).

### Subjective Findings

The health history may reveal:

- Sudden onset of symptoms in proximity to activities that increase transpulmonary pressure, such as weight-lifting or Valsalva maneuver
- Sudden onset of symptoms without discernible cause (Janahi, 2019)

### Risk Factors

The most common risk factors for spontaneous pneumothorax are:

- Male gender
- Thin, tall phenotype
- Adolescence
- Smoking
- Drug use (marijuana and cocaine inhalation)
- Underlying lung disease such as CF or asthma (Janahi, 2019; Soler et al., 2018, p. 1960)

### Review of Systems

The most common manifestations revealed during the review of systems include:

- **Respiratory:** chest tightness, cough, shortness of breath, a popping sensation, pleuritic chest pain radiating to the ipsilateral shoulder (Janahi, 2019; Soler et al., 2018)

### Objective Findings

The physical examination of the child with PSP may reveal:

- Diminished breath sounds
- Decreased chest excursion
- Hyperresonant percussion
- Signs of respiratory distress

- Decreased vocal resonance on the affected side
- Subcutaneous emphysema with crepitation (Janahi, 2019)

Large pneumothoraces and tension pneumothoraces may present with much more pronounced symptoms, including respiratory distress, cyanosis, tachycardia, and diminished heart sounds (Janahi, 2019).

### Laboratory/Diagnostic Testing

Laboratory and diagnostic testing includes:

- Expiratory chest x-ray performed upright
- Chest CT if further assessment is necessary
- Blood gas measurements for patients experiencing respiratory distress (Janahi, 2019)

▶ ALERT: A small pneumothorax may be asymptomatic and may be an incidental finding on chest x-ray.

### Differential Diagnosis

The differential diagnosis for PSP includes:

- Secondary or tension pneumothorax
- Foreign body
- Pneumonia

### Treatment/Management Plan

Treatment depends on the size of the pneumothorax and the condition of the patient. Supplemental oxygen is recommended for all patients requiring hospitalization. Treatment recommendations are adapted from evidence-based guidelines for adult patients (Janahi, 2019). Treatment can include:

- Monitoring without intervention
- Needle aspiration or chest tube placement
- Surgery (Williams et al., 2018)

With conservative management, the rate of recurrence of the pneumothorax may be as high as 57% (Soler et al., 2018). The majority of lesions recur within 1 year and require repeat hospitalization.

### Family Education

Teach the following:

- Symptoms that may indicate a recurrence of the lesion.
- Signs of respiratory distress.
- Activity limitations during healing.

### Referral

Refer as follows:

- Small pneumothoraces may be monitored by primary care providers.
- Patients should be referred for needle decompression or chest tube placement by providers experienced in performing those procedures.
- Patients with larger lesions or underlying lung disease should be referred to a pediatric pulmonologist for management.
- If surgical options are explored, patients should be referred to a pediatric surgeon for evaluation.

## OBSTRUCTIVE SLEEP APNEA SYNDROME

Obstructive sleep apnea syndrome (OSAS) is a condition characterized by prolonged partial or intermittent complete obstruction of the airway during sleep. The prevalence of OSAS in children ranges from 1.2% to 5.7% (Marcus et al., 2012). The effects of undiagnosed or untreated OSAS in children include an increase in the rate of obesity with secondary development of hypertension, heart disease, metabolic syndrome, and type 2 diabetes. Other consequences include chronic inflammatory responses, behavior problems, symptoms of attention deficit/hyperactivity, and academic underachievement (Blechner & Williamson, 2016).

### Subjective Findings

The health history may reveal:

- Snoring
- Witnessed apnea during sleep
- Gasping or labored breathing during sleep
- Chronic nasal congestion
- Hyponasal speech
- Daytime somnolence (Marcus et al., 2012; Paruthi, 2019)

### Risk Factors

The most common risk factors for OSAS are:

- Adenotonsillar hypertrophy
- Underlying neuromuscular disorders
- Craniofacial abnormalities
- Obesity (Marcus et al., 2012)

### Review of Systems

The most common manifestations revealed during the review of systems include:

- **Constitutional:** sleep arousals, failure to thrive, daytime somnolence, morning headaches
- **HEENT:** allergic rhinitis
- **Respiratory:** mouth breathing, snoring

- **Genitourinary:** nocturnal enuresis
- **Neurologic:** hyperactivity and inattention (Marcus et al., 2012; Paruthi, 2019; Wu et al., 2019)

### Objective Findings

The physical examination of the child with OSAS may reveal:

- Tonsillar hypertrophy
- High Mallampati score
- Obesity
- Poor growth
- Retrognathia, midface hypoplasia, and other craniofacial anomalies
- High-arched or narrow hard palate
- Macroglossia (Paruthi, 2019)

### Laboratory/Diagnostic Testing

The following laboratory and diagnostic testing may be performed:

- Nasopharyngoscopy may reveal adenoid hypertrophy (Wu et al., 2019).
- Attended, in-lab polysomnography (sleep study) may show evidence of sleep-disordered breathing, hypoxia, or hypoventilation (Paruthi, 2019).
- Validated sleep assessment questionnaires may help direct the need for further assessment of sleep-related disorders:
  - Pediatric Sleep Questionnaire (Chervin et al., 2000). https://bayclinicpediatrics.net/getattachment/27a261cc-b54b-413e-b22c-e3f36a37aa2f/Pediatric-Sleep-Questionnaire.aspx
  - Epworth Sleepiness Scale (Janssen et al., 2017). https://edsandosa.com/assets/pdf/epworth-sleepiness-scale-ess.pdf

**PRO TIP** Home sleep apnea testing is not currently recommended for children.

### Differential Diagnosis

The differential diagnosis for OSAS includes:

- Primary snoring
- Central sleep apnea

### Treatment/Management Plan

- Adenotonsillectomy for surgical candidates
- Weight loss for patients determined to be obese
- Continuous positive airway pressure (CPAP) for nonsurgical candidates (CPAP; Marcus et al., 2012)

### Family Education

Teach the following:

- Signs and symptoms of OSAS.
- Polysomnography procedures.

### Referral

Refer as follows:

- Sleep specialists for any child requiring ongoing evaluation or for whom CPAP may be required
- Ear, nose, and throat specialists if the patient is a candidate for surgery
- Craniofacial specialists for patients with congenital or acquired anomalies
- Nutritionists or weight loss specialists for children determined to be obese

**PRO TIP** The scoring rules for pediatric and adult sleep studies differ. Sleep specialists experienced in reading pediatric sleep studies are preferred.

## BRIEF, RESOLVED, UNEXPLAINED EVENT

A brief resolved unexplained event (BRUE) is defined as an episode that occurs in an infant under a year of age during which they experience sudden, transient, brief symptoms of neurocardiorespiratory compromise. In order to be classified as a BRUE, the duration of the event must be less than 1 minute and resolved at the time of patient presentation. These events, formerly called apparent life-threatening events (ALTEs), represent a diagnosis of exclusion following an unrevealing focused history and physical examination (Corwin, 2019a; Poets, 2017). No serious, underlying medical problems are found in the majority of infants experiencing BRUE and data do not support an association between BRUE and sudden infant death syndrome (SIDS; Corwin, 2019a). In addition, because the diagnostic criteria for BRUE are so specific, the condition should be differentiated from apnea in term infants (Patrinos & Martin, 2017).

### Subjective Findings

The health history may be normal or may reveal:

- Recent upper respiratory tract infection

- Choking episode during feeding
- Prior episodes of BRUE (Corwin, 2019a; Poets, 2017)

**PRO TIP** The history of a child presenting with BRUE should include discussion of the possibility of accidental ingestion or overdose.

### Risk Factors

The most common risk factors for BRUE are:

- Anatomic propensity toward obstructive apnea (Poets, 2017)
- Feeding difficulties
- Young infants (<2 months)
- History of previous episodes of BRUE
- Recent upper respiratory tract infection (Corwin, 2019a)

### Review of Systems

The most common manifestations revealed during the review of systems include:

- **Respiratory:** Cyanosis, apnea, decreased or irregular breathing
- **Neurologic:** hypertonia or hypotonia, altered level of responsiveness (Poets, 2017)

### Objective Findings

In order to receive a diagnosis of BRUE, the event must be resolved and the infant must be back to baseline at the time of presentation. The physical examination of the child with BRUE should reveal:

- Normal general appearance and responsiveness
- Normal vital signs
- Normal physical examination findings
- Resolved symptoms of BRUE (Tieder et al., 2019)

**PRO TIP** The physical examination for the patient with BRUE should focus on the cardiac, respiratory, and neurologic systems.

### Laboratory/Diagnostic Testing

- EKG may be performed to evaluate for a prolonged QT interval (Tieder et al., 2019).
- Pertussis testing may be performed for those infants with recent respiratory symptoms (Tieder et al., 2019).
- Patients determined to be at high risk may have testing to include CBC, electrolytes, body fluid cultures, blood gases, radiologic imaging, and polysomnography (Patrinos & Martin, 2017).

### Differential Diagnosis

The differential diagnosis for BRUE includes:

- Acute respiratory tract infection (RSV, pertussis)
- Bacterial infections (urinary tract infections, sepsis)
- Aspiration
- Gastroesophageal reflux disease (GERD)
- Cardiovascular/hematologic anomalies (arrhythmias, structural defects, channelopathies)
- Metabolic anomalies (inborn errors of metabolism)
- Neurologic disorders (seizures)
- Gastrointestinal disorders (intussusception, volvulus)
- Intentional injury (child abuse, Munchausen Syndrome by Proxy; Poets, 2017)

▶ ALERT: While rare, intentional child injury should be considered in the list of differential diagnoses for any child presenting with symptoms suggestive of BRUE.

### Treatment/Management Plan

Treatment is determined by the infant's risk stratification.

- *Low risk* is determined by the infant's current age over 2 months, gestational age over 32 weeks, and absence of concerning findings on the history and physical examination.
  - Treatment includes parental education and reassurance, shared decision-making regarding disposition, and resources for CPR training (Tieder et al., 2019).
  - Practitioners may elect to briefly monitor the patient and obtain an EKG and test for pertussis (Tieder et al., 2019).
  - Home apnea monitoring is not necessary (Tieder et al., 2019).
  - A follow-up check should be arranged within 24 hours (Corwin, 2019a).
- *High risk* is determined by age less than 2 months, prematurity less than 32 weeks, and by any concerning findings on the history and physical examination (Tieder et al., 2019).
  - Further evaluation is warranted to rule out infections, child abuse, metabolic anomalies, and abnormalities of the cardiovascular and neurological systems.
  - Treatment is guided by the potential diagnoses.

**PRO TIP** Home apnea monitoring for a diagnosis of BRUE is not indicated. In select cases, monitoring may be considered to aid in the diagnostic evaluation or to provide reassurance to parents of the absence of cardiorespiratory events. Home monitoring may be indicated for infants with known cardiopulmonary disease or in instances of prematurity (Corwin, 2019a). The endpoint of home apnea monitoring, if initiated, is variable but is generally considered safe after normal downloads have been recorded for no less than 6 to 8 weeks (Corwin, 2019b).

### Family Education

Teach the following:

- Families should be educated about the definition of BRUE and the methods by which risk is determined.
- It is important for parents to understand the lack of an association between BRUE and SIDS and that the risk of death is low (Brand & Fazzari, 2018).
- Parents should be encouraged to take an infant/child CPR class.

### Referral

Infants suspected of having GERD may be referred to speech or occupational therapy (Patrinos & Martin, 2017). Otherwise, no referrals are necessary for patients with low risk. Patients with high risk should be referred to subspecialists, as appropriate.

▶ ALERT: Apnea in term infants is not common. Etiologies include characteristics found in infants with high-risk BRUE and diagnoses found in the differential diagnosis for BRUE. A detailed laboratory and diagnostic evaluation is indicated, along with a period of inpatient observation and cardiorespiratory monitoring.

# PULMONARY FUNCTION TESTING

## TYPES OF PULMONARY FUNCTION TESTING

Pulmonary function tests (PFTs) provide an objective measure of a patient's lung function. PFTs are commonly used to assess lung function in patients with asthma, CF, and other chronic lung diseases (Rosen & Colin, 2019). PFTs may also be used to evaluate lung function in patients with neuromuscular or musculoskeletal diseases such as scoliosis, muscular dystrophy, and pectus excavatum (Koumbourlis, 2015; Rosen & Colin, 2019).

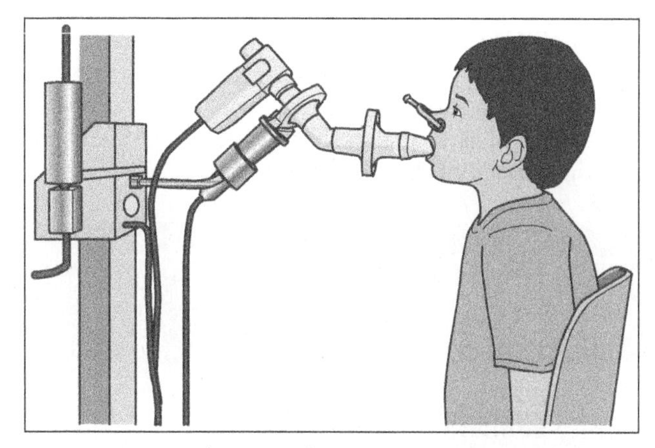

FIGURE 24.7 Pulmonary function test: Spirometry.

Two of the most common PFTs are spirometry and body plethsmography (Figure 24.7). The Global Initiative for Asthma (GINA) recommends the use of spirometry in the care and management of patients with asthma (Ayuk et al., 2017). While PFTs can guide treatment, the data should be used as a tool, in conjunction with the patient's history and physical examination, to arrive at a definitive diagnosis. Because spirometry and plethsmography require the patient to be able to follow directions involving timed respiratory maneuvers, the tests are usually recommended for children over the age of 6 years (Rosen & Colin, 2019). Patients with exacerbations of their pulmonary illness may be unable to adequately perform PFT (Welch, 2016).

Spirometry measures flow and volume over a period of time (Rosen & Colin, 2019). The test can be easily and inexpensively performed in a primary care office and is considered the "gold standard" for determining lung function (Rosen & Colin, 2019). Using forced, sustained expiration, spirometry can establish the presence of obstructive and restrictive disorders and can determine reversibility of the condition through administration of a bronchodilator during the test. Common spirometric measurements include forced vital capacity (FVC), forced expiratory volume in one second ($FEV_1$), flow between 25% and 75% of the vital capacity (FEF 25/75%), and the peak expiratory flow rate (PEFR; Rosen & Colin, 2019).

Plethsmography records breathing at rest and involves placing the child in a clear walled chamber known commonly as a body box. The box is then sealed airtight and is used to stabilize internal pressure and allow for slow pressure changes during the test. Plethsmography has the capacity to provide spirometric data as well as residual volume (RV) and total lung capacity (TLC; Rosen & Colin, 2019).

**PRO TIP** Be aware of institutional infection control practices when sanitizing equipment in between caring for patients.

### Family Education

Teach the following:

- Patients should wear loose-fitting clothing that does not restrict breathing.
- Instruct patients to refrain from eating a large meal within 2 hours prior to the test and not to engage in vigorous exercise at least 30 minutes prior to the test.
- Assure that adolescents do not smoke at least 24 hours before the test, and do not consume alcohol at least 4 hours prior to the test.

▶ ALERT: Contraindications to performing spirometry include nausea and vomiting, recent eye surgery, hemoptysis of unknown origin, pneumothorax, aneurysm, and unstable cardiovascular status (Welch, 2016).

# RESPIRATORY SPECIMEN COLLECTION

## GENERAL PRINCIPLES FOR SPECIMEN COLLECTION

On occasion, specimen collection will be needed to aid in the diagnosis and treatment of respiratory disorders. While general principles will always apply, practitioners should follow institution-specific policies and procedures to guide collection, preparation, and transportation of respiratory samples. Failure to do so may result in inadequate sampling or invalid results, which may ultimately delay patient care and treatment.

General principles for specimen collection include:

- Wearing appropriate personal protective equipment during the collection process
- Ensuring that specimens are collected prior to initiating antimicrobial therapy, if possible
- Maintaining aseptic technique
- Collecting the optimal sample (source, specimen type, amount) according to institutional or lab policies (Boruchoff & Weinstein, 2019)

The most commonly obtained respiratory sample is expectorated sputum. The quality of the lower airway sample may be affected by a predominance of secretions from the oronasopharynx, the presence of prior antimicrobial treatment, and delays in plating the specimen on the culture media (Boruchoff & Weinstein, 2019). Samples may be obtained in a variety of methods, including:

- Bronchoscopy via bronchoalveolar lavage
- Endotracheal tube suctioning
- Lung aspirate
- Sputum induction with the use of nebulized hypertonic normal saline and chest percussion (Shepherd, 2017)

Infants and young children are not capable of coughing sputum into collection containers. Therefore, sterile suctioning must be performed once the sputum has been induced.

## OBTAINING THE SPUTUM SPECIMEN

Be aware of items in the patient history that may affect specimen collection, including abnormal anatomy and underlying medical conditions. Arrive at the patient encounter with all necessary supplies to avoid having to leave the patient to retrieve missing items. Have backup supplies (extra suction catheters, etc.) in case they are needed. Request assistance from a co-worker if an extra pair of hands is necessary. When applicable, have the patient rinse out their mouth prior to specimen collection. If necessary, safely restrain the patient either in the arms of the caregiver or staff, or via the use of institution-sanctioned restraint methods. Ensure that the patient is properly monitored and appropriate emergency equipment is available in case the patient experiences distress during specimen retrieval.

The sputum sample should be collected by, or expectorated into, a sterile collection container. Whole sputum samples are far superior to sputum collection via swab. Although bulb syringes are commonly used to suction the nose and mouth of infants, they should not be used for specimen collection.

## KEY POINTS

- Avoid unnecessary lab and diagnostic testing in patients with uncomplicated bronchiolitis.
- The use of bronchodilators is generally not recommended in the treatment of bronchiolitis.
- Consider PBB in children with prolonged wet cough not responsive to bronchodilators and inhaled corticosteroids.
- Symptoms of pneumonia in young children can be atypical and subtle.
- The clinical presentation of tuberculosis in children is variable and may be subtle or nonspecific.
- When a child has CF, promoting normal growth and developmental is a key function of the primary care provider.
- Ongoing family support is needed when a child has a congenital lower airway disorders.
- Early detection and management are needed to promote optimal outcomes in children with CCH.
- Maintain a high index of suspicion for FBA in young children with cough in the absence of illness.
- A pneumothorax should be considered in children with sudden onset of pleuritic chest pain, particularly if they have the most common phenotype.
- Children with neurocognitive symptoms should be assessed for the possibility of sleep-disordered breathing.
- Spirometry is an easy, cost-effective way to evaluate lung function in primary care offices.

## REFERENCES


Adams, L. V., & Starke, J. R. (2019a). Latent tuberculosis infection in children. *UpToDate.* https://www.uptodate.com/contents/latent-tuberculosis-infection-in-children

Adams, L. V., & Starke, J. R. (2019b). Tuberculosis disease in children. *UpToDate.* https://www.uptodate.com/contents/tuberculosis-disease-in-children

Alexander, K., Cadilla, A., & Qureshi, N. (2017). Fungal infections (systemic). In T. K. McInerny, H. M. Adam, D. E. Campbell, J. M. Foy, & D. M. Kamat (Eds.), *American Academy of Pediatrics textbook of pediatric care* (2nd ed., Chapter 254). American Academy of Pediatrics.

American Academy of Pediatrics. (2014) [reaffirmed 2019]. Updated guidance for palivizumab prophylaxis among infants and young children at increased risk of hospitalization for respiratory syncytial virus infection. *Pediatrics, 134,* 415–420. https://doi.org/10.1542/peds.2014-1665

American Academy of Pediatrics Pediatric Tuberculosis Collaborative Group. (2004). Targeted tuberculin skin testing and treatment of latent tuberculosis infection in children and adolescents. *Pediatrics, 114*(4), supplement 4, 1175–1201. doi: 10.1542/peds.2004-0809

Amraoui, W. E., Bentalha, A., Hamri, H., Kettani, S. E.-C. E., & Koraichi, A. E. (2017). Congenital cystic adenomatoid malformation—Dangers of misdiagnosis: A case report. *Journal of Medical Case Reports, 11*(1), 1–5. https://doi.org/10.1186/s13256-017-1349-5

Ayuk, A. C., Uwaezuoke, S. N., Ndukwu, C. I., Ndu, I. K., Iloh, K. K., & Okoli, C. V. (2017). Spirometry in asthma care: A review of the trends and challenges in pediatric practice. *Clinical Medicine Insights: Pediatrics, 11,* 1179556517720675. https://doi.org/10.1177/1179556517720675

Bal, Z. S., Kurugöl, Z., & Özkınay, F. (2020). Clinical features of COVID-19 in children. *Journal of Pediatric Research, 7*(2), 88–91. https://doi.org/10.4274/jpr.galenos.2020.60437

Barson, W. J. (2019a). Community-acquired pneumonia in children: Clinical features and diagnosis. *UpToDate.* https://www.uptodate.com/contents/community-acquired-pneumonia-in-children-clinical-features-and-diagnosis

Barson, W. J. (2019b). Community-acquired pneumonia in children: Outpatient treatment. *UpToDate.* https://www.uptodate.com/contents/community-acquired-pneumonia-in-children-outpatient-treatment

Barson, W. J. (2020). Pneumonia in children: Epidemiology, pathogenesis, and etiology. *UpToDate.* https://www.uptodate.com/contents/pneumonia-in-children-epidemiology-pathogenesis-and-etiology

Blair, J. E., & Ampel, N. M. (2020). Primary pulmonary coccidioidal infection. *UpToDate.* https://www.uptodate.com/contents/primary-pulmonary-coccidioidal-infection

Blechner, M., & Williamson, A. A. (2016). Consequences of obstructive sleep apnea in children. *Current Problems in Pediatric and Adolescent Health Care, 46*(1), 19–26. https://doi.org/10.1016/j.cppeds.2015.10.007

Bono-Neri, F., Romano, C., & Isedeh, A. (2019). Cystic fibrosis: Advancing along the continuum. *Journal of Pediatric Health Care, 33,* 242–254. https://doi.org/10.1016/j.pedhc.2018.08.008

Boruchoff, S. E., & Weinstein, M. P. (2019). Microbiology specimen collection and transport. *UpToDate.* https://www.uptodate.com/contents/microbiology-specimen-collection-and-transport

Bourrous, M., Lahmini, W., Nouri, H., & Haimeur, N. (2019). Subcutaneous emphysema and pneumomediastinum in child with asthma revealing occult foreign body aspiration: A case report. *Journal of Medical Case Reports, 13*(157). https://doi.org/10.1186/s13256-019-2076-x

Bradley, J. S., Byington, C. L., Shah, S. S., Alverson, B., Carter, E. R., Harrison, C., Kaplan, S. L., Mace, S. E., McCracken, G. H., Moore, M. R., St. Peter, P. D., Stockwell, J. A., & Swanson, J. T. (2011). The management of community-acquired pneumonia in infants and children older than 3 months of age: Clinical practice guidelines by the Pediatric Infectious Diseases Society and the Infectious Diseases Society of America. *Clinical Infectious Diseases, 53,* e25–e76. https://doi.org/10.1093/cid/cir531

Brand, D. A., & Fazzari, M. J. (2018). Risk of death in infants who have experienced a brief resolved unexplained event: A meta-analysis. *The Journal of Pediatrics, 197,* 63–67. https://doi.org/10.1016/j.jpeds.2017.12.028

Breakell, R., Thorndyke, B., Clennett, J., & Harkensee, C. (2017). Reducing unnecessary chest x-rays, antibiotics and bronchodilators through implementation of the NICE bronchiolitis guideline. *European Journal of Pediatrics, 177*(1), 47–51. https://doi.org/10.1007/s00431-017-3034-5

Brouillette, R. T. (2019). Congenital central hypoventilation syndrome and other causes of sleep-related hypoventilation in children. *UpToDate*. https://www.uptodate.com/contents/congenital-central-hypoventilation-syndrome-and-other-causes-of-sleep-related-hypoventilation-in-children

Centers for Disease Control and Prevention. (2019a). Antibiotic prescribing and use in the U. S. https://www.cdc.gov/antibiotic-use/stewardship-report/index.html

Centers for Disease Control. (2021). *About COVID-19 vaccines*. https://www.cdc.gov/coronavirus/2019-ncov/vaccines/about-vaccines/index.html

Chervin, R. D., Hedger, K., Dillon, J. E., & Pituch, K. J. (2000). Pediatric Sleep Questionnaire (PSQ): Validity and reliability of scales for sleep-disordered breathing, snoring, sleepiness, and behavioral problems. *Sleep Medicine, 1*(1), 21–32. https://doi.org/10.1016/S1389-9457(99)00009-X

Corwin, M. J. (2019a). Acute events in infancy including brief resolved unexplained event (BRUE). *UpToDate*. https://www.uptodate.com/contents/acute-events-in-infancy-including-brief-resolved-unexplained-event-brue

Corwin, M. J. (2019b). Use of home cardiorespiratory monitors in infants. *UpToDate*. Retrieved February 2, 2020, from https://www.uptodate.com/contents/use-of-home-cardiorespiratory-monitors-in-infants

Cowger, T. L., Wortham, J. M., & Burton, D. C. (2019). Epidemiology of tuberculosis among children and adolescents in the USA, 2007–17: An analysis of national surveillance data. *The Lancet Public Health, 4*(10), e506–e516. https://doi.org/10.1016/S2468-2667(19)30134-3

Cystic Fibrosis Foundation. (n.d.). *What is CF?* https://www.cff.org

Falup-pecurariu, O. G., Diez-Domingo, J., Esposito, S., Finn, A., Rodrigues, F., Spoulou, V., Syrogiannopoulous, G. A., Usonis, V., Greenberg, D. (2018). Clinical and laboratory features of children with community-acquired pneumonia are associated with distinct radiographic presentations. *European Journal of Pediatrics, 177*, 1111–1120. https://doi.org/10.1007/s00431-018-3165-3

Federico, M. J., Baker, C. D., Deboer, E. M., Halbower, A. C., Kupfer, O., Martiniano, S. L., Sagel, S. D., Stillwell, P., Zemanick, E. T., Caraballo, M., & Hawkins, S. (2018). Respiratory tract & mediastinum. In W. W. Hay, M. J. Levin, R. R. Deterding, M. J. Abzug, & J. M. Sondheimer (Eds.), *Current diagnosis and treatment: Pediatrics* (24th ed., Chapter 19). McGraw-Hill Education.

Franklin, D., Babl, F. E., Schlapbach, L. J., Oakley, E., Craig, S., Neutze, J., Furyk, J., Fraser, J. F., Jones, M., Whitty, J. A., Dalziel, S. R., & Schibler, A. (2018). A randomized trial of high-flow oxygen therapy in infants with bronchiolitis. *New England Journal of Medicine, 378*, 1121–1131. https://doi.org/10.1056/nejmoa1714855

Gerber, J. S., Jackson, M. A., Pranita D. Tamma, P. D., Zaoutis, T. E., & Committee on Infectious Diseases, Pediatric Infectious Diseases Society. (2020). *Pediatrics, 147*(1), e2020040295. https://doi.org/10.1542/peds.2020-040295

Gilchrist, F. J. (2019). An approach to the child with a wet cough. *Pediatric Respiratory Reviews, 31*, 75–81. https://doi.org/10.1016/j.prrv.2018.11.002

Goldman, R. D., Yan, T. D., Seiler, M., Cotanda, C. P., Brown, J. C., Klein, E. J., Hoeffe, J., Gelernter, R., Hall, J. E., Davis, A. L., Griffiths, M. A., Mater, A., Manzano, S., Gualco, G., Shimizu, N., Hurt, T. L., Ahmed, S., Hansen, M., Sheridan, D., ...Staubli, G. (2020). Caregiver willingness to vaccinate their children against COVID-19: Cross sectional survey. *Vaccine, 38*, 7668–7673. https://doi.org/10.1016/j.vaccine.2020.09.084

Goldschmidt, K. (2021). COVID-19 vaccines for children: The essential role of the pediatric nurse. *Journal of Pediatric Nursing, 57*, 96–98. https://doi.org/10.1016/j.pedn.2020.12.004

Harless, J., Ramaiah, R., & Bhananker, S. (2014). Pediatric airway management. *International Journal of Critical Illness and Injury Science, 4*(1), 65–70. https://doi.org/10.4103/2229-5151.128015

Harris, C., & Homnick, D. (2011). The pulmonary physical examination. In M. J. Light, C. J. Blaisdell, & D. Homnick(Eds.), *Pediatric pulmonology* (pp. 135–146). American Academy of Pediatrics.

Hedrick, H. L., & Adzick, N. S. (2019). Congenital diaphragmatic hernia in the neonate. *UpToDate*. https://www.uptodate.com/contents/congenital-diaphragmatic-hernia-in-the-neonate

Hill, M. A. (2020). *Embryology: Respiratory system development*. https://embryology.med.unsw.edu.au/embryology/index.php/Respiratory_System_Development

Ishikawa, C. S., Matsuo, O. M., & Sarno, F. (2018). Latent tuberculosis infection and tuberculosis in children and adolescents. *Einstein (São Paulo), 16*(3), 1–6. https://doi.org/10.1590/s1679-45082018ao4090

Janahi, I. A. (2019). Spontaneous pneumothorax in children. *UpToDate*. https://www.uptodate.com/contents/spontaneous-pneumothorax-in-children

Jancelewicz, T., Brindle, M. E., Guner, Y. S., Lally, P. A., Lally, K. P., & Harting, M. T. (2019). Toward standardized management of congenital diaphragmatic hernia: An analysis of practice guidelines. *Journal of Surgical Research, 243*, 229–235. https://doi.org/10.1016/j.jss.2019.05.007

Janssen, C., Phillipson, S., O'Connor, J., & Johns, M. W. (2017). Validation of the Epworth Sleepiness Scale for Children and Adolescents using Rasch analysis. *Sleep Medicine, 33*, 30–35. https://doi.org/10.1016/j.sleep.2017.01.014

Kantar, A. (2017). Phenotypic presentation of chronic cough in children. *Journal of Thoracic Disease, 9*(4), 907–913. https://doi.org/10.21037/jtd.2017.03.53

Kasi, A., Perez, I., Kun, S., & Keens, T. (2016). Congenital central hypoventilation syndrome: Diagnostic and management challenges. *Pediatric Health, Medicine and Therapeutics, 7*, 99–107. https://doi.org/10.2147/phmt.s95054

Katkin, J. P. (2019). Cystic fibrosis: Clinical manifestations and diagnosis. *UpToDate*. https://www.uptodate.com/contents/cystic-fibrosis-clinical-manifestations-and-diagnosis

Koumbourlis, A. C. (2015). Pectus deformities and their impact on pulmonary physiology. *Paediatric Respiratory Reviews, 16*(1), 18–24. https://doi.org/10.1016/j.prrv.2014.10.009

Lewinsohn, D. M., Leonard, M. K., Lobue, P. A., Cohn, D. L., Daley, C. L., Desmond, E., Keane, J., Lewinsohn, D. A., Loeffler, A. M., Mazurek, G. H., O'Brien, R. J., Pai, M., Richeldi, L., Salfinger, M., Shinnick, T. M., Sterling, T. R., Warshauer, D. M., & Woods, G. L. (2016). Official American Thoracic Society/Infectious Diseases Society of America/Centers for Disease Control and Prevention clinical practice guidelines: Diagnosis of tuberculosis in adults and children. *Clinical Infectious Diseases, 64*(2), 1–33. https://doi.org/10.1093/cid/ciw694

Ma, H., Hu, J., Tian, J., Zhou, X., Li, H., Laws, M. T., Wesemann, L. D., Zhu, B., Chen, W., Ramos, R., Xia, J., & Shao, J. (2020). A single-center, retrospective study of COVID-19 features in children: A descriptive investigation. *BMC Medicine, 18*(1), 1–11. https://doi.org/10.1186/s12916-020-01596-9

Marcus, L., Brooks, L. J., Draper, K. A., Gozal, D., Halbower, A. C., Jones, J., Schechter, M. S., Sheldon, S. H., Spruyt, K., Ward, S. D., Lehmann, C., & Shiffman, R. N. (2012). Diagnosis and management of childhood obstructive sleep apnea syndrome. *Pediatrics, 130*, 576–584. https://doi.org/10.1542/peds.2012-1671

Mathur, S., Fuchs, A., Bielicki, J., Anker, J. V. D., & Sharland, M. (2018). Antibiotic use for community-acquired pneumonia in neonates and children: WHO evidence review. *Paediatrics and International Child Health, 38*(S1), 566–575. https://doi.org/10.1080/20469047.2017.1409455

Matlock, M., Hopfer, S., & Ogunseitan, O. A. (2019). Communicating risk for a climate-sensitive disease: A case study of valley fever in central California. *International Journal of Environmental Research and Public Health, 16*(18), 1–15. https://doi.org/10.3390/ijerph16183254

Mehta, R. M., Rashmi, N., Bajaj, P., Krishnan, S., & Srinivasan, L. (2019). Airway stenosis related to foreign body aspiration: An under-recognized long-term complication. *Clinical Medicine Insights: Case Reports, 12*, 1–4. https://doi.org/10.1177/1179547619863816

Mohakud, N. K., Mishra, M., Tripathy, R., & Mishra, M. R. (2018). Incidence and risk factors for prolonged stay in children hospitalized with pneumonia. *Journal of Clinical and Diagnostic Research, 12*(8), 12–14. https://doi.org/10.7860/jcdr/2018/35460.11944

Mozun, R., Pedersen, E. S. L., Ardura-Garcia, C. (2019). Does high-flow oxygen reduce escalation of care in infants with hypoxemic bronchiolitis? *Breathe, 15*(3), 247–249. https://doi.org/10.1183/20734735.0192-2019

Oermann, C. M. (2019). Congenital pulmonary airway (cystic adenomatoid) malformation. *UpToDate*. https://www.uptodate.com/contents/congenital-pulmonary-airway-cystic-adenomatoid-malformation

Paruthi, S. (2019). Evaluation of suspected obstructive sleep apnea in children. *UpToDate*. https://www.uptodate.com/contents/evaluation-of-suspected-obstructive-sleep-apnea-in-children

Patrinos, M. E., & Martin, R. J. (2017). Apnea in the term infant. *Seminars in Fetal and Neonatal Medicine, 22*(4), 240–244. https://doi.org/10.1016/j.siny.2017.04.003

Piedra, P. A., & Stark, A. R. (2020). Bronchiolitis in infants and children: Treatment, outcome, and prevention. *UpToDate*. https://www.uptodate.com/contents/bronchiolitis-in-infants-and-children-treatment-outcome-and-prevention

Poets, C. F. (2017). Apparent life-threatening events (ALTE) or brief resolved unexplained events (BRUE). *Paediatrics and Child Health, 27*(5), 215–221. https://doi.org/10.1016/j.paed.2017.02.004

Ralston, S. L., Lieberthal, A. S., Meissner, H. C., Alverson, B. K., Baley, J. E., Gadomski, A. M., Johnson, D. W., Light, M. J., Maraqa, N. F., Mendonca, E. A., Phelan, K. J., Zorc, J. J., Stanko-Lopp, D., Brown, M. A., Nathanson, I., Rosenblum, E., Sayles, S., & Hernandez-Cancio, S. (2015). Clinical practice guideline: The diagnosis, management, and prevention of bronchiolitis. *Pediatrics, 136*, 2015–2862. https://doi.org/10.1542/peds.2015-2862

Rosen, D. M., & Colin, A. A. (2019). Overview of pulmonary function testing in children. *UpToDate*. https://www.uptodate.com/contents/overview-of-pulmonary-function-testing-in-children

Ruiz, F. E. (2020). Airway foreign bodies in children. *UpToDate*. https://www.uptodate.com/contents/airway-foreign-bodies-in-children

Sabharwal, S., & Schwarzenberg, S. J. (2019). Cystic fibrosis: Overview of gastrointestinal disease. *UpToDate*. https://www.uptodate.com/contents/cystic-fibrosis-overview-of-gastrointestinal-disease

Shepherd, E. (2017). Specimen collection 4: Procedure for obtaining a sputum specimen. *Nursing Times, 113*(10), 49–51. https://www.nursingtimes.net/clinical-archive/assessment-skills/specimen-collection-4-procedure-for-obtaining-a-sputum-specimen-11-09-2017/

Shi, T., Balsells, E., Wastnedge, E., Singleton, R., Rasmussen, Z. A., Zar, H. J., Rath, B. A., Madhi, S. A., Campbell, S., Vaccari, L. C., Bulkow, L. R., Thomas, E. D., Barnett, W., Hoppe, C., Campbell, H., & Nair, H. (2015). Risk factors for respiratory syncytial virus associated with acute lower respiratory infection in children under five years: Systematic review and meta-analysis. *Journal of Global Health, 5*(2), 1–13. https://doi.org/10.7189/jogh.05.020416

Siegel, D. A., Jatlaoui, T. C., Koumans, E. H., Kiernan, E. A., Layer, M., Cates, J. E., Kimball, A., Weissman, D. N., Petersen, E. E., Reagan-Steiner, S., Godfred-Cato, S., Moulia, D., Moritz, E., Lehnert, J. D., Mitchko, J., London, J., Zaki, S. R., King, B. A., Jones, C. M., … the Lung Injury Response Clinical Working Group; Lung Injury Response Epidemiology/Surveillance Group. (2019). Update: Interim guidance for health care providers evaluating and caring for patients with suspected e-cigarette, or vaping, product use associated lung injury—United States, October 2019. *MMWR Morbidity and Mortality Weekly Report, 68*(41), 919–927. https://doi.org/10.15585/mmwr.mm6841e3

Simon, R. H. (2020). Cystic fibrosis: Overview of the treatment of lung disease. *UpToDate*. https://www.uptodate.com/contents/cystic-fibrosis-overview-of-the-treatment-of-lung-disease

Soler, L. M., Raymond, S. L., Larson, S. D., Taylor, J. A., & Islam, S. (2018). Initial primary spontaneous pneumothorax in children and adolescents: Operate or wait? *Journal of Pediatric Surgery, 53*(10), 1960–1963. https://doi.org/10.1016/j.jpedsurg.2017.12.014

Swain, S. K., Pattnaik, S. K., Das, A., & Sahu, M. C. (2017). Button battery aspiration in children: Our experiences in a tertiary care teaching hospital of eastern India. *Pediatria Polska, 92*, 382–388. https://doi.org/10.1016/j.pepo.2017.03.012

Tieder, J. S., Bonkowsky, J. L., Etzel, R. A., Franklin, W. H., Gremse, D. A., Herman, B., Katz, E. S., Krilov, L. R., Merritt, J. L., Norlin, C., Percelay, J., Sapién, R. E., Shiffman, R. N., Smith, M. B. H., & the Subcommittee on Apparent Life Threatening Events. (2019). Clinical practice guideline: Brief resolved unexplained events (formerly apparent life-threatening events) and evaluation of lower risk infants. *Pediatrics, 144*(1), E20160590. https://doi.org/10.1542/peds.2019-1360

University of Rochester Medical Center. (2020). *Signs of respiratory distress in children: Learning the signs of respiratory distress*. https://www.urmc.rochester.edu/encyclopedia/content.aspx?ContentTypeID=90&ContentID=P02960

Vivisenco, C. I., Farcasi, A., Iorgulescu, A., & Mertic, I. A. (2019). Foreign body aspiration—Still a challenge in pediatrics? *Romanian Journal of Pediatrics, 68*(2), 89–93. https://doi.org/10.37897/RJP.2019.2.6

Wang, Y., Hao, C., Ji, W., Lu, Y., Wu, M., Chen, S., Wang, K., & Shao, X. (2019). Detecting respiratory viruses in children with protracted bacterial bronchitis. *Respiratory Medicine, 151*, 55–58. https://doi.org/10.1016/j.rmed.2019.04.003

Welch, L. (2016). A guide to spirometry best practice for community nurses. *Journal of Community Nursing, 30*(1), 58–64.

Whittaker, E., López-Varela, E., Broderick, C., & Seddon, J. A. (2019). Examining the complex relationship between tuberculosis and other infectious diseases in children. *Frontiers in Pediatrics, 7*, 1–23. https://doi.org/10.3389/fped.2019.00233

Williams, K. B., Oyetunji, T. A., Hsuing, G., Hendrickson, R. J., & Lautz, T. B. (2018). Spontaneous pneumothorax in children: National management strategies and outcomes. *Journal of Laparoendoscopic and Advanced Surgical Techniques, 28*(2), 218–222. https://doi.org/10.1089/lap.2017.0467

World Health Organization. (2020). *Coronavirus disease (COVID-19) advice for the public: Mythbusters*. https://www.who.int/emergencies/diseases/novel-coronavirus-2019/advice-for-public/myth-busters

Wu, Y., Feng, G., Xu, Z., Li, X., Zheng, L., Ge, W., & Ni, X. (2019). Identification of different clinical faces of obstructive sleep apnea in children. *International Journal of Pediatric Otorhinolaryngology, 127*, 109621. https://doi.org/10.1016/j.ijporl.2019.109621

# Management of Cardiovascular Disorders

Tracey Cobb-Scully, Shauna di Bari, and Claire M. Rizk

## Student Learning Outcomes

**Upon completion of this chapter, the reader should be able to:**

1. Discuss pathophysiology and epidemiology for selected cardiovascular disorders in children.
2. Differentiate subjective and objective findings of selected cardiovascular disorders in children.
3. Choose appropriate laboratory or diagnostic tests for selected cardiovascular disorders in children.
4. Utilize the differential diagnosis process to determine the diagnosis of a cardiovascular disorder in children.
5. Determine treatment plan, child/family education, and need for referral for children with a cardiovascular disorder.

## INTRODUCTION

Many children with cardiovascular disease (CVD) appear healthy and thus may go undiagnosed for a period of time. Practitioners may or may not be aware that a child coming to clinic has a cardiac disorder. For those children who are undiagnosed, a meticulous history and physical examination should help to confirm suspicion of illness that may be of cardiac origin. Cardiovascular disorders in children can be divided into two main categories—congenital heart defects (CHDs) and acquired cardiac disease.

CHDs occur during the fetal period and are most often identified prenatally or within the first year of life. Some children with CHD may not be identified until later in childhood. Certain CHDs cause a child to present with a constellation of findings that reveal they are in heart failure (when the heart cannot pump well enough to meet the oxygen demand of the body). Heart failure symptoms in children differ from those in adults: children often present with feeding intolerance, respiratory distress, and behavior changes. Fortunately, advances in surgical techniques and diagnostics have improved survival rates of children with CHDs and many now live into adulthood.

CVD may also be acquired during the course of childhood. As the obesity crisis continues to affect children and teenagers, the incidence of hypertension, dyslipidemia, and other acquired heart disease continues to rise. Primary care providers are in an optimal position to determine the presence of cardiac disease by performing a comprehensive history and physical examination, in addition to counseling children and their families on healthy life choices.

Although the management of the child with CVD often requires close follow-up with a pediatric cardiologist, many CHDs, arrhythmias, and acquired cardiac diseases are first identified by the primary care provider. Therefore, it is essential to include cardiac causes in the differential diagnosis when presented with common pediatric complaints such as syncope, poor weight gain, shortness of breath, cough, wheezing, or gastrointestinal distress. Additionally, the chronic management of the child with cardiac disease will require close attention to growth, nutrition, immunization status, exercise, and psychosocial development—all of which occur most often in the primary care clinic.

The content in this chapter maps to the following areas on the Pediatric Nursing Certification Board (PNCB) Pediatric Nurse Practitioner—Primary Care certification examination:

## CLINICAL PROBLEMS: CARDIOLOGY

CONTENT AREAS:

### II. Assessment and Diagnosis

**B. History and Physical Examination**

1. Obtain history of present illness
2. Obtain a comprehensive health history for new patients
3. Complete an interval history for established patients
4. Perform a review of systems
5. Perform a complete physical examination

**C. Diagnostic Testing and Screening**

1. Order and interpret office/clinic based screening tests
2. Order and interpret diagnostic laboratory tests
3. Order and interpret the results of diagnostic imaging tests

**D. Analyzing Information**

1. Integrate health history and physical examination findings into the plan of care
2. Assimilate findings from screening and diagnostic testing into plan of care

**E. Diagnosis**

1. Develop and prioritize differential diagnoses
2. Establish a diagnosis based on evaluation of patient data

### III. Management

**A. Child and Caregiver Counseling and Education**

1. Provide condition-specific counseling and education, including treatment options
2. Educate about benefits and potential adverse reactions of pharmacological interventions
3. Discuss non-pharmacological interventions
4. Counsel regarding the threshold for seeking follow-up care
5. Review the risks of non-adherence to recommended treatment

**B. Therapeutic Interventions**

1. Prescribe pharmacologic agents
2. Recommend the use of over-the-counter pharmacologic agents
3. Order or recommend non-pharmacologic treatments for the management of symptoms
4. Discuss use of complementary and alternative therapies as appropriate

**C. Procedures**

1. Perform procedures in accordance with diagnostic guidelines and plan of care (rapid tests)
2. Initiate life-saving techniques in response to urgent or emergent situations

**D. Collaboration and Referral**

2. Refer to specialists as indicated for evaluation, counseling, and/or treatment

**E. Care Coordination**

1. Facilitate patient and family-centered care for children of all ages with acute and chronic conditions

**F. Evaluation and Follow-up**

2. Establish a plan for follow-up care

### IV. Professional Role Responsibilities

**A. Leadership and Evidence-based Practice**

4. Develop, implement, and/or modify clinical practice guidelines

## ANATOMY AND PHYSIOLOGY

The cardiovascular anatomy and physiology of the child vary greatly from those of the adult, with significant differences seen most in infants and neonates. The physiologic transition from fetal circulation to extrauterine life distinguishes the neonate from the young infant. Early in life, the cardiovascular system is assessed, diagnosed, and treated for congenital malformations. Because such diagnoses may have profound effects on a child's life course, it is vital to identify potential life-threatening cardiac conditions as early as possible.

The typical developing heart is divided into four chambers consisting of two atria and two ventricles. Blood flow is controlled by valve structures that separate the atria from the ventricles. The largest vessels—the aorta and pulmonary artery—provide pulmonary and systemic blood circulation. The aorta carries oxygenated blood for systemic circulation, while the pulmonary artery carries deoxygenated blood to the lungs.

CHDs in children are the most prevalent category of malformations diagnosed in childhood. Thus, it is imperative to gather a comprehensive history that is inclusive of both birth history as well as prenatal and genetic histories. Early identification of critical cardiac conditions in the infant and child will provide the best positive outcomes and impact on their life course. Conversely, lack or delay in diagnosis increases mortality and comorbidity factors in the developing child.

## Embryology

Because fetal circulation and development of cardiac structures begin early in pregnancy, fetal development is very important to consider when discussing congenital cardiac malformations. Transitioning from fetal to extrauterine life is necessary at birth in order to sustain and maintain independent pulmonary circulation. At birth, sudden changes occur to pressures within the fetal circulation so that fetal-maternal circulation can then transition to independent neonatal circulation. Some critical changes that occur during the transition from fetal to extrauterine life are discussed in this section.

Cardiopulmonary circulation begins as early as 8 weeks of gestation. Formation and functionality of heart structures such as the atria, ventricles, valves, and vessels have commenced at this point in pregnancy. As fetal development occurs, cardiac structures continue to become more organized and pronounced. However, it is important to remember that to sustain fetal life, the majority of the circulating blood will shunt away from the fetal pulmonary system and will instead circulate within the maternal circulatory system. This occurs due to a series of vessels that are open with other structures that allow oxygenated and deoxygenated blood to mix within this open system as blood is brought to the maternal cardiopulmonary system for oxygenation (Table 25.1).

Fetal circulation changes drastically at birth, as the fetus must transition from a dependent pulmonary circulation to an independent or closed circulatory system. This transition needs to occur within the first moments after birth for the neonate to assume a closed cardiopulmonary system. The previously elevated pulmonary vascular resistance falls starting with the baby's first breath, promoting blood flow to the neonate's lungs. Over the first few days of life, pulmonary vascular resistance continues to fall. During this period the patent foramen ovale closes, preventing mixing of oxygenated and deoxygenated blood in the atria. Within the first two weeks of life the ductus arteriosus also closes. After two weeks of life there should not be any mixing of oxygenated or deoxygenated blood. However, children with cardiac disorders may have residual mixing.

# HEART MURMURS

Heart murmurs may be found commonly in neonates, infants, and children and may be divided into two categories. Innocent murmurs (also called functional murmurs)—those that are not associated with or suspected to be associated with a structural defect—are considered a normal finding and commonly occur (Geggel, 2019). They do not require evaluation by cardiology. Other murmurs are caused by a structural defect or a defective heart valve and require evaluation and management by a pediatric cardiologist. Examples

**TABLE 25.1 Open Fetal Structures**

| Fetal Shunt | Description | Closure |
| --- | --- | --- |
| FORAMEN OVALE | Opening between the atria | Typically, this fetal shunt will close soon after birth. Blood pressure in the lungs decreases due to pulmonary vasodilation and the increase in pressures of the left side of the heart. |
| DUCTUS ARTERIOSUS | Opening between the descending aorta and the left pulmonary artery | Typically, this fetal shunt will close within the first 24 to 48 hours after birth. However, this shunt may cause bidirectional blood flow before closure. In congenital malformations, where this shunt does not close, the ductus arteriosus may also cause left to right shunt-related symptoms (increased blood flow to the lungs). |
| DUCTUS VENOSUS | Opening between umbilical vein and fetal inferior vena cava | This opening will be closed off permanently with the clamping of the umbilical cord at birth. Prior to birth, this opening allows for the mixing of maternal and fetal blood flow. |

include a hole within the heart's chambers, narrowing of cardiac vessels, and abnormal valve structures. When the opening of a heart valve is smaller than normal, it is unable to close completely and regurgitation occurs, resulting in a murmur. Other conditions such as pregnancy, fever, thyrotoxicosis, or anemia can also cause murmurs.

## SUBJECTIVE FINDINGS

The health history for a child with an innocent murmur is generally unremarkable. When a child has a pathologic murmur, the health history may reveal:

- Poor feeding
- Poor growth
- Tires easily
- Color changes (particularly with feeding)
- Diaphoresis

### Risk Factors

The most common risk factors for pathologic murmurs (typically related to a CHD) are:

- Gestational factors
  - Prematurity
  - In utero infection
- Maternal factors
  - Pre-eclampsia
  - Phenylketonuria
  - Diabetes mellitus
  - Hypertension
  - Obesity
  - Thyroid disorders
  - Systemic connective tissue disorders
  - Epilepsy and mood disorders
  - Age >40 years
  - Alcohol or substance abuse
  - Maternal medicines during pregnancy
- First- or second-degree relative with CHD

### Review of Systems

The most common manifestations revealed during the review of systems include:

- **Constitutional:** growth delay, poor feeding, easily fatigued
- **Integumentary:** sweating with feeding (especially infants)
- **Respiratory:** turning blue, difficulty breathing
- **Neurologic:** delayed development

**TABLE 25.2 Pathologic Conditions Versus Innocent Murmurs**

| Clinical Manifestations Pathological Conditions | Clinical Manifestations Innocent Murmurs |
|---|---|
| Murmur with an intensity of ≥grade 3<br>Holosystolic or diastolic murmur | Murmur with an intensity ≤grade 2<br>Short systolic duration |
| Increased intensity when child is sitting in upright position<br>Maximal intensity at left sternal border | Softer intensity when child sitting up |
| Blowing quality to murmur sound | Vibrating quality |
| May radiate | Minimal radiation |

### Objective Findings

When a child has a murmur, rigorous cardiac assessment is necessary to determine if further diagnostic testing is necessary due to a more serious condition. Table 25.2 provides an overview of the process for determining if a significant heart murmur exists in accordance with a full cardiac examination. On auscultation, be sure to focus on one aspect of the examination at a time. Remembering to distinguish between the first heart sound (S1), second heart sound (S2), third heart sound (S3), and fourth heart sound (S4) can be most helpful in a cardiac examination of a child. In addition, identifying other sounds such as an opening snap, ejection click, pericardial friction rub, and murmurs can help distinguish pathological conditions.

Additional findings associated with a pathologic murmur include:

- Respiratory rate over 40 in a child or over 60 in a comfortably resting newborn (infants with CHD are often called comfortably tachypneic, meaning they are breathing rapidly but exhibit no or minimal signs of respiratory distress
- Cyanosis
- Increased work of breathing
- Low oxygen saturation via pulse oximetry (desaturation may often be subtle and not present as visible cyanosis)

**PRO TIP** The age of the child can be critical. In the neonatal period, murmurs presenting in the first 6 hours of life are usually associated with a valve problem. Murmurs detected after 6 hours of age are more likely to stem from shunt lesions.

### Laboratory and Diagnostic Testing

All newborns should have critical CHD screening done in the newborn nursery. If results are not readily available, consider obtaining pulse oximetry on the right upper and lower extremity to evaluate for critical congenital lesions. Any saturation less than 95% should prompt further workup as well as gradients between extremities.

### Treatment/Management Plan

Children with innocent murmurs do not require treatment. Treatment for pathologic murmurs will depend upon the source of the murmur and will be determined by the pediatric cardiologist.

### Family Education

Teach the following:

- For the child with an innocent murmur, this is a normal finding, is not associated with heart disease, and may resolve independently by adulthood.

### Referral

If a pathologic murmur is suspected, refer the child to a pediatric cardiologist.

## CONGENITAL HEART DEFECTS (CHD)

CHD affects about 1% of children and is the most prevalent genetic defect (Centers for Disease Control and Prevention [CDC], 2019). Traditionally, the CHDs have been identified as either acyanotic or cyanotic, depending upon whether the structural defect itself results in cyanosis. All lesions, acyanotic and cyanotic, that require surgical or catheter intervention in the first year of life are considered critical CHDs, which comprise nearly 25% of all CHDs (CDC, 2019).

## ACYANOTIC HEART DEFECTS

Defects classified as acyanotic include atrial septal defect (ASD), ventricular septal defect (VSD), patent ductus arteriosus (PDA), atrioventricular septal defect (AVSD), coarctation of aorta (CoA), interrupted aortic arch (IAA), pulmonic stenosis (PS), aortic stenosis (AS), and critical AS.

Within this category, the defects can be further subdivided into ductal-dependent and non-ductal-dependent. The ductal-dependent lesions are coarctation of the aorta, IAA, and critical AS because with these defects, systemic blood flow is provided by the ductus arteriosus. Without limitations in pulmonary blood flow, the blood supplied to the body via the ductus will have normal oxygen saturations. The other acyanotic lesions mentioned (ASD, VSD, PDA, and AVSD) are considered volume-loading defects that place an additional strain on the heart, leading to congestive heart failure. As the pulmonary vascular resistance falls after birth and continues to decrease in the first 6 weeks of life, pulmonary blood flow increases, which results in greater pulmonary venous return to the left atrium, and overall, increased circulating volume. Along with pulmonary edema, this additional volume and atrial stretch trigger a neurohormonal cascade with activation of the sympathetic nervous system and renin-angiotensin system, leading to retention of fluid and a rise in systemic vascular resistance. This can usually be managed medically in the neonatal period, which postpones surgical intervention until later in infancy or childhood.

### Ventricular Septal Defect

VSD is the most common CHD (CDC, 2019). It is classified by its location in the ventricular septum, with severity of symptoms depending upon the size of the defect. Surgical repair is ideally performed after 6 months of age. If respiratory distress and poor growth occur, an earlier surgical repair may be indicated.

### Atrial Septal Defect

Also classified by its location in the atrial septum, ASD may not result in symptoms. Thus, many children with an ASD are asymptomatic. It may not present until later in infancy or childhood due to the high pulmonary vascular resistance in the neonatal period. As the pulmonary vascular resistance falls in the first 6 to 12 weeks of life, the left-to-right shunting will become more significant (Kannan, 2020). Over time, an ASD can cause right atrial and ventricular dilation due to the increased volume load from blood shunting across the defect from the left atrium. Over time, the ASD can cause right ventricular enlargement.

### Patent Ductus Arteriosus

The ductus arteriosus is essential to fetal circulation and usually closes in the first 24 to 48 hours of life. If it does not close in the first 6 weeks of life, it is classified as a PDA. A PDA allows for increased pulmonary blood flow, placing an increased circulatory demand on the heart. A PDA is more likely to occur in premature and low birth weight infants (Benson et al., 2020).

### Atrioventricular Septal Defect

AVSDs are also referred to as atrioventricular canal defects or endocardial cushion defects. All of these terms are used interchangeably to describe a range of defects of the atrioventricular valves and septum. Depending on which valves and part of the septum are affected, the defect is classified as complete, partial, transitional, or intermediate. These defects account for 5% of all CHDs (Puri et al., 2017). Infants usually present with signs of heart failure secondary to increased pulmonary blood flow and ventricular volume load, but might be asymptomatic in the presence of pulmonary hypertension or elevated pulmonary vascular resistance. AVSDs require initial surgical repair between the ages of 6 and 12 months; then long-term follow-up is needed, as there is a potential for development of atrioventricular valve regurgitation or stenosis.

### Coarctation of the Aorta

Coarctation of the aorta (CoA) is narrowing of the descending aorta. Depending on the severity of the narrowing, it can be mild or critical. The narrowing usually occurs at the junction of the aorta and ductus arteriosus, referred to as the *isthmus*. CoA accounts for 5%–8% of CHDs (Puri et al., 2017).

As fetal echocardiography continues to improve, an increasing number of infants are being diagnosed prenatally with CHDs. However, roughly one-third of infants and children will be diagnosed postnatally. Although some infants with a CHD will not have any clinical signs on routine examination after birth, the diagnosis prior to hospital discharge has been improved by the routine use of pulse oximetry newborn screening (Bruno & Havranek, 2015; Puri et al., 2017). Depending on the defect, infants not diagnosed prenatally or prior to hospital discharge at birth may present with rapid and life-threatening clinical decompensation within the first few days of life as the ductus arteriosus closes. The acyanotic defects that are particularly challenging to diagnose prenatally include coarctation of the aorta, IAA, and critical AS. If not diagnosed prenatally or prior to birth hospital discharge, the risk of mortality in these children increases (up to 30%) and they present with cardiogenic shock with severe metabolic acidosis and end-organ injury (Puri et al., 2017).

### Subjective Findings

The health history may reveal:

- Poor feeding—tires with feeding or becomes tachypneic or diaphoretic, decreased activity tolerance
- Irritability or inconsolability, particularly with feeding

#### Risk Factors

The most common risk factors for acyanotic CHDs include:

- Prematurity
- Genetic syndromes
  - Down syndrome is associated with a high incidence of AVSD, VSD, and ASD. In fact, half of the children with AVSD, an endocardial cushion defect, have Down syndrome
  - Williams syndrome is associated with supravalvular AS
  - DiGeorge syndrome is associated with conotruncal defects, with the most common being IAA (Puri et al., 2017)
- Familial history of sudden death in infancy, or CHD of a first-degree relative
- Maternal history of diabetes mellitus, obesity, hypertension, thyroid disease, or epilepsy
- Prenatal history positive for assistive reproductive technology infection, illicit or prescribed drug use, alcohol consumption, or smoking

#### Review of Systems

The most common manifestations revealed during the review of systems include:

- **Constitutional:** difficulty with feeding, poor weight gain, decreased activity tolerance
- **Integumentary:** diaphoresis
- **Respiratory:** exertional tachypnea
- **Genitourinary:** decreased number of wet diapers
- **Neurologic:** delayed developmental milestones (older infants and children), lethargy

### Objective Findings

The physical examination findings of the child with acyanotic CHD will depend upon whether the lesion is ductal-dependent, as well as the timing of presentation. The examination of the neonate with ductal-dependent systemic blood flow, also known as left-sided obstructive lesions, may reveal the following:

- Blood pressure differential, with the blood pressure in the right upper extremity greater than 10 mmHg higher than the lower extremities
- Weak pulses in lower extremities as compared with upper extremities
- Tachypnea, tachycardia
- Harsh systolic ejection murmur often heard at the left upper sternal border, with or without an ejection click (AS)
- Gallop, or additional heart sound, may be heard in a failing left ventricle with an elevated end-diastolic pressure
- Hepatomegaly
- Cold or cool lower extremities, particularly when temperature is compared to upper extremities
- Pallor, mottling, or dusky appearance of lower extremities

ALERT: The presence of a gallop rhythm in a neonate with an undiagnosed acyanotic defect is an ominous prognostic sign, indicating a failing left ventricle.

The physical examination of the infant or child with volume-loading defects with left to right shunting, such as VSD, ASD, PDA, or AVSD, may reveal:

- Tachypnea, intercostal retractions
- Crackles or wheezes on auscultation due to interstitial edema
- Loud and fixed S2 (ASD)
- Hyperdynamic precordium
- Holosystolic murmur at the left lower sternal border (VSD or AVSD)
- Continuous "to-fro" murmur at the left upper sternal border, often described as "machinery" (PDA)
- Hepatomegaly

**PRO TIP** The absence of a pathological murmur does not rule out a CHD. If the defect is large, there will not be sufficient turbulent flow to produce an audible murmur (Puri et al., 2017).

## Laboratory/Diagnostic Testing

The following laboratory and diagnostic testing can be used to aid in the diagnosis of the child with an acyanotic CHD:

- Chest radiograph may reveal cardiomegaly or increased pulmonary vasculature markings.
- Electrocardiogram (ECG) could demonstrate peaked P waves, indicative of right atrial enlargement, particularly in an older infant or child with an ASD or PDA. For the child with AVSD, the ECG may reveal a left axis deviation and superior QRS axis, as the conduction system travels around the large endocardial cushion defect in the center of the heart.

**PRO TIP** All children with Down syndrome should have a comprehensive cardiac evaluation due to the high incidence of AVSD, VSD, and ASD among children with the syndrome.

- Comprehensive metabolic panel may reveal elevated creatinine or transaminases, indicating end-organ injury.
- Echocardiography is essential for providing a definitive diagnosis of CHD, using two-dimensional imaging of cardiac anatomy and function.

## Differential Diagnosis

The differential diagnosis for an acyanotic CHD includes:

- Neonatal sepsis
- Respiratory viral infection
- Diaphragmatic hernia
- Airway disease
- Cardiomyopathy
- Myocarditis

## Treatment/Management Plan

Children with acyanotic heart defects are managed medically by a pediatric cardiologist with repair of the defect performed by a pediatric cardiothoracic surgeon. Table 25.3 lists specialty management of these disorders.

ALERT: In the infant with a ductal-dependent defect, closure of the ductus arteriosus is a medical, and potentially, surgical emergency. If the infant presents with cardiogenic shock with end-organ injury, that will necessitate intensive care and resuscitation with the goal of restoring systemic perfusion and reversing end-organ injury prior to surgery. All neonates with ductal-dependent systemic blood flow require surgical intervention in the first week of life.

Monitor infants with unrepaired left to right cardiac shunts for respiratory symptoms, as they have an increased risk of respiratory viral infections.

TABLE 25.3 **Management of Acyanotic Congenital Heart Defects**

| Defect | Goal | Medical Management | Surgical Treatment |
|---|---|---|---|
| Ductal-dependent systemic blood flow (CoA or IAA) | Maintain or re-establish ductus arteriosus patency until surgical repair | If the diagnosis is made prenatally, the neonate will be started on prostaglandin E1 at the time of delivery.<br>If the diagnosis is made postnatally, an infusion of prostaglandin E1 should be initiated immediately | Repair of the arch |
| Volume-loading defects with left to right shunting (VSD, ASD, PDA, AVSD) | Management of congestive heart failure | Diuresis with loop diuretics, and afterload reduction with ACE inhibitors | VSD, AVSD, ASD—patching/closure of the defect in the septum surgically or with device occlusion<br>PDA—banding or ligation |

ASD, atrial septal defect; AVSD, atrioventricular septal defect; CoA, coarctation of aorta; IAA, interrupted aortic arch; PDA, patent ductus arteriosus; PGE1, Prostaglandin E1; VSD, ventricular septal defect

When providing primary care for children with repaired acyanotic heart defects, it is important to do the following:

- Check blood pressure—the child with a repaired aorta is more prone to develop hypertension and re-coarctation can also occur (Kaza & Thiagarajan, 2016).
- Monitor for murmur—the child with repaired AVSD is at risk for atrioventricular valve regurgitation or stenosis (Puri et al., 2017).
- Follow growth and development (these should improve after surgical repairs of the defects).

▶ ALERT: Postpericardiotomy syndrome most commonly occurs after surgical ASD patch closure, and usually presents within the first week postoperatively. Clinical features include pleuritic chest pain, pericardial friction rub, and fever. Nonsteroidal anti-inflammatory drugs (NSAIDs) are the first-line treatment.

### Family Education

Teach the following:

- Signs and symptoms that would necessitate emergency medical care, as well as symptoms that would prompt a return visit to the clinic.
- Feeding and growth are of utmost importance (symptoms demonstrated during feedings are very indicative of the infant's myocardial oxygen demand [workload of the heart]).
- Encourage detailed feeding logs and weekly weights.

### Referral

Refer all infants and children with confirmed or suspected CHD to a pediatric cardiologist. Those with signs of cardiogenic shock, severe metabolic acidosis, or respiratory failure require emergent resuscitation and intensive care.

## CYANOTIC CONGENITAL HEART DEFECTS

All cyanotic CHDs are considered to be critical CHDs because they result in an inability of the heart to provide oxygenation to the remainder of the body. Visible cyanosis occurs in infants once their oxygen saturation level drops below about 85% (Adeyinka et al., 2020). Thus, blue-tinged mucous membranes or skin should be a clear indication to providers to consider a cyanotic heart defect in the child. Children with critical CHDs require surgery or catheter-based interventions within the first year of life (Rao, 2019). Many of these infants are diagnosed prenatally via fetal echocardiogram, but some present postnatally, usually within the first few days of life.

Critical CHDs constitutes about one-fourth of all CHDs (CDC, 2019). Critical and noncritical heart defects may be diagnosed during prenatal ultrasound. If not diagnosed prenatally, a critical CHD screen is generally done in the newborn nursery prior to babies being discharged home. The critical CHD screen is implemented as a way to diagnose cardiac disease, which may have been missed prenatally, and consists of using pulse oximetry measurements on the right upper extremity and a lower extremity after 24 hours of life. If there is a difference between two extremities by 3% or if the saturations are lower than 95%, then workup plus a pediatric cardiology consult are warranted (Martin et al., 2020). The test attempts to screen for seven cyanotic heart lesions but may give a false negative. Thus, newborns with suspected cardiac disease in the primary care office should still receive full workup for cardiac disease.

Cyanotic CHDs may be divided into two main categories: those resulting in decreased pulmonary blood flow or mixing lesions in which oxygenated and deoxygenated blood are able to mix within the cardiac chambers. Defects associated with decreased pulmonary blood flow have a limitation of the right ventricular outflow tract where less blood reaches the lungs, resulting in cyanosis. Children with more obstruction at the pulmonary valve are generally more cyanotic than those with less obstruction. Lesions included in this category are pulmonary valve abnormalities, tricuspid valve anomalies, Ebstein's anomaly, and tetralogy of Fallot (ToF).

The other category of cyanotic lesions (mixing lesions) includes transposition of the great arteries, truncus arteriosus, and total or partial anomalous pulmonary venous return. Mixing lesions—such as a VSD, ASD or PDA—allow oxygenated and deoxygenated blood to mix together through a connection between systemic and pulmonary systems prior to entering the systemic circulation. Without mixing of blood in the aforementioned lesions, systemic flow of oxygenated blood would be compromised and not survivable. Children with mixing lesions will present with cyanosis but may also present with symptoms of congestive heart failure depending on the amount of blood that is mixing. After the pulmonary vascular resistance falls in the first few days of life, blood preferentially flows to the lungs in the presence of a VSD or PDA.

As more blood flows through the pulmonary system, children will develop tachypnea, and pulmonary edema related to fluid overload. Furthermore, because blood flows in the path of least resistance, less blood will flow through the systemic circulation, and that blood is carrying less oxygen than in a normal circulation. Thus, children may develop feeding intolerance related to gut ischemia. If there is a restriction at the sites of mixing, children may present with cardiogenic shock. In this case prostaglandin E1 (PGE1) must be started to maintain ductal patency to allow for mixing of pulmonary and systemic circulations.

If not treated, children with cyanotic lesions are at risk for significant adverse sequelae. Lack of oxygen to organ systems may result in necrotizing enterocolitis or chronic kidney disease. Further, compensatory erythropoiesis occurs to increase red blood cell production and oxygen-carrying capacity. However, increased hemoglobin and hematocrit is directly related to increased viscosity in the blood, which puts children at risk for embolic events. Some infants with less extreme cyanosis may be medically managed to allow for growth, but generally infants with cyanotic CHD will have surgery or a catheter-based intervention to correct their heart defects in early infancy.

## Decreased Pulmonary Blood Flow: Tetralogy of Fallot

ToF is the most common cyanotic CHD, accounting for about 7%–10% of all cases (Diaz-Frias & Guillaume, 2019). ToF consists of four lesions: VSD, pulmonary stenosis, overriding aorta (aorta arises over the VSD and receives blood from both ventricles), and right ventricular hypertrophy. ToF occurs on a spectrum of cyanosis determined by the degree of pulmonary stenosis. The degree of cyanosis depends on the individual hemodynamics resulting from the four defects. If left to right blood flow across the VSD occurs, oxygen saturation may be relatively normal, yet pulmonary overcirculation may occur. With significant pulmonary stenosis, pulmonary blood flow is decreased and blood shunts right to left across the VSD, resulting in lower oxygen saturations (75%–85%). If circulation is relatively balanced, the oxygen saturation will likely be around 90% (mild hypoxia) and the infant may have few, if any, symptoms. Cyanosis may or may not be present at birth, but it progresses over time and infants generally present by 6 months of age.

## Decreased Pulmonary Blood Flow: Tricuspid Atresia

In tricuspid atresia (TA), the tricuspid valve is not patent, resulting in no direct communication between the right atrium and ventricle. In utero, the right ventricle is typically small due to blood flow bypassing the right ventricle through the foramen ovale to get to left-sided heart structures. If a VSD is present, then blood will flow from the left ventricle to the right ventricle before going to the lungs. If no VSD is present, blood will flow out of the left ventricular outflow tract and across the PDA to the pulmonary arteries leading to the lungs for oxygenation. Infants may present immediately in the neonatal period with severe cyanosis and require PGE1 infusion to maintain the PDA. In less severe cases with a large VSD, infants may have increased pulmonary blood flow. About half of these infants also have transposition of the great arteries. Outcomes in this population are generally 80% survivability at the 10-year mark and risk factors for poor outcomes are related to concomitant genetic syndromes (Alsoufi et al., 2015).

## Mixing Lesions: Transposition of the Great Arteries

Dextro-transposition of the great arteries (dTGA) is a congenital malformation that results in incomplete rotation and separation of the truncus arteriosus. The aorta arises from the right ventricle and the pulmonary artery arises from the left ventricle. Thus, the body receives deoxygenated blood from the aorta and the lungs receive oxygenated blood from the pulmonary artery. Survival relies on mixing of blood supply at some level, so this lesion is frequently seen with VSD and/or PDA. Without adequate mixing an infant will die; therefore, immediate treatment is required to increase mixing through the PDA via PGE1 infusion or balloon atrial septostomy (BAS) to create an ASD. In the first few weeks of life the infant will have corrective surgery to switch the vessel locations so the aorta arises from the left ventricle and pulmonary artery from the right ventricle. Outcomes for this lesion have found to be significantly improved with prenatal diagnosis (Ravi et al., 2018).

## Mixing Lesions: Total Anomalous Pulmonary Venous Return

Total anomalous pulmonary venous return (TAPVR), which takes place in 2% of CHD cases, occurs when the pulmonary veins do not return to the left atrium (St. Louis et al., 2019). Rather, the pulmonary veins carrying oxygenated blood return to the right side of the heart. TAPVR may be further classified in the manner by which the veins return:

- *Supracardiac*—to the superior vena cava (SVC) above the heart (50% of cases)
- *Cardiac*—to the coronary sinus or directly into the right atrium (cardiac, most likely to be associated with obstruction)
- *Infracardiac*—below the diaphragm to the portal venous system or the inferior vena cava (25%–35% of cases)
- in a *mixed fashion* (10%; St. Louis et al., 2019)

Obstruction is associated with blood backing up into the pulmonary bed, which causes pulmonary edema. Blood will flow right to left through the shunt because of elevated pressure on the right side related to increased blood volume. A level of blood mixing must exist (via ASD or PDA), otherwise there would not be systemic blood flow. Infants with severe obstruction will present as cyanotic and in shock, but those without obstruction may go undetected, with cyanosis and pulmonary edema developing over time (Shi et al., 2017).

## Subjective Findings

Many infants are diagnosed with cyanotic CHD prenatally or in the immediate postnatal period as they present with cyanosis. However, parents coming to the clinic may report the following symptoms in their children:

- Bluish tinge to mucous membranes, perioral area, or feet/hands
- Difficulty feeding or sweating during feeding

### Risk Factors

The most common risk factors for cyanotic CHD are:

- Genetic concerns: 15% to 20% related to chromosomal abnormalities (Galvis et al., 2020)
  - DiGeorge or any 22q11 deletion, velocardial-facial syndrome (ToF)
  - Trisomy 21 (ToF)
  - Noonan syndrome
  - CHARGE syndrome
  - Alagille (ToF)
- Familial history of sudden death in infancy, or CHD of a first-degree relative
- Maternal history of diabetes mellitus, obesity, hypertension, thyroid disease, or epilepsy
- Prenatal history positive for assistive reproductive technology infection, illicit or prescribed drug use, alcohol consumption, or smoking

### Review of Systems

The most common manifestations revealed during the review of systems include:

- **Constitutional:** poor weight gain, requires a long time to feed, decreased amount taken per feeding, exercise intolerance, fatigue, delayed developmental milestones
- **Respiratory:** increased work of breathing, fast breathing, frequent respiratory infections
  - Turning very blue (profound cyanosis) when agitated or with exertion (hypercyanotic spell also called a "tet spell")—may also occur with feeding, crying, or having bowel movement

- **Cardiovascular:** palpitations (older children)
- **Neurologic:** irritability, lethargy

## Objective Findings

The physical examination of the child with a cyanotic CHD may reveal:

- Poor weight gain
- Diaphoresis
- Lethargy
- Cyanosis of varying degrees
- Tachypnea
- Increased work of breathing
- Crackles
- Tachycardia
- Murmur
  - Harsh systolic ejection murmur at the upper sternal border (ToF)
  - Systolic ejection murmur at the left upper sternal border, may have S3 gallop (TAPVR)
- Hepatomegaly
- Edema (TA)

▶ ALERT: Lethargy and severe respiratory distress necessitate emergent intervention.

## Laboratory and Diagnostic Testing

The following laboratory and diagnostic testing can be useful in the diagnosis of the child with a cyanotic CHD:

- Chest X-Ray
  - ToF: a boot-shaped heart, may or may not have increased pulmonary vascular markings depending on degree of pulmonary stenosis
  - TAPVR: Snowman sign, cardiomegaly
  - TA: cardiomegaly, increased or decreased pulmonary vascular marking
  - dTGA: "egg on a string" appearance
- Pulse oximetry screening
- Echocardiogram, the primary diagnostic modality revealing blood flow and structural defects (many infants are diagnosed by fetal echo at 20 weeks' gestation)
- ECG
- Pulse oximetry screening:
  - ToF: decreased oxygen saturations with no difference on all four extremities
  - dTGA: lower oxygen saturation on right hand than lower extremities
- Complete blood count: increased hemoglobin and hematocrit occurring in response to cyanosis is directly related to increased viscosity in the blood placing infants at risk for embolic events (Zabala & Guzzetta, 2015)

## Differential Diagnosis

The differential diagnosis for a cyanotic CHD includes:

- Pulmonary disease
- Sepsis
- Inborn error of metabolism
- Hemoglobinopathy
- Pulmonary hypertension

The differential diagnosis for ToF includes:

- Pulmonary stenosis
- VSD
- Double outlet right ventricle (often associated with other CHDs)
- Primary pulmonary diseases

The differential diagnosis for TA includes:

- ToF
- Tricuspid stenosis
- Pulmonary valve atresia
- Critical valvar pulmonary stenosis

The differential diagnosis for transposition of the great arteries includes:

- Left ventricular outflow tract obstruction
- Mitral and tricuspid valve abnormalities
- Coronary artery variations

## Treatment/Management Plan

Infants with suspected cyanotic CHD will receive a PGE1 infusion at least until the cardiac defect can be identified. All children with cyanotic CHDs will require surgical repair or a catheter-based intervention during infancy to relieve the cyanosis. Some children may be managed medically with diuretics and afterload reducing agents (ACE inhibitors, beta blockers) leading up to surgical or catheter-based intervention. Children with repaired TAPVR run the risk over time of pulmonary vein stenosis and pulmonary hypertension, so close monitoring of these children is essential.

## Primary Care Activities

- Routine immunizations may be administered but live vaccines should be timed in relation to surgical planning (Galvis et al., 2020).
- Respiratory syncytial virus (RSV) prophylaxis—infants with unrepaired cyanotic defects should

receive prophylaxis during RSV season (refer to chapter 43 for additional information).

- Ensure infective endocarditis (IE) prophylaxis is prescribed for dental procedures if the child is at high risk of adverse outcomes per guidelines (refer to IE section later in this chapter).
- Prescribe increased caloric intake to promote growth
- Provide ongoing developmental screening.
- When infants with ToF have hypercyanotic spells, bring the infant's knees to the chest (to raise system vascular resistance) and provide oxygen (to decrease pulmonary vascular resistance).

## Family Education

Teach the following:

- How to provide prescribed increased calories.
- For infants with unrepaired ToF, cradle the child with the knees to the chest to relieve a tet spell.
- Even after surgical repair of the cyanotic defect, the child will need ongoing follow-up with pediatric cardiology secondary to the risk for pulmonary stenosis, obstruction, pulmonary valve regurgitation, or arrhythmia.

## Referral

Refer all children with suspected or confirmed cyanotic CHD to a pediatric cardiologist. For future family planning concerns, a genetics consultation is advised. If cyanosis or congestive heart failure symptoms are present, refer to the emergency department for stabilization. Consult a pediatric nutritionist for assistance with increasing caloric intake.

▶ ALERT: Children with cyanotic lesions may present with severe cardiogenic shock requiring resuscitation. Lethargy, respiratory distress, and poor pulses are all indications for resuscitation and emergent transfer to an intensive care setting.

# ARRHYTHMIAS

Arrhythmias in children range from normal variants to malignant or fatal rhythms. Often, arrhythmias are first detected by the primary care provider, and may be suggestive of an underlying diagnosis. Arrhythmias may be classified as fast or slow, and by the width of the QRS complex.

If the rhythm is fast, then the differential can be further divided into wide or narrow complex tachyarrhythmias. The width of the QRS complex is an indicator of where the signal, driving the rhythm, originates in the heart. A narrow QRS complex is indicative of an atrial tachyarrhythmia, such as sinus tachycardia, supraventricular tachycardia (SVT), or multifocal atrial tachycardia. The most common atrial tachyarrhythmia in pediatrics is SVT (Wackel & Cannon, 2017). SVT is usually described as having an abrupt onset and termination, the result of a reentrant mechanism via an accessory conduction pathway (Figure 25.1). A tachyarrhythmia also occurs in Wolff-Parkinson-White (WPW) syndrome. In WPW, ventricular preexcitation and the electrical impulse move along an existing accessory pathway to create the faster rate. A wide QRS complex is indicative of a rhythm originating below the atrial level, such as an accelerated junctional rhythm, junctional ectopic tachycardia, or ventricular tachycardia.

In terms of slower rhythms, the more common bradyarrhythmias in the pediatric population are sinus bradycardia (Figure 25.2), sinus node dysfunction, and atrioventricular block (Baruteau et al., 2016). Bradyarrhythmias are usually indicative of an underlying injury to the conduction system, but can also be caused by extrinsic factors affecting a normal conduction system (Wackel & Cannon, 2017). Transient bradycardia is commonly caused by an increase in parasympathetic tone via the vagus nerve. Increased vagal tone can be induced by coughing, gastric reflux, vomiting, breath-holding spells, obstructive sleep apnea, or hypothermia.

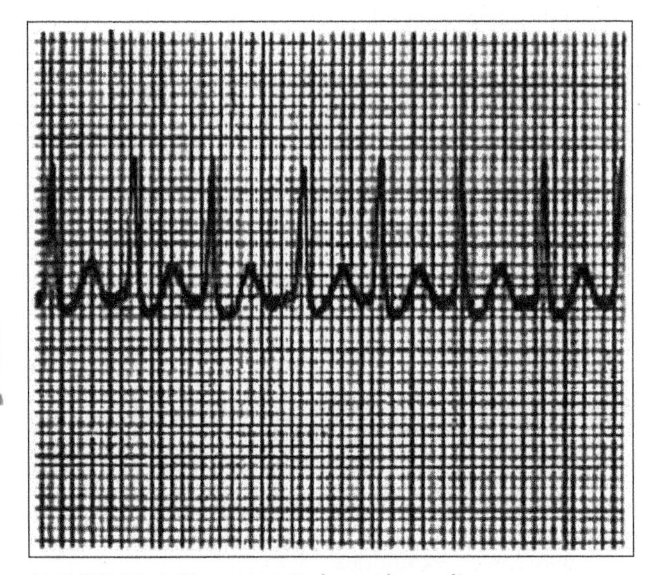

FIGURE 25.1 Supraventricular tachycardia.

*Source*: Primary Care: An Interprofessional Perspective (Singleton).

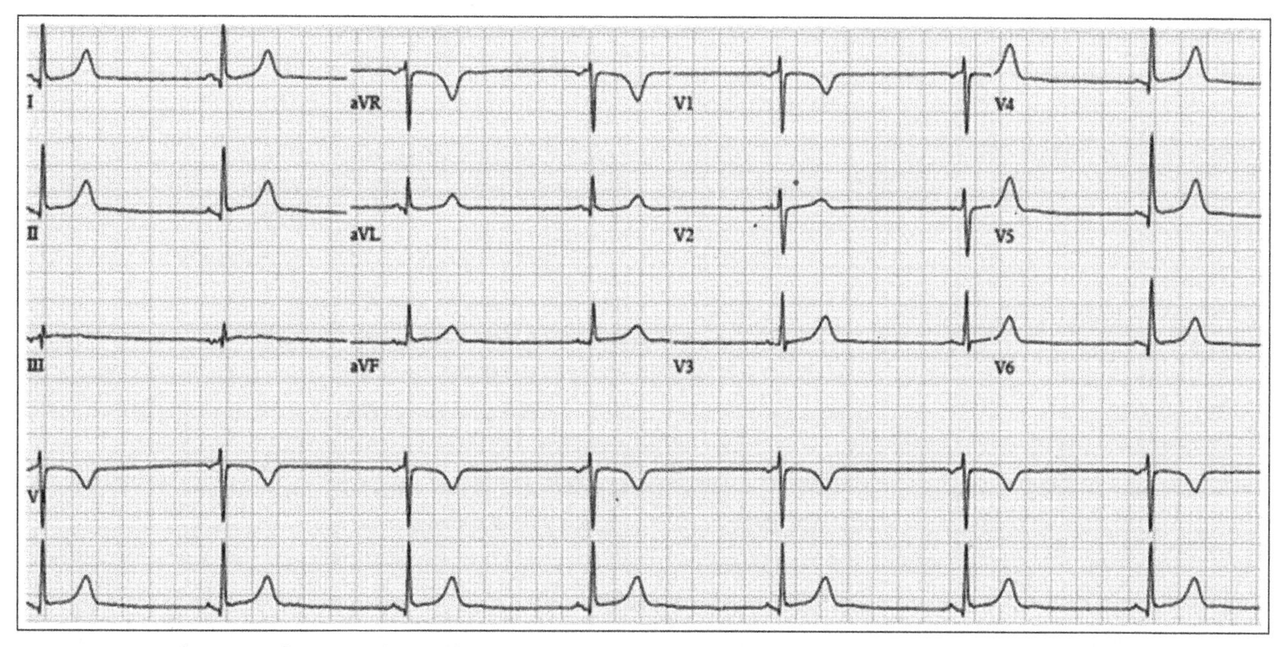


FIGURE 25.2 Electrocardiogram obtained upon admission showing sinus bradycardia at 42 beats per minute.

*Source*: Kundu, A., & Fitzgibbons, T. P. (2015). *Acute symptomatic sinus bradycardia in a woman treated with pulse dose steroids for multiple sclerosis: A case report*. https://www.ncbi.nlm.nih.gov/pmc/articles/PMC4581459/

PRO TIP It is important to recognize and manage tachyarrhythmias, as prolonged or frequent episodes of them can lead to ventricular dysfunction and heart failure.

## Subjective Findings

Although children with arrhythmias can be asymptomatic, the health history may reveal:

- Syncope
- Palpitations
- Dizziness or lightheadedness

For arrhythmias in infancy, parents may report:

- Poor feeding
- Pallor with or without cyanosis
- Loss of consciousness, or brief resolved unexplained event (BRUE)

PRO TIP When collecting data for the family history, it is important to inquire also if any relatives have died by accidental drowning. A fatal arrhythmia could have been the cause of the drowning but is unlikely to have been identified.

## Risk Factors

The most common risk factors for arrhythmias include:

- CHD
- History of cardiac surgery
- Structural coronary artery abnormalities
- Myocarditis
- WPW syndrome
- Cardiomyopathy
- Inherited channelopathy (Brugada syndrome, long QT syndrome, catecholaminergic polymorphic ventricular tachycardia)
- Family history of sudden death under the age of 50

## Review of Systems

The most common manifestations revealed during the review of systems include:

- **Constitutional:** poor feeding, fatigue, exercise intolerance
- **Cardiovascular:** palpitations, pallor, or chest pain (rare), aborted cardiac arrest
- **Neurologic:** lightheadedness, dizziness, syncope, irritability or inconsolability, unexplained seizures

ALERT: Any child or adolescent with syncope warrants a further cardiac workup and ECG.

## Objective Findings

First and foremost, it must be determined if the child with the arrhythmias is hemodynamically stable or unstable. The physical examination of the child with an arrhythmia causing hemodynamic instability may reveal:

- Pallor or mottling
- Weak or thready pulses
- Decreased level of consciousness
- Hypotension
- Cool extremities
- Diaphoresis
- Shortness of breath

In contrast, the physical examination of the child with a hemodynamically stable arrhythmia may be normal, or may reveal:

- Fussiness or agitation
- Pallor
- Diaphoresis
- Generalized weakness

▶ ALERT: Children who present with cardiogenic shock or following an aborted cardiac arrest require emergency care.

### Laboratory/Diagnostic Testing

Definitive diagnosis of the specific arrhythmia may be achieved with a 12-lead ECG to evaluate an active arrhythmia that occurs during the clinic visit. Ambulatory continuous electrocardiography may also be used to note the rhythm incidence over a multiple day period.

**PRO TIP** A classic characteristic of WPW syndrome is pre-excitation, which can be detected on a 12-lead ECG by a shortened PR interval and a delta wave with a wide QRS complex.

## Differential Diagnosis

The differential diagnosis for arrhythmias in children is focused on determining the underlying cause.
The differential diagnosis for the underlying cause of a narrow-complex tachyarrhythmia includes:

- Re-entrant arrhythmia
- CHD or worsening atrial dilation
- History of congenital heart surgery
- Wolff Parkinson White syndrome

The differential diagnosis for the underlying cause of a narrow-complex tachyarrhythmia specific to sinus tachycardia includes:

- Fever
- Pain
- Agitation or anxiety
- Medications
- Hypovolemia or shock
- Hyperthyroidism

The differential diagnosis for the underlying cause of a wide-complex tachyarrhythmia includes:

- Myocardial ischemia
- Infectious disease: myocarditis, endocarditis
- Electrolyte derangements: hypokalemia, hypomagnesemia, hypocalcemia
- Cardiomyopathy: hypertrophic cardiomyopathy (HCM), dilated cardiomyopathy (DCM), arrhythmogenic right ventricular cardiomyopathy
- Inherited channelopathy (Brugada syndrome, long QT syndrome, catecholaminergic polymorphic ventricular tachycardia; Wackel & Cannon, 2017)

The differential diagnosis for the underlying cause of sustained bradycardia includes:

- Hypothermia
- Hypoxemia
- Increased intracranial pressure
- Medications (calcium-channel blockers, beta-blockers, digoxin)
- Acquired heart disease (myocarditis, pericarditis, endocarditis, Kawasaki disease, rheumatic fever)
- Other infectious disease (Lyme disease, rubella, mumps, Chagas disease)
- Cardiac surgery
- Apnea and bradycardia of prematurity
- Long QT syndrome

## Treatment/Management Plan

The treatment of the child with bradycardia is largely dependent upon the underlying cause, as well as the degree of associated symptoms. Other reasons to intervene include the long-term risk of heart failure and sudden death (Baruteau et al., 2016). A temporary pacemaker can be placed transvenously if the underlying cause is self-limiting, such as with myocarditis. However, if the underlying cause is chronic or long-term, a permanent pacemaker may be indicated (Baruteau et al., 2016). In an acute event with hemodynamic instability, atropine is the medication of choice, as described in the pediatric advanced life support guidelines.

The treatment of the child with a tachyarrhythmia is dictated by whether the child is hemodynamically stable or unstable. If unstable, it must be determined quickly if the rhythm is sinus. If it is not sinus, urgent cardioversion is necessary. If the child is hemodynamically stable, there is time to evaluate the rhythm more closely on a 12-lead ECG to determine the appropriate treatment. For narrow complex tachyarrhythmias the best management, in order of sequence of the method that should be attempted first, includes the following:

- Vagal maneuvers
- IV adenosine
- IV calcium channel blocker

For wide complex tachyarrhythmias, the treatment pathway is also dependent upon the hemodynamic stability of the child. If the child is unconscious and pulseless, cardiopulmonary resuscitation (CPR) should be initiated immediately. If the child is conscious but severely symptomatic, synchronized cardioversion should be the first line of management. For the hemodynamically stable child with mild symptoms, the first line of management should be identifying the underlying cause, followed by IV antiarrhythmic agents (Wackel & Cannon, 2017).

### Family Education

Teach the following:

- The family should become CPR-certified if their child has a history of arrhythmias or risk factors for them.

### Referral

If a nonemergent arrhythmia or significant abnormality is detected on the initial ECG, referral to a pediatric cardiologist is warranted. Referral may also be indicated if the diagnosis is unclear, or if there is high suspicion based on the child's symptoms. A further diagnostic workup may include a Holter monitor, exercise test, echocardiogram, or electrophysiology study. If the child is hemodynamically unstable, they will require emergent and intensive care.

# ACQUIRED CARDIOVASCULAR DISEASE

Children may also experience acquired cardiovascular disorders. Some of these disorders may result secondary to lifestyle habits, whereas others may occur as a result of infection or sequela of a CHD. Acquired cardiovascular disorders in children include cardiomyopathy, chest pain, dyslipidemia, heart failure, hypertension, IE, myocarditis, pericarditis, and syncope.

## HEART FAILURE

Heart failure in children can be described as failure of the heart's pumping function. Heart failure can be further delineated as overcirculation or as pump inefficiency. *Overcirculation* means that oxygenated and deoxygenated blood is mixing somewhere in the heart's chambers, which is a problem because extra blood volume is being sent to the lungs where the resistance is lowest, resulting in pulmonary edema. Overcirculation is often related to CHDs, described earlier in this chapter. The second etiology of heart failure is pump inefficiency, which could be caused by damage to the myocardium due to infection, hereditary causes, or structural issues. Regardless of etiology, heart failure in children requires diagnosis and intervention.

### Subjective Findings

The health history may reveal:

- Cyanosis
- Lethargy
- Irritability
- Poor feeding
- Fast and/or hard breathing
- Frequent respiratory infections

### Risk Factors

The most common risk factors for heart failure include:

- Volume overload (seen with VSD, ASD, AVSD, PDA)
- Cardiomyopathy
- Myocarditis
- Supraventricular and ventricular arrhythmias, complete heart block
- Sepsis
- Chronic kidney disease
- Chemotherapy treatment

### Review of Systems

The most common manifestations revealed during the review of systems include:

- **Constitutional:** small for age, poor oral intake, poor appetite, easily fatigued, exercise intolerance (older children)

- **Integumentary:** pale color, edema, diaphoresis (especially with feedings [infants])
- **Respiratory:** increased work of breathing, tachypnea with feedings (infants), recurrent or chronic cough/wheeze
- **Cardiovascular:** cyanosis, palpitations, chest pain or syncope (older children)
- **Gastrointestinal:** abdominal pain, nausea, vomiting
- **Neurologic:** irritability, lethargy, delayed developmental milestones

### Objective Findings

Be certain to note the child's heart rate and blood pressure, comparing them with age and gender norms (refer to chapter 3). The physical examination of the child with heart failure may reveal:

- Diaphoresis
- Increased work of breathing
- Tachypnea
- Crackles
- Cyanosis
- Heart murmur
- Tachycardia
- Low blood pressure
- Poor distal perfusion, prolonged capillary refill time
- Lethargy or irritability

### Laboratory and Diagnostic Testing

Laboratory and diagnostic testing for heart failure includes:

- Chest x-ray may demonstrate pulmonary interstitial edema or pleural effusion in newly diagnosed heart failure. Chest x-ray may also be used to monitor heart failure and evaluate cardiomegaly and pulmonary congestion.
- ECG may demonstrate sinus tachycardia, or another arrhythmia commonly associated with a particular heart defect or cardiac issue.
- Echocardiogram is the primary method used for evaluating ventricular size and function, as well as the heart's structure.
- B-type natriuretic peptide (BNP) measurement assists with determining the severity of heart failure and its improvement (Singh & Singh, 2020).

### Differential Diagnosis

The differential diagnosis for heart failure includes:

- Respiratory distress
- Failure to thrive
- Gastrointestinal disorders causing feeding intolerance
- Renal failure
- Shock

### Treatment/Management

Treatment of heart failure includes:

- Increasing caloric intake to compensate for increased metabolic demand secondary to tachypnea and tachycardia
- ACE inhibitor for blood pressure control and to make pumping more efficient
- Diuretics to decrease pulmonary edema related to overcirculation (Singh & Singh, 2019)

#### Referral

Refer children with heart failure to a pediatric cardiologist for ongoing management. Consult a pediatric nutritionist for assistance with increasing calories in the diet. If blood pressure, perfusion, or oxygen saturation is compromised, refer to the emergency department.

## CARDIOMYOPATHIES

Cardiomyopathy is a disorder in which the heart muscle is functionally and structurally abnormal, yet CHD, coronary artery disease, hypertension, or valvular disease does not exist with this myocardial abnormality. The incidence is rare; about 1 to 1.5 per 100,000 children have various forms of cardiomyopathy. They include DCM (50%–60% of cases), restrictive cardiomyopathy (RCM, 5% of cases), and HCM (40% of cases; Choudhry et al., 2019). The etiology varies, but may be related to genetic causes, toxins or immune reaction, arrhythmias, and coronary artery abnormalities (Lee et al., 2017). They can be primary in nature (unrelated to other systemic disease) or secondary in nature (arising from other illnesses). DCM is associated with systolic dysfunction and increased ventricular dimensions. In about half of the cases, DCM is related to myocarditis and is the leading cause for the need for heart transplant in the pediatric population (Tunuguntla et al., 2019). The hypertrophic subtype is associated with a thickened left ventricle, which is not dilated. The HCM phenotype is significant for progressive left ventricular outflow tract obstruction, which is associated with syncope and possible cardiac arrest (Choudhry et al., 2019). Finally, restrictive morphology (RCM) is associated with diastolic dysfunction (the heart muscle has trouble relaxing), creating an enlarged atrium with normal or low normal ventricular size and preserved systolic (pumping) function (Lipschultz et al., 2019).

## Subjective Findings

The health history may reveal:

- Feeding difficulties, decreased appetite
- Diaphoresis
- Frequent respiratory illnesses
- Palpitations or chest pain in older children
- Syncope

## Risk Factors

The most common risk factors for cardiomyopathy are:

- Genetic:
  - Muscular dystrophy
  - Noonan syndrome
  - Familial history of autosomal dominant cardiomyopathy
  - Other genetic anomalies associated with inborn errors of metabolism, trisomies, neuromuscular disease and syndromes (Lee et al., 2017)
- Infectious:
  - History of myocarditis
  - Viral illness like parvovirus, Coxsackie virus, Epstein-Barr virus, human immunodeficiency virus (HIV), herpes virus, influenza, adenovirus
- Toxin exposure:
  - Chemotherapy
  - Radiation exposure

## Review of Systems

The most common manifestations revealed during the review of systems include:

- **Constitutional:** decreased energy
- **Cardiovascular:** syncope
- **Gastrointestinal:** abdominal discomfort, nausea or vomiting
- **Musculoskeletal:** muscle weakness, hypo- or hypertonia
- **Neurologic:** lethargy, seizures, developmental delay

▶ ALERT: Children presenting with syncope or history of family members who have died suddenly may have a lethal arrhythmia that is associated with cardiomyopathy.

## Objective Findings

The physical examination of the child with cardiomyopathy may reveal:

- Small-appearing, thin child
- Cool, pale, and clammy skin
- Tachypnea
- Dyspnea with crackles
- Tachycardia
- S3 gallop
- Systolic murmur
- Abdominal discomfort
- Hepatomegaly

## Laboratory and Diagnostic Testing

Perform an ECG. Lethal arrhythmias account for a significant amount of associated morbidity and mortality in individuals with cardiomyopathy (Maurizi et al., 2018). Use an echocardiogram to assess heart function. A chest x-ray may reveal cardiomegaly and pulmonary edema. Cardiac enzymes (troponin, BNP) may be elevated.

## Differential Diagnosis

The differential diagnosis for cardiomyopathy includes:

- Infectious disease
- Gastrointestinal disease
- CHD
- Arrhythmia
- Autoimmune disease

## Treatment/Management

The treatment and management of cardiomyopathy vary depending upon the morphology of the disease. The treatment of DCM includes beta blockers, aldosterone antagonists, diuretics, and afterload reduction with ACE inhibition or angiotensin receptor blockers. HCM is treated with beta blockers to slow heart rate and allow for filling. Diuretics are avoided, as volume depletion may result in decreased stroke volume, thereby inducing or worsening the left ventricular outflow tract gradient. Individuals with RCM need anticoagulation and arrhythmic therapy to address increased atrial size and the risk of embolic events. Management of arrhythmias may be achieved with medications and/or an implantable cardioversion defibrillator (ICD).

### Family Education

Teach the following:

- Prescribed exercise restriction
- Signs of progression of disease

### Referral

Refer the child with suspected cardiomyopathy to a pediatric cardiologist. Children with HCM should be referred to a geneticist for first-degree relative familial screening because of the likely genetic component.

## CHEST PAIN

Chest pain in children and adolescents usually presents as a result from a musculoskeletal structure or organ within the chest, such as ribs, intercostal muscles, sternum, diaphragm, joints, or lungs. Rarely is the source of chest pain in children of cardiac nature (Schroeder, 2017). Instead, about 20% of pediatric cases are pulmonary in nature, with other causes being from gastrointestinal or psychiatric origin (Schroeder, 2017). About 15% of cases of pediatric chest pain do not have a known cause (Schroeder, 2017).

### Subjective Findings

The health history may reveal:

- Pain with exercise
- Pain that awakens child at night

### Risk Factors

Risk factors for chest pain in the pediatric client depend largely upon the underlying cause of the chest pain. Congenital, genetic, or acquired underlying disease identification helps determine specific risk factors.

### Review of Systems

The most common manifestations revealed during the review of systems include:

- **Constitutional:** Pain—determine the onset, duration, quality (e.g., burning, cramping, aching, deep, superficial, boring, shooting), severity, exact location on chest, radiation pattern, aggravating and relieving factors, and timing (including pattern, degree of fluctuation, and frequency of remissions)

### Objective Findings

The physical examination of the child with chest pain is usually normal. If other signs are exhibited, correlate them as possible causes for the chest pain.

### Laboratory and Diagnostic Testing

A chest x-ray and ECG help rule out a cardiac cause for the chest pain.

### Differential Diagnosis

The differential diagnosis for chest pain includes:

- Musculoskeletal—chest pain related to chest wall inflammation, costochondritis, slipping rib syndrome
- Pulmonary-related chest pain syndromes derived from bronchitis, acute chest, pleurisy, exercise-induced asthma
- Gastrointestinal—peptic ulcer, gastritis, cholecystitis
- Psychological—symptoms of panic disorder or severe emotional distress

### Treatment/Management

Treatment and management of chest pain are directed toward the underlying etiology.

### Family Education

Teach the following:

- Reassure the child and family of normal cardiac findings.
- Explain that the pain is related to a noncardiac cause, providing specifics.

### Referral

If the chest pain is determined to arise from a cardiac cause, refer to a pediatric cardiologist.

## DYSLIPIDEMIA

Dyslipidemia refers to alterations in lipoprotein metabolism resulting in:

- High total cholesterol (TC)
- High low-density lipoprotein cholesterol (LDL-C)
- High non-high-density lipoprotein cholesterol (non-HDL-C)
- High triglycerides (TG)
- Low HDL-C

Hyperlipidemia is another term that is often used and refers to increased levels of lipids (fats) in the blood, including cholesterol and TG. Twenty percent of children have dyslipidemia (de Ferranti & Newburger, 2020a). Dyslipidemia results from or more of these processes:

- Excessive dietary intake of saturated and trans fats
- Diseases such as type 2 diabetes mellitus, obesity, or nephrotic syndrome
- Genetic factors such as familial hypercholesterolemia

Although dyslipidemia may not cause symptoms, it can significantly increase a child's risk of developing CVD (coronary artery disease, cerebrovascular disease, and peripheral vascular disease). Obesity in conjunction with hyperlipidemia further increases the risk of the child developing metabolic syndrome and other medical and mental conditions.

## Subjective Findings

The health history may reveal:

- Excessive dietary intake of fats
- Obesity

### Risk Factors

The most common risk factors for dyslipidemia are:

- Family history of coronary artery disease in a male first-degree relative before age 55 or a female first-degree relative before age 65

### Review of Systems

Most children and adolescents with dyslipidemia are asymptomatic and thus will not reveal symptoms during the review of systems.

## Differential Diagnosis

Differential diagnoses are not indicated for dyslipidemia, as this is a mechanism of screening for increased levels of lipids in the blood.

### Laboratory and Diagnostic Testing

According to the American Academy of Pediatrics (AAP), risk assessment should begin at age 2 years, continuing through age 8. If the risk assessment is positive, the child should be screened for hyperlipidemia with a fasting lipoprotein profile (Greer, 2017). A positive risk assessment is identified by the presence of at least one of the following:

- Obesity, diabetes, or hypertension in the child
- Parent with hyperlipidemia
- Family history of early-onset CVD
- Adolescent nicotine use

The AAP also recommends universal lipid screening at the following ages:

- Once between the age of 9 and 11 years
- Once in later adolescence (17 to 21 years; Hagan et al., 2017)

## Treatment/Management

The first step in the treatment and management of hyperlipidemia involves lifestyle modifications. Lifestyle modifications to be implemented include:

- Dietary changes—reduce intake of saturated and trans fats AND increase intake of dietary fiber (fruits, vegetables, whole grains)
- Increased physical activity—vigorous physical activity is needed daily
- Avoidance of exposure to nicotine

Prescribe statin medications for children at moderate CVD risk if after 3 months of lifestyle modifications, the target goal of LDL-C <130 mg/dL is not reached (and child is over 10 years of age). For children 10 years of age and older at severe CVD risk, begin lifestyle modifications and statin therapy simultaneously (target LDL-C goal is <100 mg/dL.). Statins are given once daily at bedtime and may be titrated upward to maximum daily dose as needed to achieve the target LDL-C goal (de Ferranti & Newburger, 2020b). Statin dosing for children 10 years and older is shown in Table 25.4.

### Family Education

Teach the following:

- Lifestyle modifications (diet and exercise)
- Adolescents should avoid all nicotine use
- How to give the prescribed medications and possible adverse effects

TABLE 25.4 **Statin Dosages for Children Age 10 and Older**

| Mediation | Initial Dose | Maximum Dose |
|---|---|---|
| Atorvastatin | 5–10 mg | 20 mg |
| Fluvastatin | 20 mg | 80 mg |
| Pravastatin | 10 mg | 20 mg until age 13, 40 mg ages 14–18 |
| Rosuvastatin | 5 mg | 20 mg |
| Simvastatin | 5 mg age 10 years; 10 mg over 10 years | 20 mg |

*Source*: Data from de Ferranti, S. D., & Newburger, J. W. (2020b). Dyslipidemia in children: Management. *UpToDate*. https://www.uptodate.com/contents/dyslipidemia-in-children-management

### Referral

Refer children with resistant hyperlipidemia to a pediatric lipid specialist.

## HYPERTENSION

The prevalence of pediatric hypertension in the United States has been increasing in the past couple of decades, and the most recent prevalence statistic in the general pediatric population is 3.5% (Flynn et al., 2017). This statistic is based only on recorded blood pressures, as a large number of children do not routinely have their blood pressure screened. Among overweight and obese children, the prevalence is as high as nearly 25% (Flynn et al., 2017).

Hypertension can be primary (essential) or secondary. In primary hypertension, no identifiable cause is found. In secondary hypertension, an underlying cause is identified. The younger the child and the higher the blood pressure, the greater the likelihood that hypertension is secondary to an identifiable cause.

A secondary cause of hypertension is most likely to be found before puberty; after puberty, hypertension is more likely to be primary due to the increased incidence of childhood obesity. Medications such as cold remedies, pressors, steroids, tricyclic antidepressants, and some attention deficit hyperactivity disorder (ADHD) medications may also contribute to the development of hypertension (Rodriguez-Cruz, 2017).

In the pediatric population, the definition of hypertension is based on frequency-distribution curves for blood pressure based on gender and length/height. These can be found at https://www.nhlbi.nih.gov/files/docs/guidelines/child_tbl.pdf. In the child age 1 to 12 years, blood pressure is considered normal if it is less than the 90th percentile for age and gender. Definitions related to elevated blood pressure in the 1- to 12-year-old are:

- Elevated blood pressure—Greater than or equal to the 90th percentile to less than the 95th percentile, or 120/80 mmHg (whichever is lower)
- Stage 1 hypertension—Greater than or equal to the 95th percentile to the 95th percentile + 12 mmHg, or 130/80 to 139/89 mmHg (whichever is lower)
- Stage 2 hypertension—Greater than or equal to the 95th percentile + 12 mmHg, or greater than or equal to 140/90 mmHg (whichever is lower; Flynn et al., 2017)

In the child age 13 years or older, blood pressure is considered normal if it is less than 120/<80 mmHg. Definitions related to elevated blood pressure in the child 13 years of age and older are:

- Elevated blood pressure—120/<80 to 129/<89 mmHg
- Stage 1 hypertension—130/80 to 139/89 mmHg
- Stage 2 hypertension—Greater than or equal to 140/90 mmHg (Flynn et al., 2017)

### Subjective Findings

The child with hypertension is usually asymptomatic, though the older child may report headache or blurred vision. It is important when gathering the history to determine caffeine, licorice, and salt consumption, history of snoring during sleep, and other habits such as smoking, drinking alcohol, and ingesting illicit substances.

#### Risk Factors

The most common risk factors for primary hypertension are:

- Genetic predisposition
- Overweight or obesity
- Sedentary lifestyle
- Exposure to first-hand or second-hand smoke

Risk factors for secondary hypertension are:

- Prematurity or bronchopulmonary dysplasia
- Congenital malformations or heritable diseases
- History of type 1 or 2 diabetes
- History of sleep disorders

#### Review of Systems

The most common manifestations revealed during the review of systems include:

- **Constitutional:** fatigue
- **HEENT:** epistaxis
- **Neurologic:** Bell palsy

### Objective Findings

The physical examination of the child with hypertension may be completely normal except for being larger than normal for age and gender. If the child has a chronic condition causing the hypertension, objective findings may correlate with that particular condition.

#### Laboratory and Diagnostic Testing

In all children and adolescents with hypertension, obtain a screening urinalysis, comprehensive metabolic panel, and lipoprotein panel (fasting or nonfasting).

In children less than 6 years of age with an abnormal urinalysis or renal function test, obtain a renal ultrasound. In addition, if the child is obese, screen for diabetes with Hgb A1c, fatty liver with aspartate transaminase (AST) and alanine transaminase (ALT), and dyslipidemia with a fasting lipid panel.

### Treatment/Management

Begin treatment of hypertension with lifestyle modifications:

- The diet should be high in fruits, vegetables, low-fat milk products, whole grains, fish, poultry, nuts, and lean red meats, with limited intake of sugar/sweets and decreased sodium intake
- Moderate to vigorous physical activity for 30 to 60 minutes, 3 to 5 days per week
- If overweight or obese, encourage weight reduction and increase moderate to vigorous physical activity to 1 hour daily
- Recommend stress reduction techniques such as mindful breathing

For children with stage 2 hypertension without a significant risk factor such as obesity, or who have symptomatic hypertension, and the blood pressure is not reduced with lifestyle modifications, begin medication therapy. Start with a low dose and titrate accordingly.

### Family Education

Teach the following:

- Lifestyle modifications
- The importance of the parental role modeling in relation to lifestyle modifications

### Referral

The child with symptomatic hypertension or stage 2 hypertension without obesity should be referred to a pediatric cardiologist and/or pediatric nephrologist for further evaluation and management.

## INFECTIVE ENDOCARDITIS

IE is a rare bacterial or fungal infection of the endocardium or heart valves that includes a vegetation of tissue and/or valves. It affects 3.3 per 100,000 children in the United States each year (Gupta et al., 2017). It is associated with significant morbidity and mortality, and thus timely diagnosis and treatment are important. The disease results from initial damage to the endothelium causing thrombus formation; a surface for pathogens to adhere to is created thereby. The offending bacterium is most frequently gram positive (staphylococcus or streptococcus) in children with or without underlying cardiac disease. Gram negative organisms associated with the oropharyngeal region (*Haemophilus parainfluenzae, Actinobacillus, Cardiobacterium, Eikenella, Kingella* [HACEK]) are also important to note. If left untreated, children may suffer permanent structural damage, heart failure, or embolic phenomena like stroke (Cao & Bi, 2019).

### Subjective Findings

The health history may reveal:

- Fever
- Fatigue
- Feeding intolerance

### Risk Factors

Risk factors for IE are:

- CHD (most significant risk with cyanotic lesions, left-sided lesions, VSD, and atrioventricular canal defects [Sun et al., 2017])
- Indwelling central venous catheter
- Rheumatic heart disease
- Immunosuppression
- Chronic parenteral nutrition—most likely to be fungal infection related to high glucose-containing fluids

### Review of Systems

The most common manifestations revealed during the review of systems include:

- **Constitutional:** fever (may be low grade or high, may be prolonged), fatigue, loss of appetite
- **Integumentary:** diaphoresis
- **Musculoskeletal:** nonspecific myalgias and arthralgias
- **Neurologic:** headache or altered mental status (if septic emboli have formed)

### Objective Findings

The physical examination of the child with IE may reveal:

- Ill appearance
- Roth spots (white centered retinal hemorrhage)
- Janeway lesions (painless red flat papules on palms and soles of feet)
- Osler nodes (painful raised red lesions on fingertips and toes)
- Respiratory distress

- Decreased oxygen saturation
- New or changed heart murmur
- Tachycardia
- Hypotension

## Laboratory and Diagnostic Testing

Blood cultures and an echocardiogram (to identify vegetation) are used to diagnose IE.

## Differential Diagnosis

The Modified Duke Criteria (Box 25.1) are the standardized criteria used to make the diagnosis of IE. The differential diagnosis for IE includes:

- Other bacterial infection

## Treatment/Management

IE necessitates treatment with intravenous antibiotics (usually vancomycin or gentamicin). Surgical removal may be indicated if it is unresponsive to medical management or if it causes hemodynamic changes (Nasser et al., 2019).

The focus of prevention of IE lies with good oral hygiene and prevention of oral disease. Certain conditions place the child at high risk for IE with dental procedures involving manipulation of the gingiva or periapical region of teeth or perforation of the oral mucosa. Candidates for antibiotic prophylaxis for dental procedures include those who have:

- Prosthetic cardiac valves, including implanted prostheses and homografts
- Prosthetic material used for cardiac valve repair, such as annuloplasty rings and chords
- Previous endocarditis
- Certain congenital heart disease
  - Unrepaired cyanotic CHD, including those with shunts and conduits
  - Completely repaired CHD with prosthetic material during first 6 months after procedure
  - Repaired CHD with residual shunts or valvular regurgitation
- Cardiac transplantation recipients with valve regurgitation due to structurally abnormal valves (American Academy of Pediatric Dentistry, 2019)

Antibiotics are given 30 to 60 minutes before a dental procedure. Recommended antibiotics with doses are:

- Amoxicillin 50 mg/kg orally (maximum dose 2 g)
- Ampicillin 50 mg/kg intravenous or intramuscular if unable to take drug orally (maximum dose 2 g)
- For penicillin-allergic children:
  - Clindamycin 20 mg/kg orally (maximum dose 600 mg) OR
  - Cephalexin 50 mg/kg orally (maximum dose 2 g) OR
  - Azithromycin or clarithromycin 15 mg/kg orally (maximum dose 500 mg)
  - If unable to take drug orally:
    - Clindamycin 20 mg/kg intravenous (maximum dose 600 mg) OR
    - Cefazolin or ceftriaxone 50 mg/kg intravenous or intramuscular (maximum dose 1 g)

BOX 25.1 **Duke Criteria for Infective Endocarditis**

| Definitive Diagnosis:<br>• 2 major criteria OR<br>• 1 major and 3 minor criteria OR<br>• 3 minor or 5 minor criteria |
|---|
| Major Criteria:<br>• Positive bacterial or fungal culture (organism consistent with IE from 2 separate specimens)<br>• Presence of pathological intracardiac lesion (vegetation or abscess)<br>• New valvular regurgitation (not just worsening of murmur)<br>Minor Criteria:<br>• Predisposing heart condition<br>• Temperature greater than or equal to 38.0 degrees Celsius<br>• Arterial embolus, pulmonary infarct, Janeway lesions, conjunctival or intracranial hemorrhage<br>• Osler nodes, Roth's spots, positive rheumatoid factor, or glomerulonephritis<br>• Positive blood culture for organism not usually associated with IE |

IE, infective endocarditis

*Source*: Data from Baltimore, R. S., Gewitz, M., Baddour, L. M., Beerman, L. B., Jackson, M. A., Lockhart, P. B., Pahl, E., Schutze, G. E., Shulman, S. T., & Willoughby, Jr., R. (2015). Infective endocarditis in childhood: 2015 update: A scientific statement from the American Heart Association. *Circulation, 132*(15), 1487–1515. https://doi.org/10.1161/CIR.0000000000000298

### Family Education

Teach the following:

- Oral hygiene and prevention of oral disease are very important.
- Information about dental procedure prophylaxis for high-risk children (Baltimore et al., 2015).

### Referral

Refer the child with IE to a pediatric cardiologist and possibly a pediatric infectious disease specialist.

## MYOCARDITIS

*Myocarditis* is inflammation of the muscular structures of the heart and is frequently associated with infections (especially viral), but may also be related to immunologic processes or toxins. Some children may have myocarditis that is mild and goes unnoticed, whereas in others it is associated with significant morbidity and mortality (Tunuguntla et al., 2019). The disease occurs in phases from acute initial injury from the virus or toxin to recovery, which may include long-term sequelae such as myocyte scarring and DCM. The initial acute phase may last only days, but immune response to initial injury can last for weeks to months and significant myocardial damage may ensue in this phase. Fulminant myocarditis is associated with hemodynamic compromise and ventricular dysfunction (Bejiqi et al., 2019). These children will require hospital care and should be referred urgently. Practitioners should use a high degree of clinical suspicion for diagnosis, as even mild cases are at risk of rapid clinical deterioration.

### Subjective Findings

The health history may reveal:

- History of flu-like or gastrointestinal viral illness in past 2 weeks
- Fever

### Risk Factors

The most common risk factors for myocarditis are:

- Recent viral illness: associated with Coxsackie B virus, enteroviruses, adenovirus, parvovirus, influenza, cytomegalovirus, varicella, mumps, HIV, RSV, rubella
- May have had a nonviral infection such as fungal or bacterial infection
- Inflammatory disorders such as rheumatic fever
- Autoimmune disorders such as Kawasaki disease
- Toxin ingestion or toxic reaction to drugs
- Hypersensitivity reactions

### Review of Systems

The most common manifestations revealed during the review of systems include:

- **Constitutional:** loss of appetite, fever
- **Integumentary:** pallor, rash, diaphoresis
- **Respiratory:** tachypnea, increased work of breathing
- **Cardiovascular:** palpitations and chest pain in older children
- **Gastrointestinal:** vomiting
- **Neurologic:** irritability

### Objective Findings

The physical examination of the child with myocarditis may reveal:

- Generally ill appearing
- Cool mottled skin in infants with mild cyanosis
- Pallor
- Respiratory distress with labored respirations and decreased pulse oximetry reading
- Tachycardia, gallop rhythm, muffled heart sounds, weak pulses
- Hepatomegaly and jugular venous distension (older children)

### Laboratory and Diagnostic Testing

Diagnostic evaluation by a pediatric cardiologist or the emergency department should include:

- Chest x-ray: moderately sensitive with cardiomegaly
- ECG: highly sensitive with ST or T wave abnormalities or axis deviation (Howard et al., 2020)
- Echocardiogram: ventricular dysfunction
- Possible cardiac magnetic resonance imaging (MRI)
- Blood work: complete blood count, inflammatory markers, cardiac enzymes (BNP, troponin T or I), liver enzymes, blood cultures, and viral cultures

### Differential Diagnosis

The differential diagnosis for myocarditis includes:

- Sepsis
- Viral illness
- Asthma
- Pneumonia
- Pericarditis

PRO TIP The five key diagnostic points for myocarditis are respiratory distress, poor perfusion, hypotension, ECG abnormalities, and abnormal chest x-ray (Chong et al., 2015)

### Treatment/Management Plan

Immunosuppression, intravenous immunoglobulin (IVIG), and antivirals are largely unproven therapies (Bejiqi et al., 2019). Yet, IVIG is often prescribed because myocarditis is associated with high risk of morbidity and IVIG is a relatively low-risk medication. If the child receives IVIG, they may need live virus vaccine updates. Corticosteroid administration shows some improvement in ventricular function, but not in survival rate (Howard et al., 2020). When the ECG is abnormal, arrhythmia management is needed. If the child does not require hospitalization, supportive care should be provided. Supportive care includes bed rest, salt/fluid restriction, possible supplemental oxygen, and correction of anemia (Howard et al., 2020). Resultant heart failure may require ongoing follow-up per cardiology recommendations.

### Family Education

Teach the following:

- Restrict exercise for 6 months.
- Follow-up with live virus vaccination updates if the child received IVIG.
- Some children will have full recovery and others may progress to having DCM with persistent ventricular dysfunction.
- Possible recurrence of disease.

### Referral

Children with suspected myocarditis should be referred to a pediatric cardiologist or sent to the emergency department, depending on the severity of symptoms.

## PERICARDITIS

Pericarditis is inflammation of the pericardium, the sac surrounding the heart. It can cause a pericardial effusion (when fluid fills within this space), making it harder for the myocardium to contract (Tunuguntla et al., 2019). It can be an emergent situation if cardiac tamponade (compression of the heart by fluid in the pericardial sac) is suspected. This fluid may also be infectious in nature and thus treatment of infection is important. It is relatively uncommon in the pediatric population, especially in those without previous history of cardiac disease, accounting for less than 0.2% of emergency room visits per year (Baskar, 2016). There is a risk for recurrence of pericarditis, so follow-up is important.

### Subjective Findings

The health history may reveal:

- Viral illness in the past 2 weeks
- In the younger child, irritability and poor feeding
- Older children may complain of chest pain

### Risk Factors

The most common risk factors for pericarditis include:

- Recent viral infection
- Bacterial infection—most frequent in children under 2
- Trauma
- Postsurgical complications (postpericardiotomy syndrome, most frequent 1 to 2 weeks postoperative, especially after ASD closure)
- Small effusion noted on postoperative echocardiogram
- Kawasaki disease
- Rheumatologic disorders
- Tuberculosis
- Bone marrow transplant

### Review of Systems

The most common manifestations revealed during the review of systems include:

- **Constitutional:** fever, loss of appetite, abdominal pain
- **Cardiovascular:** chest pain relieved when sitting, worse when supine or coughing
- **Neurologic:** lethargy

### Objective Findings

The physical examination of the child with pericarditis may reveal:

- Kussmaul breathing (slow, deep respirations)
- Jugular venous distension
- Tachycardia

- Pulsus paradoxus (decreased peripheral pulses during inspiration)
- Friction rub, muffled heart sounds
- Hepatomegaly

### Laboratory and Diagnostic Testing

Diagnostic evaluation by pediatric cardiology should include:

- Chest x-ray: enlarged cardiac silhouette
- ECG: may show ST segment elevation, T wave inversion, and PR depression
- Echocardiogram will delineate location, size of fluid collection, and extent of compression of surrounding structures (Gura, 2020)
- Fluid culture if pericardiocentesis is performed

### Differential Diagnosis

The differential diagnosis for pericarditis includes:

- Recurrent viral infection, pulmonary or gastric in nature
- Pneumonia
- Myocarditis
- Pericardial effusion

### Treatment/Management

Treatment may include:

- High-dose NSAIDs
- Colchicine has mixed recommendations for use in pediatrics (Alabed et al., 2016)
- Off-label treatment with an interleukin-1 receptor antagonist such as anakinra (Baskar, 2016)
- If pericardiocentesis is performed, antibiotics may be started if etiology is believed to have a bacterial component (Abdel-Haq et al., 2018)

### Family Education

Teach the following:

- Follow-up is important because recurrence in the pediatric population is common.

### Referral

Refer children with suspected pericarditis to a pediatric cardiologist. Referral to the pediatric cardiac surgery team may also be needed if the child had a recent surgical procedure. If hemodynamic changes occur, refer immediately to the emergency department for management.

## SYNCOPE

Syncope in children is multifaceted and can be caused by many different factors. *Syncope* is defined as a sudden, brief loss of consciousness associated with loss of postural tone from which recovery is spontaneous. Up to 15% of children experience a syncopal episode prior to the end of adolescence (Anderson et al., 2016). The vast majority of cases of syncope in the pediatric age group represent benign alterations in vasomotor tone, yet syncope can also occur as the result of a more serious disease (usually cardiac) with the potential for sudden death.

### Subjective Findings

The health history may reveal an episode of fainting or acute loss of consciousness. It is critical to obtain a thorough history surrounding the episode. Ask these questions:

- Was a trigger or precipitating event noted?
- What activity was the child involved in before the event?
- Did the child experience a positional change?
- Did the child completely lose consciousness? Was loss of consciousness complete?
- Did the loss of consciousness have rapid onset and short duration?
- Did the child wake up spontaneously and completely? Were any deficits noted upon wakening?
- Did the child fall (loss of postural tone)?

### Risk Factors

The most common risk factors for syncope include:

- Dehydration
- Emotional upset or anxiety
- Hypo- and hyperglycemia
- History of postural hypotension
- Overheating
- Cardiac disorders

### Review of Systems

A thorough review of systems for children with a suspected syncopal episode is necessary due to the variant systems from which syncope may originate. The most common manifestations revealed during the review of systems include:

- **Constitutional:** sudden increase or decrease in weight
- **Cardiovascular:** chest pain, palpitations (syncope is likely to be associated with cardiac disorder)

- **Neurologic:** loss of consciousness, increased symptoms with positional changes, unexplained and involuntary rhythmic muscle movement
- **Psychological:** recent changes to environment, stress or trauma, anxiety or depressive symptoms

▶ ALERT: Very concerning symptoms accompanying syncope include exertional onset, chest pain, dyspnea, low back pain, palpitations, or severe headache.

## Objective Findings

Determine orthostatic vital signs. A drop in systolic blood pressure of greater than 20 mm Hg or a rise in heart rate of more than 30 beats per minute when standing is consistent with the diagnosis of neurally mediated hypotension causing fainting (Anderson et al., 2016). The physical examination of the child with neurally mediated syncope is generally unremarkable. Perform a thorough cardiac examination, as murmur or arrhythmia may indicate a cardiac etiology. A comprehensive neurological examination is warranted to rule out increased intracranial pressure as a cause. A complete psychological assessment will also help in the diagnosis of any neuropsychological pathology.

▶ ALERT: Very concerning objective findings accompanying syncope include focal neurologic deficits, diplopia, dysarthria, or ataxia.

## Laboratory/Diagnostic Testing

Serum electrolytes and a complete blood count may reveal electrolyte disturbance or anemia, yet in most cases of benign syncope these values are normal. If a cardiac cause is suspected, a 12-lead ECG may be useful. An electroencephalogram is warranted when there is a suspected underlying neurological pathology. If symptoms associated with the syncopal episode are atypical, tilt-table testing may be ordered.

## Differential Diagnosis

The differential diagnosis for syncope includes:

- Cardiac disorder such as left or right ventricular outflow tract obstruction, ventricular tachycardia, congenital long QT syndrome, bradyarrhythmia
- Hypotension
- Hypovolemia
- Vasovagal response
- Migraine
- Panic attack
- Seizure

## Treatment/Management Plan

As the most prevalent cause of syncope in children is related to neurally mediated syncope, treatment should include:

- Ensuring adequate fluid intake
- Ensuring adequate sodium intake
- Encouragement of regular exercise that is consistent

In some cases, use of medications (such as beta blockers, fludrocortisone, midrodrine) may also be required.

### Family Education

Teach the following:

- Manage these symptoms with nutrition and exercise.
- Follow up with adherence to lifestyle changes.

### Referral

Refer to specialists when the presenting symptoms are atypical. With suspected underlying cardiac pathology, refer to a pediatric cardiologist. If serious neurological pathology is being considered, refer to a pediatric neurologist. Although these incidences are rarer, caution should be taken when concerns regarding these disease processes arise.

## KEY POINTS

- Acyanotic cardiac defects can be further subdivided into left-to-right volume-loading lesions and ductal-dependent lesions with left-sided obstruction.
- If undiagnosed, ductal-dependent lesions with left-sided obstruction will present with cardiogenic shock.
- Left-to-right volume-loading lesions present with signs of congestive heart failure that require medical management with diuretics and systemic afterload reduction following surgical intervention, ideally after 6 months of age.
- Cyanotic cardiac defects are classified as resulting in pulmonary blood flow or as mixing lesions.
- Hypercyanosis or "tet spells" may occur when the infant experiences profound and sometimes sudden changes in pulmonary blood flow.

- Prevention of further complications or sequelae due to dyslipidemia are major goals for the management of pediatric dyslipidemia.
- Family education and support for lifestyle changes are needed to maintain a healthy lifestyle and prevent CVD.
- Cardiomyopathy may present with mild symptoms following viral illness or as fulminant cardiogenic shock.
- Resting tachycardia, abdominal discomfort, and/or vomiting are subtle signs that should be investigated further as early signs of acute or subacute myocarditis.
- Antibiotic prophylaxis for IE for dental procedures is required for a particular subset of children with cardiac disease.
- Arrhythmias are usually an indication of an underlying disease process and the hemodynamic stability of the child will dictate the need for emergent treatment.

## REFERENCES


Abdel-Haq, N., Moussa, Z., Farhat, M. H., Chandrasekar, L., & Asmar, I. B. (2018). Infectious and noninfectious acute pericarditis in children: An 11-year experience. *International Journal of Pediatrics, 2018,* 5450697. https://doi.org/10.1155/2018/5450697

Adeyinka, A., Samanapally, H., & Kondamudi, N. P. (2020). Cyanosis. *StatPearls.* https://www.ncbi.nlm.nih.gov/books/NBK482247/

Alabed, S., Pérez-Gaxiola, G., & Burls, A. (2016). Colchicine for children with pericarditis: Systematic review of clinical studies. *Archives of Disease in Childhood, 101*(10). http://dx.doi.org/10.1136/archdischild-2015-310287

Alsoufi, B., Schlosser, B., Mori, M., McCracken, C. Slesnick, T., Kogon, B., Petit, C., Sachdeva, R., & Kanter, K. (2015). Influence of morphology and initial surgical strategy on survival of infants with tricuspid atresia. *Annals of Thoracic Surgery, 100*(4), 1403–1409. https://doi.org/10.1016/j.athoracsur.2015.05.037

American Academy of Pediatric Dentistry. (2019). Antibiotic prophylaxis for dental patients at risk for infection. In *AAPD Review Council, the reference manual of pediatric dentistry 2019–2020* (pp. 416–421).

Anderson, J. B., Willis, M., Lancaster, H., Leonard, K., & Thomas, C. (2016). The evaluation and management of pediatric syncope. *Pediatric Neurology, 55,* 6–13. https://doi.org/10.1016/j.pediatrneurol.2015.10.018

Baltimore, R. S., Gewitz, M., Baddour, L. M., Beerman, L. B., Jackson, M. A., Lockhart, P. B., Pahl, E., Schutze, G. E., Shulman, S. T., & Willoughby, Jr., R. (2015). Infective endocarditis in childhood: 2015 update: A scientific statement from the American Heart Association. *Circulation, 132*(15), 1487–1515. https://doi.org/10.1161/CIR.0000000000000298

Baruteau, A., Perry, J. C., Sanatani, S., Horie, M., & Dubin, A. M. (2016). Evaluation and management of bradycardia in neonates and children. *European Journal of Pediatrics, 175,* 151–161. https://doi.org/10.1007/s00431-015-2689-z

Baskar, S. (2016). *Pediatric pericarditis.* https://www.acc.org/latest-in-cardiology/articles/2016/06/08/11/43/pediatric-pericarditis

Bejiqi, R., Retkoceri, R., Maloku, A., Mustafa, A., Bejiqi, H., & Bejiqi, R. (2019). The diagnostic and clinical approach to pediatric myocarditis: A review of the current literature. *Open Access Macedonian Journal of Medical Sciences, 7*(1), 162–173. https://doi.org/10.3889/oamjms.2019.010

Benson, L. N., Spicer, D. E., & Anderson, R. H. (2020). Arterial duct: Its persistence and its patency. In G. Wernovsky, R. H. Anderson, K. Kumar, K. Mussatto, A. N. Redington, J. S. Tweddell, & J. T. Tretter (Eds.), *Anderson's pediatric cardiology* (4th ed., Chapter 41). Elsevier.

Bruno, C., & Havranek, T. (2015). Screening for critical congenital heart disease in newborns. *Advances in Pediatrics, 62*(1), 211–226. https://doi.org/10.1016/j.yapd.2015.04.002

Cao, G. F., & Bi, Q. (2019). Pediatric infective endocarditis and stroke: A 13-year single-center review. *Pediatric Neurology, 90,* 56–60. https://doi.org/10.1016/j.pediatrneurol.2018.07.001

Centers for Disease Control and Prevention. (2019). *Data and statistics on congenital heart defects.* https://www.cdc.gov/ncbddd/heartdefects/data.html

Chong, S.-L., Bautista, D., & Ang, A. S.-Y. (2015). Diagnosing paediatric myocarditis: What really matters. *Emergency Medical Journal, 32*(2). http://dx.doi.org/10.1136/emermed-2013-202926

Choudhry, S., Puri, K., & Denfield, S. W. (2019). An update on pediatric cardiomyopathy. *Current Treatment Options in Cardiovascular Medicine, 21*(8), 36. https://doi.org/10.1007/s11936-019-0739-y

de Ferranti, S. D., & Newburger, J. W. (2020a). Dyslipidemia in children: Definition, screening, and diagnosis. *UpToDate.* https://www.uptodate.com/contents/dyslipidemia-in-children-definition-screening-and-diagnosis

de Ferranti, S. D., & Newburger, J. W. (2020b). Dyslipidemia in children: Management. *UpToDate.* https://www.uptodate.com/contents/dyslipidemia-in-children-management

Diaz-Frias, J., & Guillaume, M. (2019). Tetralogy of Fallot. *StatPearls.* https://www.ncbi.nlm.nih.gov/books/NBK513288/

Flynn, J. T., Kaelber, D. C., Baker-Smith, C. M., Blowey, D., Carroll, A. E., Daniels, S. R., de Ferranti, S. D., Dionne, J. M., Falkner, B., Flinn, S. K., Gidding, S. S., Goodwin, C., Leu, M. G., Powers, M. E., Rea, C., Samuels, J., Simasek, M., Thaker, V. V., Urbina, E. M., & Subcommittee on Screening and Management of High Blood Pressure in Children. (2017). Clinical practice guideline for screening and management of high blood pressure in children and adolescents. *Pediatrics, 140*(3), e20171904. https://doi.org/10.1542/peds.2017-1904

Galvis, M. M. O., Bhakta, R. T., Tarmahomed, A., & Mendez, M. D. (2020). Cyanotic heart disease. *StatPearls.* https://www.ncbi.nlm.nih.gov/books/NBK500001

Geggel, R. L. (2019). Approach to the infant or child with a cardiac murmur. *UpToDate.* Retrieved July 15, 2020, from https://www.uptodate.com/contents/approach-to-the-infant-or-child-with-a-cardiac-murmur

Greer, F. R. (2017). Healthy nutrition, children. In T. K. McInerny, H. M. Adam, D. E. Campbell, J. M. Foy, & D. M. Kamat (Eds.), *American Academy of Pediatrics textbook of pediatric care* (2nd ed., Chapter 37). American Academy of Pediatrics.

Gupta, S., Sakhuja, A., McGrath, E., & Asmar, B. (2017). Trends, microbiology, and outcomes of infective endocarditis in children during 2000–2010 in the United States. *Congenital Heart Disease, 12*(2), 196–201. https://doi.org/10.1111/chd.12425

Gura, G. F. (2020). Pediatric pericarditis case report. *Journal of Pediatric Health Care, 34*(1), 67–70. https://doi.org/10.1016/j.pedhc.2019.09.007

Hagan, J. F., Shaw, J. S., & Duncan, P. M. (2017). *Bright futures: Guidelines for health supervision of infants, children, and adolescents* (4th ed.). American Academy of Pediatrics.

Howard, A., Hasan, A., Brownlee, J., Mehmood, N., Ali, M., Mehta, S., & Fergie, J. (2020). Pediatric myocarditis protocol: An algorithm for early identification and management with retrospective analysis for validation. *Pediatric Cardiology, 41*(2), 316–326. https://doi.org/10.1007/s00246-019-02258-1

Kannan, B. R. J. (2020). Clinical diagnostic approach to congenital acyanotic congenital heart disease in infants and children. *Indian Journal of Pediatrics, 87*(5), 381–384. https://doi.org/10.1007/s12098-020-03251-w

Kaza, A., & Thiagarajan, R. (2016). Left ventricular outflow tract obstruction: Coarctation of the aorta, interrupted aortic arch, and borderline left ventricle. *Pediatrics Critical Care Medicine, 17*(8 Suppl. 1), S315–S317. https://doi.org/10.1097/PCC.0000000000000826

Lee, T. M., Hsu, D. T., Kantor, P., Towbin, J. A., Ware, S. M., Colan, S. D., Chung, W. K., Jefferies, J. L., Rossano, J. W., Castleberry, C. D., Addonizio, L. J., Lal, A. K., Lamour, J. M., Miller, E. M., Thrush, P. T., Czachor, J. D., Razoky, H., Hill, A., & Lipshultz, S. E. (2017). Pediatric cardiomyopathies. *Circulation Research, 121*, 855–873. https://doi.org/10.1161/CIRCRESAHA.116.309386

Lipshultz, S. E., Law, Y. M., Asante-Korang, A., Austin, E. D., Dipchand, A. I., Everitt, M. D., Hsu, D. T., Lin, K. Y., Price, J. F., Wilkinson, J. D., & Colan, S. D. (2019). Cardiomyopathy in children: Classification and diagnosis: A scientific statement from the American Heart Association. *Circulation, 140*(1), e9–e68. https://doi.org/10.1161/CIR.0000000000000682

Martin, G. R., Ewer, A. K., Gaviglio, A., Hom, L. A., Saarinen, A., Marci Sontag, M., Burns, K. M., Alex R. Kemper, A. R., & Oster, M. E. (2020). Updated strategies for pulse oximetry screening for critical congenital heart disease. *Pediatrics, 146*(1), e20191650. https://doi.org/10.1542/peds.2019-1650

Maurizi, N., Passantino, S., Spaziani, G., Girolami, F., Arretini, A., Targetti, M., Pollini, I., Tomberli, A., Pradella, S., Calabri, G. B., Vinattieri, V., Bertaccini, B., Leone, O., De Simone, L., Rapezzi, C., Marchionni, N., Cecchi, F., Favilli, S., & Olivotto, I. (2018). Long-term outcomes of pediatric-onset hypertrophic cardiomyopathy. *JAMA Cardiology, 3*(6), 520–525. https://doi.org/10.1001/jamacardio.2018.0789

Nasser, B. A., Al Qwaee, A., Almesned, A. R., Akhfash, A., Mohamad, T., Chaikhouni, F., Alhabshan, F., & Kabbani, M. S. (2019). Infective endocarditis in children with normal heart: Indication for surgical intervention. *Journal of the Saudi Heart Association, 31*(2), 51–56. https://doi.org/10.1016/j.jsha.2018.11.003

Puri, K., Allen, H. D., & Qureshi, A. M. (2017). Congenital heart disease. *Pediatrics in Review, 38*(10), 471–486. https://doi.org/10.1542/pir.2017-0032

Rao, P. S. (2019). Management of congenital heart disease: State of the art—Part II—Cyanotic heart defects. *Children, 6*, 54. https://doi.org/10.3390/children6040054

Ravi, P., Mills, L., Fruitman, D., Savardi, W., Colen, T., Khoo, N., Serrano-Lomelini, J., & Hornberger, L. K. (2018). Population trends in prenatal detection of transposition of great arteries: Impact of obstetric screening ultrasound guidelines. *Ultrasound in Obstetrics and Gynecology, 51*, 659–664. https://doi.org/10.1002/uog.17496

Rodriguez-Cruz, E. (2017). Pediatric hypertension. *eMedicine*. https://emedicine.medscape.com/article/889877-overview

Schroeder, S. A. (2017). Chest pain. In T. K. McInerny, H. M. Adam, D. E. Campbell, J. M. Foy, & D. M. Kamat (Eds.), *American Academy of Pediatrics textbook of pediatric care* (2nd ed., Chapter 133). American Academy of Pediatrics.

Shi, G.,Zhu, Z., Chen, J., Ou, Y., Hong, H., Nie, Z., Zhang, H., Liu, X., Zheng, J., Sun, Q., Liu, J., Chen, H., & Zhuang, J. (2017). Total anomalous pulmonary venous connection: The current management strategies in a pediatric cohort of 768 patients. *Circulation, 135*(1), 48–58. https://doi.org/10.1161/CIRCULATIONAHA.116.023889

Singh, R. K., & Singh, T. P. (2019). Heart failure in children: Management. *UpToDate*. https://www.uptodate.com/contents/heart-failure-in-children-management

Singh, R. K., & Singh, T. P. (2020). Heart failure in children: Etiology, clinical manifestations, and diagnosis. *UpToDate*. https://www.uptodate.com/contents/heart-failure-in-children-etiology-clinical-manifestations-and-diagnosis

St. Louis, J., Molitor-Kirsch, E., Shaha, S., & O'Brien, J. (2019). Total anomalous pulmonary venous return. In R. M. Ungerleider, J. N. Mcliones, K. N. McMillan, D. S. Cooper, & J. P. Jacobs (Eds.), *Critical heart disease in infants and children* (3rd ed., pp. 587–596). Elsevier.

Sun, L.-C., Lai, C.-C., Wang, C.-Y., Wang, Y.-H., Wang, J.-Y., Hsu, Y.-L., Hu, Y.-L., Wu, E.-T., Lin, M.-T., Sy, L. B., & Cheng, L. (2017). Risk factors for infective endocarditis in children with congenital heart diseases—A nationwide population-based case control study. *International Journal of Cardiology, 248*, 126–130. https://doi.org/10.1016/j.ijcard.2017.08.009

Tunuguntla, H., Jeewa, A., & Denfield, S. W. (2019). Acute myocarditis and pericarditis in children. *Pediatrics in Review, 40*(1), 14–25. https://doi.org/10.1542/pir.2018-0044

Wackel, P., & Cannon, B. (2017). Heart rate and rhythm disorders. *Pediatrics in Review, 38*(6), 243–253. https://doi.org/10.1542/pir.2016-0119

Zabala, L. M., & Guzzetta, N. A. (2015). Cyanotic congenital heart disease (CCHD): Focus on hypoxemia, secondary erythrocytosis, and coagulation alterations. *Pediatric Anesthesia, 35*(10), 981–989. https://doi.org/10.1111/pan.12705

# Management of Gastrointestinal Disorders

Megan Gentry, Melissa Nunn, and Graciela Sanabria

## Student Learning Outcomes

**Upon completion of this chapter the reader should be able to:**

1. Discuss pathophysiology and epidemiology of selected gastrointestinal (GI) disorders in children.
2. Differentiate subjective and objective findings for selected GI disorders in children.
3. Choose appropriate laboratory or diagnostic tests for selected GI disorders in children.
4. Utilize the differential diagnosis process to determine the diagnosis of GI disorders in children.
5. Determine treatment plan, child/family education, and need for referral for children with a GI disorder.

## INTRODUCTION

The gastrointestinal (GI) system is responsible for the digestion and absorption of nutrients needed for proper growth and function. Organs within the GI system are also responsible for endocrinologic and immune function. Although some GI conditions are present at birth, others may not present until late adolescence. Both medical and surgical interventions can be required when dealing with this body system, which can present with both acute and chronic conditions. Further, the need for prompt referrals at times requires a comprehensive understanding of the GI system. While there are some insidious conditions associated with the GI system, the majority of complaints are common conditions requiring the sometimes continuous care of a primary care practitioner.

The content in this chapter maps to the following areas on the Pediatric Nursing Certification Board (PNCB) Pediatric Nurse Practitioner—Primary Care certification examination:

**CLINICAL PROBLEMS: GASTROINTESTINAL**

CONTENT AREAS:

**II. Assessment and Diagnosis**

**B. History and Physical Examination**

1. Obtain history of present illness
2. Obtain a comprehensive health history for new children
3. Complete an interval history for established children
4. Perform a review of systems
5. Perform a complete physical examination

**C. Diagnostic Testing and Screening**

1. Order and interpret office/clinic based screening tests
2. Order and interpret diagnostic laboratory tests
3. Order and interpret the results of diagnostic imaging tests

**D. Analyzing Information**

1. Integrate health history and physical examination findings into the plan of care
2. Assimilate findings from screening and diagnostic testing into plan of care

**E. Diagnosis**

1. Develop and prioritize differential diagnoses
2. Establish a diagnosis based on evaluation of child data

## III. Management

**A. Child and Caregiver Counseling and Education**

1. Provide condition-specific counseling and education, including treatment options
2. Educate about benefits and potential adverse reactions of pharmacological interventions
3. Discuss non-pharmacological interventions
4. Counsel regarding the threshold for seeking follow-up care
5. Review the risks of non-adherence to recommended treatment

**B. Therapeutic Interventions**

1. Prescribe pharmacologic agents
2. Recommend the use of over-the-counter pharmacologic agents
3. Order or recommend non-pharmacologic treatments for the management of symptoms
4. Discuss use of complementary and alternative therapies as appropriate

**C. Procedures**

1. Perform procedures in accordance with diagnostic guidelines and plan of care (rapid tests)

**D. Collaboration and Referral**

1. Refer to specialists as indicated for evaluation, counseling, and/or treatment

**E. Care Coordination**

1. Facilitate child and family-centered care for children of all ages with acute and chronic conditions

**F. Evaluation and Follow-up**

1. Establish a plan for follow-up care

## IV. Professional Role Responsibilities

**A. Leadership and Evidence-based Practice**

1. Develop, implement, and/or modify clinical practice guidelines

# STRUCTURAL ANOMALIES

There are a number of GI conditions that can affect children due to an alteration in anatomy or structure. Some may be present at birth, others progress through childhood, but most can lead to a functional obstruction and progress to severe malnutrition and death. While many of these conditions can be diagnosed clinically, imaging modalities can be employed to confirm and classify a diagnosis. Although these conditions will be surgically treated, the primary care nurse practitioner will be responsible for the identification and management of these conditions and for rendering follow-up care. In this section, pyloric stenosis, umbilical hernias, intussusception, and Hirschsprung disease are covered.

## PYLORIC STENOSIS

Pyloric stenosis, also known as infantile hypertrophic pyloric stenosis, is a progressive disorder in which the pylorus, or the junction of the stomach to the duodenum, becomes hypertrophic and can lead to outlet obstruction. Progression can lead to emesis, electrolyte imbalances, and malnutrition. Pyloric stenosis occurs in approximately 2 per 1,000 live births (Costanzo et al., 2017). This condition can be familial and is seen more often in first-born children.

### Subjective Findings

The health history may reveal:

- Postprandial regurgitation and vomiting that becomes projectile between 2–8 weeks old
- Hunger immediately after emesis
- Weight loss

### Risk Factors

The most common risk factor for pyloric stenosis is macrolide antibiotic usage (especially erythromycin and azithromycin usage) before the child is 2 weeks of age (Eberly et al., 2015).

### Review of Systems

The most common manifestations revealed during the review of systems include:

- **Constitutional:** weight loss (if progressed)
- **HEENT:** lack of tears, dry mouth

- **Gastrointestinal:** forceful emesis immediately after meals, nonbilious emesis, constipation
- **Genitourinary:** decreased urinary output (due to dehydration)

### Objective Findings

The physical examination of the child with pyloric stenosis may reveal:

- Palpable pylorus in the right upper quadrant (similar in size to an olive)
- Peristalsis in the upper abdomen from left to right before vomiting
- Weight loss
- Sunken fontanelle, dry mucous membranes (alludes to dehydration)

### Laboratory/Diagnostic Testing

The diagnosis of pyloric stenosis is based upon the clinical findings, but can be confirmed with an ultrasound, which allows the measurement of pylorus thickness. If inconclusive, ultrasound may be repeated in a few days, or an upper GI series can be performed to visualize the thinned pyloric canal due to the hypertrophy of the pylorus.

Infants with suspected or confirmed pyloric stenosis should also receive fluid and electrolyte assessment, including an electrolyte panel. Infants with a prolonged course of pyloric stenosis usually present with laboratory results consistent with decreased chloride and potassium levels and an elevated bicarbonate level.

### Differential Diagnosis

The differential diagnosis for pyloric stenosis includes:

- Gastroesophageal reflux (GER)
- Gastroenteritis
- Intestinal obstruction

### Treatment/Management Plan

Confirmed pyloric stenosis requires surgical intervention, usually a pyloromyotomy. This is performed after correction of any fluid or electrolyte imbalances. Infants can still present with emesis after surgical repair; however, most can resume feedings shortly after surgery. Complication risks are very low, and most infants have an excellent prognosis following treatment.

### Family Education

Teach the following:

- Families need to continue routine medical care after treatment (to assess for feeding and growth).
- GER and emesis are common after treatment and usually will not warrant further treatment or testing.

### Referral

If pyloric stenosis is suspected or confirmed, referral to a pediatric surgeon is needed.

## UMBILICAL HERNIA

The umbilical ring is a fibrous band that surrounds the umbilicus during fetal development. Congenital umbilical hernias occur when the abdominal fascia does not close, allowing the umbilical ring to remain open after separation of the umbilical cord. Umbilical hernias usually self-resolve by the age of 5. Although there is minimal risk associated with umbilical hernias, monitoring is warranted, and referral is indicated in the case of a persistent hernia.

### Subjective Findings

The health history may reveal:

- Fluctuating swelling or mass at the level of the umbilicus, especially during crying or straining

### Risk Factors

The most common risk factors for delayed umbilical hernia closure include:

- openings greater than 1.5 centimeters
- being older than 5 years old

### Review of Systems

Children with umbilical hernias are usually asymptomatic unless strangulation or incarceration occurs (unable to reduce with or without signs of vascular damage).

### Objective Findings

The physical examination of the child with hernia may reveal:

- Soft, nontender swelling at the level of the umbilicus that reduces without difficulty (child will need to be relaxed for reduction)
  - Swelling may enlarge if child is supine, coughing, crying, or bearing down

### Laboratory/Diagnostic Testing

The diagnosis of an umbilical hernia is based upon the clinical findings. No laboratory or diagnostic testing is needed.

### Differential Diagnosis

The differential diagnosis for umbilical hernia includes:

- Umbilical mass
- Gastroschisis

### Treatment/Management Plan

Management of umbilical hernia includes monitoring for spontaneous resolution. If closure does not occur by 5 years of age, referral to a pediatric surgeon is recommended for further evaluation and potential surgical closure. Spontaneous closure usually occurs by the time the child is 5 years old, and waiting until this age to utilize surgical closure results in fewer complications and a lower risk of recurrence (Helleran et al., 2020).

### Family Education

Teach the following:

- Counsel on signs of incarceration and strangulation and, if that occurs, instruct to seek immediate care.
- Do not tape coins or other occlusive dressings or objects over the umbilicus, as this can create an infection risk.

### Referral

If an umbilical hernia does not resolve by 5 years of age or becomes symptomatic, referral to a pediatric surgeon is warranted.

## INTUSSUSCEPTION

Intussusception is an acute condition involving a portion of the intestine telescoping or being pulled into the section of intestine adjacent to it. In intussusception, the proximal portion of intestine is trapped within the distal portion. The most common site is the ileocecal junction, but intussusception can occur at other junctions. Intussusception is the leading cause of pediatric intestinal obstruction and can lead to ischemia, perforation, and peritonitis.

Intussusception most commonly occurs in children between the ages of 3 months and 3 years old. The peak occurrence is between 5 to 9 months and is seen more frequently in males (Laquerre, 2020). Most cases (approximately 75%) are idiopathic, but some children may be predisposed to intussusception because of viral illness such as adenovirus, rotavirus, enterovirus, and cytomegalovirus, due to the enlargement of intestinal lymph tissue. In the other 25% of cases, intussusception may be a result of a lead point or variation in intestinal tissue due to a condition such as Meckel diverticulum, lymphoma, vascular malformation, polyps, or cystic fibrosis (Ntoulia et al., 2016).

### Subjective Findings

The health history may reveal:

- Recent viral illness
- Episodic periods of severe progressive pain (lasting between 10–20 minutes)
- Vomiting
- Bloody stool that may be described as loose, like diarrhea or mucoid

### Risk Factors

The most common risk factors for intussusception are:

- Recent viral illness or contributing condition.
- Association of intussusception and rotavirus vaccine administration with an incidence of 1 to 5 in 100,000. However, the risk of severe dehydration due to rotavirus infection outweighs the risk of immunization (Haber et al., 2015).

### Review of Systems

The most common manifestations revealed during the review of systems include:

- **Constitutional:** progressive, intermittent abdominal pain with reports of drawing the legs inward. Fever is not common, but can occur if concurrent infection or perforation is present.
- **Gastrointestinal:** vomiting (starts nonbilious and then progresses toward bilious as the obstruction worsens), bloody stool that may also be mucoid (sometimes described as "currant jelly" stool)
- **Neurologic:** lethargy or altered mental status

### Objective Findings

The physical examination of the child with intussusception may reveal:

- Palpable sausage-like mass in the right middle to upper quadrant of the abdomen
  - May only be palpable while child is calm
  - Right lower quadrant (RLQ) may appear empty (Dance's sign)

- Periods of crying and distress interspaced with periods of being pain-free
  - Pain becomes more frequent and severe as the condition progresses
  - Child may behave normally during periods of pain or be withdrawn
- Abdominal distention and focal tenderness to palpation
- Rectal bleeding and or lethargy in progressive cases

### Laboratory/Diagnostic Testing

The diagnosis of intussusception is based upon the clinical findings and usage of ultrasound or plain radiography. On ultrasound, intussusception can be identified though visualization of a target sign. Ultrasound is the preferred method of visualization and can also be used to identify other causes of abdominal pain such as appendicitis. Target signs can sometime be visualized on plain radiographs and plain films can help identify intestinal obstructions through a lack of air in the rectum and distended loops of bowel.

### Differential Diagnosis

The differential diagnosis for intussusception includes:

- Gastroenteritis
- Malrotation and volvulus
- Appendicitis
- Ovarian torsion
- Incarcerated hernia
- Peritonitis
- Testicular torsion
- Colic

### Treatment/Management Plan

Children with confirmed or suspected intussusception should be emergently referred to a pediatric radiologist or surgeon for an air contrast enema. This is done under fluoroscopy and can confirm diagnosis and also reduce the telescoped section of intestine. If reduction is not successful, surgical intervention will be necessary. Intravenous fluids may be required if there are signs of dehydration, and intravenous antibiotics may be warranted if there is risk of infection or perforation. After reduction or repair, the child may be observed for between 12 and 24 hours for recurrence.

### Family Education

Teach the following:

- After correction, recurrence may occur in approximately 10% of cases.
- Signs of recurrence and complications (such as lethargy, sepsis, and shock).
- How to slowly advance the diet.

### Referral

If intussusception is suspected or confirmed, emergent referral to a pediatric radiologist and surgeon is needed.

## HIRSCHSPRUNG DISEASE

Hirschsprung disease, also known as congenital aganglionic megacolon, is a motility condition of the colon due to a lack of ganglion cells. It usually involves the rectosigmoid colon and can lead to obstruction within the intestine due to loss of peristalsis. A majority of cases are diagnosed during the neonatal period, but milder cases may not be diagnosed until early childhood.

Incidence is between 1 to 2 cases per 10,000 births and has a higher incidence in males than females. There is a correlation with Down syndrome or trisomy 21 and there is a familial aspect to Hirschsprung disease (Pathak et al., 2018).

### Subjective Findings

The health history may reveal:

- Failure to pass meconium within 48 hours after birth
- Poor growth
- Chronic constipation
- Abdominal distention

### Risk Factors

The most common risk factors for Hirschsprung disease are:

- Having a sibling with Hirschsprung disease
- Having a related genetic mutation or an associated syndrome such as trisomy 21

### Review of Systems

The most common manifestations revealed during the review of systems include:

- **Constitutional:** poor growth or weight loss, malnutrition, fever (if presenting with enterocolitis or toxic megacolon too)
- **Gastrointestinal:** constipation (can be long-standing and refractory if not diagnosed in the neonatal period), emesis progressing to bilious

### Objective Findings

The physical examination of the child with Hirschsprung disease may reveal:

- Abdominal distention
- Explosive gas or stool after digital rectal exam
- Tight anal sphincter

### Laboratory/Diagnostic Testing

The diagnosis of Hirschsprung disease is based upon the clinical findings. Strong suspicion is warranted if there is no passage of meconium or if an infant or child presents with signs of obstruction and a family history. Diagnosis is confirmed through rectal biopsy to demonstrate lack of ganglion cells. If a plain radiograph is obtained, dilated loops of bowel and absence of air in the rectum may be noted.

### Differential Diagnosis

The differential diagnosis for Hirschsprung disease includes:

- Malrotation
- Idiopathic constipation
- Meconium ileus due to cystic fibrosis
- Meconium plug syndrome
- Small left colon syndrome

### Treatment/Management Plan

After confirmation of Hirschsprung disease, treatment consists of surgical repair and resecting the section of colon without ganglionic cells. Constipation and fecal incontinence are common outcomes after surgery repair and may require further management.

### Family Education

Teach the following:

- Treatment of postoperative complications such as constipation and encopresis.
- Signs of intestinal infection such as fever, distention, and pain require immediately seeking of care if warranted.

### Referral

If Hirschsprung disease is suspect or confirmed, emergent referral to a pediatric gastroenterologist and surgeon is needed.

# ACUTE DISORDERS

Children are susceptible to numerous acute GI disorders, which are common complaints in primary care. Although most cases are benign, other cases can become progressive and lead to dehydration, disability, and even death. Close physical examination, along with a thorough history of present illness, can lead to prompt diagnosis. A large percentage of these cases can be managed successfully in a primary care setting, but severe cases should be referred as needed. In this section, vomiting, diarrhea, dehydration, acute gastroenteritis, acute abdominal pain, appendicitis, and foreign body ingestion are discussed.

## VOMITING

Vomiting (emesis) is the forceful expulsion of stomach and sometimes intestinal contents. It occurs due to the interaction of the gut and brain receptors, including the chemoreceptor trigger zone and vomiting center. Vomiting is a common condition in childhood and can present as part of the presentation of another disorder. Vomiting can be acute or chronic in nature and its character can further lead to a diagnosis. For example, projectile emesis is encountered with increased intracranial pressure, bloody vomiting can be associated with an upper GI bleeding issue such as esophageal ulceration, and bilious vomiting can be indicative of intestinal obstruction.

This section focuses on acute causes and presentations of emesis as seen with systemic infections (acute gastroenteritis, strep pharyngitis, urinary tract infection (UTI), appendicitis), structural anomalies or obstructions (foreign body, strictures, pyloric stenosis, intussusception, tracheoesophageal fistula, malrotation, ileus, and constipation), central nervous system issues (hydrocephalus, space-occupying lesions, traumatic brain injuries, migraines), pregnancy, metabolic conditions (inborn errors of metabolism, diabetes mellitus), food intolerance or allergy, and toxin exposure or drug ingestion.

### Subjective Findings

Be sure to ask about the features of the emesis (timing, onset, duration, alleviating or aggravating factors). Obtain information about onset and timing (with meals, after certain activities, early morning), as well as the characteristics of emesis (forceful, bloody, bilious). The health history may reveal:

- Recent illness, injury, travel, stress
- Exposure to spoiled food or toxin
- Sick contacts
- New or change in medication
- Ingestion (of a drug or toxin)

### Risk Factors

The most common risk factors for vomiting are exposure to infected individuals, food, or toxins.

### Review of Systems

The most common manifestations revealed during the review of systems include:

- **Constitutional:** fever, polydipsia, lethargy
- **HEENT:** sore throat, change in vision
- **Respiratory:** cough
- **Gastrointestinal:** concurrent abdominal pain, nausea, constipation, diarrhea
- **Neurologic:** headache, injury/trauma

### Objective Findings

The physical examination of the child with vomiting may be nonspecific or may reveal:

- Abdominal tenderness or distention (GI etiology such as obstruction or infection)
- Hypoactive or no bowel sounds (possible obstructive process)
- Increased bowel sounds (gastroenteritis)
- Lethargy or irritability may occur with dehydration, sepsis, or intracranial processes
- Lack of tears, sunken fontanelle, decreased skin turgor (signal dehydration)
- Tachypnea or decreased oxygen saturation may be present with pneumonia or airway anomaly

### Laboratory/Diagnostic Testing

When vomiting is the presenting symptom, diagnostics and laboratory testing are directed based on the possible etiology. Laboratory testing can include complete blood count, comprehensive metabolic panel, amylase, lipase, blood culture, inflammatory markers (C-reactive protein, erythrocyte sedimentation rate [ESR]), blood culture, urinalysis, urine toxicology, urine pregnancy test, urine culture, rapid strep test or throat culture, and stool studies (fecal occult blood, WBC count, ova and parasite, culture).

Imaging can include plain radiographs including kidney-ureter-bladder (KUB), lateral decubitus, chest views, upper GI series (can access for reflux or foreign bodies), ultrasound, computed tomography (CT) scan, and pH probe.

### Differential Diagnosis

The differential diagnosis for vomiting includes:

- *Infants*: GER, gastroenteritis, overfeeding, infection (sepsis, UTI), hydrocephalus, congenital anomalies
- *Toddlers and school-age children*: gastroenteritis, gastritis, GI obstruction, constipation, toxin or medication ingestion, infection (UTI, pneumonia, strep pharyngitis, otitis media, appendicitis), migraines
- *Adolescents:* gastroenteritis, gastritis, infection (UTI, pancreatitis, appendicitis, hepatitis), pregnancy, drug intoxication, migraines

### Treatment/Management Plan

Treatment of vomiting begins with the identification of cause or etiology and alleviating the cause if possible. Constipation may require disimpaction; otitis media or strep pharyngitis may require antibiotic treatment. Antiemetic medications may be utilized to stop emesis and prevent dehydration and nutritional deficits. However, these medications should not be used in infants or when the causative agent is not identifiable. The most common medications used are 5-$HT_3$ receptor antagonists, which can reduce nausea and vomiting without much sedation. Restricting diet to clear liquids with the administration of frequent but small volumes can be helpful until a full diet can be tolerated. While managing emesis, it is also important to monitor for signs of dehydration and treat appropriately as needed.

### Family Education

Teach the following:

- Diet restriction during periods of emesis and how to restart diet first with clear liquids.
- Signs of dehydration (including lack of tears, dry mouth, decreased urine output, lethargy).

### Referral

Referral to a pediatric gastroenterologist may be warranted if emesis is progressive or recurrent. Further specialty referral is needed if a concurrent underlying condition is present. Worsening emesis, especially in the setting of severe dehydration or severe systemic illness, requires an emergent referral to a pediatric emergency department.

## DIARRHEA

Diarrhea is classified as having three or more episodes of stool in one day. Often the stool is described as watery or loose and can be a larger volume than usual (at least 10 mL/kg of stool in infants and toddlers). Diarrhea can be due to increased intestinal peristalsis, increased secretory mechanisms of the GI tract, or damage to intestinal mucosa from infection or inflammation. Although there are common parameters for classifying diarrhea, the practitioner should be sensitive to any deviation in a child's stooling pattern. Extra consideration should be given in the context of concerning symptoms such as high fever, bloody stool, signs of dehydration, or lethargy.

Acute diarrhea is usually less than 1 month in duration. Common causes of acute diarrhea include viral, bacterial, or parasitic GI infections; systemic infections (otitis media, UTI, sepsis); and antibiotic use. Other causes include GI conditions such as intussusception, partial obstruction, malabsorption, and constipation (fecal overflow), along with feeding issues (starvation stool, ingestion of contaminated water, or overingestion of fruit juices). Diarrhea can quickly lead to dehydration and electrolyte imbalance, which can progress to malnutrition, coma, and death. There are more than 1.7 billion cases of pediatric diarrheal diseases each year, and for children under 5 it is the second leading cause of death globally (World Health Organization, 2017).

### Subjective Findings

Ask about the amount and character of the stool (bloody stool may indicate bacterial infection). Verify the child's diet (including amount of formula or fruit juice ingested). The health history may reveal:

- Recent travel and/or contact with contaminated water sources (drinking water, rivers /streams/pools)
- Recent sick contacts
- Day care or school attendance (increased risk of exposure)
- Recent medications (antibiotics, laxatives, stool softeners)
- Recent weight loss

### Risk Factors

The most common risk factors for diarrhea include:

- History of GI conditions such as inflammatory bowel disease (IBD) and/or immunocompromised status, as this increases the risk for infection, especially from a less common organism
- Unimmunized against rotavirus (leading cause of viral gastroenteritis)
- Recent antibiotic usage (increased risk of *Clostridium difficile* [*C. diff*] or alterations in intestinal biome)
- Poor sanitary conditions
- Exposure to contaminated water
- Travel (increased exposure to viral, bacterial, and parasitic agents)

### Review of Systems

The most common manifestations revealed during the review of systems include:

- **Constitutional:** fever (viral or bacterial cause), abdominal pain (encountered with infectious causes, partial obstructions, and intussusception)
- **HEENT:** lack of tears, dry mouth (dehydration), ear pain (associated symptom)
- **Gastrointestinal:** nausea and/or vomiting
- **Genitourinary:** decreased urine output (dehydration), urinary frequency/dysuria
- **Neurologic:** irritability

### Objective Findings

The physical examination of the child with diarrhea may reveal:

- Abdominal distention, hyperactive bowel sounds, tenderness, palpable mass
- Signs of dehydration
- Lethargy, irritability (intussusception, sepsis)

### Laboratory/Diagnostic Testing

The diagnosis of diarrhea is based on the history and clinical examination. Electrolytes can be assessed if there is a concern for dehydration or metabolic imbalance. Stool studies can be utilized to determine disease etiology. The presence of stool leukocytes is indicative of a bacterial infection, while reducing substances can be encountered in viral infections. Stool cultures can identify bacterial causes and should be considered when diarrhea is bloody, occurs with high fevers, or there is a recent travel history. Stool studies can also include specific testing for *C. diff*, if there is recent antibiotic usage, or tested for ova and parasites if indicated (immunocompromised, travel history, contaminated water).

Abdominal plain films can be utilized to reveal perforation or peritonitis. An abdominal ultrasound is used to assess for findings of intussusception or abdominal infections including appendicitis.

### Differential Diagnosis

The differential diagnosis for diarrhea includes:

- Acute gastroenteritis
- Recent antibiotic usage
- Food poisoning
- Systemic infection (acute otitis media, sepsis, UTI)
- Diet issues (overfeeding, excessive fruit juice, starvation)
- Bacterial colitis
- Toxin ingestion

### Treatment/Management Plan

The primary goal with diarrhea is to maintain or restore hydration. This can be achieved through oral rehydration solutions (ORSs) if dehydration is mild to moderate. The child should receive 50 to 100 ml/kg over a 4-hour period in small, frequent volumes. Additional hydration should be given with each episode of diarrhea. Once rehydration is complete, regular feeding should be resumed to prevent starvation diarrhea. In children, antidiarrheals are not recommended due to the risk of increasing viral load or toxin. Antidiarrheals should be withheld in dehydrated children and those with bloody diarrhea or signs of systemic infection (fever). Antibiotics should only be utilized if a bacterial cause is confirmed and/or the clinical findings result in a strong suspicion. Diet changes are recommended if diarrhea is caused by overfeeding, ingestion of excessive fruit juice or sorbitol, or a very restricted diet. Finally, probiotics can be utilized to restore the intestinal biome after a viral illness or antibiotic usage.

### Family Education

Teach the following:

- Amount and how to administer ORSs and when to resume a regular diet.
- Worsening signs such as high fever, decreased urinary output, and bloody stool and when to seek routine and emergency care.
- How to prevent diarrheal diseases (proper and frequent handwashing, proper food handling and fully cooking meat products, access to clean water, decreasing antibiotic usage, rotavirus vaccination, proper handling of soiled diapers).

### Referral

Referral can be made to a pediatric gastroenterologist if diarrhea is persistent. Refer to a pediatric surgeon if diarrhea is due to intussusception. If symptoms become severe or there are signs of sepsis or severe dehydration, the child should be referred to a pediatric emergency department.

## DEHYDRATION

Dehydration involves the loss of either water and/or electrolytes and can be caused by multiple means, including GI losses (bleeding, vomiting, diarrhea), diabetes, and when excretion or loss is greater than intake. Dehydration can be categorized by the relationship between water and electrolytes, namely sodium. Most pediatric dehydration is caused by an equal loss of water and electrolytes and is termed *isotonic* or *isonatremic dehydration*. Other types of dehydration include hypertonic (hypernatremic) and hypotonic (hyponatremic). Infants and younger children are further susceptible to hypotonic dehydration if feeds or oral rehydration is attempted with free water instead of formula, breastmilk, or oral rehydration fluid.

Dehydration is classified as mild (loss of 3%–5% volume loss), moderate (loss of 6%–9% volume loss), and severe (more than 10% volume loss). Proper classification leads to prompt assessment and appropriate treatment. Children, especially infants, have the highest risk of dehydration, due to a higher body surface ratio along with being unable to actively hydrate and correct any imbalance.

### Subjective Findings

The health history may reveal:

- Recent illness with fever, vomiting, and/or diarrhea
- Increased fluid loss as seen with excessive sweating and hyperthermia
- Thirst (sign of moderate dehydration) or refusal of fluids (sign of mild dehydration)

### Risk Factors

The most common risk factors for dehydration are:

- Fever
- Vomiting
- Diarrhea
- Decreased oral fluid intake

### Review of Systems

The most common manifestations revealed during the review of systems include:

- **Constitutional:** fever (bacterial or viral cause)
- **Gastrointestinal:** vomiting and/or diarrhea
- **Genitourinary:** decreased urinary output
- **Neurologic:** lethargy, irritability

### Objective Findings

The physical examination of the child with dehydration may reveal:

- Tachycardia, tachypnea (moderate to severe)
- Decreased blood pressure (severe)
- Poor skin turgor (moderate to severe)
- Sunken fontanelle (moderate to severe)
- Dry mucus membranes (moderate to severe)
- Decreased perfusion as evidenced by cool extremities, decreased pulses, and prolonged capillary refill (moderate to severe)
- Obtundation (diminished awareness)

> **PRO TIP** It can be difficult to assess urinary output in diapered children.

### Laboratory/Diagnostic Testing

The diagnosis and classification of dehydration are based upon the clinical findings. Laboratory evaluation of dehydration is warranted in moderate and severe dehydration or if the child presents with altered mental status or concern for severe systemic infection. Common laboratory evaluation includes a comprehensive metabolic panel to assess sodium, $CO_2$, and glucose levels (hypoglycemia can be seen with dehydration).

### Differential Diagnosis

The differential diagnosis for dehydration includes:

- Diabetes insipidus
- Diabetic ketoacidosis
- Oliguria
- Shock

### Treatment/Management Plan

Mild to moderate dehydration can first be treated with ORSs if the child is alert and aware. ORSs consist of water with glucose, sodium, potassium, and chloride. The solution may be prepared at home (use a clean water source) or be purchased commercially. Fruit juices and sports drinks are not recommended due to inappropriate levels of sugar and electrolytes. Oral rehydration should never be attempted with plain water or with soda.

Rehydration should focus on replenishment first, by giving the child 50 to 100 mL/kg over 4 hours. This should be given in small, frequent feeds such as 5 to 15 mL every 2 to 5 minutes. During this time ORSs or breast milk can be utilized. Concurrent treatment of vomiting with antiemetics or fever with antipyretics may be warranted. The provider should also monitor intake and urinary output during rehydration.

### Family Education

Teach the following:

- The signs of dehydration (decreased urinary output, decreased tears, dry mouth, change in mental status /behavior).
- Proper ORSs as well as how to prepare and give the solution.
- Prevention (proper feeding and formula mixing, not giving free water to infants, handwashing).

### Referral

Children with moderate to severe dehydration or failed attempts at oral rehydration require emergent referral to a pediatric emergency department for evaluation and treatment (intravenous fluids, electrolytes).

## GASTROENTERITIS

*Acute gastroenteritis* is defined as diarrhea (three or more episodes of loose stool in a single day) and can occur with fever, vomiting, nausea, and abdominal pain. Acute cases last less than 2 weeks and usually self-resolve. Supportive care and monitoring for dehydration and worsening symptoms are warranted. The most common etiology is a virus (rotavirus, adenovirus, norovirus), but acute gastroenteritis can also be due to bacterial and parasitic agents. Diarrhea is caused by increased intestinal fluid in the GI tract after damage of intestinal mucosa due to pathogens. This can lead to dehydration, malabsorption of nutrients, coma, and death.

### Subjective Findings

The health history may reveal:

- Three or more episodes of loose stool in 1 day (usually not bloody or mucous)

- Vomiting (usually resolves before diarrhea)
- Fever

### Risk Factors

The most common risk factors for gastroenteritis are:

- Lack of immunization against rotavirus (leading cause of viral gastroenteritis)
- Recent antibiotic usage (increased risk of *Clostridium difficile* or alterations in intestinal biome)
- Poor sanitary conditions
- Exposure to contaminated water
- Travel (increased exposure to viral, bacterial, and parasitic agents)

### Review of Systems

The most common manifestations revealed during the review of systems include:

- **Constitutional:** anorexia, abdominal pain (usually crampy)
- **HEENT:** conjunctivitis or sore throat (with adenovirus infection)
- **Respiratory:** tachypnea (if dehydrated)
- **Cardiovascular:** tachycardia (if dehydrated)
- **Gastrointestinal:** diarrhea and/or vomiting

### Objective Findings

The physical examination of the child with gastroenteritis may be nonspecific if mild but may reveal:

- Abdominal distention and/or tenderness
- Signs of dehydration
- Altered mental status (if severe dehydration, sepsis)

### Laboratory/Diagnostic Testing

The diagnosis of acute gastroenteritis is based upon the clinical findings. Laboratory and diagnostic testing can be used in severe cases to determine if there is another etiology other than a viral pathogen. Testing includes comprehensive metabolic panel, complete blood count (elevated neutrophils can signal bacterial infections), and stool studies (especially fecal occult blood, stool white blood cell count, viral antigen tests, and cultures).

### Differential Diagnosis

The differential diagnosis for viral gastroenteritis includes:

- Bacterial or parasitic gastroenteritis
- Bacterial sepsis
- UTI
- Pneumonia
- Otitis media
- Overfeeding or excessive fruit juice intake

### Treatment/Management Plan

Because viral gastroenteritis is a self-limiting process, management is based on supportive care, including maintainance of hydration with ORSs or other clear liquids. Children should continue age-appropriate regular diets, as prolonged clear liquid diets can lead to malnutrition and further diarrhea. Concurrent fever or emesis can be treated with appropriate pharmacotherapeutic agents. Antidiarrheal and antibiotic agents are not routinely indicated for viral gastroenteritis. If there is concern for moderate or severe dehydration, emergent referral is needed for further evaluation and treatment.

### Family Education

Teach the following:

- Concerning signs for dehydration and worsening gastroenteritis.
- Constructing and administering ORSs when warranted.
- Prevention including proper handwashing, appropriate handling of soiled diapers, clean drinking water and sanitation, and proper food handling.

### Referral

Referral to a pediatric emergency department is warranted in severe cases or those with signs of dehydration. Referral may also be necessary to a pediatric gastroenterologist if diarrhea becomes recurrent or chronic without identification of a source.

## ABDOMINAL PAIN

Acute abdominal pain can have a multitude of causes and accounts for approximately 9% of pediatric primary care visits (Reust & Amy, 2016). This can range from surgical issues such as appendicitis and ovarian torsion to medical processes such as pancreatitis and hepatitis. Additionally, abdominal pain can be referred pain from a condition like pneumonia or testicular torsion. Trauma and psychiatric issues can also be the cause of abdominal pain. Concurrent symptoms can lead to a potential diagnosis, as in the case of fever, emesis, and anorexia in appendicitis. Using the child's age to guide one to the most common etiologies is appropriate. In the end, the task of the practitioner is to use a careful history and thorough exam to determine the cause of acute abdominal pain.

## Subjective Findings

Ascertain the characteristics of current pain (onset, duration, factors) and the location of pain (poorly localized pain or umbilical pain is less likely to be surgical, right-lower-quadrant (RLQ) pain is associated with appendicitis). Determine if the adolescent is sexually active. The health history may reveal:

- History of GI conditions or surgeries, previous history of abdominal pain
- Injury/trauma
- New stressors

## Risk Factors

The most common risk factors for abdominal pain are:

- Constipation
- Other GI illness or infection
- Trauma

## Review of Systems

The most common manifestations revealed during the review of systems include:

- **Constitutional:** fever (usually due to infectious process), anorexia (appendicitis)
- **HEENT:** sore throat (*Streptococcus*, e.g., group A strep) or viral pharyngitis)
- **Respiratory:** cough or shortness of breath
- **Gastrointestinal:** vomiting, diarrhea, constipation, abdominal rigidity
- **Genitourinary:** dysuria, hematuria, urinary frequency, vaginal discharge, menstrual changes, testicular pain

## Objective Findings

The physical examination of the child with abdominal pain may reveal:

- Lethargy, irritability (signs of sepsis or perforation)
- Tonsillar swelling and exudate (pharyngitis)
- Focal abnormal lung sounds (pneumonia)
- Diminished or absent bowel sounds (ileus)
- Yyperactive bowel sounds (gastroenteritis)
- Abdominal tenderness (palpate area of identified pain last, can place the child's hands on abdomen with the practitioner's on top if child is sensitive to touch)
- Guarding or rebound tenderness (signs of peritonitis)
- Abdominal distention (obstruction, mass, or constipation)
- Cervical motion tenderness (pelvic inflammatory disease [PID], sexually transmitted infections [STIs]; only assess in sexually active females)
- Lack of cremasteric reflex (testicular torsion)

## Laboratory/Diagnostic Testing

Laboratory or diagnostic testing is directed toward the potential cause of the abdominal pain. This may include laboratory testing such as complete blood count, inflammatory markers (C reactive protein, ESR), comprehensive metabolic panel, blood culture, urinalysis, urine pregnancy, urine culture, STI testing, rapid strep testing or throat culture, and stool testing (fecal occult blood, WBC count, culture).

Radiographic modalities may also be utilized, such as plain radiographs (KUB and lateral decubitus views to access stool load and signs of obstruction or peritonitis) and ultrasound. Ultrasound is recommended over CT because of the decreased exposure of radiation and lower expense. Ultrasound can be used to access bowel thickness, signs of intussusception, appendicitis, and ovarian torsion (Reust & Amy, 2016).

## Differential Diagnosis

The differential diagnosis for abdominal pain includes:

*Urgent causes:*

- Appendicitis
- Intra-abdominal trauma
- Intussusception
- Malrotation
- Incarcerated hernia
- Intestinal obstruction
- Ovarian torsion
- Ectopic pregnancy
- PID
- Testicular torsion
- Magnet or battery ingestion
- Toxin ingestion (dependent on toxin and dose)

*Other causes:*

- Constipation
- Acute gastroenteritis
- UTI
- STI
- Strep pharyngitis

- Pneumonia
- Viral illnesses
- Colic
- Ovarian cysts
- Renal calculi
- Henoch-Schonlein purpura

### Treatment/Management Plan

Treatment is based on presumed or confirmed etiology of abdominal pain.

### Family Education

Teach the following:

- Counseling is based on cause of abdominal pain and should include a discussion on concerning signs and when to seek care.

### Referral

Referral to a pediatric emergency department is warranted if there is concern for surgical or urgent cause. Referral can also be made to a pediatric gastroenterologist if pain becomes chronic. Specialty referral may also be warranted if the cause is not GI-related, such as a referral to a pediatric urologist in the case of testicular torsion or hydrocele.

## APPENDICITIS

Appendicitis is the inflammation of the appendix, a sac-like structure located in the first part of the cecum in the RLQ of the abdomen. There is no singular etiology for appendicitis, but some cases are due to obstruction of the appendix by fecal matter, lymphoid tissue, neoplasm, or appendicoliths. The highest incidence of appendicitis is between 10 and 19 years of age and occurs in approximately one per 1,000 children (Rentea et al., 2017). Appendicitis can lead to intra-abdominal abscess formation, peritonitis, and perforation, which can occur within a few days and result in sepsis and death. Acute appendicitis, therefore, requires rapid detection and emergent intervention.

### Subjective Findings

The health history may reveal:

- Abdominal pain (may start general and then localize to RLQ)
- Fever
- Nausea and/or vomiting

### Risk Factors

The most common risk factors for appendicitis are:

- Familial history
- Recent bacterial, viral, or parasitic infections (Rentea et al., 2017)

### Review of Systems

The most common manifestations revealed during the review of systems include:

- **Constitutional:** anorexia, fever (usually low-grade, high-grade fever more consistent with perforation)
- **Gastrointestinal:** focal abdominal pain (resolution of pain can occur with perforation), lack of stool, abdominal guarding and not wanting to move
- **Neurologic:** fussiness, irritability

### Objective Findings

The physical examination of the child with appendicitis may reveal:

- Guarding and rebound tenderness
- Maximal pain over McBurney point (area between umbilicus and right anterior superior iliac crest)
- Positive psoas or obturator sign
- Rovsing sign (pain in RLQ when there is deep palpation and release in left lower quadrant [LLQ])
- Heel-drop jarring test or pain in RLQ when striking heels
- Difficulty moving onto examination table or walking around

### Laboratory/Diagnostic Testing

The diagnosis of appendicitis is based upon the clinical findings and can be confirmed with laboratory or diagnostic testing. WBC and neutrophil counts can be increased during acute appendicitis. C-reactive protein levels may also be evaluated in appendicitis. Ultrasound should be utilized first to visualize the appendix and may identify enlargement and thickening of the appendix wall. Abscess formation or free fluid may also be identified. If the ultrasound is inconclusive and there is high suspicion, a CT scan can be used to evaluate the appendix. A urine pregnancy test is usually needed before a CT scan or surgery and will rule out pregnancy or ectopic pregnancy and, possibly, the source of pain.

### Differential Diagnosis

The differential diagnosis for appendicitis includes:

- Bowel obstruction
- Intestinal malrotation

- Intussusception
- Ovarian torsion
- Ectopic pregnancy
- Testicular torsion
- Diabetic ketoacidosis
- Peritonitis
- Hemolytic uremic syndrome
- Nephrolithiasis
- PID
- Ovarian cyst
- Gastroenteritis
- UTI
- Constipation

### Treatment/Management Plan

Laboratory and diagnostic testing along with the physical examination findings can direct further management. There are multiple scoring systems that can be used to diagnosis appendicitis. One of them is the Pediatric Appendicitis Score (PAS), which is highly specific when multiple parameters are met (Rentea et al., 2017). Children receive 2 points if there is migration of pain or tenderness in the RLQ with coughing, hopping, or percussion. Children receive 1 point if there is anorexia, nausea or vomiting, tenderness on palpitation, fever (over 100.4 °F), leukocytosis (>10,000/µL), or left shift on WBC count. These points are added together and if the score is equal to 3 or less than 3, there is low risk for appendicitis. These children can be monitored at home and are instructed to return if there are new or worsening symptoms. PAS scores from 4 to 7 are considered indeterminate. The child should receive serial examination and surgical consult and imaging may be warranted. PAS scores of 7 or higher are highly suspicious of appendicitis and warrant emergent referral for a surgical consult and further imaging.

Surgical intervention may be needed for acute appendicitis, along with antibiotic administration and pain control.

### Family Education

Teach the following:

- Education is focused on signs of appendicitis and when to seek emergent care.
- Reinforcement of postoperative teaching (activity restriction, pain mediation administration, advancing diet) may be needed.

### Referral

If appendicitis is suspected or diagnosed, emergent referral to a pediatric emergency department or pediatric surgeon is warranted.

## FOREIGN BODY INGESTION

Foreign body ingestions are common in children between 6 months old and 3 years old and result in 100,000 cases per year. Most ingestions are benign and transient, with 80% to 93% of objects passing through the stomach without issue, negating the need for intervention (Brown et al., 2019). Furthermore, most cases are only caught due to a witnessed ingestion by a parent or caregiver. Common items ingested include organic items such as rocks, small toys, screws, magnets, coins, and batteries. Urgent intervention is needed when there are signs of obstruction, intestinal perforation, or ingestion of a dangerous object (magnets, batteries, sharp objects such as needles or broken glass).

### Subjective Findings

The health history may reveal:

- Witnessed or reported ingestion of foreign body
- Difficulty breathing or stridor
- Difficulty swallowing or refusing foods and liquids
- Vomiting
- Constipation

### Risk Factors

The most common risk factors for foreign body ingestion are:

- Young age, due to oral exploration
- Unsupervised playtime, especially with other siblings
- Developmental or sensory delay
- Having a small esophagus

### Review of Systems

The most common manifestations revealed during the review of systems include:

- **Constitutional:** anorexia, refusing fluid, chest pain (when at esophageal level)
- **Respiratory:** trouble breathing, cyanosis, wheezing (when at esophageal level)
- **Gastrointestinal:** dependent on level of foreign body:

- Esophageal
  - Dysphagia
  - Drooling
- Stomach
  - Vomiting (if obstructive)
  - Gastric distention
- Intestinal
  - Bilious vomiting
  - Constipation
  - Abdominal pain (if perforation or peritonitis)

### Objective Findings

The physical examination of the child with foreign body ingestion is usually unremarkable but may reveal:

- Stridor or wheezing if located in the esophagus
- Abdominal tenderness or distention if obstruction or perforation

### Laboratory/Diagnostic Testing

In witnessed or suspected foreign body ingestions, plain radiograph is warranted, as the most concerning objects are usually radiopaque. Single views can be utilized if the location is known, or multiple views can be obtained to see the entire digestive tract. Views should include chest anterior-posterior (AP), lateral neck, and KUB. If the object is not identified or more definite imaging is needed, CT or magnetic resonance imaging (MRI) can be used. Additionally, an upper GI study with oral contrast can be used to identify location or radiolucent foreign bodies.

### Differential Diagnosis

The differential diagnosis for foreign body ingestion includes:

- Tracheal foreign body

### Treatment/Management Plan

As discussed, most ingested foreign bodies will pass harmlessly without intervention. Objects requiring emergent removal include button batteries, due to risk of ulceration or leakage of contents and subsequent perforation; and magnets, due to the risk of connecting between mucosa resulting in necrosis. Any object will also have to be removed if there are signs of airway compromise, obstruction, or symptoms of intestinal inflammation (fever, pain). Additionally, sharp (such as needles) and long (>5 cm) objects in the esophagus or stomach warrant removal. Emergent endoscopy is needed and requires a referral to either a pediatric gastroenterologist or surgeon.

### Family Education

Teach the following:

- Prevention (removal of small objects and toys from play areas, continuous supervision).
- Families can monitor stools for passage of item.
- Counsel on signs of obstruction or perforation and the need for immediate care.

### Referral

Referral to a pediatric gastroenterologist or surgeon may be required for removal of the ingested foreign body.

## HELMINTHIC AND PARASITIC INFECTIONS

Three groups of nematodes (roundworms), trematodes (flukes), and cestodes (tapeworms)---which are both types of flatworms---comprise parasitic helminths. All three types of helminths, which include pinworms (*Enterobius vermicularis*), hookworms (*Ancylostoma duodenale* and *Necator americanus*), and ascariases (*Ascaris lumbricoides*), infect the GI tract. Infection occurs most commonly by larvae traveling through the skin or by ingestion of eggs or larvae, often through raw or undercooked meat, and some cause infection through fecal-oral transmission. Symptoms are often caused by irritation and inflammation at the site of larvae or eggs (Kronman et al., 2019).

Two other parasitic infections to note are *Giardia lamblia*, a flagellated protozoan, and *Entamoeba histolytica*, an amoeba. *Giardia* is transmitted in its cyst state from contaminated water or stool and causes symptoms in its motile phase as a trophozoite; the cysts are ingested and once exposed to acid in the stomach, excystation follows and the trophozoites are released, becoming stuck to duodenal and jejunal enterocytes. *Entamoeba histolytica* is similarly transmitted in its cyst form via contaminated food or water or sexual contact, and *E. histolytica* also causes symptoms in its trophozoite form. Excystation occurs in the small intestine and adherence to the large intestine can cause invasive colitis (Herman & Surawicz, 2016).

### Subjective Findings

The health history may reveal:

- Abdominal pain, bloating, distention, anorexia, indigestion (hookworm), nausea, flatulence, diarrhea (Herman & Surawicz, 2016; Kronman et al., 2019)
- Pruritus ani or nocturnal anal itching (pinworms)

### Risk Factors

The most common risk factors for helminthic and parasitic infections are:

- Immunocompromised state
- Areas of contaminated water sources
- Raw or undercooked meats

### Review of Systems

The most common manifestations revealed during the review of systems include:

- **Constitutional:** fever (visceral larva migrans [VLM], schistosomiasis), fatigue, weight loss, pica (VLM), difficulty sleeping (pinworms), malaise (schistosomiasis)
- **Integumentary:** rash (schistosomiasis)
- **HEENT:** decreased vision (VLM), cough, seizures, pica (VLM)
- **Respiratory:** cough (echinococcosis, schistosomiasis), hemoptysis (echinococcosis), dyspnea (echinococcosis)
- **Gastrointestinal:** nausea, vomiting, and/diarrhea; pain
- **Neurologic:** seizures (neurocysticercosis)

### Objective Findings

The physical examination of the child with helminthic and parasitic infections may reveal unremarkable findings, although it may include:

- Abdominal tenderness or distention
- Hepatomegaly
- Lymphadenopathy
- Granulomatous lesions on eye examination near disc or macula (VLM)

### Laboratory/Diagnostic Testing

The diagnosis of helminthic and parasitic infections is based upon the clinical findings. Many of the helminths will leave visible eggs in the stool, specifically the nematodes (hookworms and ascariasis), and pinworm eggs are commonly seen near the anus in the morning (Kronman et al., 2019). No laboratory or diagnostic testing is needed unless disease is more severe or disseminated. For *Giardia* and *E. histolytica*, a stool antigen test or stool microscopy may be obtained; in addition, serology may be obtained for *E. histolytica* (Herman & Surawicz, 2016).

### Differential Diagnosis

The differential diagnosis for helminthic and parasitic infections includes:

- Other infectious (bacterial, viral) diarrhea
- Traveler's diarrhea
- Toxic megacolon
- IBD

### Treatment/Management Plan

Pharmacologic therapy is dependent on the type of helminth, although sanitary measures are recommended in all cases. For nematodes, an antihelminthic (e.g., albendazole, mebendazole, or thiabendazole) or an antiparasitic (e.g., ivermectin or pyrantel pamoate) is recommended for therapy. For parasitic trematodes or cestodes, praziquantel is often recommended. Other considerations include deworming household pets to minimize spread and ensuring that foods are fully cooked prior to eating (Kronman et al., 2019).

Treatment for *Giardia* includes nitroimidazoles, as well as antiparasitics such as albendazole and nitazoxanide. Therapy for *E. histolytica* is dependent on the severity of the disease: invasive disease evidenced by liver abscesses or invasive colitis is treated with nitroimidazoles, and asymptomatic individuals who are found to be carriers are treated with iodoquinol, a luminal amebicide, or the antiparasitic paromomycin (Herman & Surawicz, 2016).

### Family Education

Teach the following:

- Maintain good hand hygiene.
- Ensure that meat is fully cooked before consumption.
- If planning for foreign travel, ensure prior review of possible prevalent infectious etiologies, including parasites.

## ANAL FISSURE

An *anal fissure* is a tear in the lining of the anal canal below the mucocutaneous junction. The usual form is due to trauma. In the pediatric population, this is usually due to passage of large hard stool that tears the mucosal lining. Due to pain with defecation, a child may hold stool, leading to worsening constipation; therefore, there is continued damage to the anal mucosa and continued pain (Shanti, 2020). It becomes a vicious cycle.

### Subjective Findings

The health history may reveal:

- Pain with defecation
- Blood-streaked stool
- Constipation

### Risk Factors

The most common risk factor for anal fissure is constipation. Fissures can also develop at the initiation of solid food, starting of school, or with potty training.

### Review of Systems

The most common manifestations revealed during the review of systems include:

- **Constitutional:** rectal pain
- **Gastrointestinal:** retention of stool, anal skin tag due to repetitive healing and tearing

### Objective Findings

The physical examination of the child with anal fissure may reveal:

- Direct visualization will show tear in skin-anus junction.
- Posterior or anterior midline tear.
- Multiple anal tears should be concerning for sexual abuse. Refer to authorities for further investigation according to local regulations.

### Laboratory/Diagnostic Testing

The diagnosis of anal fissure is based upon the clinical findings. No laboratory or diagnostic testing is needed. Rectal examination is not needed.

### Differential Diagnosis

The differential diagnosis for anal fissure includes:

- Anal fistula
- Anal anomalies
- Crohn's disease

### Treatment/Management Plan

Treating constipation is key to allowing for proper healing of the fissure. Conservative measures include increasing water intake and adding fiber to diet. St[illegible]ing a bowel regimen with a stool softener rather th[illegible] a stimulant is preferred. The stimulant will promot[illegible] passage of hard stool, leading to more pain. Enemas should be avoided. Petroleum jelly can be used to protect the skin. Keeping the area clean and dry is also important for healing. Topical agents such as lidocaine and nitroglycerin can be used in older children.

Surgery is very rarely done for children. A sphincterotomy would be performed to lower high anal resting pressure. It runs the risk of causing permanent sphincter damage; therefore, surgery would only be done for children who fail medical management and about whom there is concern for high anal resting pressure.

### Family Education

Teach the following:

- Treat constipation with higher fiber diet, increase water intake.
- It is all right to use a stool softener such as oral polyethylene glycol (PEG), but avoid stimulants.
- Acetaminophen or ibuprofen for pain control
- Place the child in warm sitz baths for cleaning and healing.

### Referral

Refer to a pediatric gastroenterologist if there is a concern for IBD in older children.

# CHRONIC DISORDERS

## CONSTIPATION/ENCOPRESIS

Frequency of bowel movements will vary with age. Newborn infants may have four to eight bowel movements per day. This will change as they grow and formula/milk is introduced into their diet. By toddler years, GI transit time has increased and on average a toddler may have one bowel movement per day. Constipation is defined by a delay or difficulty in passing stool. Children may hold their stool, which leads to continued hardening of the stool. Softer stool may seep around the hard stool, leading to encopresis, or fecal incontinence.

In evaluating a child with constipation, the practitioner needs to distinguish between functional and organic causes of constipation. Functional constipation is the most common type of constipation and is based on criteria that evaluate stool frequency, hardness, and size (Sood, 2021). Organic constipation is

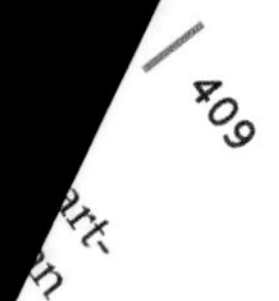



, associated with other disorders: ...sease, spinal cord injury, neuromus- ...rs, metabolic disorders, or cystic fibrosis.

## ...jective Findings

...he health history may reveal:

- *Newborn*: delayed passing of meconium; this can indicate underlying structural issues
- *Infants/Toddlers/Children*: onset of constipation, quality of appearance of stool, frequency of stools, urinary incontinence
- Poor weight gain
- Pebble-like stool, ribbon-like stool
- Encopresis—leakage of liquid stool (around hard stool mass), usually into the underpants

## Risk Factors

For functional constipation, dietary factors such as low fiber and low fluid intake may contribute to constipation. Additionally, some young children struggle with defecating in a public bathroom, so day care and school attendance place them at further risk. The most common risk factors for organic constipation are lead poisoning, developmental delay, and associated disorders that may increase risk (i.e., hypothyroidism, celiac disease, neuromuscular disorders).

## Review of Systems

The most common manifestations revealed during the review of systems include:

- **Constitutional:** poor oral intake, abdominal pain
- **Gastrointestinal:** painful defecation, nausea, vomiting, rectal bleeding
- **Neurologic:** fussiness, irritability

## Objective Findings

When a child is constipated, also evaluate the sensory and motor function. The physical examination of the child with constipation may reveal:

- Distended abdomen
- Palpable stool mass
- Anal fissure
- Perianal examination: anteriorly displaced anus

A digital rectal examination is not required and should be reserved for cases where there is concern for fecal impaction. If a rectal examination is performed, a sample should be sent for occult blood.

## Laboratory/Diagnostic Testing

The diagnosis of constipation is based on at least two of the following symptoms being present for at least 1 month:

- Two or fewer defecations per week
- History of excessive stool retention
- History of painful or hard bowel movements
- History of large-diameter stools
- Presence of a large fecal mass in the rectum (Maqbool & Liacouras, 2020)

## Differential Diagnosis

The differential diagnosis for constipation includes:

- Hirschsprung disease
- Celiac disease
- Spinal dysraphism
- Lactulose intolerance
- Anal fissure

## Treatment/Management Plan

Treatment will vary based on age. However, in general, treatment for functional constipation begins with diet modifications. Introduce additional fiber into the child's diet and increase their fluid intake.

### Younger Than 4 Months

- 1–2 oz. of diluted prune juice daily

### Older Than 4 Months

- 3–4 oz. of 100% fruit juice daily
- Lactulose 1 mg/kg daily
- Glycerin suppository if persistent constipation despite a stool softener

### Toddlers/Children

Either an oral stool softener or laxative can be started. Oral medications are preferred over rectal medications, as administration will be less traumatic for the child. PEG is an odorless, tasteless powder that may be added to water or juice and administered daily to keep the stool soft enough for easier passage. If a fecal impaction is present, disimpaction is needed before a maintenance bowel regimen is initiated. For organic constipation, the underlying disease process must be addressed.

### Family Education

Teach the following:

- Children may develop fecal incontinence due to chronic constipation. This is not a behavioral issue and a child should not be reprimanded.
- Toilet teaching may have to be postponed until the constipation is resolved.
- Children who had already achieved stool continence may benefit from a bowel behavior program.
  - Have the child sit on the toilet for 15 minutes twice a day (the best times for stool evacuation success are after a meal—such as after breakfast and after dinner)
  - A younger child may be incentivized by a sticker chart for completing the required amount of toilet sitting (whether or not a bowel movement is passed)
- It may take months to fully retrain the bowel and the child. Be patient and stay with the plan.
- PEG preparation: Mix 17 gm (marked on inside of cap) with 8 ounces of water or diluted fruit juice. Store the unused portion in the refrigerator. Give your child the following amount of prepared PEG daily:
  - 20 lb.—3 ounces
  - 30 lb.—4 ounces
  - 40 lb.—5 ounces
  - 50 lb.—6 ounces
  - 60 lb.—8 ounces
  - 70 lb.+—8–16 ounces

### Referral

Alarming symptoms such as delayed passage of meconium, fever, vomiting, diarrhea, rectal bleeding, or abdominal distention should prompt the provider to refer to a pediatric gastroenterologist for further evaluation.

## GASTROESOPHAGEAL REFLUX DISEASE

GER is the passage of gastric contents from the stomach into the esophagus. This is a normal physiologic process that occurs several times per day. It becomes problematic, however, when children start having symptoms or mucosal changes. This is when it is considered GER disease (GERD). The reflux of gastric content is due to the lower esophageal sphincter (LES) pressure being lower than gastric pressure.

About 1.8% to 8.2% of children have GER symptoms (Winter, 2020). Higher rates are seen in children with prematurity, developmental delays, neuromuscular disorders, obesity, or pulmonary disease. Some long-term complications include respiratory disease, Barrett esophagus, or esophageal strictures. In general, infants who suffer from GERD have a decrease in their symptoms within the first year of life.

### Subjective Findings

The health history may reveal:

- *Infants:* regurgitation, poor weight gain, irritability, failure to thrive
- *Toddlers:* regurgitation, decreased food intake
- *School-age children*: heartburn, regurgitation, dysphagia

### Risk Factors

The most common risk factors for GERD are:

- Prematurity
- Developmental delays
- Neuromuscular disorders
- Obesity
- Pulmonary disease

### Review of Systems

The most common manifestations revealed during the review of systems include:

- **Constitutional:** poor growth, chronic epigastric pain, chest pain
- **HEENT:** bad breath, hoarseness, gagging
- **Respiratory:** cough, wheeze, recurrent infection
- **Gastrointestinal:** nausea, vomiting, dysphagia

### Objective Findings

The physical examination of the child with GERD may reveal:

- Soft abdomen

### Laboratory/Diagnostic Testing

The diagnosis of GERD is based upon the clinical findings. No laboratory or diagnostic testing is needed. However, some children with chronic constipation may present with GERD symptoms. A rectal examination may be done evaluating for hard stool.

### Differential Diagnosis

The differential diagnosis for GERD includes:

- Esophagitis
- Peptic ulcer disease (PUD)

- Pneumonia
- Esophageal stricture
- Gastroparesis
- Rumination syndrome

### Treatment/Management Plan

Nonmedical management should be tried before any medications are initiated. This includes diet and lifestyle modifications. In infants, maintaining the baby upright after feeding or using a slower-flowing nipple may be helpful. In older children and adolescents, weight loss and cessation of smoking/alcohol can help with symptoms. Avoidance of spicy foods, chocolate, or caffeine may be tried. Finally, keeping the head of bed elevated and avoiding going to bed after a meal can also be considered.

An H2 receptor antagonist can be started for short-term relief of symptoms. For children whose symptoms persist despite diet and lifestyle modifications or who have severe to moderate symptoms, a proton pump inhibitor is recommended.

### Family Education

Teach the following:

- In infants, regurgitation usually resolves around age 18 months.
- Advise about first-line treatment of lifestyle and diet modification.

### Referral

If a child presents with fever, weight loss, abdominal tenderness, and bilious vomiting, they should have a more thorough workup, because these are not symptoms associated with GERD. Children whose symptoms do not improve with initiation of a proton pump inhibitor should be referred to a pediatric gastroenterologist for possible endoscopic evaluation.

## FUNCTIONAL ABDOMINAL PAIN

Functional abdominal pain (FAP) is included in functional GI disorders (FGID) that are characterized by a set of criteria, Rome IV, from the nonprofit Rome Foundation (https://theromefoundation.org). The Rome Criteria originated in 1988 and have had two iterations since then (Schmulson & Drossman, 2017). These criteria help diagnose FGID using guidelines that are based on symptomatology (Hyams et al., 2016). FAP specifically has now been named FAP-not otherwise specified (FAP-NOS), where functional dyspepsia, abdominal migraine, and irritable bowel syndrome (IBS) criteria are not met (Hyams et al., 2016).

Children with FAP-NOS seem to show alteration of their GI tract physiology, including decreased gastric motility of liquids, decrease in contractions of the gastric antrum, and a rectum that is not hypersensitive (Hyams et al., 2016). There is also a component of psychosocial stress that seems to contribute to chronic abdominal pain (Hyams et al., 2016). Furthermore, according to Schmulson and Drossman, FAP-NOS is also thought to have a component of pain related to central dysregulation that contributes to the disorder, whereby symptoms may originate centrally (2017).

### Subjective Findings

The health history may reveal:

- Nearly daily pain
- Mornings are when the pain is at its worst
- Defecation does not provide relief
- No association with eating (Bishop & Ebach, 2019)

Other important components of the health history should include:

- Characterization of the pain
- Location of the pain
- Frequency and duration
- Home, Education, Activities, Drugs, Sexuality, Suicide (HEADSS) screening for psychosocial concerns
- Family history of IBS or IBD

### Risk Factors

The most common risk factors for FAP are recent stressors, including school or new environments, abuse, bullying, or parental divorce (Bishop & Ebach, 2019; Hyams et al., 2016).

### Review of Systems

The most common manifestations revealed during the review of systems include:

- **Constitutional:** food triggers (dietary history may be helpful), previous therapies for similar pain
- **Gastrointestinal:** changes in stool pattern (Korterink et al., 2015)

Alarming symptoms that should be explored include:

- **Constitutional:** fever, unintentional weight loss, lack of consistent growth or not maintaining on the growth curve

- **Gastrointestinal:** severe vomiting (including bilious, prolonged, or cyclical), GI bleeding, severe diarrhea, RUQ or RLQ pain that is persistent (Fishman et al., 2020)

These symptoms may be indicative of an organic cause and should be explored further, including consideration of further diagnostic testing.

### Objective Findings

The physical examination of the child with FAP may not reveal focal findings. The examination should focus on abnormal findings such as:

- Tenderness that is localized, specifically in the right lower or right upper quadrants
- Hepatosplenomegaly
- Palpation of a mass
- Spinal tenderness
- Tenderness of the costovertebral angle
- Abnormalities of the anorectal area

### Laboratory/Diagnostic Testing

The diagnosis of FAP is based upon the history and symptoms. No laboratory or diagnostic testing is needed. The Rome IV Diagnostic Criteria include the following, which must be met 2 months or more prior to diagnosis and must occur a minimum of four times per month:

- Episodic or continuous abdominal pain that does not occur solely during physiologic events (e.g., eating, menses)
- Insufficient criteria for IBS, functional dyspepsia, or abdominal migraine
- After appropriate evaluation, the abdominal pain cannot be fully explained by another medical condition (Hyams et al., 2016)

Obtain a stool sample to assess for occult blood (Fishman et al., 2020). Blood samples and urinalysis may be sent if there is concern for other or organic causes of abdominal pain (Korterink et al., 2015).

### Differential Diagnosis

The differential diagnosis for FAP includes:

- Constipation
- IBS
- Lactose intolerance
- IBD
- Celiac disease (Bishop & Ebach, 2019)

### Treatment/Management Plan

Amitriptyline or a selective serotonin reuptake inhibitor (SSRI) could be used for more challenging or unrelenting cases (Bishop & Ebach, 2019). Other considerations include use of cognitive-behavioral therapy or hypnotherapy as treatment options (Hyams et al., 2016). In addition, probiotics may be considered if symptoms are persistent (Rutten et al., 2015).

#### Family Education

Teach the following:

- Encourage normal routines and activities.
- Rather than encourage absence from school, ask that short breaks be permitted during the school day to allow for pain alleviation (Bishop & Ebach, 2019).

Other considerations include:

- Encouragement of healthy sleep patterns
- Extracurricular activity participation
- Individualization of the child's therapy (Korterink et al., 2015)

#### Referral

Consider referral to a pediatric mental health professional if there is continued concern for increasing social dysfunction or anxiety (Bishop & Ebach, 2019).

## CYCLIC VOMITING SYNDROME

Cyclic vomiting syndrome is considered a functional vomiting disorder that is defined by acute, recurrent episodes of severe vomiting with nausea with return to baseline health in between episodes (Li, 2018). It can occur in infants to those in middle-age adulthood, although the prevalence peaks in younger children approximately 2 to 7 years of age (Zeevenhooven et al., 2017). Females are more frequently found to have pediatric onset of cyclic vomiting syndrome (Donnet & Redon, 2018).

### Subjective Findings

The health history may reveal:

- Inconsistent or regular intervals of episodes
- Episodes lasting hours to days
- Episodes occurring at consistent time of day, most frequently early morning or late at night (Zeevenhooven et al., 2017)

Additionally,

- Resolution is complete between episodes
- Episodes are stereotypical for each child (Donnet & Redon, 2018)

### Risk Factors

The most common risk factors for cyclic vomiting syndrome are best described as triggers which for some children include sleep deprivation, stress, exercise, and menstruation as well as certain foods (Donnet & Redon, 2018).

### Review of Systems

The most common manifestations revealed during the review of systems may include:

- **Constitutional:** fatigue, loss of appetite, abdominal pain
- **Integumentary:** pallor
- **HEENT:** phono- or photophobia
- **Gastrointestinal:** severe nausea
- **Neurologic:** headache
- **Psychiatric:** changes in mood (Donnet & Redon, 2018)

### Objective Findings

The physical examination of the child with cyclic vomiting syndrome may reveal:

- Signs of dehydration, including dry mucous membranes, decreased skin turgor, or delayed capillary refill

The child should also be examined for:

- Pulmonary involvement by chest auscultation
- Abdominal distention
- Bowel sound activity
- Organomegaly
- Guarding
- Abdominal tenderness (Bishop & Ebach, 2019)

### Laboratory/Diagnostic Testing

The diagnosis of cyclic vomiting syndrome is based upon the history and presentation without need for laboratory testing. The Rome IV Diagnostic Criteria include the following, all four of which must be met (Hyams et al., 2016):

1. Two or more intervals of persistent, extreme nausea and paroxysmal vomiting that last hours to days over a 6-month time frame
2. Stereotypical episodes for each child
3. Weeks to months separate episodes, and child is able to return to baseline between intervals
4. Symptoms are unable to be ascribed to another diagnosis or condition with appropriate medical evaluation

### Differential Diagnosis

The differential diagnosis for cyclic vomiting syndrome includes:

- Acute causes of vomiting, including infectious etiology, congenital or other obstructive lesions, pyloric stenosis, metabolic disorders, or central nervous system disorders such as migraine, increased intracranial pressure, or other intracranial abnormality (Bishop & Ebach, 2019)
- Postural orthostatic tachycardia syndrome (POTS; Li, 2018)
- Cannabinoid hyperemesis syndrome (particularly in adolescents; Hyams et al., 2016)

### Treatment/Management Plan

The focus of treatment in cyclic vomiting syndrome is prevention of and decrease in severity of episodes via prophylaxis. Age range determines choice of pharmacologic therapy. For children less than 5 years of age, cyproheptadine is recommended as first-line preventive therapy. For those 5 years or older, amitriptyline is the drug of choice, with propranolol as second-line prevention (Li, 2018). Stress reduction techniques should also be employed. Considerations for reduction in severity of episodes include oral acid-inhibiting medications to protect the esophageal mucosa, and lorazepam for antiemetic and anxiolytic effects (Zeevenhooven et al., 2017).

### Family Education

Teach the following:

- In addition to pharmacologic therapies, changes in habits of daily living and finding adequate methods. of reducing stress for the individual child are needed
- Contact the healthcare provider if the child is unable to retain fluids.

## IRRITABLE BOWEL SYNDROME

IBS is considered a FGID that is characterized by chronic abdominal pain and bowel habits that are altered without evidence of a different medical condition (Hyams et al., 2016). IBS is considered a disorder of the brain-gut axis in which the pain is processed differently and a hypersensitivity in the viscera exists, combined with inflammation of the gut and dysmotility. Psychosocial factors may contribute to the visceral hypersensitivity. Similar to adult IBS, children with IBS can also have subtypes that are characterized by the predominant stool pattern: IBS with constipation, IBS with diarrhea, IBS with constipation and diarrhea, and unspecified IBS. With the Rome IV Criteria, IBS and its subtypes are on a spectrum with functional constipation and functional diarrhea rather than being separate disorders (Schmulson & Drossman, 2017).

### Subjective Findings

The health history may reveal:

- Bloating
- Distention
- Change in frequency and/or consistency of stools
- Abdominal pain that does not improve with defecation (Schmulson & Drossman, 2017)

#### Risk Factors

A noted risk factor for IBS includes surgery or other traumatic event early in life, as well as demonstration of increased mental health or emotional issues including depression or anxiety.

#### Review of Systems

The most common manifestations revealed during the review of systems include:

- **Psychiatric:** school avoidance, poor coping skills, peer relationship difficulty, imaginary causes of anxiety (Bishop & Ebach, 2019)

Manifestations that may be indicative of an organic or more concerning cause include:

- **Constitutional:** fever, decreased growth rate, unintentional weight loss, nocturnal pain arousing the child from sleep
- **Gastrointestinal:** severe vomiting, particularly if bilious or bloody
- **Endocrine:** impeded puberty

### Objective Findings

Similar to FAP, the physical examination of the child with IBS may not reveal acute findings. Abnormalities found during the examination should be noted, such as:

- Tenderness that is localized, specifically in the right lower or right upper quadrants
- Hepatosplenomegaly
- Palpation of a mass
- Localized fullness
- Costovertebral angle tenderness
- Abnormalities of the perianal area

#### Laboratory/Diagnostic Testing

The diagnosis of IBS is based on symptomatology. Rome IV Diagnostic Criteria include the following, where symptoms must have begun 2 months prior to diagnosis:

- Recurrent abdominal pain averaging at least 4 days each month associated with one or more of the following:
  - Pain is related to defecation
  - Associated with a change in the stool frequency
  - Associated with a change in the stool consistency
- If children have constipation, pain is not resolved even if constipation resolves (sign of functional constipation if pain resolves)
- Symptoms cannot be fully explained by another medical condition after appropriate evaluation (Hyams et al., 2016)

### Differential Diagnosis

The differential diagnosis for IBS includes:

- Functional diarrhea
- Functional constipation
- Infectious etiology
- Celiac disease
- Malabsorption of carbohydrates
- IBD

### Treatment/Management Plan

A multifaceted approach may be helpful in the treatment of IBS. Supplementation with fiber may be helpful in symptom management, and in cases that are more prolonged or severe, use of an SSRI could be considered. Modification of diet, specifically a decrease in the intake of fermentable oligosaccharides, disaccharides, monosaccharides, and polyols (FODMAPs) and addition of probiotics may be helpful. Similar to FAP, addition of mental health and behavioral therapy is recommended, with particular emphasis on skills for coping with symptoms (Hyams et al., 2016).

#### Family Education

Teach the following:

- Modification of diet if recommended.
- Encourage normalcy of daily routines, patterns, and activities (see "Family Education" section under FAP).

#### Referral

As with FAP, referral to a mental health professional should be considered if there is an increase in anxiety or social dysfunction.

## PEPTIC ULCER DISEASE

PUD is less common in children than in adults, but can still cause complications. Different from GERD, PUD is an imbalance of the protective and damaging mechanisms within the upper GI tract. Essentially, it occurs when mucus and bicarbonate secretion from GI mucosa, the protective features, are overwhelmed by the damaging effects of gastric acid and pepsin. This imbalance leads to damage in the lining of the stomach and duodenum. In children, the most likely cause is medications. Another common cause is *H. pylori* infection, although some cases are idiopathic (Blanchard & Czinn, 2020).

### Subjective Findings

In younger children, the mostly likely symptoms are vomiting and/or abdominal pain. Older children are more likely to present with symptoms similar to those of adults, with epigastric pain several hours after eating. Other associated symptoms are hematemesis, bloating, poor appetite, weight loss, anemia, or early satiety. The health history may reveal:

- Corticosteroid, nonsteroidal anti-inflammatory drug (NSAID) use
- *H. pylori* infection
- Physical stress: recent surgery, major infection, shock
- Alcohol use or smoking in adolescents
- Positive family history of PUD or *H. pylori* infection

#### Risk Factors

The most common risk factors for PUD are NSAID use, steroid use, and *H. pylori* infection.

#### Review of Systems

The most common manifestations revealed during the review of systems include:

- **Constitutional:** abdominal pain in the early morning or in between meals, weight loss, poor growth, early satiety, poor appetite, anorexia, fatigue
- **Gastrointestinal:** nausea, vomiting

### Objective Findings

The physical examination of the child with PUD may reveal:

- Epigastric tenderness
- Succussion splash—advancement of disease may lead to gastric outlet obstruction

#### Laboratory/Diagnostic Testing

The diagnosis of PUD is based upon the clinical findings as well as endoscopy. Endoscopy will assist in visualizing an ulcer or bleeding. It will also aid in diagnosing an *H. pylori* infection.

### Differential Diagnosis

The differential diagnosis for PUD includes:

- Zollinger–Ellison syndrome
- Crohn's disease
- Pancreatitis
- Gallbladder disease
- Functional dyspepsia

### Treatment/Management Plan

The key to treating PUD is to treat the underlying cause. For positive *H. pylori* cases, treatment of the infection is necessary. It is recommended that children be treated with a proton-pump inhibitor and two antibiotics: metronidazole plus amoxicillin or amoxicillin plus clarithromycin. For non-*H. pylori* cases, acid suppression with an H2 inhibitor or proton-pump inhibitor should be tried. If the child is on NSAIDs or steroids, they should be stopped. If they cannot be stopped, then an H2 blocker or proton-pump inhibitor should be started. A bleeding ulcer can be treated via endoscopy with epinephrine injections. Surgery is reserved for acute bleeding or perforation.

#### Family Education

Teach the following:

- Avoid close contact with someone who is positive for *H. pylori*.
- Good handwashing is important.
- Avoid contaminated food.
- Stop smoking/alcohol use.
- Diet does not stop disease progression, as previously thought.

#### Referral

Refer to a pediatric gastroenterologist if endoscopy is needed to aid in diagnosis.

## VIRAL HEPATITIS

Viral hepatitis is liver inflammation resulting from infectious hepatitis, A, B, C, D, or E virus, or others such as cytomegalovirus, Epstein–Barr virus, or

**TABLE 26.1 The Hepatitis Viruses**

| Virus | Transmission | Incubation |
|---|---|---|
| Hepatitis A | Oral-fecal, waterborne, poor sanitation | 15–30 days |
| Hepatitis B | Perinatally mother to infant, sexual intercourse, contaminated needles (intravenous drug use, tattoo, acupuncture), blood product transfusion | 50–150 days |
| Hepatitis C | Contaminated needles (intravenous drug use, tattoo, acupuncture), blood product transfusion | 30–60 days |
| Hepatitis D | Perinatally mother to infant, sexual intercourse, contaminated needles (intravenous drug use, tattoo, acupuncture), blood product transfusion | 50–150 days |
| Hepatitis E | Oral-fecal | 15–65 days |

*Source*: Data from Sokol, R. J., Narkewicz, M. R., Mark, J. A., Mack, C. L., Feldman, A. G., & Sundaram, S. S. (2020) Liver & pancreas. In W. W. Hay Jr., M. J. Levin, M. J. Abzug, & M. Bunik (Eds.), *Current diagnosis & treatment: Pediatrics* (25th ed., Chapter 22). McGraw-Hill Education.

adenovirus (Jensen & Balistreri, 2020). Other causes of hepatitis also exist. It may occur as an acute fulminant state or may present as a chronic disease. Children may be asymptomatic or may experience the common clinical manifestations of flu-like symptoms, abdominal pain, anorexia, and eventually jaundice, icteric sclera, and hepatomegaly. Table 26.1 provides incubation periods and transmission routes for hepatitis viruses A–E. It is important to note that hepatitis A and B infection are both vaccine-preventable.

The diagnostic workup includes complete blood count, comprehensive metabolic panel, liver function tests, and viral titers. Due to the complexity of hepatitis, early referral to a pediatric gastroenterologist for evaluation and treatment should occur.

## INFLAMMATORY BOWEL DISEASE

IBD consists of two chronic disorders, Crohn's disease and ulcerative colitis, each of which is defined by their location of involvement: Crohn's disease is located throughout the entire gut, whereas ulcerative colitis only affects the colon. About 25% of individuals with IBD present prior to age 20 (Stein & Baldassano, 2020). The presentation includes concerning signs and symptoms: fever, fatigue, unintentional weight loss, abdominal pain, and blood from the rectum warranting a diagnostic workup. The workup should include a complete blood count, inflammatory markers (C-reactive protein and ESR), and fecal calprotectin. Due to possible severity, chronicity, complications, and therapy needed for children with IBD, early referral to pediatric gastroenterology for evaluation and treatment should occur.

## KEY POINTS

- The majority of parasitic infections are transmitted through ingestion or penetration of the skin.
- Intestinal parasitic infections are treatable, though complications can occur, so a thorough history should be obtained.
- FAP, cyclic vomiting syndrome, and IBS are diagnosed based on the Rome IV Criteria.
- Inclusion of mental health and psychosocial resources should be considered in the treatment of FAP.
- Ensure that there is no evidence of dehydration upon physical examination of the child with cyclic vomiting syndrome.
- Refer children and adolescents with suspected hepatitis or IBD early to a pediatric gastroenterologist.

## REFERENCES

Bishop, W. P., & Ebach, D. R. (2019). Digestive system. In K. J. Marcdante & R. M. Kliegman (Eds.), *Nelson's essentials of pediatrics* (8th ed., Section 17). Elsevier.

Blanchard, S. S., & Czinn, S. J. (2020). Peptic ulcer disease in children. In R. M. Kliegman, J. St. Geme, N. J. Blum, S. S. Shah, R. C. Tasker, K. M. Wilson, & R. E. Behrman (Eds.), *Nelson textbook of pediatrics* (21st ed., Chapter 361). Elsevier.

Brown, J., Kidder, M., Fabbrini, A., deVries, J., Robertson, J., Chandler, N., & Wilsey, M. (2019). Down the rabbit hole—Considerations for ingested foreign bodies. *Pediatric Gastroenterology, Hepatology, and Nutrition, 22*(6), 619–623. https://doi.org/10.5223/pghn.2019.22.6.619

Costanzo, C. M., Vinocur, C., & Berman, L. (2017). Prematurity affects age of presentation of pyloric stenosis. *Clinical Pediatrics, 56*(2), 127–131. https://doi.org/10.1177/0009922816641367

Donnet, A., & Redon, S. (2018). Cyclic vomiting syndrome in children. *Current Pain and Headache Reports, 22*(30). https://doi.org/10.1007/s11916-018-0684-6

Eberly, M. D., Eide, M. B., Thompson, J. L., & Nylund, C. M. (2015). Azithromycin in early infancy and pyloric stenosis. *Pediatrics, 135*(3), 483–488. https://doi.org/10.1542/peds.2014-2026

Fishman, M. B., Aronson, M. D., & Chacko, M. R. (2020). Chronic abdominal pain in children and adolescents:

Approach to the evaluation. *UpToDate*. Retrieved October 11, 2020, from https://www.uptodate.com/contents/chronic-abdominal-pain-in-children-and-adolescents-approach-to-the-evaluation

Haber, P., Parashar, U. D., Haber, M., & DeStefano, F. (2015). Intussusception after monovalent rotavirus vaccine—United States, Vaccine Adverse Event Reporting System (VAERS), 2008–2014. *Vaccine, 33*, 4873–4877. https://doi.org10.1016/j.vaccine.2015.07.054

Helleran, D. R., Minneci, P. C., & Cooper, J. N. (2020). Association between age and umbilical hernia repair outcomes in children: A multistate population-based cohort study. *The Journal of Pediatrics, 217*, 125–130.e4. https://doi.org/10.1016/j.jpeds.2019.10.035

Herman, M. L., & Surawicz, C. M. (2016). Intestinal parasites. In S. Guandalini, A. Dhawan, & D. Branski (Eds.), *Textbook of pediatric gastroenterology, hepatology and nutrition: A comprehensive guide to practice* ( pp. 185–194). Springer International Publishing.

Hyams, J., Di Lorenzo, C., Saps, M., Shulman, R., Staiano, A., & van Tilburg, M. (2016). Childhood functional gastrointestinal disorders: Child/adolescent. *Gastroenterology, 150*(6), 1456–1468.e2. https://doi.org/10.1053/j.gastro.2016.02.015

Jensen, M. K., & Balistreri, W. F. (2020). Viral hepatitis. In R. M. Kliegman, J. St. Geme, N. J. Blum, S. S. Shah, R. C. Tasker, K. M. Wilson, & R. E. Behrman (Eds.), *Nelson textbook of pediatrics* (21st ed., Chapter 385). Elsevier.

Korterink, J., Devanarayana, N. M., Rajindrajith, S., Vlieger, A., & Benninga, M. A. (2015). Childhood functional abdominal pain: Mechanisms and management. *Nature Reviews Gastroenterology & Hepatology, 12*, 159–171. https://doi.org/10.1038/nrgastro.2015.21

Kronman, M. P., Crowell, C. S., & Vora, S. B. (2019). Infectious diseases. In K. J. Marcdante & R. M. Kliegman (Eds.), *Nelson's essentials of pediatrics* (8th ed., Section 16). Elsevier.

Laquerre, J. N. (2020). Intussusception: Sonographic findings to fluoroscopic reduction in pediatrics. *Radiologic Technology, 91*(4), 380–384.

Li, B. (2018). Managing cyclic vomiting syndrome in children: Beyond the guidelines. *European Journal of Pediatrics, 177*, 1435–1442. https://doi.org/10.1007/s00431-018-3218-7

Maqbool, A., & Liacouras, C. A. (2020). Encopresis and functional constipation. In R. M. Kliegman, J. St. Geme, N. J. Blum, S. S. Shah, R. C. Tasker, K. M. Wilson, & R. E. Behrman (Eds.), *Nelson textbook of pediatrics* (21st ed., Chapter 358.3). Elsevier.

Ntoulia, A., Tharakan, S. J., Reid, J. R., & Mahboubi, S. (2016). Failed intussusception reduction in children: Correlation between radiologic, surgical, and pathologic findings. *American Journal of Roentgenology, 207*(2), 424–433. https://doi.org/10.2214/AJR.15.15659

Pathak, M., Saxena, R., Sinha, A., & Singh, V. (2018). Hirschsprung's disease and neonatal intestinal obstruction: Where does it lie in the spectrum? *Journal of Clinical Neonatology, 7*(4), 231–236. https://doi.org/10.4103/jcn.JCN_48_18

Rentea, R. M., St. Peter, S. D., & Snyder, C. L. (2017). Pediatric appendicitis: State of the art review. *Pediatric Surgery International, 33*(3), 269–283. https://doi.org/10.1007/s00383-016-3990-2

Reust, C. E., & Amy, W. (2016). Acute abdominal pain in children. *American Family Physician, 93*(10), 830–837. https://www.aafp.org/afp/2016/0515/p830.html

Rutten, J., Korterink, J., Venmans, L., Benninga, M., & Tabbers, M. (2015). Nonpharmacologic treatment of functional abdominal pain disorders: A systematic review. *Pediatrics, 135*(3), 522–535. https://doi.org/10.1542/peds.2014-2123

Schmulson, M., & Drossman, D. (2017). What is new in Rome IV. *Journal of Neurogastroenterology and Motility, 23*(2), 151–163. https://doi.org/10.5056/jnm16214

Shanti, C. M. (2020). Anal fissure. In R. M. Kliegman, J. St. Geme, N. J. Blum, S. S. Shah, R. C. Tasker, K. M. Wilson, & R. E. Behrman (Eds.), *Nelson textbook of pediatrics* (21st ed., Chapter 371.2). Elsevier.

Sood, M. (2021). Constipation in infants and children: Evaluation. *UpToDate*. https://www.uptodate.com/contents/constipation-in-infants-and-children-evaluation

Stein, R. E., & Baldassano, R. N. (2020). Chapter 362: Inflammatory bowel disease. In R. M. Kliegman, J. St. Geme, N. J. Blum, S. S. Shah, R. C. Tasker, K. M. Wilson, & R. E. Behrman (Eds.), *Nelson textbook of pediatrics* (21st ed.). Elsevier.

Winter, H. S. (2020). Clinical manifestations and diagnosis of gastroesophageal reflux disease in children and adolescents. *UpToDate*. Retrieved July 7, 2020, from https://www.uptodate.com/contents/clinical-manifestations-and-diagnosis-of-gastroesophageal-reflux-disease-in-children-and-adolescents

World Health Organization. (2017). *Diarrhoeal disease*. https://www.who.int/en/news-room/fact-sheets/detail/diarrhoeal-disease

Zeevenhooven, J., Koppen, I., & Benninga, M. (2017). The New Rome IV criteria for functional gastrointestinal disorders in infants and toddlers. *Pediatric Gastroenterology Hepatology Nutrition, 20*(1), 1–13. https://doi.org/10.5223/pghn.2017.20.1.1

## FURTHER READING

Vandenplas, Y. (2017). *Gastroesophageal reflux in children*. Springer Publishing Company. https://doi.org/10.1007/978-3-319-60678-1

# Management of Nutritional Disorders

Janine M. Bamberger, Cynthia S. Nelson, and Maria Fatima G. Westry

## Student Learning Outcomes

**Upon completion of this chapter the reader should be able to:**

1. Discuss pathophysiology and epidemiology of selected nutritional disorders in children.
2. Differentiate subjective and objective findings of selected nutritional disorders in children.
3. Choose appropriate laboratory or diagnostic tests for particular nutritional disorders in children.
4. Utilize the differential diagnosis process to determine the diagnosis of nutritional disorders in children.
5. Determine treatment plan, child/family education, and need for referral for children with a nutritional disorder diagnosis.

The content in this chapter maps to the following areas on the Pediatric Nursing Certification Board (PNCB) Pediatric Nurse Practitioner—Primary Care certification examination: Clinical Problems: Nutrition

### CONTENT AREAS:

### II. Assessment and Diagnosis

**A. History and Physical Examination**

1. Obtain history of present illness
2. Obtain a comprehensive health history for new patients
3. Complete an interval history for established patients
4. Perform a review of systems
5. Perform a complete physical examination

**B. Diagnostic Testing and Screening**

1. Order and interpret office/clinic based screening tests
2. Order and interpret diagnostic laboratory tests
3. Order and interpret the results of diagnostic imaging tests

**C. Analyzing Information**

1. Integrate health history and physical examination findings into the plan of care
2. Assimilate findings from screening and diagnostic testing into plan of care

**D. Diagnosis**

1. Develop and prioritize differential diagnoses
2. Establish a diagnosis based on evaluation of patient data

## INTRODUCTION

Adequate and appropriate nutrition is required by infants, children, and adolescents to support normal growth and development. Extremely rapid growth occurs during infancy, and the highest-risk period for impaired linear growth is between 4 and 24 months of age (Maqbool et al., 2020). Childhood nutritional disorders include lactose intolerance, food allergy, celiac disease, malnutrition/undernutrition, metabolic syndrome, and obesity. The goal for childhood nutrition is to promote adequacy of the diet, prevent deficiencies, and reduce the risk of developing diseases associated with excess intake. Identifying nutritional alterations and appropriately treating them in infancy and childhood are essential not only for supporting normal growth and development but also as the foundation for lifelong health.

## III. Management

**A. Child and Caregiver Counseling and Education**

1. Provide condition-specific counseling and education, including treatment options
2. Educate about benefits and potential adverse reactions of pharmacological interventions
3. Discuss non-pharmacological interventions
4. Counsel regarding the threshold for seeking follow-up care
5. Review the risks of non-adherence to recommended treatment

**B. Therapeutic Interventions**

1. Prescribe pharmacologic agents
2. Recommend the use of over-the-counter pharmacologic agents
3. Order or recommend non-pharmacologic treatments for the management of symptoms
4. Discuss use of complementary and alternative therapies as appropriate

**C. Procedures**

1. Perform procedures in accordance with diagnostic guidelines and plan of care (rapid tests)
2. Initiate life-saving techniques in response to urgent or emergent situations

**D. Collaboration and Referral**

2. Refer to specialists as indicated for evaluation, counseling, and/or treatment

**E. Care Coordination**

1. Facilitate patient and family-centered care for children of all ages with acute and chronic conditions

**F. Evaluation and Follow-up**

2. Establish a plan for follow-up care

## IV. Professional Role Responsibilities

**A. Leadership and Evidence-based Practice**

4. Develop, implement, and/or modify clinical practice guidelines

# ANATOMY AND PHYSIOLOGY

While it may seem that children are just small versions of adults, that is not exactly the case. Adolescent anatomy and physiology are similar to those of adults, but on the other end of the spectrum, infants and young children are rather different from grown-ups. The smaller the child, the faster the metabolism and therefore, the more calories needed per kilogram. The smaller the child, the more difficult it is for the individual to consume the same foods and beverages ingested by adults. Infants and small children do not yet have the teeth or physical abilities required to safely chew and swallow large food pieces or fibrous or hard foods. A child's stomach capacity and kidney size are smaller than those of an adult. In the typical adult, gastric emptying is biphasic, with the first phase taking only 10 to 20 minutes and the second phase being quite a bit slower. For preterm infants, gastric emptying is slow and typically linear. The gastric emptying reaches adult values around the age of 6 to 8 months of life. The liver at birth is about 5% of the birth weight but only about 2% of the weight of the adult. Kidney blood flow typically reaches that of adults by age 2 (Fernandez et al., 2011). The proportion of body fat and water are greater in the child as well.

Nutrient requirements to support growth and development also vary with age and body size. Compared with adults, infants require more protein on a per-kilogram basis, because growth (anabolism) requires more protein than does maintenance. Developmentally, a child or adolescent may not be a good historian, so understanding the sequence of events around a potential condition may be difficult. Thus, when considering how to support infants, children, and adolescents who are faced with nutritional disorders, the ability to meet growth needs as they relate to anatomy, and possibly physiology, is critical (Milla, 2002; World Health Organization [WHO], 2019).

# GENERAL APPROACH TO CHILD WITH A NUTRITIONAL DISORDER

Children are different from adults in that they are expected to spend all of childhood and adolescence growing and maturing. It is critical, therefore, that children with nutritional disorders are supported by family, caregivers, and the healthcare team in a manner that allows them access to all nutrients required for growth. Such nutrients have to be provided in amount, form, and frequency appropriate to the medical condition, layered on top of developmental and chronological age and size and ability, so that growth and development are continually maximized. Because this entire period is one of constant change, reassessment of needs and review of the feeding plan are ongoing and must occur both routinely and as new concerns arise. In addition to the primary care providers, children with nutritional disorders may also benefit from working with a dietitian, gastroenterologist, psychologist, occupational therapist, physical therapist, speech pathologist, social worker, or others.

## Subjective Findings

The health history may reveal:

- Swallowing difficulties
- Chewing difficulties
- Poor appetite
- Fatigue
- Weakness
- Abdominal discomfort/pain
- Inability to concentrate

## Risk Factors

The most common risk factors for nutritional disorders are:

- Inadequate nutrient intake
- Chronic illness

## Review of Systems

The most common manifestations revealed during the review of systems include:

- **Constitutional:** weight loss or gain, fatigue, anorexia, change in appetite/thirst
- **Integumentary:** rash, dryness, slow wound healing, itching, hives, abnormal color, hair and nail changes
- **HEENT:** poor head growth (infant); eye color changes or spots; nasal stuffiness/discharge/itching; abnormalities of mouth, lips, tongue, gums, teeth, throat, taste; neck swelling
- **Respiratory:** coughing, wheezing
- **Cardiovascular:** blood pressure (BP) changes
- **Gastrointestinal:** nausea, vomiting, flatulence, diarrhea, constipation
- **Genitourinary:** frequent urination
- **Musculoskeletal:** weakness, cramps, twitching, tingling, pain or tenderness
- **Neurologic/Behavioral:** weakness, numbness, memory/concentration/cognitive impairment, disorientation, behavioral disturbances
- **Hematologic:** bruising, bleeding (Leonberg, 2020; Mordarski & Wolff 2018; Phillips et al., 2017)

## Objective Findings

Nutritional disorders can occur in relation to every system in the body. Objective findings relate to the system affected and specific nutrient deficiency or excess, as well as timing during physical development, and duration. The physical examination of the child with a nutritional disorder may reveal:

- Weight loss or gain
- Poor or excessive growth (weight, length/height, occipital frontal circumference [under age 2 to 3 years], mid upper arm circumference, skinfold thickness)
- Thyroid enlargement
- Muscle wasting
- Bone deformities (Litchford, 2020; Pediatric Nutrition Practice Group of the Academy of Nutrition and Dietetics [PNPGAND], 2020)

## Laboratory/Diagnostic Testing

When a nutritional disorder is suspected, the following laboratory tests may be considered:

- Clinical chemistry panels (basic and comprehensive metabolic panel)
- Complete blood count (CBC) with differential
- Stool testing for parasites, infections, occult blood
- Urinalysis
- Inflammatory markers—positive (C-reactive protein, ferritin) and negative (albumin, transthyretin, retinol-binding protein, transferrin) acute phase reactants
- Tests for anemias (hematocrit/hemoglobin, serum ferritin and iron, total iron-binding capacity, folate, Vitamin B12)
- Markers of body composition (creatinine, nitrogen balance)
- Lipid indices for cardiovascular risk
- Hemoglobin $A_1C$
- Vitamins and trace minerals (Litchford, 2020; PNPGAND, 2020)

Nutritional disorders may occur in, or affect, every area of the gastrointestinal (GI) tract. Nutrition excesses and deficiencies can also affect every system outside of the GI tract. The following sections address six specific nutrition disorders: lactose intolerance, celiac disease, food allergy, pediatric malnutrition/undernutrition, metabolic syndrome, and obesity. Each is complex in its own way, and each may exist alone or along with another nutrition or non-nutrition disorder.

# LACTOSE INTOLERANCE

*Lactose intolerance* is a term that is used to describe a group of symptoms that result when an individual is unable to digest or absorb the disaccharide lactose effectively. Although neonates typically possess the enzyme needed to digest lactose (lactase), the carbohydrate in breast milk, most adults (except those primarily of European descent) have limited intestinal activity of lactase. Lactose intolerance is, in fact, the most common adverse food reaction. The condition is known by other names, such as milk sugar intolerance and dairy product intolerance, and is associated with lactose malabsorption, lactase maldigestion, alactasia, hypolactasia, and lactose nonpersistence (Fassio et al., 2018; Genetics Home Reference, 2010; Litchford, 2020). The definition of lactose intolerance is a clinical syndrome characterized by abdominal distention and pain, flatulence, and diarrhea occurring after consumption of lactose (Bass III, 2017; Fassio et al., 2018). It is an inability to digest and absorb lactose (Fassio et al., 2018; Heyman & the Committee on Nutrition [CON], 2006; Silberman & Jin, 2019).

Lactose intolerance occurs in 65% to 75% of individuals worldwide. In the United States, 6% to 22% of Whites are lactose intolerant, while the rate for American Indians/Alaskan Natives is 80% to 100%. Persons of Asian, African, and Hispanic descent display a significantly increased incidence of lactose intolerance as compared with whites (Fassio et al., 2018; Harvey et al., 2018; Heyman & CON, 2006; Kleinman & Greer, 2020; Mahan & Swift, 2020). Lactose intolerance results from deficiency of the lactase enzyme that is required to break lactose down into glucose and galactose. GI symptoms occur when lactose is consumed in amounts greater than the body can absorb. Unabsorbed lactose pulls water into the stool, causing the stool to be looser than normal and more watery. The unabsorbed sugar (lactose) can function as a substrate for fermentation by intestinal (colonic) bacteria, yielding short-chain fatty acids, carbon dioxide, and hydrogen (VanReken et al., 2020).

Primary lactase deficiency is due to nonpersistence of lactase starting at 2 to 5 years of age depending on ethnicity. Secondary lactase deficiency (hypolactasia) is due to loss of the lactase enzyme as a result of clinical conditions in the GI tract, such as acute gastroenteritis, infectious diarrhea, cancer chemotherapy, and celiac disease. It may occur at any age, but is more common in infancy. *Developmental lactase deficiency* refers to a relative lactase deficiency in preterm infants less than 34 weeks' gestation. Congenital lactase deficiency (alactasia) is inherited and extremely rare. Comorbidities associated with lactose intolerance include weight loss, eating disorder, anxiety, and depression.

## Subjective Findings

The health history may reveal:

- Abdominal discomfort after eating
- Abdominal discomfort after consuming milk-containing products, although less pronounced discomfort after consuming cultured dairy products such as hard or soft cheese (Parmesan or cottage cheese, for example), yogurt, buttermilk, kefir, or acidophilus (e.g., LACTAID®) milk
- Gas, loose stools, or diarrhea after eating
- Borborygmi (rumbling or gurgling noise made by gas or fluid movement in the intestines)
- Nausea or vomiting after eating (Hertzler et al., 2014)

### Risk Factors

The most common risk factors for lactose intolerance are:

- Increasing age, particularly after age 3 to 5 years
- Ethnicity based on lactase nonpersistence, from most to least intolerant: Asian, Native American, Black American, African American, Ashkenazi Jews, Hispanics, and from Indian subcontinent
- Enteritis (bacterial or viral, radiation, chemotherapy)
- Parasitic disease
- Celiac disease
- Inflammatory bowel syndrome (IBS; ulcerative colitis, Crohn's disease)
- Severe malnutrition
- Short bowel syndrome; postsurgical conditions
- Medications (Hertzler et al., 2014; VanReken et al., 2020)

### Review of Systems

The most common manifestations revealed during the review of systems include:

- **Gastrointestinal:** nausea, vomiting, constipation, abdominal pain, excessive flatus
- **Musculoskeletal:** joint and/or muscle pain
- **Neurologic:** headache, difficulties concentrating, tiredness (Fassio et al., 2018)

## Objective Findings

The physical examination of the child with lactose intolerance may reveal

- Abdominal fullness or bloating
- Hyperactive bowel sounds
- Diarrhea
- Flatulence (Fassio et al., 2018; Hertzler et al., 2014)

### Laboratory/Diagnostic Testing

The diagnosis of lactose intolerance is based upon the clinical findings and results of laboratory and diagnostic testing:

- The primary method for determining lactose intolerance is through an exclusion-diet. All sources of lactose should be eliminated, and a strict 2-week trial should be done. If resolution of symptoms occurs and subsequent reintroduction of dairy causes return of symptoms, then a diagnosis can be made (Heyman & CON, 2006).
- Lactose tolerance test: blood glucose level does not increase.
- Hydrogen breath test (HBT): hydrogen gas increases after lactose intake. This is the least invasive of tests, is good for those with more subtle cases, and has been shown to be more reliable than clinical history taking.
- Fecal pH: acidic.
- Stool for reducing substances: increased.
- Genetic testing: 13910C>T lactase nonpersistence gene polymorphism (Fassio et al., 2018; Hertzler et al., 2014; Rojo et al., 2018).

### Differential Diagnosis

Prior to making a definitive diagnosis of lactose intolerance, invite the child and family to document symptoms as part of a detailed food diary (3–7 days or more). The differential diagnosis for lactose intolerance includes:

- Sucrase deficiency.
- Diabetic diarrhea.
- Disorders associated with secondary lactose intolerance (acquired, or secondary lactase deficiency or hypolactasia), which are a result of small bowel injury. This is possible in disorders such as gastroenteritis, giardiasis, inflammatory bowel disease, irritable bowel syndrome, celiac disease, and severe malnutrition.
- Food poisoning (Fassio et al., 2018; Roy & Cagir, 2019).

### Treatment/Management Plan

Standard treatments include reduction or elimination of lactose-containing foods and beverages, use of lactase enzyme (e.g., LACTAID®), and use of lactose-free formula (beverage; Fassio et al., 2018; Hertzler et al., 2014; VanReken et al., 2020). Follow up within 1 month to confirm that symptoms have subsided or been eliminated with expected dietary changes. Potential treatments (still being researched) include lactose challenge with increasing amounts of lactose/colonic adaptation, introduction of probiotics to modulate the intestinal microbiota and thus improve tolerance to small amounts of lactose (currently under review), and gene therapy (Fassio et al., 2018; Hertzler et al., 2014; Silberman & Jin, 2019).

### Family Education

Teach the following, particularly to those who grocery shop and prepare food:

- Symptoms of lactose intolerance.
- Sources of dietary lactose.
- The plan for reducing or eliminating lactose-containing foods and beverages.
- Substitutions for lactose.
- Names of lactase enzyme tablets, liquids, and milk products pretreated with lactase enzyme, as well as purchase locations.

**PRO TIP** Once a diagnosis of lactose intolerance is confirmed, be clear with the child/parent(s)/caregivers that the diagnosis is an intolerance rather than an allergy; the two are often confused, but allergy requires a higher level of safety precautions.

### Referral

For additional care and education, refer the child with lactose intolerance to a registered dietitian nutritionist and/or pediatric gastroenterologist.

## FOOD ALLERGY

Food allergy is a very broad topic that is included under the even broader subject heading of adverse reactions to food. Adverse reactions to food are divided into toxic and nontoxic reactions. Toxic compounds (such as fertilizers, insecticides, and bacterial toxins) can trigger a reaction in any individual. They can occur naturally, or they can be induced by food processing or contaminants, and toxic food reactions (which are predictable because they depend on the dose of a compound rather than individual susceptibility) can be indistinguishable from food allergy reactions because symptoms may be similar in both cases. Nontoxic adverse reactions to food, however, are either immune-mediated (called food allergy) or non-immune mediated (called food intolerance). Furthermore, food allergy is divided into IgE-mediated and non-IgE–mediated reactions (Bruijnzeel-Koomen et al., 1995; Mahan & Swift, 2020; Montalto et al., 2008). This section focuses on immune-mediated food allergies.

A *food allergy* is defined as an adverse health effect arising from a specific immune response that occurs reproducibly on exposure to a given food (food antigen) that is normally harmless to the healthy population, with *food* being defined as any substance intended for human consumption (Boyce et al., 2010; De Martinis et al., 2020). Sensitization occurs through the GI tract, oral route, skin or skin barrier dysfunction, or the respiratory tract (Mahan & Swift, 2020; Sampson et al., 2018). IgE-mediated reactions have been linked to more than 170 foods and after consumption of or contact with (sensitization to) the allergen, signs and symptoms develop (Boyce et al., 2010; Mahan & Swift, 2020; National Institute of Allergy and Infectious Diseases [NIAID], 2011; Waserman et al., 2018). *Cell-mediated (non-IgE-mediated) food allergy* refers to development of reproducible signs and symptoms that result from exposure to a food and resolve when the food is avoided. Factors influencing the antigenic response (tissue and immune) include genetics, epigenetics, age, immune status/disease state, microbiome, epidermal barrier defects, and medications (Mahan & Swift, 2020; Sampson et al., 2018; Sicherer & Sampson, 2018).

Food allergy occurs more often in children than in adults (De Martinis et al., 2017). It affects people in industrialized/westernized regions more than in other regions and has increased in prevalence in the past 2 to 3 decades. The prevalence ranges from 5.8% in younger children to 8.5% in adolescents (Moen et al., 2019). Up to 40% of children with food allergies have multiple food allergies (R. Gupta et al., 2018). Based on current health status, food allergies affect 5.8% of children in excellent or very good health, 9.1% of children in good health, and 25.4% of children in fair or poor health. It is not understood why food allergy incidence has been increasing, how to best diagnose food allergies, or even how to "maximize safety or quality of life during management" (Sicherer & Sampson, 2018). Comorbidities or factors that may increase risk of food-induced anaphylaxis include asthma and other atopic disorders (e.g., atopic dermatitis, eosinophilic esophagitis), respiratory allergies, chronic lung disease (e.g., chronic obstructive pulmonary disease or recurrent pneumonia), anatomic airway obstruction (e.g., airway hemangioma or laryngotracheomalacia), and cardiovascular disease (CVD; Boyce et al., 2010).

## Subjective Findings

Complete a basic nutrition assessment to review for symptoms of food allergy, as well as poor growth and nutrient deficiencies that could relate to food allergies. Investigate symptoms, time of onset, age of onset, circumstances before symptom onset, comorbidities, family history of allergy, detailed food history, and previous food elimination or therapeutic interventions (Gomes-Belo et al., 2018). The health history may reveal:

- Itchy mouth or eyes
- Difficulty swallowing
- Throat tightness
- Mouth or throat tingling
- Nasal congestion (Bunyavanich & Berin, 2019; Feehley et al., 2019; Gomes-Belo et al., 2018; M. Gupta et al., 2018; Mahan & Swift, 2020)

## Risk Factors

The most common risk factors for food allergy are:

- Family history
- Nonfood allergies
- Unintentional exposure to food allergens
- Asthma
- Atopic dermatitis
- Non-Hispanic African American
- Dysbiosis (Bunyavanich & Berin, 2019; Feehley et al., 2019; Gomes-Belo et al., 2018; M. Gupta et al., 2018)

## Review of Systems

The most common manifestations revealed during the review of systems include:

- **Constitutional:** abdominal pain
- **Integumentary:** rash, flushing, hives
- **HEENT:** oral itching, throat tightness
- **Respiratory:** chest tightness, dyspnea
- **Gastrointestinal:** nausea, vomiting, abdominal cramping or pain, belching, oral itching
- **Neurologic/Behavioral:** dizziness, sense of impending gloom (Mahan & Swift, 2020)

## Objective Findings

The physical examination of the child with a food allergy may reveal:

- Rash, acute urticaria, angioedema
- Eye tearing, periorbital edema, conjunctival erythema
- Rhinorrhea, sneeze, cough, wheeze, hoarse voice, cyanosis

- Bradycardia, tachycardia, hypotension, cardiac arrest (Boyce et al., 2010; Gomes-Belo et al., 2018; M. Gupta et al., 2018; Mahan & Swift, 2020; Sampson et al., 2014)

## Laboratory/Diagnostic Testing

The diagnosis of food allergy is based on a comprehensive client history and review of clinical findings. Identify causative food(s) through one or more of the following methods:

- Food elimination diet, beginning with elimination of one or more of the primary allergens:
  - Milk, egg, peanut, tree nuts, crustacean shellfish, fish, wheat, and soy (Boyce et al., 2010; Sampson et al., 2014).
  - This should be reserved for patients with mild or moderate symptoms. Those with severe symptoms should have further, more intensive testing done, especially with a history of anaphylaxis.
- Oral food challenge—double-blind placebo-controlled (gold standard), single-blind, or open-food challenge, of the suspected food(s).
- Allergen-specific serum IgE (in conjunction with other testing).
- Skin testing (scratch, prick, puncture)—complete in combination with thorough food-symptom history (Boyce et al., 2010; Gomes-Belo et al., 2018; Mahan & Swift, 2020).

**PRO TIP** Tree nuts of allergy concern include almonds, Brazil nuts, cashews, hazelnuts, macadamia nuts, pecans, pistachios, Queensland nuts, walnuts, and other non-peanut tree nuts.

## Differential Diagnosis

The differential diagnosis for food allergy includes:

- Food intolerance (e.g., lactase or sulfites)
- Spicy food-related gustatory rhinitis (e.g., hot peppers, chili powder, onions, black pepper, curry)
- Food poisoning (such as with *Escherichia coli*) or toxic reactions (e.g., ciguatoxin from fish, toxins from wild mushrooms, or mycotoxins on nuts, spices, or cereals; (WHO, 2018)
- Pharmacologic reactions to products such as caffeine, theobromine (in tea, for example), or alcohol
- Allergic reactions to drugs, inhalants, or venom
- Panic reaction
- Eating disorders (M. Gupta et al., 2018; Sampson et al., 2014)

## Treatment/Management Plan

Treatment of food allergies can be very challenging due to the complicated nature of ingredient identification in foods and the fact that infants and young children may not be able to describe symptoms although they depend fully on adults for diet modification. The general approach to treatment is simple, however: avoid offending allergens in the form of foods and beverages. Most children will outgrow food allergy to milk, egg, soy, and wheat (Boyce et al., 2010; Kleinman & Greer, 2020; Mahan & Swift, 2020; Togias et al., 2017; Waserman et al., 2018). Follow up within 1 month to confirm that symptoms have subsided or been eliminated with expected dietary changes.

In a recent report from the American Academy of Pediatrics (AAP), it was indicated that no conclusions could be made regarding duration of breastfeeding as it relates to either prevention or delay of the onset of specific food allergies (Greer et al., 2019). Additionally, there is a lack of evidence to support giving infants partially or extensively hydrolyzed formula to prevent atopic disease (Greer et al., 2019). There is evidence to support the early introduction of infant-safe forms of peanuts to reduce risk of peanut allergies; therefore, follow the addendum guidelines for the prevention of peanut allergy in the United States (see chapter 32 for additional information) (Greer et al., 2019; Togias et al., 2017). Evidence is emerging to support the concept that maintenance of a healthy intestinal microbiome may offer protection against food allergy (Bunyavanich & Berin, 2019; Feehley et al., 2019).

## Family Education

Teach the following:

- Until identification of a suspected food allergen is definitive, request maintenance of a food and symptom diary (for 7 to 14 days or more) in order to link food with reaction. Include:
  - Time food [or beverage] was consumed
  - Type of food, including all ingredients and preparation method if appropriate
  - Quantity of food consumed
  - Time symptoms occurred in relation to when food was consumed
  - Other information pertinent around the time of the symptoms, such as environmental factors, stress, physical activity, urine and bowel elimination as well as nausea or vomiting, sleep patterns, pain, and reactions such as itching, sneezing, or rash.
- If an elimination diet is prescribed, encourage strict adherence for the designated time period.

- Once an allergen is identified, advise avoidance of offending foods, alone or in combination with other food (e.g., tomatoes in pizza sauce) or beverage (e.g., chocolate in milk).
- Advise careful food label reading as a key tool for food allergen avoidance.
- Advise dietary approaches that help maintain a healthy microbiome.
- Be sure that all regular caregivers are also educated, including grandparents and extended family members and friends, babysitters, daycare workers, and teachers—anyone who may provide food to or prepare food for the child.
- Always seek prompt and rapid treatment if symptoms of anaphylaxis are present.

### Referral

Refer the child and family for allergy education to a registered dietitian, nutritionist, or other specialist trained in food allergy management. Topics to be taught should include label and recipe reading, food substitutions, dining out and eating away from home, special occasions, and grocery shopping. Referral to pediatric allergy/immunology or pediatric gastroenterology may also be needed depending upon the child.

▶ ALERT: Call 911 (or local emergency number) or seek care immediately at an emergency or urgent care facility in the case of a serious or life-threatening reaction to food (difficulty breathing, or reduced BP as indicated by pale skin, weak pulse, confusion, or loss of consciousness).

## CELIAC DISEASE

The clinical presentation, definition, and epidemiology of celiac disease (CD) has changed in the past 50 years. The disease was usually recognized in young children with malabsorption, failure to thrive, and loose stools and found to be related to dietary gluten. Now the disease is recognized as an autoimmune inflammatory disorder of the small intestine triggered by gluten in genetically susceptible individuals that has multiple manifestations presenting throughout childhood or adulthood (Ludvigsson & Murray, 2019; Popp & Mäki, 2019). CD occurs worldwide, with incidence increasing among children and adults in the last few decades (King et al., 2020; Lionetti et al., 2015). Reasons for the increase are unclear but likely related to increased awareness of, availability of, and recommendations for diagnostic testing and screening, and environmental factors (Almallouhi et al., 2017; King et al., 2020; Lionetti et al., 2015).

CD is a gluten-induced enteropathy which is immune-mediated in nature (Leonard et al., 2017). It is related to an inappropriate adaptive immune response accompanied by an innate immune reaction to gluten in the small intestines in genetically predisposed individuals. Exposure to dietary gluten causes release of tissue transglutaminase that deamidates gliadin, increasing its immunogenicity (Leonard et al., 2017; McAllister et al., 2019). This process facilitates binding of gliadin fragments to the HLA-DQ2/DQ8 molecules expressed on antigen-presenting cells, activating CD4+ T cells and subsequent Th2 and Th1 immune response, leading to activation of B cells and production of pro-inflammatory cytokines, migration of natural killer cells, and increased intraepithelial lymphocytes. This cascade culminates in tissue destruction, cryptal hyperplasia, and likely increased permeability of the gut wall (Caio et al., 2019; Leonard et al., 2017; McAllister et al., 2019). During this process, antibodies to tissue transglutaminase, gliadin, and actin are produced (Lebwohl et al., 2018).

The prevalence of CD in the United States is 0.3% to 0.9%. Having a first-degree relative with CD results in a 10% chance that the individual will develop CD (Celiac Disease Foundation, 2020). The major histocompatibility complex class 2 human leukocyte antigen (HLA) genes, particularly the HLA-DQ2 and DQ8 types, are strongly associated with CD. About 90% of children with CD carry HLA-DQ2 and 5%–7% carry DQ8 (Almallouhi et al., 2017; King et al., 2020; Lionetti et al., 2015; McAllister et al., 2019). Approximately 40% of the Western population have one or more of the HLA-DQ2/DQ8 alleles, but only about 0.5% to 1% of the population has CD (Caio et al., 2019; Hill et al., 2016). Having DQ2 or DQ8 haplotypes is necessary but not sufficient for disease development, and most individuals will not develop CD (McAllister et al., 2019).

Infections have been considered possible risk factors for the onset of CD in predisposed children. Prospective studies have shown bacterial and viral infections such as rotavirus and enterovirus in early life to be associated with later CD, with a protective effect of rotavirus vaccination (Kahrs et al., 2019; Kemppainen Lynch, et al., 2017; Mårild et al., 2015; Meijer et al., 2018; Szajewska et al., 2016). The association between early-life antibiotic exposure and risk of CD or CDA is unclear with conflicting evidence (Dydensborg Sander et al., 2019; Kemppainen, Vehik, et al., 2017; Kołodziej et al., 2019). Disruption of the intestinal microbiome has also been hypothesized to increase risk of autoimmune diseases such as CD (Popp & Mäki, 2019; Tye-Din et al., 2018). It is unclear, however, whether differences in the microbiota of children with CD and those without CD are a causative factor or a consequence of the disease (Chmielewska et al., 2015; Serena et al., 2019). Further studies are needed to investigate the contribution of infections, antibiotics, and the microbiome to CD pathogenesis (Kemppainen, Lynch, et al., 2017; Kemppainen, Vehik, 2017; Serena et al., 2019; Tye-Din et al., 2018).

## Subjective Findings

Celiac disease can be diagnosed at any age with a highly variable presentation. Subjective findings may include chronic diarrhea, abdominal distention, poor growth, weight loss, fatigue, or malaise (VanReken et al., 2020).

### Risk Factors

The most common risk factors for CD are:

- Diet containing wheat, barley or rye
- 1st-degree relative with CD
- Genetic predisposition (presence of HLA-DQ2 or DQ8 is necessary)
- Type 1 diabetes mellitus
- IgA deficiency
- Autoimmune thyroiditis
- Autoimmune hepatitis
- Trisomy 21
- Williams syndrome
- Turner syndrome
- Infant diet: Early studies suggested age at gluten introduction, amount of gluten consumption, breastfeeding at time of gluten introduction, and breastfeeding itself may influence development of CD. Current evidence has shown that duration of breastfeeding, breastfeeding at time of gluten introduction, and type of gluten at introduction do not affect the development of CD or CD autoimmunity (Al-Toma et al., 2019; Hyytinen et al., 2017; Ludvigsson & Murray, 2019; Szajewska et al., 2016). Early or late introduction of gluten to the infant's diet has been implicated as a risk factor for CD or CDA; however, it remains unclear if introduction of gluten at age less than 3 to 4 months compared with more than 6 months has an effect on the development of CD or CDA (Szajewska et al., 2016). Similarly, the amount of gluten in the infant's diet may influence the risk for CD at a young age, although the quantity of gluten that has such effect is unclear (Meijer et al., 2018; Szajewska et al., 2016).

### Review of Systems

The most common manifestations revealed during the review of systems include:

- **Constitutional:** poor weight gain and growth, short stature, unexpected weight loss, chronic fatigue, abdominal pain, anorexia, headaches
- **HEENT:** mouth ulcers
- **Gastrointestinal:** chronic diarrhea, abdominal distention, weight loss (infants and young children), bloating, constipation, nausea or vomiting. When CD presents later in childhood, GI symptoms are usually mild and may not be present (Krauthammer et al., 2020; Popp & Mäki, 2019)
- **Musculoskeletal:** muscle wasting, joint pain
- **Neurologic:** numbness or tingling, altered gait, seizure
- **Reproductive:** delayed puberty
- **Psychiatric/behavioral:** attention deficit hyperactivity disorder, anxiety, depression

## Objective Findings

The physical examination of the child with CD may reveal:

- Wasted appearance
- Aphthous stomatitis
- Dental enamel hypoplasia
- Dermatitis herpetiformis
- Distended abdomen

### Laboratory/Diagnostic Testing

Testing is recommended for two groups of children: (1) children with symptoms suggestive of CD not otherwise explained, and (2) children belonging to a high-risk group with or without symptoms (Hill et al., 2016). Complete blood count (CBC) with differential and iron studies may reveal anemia. Serologic testing should be performed while the child is on a gluten-containing diet. The North American Society for Pediatric Gastroenterology, Hepatology & Nutrition (NASPGHAN) recommends ingestion of 10g of gluten (2 slices of wheat bread) per day for 8 weeks, although the amount and duration of gluten consumption for accurate testing is not known (Hill et al., 2016). Serologic testing is explained in Table 27.1.

- Total IgA and TTG-IgA (initial step): For children younger than 2 years of age, both TTG-IgA and DGP-IgG can be used (Hill et al., 2016). If the IgA is normal and the tests are positive, the child should be referred to a pediatric gastroenterologist to confirm CD, usually with a biopsy. NASPGHAN suggests a no-biopsy option for diagnosis (see following).

**TABLE 27.1 Serologic Testing for Celiac Disease**

| Test | Explanation | Comments |
|---|---|---|
| Tissue transglutaminase antibodies (TTG) | Highly sensitive and specific<br>May not be as accurate in children younger than age 2 years<br>For children with IgA deficiency, TTG-IgG tests are necessary | Cost-effective test to screen children for CD |
| Endomysial antibodies (EMA) | Based on antibody reactivity to tissue-bound transglutaminase 2<br>Less sensitive but more specific than the TTG-IgA test<br>Associated with high likelihood for CD | More expensive<br>Is an immunofluorescent test, thus subject to interobserver variation<br>Useful as a second-line test for equivocal results of anti-TTG or for a no-biopsy diagnosis in children |
| Deamidated gliadin peptide (DGP) | Anti-DPG tests detect antibodies against synthetically derived peptides | DPG-IgA test has lower sensitivity and specificity compared to TTG-IgA and EMA-IgA test<br>DPG-IgG has comparable specificity<br>For children younger than 2 years of age, recommendation is sending DPG-IgG in conjunction with TTG-IgA for initial testing |
| Genetic testing | HLA-DQ2 and HLA-DQ8 testing are used for diagnostic dilemmas | Negative predictive value of almost 99% (if negative for HLA-DQ2/DQ8, CD is highly unlikely)<br>A positive result does not confirm CD diagnosis |

*Sources*: Data from Hill et al., 2016; Husby, S., Koletzko, S., Korponay-Szabó, I., Kurppa, K., Mearin, M. L., Ribes-Koninckx, C., Shamir, R., Troncone, R., Auricchio, R., Castillejo, G., Christensen, R., Dolinsek, J., Gillett, P., Hróbjartsson, A., Koltai, T., Maki, M., Nielsen, S. M., Popp, A., Størdal, K., ... Wessels, M. (2020). European Society Paediatric Gastroenterology, Hepatology, and Nutrition guidelines for diagnosing coeliac disease 2020. *Journal of Pediatric Gastroenterology and Nutrition*, *70*(1), 141–156. https://doi.org/10.1097/MPG.0000000000002497; Lebwohl, B., Sanders, D. S., & Green, P. H. R. (2018). Coeliac disease. *Lancet (London, England)*, *391*(10115), 70–81. https://doi.org/S0140-6736(17)31796-8

- Evaluate for a possible false negative serology test (low gluten diet, immunosuppressive therapy) if the IgA is normal and the CD antibody tests are negative in a symptomatic child.
  - If there is no risk for a false negative serology test, the child likely does not have CD.
  - If a risk for false negative serology tests exists, HLA testing could be sent; a positive HLA-DQ2/DQ8 test warrants retesting on a high-gluten diet, or consider a biopsy. If the HLA testing is negative, other causes for symptoms should be investigated.
  - If there is a strong clinical suspicion for CD, an intestinal biopsy can be pursued (Al-Toma et al., 2019; Hill et al., 2016; Husby et al., 2020).
- For children with IgA deficiency, IgG testing for TTG, EMA, or DGP is required. For positive IgG results, biopsy should be done (Husby et al., 2020).
- Asymptomatic children in a high-risk group with negative antibody testing likely do not have CD. If HLA testing is not done, observing the child for development of symptoms is recommended, or serology can be monitored every 2 to 3 years (Hill, 2020; Husby et al., 2012).
- For children with autoimmune disease and low TTG-IgA (<3× upper limit of normal), EMA-IgA can be tested and if positive, move forward with biopsy. If EMA-IgA is negative and the child has no symptoms, repeat serology testing can be done in 6–12 months (Hill et al., 2016; Snyder et al., 2016).
- In children already on a gluten-free diet, standard serology tests (TTG-IgA or EMA-IgA) may be negative depending on the duration of the gluten-free diet. HLA testing can be done prior to trying a gluten challenge to diagnose CD. No further workup is necessary if HLA-DQ2/DQ8 is negative, as CD is unlikely (Rubio-Tapia et al., 2013; Snyder et al., 2016).
- Histology testing is an important step for diagnosing celiac disease. The pediatric gastroenterologist may perform an endoscopy to visualize the small intestine and/or a biopsy to evaluate the duodenum (Hill et al., 2016).

### Gluten Challenge

A gluten challenge with repeat serology and biopsy is reserved for children for whom diagnosis is in doubt, such as children already on a gluten-free diet or with discrepant serology and histology results. An

HLA-DQ2/DQ8 test should be done first. A gluten challenge should be discouraged in children younger than 5 years or during puberty unless the child was placed on a gluten-free diet without proper testing. A child is considered to have CD if CD-specific antibodies become positive and a clinical and/or histologic relapse is observed when the child eats more than 5 g/day of gluten. CD can be excluded if antibodies remain negative and no histologic changes are noted; however, future evaluation may be required for delayed development of disease (Al-Toma et al., 2019; Hill et al., 2016; Husby et al., 2012).

## Differential Diagnosis

The differential diagnosis for CD includes:

- Non-celiac gluten sensitivity
- Wheat allergy
- Milk or soy protein allergy
- Autoimmune enteropathy
- Inflammatory bowel disease
- Viral, parasitic, or bacterial infections, such as *Giardia* or *Helicobacter pylori*
- Bacterial overgrowth
- Pancreatic insufficiency
- Eosinophilic gastroenteritis
- Drug-induced enteropathy (nonsteroidal anti-inflammatory drugs, sartans, mycophenolate)
- Lymphocytic colitis
- Peptic duodenitis
- Malnutrition (Caio et al., 2019; Hill et al., 2016; Hujoel et al., 2019)

## Classifications of Celiac Disease

CD may be classified using uniform definitions (the Oslo definitions):

- *Gastrointestinal and Classic CD:* Commonly seen in children, CD presenting with GI signs and symptoms. Classical CD refers to presentation with signs and symptoms of malabsorption and failure to thrive (FTT), typically in young children. CD is confirmed with serologic antibody/genetic testing and characteristic histologic findings, and symptoms should resolve with a gluten-free diet (Caio et al., 2019; Ludvigsson et al., 2013).
- *Extraintestinal CD:* CD presenting with extraintestinal symptoms such as anemia or short stature with few or no GI symptoms; diagnosis requires serologic and histologic testing and symptom improvement on a gluten-free diet.
- *Subclinical CD:* Also referred to as silent or asymptomatic disease, this form includes children with positive CD antibodies or HLA testing and biopsy findings consistent with CD but GI or extraintestinal signs/symptoms below the threshold of clinical suspicion. These children are usually identified from screening due to risk factors (Caio et al., 2019; Ludvigsson et al., 2013).
- *Potential CD:* Children who have positive CD antibodies and genetic markers but have not had a biopsy, have no intestinal histologic abnormalities, or have modified Marsh-Oberhuber grade 0 to 1 biopsy results (Ludvigsson et al., 2013). Children may or may not have GI or extraintestinal symptoms. These children are at increased risk for developing CD (Ludvigsson et al., 2013).
- *Latent CD:* Oslo definitions discourage the use of the term "latent CD" as there are various definitions, and the term has been used interchangeably with potential CD. Latent disease can refer to children who are serum antibody positive with normal intestinal mucosa and may become serum antibody negative or develop disease at a later time. Latent CD has also been used to describe children who have met criteria for CD at some point in life but have recovered and now have normal intestinal mucosa, may or may not have abnormal serum antibodies, and may or may not have symptoms (Husby et al., 2012; Popp & Mäki, 2019).
- *Seronegative CD:* A rare diagnostic challenge has emerged for children who have negative CD-antibody serology and histologic findings of duodenal villous atrophy. HLA DQ2/DQ8 haplotype can help rule out CD. Truly seronegative CD seems to be exceptional in children, and it is important to investigate for alternative etiologies of villous atrophy (Caio et al., 2019; Gustafsson et al., 2020; McAllister et al., 2019).
- *Non-Celiac Gluten Sensitivity:* Children who have intestinal or extraintestinal celiac-like symptoms precipitated by ingestion of gluten-containing foods, clinical improvement with gluten withdrawal, and in whom CD and wheat allergy have been excluded (Bathrellou et al., 2018; Hill et al., 2016; McAllister et al., 2019).

## Treatment/Management Plan

The treatment for CD is lifelong exclusion of gluten (wheat, barley, and rye) from the diet, i.e., a gluten-free diet. Oats are tolerated by a majority of children and can be introduced to the diet slowly with monitoring for symptoms (Al-Toma et al., 2019). Some children also omit oats due to potential contamination of oats by wheat, barley, or rye in the oat processing plant. Children who adhere to a gluten-free diet can have resolution of symptoms, maintain normal growth and development, achieve intestinal repair, and prevent CD-related complications. New therapeutic approaches including pharmaceuticals are under development, but have not been tested in children (Tye-Din et al., 2018).

Address the potential for nutritional deficiencies, such as in iron, folate, Vitamin B12, and Vitamin D, that are known to exist in individuals with CD (Leonard et al., 2017). In addition, children should be instructed on age-appropriate daily intake of calcium and vitamin D, routine vitamin supplementation, and signs and symptoms of diabetes. Bone mineral density testing is not necessary unless children have severe presentation, prolonged diagnosis, signs of rickets, or a history of bone fractures. Routine screening for zinc and other trace elements is not recommended except in children with severe malabsorption or prolonged delay in diagnosis (Snyder et al., 2016).

NASPGHAN recommends that children have repeat serology (TTG-IgA or DGP-IgG) tests at 3 to 6-month intervals until levels normalize (Hill et al., 2016). Once symptoms resolve and serology normalizes, children can be followed annually. CBC and thyrotropin levels should be routinely done at follow-up, and children with initial abnormal transaminases, bone density, trace elements, or vitamin D deficiency require follow-up evaluation (Snyder et al., 2016). Some children with CD may not respond to the hepatitis B virus vaccine prior to starting a gluten-free diet; children with inadequate titers will need revaccination after CD-specific antibodies decline (Anania et al., 2017). Individuals with CD may also be at increased risk for bacterial pneumonia and pneumococcal infections, possibly due to hyposplenism seen in adults, so it is important that children receive recommended pneumococcal immunizations (Canova et al., 2019; Simons et al., 2018). In addition, a gluten-free diet can be deficient in fiber, B vitamins, folate, and iron and have an imbalance in macronutrients; therefore, monitoring for micronutrient deficiency and advising about proper energy intake and weight monitoring should be considered (Al-Toma et al., 2019; Hill et al., 2016). A repeat biopsy is not necessary unless symptoms and abnormal serology tests persist despite adherence to a gluten-free diet (Hill et al., 2016).

For children with continued symptoms, persistent presence of serologic antibodies, or subsequent increase in antibodies, review of the diet is required to assess for inadvertent gluten intake or nonadherence to the gluten-free diet (Nardecchia et al., 2019). Children with apparent adherence to diet and continued signs of CD should also be evaluated for other diagnoses.

A gluten-free diet can be difficult to maintain due to hidden sources of gluten in commercially produced foods and medications, expense, availability of gluten-free products, time for meal preparation, social difficulties such as stigma and isolation, and level of knowledge about CD and gluten-free diets among children and parents (Myléus et al., 2020; White et al., 2016). Adolescence appears to be a risk factor for nonadherence to a gluten-free diet: teens are more likely to intentionally break from it, reporting lack of symptoms with consumption of small amounts of gluten. Younger children are more likely to have nonintentional gluten-free diet failure, often due to parental knowledge of CD, gluten-free diets, and reading labels (Czaja-Bulsa & Bulsa, 2018; Myléus et al., 2020). Being involved with a group of people who have CD and having social support may foster adherence to a gluten-free diet (Myléus et al., 2020; White et al., 2016).

In general, CD has been associated with increased mortality compared with the general population, although data can be contradictory with common causes related to CVD, respiratory disease, and cancer (Bathrellou et al., 2018; Lebwohl et al., 2020; McAllister et al., 2019). Malignancies, particularly lymphoproliferative and GI cancers, have been associated with CD. Long-term adherence to a gluten-free diet can reduce the risk for other morbidities associated with CD, such as impaired bone health, reproductive abnormalities, neuropsychiatric disorders, and GI problems (Bathrellou et al., 2018). It is important to provide families and children with support and access to dietitians and physicians familiar with CD to optimize management and reduce risks for morbidity and mortality.

**PRO TIP** Encourage diet adherence by helping the child/family notice improvement in comfort as symptoms decrease.

## Family Education

Teach the following:

- The role of gluten in CD and which foods contain gluten.
- How to read labels.
- How to prepare gluten-free meals.
- Organizations such as the North American Society for Pediatric Gastroenterology, Hepatology and

Nutrition (www.gikids.org), National Celiac Association (www.nationalceliac.org), and Celiac Disease Foundation (www.celiac.org) offer additional materials and support for children and families.

**PRO TIP** Allow plenty of time for education and follow-up education. There is a significant amount of information for children (and their families/caregivers) to learn and understand with a new diagnosis of CD. As they settle into managing the condition, new questions will arise for an extended time. Be sure they have an opportunity to easily pose questions and receive answers. CD support groups and discussion boards, moderated by a professional, can be invaluable.

### Referral

Refer children who have clinical manifestations of CD and positive CD-specific antibodies to pediatric gastroenterology and a registered dietitian or nutritionist specially trained in CD. Referral to pediatric allergy/immunology may be helpful in some children.

▶ ALERT: In the case of celiac crisis, which may include explosive diarrhea, dehydration, and severe electrolyte disturbances, as well as possibly cerebellar ataxia, consider the need for hospitalization.

## PEDIATRIC MALNUTRITION/UNDERNUTRITION

In the past, pediatric malnutrition, specifically undernutrition, was thought to be a problem only outside of developed countries, with direct relation to the lack of a nutritional, well-balanced diet. However, it has become more widely recognized that pediatric malnutrition also occurs within the United States and other developed countries. Food insecurity contributes to malnutrition, and food insecurity rates remained elevated during the COVID pandemic in 2020 (Bauer, 2020). In 2013, the Academy of Nutrition and Dietetics and American Society for Parenteral and Enteral Nutrition (ASPEN) published a new definition for malnutrition in relation to the pediatric population of developed countries. It recognized the fact that in developed countries, malnutrition is predominantly related to chronic illnesses/conditions, disease, trauma, and surgery (Mehta et al., 2013). Because malnutrition can progress rapidly in the pediatric population, timely recognition and treatment of malnutrition is essential in decreasing or preventing the adverse outcomes of malnutrition, including developmental and growth issues.

The term *malnutrition* encompasses both obesity and undernutrition; however, it refers most commonly to undernutrition, which is the primary focus of this section. Note that FTT is sometimes used inappropriately interchangeably with malnutrition or undernutrition. Homan (2016) points out that "failure to thrive (FTT) is an abnormal pattern of weight gain defined by the lack of sufficient usable nutrition and documented by inadequate weight gain over time." FTT is a clinical finding more than a diagnostic term. Pediatric malnutrition/undernutrition is defined as an imbalance between nutrient requirements and intake that results in cumulative deficits of energy, protein, or micronutrients that may negatively affect growth, development, and other relevant outcomes (Mehta et al., 2013). This definition, as outlined by ASPEN, addresses five key domains that were relevant in the evaluation (diagnosis) and management of malnutrition in children between 1 month to 18 years old: (1) anthropometric variables, (2) growth, (3) chronicity, (4) etiology, and (5) impact on functional status. Figure 27.1 provides a summarized chart to enhance understanding of the relationship between the key domains that have to be considered.

Growth is the primary outcome measure of a child's nutritional status. Serial anthropometric measurements such as weight, height, body mass index (BMI) and mid-upper-arm circumference are plotted on growth charts. This outlines a report of the child's growth status in comparison with a population data and reference curve. If the child's plotted growth chart or curve is below the comparison data, then the child is diagnosed as malnourished. As stated earlier, defining malnutrition also requires determining its chronicity, etiology, and impact on functional status. The chronicity of malnutrition is divided into acute (less than 3 months duration) and chronic (greater than 3 months duration). Etiology can be simplified into illness-related and non-illness-related malnutrition (Table 27.2). *Illness-related malnutrition* refers to one or more diseases that result in nutrient imbalance losses, hypermetabolism not matched by intake, and altered utilization (Mehta et al., 2013). Contrastingly, *non-illness-related malnutrition* takes into consideration environmental, socioeconomic, and behavioral factors that may lead to decreased nutrient intake and/or delivery. The degree of impact of malnutrition on functional and developmental outcome varies with each child and determines the severity of the illness.

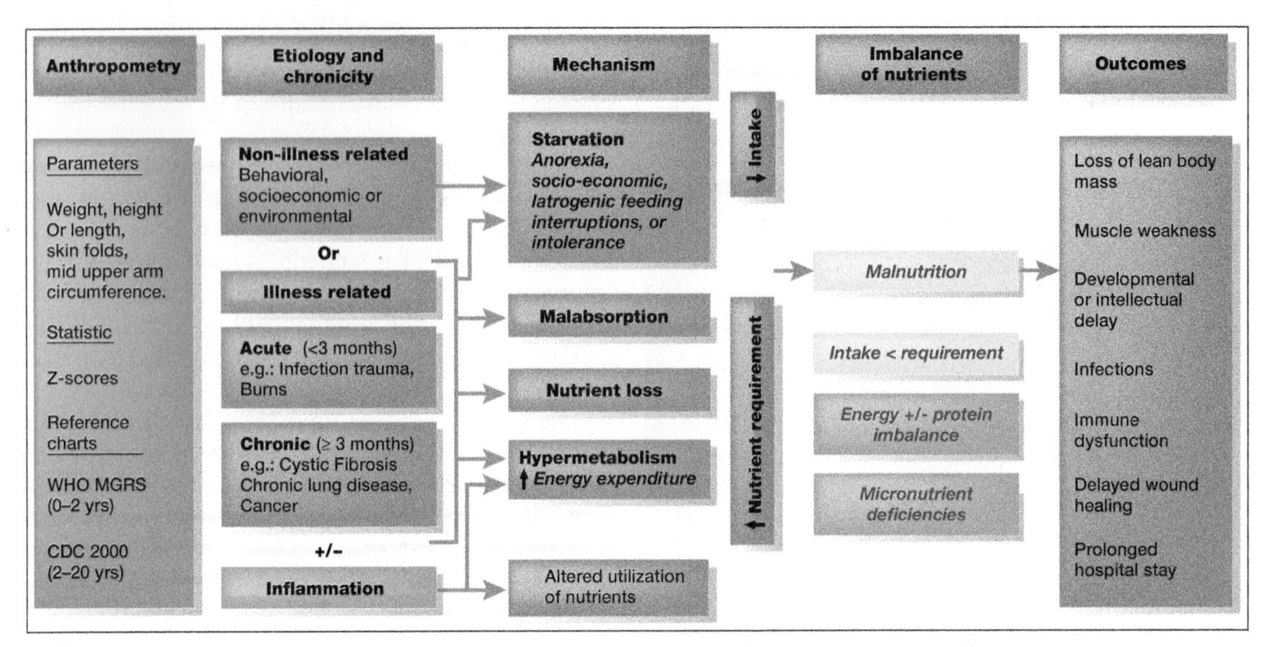


FIGURE 27.1 Defining pediatric malnutrition: a paradigm shift toward etiology-related definitions.

*Source*: Reproduced with permission from Mehta, N. M., Corkins, M. R., Lyman, B., Malone, A., Goday, P. S., Carney, L. N., Monczka, J. L., Plogsted, S. W., Schwenk, W. F., & American Society for Parenteral and Enteral Nutrition Board of Directors. (2013). Defining pediatric malnutrition: A paradigm shift toward etiology-related definitions. *JPEN Journal of Parenteral Enteral Nutrition, 37*(4), 460. https://doi.org/10.1177/0148607113479972

TABLE 27.2 Etiology of Malnutrition

| Illness-Related | Non-Illness-Related |
|---|---|
| Acute illness/diseases | Parental depression, stress, divorce |
| Infection | Parental developmental delay |
| Chronic conditions (i.e., cancer, inflammatory bowel disease, hypothyroidism, etc.) | Parenteral psychological problems |
| Trauma | Young and single parents, especially lack of social support |
| Surgery | Domestic violence |
| Burns | Alcohol or other substance abuse |
| | History of child abuse (parental or child) |
| | Poverty |
| | Social isolation |

*Source*: Data from Kleinman, R. E., & Greer, F. R. (2020). *Pediatric nutrition*. American Academy of Pediatrics.

This may include findings such as decreased mobility, muscle loss and weakness, cognitive or developmental delays, immune dysfunction, and delayed wound healing (Mehta et al., 2013). Some of these may resolve once malnutrition has corrected; however, other outcomes may be permanent.

The prevalence of undernutrition in children in the United States is 2.6% to 24.5%. The low caloric reserves and higher-than-adult nutrient requirements of children (per unit of body weight) make them particularly vulnerable to undernutrition (McCarthy et al., 2019). The pathophysiology of pediatric undernutrition typically involves the following conditions:

- Decreased nutrient intake
- Excessive losses such as through vomiting and diarrhea
- Increased requirements, hypermetabolism, or catabolism
- Altered utilization/malabsorption (Beer et al., 2015)

Comorbidities associated with pediatric malnutrition may include:

- Diarrhea, acute gastroenteritis
- Anemia
- Acute respiratory infections, pneumonia
- HIV/AIDS
- Tuberculosis

- Rickets
- Cancer
- Preterm birth (Derseh et al., 2018; Kumar et al., 2018; Revuelta Iniesta et al., 2019; Ziegler, 1991)

> **PRO TIP** Measure and plot accurate anthropometric measurements at each ambulatory visit, and per facility protocol if hospitalized. Watch for early signs of poor growth.

## Subjective Findings

The health history may reveal:

- Previous diagnosis of chronic illnesses or nutrition-related illnesses
- Pre-term birth
- Delayed Tanner stage
- Changes in body weight
- Inadequacy of dietary intake:
  - Child's appetite
  - Frequency of intake
  - Foods eaten
  - Feeding/eating problems
  - Dietary restrictions that interfere with ability to meet nutritional requirements
- Presence of GI symptoms:
  - May indicate intolerance of a normal diet
  - Inquire about presence, severity, and duration of symptoms: anorexia, nausea, abdominal pain, vomiting/gastroesophageal reflux, diarrhea, constipation
- Presence of functional impairment (i.e., developmental and/or cognitive delays, decreased muscle function/strength, behavioral issues, abnormal growth and development)
- Presence of metabolic stress (e.g., surgery, trauma, infections, pressure sores/ulcers, shock, inflammation; Corkins & Teague, 2017)

## Risk Factors

The most common risk factors for malnutrition are:

- Hospitalization
- Recurrent febrile illness
- Malignancy
- Developmental disability
- Presence of underlying illness or environmental or behavioral issues (i.e., low income, chronic eating disorders)
- Mechanisms that reduce nutrient intakes relative to nutrient requirements (food depravation, hypermetabolism, malabsorption; Corkins & Teague, 2017)

## Review of Systems

The most common manifestations revealed during the review of systems include:

- **Constitutional:** change in activity, lack of appetite, fatigue
- **Integumentary:** dry skin, changes in hair or nails
- **HEENT:** dry mouth/lips, difficulty swallowing, altered/loss of taste and smell, facial swelling, delayed teeth eruption
- **Respiratory:** breathing difficulties, increased respiratory infections
- **Cardiovascular:** palpitations
- **Gastrointestinal:** nausea, diarrhea, constipation
- **Musculoskeletal:** reduced muscle and tissue mass
- **Neurologic:** altered mental status
- **Endocrine:** difficulty staying warm, hypothermia
- **Psychiatric:** anorexia nervosa, bulimia nervosa, depression, anxiety

## Objective Findings

The physical examination of the child with malnutrition may reveal:

- Anthropometric measurements plotted on growth charts are below the standard mean deviation (Z-score). In children less than 2 years of age, the anthropometric measurements should be plotted using the WHO charts. Similarly, for children 2 to 20 years old, the use of the Centers for Disease Control and Prevention (CDC) charts is recommended. Specialty growth charts are also available online for various different diseases and disorders, including Down syndrome, Turner syndrome, and cerebral palsy. The standard deviation or Z-score calculation along these growth-chart curves provides a comparable measurement from the median population and allows for determination of a growth problem and its severity.
  - Length or height
    - Length: obtained from children 0 to 24 months of age
    - Height: obtained from children older than 24 months who are able to stand
    - Alternative height measurements may be used for nonmobile children, such as knee height, arm span, and tibial length. Each measurement uses its respective equations to determine the child's height.
  - Weight
  - Head circumference, obtained on children <36 months of age
  - Mid-arm/mid-upper-arm circumference

- Weight/Length: measurement to determine proportionality in pediatric population <2 years old
- BMI: compares proportionality of weight for height in children >2 years old
- Mid-parental height: an equation that is not plotted on a growth chart but may be used to assist with determining children who have short stature versus children with stunted growth
- Evidence of loss of subcutaneous fat and muscle stores (Table 27.3)
- Poor-quality hair or alopecia
- Dull, dry eyes
- Dry, swollen lips and/or mouth
- Dry mucous membranes
- Magenta and edematous tongue
- Evidence of lesions or thrush in mouth
- Bleeding and inflamed gums
- Presence of dental caries
- Dry, scaly skin or dermatitis
- Abnormal nails: presence of transverse lines, flaky or poorly blanched (Corkins & Teague, 2017)

**TABLE 27.3 How to Evaluate Subcutaneous Fat, Muscle Stores, and Edema**

| Subcutaneous Fat | Special Tips | Severe Malnutrition | Moderate Malnutrition | Well Nourished |
|---|---|---|---|---|
| Facial cheeks (buccal pads) | Gently palpate pads over cheek | Hollow, narrow face | Flat | Full, round, filled out |
| Biceps and triceps | Arm bent; be careful not to include muscle; pinch fat stores and roll between fingers | Very little space between fingers, or fingers touch | Some space between fingers | Ample or thick fold of fat tissue between fingers |
| Ribs<br>– Lower back<br>– Midaxillary line | With child pressing hand against solid object | Depressions between the ribs very apparent | Ribs can be apparent. Depressions less pronounced | Chest is full, round; ribs do not show |
| Buttocks | Infant upright or child standing | Wasted, flat or "baggy." Skin may appear wrinkled | Slight curve but not round | Full, round |
| After examining all of these subcutaneous fat areas, subjectively rate the degree of fat loss. Is the amount of fat loss severe in each area? If yes, then the child should be placed in the severe category. If there is no subcutaneous fat loss, the child should be classified as normal. If the child shows some signs in some areas, but not others, the inconsistency would place the child in the moderate category. | | | | |
| **Muscle Wasting** | | | | |
| Clavicle | Look along line of the clavicle. The smaller the muscles' mass, the more prominent the bone | Protruding, prominent bone | Some protrusion | May be visible but not prominent |
| Shoulder (deltoid muscles) | Position arms at sides and look for prominent bones, shape | Shoulder-to-arm joint looks square. Bones prominent. Acromion protrusion quite prominent | Shoulders not square but acromion process may protrude slightly | Rounded, curved at junction between neck and shoulder and at shoulder joint. Able to grasp muscle tissue at shoulder joint |
| Scapula<br>– As the muscle groups around the scapula waste, this bone becomes more apparent | Look for prominent bones. Have child push hands forward against a solid object | Prominent, visible bone. Depressions above the scapula, between the scapula and the shoulder joint, and between the scapula and the spine | Degree of wasting variable, in both location and depth. Mild depressions or bone may show slightly in some but not all areas | Scapula bone is not prominent. No depressions around the bone |

(continued)

**TABLE 27.3 How to Evaluate Subcutaneous Fat, Muscle Stores, and Edema** (*continued*)

| | | | | |
|---|---|---|---|---|
| **Muscle Wasting** | | | | |
| Thigh (quadriceps muscle; Note: lower body is less sensitive to change) | Have child sit; prop leg up on low furniture. Grasp quads to differentiate amount of muscle tissue from amount of fat tissue | Quads can be significantly reduced (squeezed). Depression on inner thigh, obviously thin | Slight depressions along inner thigh, thin | Not able to reduce. Well rounded, no depressions |
| Knee | Knee propped as above | Knee bone is square and prominent, no muscle mass | Slight depressions along inner thigh, thin | Not able to reduce. Well rounded, no depressions |
| Calf (gastrocnemius muscle) | Grasp the calf muscle to determine amount of tissue | Definite tissue reduction. Thin, flat, no muscle definition | Some shape and firmness to tissue | "Bulb" shape, firm and well developed |
| After examining all of these muscle groups, subjectively rate the degree of wasting. Is the amount of muscle loss severe in all or most areas? If yes, the child should be placed in the severe category. If there is no muscle tissue loss, the child should be classified as normal. If the child shows signs in some areas but not others, the inconsistency would place the child in the moderate category. | | | | |
| **Edema** | | | | |
| Try to rule out causes other than malnutrition (renal, liver, heart)<br>– Ankle (mobile child), sacrum (activity-restricted child) | Press on middle to latter third or distal anterior surface of foot (or over sacrum) for 5 seconds to move fluid out of the subcutaneous tissue. Observe for pitting. | Rounded contour with a deep depression or pit that persists | Fairly normal to moderately swollen contour with a moderately deep pit that persists | Normal contour with a barely perceptible pit |

*Source*: From Secker, D. J., & Jeejeebhoy, K. N. (2012). How to perform subjective global nutritional assessment in children. *Journal of the Academy of Nutrition and Dietetics, 112*(3), 424–431.e6. https://doi.org/10.1016/j.jada.2011.08.039

**PRO TIP** Utilize all available evidence (including evidence of muscle loss and diminished fat stores), not just anthropometric values, to diagnose pediatric undernutrition/malnutrition.

## Laboratory/Diagnostic Testing

Laboratory tests to evaluate malnutrition are used in conjunction with the history and physical examination. These tests are useful to identify nutritional deficiencies associated with undernutrition before clinical findings are evident, to confirm the presence of nutrient deficiencies that are commonly seen with specific diseases, or to monitor recovery from malnutrition that occurs as a complication of illness.

- Hemoglobin and red blood cell indices: can be used to identify nutritional deficiencies of iron, folate, or vitamin B12 or with anemia of chronic disease
- Transthyretin (prealbumin) and albumin: markers of adequacy of the diet over the short and long term, respectively. Of note, these markers will not give an accurate representation of nutritional status in children with acute inflammatory response or diseases.
- Vitamin deficiencies, including vitamin D and vitamin B
- Mineral deficiencies
- Electrolyte deficiencies

## Differential Diagnosis

The differential diagnosis for malnutrition includes:

- Mechanical feeding difficulties (due to oromotor dysfunction, congenital anomalies, central nervous system damage, severe reflux)
- Psychiatric disorders (depression)
- Inflammatory bowel disease
- CD
- Cystic fibrosis
- Milk protein allergy
- Liver disease
- Chronic kidney disease
- Cardiac disease

- Genetic anomalies
- Metabolic disorders

## Treatment/Management Plan

Management of pediatric malnutrition varies depending on the severity of malnutrition and other underlying medical problems. Mild and moderate malnutrition can usually be managed in an outpatient setting by the child's primary care physician, which involves psychosocial support and education regarding a well-balanced diet depending on the child's age. If the child has moderate malnutrition or has an underlying medical disorder, a multidisciplinary approach may be warranted, including involvement of a dietitian to assist with formulating an appropriate nutritional plan. It is important to have regular follow-up visits to monitor weight gain.

For children with severe malnutrition, the initial management includes hospitalization with involvement of a multidisciplinary team including dietitian, social worker, nurses, occupational or speech therapists, child-life workers, and other medical subspecialists as needed. Inpatient management will allow for safe implementation of a feeding regimen, as a number of complications may occur with the introduction of feeds. These adverse side effects include malabsorption, diarrhea, or "refeeding" syndrome. Hospitalization will also allow for daily monitoring of catch-up growth and provide an environment for support and hands-on education for the family using an appropriate nutritional plan depending on the child's age.

### Nutritional Therapy

The mainstay treatment of pediatric malnutrition is nutritional therapy. This process includes determining a nutrition plan that takes into account the child's age, severity of malnutrition, estimated energy expenditure, and caloric, protein, fat, and fluid requirements that allow for catch-up growth. Strategies to increase intake include:

*Infants:*

- Increase caloric density of human milk by adding infant formula powder to pumped breast milk
- Supplement breastfeeding with infant formula
- Increase caloric density of formula by concentrating the formula or adding supplement

*Toddlers and older children:*

- Add rice cereal or formula powder to pureed foods to increase caloric density
- Add high-fat ingredients to meals, including cheese, butter, sour cream
- Vitamin and mineral supplementation

### *Management of Medical, Developmental, and Behavioral Factors*

Manage the following medical, developmental/behavioral, psychosocial, and pharmacologic factors associated with malnutrition:

- Medical: Recognize underlying medical conditions that may contribute to malnutrition and address as indicated
- Developmental and behavioral: A multidisciplinary approach will be most beneficial in the overall management of these children, including occupational therapists and referrals to developmental-behavioral pediatricians or behavioral psychologists
- Psychosocial support: Address any psychosocial needs and provide support as needed, including assistance by social workers or assistance with obtaining basic necessities (e.g., Women and Infants/Children [WIC] and the Supplemental Nutrition Assistance Program [SNAP, formerly known as the food stamp program])
- Pharmacologic treatment: Appetite stimulants may be considered in older children who have not exhibited adequate catch-up weight gain despite optimizing nutritional intake

ALERT: Once management for malnutrition has been initiated, some children may encounter refeeding syndrome. This is a potentially fatal syndrome in which the introduction of nutritional intake, usually in a severely malnourished child, causes electrolyte and fluid shifts. Findings include hypophosphatemia, hypokalemia, congestive heart failure, peripheral edema, rhabdomyolysis, seizures, and hemolysis. The risk of development usually occurs in the first 1–2 weeks of steady nutritional intake. Treatment involves decreasing the amount of nutritional intake, correcting electrolyte deficiencies, and managing its related abnormalities.

### Family Education

Teach the following:

- Importance of an optimal feeding environment, including:
  - Decreased consumption of excessive fluid intake (offer solids before liquids)
  - Limit sweetened or carbonated beverages
  - Limit junk foods, as these provide limited calories and protein

- Offer three meals and two–three snacks a day. Time snacks in between meals so as to not spoil mealtimes
- Mealtimes should be pleasant and positive for everyone
- Recognize hunger and satiety cues
- Try to eat together as a family and limit distractions during mealtimes

### Referral

Children who have an underlying diagnosis that is contributing to the child's malnourished state should be referred to the appropriate specialist that manages it. For example, if an infant is found to have a congenital heart condition while undergoing diagnostic workup for malnutrition, the infant should be referred to pediatric cardiology.

## METABOLIC SYNDROME

With the prevalence of adult and pediatric obesity on the rise globally, so is the concern for its comorbidities. Metabolic syndrome (MetS, also known as syndrome X, Reavan syndrome, "the deadly quartet," and insulin resistance syndrome) refers to a constellation of cardiometabolic risk factors associated with obesity that, when occurring together, increases the risk for development of CVD and type 2 diabetes mellitus in adults (Magge et al., 2017). These cardiometabolic risk factors include dyslipidemia, abnormal glucose regulation, central adiposity, and hypertension.

The primary treatment for MetS involves lifestyle modification through diet and exercise. However, it has been difficult to construct a set of clinical criteria to clinically define MetS in pediatrics. Instead, the AAP recommends that clinicians focus assessment and management on the clustering of the cardiometabolic risk factors (Magge et al., 2017).

Metabolic syndrome occurs in 0.2% to 38.9% of children with the following distribution:

- Mexican Americans 12.9%
- Non-Hispanic Whites 10.9%
- Non-Hispanic Blacks 2.5%
- Overweight/obese adolescents 31.2% (Al-Hamad & Raman, 2017; de Ferranti et al., 2004; Magge et al., 2017)

The pathophysiology of MetS is not fully understood, but the most widely accepted explanation stems from insulin resistance (Higgins & Adeli, 2017). Insulin is a hormone responsible for maintaining glucose homeostasis in various organs such as the liver, skeletal muscle, adipocytes, and pancreas. Once the liver is in an insulin-resistant state, there is no longer a control of glucose production;, thus hyperglycemia ensues (Magge et al., 2017). This in turn could lead to type 2 diabetes mellitus if not controlled. However, for undetermined reasons, the presence of insulin in the liver's lipogenesis is not impaired, which causes a release of free fatty acids and triglycerides, leading to dyslipidemia and adipose disposition.

Since the concept was first introduced in the 1980s, many organizations, including the WHO, the International Diabetes Foundation (IDF), the American Heart Association (AHA), and the National Heart, Lung, and Blood Institute (NHLBI), have introduced varying diagnostic criteria to define MetS (Alberti et al., 2009). In 2009, the IDF, AHA, NHLBI, and other organizations came together and proposed a universal set of clinical criteria in order to provide clinical providers a unified diagnostic definition (Table 27.4).

**TABLE 27.4 Criteria for Clinical Diagnosis of the Metabolic Syndrome in Adults**

| More than 3 of the following 5 criteria are required for a clinical diagnosis of MetS in adults: | |
|---|---|
| **Measure** | **Categorical Cut Points** |
| Elevated waist circumference | Population- and country-specific definitions<br>For United States: ≥102 cm for males; ≥88 cm for females (AHA/NHLBI) |
| Elevated triglycerides | ≥150 mg/dL (1.7 mmol/L)<br>or receiving treatment for elevated triglycerides |
| Reducing HDL-C | <40 mg/dL (1.0 mmol/L) in males;<br><50 mg/dL (1.3 mmol/L) in females<br>Or receiving treatment to reduce HDL-C |
| Elevated blood pressure | Systolic ≥130 and/or diastolic ≥ 85 mmHg<br>Or receiving antihypertensive treatment |
| Elevated fasting glucose | ≥100 mg/dL<br>Or receiving treatment for hyperglycemia |

*Source*: Data from Magge, S. N., Goodman, E., & Armstrong, S. C. (2017). The metabolic syndrome in children and adolescents: Shifting the focus to cardiometabolic risk factor clustering. *Pediatrics, 140*(2). https://doi.org/10.1542/peds.2017-1603

Unfortunately, unlike the adult counterparts, there is a lack of consensus on a clinical definition for the pediatric population. This is largely due to the fact that numerous physiological changes occur while children undergo growth and development. Reasons making it difficult to produce a pediatric definition for MetS include:

- Metabolism and weight gain can be affected by the increase in insulin resistance during puberty (Wittcopp & Conroy, 2016)
- Varying ranges of acceptable lipid values depend on age and race, so it is difficult to use a single set of criteria for a definition such as in adults (Lee & Sanders, 2012)
- Lack of consensus on defininge central adiposity, as the criteria for weight circumference vary with age (Lee & Sanders, 2012)

Despite the lack of definition of MetS in pediatrics, it is clear that obesity, CVD, and diabetes are on the rise in children and adolescents (Magge et al., 2017). Thus, the AAP has recommended a focus on the assessment and management of children relative to the cardiometabolic risk factors, which include obesity, hypertension, dyslipidemia, and hyperglycemia.

## Subjective Findings

Although MetS is a diagnosis largely based on physical and laboratory findings, it is still important to obtain a history from the parent and child (as age allows), which may reveal symptoms of any of its components. The health history may reveal:

- Family history of obesity, CVD, dyslipidemia, and insulin resistance
- Dietary history, including eating patterns, types of food consumed, mealtime schedule
- Sleep-disordered breathing (e.g., snoring, OSA, enlarged tonsils)
- Social history, including socioeconomic stressors (e.g., low income)
- Psychosocial history, including mental diseases, sexual or physical abuse, bullying
- Lack of physical activity

### Risk Factors

The most common risk factors for MetS in children are:

- Familial influences, including genetic and environmental factors
- Ethnicity
- Increased sedentary behavior (e.g., excessive screen time)
- Lack of physical activity
- Unbalanced dietary intake (lack of whole grain and fiber intake)
- Presence of maternal gestational diabetes
- Tobacco smoke exposure
- Abnormal sleep patterns (Steinberger et al., 2009)

### Review of Systems

The most common manifestations revealed during the review of systems include:

- **Constitutional:** change in activity, change in appetite, fatigue
- **Integumentary:** dry skin, changes in hair or nails, hirsutism, acne, acanthosis nigricans (especially around the neck and axillary regions)
- **HEENT:** blurry vision
- **Respiratory:** shortness of breath, apnea, snoring, wheezing
- **Cardiovascular:** palpitations, arrhythmia, swelling in the lower extremities
- **Gastrointestinal:** abdominal pain, reflux, constipation, nausea
- **Genitourinary:** dysmenorrhea
- **Musculoskeletal:** arthralgias, back pain, trouble walking
- **Neurologic:** headaches
- **Endocrine:** polydipsia, polyuria, polyphagia
- **Psychiatric:** anxiety, binge eating disorder, depression, teasing/bullying (Barlow & Expert Committee, 2007)

## Objective Findings

The physical examination of the child with MetS may reveal (Barlow & Expert Committee, 2007):

- Obesity: the gold standard in diagnosing obesity is to calculate the BMI and plot it on a standard growth curve
- Increased visceral adiposity
- Hypertension
- Acanthosis nigricans (darkened skin patches over the neck or armpits), excessive acne, hirsutism, irritation or inflammation
- Hepatomegaly
- Violaceous striae
- Papilledema
- Tonsillar hypertrophy
- Goiter
- Hepatomegaly
- Female: irregular menstrual cycles
- Male: apparent micropenis, undescended testes
- Abnormal gait or bowing of tibia

### Laboratory/Diagnostic Testing

The assessment for cardiometabolic risk factors is based upon clinical findings and laboratory testing. According to the evidence-based 2007 AAP guidelines, laboratory testing is recommended based on the child's BMI percentile and if there are any known risk factors for CVD:

- For children with a BMI between 5th to 84th percentile with no known risk factors, a nonfasting lipid profile should be obtained between ages of 9 and 11 and again between 18 and 21 to evaluate for genetic dyslipidemia.
- For those who are overweight (BMI 85%–94%) without risk factors, a lipid profile should be obtained.
- For children with BMI 85% to 94% *with* risk factors present, a fasting glucose, fasting lipid profile, and serum alanine transaminase and aspartate transaminase should be obtained.
- For children with BMI ≥95%, the same laboratory work should be done as above plus evaluation of blood urea nitrogen and creatinine (Daniels et al., 2008).

### Differential Diagnosis

The differential diagnosis for MetS includes:

- Sleep-disordered breathing
- Revovascular diseases (diseases of the arteries to the kidneys)
- Hyperglycemia due to glucocorticoid use
- Hormonal tumors
- Thyroid disorders (e.g., Graves disease, Hashimoto thyroiditis)
- Medication side effect

Comorbidities associated with MetS or conditions that may share overlapping features include:

- Nonalcoholic fatty liver disease: liver disease that can range in severity and involves intrahepatic fat accumulation
- Polycystic ovary syndrome: disorder that may be seen in obese, adolescent females, characterized by hyperandrogenism, menstrual dysfunction, or polycystic ovaries
- Sleep-disordered breathing, including OSA
- Gout
- Chronic kidney disease

### Treatment/Management Plan

Lifestyle modification targeting weight reduction or decrease in BMI is the mainstay treatment of MetS. This includes dietary modification and increased physical activity. In 2011, the NHLBI published an evidence-based recommendation for diet and nutrition that integrates positive cardiovascular health. Additionally, there are also behavioral modification programs available that may be beneficial for children. Overall focus of dietary modification involves decreasing total caloric consumption while maintaining an appropriate well-balanced diet (Expert Panel on Integrated Guidelines for Cardiovascular Health and Risk Reduction in Children and Adolescents, 2011).

In regard to physical activity, evidence shows that any movement that increases energy expenditure improves insulin sensitivity in children. There are a range of physical activities in which children may participate, but studies in adults show that aerobic activity has shown up to 30% reduction in MetS (Wittcopp & Conroy, 2016).

As MetS comprises multiple metabolic disorders, it is also important to treat each of these specific disorders. The NHLBI gave further recommendations on the treatment of hypertension, dyslipidemia, and insulin resistance (Wittcopp & Conroy, 2016). If lifestyle modifications are insufficient to produce results of weight reduction in adolescents and subsequent cardiometabolic risk factors, medications may be used as adjunct therapy to treat individual risk factors.

### Family Education

Teach the following:

- Limit intake of sugar-sweetened beverages.
- Encourage consumption of diet as outlined by the U.S. Department of Agriculture (www.mypyramid.gov).
- Encourage a diet that is high in fiber and calcium.
- Encourage exclusive breastfeeding to 6 months of age as recommended by the AAP and continue breastfeeding after introduction of solid food to 12 months and beyond.
- Eat a healthy breakfast daily.
- Limit eating out at restaurants and most especially at fast-food chains.
- Encourage family meals.
- Limit screen time. The AAP recommends no screen time for children <2 years of age and up to 2 hours per day for children older than 2 years old.
- Encourage moderate to vigorous physical activity for at least 60 minutes each day.

### Referral

Children with evidence of prediabetes or type 2 diabetes on screening should be referred to pediatric endocrinology, a registered dietitian/nutritionist specializing in children with diabetes mellitus, and/or a pediatric certified diabetes educator.

## OBESITY

Pediatric obesity poses a serious public health challenge for the United States and other countries around the world. Without intervention, obesity can lead to medical and psychological complications persisting into adulthood (WHO, 2017). Children who are obese are five times more likely to be obese as adults (Simmonds et al., 2016). In the United States, data from the 2015–2016 National Health and Nutrition Examination Survey (NHANES) showed that 18.5% of children and adolescents ages 2 to 19 years were obese, with a significant increase in the prevalence of severe obesity among children ages 2 to 5 years from the previous 2013–2014 NHANES cycle (Skinner et al., 2018).

Pediatric obesity is a complex disease that involves the interaction of genetic, biologic, environmental, and social factors affecting the physiology of energy regulation leading to positive energy balance and excess weight gain (Kohut et al., 2019; Kumar & Kelly, 2017). In 2007, the Expert Committee, made up of experienced scientists and clinicians as well as representatives of 15 professional organizations, issued a report that defined obesity in children 2 to 19 years old as BMI greater than 95th percentile, and overweight as BMI 85th to 94th percentile (Barlow & Expert Committee, 2007).

The majority of pediatric obesity cases is due to primary obesity that results from the complex interplay of genetic susceptibility and the environment (Kumar & Kelly, 2017). *Polygenic obesity* refers to multiple gene defects with modest effects that are amplified by lifestyle and environmental factors (Pigeyre et al., 2016). The obesogenic environment has been used to describe

**BOX 27.1 Genetic and Secondary Causes of Obesity**

| | |
|---|---|
| **Endocrine**<br>• Cushing syndrome<br>• Growth hormone deficiency<br>• Hypothyroidism<br>• Polycystic ovary syndrome (PCOS)<br>• Pseudohypoparathyroidism<br><br>**Neurologic**<br>• Traumatic brain injury (TBI)<br>• Brain or hypothalamic lesions<br>• History of brain surgery<br>• History of radiation<br>• ROHHAD/ROHHADNET* syndrome<br><br>**Medications**<br>• Antiepileptics<br>• Antidepressants<br>• Antipsychotics<br>• Glucocorticoids<br>• Gabapentin<br>• Migraine treatments<br>• Sulfonylureas | **Monogenic Obesity**<br>• Adenylate cyclase 3 (ADCY3)<br>• Brain-derived neurotrophic factor (BDNF)<br>• Kinase suppressor of ras 2 (KSR2)<br>• Leptin and leptin receptor (LEP, LEPR)<br>• Melanocortin 4 receptor (MCR4)<br>• Proopiomelanocortin (POMC)<br>• Proprotein convertase type 1 (PCSK1)<br>• Src homology 2B adaptor protein (SH2B1)<br><br>**Genetic Syndromes**<br>• Alström<br>• Albright hereditary osteodystrophy<br>• Bardet-Biedl<br>• Beckwith-Wiedemann<br>• Carpenter<br>• Cohen<br>• Prader-Willi<br>• 16p11.2 microdeletion<br><br>**Psychiatric**<br>• Depression<br>• Eating disorders |

*ROHHAD(T) = rapid onset obesity with hypothalamic dysfunction, hypoventilation, autonomic dysregulation (with neural crest tumors)

*Sources*: Data from Cuda, S. E., & Censani, M. (2019). Pediatric obesity algorithm: A practical approach to obesity diagnosis and management. *Frontiers in Pediatrics, 6*, 431. https://www.frontiersin.org/article/10.3389/fped.2018.00431; Fairbrother, U., Kidd, E., Malagamuwa, T., & Walley, A. (2018). Genetics of severe obesity. *Current Diabetes Reports, 18*(10), 85. https://doi.org/10.1007/s11892-018-1053-x; Hamed, S. A. (2015). Antiepileptic drugs influences on body weight in people with epilepsy. *Expert Review of Clinical Pharmacology, 8*(1), 103–114. https://doi.org/10.1586/17512433.2015.991716; Kumar, S., & Kelly, A. S. (2017). Review of childhood obesity: From epidemiology, etiology, and comorbidities to clinical assessment and treatment. *Mayo Clinic Proceedings, 92*(2), 251–265. https://doi.org/10.1016/j.mayocp.2016.09.017; Reekie, J., Hosking, S. P., Prakash, C., Kao, K. T., Juonala, M., & Sabin, M. A. (2015). The effect of antidepressants and antipsychotics on weight gain in children and adolescents. *Obesity Reviews, 16*(7), 566–580. https://doi.org/10.1111/obr.12284; Sheikh, A. B., Nasrullah, A., Haq, S., Akhtar, A., Ghazanfar, H., Nasir, A., Afzal, R. M., Bukhari, M. M., Chaudhary, A. Y., & Naqvi, S. W. (2017). The interplay of genetics and environmental factors in the development of obesity. *Cureus, 9*(7), e1435. https://doi.org/10.7759/cureus.1435

modern local environments that promote sedentary lifestyles and easy availability of high-calorie foods that contribute to obesity (Rendina et al., 2019).

Secondary causes of childhood obesity include potentially treatable underlying conditions that affect appetite, metabolism, and adipose distribution. Medical causes of obesity in children can include endocrinopathies, genetic syndromes, chronic conditions, and medications (Cuda & Censani, 2019; Greydanus et al., 2018). Monogenic obesity, caused by a single gene, is often associated with severe obesity and most of the genes involved relate to the leptin-melanocortin pathway (Cuda & Censani, 2019; Fairbrother et al., 2018; Greydanus et al., 2018; Thaker, 2017). Genetic and secondary causes of pediatric obesity can be found in Box 27.1.

## Subjective Findings

Clinic visits for all infants, children, and adolescents begin with a thorough history to identify children at risk or already meeting criteria for overweight or obesity, detect potential modifiable behaviors, and assess the child's and family's readiness for behavioral change (Hagan et al., 2017).

### Talking to Families About Obesity

Remaining nonjudgmental and sensitive to cultural and family perceptions is important when talking with families and children. Many parents do not accurately recognize their child as overweight or obese (Faircloth et al., 2019). Using sensitive language, discussing the facts, and using terms such as "unhealthy weight," acknowledging the complex etiology of obesity, refraining from placing blame, and emphasizing healthy habits in relation to healthy weight can help maintain a supportive therapeutic relationship with children and families (Faircloth et al., 2019; Hagan et al., 2017; Pont et al., 2017).

### Health History

Update child health histories regularly, reviewing for factors known to predispose the child to or associated with obesity (also refer to conditions in Box 27.1 or factors in Box 27.2 and Table 27.5). The health history may reveal:

**BOX 27.2 Potential Risk Factors for Obesity**

| Perinatal | Childhood behaviors |
|---|---|
| • Maternal obesity<br>• Maternal smoking during pregnancy<br>• Maternal excess gestational weight gain<br>• High birth weight<br>• Accelerated weight gain after birth | • Inadequate sleep<br>• Skipping breakfast<br>• Dietary pattern<br>• Drinking sugar-sweetened beverages<br>• Watching television while eating<br>• Watching television for >1–2 hours/day<br>• Inadequate physical activity |
| **Family** | **Other** |
| • Parental obesity<br>• Parental smoking<br>• Parental, family stress<br>• Family dysfunction<br>• Socioeconomic status (SES), household education level | • Personal stress, history of abuse<br>• Poor coping, junk food self-medication habits<br>• Race/ethnicity |

*Sources*: Data from Anderson, K. L. (2018). A review of the prevention and medical management of childhood obesity. *Child and Adolescent Psychiatric Clinics of North America, 27*(1), 63–76. https://doi.org/10.1016/j.chc.2017.08.003; Avery, A., Anderson, C., & McCullough, F. (2017). Associations between children's diet quality and watching television during meal or snack consumption: A systematic review. *Maternal and Child Nutrition, 13*(4), e12428. https://doi.org/10.1111/mcn.12428; Baidal, J. A. W., Locks, L. M., Cheng, E. R., Blake-Lamb, T. L., Perkins, M. E., & Taveras, E. M. (2016). Risk factors for childhood obesity in the first 1,000 days: A systematic review. *American Journal of Preventive Medicine, 50*(6), 761–779. https://doi.org/10.1016/j.amepre.2015.11.012; Brown, C. L., Halvorson, E. E., Cohen, G. M., Skelton, J. A., & Lazorick, S. (2015). Addressing childhood obesity: Opportunities for prevention. *Pediatric Clinics of North America, 67*(5), 1241–1261. https://doi.org/10.1016/j.pcl.2015.05.013; Daniels, S. R., Greer, F. R., & Committee on Nutrition. (2008). Lipid screening and cardiovascular health in childhood. *Pediatrics, 101*(1), 141. https://doi.org/10.1542/peds.2008-1349; Hemmingsson, E. (2018). Early childhood obesity risk factors: Socioeconomic adversity, family dysfunction, offspring distress, and junk food self-medication. *Current Obesity Reports, 7*(2), 204–209. https://doi.org/10.1007/s13679-018-0310-2; Heyman, M. B., Abrams, S. A., & Section on Gastroenterology, Hepatology, and Nutrition, Committee on Nutrition. (2017). Fruit juice in infants, children, and adolescents: Current recommendations. *Pediatrics, 139*(6), e20170967. https://doi.org/10.1542/peds.2017-0967; Poorolajal, J., Sahraei, F., Mohamdadi, Y., Doosti-Irani, A., & Moradi, L. (2020). Behavioral factors influencing childhood obesity: A systematic review and meta-analysis. *Obesity Research & Clinical Practice, 14*(2), 109–118. https://doi.org/10.1016/j.orcp.2020.03.002; Sanyaolu, A., Okorie, C., Qi, X., Locke, J., & Rehman, S. (2019). Childhood and adolescent obesity in the United States: A public health concern. *Global Pediatric Health*. https://doi.org/10.1177/2333794X19891305; Williams, A. S., Ge, B., Petroski, G., Kruse, R. L., McElroy, J. A., & Koopman, R. J. (2018). Socioeconomic status and other factors associated with childhood obesity. *The Journal of the American Board of Family Medicine, 31*(4), 514–521. https://doi.org/10.3122/jabfm.2018.04.170261.

TABLE 27.5 **Potential Underlying Etiologies or Associated Comorbidities for Obesity Based on Symptoms**

| Symptom | Potential Etiology of Comorbidity |
|---|---|
| Daytime sleepiness, snoring, apnea, nocturnal enuresis | Sleep disorder |
| Anxiety, isolation, school avoidance | Depression, bullying |
| Severe recurrent headaches, blurred vision, nausea, vomiting | Pseudotumor cerebri |
| Wheezing, shortness of breath | Asthma, physical deconditioning |
| Polyuria, polydipsia, nocturia | Type 2 diabetes mellitus (T2DM), insulin resistance |
| Weight loss | Type 2 diabetes mellitus (T2DM), insulin resistance, eating disorder |
| Hyperphagia | Genetic syndrome (e.g., Prader-Willi), hypothalamic pituitary lesion |
| Abdominal pain, indigestion | Gastroesophageal reflux disease (GERD), constipation, gallbladder disease, Non-alcoholic fatty liver disease (NAFLD) |
| Binge eating, loss of control eating, food restriction, self-induce vomiting | Eating disorder |
| Fatigue and muscle aches | Vitamin D deficiency |
| Hip and/or knee pain, limp | Slipped capital femoral epiphysis, Blount's disease, stress on weight-bearing joints |
| Irregular menses or amenorrhea | Polycystic ovary syndrome (PCOS), genetic syndrome |

*Sources*: Data from Barlow, S. E., & Expert Committee. (2007). Expert Committee recommendations regarding the prevention, assessment, and treatment of child and adolescent overweight and obesity: Summary report. *Pediatrics, 120*(Suppl. 4), S164–S192. https://doi.org/10.1542/peds.2007-2329C; Cuda, S. E., & Censani, M. (2019). Pediatric obesity algorithm: A practical approach to obesity diagnosis and management. *Frontiers in Pediatrics, 6*, 431. https://www.frontiersin.org/article/10.3389/fped.2018.00431; Kumar, S., & Kelly, A. S. (2017). Review of childhood obesity: From epidemiology, etiology, and comorbidities to clinical assessment and treatment. *Mayo Clinic Proceedings, 92*(2), 251–265. https://doi.org/10.1016/j.mayocp.2016.09.017

- Family history: First- and second-degree relatives with obesity or comorbidities (e.g., cardiovascular disease, hyperlipidemia, type 2 diabetes mellitus, hypertension, liver or gallbladder disease, sleep apnea)
- Medical and surgical history: Developmental history; medications; neurologic or psychologic disorders; hypertension or insulin resistance; cholecystectomy or tonsillectomy
- Dietary history: Routinely consumed food and beverages; portion sizes, fat content of milk, daily volume of sugar-sweetened beverages, juice, and water; typical eating patterns and settings
- Physical activity: Duration and types of physical activity and nonhomework sedentary behaviors
- Sleep history:- Sleep duration and quality, snoring or daytime sleepiness (Kumar & Kelly, 2017)
- Psychosocial history: Socioeconomic and family stressors; sexual or physical abuse (Hemmingsson, 2018); anxiety, depression, low self-esteem, and experience being bullied or socially isolated (Pont et al., 2017)

## Risk Factors

In addition to genetic and medical conditions, demographic, environmental, and behavioral factors can contribute to a higher risk of developing obesity. Awareness of these factors, along with demographic features, can help clinicians identify children at risk for obesity and provide important preventive and treatment strategies.

### *Prenatal and Perinatal Factors*

Higher pre-pregnancy BMI, maternal smoking, excess gestational weight gain, high infant birth weight, and accelerated infant weight gain have been associated with later childhood obesity, whereas breastfeeding may be protective against developing obesity (Baidal et al., 2016; Ortega-García et al., 2018; Rito et al., 2019).

### *Demographic Factors/Prevalence*

The prevalence of pediatric obesity and severe obesity increases with advancing age and is higher in Hispanic and non-Hispanic black youth than non-Hispanic white and Asian youth (Skinner et al., 2018). Nearly half of Hispanic children were overweight or obese according to NHANES 2015–2016 data, and Native American children may have almost double the odds of being overweight or obese compared with white children

(Skinner et al., 2018; Williams et al., 2018). From 2013 to 2016, the prevalence of obesity was similar across levels of urbanization, but severe obesity was higher in less urbanized areas (Ogden, Fryar et al., 2018).

Association of levels of income and childhood obesity is complex and varies by sex and race/ethnicity. For example, prevalence of obesity among non-Hispanic black females did not differ by income level, whereas obesity was lower in the highest income groups for Hispanic, non-Hispanic white, and non-Hispanic Asian females (Ogden, Carroll et al., 2018). Obesity and prevalence of severe obesity are more consistent across race/ethnicity groups in relation to education of the head of household, with prevalence of obesity decreased with a higher level of education of the head of the household (Ogden, Carroll et al., 2018).

### *Environment, Nutrition, and Lifestyle Factors*

Potentially modifiable factors that can lead to energy imbalance and increased risk for becoming overweight or obese continue to be studied (Box 27.2).

### Review of Systems

Reviewing systems is important for assessing children for comorbidities associated with obesity or medical etiologies of obesity (see Table 27.5).

## Objective Findings

The clinical examination should be directed at identifying overweight or obese children and identifying the cause or related condition. Weight-for-length (WFL) for infants should be plotted on growth charts and BMI should be measured and plotted at least annually for children 2 years and older (Hagan et al., 2017). Most obese children have consistent or accelerated linear growth; thus, overweight or obese children with poor linear growth, deceleration of growth, or short stature should be evaluated for rare endocrinopathies or genetic syndromes (Cuda & Censani, 2019; Greydanus et al., 2018). Children with obesity related to a genetic syndrome usually have hyperphagia and coexisting dysmorphic features, developmental and cognitive delay, short stature, and hearing and vision impairment (Pigeyre et al., 2016). Physical examination findings suggestive of etiologies or comorbid conditions are included in Table 27.6.

Detailed body composition measurements are not feasible in a clinical setting, thus other anthropometric measures are used as a proxy and screening tool for adiposity and weight status in infants, children, adolescents, and adults. BMI is an anthropometric index of body weight adjusted for height that is generally used to classify overweight and obesity (Tyson & Frank, 2018). BMI is calculated by dividing weight in kilograms by the height in meters squared (Sanyaolu et al., 2019). For children and adolescents, the WHO developed child growth standards that include length/height-for-age, weight-for-age, weight-for-length/height, and BMI-for-age (WHO Multicentre Growth Reference Study Group, 2006). Overall, these standards have been adopted worldwide for child growth assessment and monitoring (de Onis et al., 2012).

### Infants and Children Younger Than 24 Months

In the United States, the WHO weight-for-length (WFL) is the standard anthropometric measurement for infants and children younger than 2 years of age (Daniels et al., 2015; Grummer-Strawn et al., 2010). The WHO charts establish growth parameters for infants in optimal conditions and predominantly breastfed for at least 4 months (Grummer-Strawn et al., 2010). In this age group, there is not a consensus definition for obesity. WFL greater than the 95th percentile or persistently climbing across percentiles rather than maintaining growth along the same percentile are indicators for overweight (Barlow & Expert Committee, 2007; Cuda & Censani, 2019; Styne et al., 2017).

### Children and Adolescents Ages 2–20 Years

Adiposity varies with age and sex during childhood and adolescence; therefore, the norms for BMI vary by age and sex. The CDC BMI-for-age and sex charts published in 2000 are the standard tools used to assess weight status for children and adolescents between the ages of 2 and 20 years (Kuczmarski et al., 2002). The following BMI percentile ranges are used for pediatric weight classification (CDC, 2018; Skinner et al., 2018):

- Underweight: BMI less than 5th percentile for age and gender
- Normal or healthy weight: BMI 5th to 84th percentile for age and gender
- Overweight: BMI >85th to 94th percentile for age and gender
- Obesity (Class I): BMI >95th percentile for age and gender
- Severe obesity
  - Class II Obesity: BMI >120% of the 95th percentile or BMI >35 (whichever is lowest) for age and gender
  - Class III Obesity: BMI >140% of the 95th percentile or BMI 40 (whichever is lowest) for age and gender

**TABLE 27.6 Examination Findings and Possible Related Underlying Etiology or Comorbidity for Obesity**

| Body System | Exam Finding Short Stature | Possible Etiology or Comorbidity |
|---|---|---|
| Vital Signs | Elevated blood pressure<br>Short stature | Hypertension<br>Endocrinopathy, genetic syndrome |
| Skin, Hair, Nails | Acanthosis nigricans<br>Severe acne<br>Hirsutism<br>Violaceous striae<br>Intertrigo<br>Dry, coarse hair, brittle nails<br>Dorsal finger calluses | Type 2 diabetes mellitus, insulin resistance<br>PCOS<br>PCOS, Cushing syndrome<br>Cushing syndrome<br>Severe obesity<br>Hypothyroidism<br>Self-induced vomiting |
| Eyes | Papilledema, optic disc blurred<br>Nystagmus | Pseudotumor cerebri<br>Hypothalamic injury |
| HENT | Microcephaly<br>Dysmorphic features<br>Goiter<br>Tonsillar hypertrophy, neck circumference | Genetic disorder (e.g., Cohen)<br>Genetic disorder<br>Hypothyroidism<br>Obstructive sleep apnea |
| Chest | Wheeze | Asthma |
| Abdomen | Tenderness<br>Hepatomegaly | GERD, NAFLD, gallbladder disease<br>NAFLD |
| Genitourinary | Tanner stage<br>Apparent micropenis<br>Undescended testes | Premature puberty<br>May be normal due to adiposity<br>Genetic syndrome (e.g., Prader-Willi) |
| Extremities | Abnormal gait, limited hip range of motion<br>Bowing of tibia<br>Small hands, feet; polydactyly | Slipped capital femoral epiphysis<br>Blount disease<br>Genetic syndrome (e.g., Bardet-Biedel, Prader-Willi) |
| Psychosocial | Flat affect, withdrawn | Depression |

GERD, gastroesophageal reflux disease; NAFLD, nonalcoholic fatty liver disease; PCOS, polycystic ovarian syndrome.

*Sources:* Data from Barlow, S. E., & Expert Committee. (2007). Expert Committee recommendations regarding the prevention, assessment, and treatment of child and adolescent overweight and obesity: Summary report. *Pediatrics, 120*(Suppl. 4), S164–S192. https://doi.org/10.1542/peds.2007-2329C; Cuda, S. E., & Censani, M. (2019). Pediatric obesity algorithm: A practical approach to obesity diagnosis and management. *Frontiers in Pediatrics, 6*, 431. https://www.frontiersin.org/article/10.3389/fped.2018.00431; Kumar, S., & Kelly, A. S. (2017). Review of childhood obesity: From epidemiology, etiology, and comorbidities to clinical assessment and treatment. *Mayo Clinic Proceedings, 92*(2), 251–265. https://doi.org/10.1016/j.mayocp.2016.09.017

## Laboratory/Diagnostic Testing

Obesity is a clinical diagnosis. Although there is no consensus on routine laboratory testing for children with obesity, screening for associated comorbidities is recommended.

- Type 2 diabetes mellitus screening: The American Diabetes Association recommends testing children after the onset of puberty or age >10 years who are overweight or obese and have at least 1 additional risk factor (maternal history of diabetes or gestational diabetes during the child's gestation; family history of type 2 diabetes mellitus in first- or second-degree relative; race/ethnicity Native American, African American, Latino, Asian American or Pacific Islander; signs of or conditions associated with insulin resistance). A fasting blood glucose level, 2-hour plasma glucose 75 g oral glucose tolerance test or A1c level may be used for screening (Arslanian et al., 2018).
- CVD risk factor screening: BP is usually measured annually starting at age 3 years; for obese children, BP should be measured at each visit to screen for hypertension (BP 95th percentile at three different visits; Flynn et al., 2017). The Expert Panel on Integrated Guidelines for Cardiovascular Health and Risk Reduction in Children and Adolescents (2011) recommends universal lipid screening for children between the ages of 9 and 11 years and again for adolescents and young adults ages 17 to 21 years regardless of weight or CVD risk factors. For children

with obesity, the AHA recommends yearly screening with a nonfasting lipid profile followed by fasting lipid profile for abnormal initial screening (de Ferranti et al., 2019).

- Nonalcoholic fatty liver disease (NAFLD) screening: The Expert Committee on NAFLD and North American Society of Pediatric Gastroenterology, Hepatology and Nutrition (NASPGHAN) recommend screening using the alanine aminotransferase test beginning at age 9 to 11 years in children who are obese or who are overweight with additional risk factors (insulin resistance; prediabetes or diabetes; sleep apnea; family history of NAFLD/nonalcoholic steatohepatitis (NASH); dyslipidemia; central adiposity). Children with severe obesity, family history of NAFLD/NASH, or hypopituitarism may be screened before age 9 years (Vos et al., 2017).
- Pseudotumor cerebri (Faz et al., 2010).
- Obstructive sleep apnea (Marcus et al., 2012).
- Polycystic ovarian syndrome (PCOS; Anderson et al., 2014).

## Differential Diagnosis

The differential diagnosis for obesity includes:

- Hypothyroidism
- Growth hormone deficiency
- Fatty liver
- Cushing syndrome
- PCOS (Crocker & Yanovski, 2009)

## Treatment/Management Plan

### Prevention

Obesity prevention at the society and community levels includes advocacy for changing the obesogenic environment, providing safe environments for children to play and engage in organized or unorganized physical activity, and providing food security and developing school programs offering education, physical education, and healthy school meals (Anderson, 2018; Barlow & Expert Committee, 2007; Styne et al., 2017).

- Primary prevention should be family-oriented, begin in infancy and target all children (Barlow & Expert Committee, 2007; Brown et al., 2015).
- Secondary prevention for children who are overweight or identified as at high risk for obesity may need an individualized approach to reduce risk (Brown & Perrin, 2018; Taylor et al., 2016).

Providing education and anticipatory guidance to parents and children about nutrition and healthy eating and lifestyle behaviors is key to preventing obesity (Brown & Perrin, 2018; Sanyaolu et al., 2019). Clinicians should encourage parents to model healthy behaviors; families may need to make changes for the entire household to help children maintain a healthy weight.

Motivational interviewing has been used in the primary care setting for the prevention and management of pediatric obesity (Resnicow et al., 2015). Motivational interviewing is a child-centered communication style in which providers utilize techniques such as reflective listening, open-ended questions, expressions of acceptance and affirmation, and eliciting change-talk to help children and parents identify their motivation to change and implement a plan of action (Desai, 2019; Resnicow et al., 2015). Additional research is needed to determine the clinical significance, feasibility, and generalized applicability of using motivational interviewing for long-term weight management (Enö Persson et al., 2017; Resnicow et al., 2015; Vallabhan et al., 2018). Box 27.3 lists behaviors that clinicians can recommend for promotion of healthy nutrition and energy balance to prevent childhood obesity.

### Treatment

Treatment for pediatric obesity consists of lifestyle and behavior modification to decrease caloric intake, decrease in sedentary behaviors, and increase in physical activity. Pharmacotherapy and weight loss surgery are reserved for severe obesity in adolescents. Strategies depend on the age of the child and degree of obesity and can be tailored to modifiable behaviors and factors identified in the assessment of the child. In general, guiding principles involve:

- Family- and child-based interventions (Styne et al., 2017; Tyson & Frank, 2018)
  - Focus on adoption of healthy lifestyle habits and healthy diets for long-term changes (Brown & Perrin, 2018)
  - Multicomponent interventions that include dietary and physical activity education and modification (Styne et al., 2017)
  - Referral to comprehensive multidisciplinary pediatric clinics for children with severe obesity and comorbidities who need intensive therapy and may benefit from weight loss surgery (Taylor et al., 2016)

## BOX 27.3 Healthy Habits to Promote a Healthy Weight

**Infancy to 24 months**

Encourage exclusive breastfeeding for 6 months and continue breastfeeding as foods are introduced, with continuation of breastfeeding for 1 year or longer
No juice or sugar-sweetened beverages before age 12 months
Limit juice (100% fruit juice) intake to 4 ounces per day for children 12–24 months; no sugar-sweetened beverages
Whole milk starting at age 12 months until age 24 months; can use reduced-fat milk for children with concern for or family history of obesity and comorbidities
No television or screen time before age 24 months*
Allow infants to move freely, have tummy time and toddlers to have free play time

**Children and Adolescents**

**Diet and Nutrition**
Eat breakfast every day
Provide age-appropriate serving sizes for meals and snacks
Transition to low fat or fat free milk after age 2 years
Encourage nutrient-rich foods
Limit high-fat, calorie-dense, nutrient-poor foods (candy, chips, desserts)
Limit eating at restaurants or fast-food restaurants

**100% Fruit Juice and Sugar Sweetened Beverages**
Limit fruit juice to 4 ounces/day for toddlers ages 1–3 years
Limit fruit juice to 4–6 ounces/day for children ages 4–6 years
Limit fruit juice to 8 ounces/day for children and adolescents ages 7–18 years
Avoid or limit other sugar sweetened beverages like sodas, sports drinks, sugar-added juices

**Physical and Sedentary Activity**
Children ages 3–5 years: aim for 3 hours a day of physical activity
Children 6–12 years: at least 60 minutes of moderate to vigorous physical activity per day and muscle- and bone-strengthening activities 3 days a week (jumping, climbing, push-ups, running)
Limit television and screen time to 1 hour per day for ages 2–5 years
No televisions or other types of screens in bedrooms
Avoid eating meals or snacking while watching television

**Other Lifestyle Behaviors**
Promote healthy sleeping habits
Encourage family mealtimes without distractions
Keep healthy foods easily available
Purchase healthy food choices

*The AAP recommends that, for children 18–24 months, parents should choose high-quality programs and use screen devices with the child.

*Sources*: Data from American Academy of Pediatrics. (2018). *Children and media tips from the American Academy of Pediatrics.* http://www.aap.org/en-us/about-the-aap/aap-press-room/news-features-and-safety-tips/Pages/Children-and-Media-Tips.aspx; American Academy of Pediatrics. (2020). *Where we stand: Screen time.* https://www.healthychildren.org/English/family-life/Media/Pages/Where-We-Stand-TV-Viewing-Time.aspx; Anderson, K. L. (2018). A review of the prevention and medical management of childhood obesity. *Child and Adolescent Psychiatric Clinics of North America, 27*(1), 63–76. https://doi.org/10.1016/j.chc.2017.08.003; Centers for Disease Control and Prevention. (2018). *Defining childhood obesity: BMI for children and teens.* https://www.cdc.gov/obesity/childhood/defining.html; Centers for Disease Control and Prevention. (2020a). *How much physical activity do children need? Physical activity/CDC.* https://www.cdc.gov/physicalactivity/basics/children/index.htm; Centers for Disease Control and Prevention. (2020b). *Tips for parents—Ideas to help children maintain a healthy weight.* https://www.cdc.gov/healthyweight/children/index.html; Daniels, S. R., Greer, F. R., & Committee on Nutrition. (2008). Lipid screening and cardiovascular health in childhood. *Pediatrics, 101*(1), 141. https://doi.org/10.1542/peds.2008-1349; Hagan, J. F. J., Shaw, J. S., Duncan, P. M., & American Academy of Pediatrics. (2017). *Bright futures: Guidelines for health supervision of infants, children, and adolescents* (4th ed.). Bright Futures/American Academy of Pediatrics; Heyman, M. B., Abrams, S. A., & Section on Gastroenterology, Hepatology, and Nutrition, Committee on Nutrition. (2017). Fruit juice in infants, children, and adolescents: Current recommendations. *Pediatrics, 139*(6), e20170967. https://doi.org/10.1542/peds.2017-0967; Holt, K., Wooldridge, N., Story, M., & Sofka, D. (2011). *Bright futures nutrition* (3rd ed.). American Academy of Pediatrics; Styne, D. M., Arslanian, S. A., Connor, E. L., Farooqi, I. S., Murad, M. H., Silverstein, J. H., & Yanovski, J. A. (2017). Pediatric obesity—Assessment, treatment, and prevention: An Endocrine Society clinical practice guideline. *The Journal of Clinical Endocrinology & Metabolism, 102*(3), 709–757. https://doi.org/10.1210/jc.2016-2573

- The AAP recommends a stepwise approach for management with children, starting at the least intensive stage and advancing through the stages depending on response to treatment (Barlow & Expert Committee, 2007):
  - Stage 1 (Prevention Plus): Specific dietary or activity interventions provided by the primary care provider with the goal of positive behavior change and maintenance or improvement in BMI.
  - Stage 2 (Structured Weight Management): Similar focus on behaviors targeted in Stage 1 with increased support and structure, including more frequent visits and involvement of a dietitian with the same goals which, if not achieved in 3 to 6 months, results in an advance to the next stage.
  - Stage 3 (Comprehensive Multidisciplinary Intervention): Intensive and structured behavior modification requiring parental participation and weekly visits with a multidisciplinary team with expertise in pediatric obesity (dietitians, counselors, exercise therapist), usually requiring referral to a weight management program. If the goal BMI is not achieved in 3 to 6 months, consider advancing to the next stage.
  - Stage 4 (Tertiary Care Intervention): For severely obese children or children who have not achieved goals advancing through the first three stages, referral to a pediatric weight management center for the addition of medical diets, medication, or weight loss surgery to the therapy plan.
- Weight loss goals are determined by age and degree of obesity; some children may need to maintain weight, as BMI will decrease with growth in height. Guidelines for weight loss include:
  - For children younger than age 2 years, weight loss interventions are not recommended. Clinicians can help parents implement healthy habits to promote a healthy weight and prevent obesity.
  - Children ages 2 to 5 years should not lose more than 1 pound per month.
  - Children and adolescents older than age 5 years should not lose more than 2 pounds per month (Hagan et al., 2017).

### Health Promotion Guidelines

Although no consensus exists for a single formula for an ideal lifestyle modification intervention to treat pediatric obesity, common behavior-modification techniques include self-monitoring, motivational interviewing, positive reinforcement, goal setting, stimulus control, coping skills training, and prevention of relapse (Rijks et al., 2015; Zolotarjova et al., 2018). The U.S. Preventive Services Task Force found that multicomponent, intensive behavioral interventions with at least 26 contact hours over a period of 6 to 12 months resulted in weight loss, and interventions with 52 or more contact hours resulted in greater weight loss and improvement in metabolic and cardiovascular risk factors. Interventions involved both parents and children, including individual and group sessions (US Preventive Services Task Force et al., 2017). Information technology and mobile applications for health promotion can also assist with behavior change, although further research is needed to determine the effectiveness for treatment and prevention of childhood obesity (Schoeppe et al., 2017; Sutherland et al., 2019).

### Pharmacologic Therapy

Pharmacologic treatment is limited for pediatrics. Weight loss medications function by reducing appetite and caloric intake, increasing energy expenditure, or decreasing fat absorption (Pilitsi et al., 2019). Pharmacotherapy should only be used as an adjunct for adolescents with severe obesity or overweight with severe comorbidities that persist despite intensive lifestyle modification therapy, and children should be closely followed by a multidisciplinary team (Ryder et al., 2018; Srivastava et al., 2019; Styne et al., 2017). The Endocrine Society Clinical Guidelines Subcommittee Task Force recommends against using pharmacotherapy in adolescents younger than age 16 years who are overweight but not obese (Styne et al., 2017). Further research on the safety and efficacy of pharmacologic therapy will guide future options for therapy for severe pediatric obesity. FDA-approved and non-FDA–approved medications for pediatric obesity include:

- Orlistat: The only FDA-approved weight loss medication for adolescents 12 to 16 years old; inhibits gastric and pancreatic lipases, thus reducing fat absorption; can produce a small amount of weight loss but associated with common gastrointestinal side effects (Cuda & Censani, 2019).
- Phentermine: A noradrenergic appetite suppressant FDA-approved for short-term therapy (about 12 weeks) in adolescents and adults older than 16 years of age (Srivastava et al., 2019).
- Metformin: FDA-approved to treat Type 2 diabetes mellitus in children ages 10 years and older; has been used off-label for weight loss but is not FDA-approved as a weight loss medication (Srivastava et al., 2019).
- Topiramate: Primarily used as an antiepileptic medication, it has been used off-label for weight loss and binge eating disorder (Srivastava et al., 2019).

- Phentermine/topiramate: FDA-approved for obesity in adults older than age 18 years.
- Liraglutide: A glucagon-like 1 receptor agonist used for weight loss in adults, has been used off-label for adolescents (Srivastava et al., 2019).

### *Surgery*

Metabolic and bariatric surgery (MBS) is safe and effective for children with severe obesity (class II or class III obesity) and comorbidities that persist despite intensive lifestyle therapy with or without pharmacotherapy (Armstrong et al., 2019). MBS can provide sustained weight loss and improvement or resolution of comorbid diseases (Ahn, 2020; Inge et al., 2016). Three common weight loss procedures include the Roux-en-Y gastric bypass, vertical sleeve gastrectomy, and adjustable gastric band. Vertical sleeve gastrectomy is the most common operation in adults and adolescents and involves removal of about 80% of the stomach, creating a gastric sleeve resulting in appetite suppression and enhanced satiety (Bolling et al., 2019; Pratt et al., 2018). In Roux-en-Y gastric bypass, a small pouch in the upper stomach is created and connected directly to the second portion of the small intestine, thereby altering appetite, satiety, and absorption (Bolling et al., 2019). The adjustable gastric bypass is a reversible procedure in which a silicone band is placed around the proximal portion of the stomach that can be adjusted to control the size of the pouch, limiting food intake without affecting satiety; it is approved for children age 18 years and older and is not the preferred procedure for adolescents seeking satiety (Bolling et al., 2019; Pratt et al., 2018). Some of the risks and complications associated with these surgeries include surgical site infections, micronutrient deficiencies, and potential need for reoperation due to conditions such as anastomosis leak, strictures, gallstones, or intestinal obstruction (Bolling et al., 2019; Pratt et al., 2018).

Although these surgeries are effective, barriers such as provider understanding of the role of MBS for severe obesity, unsubstantiated exclusion criteria, access to appropriate care, and inadequate insurance coverage prevent eligible children from receiving these surgeries. The AAP recommends that providers identify pediatric patients with severe obesity who meet criteria for weight loss surgery and refer them to high-quality multidisciplinary centers experienced in pediatric metabolic and bariatric surgery programs. The adolescent child must be included in the decision-making process, with realistic discussions about the risks and benefits of the procedures, expected outcomes, and postoperative care requirements (Armstrong et al., 2019).

Indications for MBS in adolescents ages 10 to 19 years according to the 2018 American Society for Metabolic and Bariatric Surgery (AMSBS) guidelines include:

- BMI >35 kg/m$^2$ or 120% of the 95th percentile with clinically significant comorbidities (obstructive sleep apnea [OSA], hypertension, pseudotumor cerebri, T2DM, NAFLD, Blount's disease, slipped capital femoral epiphysis, depressed quality of life [QOL])
- BMI >40 kg/m$^2$ or >40% of the 95th percentile (whichever is lower)
- Disability, Tanner stage or bone age, history of mental illness or eating disorders that are treated, unstable family environments, or history of trauma/abuse should not be considered absolute contraindications, but warrant thorough discussion and consideration with a multidisciplinary team
- Ability and motivation for the child and family to adhere to recommendations for preoperative and postoperative care (Pratt et al., 2018)

Contraindications for MBS include:

- Medically correctable cause of obesity
- Ongoing substance abuse problem (within preceding 1 year)
- Medical, psychiatric, psychosocial, or cognitive condition that prevents adherence to postoperative dietary and medication regimens
- Current or planned pregnancy within 12 to 18 months of the procedure(Pratt et al., 2018)

As new technologies and procedures are developed and as MBS is performed for adolescents, studies will continue to evaluate optimal timing for surgery, perioperative effects, and long-term outcomes of these procedures.

## Family Education

Teach the following:

In addition to the prevention and management strategies outlined, providing easy-to-understand educational materials and resources can help educate and reinforce guidance delivered in the office setting:

- AAP Institute for Healthy Childhood Weight www.ihcw.aap.org
- AAP Healthy Active Living for Families www.aap.org/en-us/advocacy-and-policy/aap-health-initiatives/HALF-Implementation-Guide/Pages/HALF-Implementation-Guide.aspx
- AAP Healthychildren.org

- ChooseMyPlate.gov
- Dietary Guidelines for Americans at HHS.gov
- CDC website for overweight, obesity, and physical activity tools
- Traffic Light system for food choices https://heas.health.vic.gov.au/healthy-choices/guidelines/traffic-light-system
- WHO Commission on Ending Childhood Obesity www.who.int/end-childhood-obesity/en/

### Referral

Children who do not respond to brief clinical interventions in the primary care center or have severe obesity and comorbidities require multidisciplinary care or referral to tertiary care centers or specialized weight management programs. Families or children with unhealthy intrafamily communication patterns or psychosocial comorbidities may need referral to counseling or psychiatric care.

> **PRO TIP** Caring for a child or adolescent with an obesity diagnosis typically requires the support of multiple members of the healthcare team over an extended period of time. Support is important for the child as well as the parent(s) and potentially for primary caregivers.

## KEY POINTS

- Lactose intolerance results from a deficiency in lactase resulting in numerous GI symptoms.
- Lactose intolerance is not an allergy and may be managed with avoidance of lactose-containing foods.
- Food allergy is mainly an IgE-mediated response to an allergenic food, resulting in itching, swelling, and potentially anaphylaxis.
- Avoidance of the offending foods prevents the allergic reaction from occurring.
- CD is an autoimmune inflammatory disorder of the small intestine, triggered by gluten in genetically susceptible individuals, that has multiple manifestations.
- Diagnosis of CD in pediatric patients requires clinical suspicion or belonging to a high-risk group, CD-specific antibody serology testing, genetic testing in certain circumstances, duodenal histology for some children, and response to a gluten-free diet.
- Children with positive CD-specific serology testing and abnormal duodenal histologic changes should be started on a gluten-free diet, which may result in symptom resolution.
- Children with CD should be followed by a pediatric gastroenterologist and a dietitian.
- Early recognition of undernutrition/malnutrition, using a variety of data types, is key to improving outcomes in children.
- Pediatric undernutrition/malnutrition may be related to illness (or injury), or non-illness, such as in the case of environmental/behavioral factors.
- Watch for risk factors and symptoms of MetS in order to diagnose and treat early.
- Accurate interpretation of anthropometric assessment data requires use of the most appropriate growth graphs, considering age, gender, condition, and ethnicity. Use of z-scores for comparison with norms is now standard practice.
- Pediatric obesity is a complex disease that involves the interaction of genetic, biologic, environmental, behavioral, and social factors and without intervention can lead to medical and psychological complications persisting into adulthood.
- Assessment of obese children involves evaluation for possible etiologies (although rare) such as endocrinopathies, genetic syndromes, or chronic medical conditions and identification of comorbidities associated with obesity.
- Prevention begins in infancy, consisting of counseling about healthy nutrition and physical activity, regularly monitoring weight at clinic visits, and providing guidance to reduce risk behaviors that contribute to the development of obesity.
- Treatment for pediatric obesity requires lifestyle modifications to decrease caloric intake and increase physical activity. The AAP recommends a staged approach with management that begins in the primary care office. No single intervention exists; strategies require tailored interventions for specific targeted behaviors according to age of the child, degree of obesity, and family motivation.
- Pharmacology and weight loss surgery are recommended for older children with severe obesity, and require care from a multidisciplinary team with expertise in pediatric obesity.

## REFERENCES

Ahn, S. M. (2020). Current issues in bariatric surgery for adolescents with severe obesity: Durability, complications, and timing of intervention. *Journal of Obesity and Metabolic Syndrome, 29*(1), 4–11. https://doi.org/10.7570/jomes19073

Alberti, K. G. M. M., Eckel, R. H., Grundy, S. M., Zimmet, P. Z., Cleeman, J. I., Donato, K. A., Fruchart, J.-C., James, W. P. T., Loria, C. M., & Smith, S. C., Jr. (2009). Harmonizing the metabolic syndrome: A joint interim statement of the International Diabetes Federation Task Force on Epidemiology and Prevention; National Heart, Lung, and Blood Institute; American Heart Association; World Heart Federation; International Atherosclerosis Society; and International Association for the Study of Obesity. *Circulation, 120,* 1640–1645. https://doi.org/10.1161/CIRCULATIONAHA.109.192644

Al-Hamad, D., & Raman, V. (2017). Metabolic syndrome in children and adolescents. *Translational Pediatrics, 6*(4), 397–407. https://doi.org/10.21037/tp.2017.10.02 [doi]

Almallouhi, E., King, K. S., Patel, B., Wi, C., Juhn, Y. J., Murray, J. A., & Absah, I. (2017). Increasing incidence and altered presentation in a population-based study of pediatric celiac disease in North America. *Journal of Pediatric Gastroenterology and Nutrition, 65*(4), 432–437. https://doi.org/10.1097/MPG.0000000000001532

Al-Toma, A., Volta, U., Auricchio, R., Castillejo, G., Sanders, D. S., Cellier, C., Mulder, C. J., & Lundin, K. E. A. (2019). European Society for the Study of Coeliac Disease (ESsCD) guideline for coeliac disease and other gluten-related disorders. *United European Gastroenterology Journal, 7*(5), 583–613. https://doi.org/10.1177/2050640619844125

American Academy of Pediatrics. (2018). *Children and media tips from the American Academy of Pediatrics.* http://www.aap.org/en-us/about-the-aap/aap-press-room/news-features-and-safety-tips/Pages/Children-and-Media-Tips.aspx

American Academy of Pediatrics. (2020). *Where we stand: Screen time.* https://www.healthychildren.org/English/family-life/Media/Pages/Where-We-Stand-TV-Viewing-Time.aspx

Anania, C., Olivero, F., Spagnolo, A., Chiesa, C., & Pacifico, L. (2017). Immune response to vaccines in children with celiac disease. *World Journal of Gastroenterology, 23*(18), 3205–3213. https://doi.org/10.3748/wjg.v23.i18.3205

Anderson, A. D., Solorzano, C. M., & McCartney, C. R. (2014). Childhood obesity and its impact on the development of adolescent PCOS. *Seminars in Reproductive Medicine, 32*(3), 202–213. https://doi.org/10.1055/s-0034-1371092

Anderson, K. L. (2018). A review of the prevention and medical management of childhood obesity. *Child and Adolescent Psychiatric Clinics of North America, 27*(1), 63–76. https://doi.org/10.1016/j.chc.2017.08.003

Armstrong, S. C., Bolling, C. F., Michalsky, M. P., Reichard, K. W., & Section on Obesity, Section on Surgery. (2019). Pediatric metabolic and bariatric surgery: Evidence, barriers, and best practices. *Pediatrics, 144*(6), e20193223. https://doi.org/10.1542/peds.2019-3223

Arslanian, S., Bacha, F., Grey, M., Marcus, M. D., White, N. H., & Zeitler, P. (2018). Evaluation and management of youth-onset type 2 diabetes: A position statement by the American Diabetes Association. *Diabetes Care, 41*(12), 2648–2668. https://doi.org/10.2337/dci18-0052

Avery, A., Anderson, C., & McCullough, F. (2017). Associations between children's diet quality and watching television during meal or snack consumption: A systematic review. *Maternal and Child Nutrition, 13*(4), e12428. https://doi.org/10.1111/mcn.12428

Baidal, J. A. W., Locks, L. M., Cheng, E. R., Blake-Lamb, T. L., Perkins, M. E., & Taveras, E. M. (2016). Risk factors for childhood obesity in the first 1,000 days: A systematic review. *American Journal of Preventive Medicine, 50*(6), 761–779. https://doi.org/10.1016/j.amepre.2015.11.012

Barlow, S. E., & Expert Committee. (2007). Expert Committee recommendations regarding the prevention, assessment, and treatment of child and adolescent overweight and obesity: Summary report. *Pediatrics, 120*(Suppl. 4), S164–S192. https://doi.org/10.1542/peds.2007-2329C

Bass III, P. F. (2017). *Lactose intolerance: Diagnosis and diet strategies.* MJH Life Sciences.

Bathrellou, E., Kontogianni, M. D., & Panagiotakos, D. B. (2018). Celiac disease and non-celiac gluten or wheat sensitivity and health in later life: A review. *Maturitas, 112,* 29–33. https://doi.org/S0378-5122(18)30029-X

Bauer, E. (2020). *About 14 million children in the US are not getting enough to eat.* https://www.brookings.edu/blog/up-front/2020/07/09/about-14-million-children-in-the-us-are-not-getting-enough-to-eat

Beer, S. S., Juarez, M. D., Vega, M. W., & Canada, N. L. (2015). Pediatric malnutrition: Putting the new definition and standards into practice. *Nutrition in Clinical Practice, 30*(5), 609–624. https://doi.org/10.1177/0884533615600423

Bolling, C. F., Armstrong, S. C., Reichard, K. W., Michalsky, M. P., & Section on Obesity, Section on Surgery. (2019). Metabolic and bariatric surgery for pediatric children with severe obesity. *Pediatrics, 144*(6), e20193224. https://doi.org/10.1542/peds.2019-3224

Boyce, J. A., Assa'ad, A., Burks, A. W., Jones, S. M., Sampson, H. A., Wood, R. A., Plaut, M., Cooper, S. F., Fenton, M. J., Arshad, S. H., Bahna, S. L., Beck, L. A., Byrd-Bredbenner, C., Camargo, C. A., Jr., Eichenfield, L., Furuta, G. T., Hanifin, J. M., Jones, C., Kraft, M., ... Schwaninger, J. M. (2010). Guidelines for the diagnosis and management of food allergy in the United States: Summary of the NIAID-sponsored expert panel report. *The Journal of Allergy and Clinical Immunology, 126*(6), 1105–1118. https://doi.org/10.1016/j.jaci.2010.10.008

Brown, C. L., Halvorson, E. E., Cohen, G. M., Skelton, J. A., & Lazorick, S. (2015). Addressing childhood obesity: Opportunities for prevention. *Pediatric Clinics of North America, 67*(5), 1241–1261. https://doi.org/10.1016/j.pcl.2015.05.013

Brown, C. L., & Perrin, E. M. (2018). Obesity prevention and treatment in primary care. *Academic Pediatrics, 18*(7), 736–745. https://doi.org/10.1016/j.acap.2018.05.004

Bruijnzeel-Koomen, C., Ortolani, C., Aas, K., Bindslev-Jensen, C., Björkstén, B., Moneret-Vautrin, D., & Wüthrich, B. (1995). Adverse reactions to food. European Academy of Allergology and Clinical Immunology Subcommittee. *Allergy, 50*(8), 623–635. https://doi.org/10.1111/j.1398-9995.1995.tb02579.x

Bunyavanich, S., & Berin, M. C. (2019). Food allergy and the microbiome: Current understandings and future directions. *Journal of Allergy and Clinical Immunology, 144*(6), 1468–1477. https://doi.org/10.1016/j.jaci.2019.10.019

Caio, G., Volta, U., Sapone, A., Leffler, D. A., De Giorgio, R., Catassi, C., & Fasano, A. (2019). Celiac disease: A comprehensive current review. *BMC Medicine, 17*(1), 142. https://doi.org/10.1186/s12916-019-1380-z

Canova, C., Ludvigsson, J., Baldo, V., Barbiellini Amidei, C., Zanier, L., & Zingone, F. (2019). Risk of bacterial pneumonia and pneumococcal infection in youths with celiac disease: A population-based study. *Digestive and Liver Disease, 51*(8), 1101–1105. https://doi.org/10.1016/j.dld.2019.02.010

Celiac Disease Foundation. (2020). *What is celiac disease?* https://celiac.org/about-celiac-disease/what-is-celiac-disease

Centers for Disease Control and Prevention. (2018). *Defining childhood obesity: BMI for children and teens.* https://www.cdc.gov/obesity/childhood/defining.html

Centers for Disease Control and Prevention. (2020a). *How much physical activity do children need? Physical activity/CDC.* https://www.cdc.gov/physicalactivity/basics/children/index.htm

Centers for Disease Control and Prevention. (2020b). *Tips for parents—Ideas to help children maintain a healthy weight.* https://www.cdc.gov/healthyweight/children/index.html

Chmielewska, A., Pieścik-Lech, M., Szajewska, H., & Shamir, R. (2015). Primary prevention of celiac disease: Environmental factors with a focus on early nutrition. *Annals of Nutrition and Metabolism, 67*(Suppl. 2), 43–50. https://doi.org/10.1159/000440992

Corkins, K. G., & Teague, E. E. (2017). Pediatric nutrition assessment: Anthropometrics to zinc. *Nutrition in Clinical Practice, 32*(1), 40–51. https://doi.org/10.1177/0884533616679639

Crocker, M. K., & Yanovski, J. A. (2009). Pediatric obesity: Etiology and treatment. *Endocrinology and Metabolism Clinics of North America, 38*(3), 525–548. https://doi.org/10.1016/j.ecl.2009.06.007

Cuda, S. E., & Censani, M. (2019). Pediatric obesity algorithm: A practical approach to obesity diagnosis and management. *Frontiers in Pediatrics, 6*, 431. https://www.frontiersin.org/article/10.3389/fped.2018.00431

Czaja-Bulsa, G., & Bulsa, M. (2018). Adherence to gluten-free diet in children with celiac disease. *Nutrients, 10*(10), 1424. https://doi.org/10.3390/nu10101424

Daniels, S. R., Greer, F. R., & Committee on Nutrition. (2008). Lipid screening and cardiovascular health in childhood. *Pediatrics, 101*(1), 141. https://doi.org/10.1542/peds.2008-1349

Daniels, S. R., Hassink, S. G., & Committee on Nutrition. (2015). The role of the pediatrician in primary prevention of obesity. *Pediatrics, 136*(1), e275. https://doi.org/10.1542/peds.2015-1558

de Ferranti, S. D., Gauvreau, K., Ludwig, D. S., Neufeld, E. J., Newburger, J. W., & Rifai, N. (2004). Prevalence of the metabolic syndrome in American adolescents: Findings from the third national health and nutrition examination survey. *Circulation, 110*(16), 2494–2497. https://doi.org/10.1161/01.CIR.0000145117.40114.C7

de Ferranti, S. D., Julia, S., Rebecca, A., Annette, B., Holly, G., Kelly, A. S., Mietus-Snyder, M., Mitsnefes, M. M., Peterson, A. L., St-Pierre, J., Urbina, E. M., Zachariah, J. P., & Zaidi, A. N. (2019). Cardiovascular risk reduction in high-risk pediatric children: A scientific statement from the American Heart Association. *Circulation, 139*(13), e603–e634. https://doi.org/10.1161/CIR.0000000000000618

De Martinis, M., Sirufo, M. M., & Ginaldi, L. (2017). Allergy and aging: An old/new emerging health issue. *Aging and Disease, 8*(2), 162–175. https://doi.org/10.14336/AD.2016.0831

De Martinis, M., Sirufo, M. M., Suppa, M., & Ginaldi, L. (2020). New perspectives in food allergy. *International Journal of Molecular Sciences, 21*(4), 1474. https://doi.org/10.3390/ijms21041474

de Onis, M., Onyango, A., Borghi, E., Siyam, A., Blössner, M., & Lutter, C. (2012). Worldwide implementation of the WHO child growth standards. *Public Health Nutrition, 15*(9), 1–8. https://doi.org/10.1017/S136898001200105X

Derseh, B., Mruts, K., Demie, T., & Gebremariam, T. (2018). Co-morbidity, treatment outcomes and factors affecting the recovery rate of under-five children with severe acute malnutrition admitted in selected hospitals from Ethiopia: Retrospective follow up study. *Nutrition Journal, 17*(1), 116. https://doi.org/10.1186/s12937-018-0423-1

Desai, N. (2019). The role of motivational interviewing in children and adolescents in pediatric care. *Pediatric Annals, 48*(9), e376–e379. https://doi.org/10.3928/19382359-20190816-01

Dydensborg Sander, S., Nybo Andersen, A. M., Murray, J. A., Karlstad, Ø., Husby, S., & Størdal, K. (2019). Association between antibiotics in the first year of life and celiac disease. *Gastroenterology, 156*(8), 2217–2229. https://doi.org/10.1053/j.gastro.2019.02.039

Enö Persson, J., Bohman, B., Tynelius, P., Rasmussen, F., & Ghaderi, A. (2017). Prevention of childhood obesity in child health services: Follow-up of the PRIMROSE trial. *Childhood Obesity, 14*(2), 99–105. https://doi.org/10.1089/chi.2017.0117

Expert Panel on Integrated Guidelines for Cardiovascular Health and Risk Reduction in Children and Adolescents. (2011). Expert Panel on Integrated Guidelines for Cardiovascular Health and Risk Reduction in Children and Adolescents: Summary report. *Pediatrics, 128*(Suppl. 5), S213–S256. https://doi.org/10.1542/peds.2009-2107C

Fairbrother, U., Kidd, E., Malagamuwa, T., & Walley, A. (2018). Genetics of severe obesity. *Current Diabetes Reports, 18*(10), 85. https://doi.org/10.1007/s11892-018-1053-x

Faircloth, R. S., Brooks, D. I., Vogt, K. S., & Emerick, J. E. (2019). Talking about childhood obesity: A survey of what parents want. *Academic Pediatrics, 19*(7), 756–763. https://doi.org/10.1016/j.acap.2019.03.003

Fassio, F., Facioni, M. S., & Guagnini, F. (2018). Lactose maldigestion, malabsorption, and intolerance: A comprehensive review with a focus on current management and future perspectives. *Nutrients, 10*(11), 1599. https://doi.org/10.3390/nu10111599

Faz, G., Butler, I. J., & Koenig, M. K. (2010). Incidence of papilledema and obesity in children diagnosed with idiopathic "benign" intracranial hypertension: Case series and review. *Journal of Child Neurology, 25*(11), 1389–1392. https://doi.org/10.1177/0883073810364853

Feehley, T., Plunkett, C. H., Bao, R., Choi Hong, S. M., Culleen, E., Belda-Ferre, P., Campbell, E., Aitoro, R., Nocerino, R., Paparo, L., Andrade, J., Antonopoulos, D. A., Canani, R. B., & Nagler, C. R. (2019). Healthy infants harbor intestinal bacteria that protect against food allergy. *Nature Medicine, 25*(3), 448–453. https://doi.org/10.1038/s41591-018-0324-z

Fernandez, E., Perez, R., Hernandez, A., Tejada, P., Arteta, M., & Ramos, J. T. (2011). Factors and mechanisms for pharmacokinetic differences between pediatric population and adults. *Pharmaceutics, 3*(1), 53–72. https://doi.org/10.3390/pharmaceutics3010053

Flynn, J. T., Kaelber, D. C., Baker-Smith, C., Blowey, D., Carroll, A. E., Daniels, S. R., de Ferranti, S. D., Dionne, J. M., Falkner, B., Flinn, S. K., Gidding, S. S., Goodwin, C., Leu, M. G., Powers, M. E., Rea, C., Samuels, J., Simasek, M., Thaker, V. V., Urbina, E. M., & Subcommittee on Screening and Management of High Blood Pressure in Children. (2017). Clinical practice guideline for screening and management of high blood pressure in children and adolescents. *Pediatrics, 140*(3), e20171904. https://doi.org/10.1542/peds.2017-1904

Genetics Home Reference, National Library of Medicine, National Institutes of Health. (2010). *Lactose intolerance.* https://ghr.nlm.nih.gov/condition/lactose-intolerance

Gomes-Belo, J., Hannachi, F., Swan, K., & Santos, A. F. (2018). Advances in food allergy diagnosis. *Current Pediatric*

*Reviews, 14*(3), 139–149. https://doi.org/10.2174/15733963 14666180423105842

Greer, F. R., Sicherer, S. H., Burks, A. W., & Committee on Nutrition and Section on Allergy and Immunology. (2019). The effects of early nutritional interventions on the development of atopic disease in infants and children: The role of maternal dietary restriction, breastfeeding, hydrolyzed formulas, and timing of introduction of allergenic complementary foods. *Pediatrics, 143*(4). https://doi.org/10.1542/peds.2019-0281

Greydanus, D. E., Agana, M., Kamboj, M. K., Shebrain, S., Soares, N., Eke, R., & Patel, D.R. (2018). Pediatric obesity: Current concepts. *Disease-a-Month, 64*(4), 98–156. https://doi.org/10.1016/j.disamonth.2017.12.001

Grummer-Strawn, L. M., Reinold, C., & Krebs, N. F. (2010). Use of World Health Organization and CDC growth charts for children aged 0–59 months in the United States. *Morbidity and Mortality Weekly Report: Recommendations and Reports, 59*(RR-9), 1–14.

Gupta, M., Cox, A., Nowak-Węgrzyn, A., & Wang, J. (2018). Diagnosis of food allergy. *Immunology and Allergy Clinics of North America, 38*(1), 39–52. https://doi.org/10.1016/j.iac.2017.09.004

Gupta, R. S., Warren, C. M., Smith, B. M., Blumenstock, J. A., Jiang, J., Davis, M. M., & Nadeau, K. C. (2018). The public health impact of parent-reported childhood food allergies in the United States. *Pediatrics, 142*(6). https://doi.org/10.1542/peds.2018-1235

Gustafsson, I., Repo, M., Popp, A., Kaukinen, K., Hiltunen, P., Arvola, T., Taavela, J., Vornanen, M., Kivelä, L., & Kurppa, K. (2020). Prevalence and diagnostic outcomes of children with duodenal lesions and negative celiac serology. *Digestive and Liver Disease, 52*(3), 289–295. https://doi.org/10.1016/j.dld.2019.11.011

Hagan, J. F. J., Shaw, J. S., Duncan, P. M., & American Academy of Pediatrics. (2017). *Bright futures: Guidelines for health supervision of infants, children, and adolescents* (4th ed.). Bright Futures/American Academy of Pediatrics.

Hamed, S. A. (2015). Antiepileptic drugs influences on body weight in people with epilepsy. *Expert Review of Clinical Pharmacology, 8*(1), 103–114. https://doi.org/10.1586/17512433.2015.991716

Harvey, L., Ludwig, T., Hou, A. Q., Hock, Q. S., Tan, M. L., Osatakul, S., Bindels, J., & Muhardi, L. (2018). Prevalence, cause and diagnosis of lactose intolerance in children aged 1–5 years: A systematic review of 1995–2015 literature. *Asia Pacific Journal of Clinical Nutrition, 27*(1), 29–46. https://doi.org/10.6133/apjcn.022017.05

Hemmingsson, E. (2018). Early childhood obesity risk factors: Socioeconomic adversity, family dysfunction, offspring distress, and junk food self-medication. *Current Obesity Reports, 7*(2), 204–209. https://doi.org/10.1007/s13679-018-0310-2

Hertzler, S., Kim, Y., Khan, R., Asp, M., & Savaiano, D. (2014). Diet and intestinal disaccharidases. In C. A. Ross, B. Caballero, R. J. Cousins, K. L. Tucker, & T. R. Ziegler (Eds.), *Modern nutrition in health and disease* (11th ed., pp. 1058–1069). Wolters Kluwer Health.

Heyman, M. B., Abrams, S. A., & Section on Gastroenterology, Hepatology, and Nutrition, Committee on Nutrition. (2017). Fruit juice in infants, children, and adolescents: Current recommendations. *Pediatrics, 139*(6), e20170967. https://doi.org/10.1542/peds.2017-0967

Heyman, M. B., & Committee on Nutrition. (2006). Lactose intolerance in infants, children, and adolescents. *Pediatrics, 118*(3), 1279–1286.

Higgins, V., & Adeli, K. (2017). Pediatric metabolic syndrome: Pathophysiology and laboratory assessment. *EJIFCC, 28*(1), 25–42. https://www.ifcc.org/media/450787/eJIFCC2017Vol28No1.pdf

Hill, I. D. (2020). Diagnosis of celiac disease in children. *UpToDate*. Retrieved October 25, 2020, from https://www.uptodate.com/contents/diagnosis-of-celiac-disease-in-children

Hill, I. D., Fasano, A., Guandalini, S., Hoffenberg, E., Levy, J., Reilly, N., & Verma, R. (2016). NASPGHAN clinical report on the diagnosis and treatment of gluten-related disorders. *Journal of Pediatric Gastroenterology and Nutrition, 63*(1), 156–165. https://doi.org/10.1097/MPG.0000000000001216

Holt, K., Wooldridge, N., Story, M., & Sofka, D. (2011). *Bright futures nutrition* (3rd ed.). American Academy of Pediatrics.

Homan, G. J. (2016). Failure to thrive: A practical guide. *American Family Physician, 94*(4), 295–299.

Hujoel, I. A., Reilly, N. R., & Rubio-Tapia, A. (2019). Celiac disease: Clinical features and diagnosis. *Gastroenterology Clinics of North America, 48*(1), 19–37. https://doi.org/10.1016/j.gtc.2018.09.001

Husby, S., Koletzko, S., Korponay-Szabó, I., Kurppa, K., Mearin, M. L., Ribes-Koninckx, C., Shamir, R., Troncone, R., Auricchio, R., Castillejo, G., Christensen, R., Dolinsek, J., Gillett, P., Hróbjartsson, A., Koltai, T., Maki, M., Nielsen, S. M., Popp, A., Størdal, K., … Wessels, M. (2020). European Society Paediatric Gastroenterology, Hepatology, and Nutrition guidelines for diagnosing coeliac disease 2020. *Journal of Pediatric Gastroenterology and Nutrition, 70*(1), 141–156. https://doi.org/10.1097/MPG.0000000000002497

Husby, S., Koletzko, S., Korponay-Szabó, I. R., Mearin, M. L., Phillips, A., Shamir, R., Troncone, R., Giersiepen, K., Branski, D., Catassi, C., Lelgeman, M., Mäki, M., Ribes-Koninckx, C., Ventura, A., & Zimmer, K. P. (2012). European Society for Pediatric Gastroenterology, Hepatology, and Nutrition guidelines for the diagnosis of coeliac disease. *Journal of Pediatric Gastroenterology and Nutrition, 54*(1), 136–160. https://doi.org/10.1097/MPG.0b013e31821a23d0

Hyytinen, M., Savilahti, E., Virtanen, S. M., Härkönen, T., Ilonen, J., Luopajärvi, K., Uibo, R., Vaarala, O., Åkerblom, H. K., & Knip, M. (2017). Avoidance of cow's milk-based formula for at-risk infants does not reduce development of celiac disease: A randomized controlled trial. *Gastroenterology, 153*(4), 961–970.e3. https://doi.org/10.1053/j.gastro.2017.06.049

Inge, T. H., Courcoulas, A. P., Jenkins, T. M., Michalsky, M. P., Helmrath, M. A., Brandt, M. L., Harmon, C. M., Zeller, M. H., Chen, M. K., Xanthakos, S. A., Horlick, M., & Buncher, C. R. (2016). Weight loss and health status 3 years after bariatric surgery in adolescents. *New England Journal of Medicine, 374*(2), 113–123. https://doi.org/10.1056/NEJMoa1506699

Kahrs, C. R., Chuda, K., Tapia, G., Stene, L. C., Mårild, K., Rasmussen, T., Rønningen, K. S., Lundin, K. E. A., Kramna, L., Cinek, O., & Størdal, K. (2019). Enterovirus as trigger of coeliac disease: Nested case-control study within prospective birth cohort. *BMJ, 364*, l231. https://doi.org/10.1136/bmj.l231

Kemppainen, K. M., Lynch, K. F., Liu, E., Lönnrot, M., Simell, V., Briese, T., Koletzko, S., Hagopian, W., Rewers, M., She, J.-X., Simell, O., Toppari, J., Ziegler, A.-G., Akolkar, B., Krischer, J. P., Lernmark, A., Hyöty, H., Triplett, E. W., & Agardh, D. (2017). Factors that increase risk of celiac disease autoimmunity after a gastrointestinal infection in early life. *Clinical Gastroenterology and Hepatology, 15*(5), 694–702.e5. https://doi.org/10.1016/j.cgh.2016.10.033

Kemppainen, K. M., Vehik, K., Lynch, K. F., Larsson, H. E., Canepa, R. J., Simell, V., Koletzko, S., Liu, E., Simell, O. G., Toppari, J., Ziegler, A. G., Rewers, M. J., Lernmark, A., Hagopian, W. A., She, J.-X., Akolkar, B., Schatz, D. A., Atkinson, M. A., Blaser, M. J., ... Triplett, E. W. (2017). Association between early-life antibiotic use and the risk of islet or celiac disease autoimmunity. *JAMA Pediatrics, 171*(12), 1217–1225. https://doi.org/10.1001/jamapediatrics.2017.2905

King, J. A., Jeong, J., Underwood, F. E., Quan, J., Panaccione, N., Windsor, J. W., Coward, S., deBruyn, J., Ronksley, P. E., Shaheen, A.-A., Quan, H., Godley, J., van Zanten, S. V., Lebwohl, B., Ng, S. C., Ludvigsson, J. F., & Kaplan, G. G. (2020). Incidence of celiac disease is increasing over time: A systematic review and meta-analysis. *American Journal of Gastroenterology, 115*(4). https://doi.org/10.14309/ajg.0000000000000523

Kleinman, R. E., & Greer, F. R. (2020). *Pediatric nutrition*. American Academy of Pediatrics.

Kohut, T., Robbins, J., & Panganiban, J. (2019). Update on childhood/adolescent obesity and its sequela. *Current Opinion in Pediatrics, 31*(5). https://doi.org/10.1097/MOP.0000000000000786

Kołodziej, M., Patro-Gołąb, B., Gieruszczak-Białek, D., Skórka, A., Pieścik-Lech, M., Baron, R., & Szajewska, H. (2019). Association between early life (prenatal and postnatal) antibiotic administration and coeliac disease: A systematic review. *Archives of Disease in Childhood, 104*(11), 1083–1089. https://doi.org/10.1136/archdischild-2019-317174

Krauthammer, A., Guz-Mark, A., Zevit, N., Marderfeld, L., Waisbourd-Zinman, O., Silbermintz, A., Mozer-Glassberg, Y., Friedler, V. N., Bar Lev, M. R., Matar, M., Assa, A., & Shamir, R. (2020). Two decades of pediatric celiac disease in a tertiary referral center: What has changed? *Digestive and Liver Disease, 52*(4), 457–461. https://doi.org/10.1016/j.dld.2020.02.001

Kuczmarski, R. J., Ogden, C. L., Guo, S. S., Grummer-Strawn, L. M., Flegal, K. M., Mei, Z., Wei, R., Curtin, L. R., Roche, A. F., & Johnson, C. L. (2002). 2000 CDC growth charts for the United States: Methods and development. *Vital and Health Statistics. Series 11, Data from the National Health Survey*, (246), 1–190.

Kumar, P., Singh, A., & Nidhi, N. (2018). Outcome and co-morbidities associated with severe acute malnutrition: Admitted at nutrition rehabilitation centre (NRC) of a tertiary care centre. *Journal of Evidence Based Medicine and Healthcare, 5*(14), 1258–1261. https://doi.org/10.18410/jebmh/2018/260

Kumar, S., & Kelly, A. S. (2017). Review of childhood obesity: From epidemiology, etiology, and comorbidities to clinical assessment and treatment. *Mayo Clinic Proceedings, 92*(2), 251–265. https://doi.org/10.1016/j.mayocp.2016.09.017

Lebwohl, B., Green, P. H. R., Söderling, J., Roelstraete, B., & Ludvigsson, J. F. (2020). Association between celiac disease and mortality risk in a Swedish population. *JAMA, 323*(13), 1277–1285. https://doi.org/10.1001/jama.2020.1943

Lebwohl, B., Sanders, D. S., & Green, P. H. R. (2018). Coeliac disease. *Lancet (London, England), 391*(10115), 70–81. https://doi.org/S0140-6736(17)31796-8

Lee, L., & Sanders, R. A. (2012). Metabolic syndrome. *Pediatrics in Review, 33*(10), 459–466; quiz 467–468. https://doi.org/10.1542/pir.33-10-459

Leonard, M. M., Sapone, A., Catassi, C., & Fasano, A. (2017). Celiac disease and nonceliac gluten sensitivity: A review. *JAMA, 318*(7), 647–656. https://doi.org/10.1001/jama.2017.9730

Leonberg, B. L. (2020). *Pocket guide to pediatric nutrition assessment* (3rd ed.). Academy of Nutrition and Dietetics.

Lionetti, E., Gatti, S., Pulvirenti, A., & Catassi, C. (2015). Celiac disease from a global perspective. *Best Practice & Research: Clinical Gastroenterology, 29*(3), 365–379. https://doi.org/S1521-6918(15)00058-X

Litchford, M. D. (2020). Clinical: Biochemical, physical, and functional assessment. In K. Morrow & J. L. Raymond (Eds.), *Krause and Mahan's food and the nutrition care process E-book* (15th ed., pp. 57–80). Elsevier.

Ludvigsson, J. F., Leffler, D. A., Bai, J. C., Biagi, F., Fasano, A., Green, P. H. R., Hadjivassiliou, M., Kaukinen, K., Kelly, C. P., Leonard, J. N., Lundin, K. E. A., Murray, J. A., Sanders, D. S., Walker, M. M., Zingone, F., & Ciacci, C. (2013). The Oslo definitions for coeliac disease and related terms. *Gut, 62*(1), 43. https://doi.org/10.1136/gutjnl-2011-301346

Ludvigsson, J. F., & Murray, J. A. (2019). Epidemiology of celiac disease. *Gastroenterology Clinics of North America, 48*(1), 1–18. https://doi.org/10.1016/j.gtc.2018.09.004

Magge, S. N., Goodman, E., & Armstrong, S. C. (2017). The metabolic syndrome in children and adolescents: Shifting the focus to cardiometabolic risk factor clustering. *Pediatrics, 140*(2). https://doi.org/10.1542/peds.2017-1603

Mahan, L. K., & Swift, K. M. (2020). Medical nutrition therapy for adverse reactions to food: Allergies and intolerances. In K. Morrow & J. L. Raymond (Eds.), *Krause and Mahan's food & the nutrition care process E-book* (15th ed., pp. 494–524). Elsevier.

Maqbool, A., Parks, E. P., Shaikhkhalil, A., Panganiban, J., Mitchell, J. A., & Stallings, V. A. (2020). Nutritional requirements. In R. M. Kliegman, J. W. St. Geme III, N. J. Blum, S. S. Shah, R. C. Tasker, K. M. Wilson, & R. E. Behrman (Eds.), *Nelson textbook of pediatrics* (21st ed., Chapter 55). Elsevier.

Marcus, C. L., Brooks, L. J., Draper, K. A., Gozal, D., Halbower, A. C., Jones, J., Schechter, M S., Ward, S. D., Sheldon, S. H., Shiffman, R. N., Lehmann, C., Spruyt, K., & American Academy of Pediatrics. (2012). Diagnosis and management of childhood obstructive sleep apnea syndrome. *Pediatrics, 130*(3), 714–755. https://doi.org/10.1542/peds.2012-1672

Mårild, K., Kahrs, C. R., Tapia, G., Stene, L. C., & Størdal, K. (2015). Infections and risk of celiac disease in childhood: A prospective nationwide cohort study. *American Journal of Gastroenterology, 110*(10). https://doi.org/10.1038/ajg.2015.287

McAllister, B. P., Williams, E., & Clarke, K. (2019). A comprehensive review of celiac disease/gluten-sensitive enteropathies. *Clinical Reviews in Allergy and Immunology, 57*(2), 226–243. https://doi.org/10.1007/s12016-018-8691-2

McCarthy, A., Delvin, E., Marcil, V., Belanger, V., Marchand, V., Boctor, D., Rashid, M., Noble, A., Davidson, B., Groleau, V., Spahis, S., Roy, C., & Levy, E. (2019). Prevalence of malnutrition in pediatric hospitals in developed and in-transition countries: The impact of hospital practices. *Nutrients, 11*(2), 236. https://doi.org/10.3390/nu11020236

Mehta, N. M., Corkins, M. R., Lyman, B., Malone, A., Goday, P. S., Carney, L. N., Monczka, J. L., Plogsted, S. W., Schwenk, W. F., & American Society for Parenteral and Enteral Nutrition Board of Directors. (2013). Defining pediatric malnutrition: A paradigm shift toward etiology-related definitions. *JPEN Journal of Parenteral Enteral Nutrition, 37*(4), 460. https://doi.org/10.1177/0148607113479972

Meijer, C., Shamir, R., Szajewska, H., & Mearin, L. (2018). Celiac disease prevention. *Frontiers in Pediatrics, 6*, 368. https://www.frontiersin.org/article/10.3389/fped.2018.00368

Milla, P. (2002). Children are not just little adults. *Clinical Nutrition, 21*, 137–139. https://doi.org/10.1016/S0261-5614(02)80031-0

Moen, Ø. L., Opheim, E., & Trollvik, A. (2019). Parents' experiences raising a child with food allergy: A qualitative review. *Journal of Pediatric Nursing, 46*, 52.

Montalto, M., Santoro, L., D'Onofrio, F., Curigliano, V., Gallo, A., Visca, D., Cammarota, G., Gasbarrini, A., & Gasbarrini, G. (2008). Adverse reactions to food: Allergies and intolerances. *Digestive Diseases, 26*(2), 96–103. https://doi.org/10.1159/000116766

Mordarski, B., & Wolff, J. (2018). *Pediatric nutrition focused physical exam pocket guide* (2nd ed.). Academy of Nutrition and Dietetics.

Myléus, A., Reilly, N. R., & Green, P. (2020). Rate, risk factors, and outcomes of nonadherence in pediatric children with celiac disease: A systematic review. *Clinical Gastroenterology and Hepatology, 18*(3), 562–573. https://doi.org/10.1016/j.cgh.2019.05.046

Nardecchia, S., Auricchio, R., Discepolo, V., & Troncone, R. (2019). Extra-intestinal manifestations of coeliac disease in children: Clinical features and mechanisms. *Frontiers in Pediatrics, 7*, 56. https://doi.org/10.3389/fped.2019.00056

National Institute of Allergy and Infectious Diseases. (2011). *Guidelines for the diagnosis and management of food allergy in the United States: Summary for children, families, and caregivers.* U.S. Department of Health and Human Services, National Institute of Health, National Institute of Allergy and Infectious Diseases.

Ogden, C. L., Carroll, M. D., Fakhouri, T. H., Hales, C. M., Fryar, C. D., Li, Z., & Freedman, D. S. (2018). Prevalence of obesity among youths by household income and education level of head of household—United States 2011–2014. *MMWR. Morbidity and Mortality Weekly Report, 67*. https://doi.org/10.15585/mmwr.mm6706a3

Ogden, C. L., Fryar, C. D., Hales, C. M., Carroll, M. D., Aoki, Y., & Freedman, D. S. (2018). Differences in obesity prevalence by demographics and urbanization in US children and adolescents, 2013–2016. *JAMA, 319*(23), 2410–2418. https://doi.org/10.1001/jama.2018.5158

Ortega-García, J. A., Kloosterman, N., Alvarez, L., Tobarra-Sánchez, E., Cárceles-Álvarez, A., Pastor-Valero, R., López-Hernández, F. A., Sánchez-Solis, M., & Claudio, L. (2018). Full breastfeeding and obesity in children: A prospective study from birth to 6 years. *Childhood Obesity (Print), 14*(5), 327–337. https://doi.org/10.1089/chi.2017.0335

Pediatric Nutrition Practice Group of the Academy of Nutrition and Dietetics. (2020). *Pediatric nutrition care manual.* https://www.nutritioncaremanual.org

Phillips, A., Frank, A., Loftin, C., & Shepherd, S. (2017). A detailed review of systems: An educational feature. *The Journal for Nurse Practitioners, 13*(10), 681–686. https://doi.org/10.1016/j.nurpra.2017.08.012

Pigeyre, M., Yazdi, F. T., Kaur, Y., & Meyre, D. (2016). Recent progress in genetics, epigenetics and metagenomics unveils the pathophysiology of human obesity. *Clinical Science, 130*(12), 943–986. https://doi.org/10.1042/CS20160136

Pilitsi, E., Farr, O. M., Polyzos, S. A., Perakakis, N., Nolen-Doerr, E., Papathanasiou, A. E., & Mantzoros, C. S. (2019). Pharmacotherapy of obesity: Available medications and drugs under investigation. *Metabolism: Clinical and Experimental, 92*, 170–192. https://doi.org/10.1016/j.metabol.2018.10.010

Pont, S. J., Puhl, R., Cook, S. R., Slusser, W., & Section on Obesity, Obesity Society. (2017). Stigma experienced by children and adolescents with obesity. *Pediatrics, 140*(6), e20173034. https://doi.org/10.1542/peds.2017-3034

Poorolajal, J., Sahraei, F., Mohamdadi, Y., Doosti-Irani, A., & Moradi, L. (2020). Behavioral factors influencing childhood obesity: A systematic review and meta-analysis. *Obesity Research & Clinical Practice, 14*(2), 109–118. https://doi.org/10.1016/j.orcp.2020.03.002

Popp, A., & Mäki, M. (2019). Changing pattern of childhood celiac disease epidemiology: Contributing factors. *Frontiers in Pediatrics, 7*, 357. https://doi.org/10.3389/fped.2019.00357

Pratt, J. S. A., Browne, A., Browne, N. T., Bruzoni, M., Cohen, M., Desai, A., Inge, T., Linden, B. C., Mattar, S. G., Michalsky, M., Podkameni, D., Reichard, K. W., Stanford, F. C., Zeller, M. H., & Zitsman, J. (2018). ASMBS pediatric metabolic and bariatric surgery guidelines, 2018. *Surgery for Obesity and Related Diseases, 14*(7), 882–901. https://doi.org/10.1016/j.soard.2018.03.019

Reekie, J., Hosking, S. P., Prakash, C., Kao, K. T., Juonala, M., & Sabin, M. A. (2015). The effect of antidepressants and antipsychotics on weight gain in children and adolescents. *Obesity Reviews, 16*(7), 566–580. https://doi.org/10.1111/obr.12284

Rendina, D., Campanozzi, A., & De Filippo, G. (2019). Methodological approach to the assessment of the obesogenic environment in children and adolescents: A review of the literature. *Nutrition, Metabolism and Cardiovascular Diseases, 29*(6), 561–571. https://doi.org/10.1016/j.numecd.2019.02.009

Resnicow, K., McMaster, F., Bocian, A., Harris, D., Zhou, Y., Snetselaar, L., Schwartz, R., Myers, E., Gotlieb, J., Foster, J., Hollinger, D., Smith, K., Woolford, S., Mueller, D., & Wasserman, R. C. (2015). Motivational interviewing and dietary counseling for obesity in primary care: An RCT. *Pediatrics, 135*(4), 649–657. https://doi.org/10.1542/peds.2014-1880

Revuelta Iniesta, R., Paciarotti, I., Davidson, I., McKenzie, J. M., Brougham, M. F. H., & Wilson, D. C. (2019). Nutritional status of children and adolescents with cancer in Scotland: A prospective cohort study. *Clinical Nutrition ESPEN, 32*, 96–106. https://doi.org/10.1016/j.clnesp.2019.04.006

Rijks, J. M., Plat, J., Mensink, R. P., Dorenbos, E., Buurman, W. A., & Vreugdenhil, A. C. E. (2015). Children with morbid obesity benefit equally as children with overweight and obesity from an ongoing care program. *The Journal of Clinical Endocrinology & Metabolism, 100*(9), 3572–3580. https://doi.org/10.1210/jc.2015-1444

Rito, A. I., Buoncristiano, M., Spinelli, A., Salanave, B., Kunešová, M., Hejgaard, T., Solano, M. G., Fijałkowska, A., Sturua, L., Hyska, J., Kelleher, C., Duleva, V., Milanović, S. M., Sant'Angelo, V. F., Abdrakhmanova, S., Kujundzic, E., Peterkova, V., Gualtieri, A., … Breda, J. (2019). Association between characteristics at birth, breastfeeding and obesity in 22 countries: The WHO European childhood obesity surveillance initiative–COSI 2015/2017. *Obesity Facts, 12*(2), 226–243. https://doi.org/10.1159/000500425

Rojo, C., Jaime, F., Azócar, L., Hernández, C., Villagrán, A., Miquel, J. F., & Arancibia, G. (2018). Concordance between lactose quick test, hydrogen–methane breath test and genotyping for the diagnosis of lactose malabsorption in

children. *Neurogastroenterology & Motility, 30*(5), e13271. https://doi.org/10.1111/nmo.13271
Roy, P. K., & Cagir, B. (2019). *Lactose intolerance differential diagnoses.* https://emedicine.medscape.com/article/187249-differential
Rubio-Tapia, A., Hill, I. D., Kelly, C. P., Calderwood, A. H., Murray, J. A., & American College of Gastroenterology. (2013). ACG clinical guidelines: Diagnosis and management of celiac disease. *The American Journal of Gastroenterology, 108*(5), 656–676. https://doi.org/10.1038/ajg.2013.79
Ryder, J. R., Fox, C. K., & Kelly, A. S. (2018). Treatment options for severe obesity in the pediatric population: Current limitations and future opportunities. *Obesity, 26*(6), 951–960. https://doi.org/10.1002/oby.22196
Sampson, H. A., Aceves, S., Bock, S. A., James, J., Jones, S., Lang, D., Nadeau, K., Nowak-Wegrzyn, A., Oppenheimer, J., Perry, T. T., Randolph, C., Sicherer, S. H., Simon, R. A., Vickery, B. P., Wood, R., Bernstein, D., Blessing-Moore, J., Khan, D., Lang, D., … Wood, R. (2014). Food allergy: A practice parameter update—2014. *The Journal of Allergy and Clinical Immunology, 134*(5), 1016–1025. https://doi.org/10.1016/j.jaci.2014.05.013
Sampson, H. A., O'Mahony, L., Burks, A. W., Plaut, M., Lack, G., & Akdis, C. A. (2018). Mechanisms of food allergy. *The Journal of Allergy and Clinical Immunology, 141*(1), 11–19. https://doi.org/10.1016/j.jaci.2017.11.005
Sanyaolu, A., Okorie, C., Qi, X., Locke, J., & Rehman, S. (2019). Childhood and adolescent obesity in the United States: A public health concern. *Global Pediatric Health.* https://doi.org/10.1177/2333794X19891305
Schoeppe, S., Alley, S., Rebar, A. L., Hayman, M., Bray, N. A., Van Lippevelde, W., Gnam, J.-P., Bachert, P., Direito, A., & Vandelanotte, C. (2017). Apps to improve diet, physical activity and sedentary behaviour in children and adolescents: A review of quality, features and behaviour change techniques. *International Journal of Behavioral Nutrition and Physical Activity, 14*(1), 83. https://doi.org/10.1186/s12966-017-0538-3
Secker, D. J., & Jeejeebhoy, K. N. (2012). How to perform subjective global nutritional assessment in children. *Journal of the Academy of Nutrition and Dietetics, 112*(3), 424–431.e6. https://doi.org/10.1016/j.jada.2011.08.039
Serena, G., Lima, R., & Fasano, A. (2019). Genetic and environmental contributors for celiac disease. *Current Allergy and Asthma Reports, 19*(9), 40. https://doi.org/10.1007/s11882-019-0871-5
Sheikh, A. B., Nasrullah, A., Haq, S., Akhtar, A., Ghazanfar, H., Nasir, A., Afzal, R. M., Bukhari, M. M., Chaudhary, A. Y., & Naqvi, S. W. (2017). The interplay of genetics and environmental factors in the development of obesity. *Cureus, 9*(7), e1435. https://doi.org/10.7759/cureus.1435
Sicherer, S. H., & Sampson, H. A. (2018). Food allergy: A review and update on epidemiology, pathogenesis, diagnosis, prevention, and management. *The Journal of Allergy and Clinical Immunology, 141*(1), 41–58. https://doi.org/10.1016/j.jaci.2017.11.003
Silberman, E. S., & Jin, J. (2019). Lactose intolerance. *JAMA, 322*(16), 1620. https://doi.org/10.1001/jama.2019.9608
Simmonds, M., Llewellyn, A., Owen, C. G., & Woolacott, N. (2016). Predicting adult obesity from childhood obesity: A systematic review and meta-analysis. *Obesity Reviews, 17*(2), 95–107. https://doi.org/10.1111/obr.12334
Simons, M., Scott-Sheldon, L., Risech-Neyman, Y., Moss, S. F., Ludvigsson, J. F., & Green, P. (2018). Celiac disease and increased risk of pneumococcal infection: A systematic review and meta-analysis. *The American Journal of Medicine, 131*(1), 83–89. https://doi.org/10.1016/j.amjmed.2017.07.021
Skinner, A. C., Ravanbakht, S. N., Skelton, J. A., Perrin, E. M., & Armstrong, S. C. (2018). Prevalence of obesity and severe obesity in US children, 1999–2016. *Pediatrics, 141*(3), e20173459. https://doi.org/10.1542/peds.2017-3459
Snyder, J., Butzner, J. D., DeFelice, A. R., Fasano, A., Guandalini, S., Liu, E., & Newton, K. P. (2016). Evidence-informed expert recommendations for the management of celiac disease in children. *Pediatrics, 138*(3), e20153147. https://doi.org/10.1542/peds.2015-3147
Srivastava, G., Fox, C. K., Kelly, A. S., Jastreboff, A. M., Browne, A. F., Browne, N. T., Pratt, J. S. A., Bolling, C., Michalsky, M. P., Cook, S., Lenders, C. M., & Apovian, C. M. (2019). Clinical considerations regarding the use of obesity pharmacotherapy in adolescents with obesity. *Obesity, 27*(2), 190–204. https://doi.org/10.1002/oby.22385
Steinberger, J., Daniels, S. R., Eckel, R. H., Hayman, L., Lustig, R. H., McCrindle, B., & Mietus-Snyder, M. L. (2009). Progress and challenges in metabolic syndrome in children and adolescents. A scientific statement from the American Heart Association Atherosclerosis, Hypertension, and Obesity in the Young Committee of the Council on Cardiovascular Disease in the Young; Council on Cardiovascular Nursing; and Council on Nutrition, Physical Activity, and Metabolism. *Circulation, 119*(4), 628–647. https://doi.org/10.1161/CIRCULATIONAHA.108.191394
Styne, D. M., Arslanian, S. A., Connor, E. L., Farooqi, I. S., Murad, M. H., Silverstein, J. H., & Yanovski, J. A. (2017). Pediatric obesity—Assessment, treatment, and prevention: An Endocrine Society clinical practice guideline. *The Journal of Clinical Endocrinology & Metabolism, 102*(3), 709–757. https://doi.org/10.1210/jc.2016-2573
Sutherland, R., Brown, A., Nathan, N., Janssen, L., Reynolds, R., Walton, A., Hudson, N., Chooi, A., Yoong, S., Wiggers, J., Bailey, A., Evans, N., Gillham, K., Oldmeadow, C., Searles, A., Reeves, P., Rissel, C., Davies, M., Reilly, K., … Wolfenden, L. (2019). Protocol for an effectiveness-implementation hybrid trial to assess the effectiveness and cost-effectiveness of an m-health intervention to decrease the consumption of discretionary foods packed in school lunchboxes: The 'SWAP IT' trial. *BMC Public Health, 19*(1), 1510. https://doi.org/10.1186/s12889-019-7725-x
Szajewska, H., Shamir, R., Mearin, L., Ribes-Koninckx, C., Catassi, C., Domellöf, M., Fewtrell, M. S., Husby, S., Papadopoulou, A., Vandenplas, Y., Castillejo, G., Kolacek, S., Koletzko, S., Korponay-Szabó, I. R., Lionetti, E., Polanco, I., & Troncone, R. (2016). Gluten introduction and the risk of coeliac disease: A position paper by the European Society for Pediatric Gastroenterology, Hepatology, and Nutrition. *Journal of Pediatric Gastroenterology and Nutrition, 62*(3), 507–513. https://doi.org/10.1097/MPG.0000000000001105
Taylor, S. A., Borzutsky, C., Jasik, C. B., Mihalopoulos, N. L., Smith-Barron, K., Woolford, S. J., Garber, A., McPherson, M., AlBuhairan, F. S., Kohn, M., Garland, B. H., & Dixon, A. (2016). Preventing and treating adolescent obesity: A position paper of the Society for Adolescent Health and Medicine. *Journal of Adolescent Health, 59*(5), 602-606. https://doi.org/10.1016/j.jadohealth.2016.08.020
Thaker, V. V. (2017). Genetic and epigenetic causes of obesity. *Adolescent Medicine: State of the Art Reviews, 28*(2), 379–405. https://www.ncbi.nlm.nih.gov/pmc/articles/PMC6226269/
Togias, A., Cooper, S. F., Acebal, M. L., Assa'ad, A., Baker, J. R., Beck, L. A., Block, J., Byrd-Bredbenner, C., Chan, E. S., Eichenfield, L. F., Fleischer, D. M., Fuchs, G. J., Furuta, G.

T., Greenhawt, M. J., Gupta, R. S., Habich, M., Jones, S. M., Keaton, K., Muraro, A., ... Boyce, J. A. (2017). Addendum guidelines for the prevention of peanut allergy in the United States: Summary of the National Institute of Allergy and Infectious Diseases-sponsored expert panel. *Journal of the Academy of Nutrition and Dietetics, 117*(5), 788–793. https://doi.org/10.1016/j.jaci.2016.10.010

Tye-Din, J., Galipeau, H. J., & Agardh, D. (2018). Celiac disease: A review of current concepts in pathogenesis, prevention, and novel therapies. *Frontiers in Pediatrics, 6*, 350. https://www.frontiersin.org/article/10.3389/fped.2018.00350

Tyson, N., & Frank, M. (2018). Childhood and adolescent obesity definitions as related to BMI: Evaluation and management options. *Best Practice & Research. Clinical Obstetrics & Gynecology, 48*, 158–164. https://doi.org/10.3389/fped.2018.00350

US Preventive Services Task Force; Grossman, D. C., Bibbins-Domingo, K., Curry, S. J., Barry, M. J., Davidson, K. W., Doubeni, C. A., Epling, J. W., Jr., Kemper, A. R., Krist, A. H., Kurth, A. E., Landefeld, C. S., Mangione, C. M., Phipps, M. G., Silverstein, M., Simon, M. A., & Tseng, C.-W. (2017). Screening for obesity in children and adolescents: US Preventive Services Task Force recommendations statement. *JAMA, 317*(23), 2417–2426. https://doi.org/10.1001/jama.2017.6803

Vallabhan, M. K., Jimenez, E. Y., Nash, J. L., Gonzales-Pacheco, D., Coakley, K. E., Noe, S. R., DeBlieck, C. J., Summers, L. C., Feldstein-Ewing, S. W., & Kong, A. S. (2018). Motivational interviewing to treat adolescents with obesity: A meta-analysis. *Pediatrics, 142*(5), e20180733. https://doi.org/10.1542/peds.2018-0733

VanReken, D. W., Kay, R. E., & Ireton-Jones, C. S. (2020). Medical nutrition therapy for lower gastrointestinal tract disorders. In K. Morrow & J. L. Raymond (Eds.), *Krause and Mahan's food and the nutrition care process E-book* (15th ed., pp. 544–578). Elsevier.

Vos, M. B., Abrams, S. H., Barlow, S. E., Caprio, S., Daniels, S. R., Kohli, R., Mouzaki, M., Sathya, P., Schwimmer, J. B., Sundaram, S. S., & Xanthakos, S. A. (2017). NASPGHAN clinical practice guideline for the diagnosis and treatment of nonalcoholic fatty liver disease in children: Recommendations from the expert committee on NAFLD (ECON) and the North American Society of Pediatric Gastroenterology, Hepatology and Nutrition (NASPGHAN). *Journal of Pediatric Gastroenterology and Nutrition, 64*(2). https://doi.org/10.1097/MPG.0000000000001482

Waserman, S., Bégin, P., & Watson, W. (2018). IgE-mediated food allergy. *Allergy, Asthma, and Clinical Immunology, 14*(Suppl. 2), 55. https://doi.org/10.1186/s13223-018-0284-3

White, L. E., Bannerman, E., & Gillett, P. M. (2016). Coeliac disease and the gluten-free diet: A review of the burdens; factors associated with adherence and impact on health-related quality of life, with specific focus on adolescence. *Journal of Human Nutrition and Dietetics, 29*(5), 593–606. https://doi.org/10.1111/jhn.12375

Williams, A. S., Ge, B., Petroski, G., Kruse, R. L., McElroy, J. A., & Koopman, R. J. (2018). Socioeconomic status and other factors associated with childhood obesity. *The Journal of the American Board of Family Medicine, 31*(4), 514–521. https://doi.org/10.3122/jabfm.2018.04.170261

Wittcopp, C., & Conroy, R. (2016). Metabolic syndrome in children and adolescents. *Pediatrics in Review, 37*(5), 193–202. https://doi.org/10.1542/pir.2014-0095

World Health Organization. (2017). *Report of the Commission on Ending Childhood Obesity: Implementation plan executive summary.* http://www.who.int/end-childhood-obesity/en/

World Health Organization. (2018). *Natural toxins in food.* https://www.who.int/news-room/fact-sheets/detail/natural-toxins-in-food

World Health Organization. (2019). *Children are not little adults.* https://www.who.int/ceh/capacity/Children_are_not_little_adults.pdf

World Health Organization, Multicentre Growth Reference Study Group. (2006). *WHO child growth standards: Methods and development: Length/height-for-age, weight-for-age, weight-for-length, weight-for-height and body mass index-for-age: Methods and development.* https://www.who.int/childgrowth/standards/technical_report/en

Ziegler, E. E. (1991). Malnutrition in the premature infant. *Acta Paediatrica Scandinavica, 80*(Suppl. 374), 58–66. https://doi.org/10.1111/j.1651-2227.1991.tb12008.x

Zolotarjova, J., Ten Velde, G., & Vreugdenhil, A. C. E. (2018). Effects of multidisciplinary interventions on weight loss and health outcomes in children and adolescents with morbid obesity. *Obesity Reviews, 19*(7), 931–946. https://doi.org/10.1111/obr.12680

# Management of Genitourinary Disorders

Chrisla Key, Jill Travis, and Elizabeth A. Paton

## Student Learning Outcomes

Upon completion of this chapter the reader should be able to:

1. Discuss pathophysiology and epidemiology of selected genitourinary (GU) disorders in children.
2. Differentiate subjective and objective findings of selected GU disorders in children.
3. Choose appropriate laboratory or diagnostic tests for particular GU disorders in children.
4. Utilize the differential diagnosis process to determine GU diagnosis in children.
5. Determine treatment plan, child/family education, and need for referral in children with a GU diagnosis.

## INTRODUCTION

Genitourinary (GU) conditions in infants and children can cross all age groups and include infectious disorders, noninfectious disorders, and problems specific to the female and male genitalia. The severity of these conditions can range from common childhood conditions that can be managed with patient and family education to surgical emergencies that require immediate intervention.

The content in this chapter maps to the following areas on the Pediatric Nursing Certification Board (PNCB) Pediatric Nurse Practitioner—Primary Care certification examination:

**CLINICAL PROBLEMS: GENITOURINARY**

CONTENT AREAS:

**II. Assessment and Diagnosis**

**B. History and Physical Examination**

1. Obtain history of present illness
2. Obtain a comprehensive health history for new patients
3. Complete an interval history for established patients
4. Perform a review of systems
5. Perform a complete physical examination

**C. Diagnostic Testing and Screening**

1. Order and interpret office/clinic based screening tests
2. Order and interpret diagnostic laboratory tests
3. Order and interpret the results of diagnostic imaging tests

**D. Analyzing Information**

1. Integrate health history and physical examination findings into the plan of care
2. Assimilate findings from screening and diagnostic testing into plan of care

**E. Diagnosis**

1. Develop and prioritize differential diagnoses
2. Establish a diagnosis based on evaluation of patient data

## III. Management

### A. Child and Caregiver Counseling and Education

1. Provide condition-specific counseling and education, including treatment options
2. Educate about benefits and potential adverse reactions of pharmacological interventions
3. Discuss non-pharmacological interventions
4. Counsel regarding the threshold for seeking follow-up care
5. Review the risks of non-adherence to recommended treatment

### B. Therapeutic Interventions

1. Prescribe pharmacologic agents
2. Recommend the use of over-the-counter pharmacologic agents
3. Order or recommend non-pharmacologic treatments for the management of symptoms
4. Discuss use of complementary and alternative therapies as appropriate

### C. Procedures

1. Perform procedures in accordance with diagnostic guidelines and plan of care (rapid tests)
2. Initiate life-saving techniques in response to urgent or emergent situations

### D. Collaboration and Referral

2. Refer to specialists as indicated for evaluation, counseling, and/or treatment

### E. Care Coordination

1. Facilitate patient and family-centered care for children of all ages with acute and chronic conditions

### F. Evaluation and Follow-up

2. Establish a plan for follow-up care

## IV. Professional Role Responsibilities

### A. Leadership and Evidence-based Practice

4. Develop, implement, and/or modify clinical practice guidelines

## ANATOMY AND PHYSIOLOGY

The GU system consists of the upper and lower urinary tract (Figure 28.1). The upper urinary tract consists of two kidneys and two ureters. The components of the lower urinary tract are the bladder and the urethra. The kidneys are complex structures with three layers: a tough outer renal capsule, a cortex, and an inner medulla. The blood supply to the kidneys is via the renal vein and artery. The renal wastes drain through the renal pelvis and into the ureters. Within the ureters are valves that keep urine from refluxing into the kidneys. Finally, urine drains into the bladder and is excreted out of a single urethra. Functions of the GU system include acid-base balance, fluid regulation, electrolyte regulation, elimination of cellular waste products, and blood pressure regulation.

In females, the GU system also comprises reproductive organs: the ovaries, uterine (fallopian) tubes, uterus, cervix, and vagina (Figure 28.2B). In males, the reproductive organs include the penis, scrotum, testicles, vas deferens, seminal vesicles, prostate gland, and urethra (Figure 28.2A). The testicles are found within the scrotal sac. Testosterone and sperm are produced in the testicles. Once sperm is produced, it travels through the epididymis and the vas deferens into the seminal vesicles. The seminal vesicles are found behind the prostate and bladder.

## URINARY TRACT INFECTION

Urinary tract infection (UTI) is a blanket term for bacterial infection within the lower urinary tract or upper urinary system. The younger child with a UTI often presents with fever, whereas in the older child, an infection in the bladder alone will most often cause irritating symptoms, without fever. When the child presents as acutely ill with fever, nausea, and/or vomiting, then pyelonephritis (infection in the kidney) must be suspected.

The most common pathogen associated with UTIs in children is *Escherichia coli* (E. coli). There is a greater chance of renal scarring when bacteria other than E. coli are present. Most diagnosed UTIs can be managed on an outpatient basis with oral antibiotics. Children who are less than 2 months old, immunocompromised, or do not respond to oral antibiotics may need admission for intravenous antibiotic treatment (Shaikh & Hoberman, 2021).

Cystitis (bladder inflammation) can be present without an active infection of the urinary tract. This can occur after recent treatment of an infection or as a stand-alone illness. Children with cystitis may present with urinary symptoms that mimic symptoms of a UTI.

Children with pyelonephritis typically have an ill appearance and present with high fever, nausea, and/or vomiting. Some children have other vague complaints, including fatigue, decreased appetite,

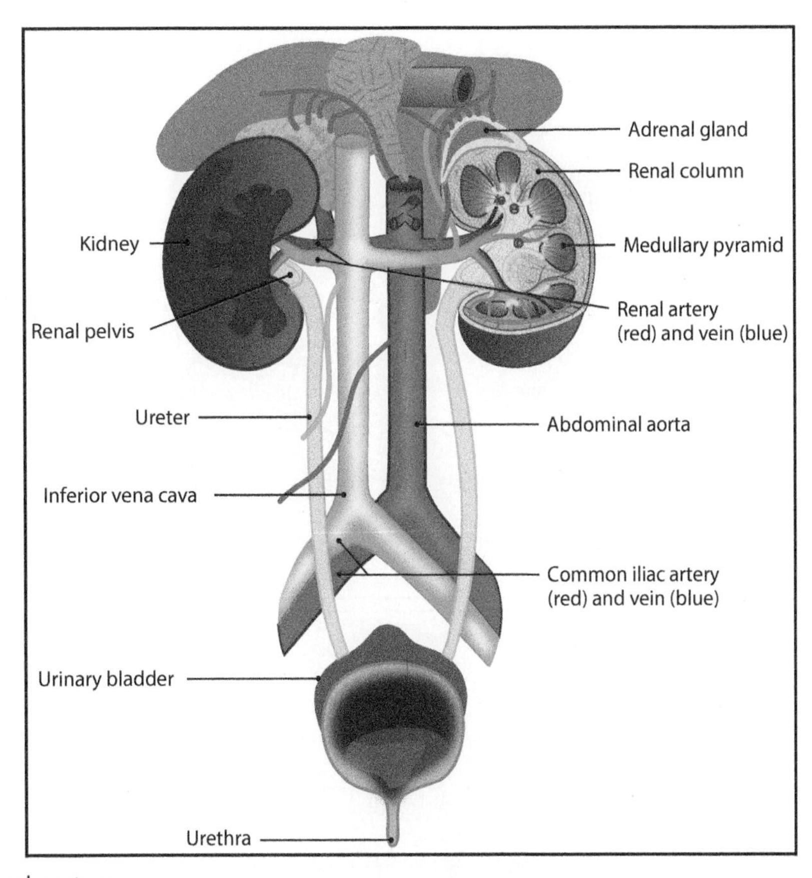


FIGURE 28.1 The renal system.

*Source:* Gawlik, K. S., Melnyk, B. M., & Teall, A. M. (Eds). (2021). *Evidence-based physical assessment: Best practices for health and well-being assessment*. Springer Publishing.

back and/or abdominal pain. Kidney involvement is the differentiating factor between pyelonephritis and standard UTI. Pyelonephritis in children increases suspicion of vesicoureteral reflux (VUR), an abnormal back-flow of urine (Shaikh & Hoberman, 2021).

## Subjective Findings

The health history may reveal:

- Dysuria
- Urinary incontinence, urgency, or frequency
- Malodorous urine
- Fever (particularly with pyelonephritis)

## Risk Factors

The most common risk factors for UTIs are:

- Age/Gender: Girls are more likely to have a UTI than boys. Girls younger than 4 years of age are of increased risk with the most common age being infancy. Although UTIs in boys are uncommon, boys who are uncircumcised and less than one year are at greatest risk.
- Ethnicity: For unknown reasons, infection in Caucasian children is more common that in African-American children.
- Family history of a parent or sibling having an infection
- Constipation
- Voiding postponement
- Poor hygiene
- Labial adhesions
- Previous infections
- Conditions resulting in urinary obstruction
- Neurogenic bladder, especially those requiring intermittent catheterization
- Sexual activity

## Review of Systems

The most common manifestations revealed during the review of systems include:

- **Constitutional:** fever or chills, weight loss, polydipsia, poor perineal hygiene
- **Gastrointestinal:** abdominal pain, nausea and/or vomiting, constipation, encopresis

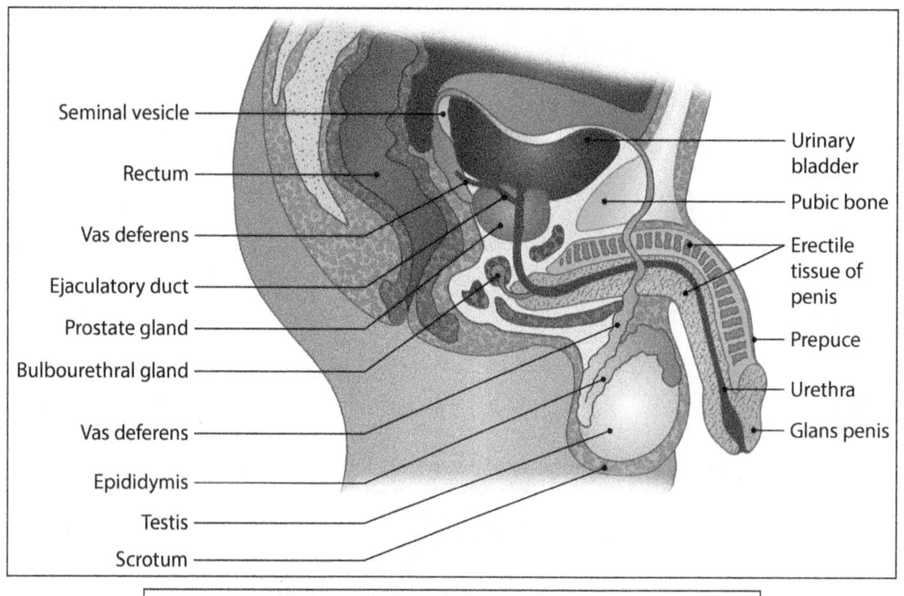


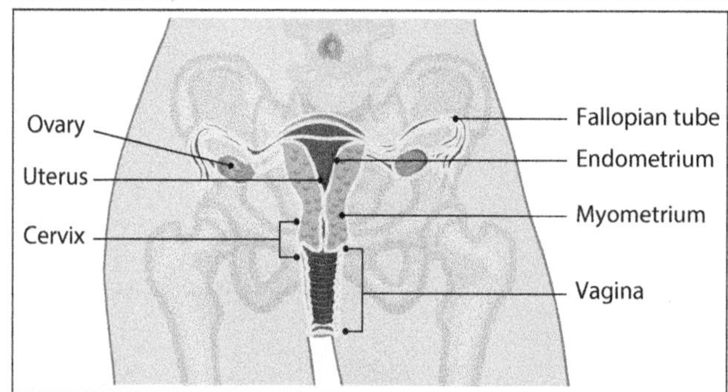


FIGURE 28.2 Reproductive system. (A) Male child. (B) Female child.

*Source*: Gawlik, K. S., Melnyk, B. M., & Teall, A. M. (Eds). (2021). *Evidence-based physical assessment: Best practices for health and well-being assessment*. Springer Publishing.

- **Genitourinary:** dysuria, urinary urgency or frequency, malodorous urine, voiding postponement
- **Musculoskeletal:** back or flank pain
- **Lymphatic:** swollen lymph nodes
- **Dermatologic:** rash to genitalia

## Objective Findings

The physical examination of the child with a UTI may reveal:

- Vaginal erythema/swelling
- Penile irritation/balanitis
- Abdominal or pelvic tenderness
- Fever
- Ill appearance (pyelonephritis)
- Back or flank (costovertebral angle or CVA) tenderness (pyelonephritis)

## Laboratory/Diagnostic Testing

The diagnosis of a UTI is presumed based on initial clinical findings and the results of urinalysis. Urine samples (including culture) should be obtained via the clean-catch method in toilet-trained children and via sterile catheterization or suprapubic aspiration in infants and non-toilet-trained children. A dipstick urinalysis may be performed in most outpatient settings, while few of those settings are equipped for microscopic analysis of urine. Laboratory findings helpful in diagnosis of UTI include:

- Urinalysis: although not sufficient to diagnose UTI, results suggestive of UTI include:
  - Positive for leukocyte esterase
  - Positive for nitrites
  - Microscopic analysis revealing white blood cells or bacteria (American Academy of Pediatrics [AAP], 2011)

- Urine culture is the gold standard for diagnosis of UTI and takes two to three days to provide a result. A urine culture is considered positive in:
  - Sample obtained via sterile catheterization or suprapubic aspiration: >50,000 colony forming units/mL
  - Clean-catch sample: positive urine culture has >100,000 colony forming units/ mL.
  - Urine cultures returning two or more pathogens are generally considered to be contaminated.
  - Immediate imaging is not standard practice. Pyelonephritis is the assumed diagnosis in ill-appearing, febrile children with a positive urine culture (AAP, 2011).

## Differential Diagnosis

The differential diagnosis for a UTI includes:

- Vulvovaginitis or vaginitis
- Urethritis
- Insulin-dependent diabetes
- Primary or secondary enuresis
- Detrusor instability/contractions
- Cystitis

The differential diagnosis for pyelonephritis includes:

- Uncomplicated UTI
- Pelvic inflammatory disease (PID)
- Intraabdominal infection such as appendicitis, colitis, or gastroenteritis
- Nephrolithiasis

> **PRO TIP** An online tool to assist with clinical decision making for the child 2 to 23 months of age is UTICalc (https://uticalc.pitt.edu).

## Treatment/Management Plan

Supportive care includes increased water intake, timed voiding, and treatment of underlying causes such as constipation. Children with fever may be given antipyretics. Initiate empiric antibiotics based on the presence of fever, suspicion of UTI, and the child's other risk factors (Figure 28.3). It is important to start antibiotics when suspicion of UTI is high, prior to receiving results of the urine culture, in order to avoid renal scarring (Nanda et al., 2017). High resistance to trimethoprim-sulfamethoxazole and amoxicillin is seen in some areas. Antibiotics to consider include:

- In low-risk children—cephalexin—50 to 100 mg/kg/day orally in two divided doses
- In high-risk children—cefdinir—14 mg/kg/day orally once daily
- cefixime—16 mg/kg orally on the first day, then 8 mg/kg orally once daily for the duration
- cefuroxime—30 mg/kg/day orally in two divided doses

The American Academy of Pediatrics (AAP) clinical guidelines advocate for 7 to 14 days of treatment. Nitrofurantoin (5–7 mg/kg/day orally, divided every 6 hours) may also be used but is known to result in gastrointestinal upset (Shaikh & Hoberman, 2021). Review urine culture results to ensure that the identified pathogen is susceptible to the prescribed antibiotic. It is important to note extended spectrum beta-lactamase (ESBL)-producing bacteria on the urine culture. When ESBL is positive, antibiotic treatment should be chosen that will penetrate the enzyme. If the urine culture result is negative, parents should be informed and antibiotics should be discontinued (AAP, 2011).

The AAP recommends a renal bladder ultrasound following a first UTI in children 2 to 24 months of age. Renal bladder ultrasound (RBUS) allows assessment of the renal and bladder anatomy. If the renal bladder ultrasound demonstrates obstructive uropathy, hydronephrosis, high-grade vesicoureteral reflux (VUR), or renal scarring, then a voiding cystourethrogram should be obtained as well (American Urological Association [AUA], 2017). Following a second UTI in children age 2 to 24 months, a voiding cystourethrogram should be performed to rule out VUR. Recommendations for older children are not established. A voiding cystourethrogram should never be performed when a child has an active infection.

> **PRO TIP** Always confirm UTI diagnosis with urine culture with sensitivities, as a negative urinalysis does not always completely rule out UTI. In contrast, a positive urinalysis does not differentiate between normal flora and a pathologic UTI.

### Family Education

Teach the following:

- Complete antibiotics as prescribed.
- Prevent additional UTIs by:
  - Having the toilet-trained child practice timed voiding.
  - Teaching proper wiping techniques (wiping anteriorly to posteriorly).
  - Treating constipation. If the child has been diagnosed with constipation, they will need to start a daily stool management such as polyeth-

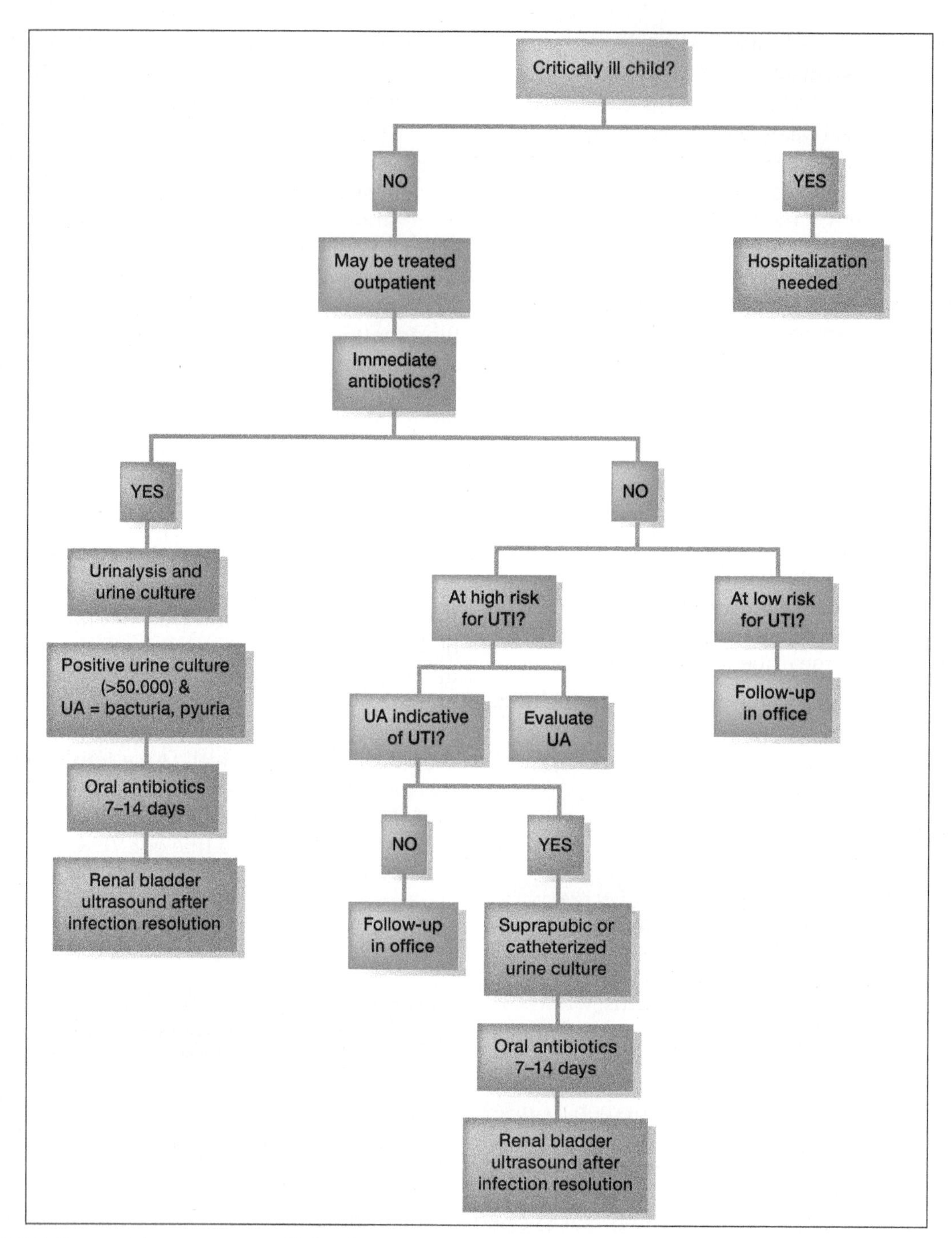


FIGURE 28.3 Fever without a source of infection

*Source*: Adapted from Nanda, G., Jahnukainen, T., & Vats, A. (2017). Urinary tract infections. In T. K. McInerny, H. M. Adam, D. E. Campbell, J. M. Foy, & D. M. Kamat (Eds.), American Academy of Pediatrics textbook of pediatric care (2nd ed., Chapter 344). American Academy of Pediatrics.

ylene glycol to prevent future episodes. Once the child reports pain with defecation or the inability to pass stool, the bladder has already been affected.

- Avoiding bladder-irritating foods and drinks in the diet such as citrus, artificial dyes, sugars/artificial sweeteners, caffeine (including chocolate), tea, and soda.

- Return for a recheck in 2 to 3 weeks.
- Ensure the child has prompt medical evaluation upon onset of fever if child has a history of pyelonephritis, febrile UTIs, or history of known VUR.

### Referral

Refer febrile infants younger than 2 months of age suspected of having UTIs to the hospital for admission to receive parenteral antibiotics. Children over 2 months of age who are febrile and toxic in appearance should also be reffered for parenteral antibiotics. Refer children with recurrent UTIs to a pediatric urologist.

# NONINFECTIOUS DISORDERS

Noninfectious urinary disorders occurring in children include VUR and nocturnal enuresis (NE).

## VESICOURETERAL REFLUX

VUR, also known as kidney reflux, is the retrograde flow of urine. Normally urine is produced in the kidneys and drains into the ureters, then into the bladder where it is stored. Once the bladder contracts, the urine is evacuated from the bladder by way of voiding. With VUR, the urine flows back into the mid- and/or upper-urinary tract.

Etiologies of VUR include abnormalities at the ureterovesical junction and diagnoses that disturb the bladder dynamics, including neurogenic bladder (Khoury & Bägli, 2021). The ureterovesical junction should have a valve to allow for antegrade flow of urine into the bladder; however, with VUR there can be incompetence of this valve allowing for the retrograde flow of urine back into the ureters and into the renal collecting system. When patients with VUR develop cystitis, the infected urine has a vehicle to reach the kidneys and can lead to pyelonephritis, which can then lead to irreversible renal scarring. VUR has a familial tendency; the prevalence of siblings with VUR is as high as >30% (Khoury & Bägli, 2021).

### Subjective Findings

The health history may reveal:

- Recurrent UTIs associated with fever
- Family history of recurrent UTIs (more importantly kidney infections) or VUR

### Risk Factors

The most common risk factors for VUR are:

- Family history of VUR
- Bladder and bowel dysfunction, including voiding postponement
- Complete ureteral duplication
- Paraureteral diverticulum
- Abnormal bladder dynamics due to neurogenic bladder
- Bladder outlet obstruction such as males with posterior urethral valves
- Multicystic dysplastic kidney (MCDK)—26% of patients with MCDK have VUR of the contralateral kidney
- Renal agenesis—46% of patients with renal agenesis have VUR of the contralateral kidney (Khoury & Bägli, 2021)

### Review of Systems

The most common manifestations revealed during the review of systems include:

- **Constitutional:** fever, flank pain
- **Genitourinary:** voiding postponement, CVA tenderness

### Objective Findings

The physical examination of the child with VUR will most likely be normal unless he or she has an acute UTI. In the case of an acute UTI, the patient may have the following on physical examination:

- Suprapubic tenderness
- CVA tenderness
- Malodorous urine
- Fever

### Laboratory/Diagnostic Testing

VUR is typically detected on a voiding cystourethrogram (VCUG). VCUG allows for the detection of VUR as well as grading of its severity. VUR is categorized as grade I, II, III, IV, or V (Khoury & Bägli, 2021):

- Grade I—retrograde flow of urine into a nondilated ureter, but does not reach the collecting system
- Grade II—retrograde flow of urine into the renal pelvis and calyces, no dilation
- Grade III—retrograde flow of urine into the renal pelvis and calyces, mild to moderate degree of ureteral dilation, fornices are blunted
- Grade IV—retrograde flow of urine into renal dilated pelvis and calyces, moderate tortuosity of ureter
- Grade V—retrograde flow of urine into markedly dilated ureter, renal pelvis, and calyces with severe ureteral tortuosity and loss of papillary impressions

Findings important to note with VUR are the presence or absence of renal parenchymal scarring due to a previous episode of pyelonephritis, duplicated renal collecting system, or the presence or absence of hydronephrosis. Fluctuating hydronephrosis may occur with VUR and is not directly indicative of the significance of VUR.

Prior to obtaining a VCUG, it is important to ensure that the patient does not have an acute UTI, because the VCUG is a retrograde study. If the patient has acute cystitis, a retrograde urinary tract study can cause pyelonephritis. At least 3 days of culture-specific antibiotic treatment is recommended prior to performing a retrograde urinary tract study.

### Differential Diagnosis

The differential diagnosis for VUR includes:

- Hydronephrosis
- Ureteropelvic junction obstruction
- Ureterovesical junction obstruction
- Neurogenic bladder
- Congenital megaureter
- UTI

### Treatment/Management Plan

Management of VUR can be classified into two categories: medical and surgical. The nonsurgical approach includes medical observation. Some patients experience spontaneous resolution of the VUR. The rate of spontaneous resolution is inversely related to the initial grade of the VUR (Khoury & Bägli, 2021). Bladder and bowel dysfunction can cause VUR that possibly would have spontaneously resolved to persist. Therefore, management of bowel and bladder dysfunction (including neurogenic bladder) in patients with VUR is important.

- With medical observation, obtain an annual RBUS and VCUG. Educate the family about prevention of UTI (see "Family Education" section following). For prevention of recurrent UTI in the child with VUR, antibiotic prophylaxis is suggested for all non-toilet–trained children and children with bowel or bladder dysfunction, regardless of severity of VUR, and all children with high-grade VUR (grades III–V). Suggested antibiotics include:
  - Infants 2 months of age and younger—either amoxicillin or cephalexin 25 mg/kg/day once daily in the evening (to maximize exposure with overnight urinary stasis; Khoury & Bägli, 2021).
- Children over 2 months of age—trimethoprim/sulfamethoxazole 2 mg/kg/day of each component or nitrofurantoin 1 to 2 mg/kg/day, once daily in the evening.

Surgical intervention is also a treatment option for patients. Ureteral reimplantation is a highly effective surgical approach for VUR. For lower grades of VUR, an endoscopic approach with subureteral dextranomer hyaluronic copolymer (Deflux) injections is effective as well (Khoury & Bägli, 2021).

#### Family Education

Teach the following:

- Discourage voiding postponement by placing the child on a timed-voiding regimen every 2–3 hours while awake (Williams et al., 2019).

#### Referral

If high-grade (III to V) VUR is diagnosed, refer to pediatric urology for further evaluation and possible surgical treatment.

> ALERT: Do not perform retrograde urinary tract diagnostic studies (e.g., VCUG) while the patient has an acute UTI, as infected urine may cause temporary VUR, which resolves with bacterial eradication (could result in erroneous diagnosis of VUR).

## NOCTURNAL ENURESIS

Nocturnal enuresis (NE) is involuntary wetting during the night in a toilet-trained child. Occasionally, a child with night wetting will become wet when napping during day hours. NE is described as either primary (no spans of dryness for 6 months since toilet training) or secondary. NE is further divided into monosymptomatic and nonmonosymptomatic NE. Nonmonosymptomatic NE is associated with day symptoms as well, including incontinence, urinary urgency, difficulty voiding, and urinary frequency.

NE is a common condition, with an estimated 10% of 7-year-olds still wetting their beds. The prevalence decreases with age, with 3% of teens and less than 1% of adults still having NE. It is a very stressful condition for the child and family. Early management helps prevent poor self-esteem, limitations of participation in age-appropriate activities, and family discord. Research shows that treatment also has positive effects on daytime behavior (Neveus, 2019).

### Subjective Findings

The health history may reveal:

- Night wetting
- Heavy sleep patterns

## Risk Factors

The most common risk factors for NE are:

- Family history
- Heavy sleep patterns (snoring, sleep apnea)
- Consuming fluids until bedtime
- Failure to void prior to bed
- Constipation
- Detrusor instability or spasms
- Small bladder capacity
- Attention deficit hyperactivity disorder (ADHD)
- Stress
- UTI
- Meatal stenosis
- Neurogenic bladder

## Review of Systems

The most common manifestations revealed during the review of systems include:

- **Constitutional:** consumption of dietary irritants (citrus, dye, and flavor additives, sugar/artificial sweeteners, caffeine [including chocolate], spicy foods, tea), smoking
- **Gastrointestinal:** constipation, encopresis
- **Genitourinary:** dysuria, urinary urgency, urinary frequency, voiding postponement
- **Musculoskeletal:** back or flank pain
- **Lymphatic:** swollen lymph nodes
- **Dermatologic:** rash to genitalia
- **Psychologic:** ADHD, stress, recent major life event

## Objective Findings

The physical examination of the child with NE may reveal:

- Abdominal distention
- Palpable stool in the abdomen
- Vulvovaginitis/vaginitis/perineal and gluteal rashes
- Abnormal lower spine (sacral dimples, hair tufts) and lower extremities (muscle atrophy)

## Laboratory/Diagnostic Testing

Obtaining a urinalysis to monitor for urine glucose and potential UTI is reasonable. For reports of foul-smelling urine or an abnormal urinalysis, a urine culture is warranted. For suspected constipation, a plain abdominal film of the kidneys, ureter, and bladder can help with diagnosis.

## Differential Diagnosis

The differential diagnosis for NE includes:

- Neurogenic bladder
- UTI
- Sleep apnea
- Diabetes

## Treatment/Management Plan

There are three categories of treatment for NE: behavioral modifications, use of a bed-wetting alarm, and pharmacologic management.
First-line treatment is behavioral modifications:

- Timed voiding every 2 hours throughout the day
- Monitoring and management of defecation with a goal of a soft, easy-to-pass, Bristol 4 stool daily
- Avoidance of bladder-irritating food/drinks in the diet
- Structured nightly routines: no excessive drinking prior to bed, always void prior to bed
- Evaluate and manage underlying stressors/ADHD (Tu & Baskin, 2020)

Second-line treatment is the use of a bedwetting alarm:

- Bedwetting alarms are only successful in well-motivated families. They are to be used in conjunction with all of the established bowel and bladder routines.
- Alarms must be used consistently for 3 to 6 months before deemed unsuccessful; heavy sleepers may have to use them longer.
- They are most successful when used in children >8 years old who can dress and undress themselves with ease and take themselves to the toilet (Tu & Baskin, 2020).

Third-line treatment is pharmacological management:

- Desmopressin (Vasopressin): A synthetic of the antidiuretic hormone (ADH) has been shown to be helpful in treating NE. Prescribe 0.2 mg orally, 1 hour before bedtime; after 10 to 14 days may increase dose as needed to a maximum of 0.4 mg (Desmopressin, 2021).
- Oxybutynin: An anticholinergic medication may be used in combination with desmopressin in children thought to have detrusor overactivity. Prescribe 25 to 50 mg orally, at bedtime. Children should have no post-void residual or constipation prior to use of this medication (Oxybutynin, 2021).

**PRO TIP** Encourage parents to begin treatment of NE only when the child is fully motivated and willing to be an active participant in care.

### Family Education

Teach the following:

- Avoid punishment for night wetting.
- Place a plastic pad over the mattress.
- Use disposable or washable bed pads.
- Avoid using night diapers, especially in children who are opposed to wearing them (in families with extreme discord as a result of the NE, this can be adjusted to meet the situation).
- Waking the child at night is neither medically supported nor curative.
- Proper use of bed-wetting alarms if they are used.
- If medications are prescribed, they must be properly used and stored (do not allow children to store and administer their own medications).

Teaching specific to particular medications:

- *Desmopression*: Rarely can lead to hyponatremia secondary to water intoxication when children are allowed to consume large amounts of water after it has been administered. Behavior modifications with consistent limitations of drinking at bedtime should be established before the medication is prescribed. Cases of seizures and death have been reported.
- *Oxybutynin*: may cause the side effects of anticholinergics (dry mouth, constipation, nose bleeds, etc.).

### Referral

Referral to a pediatric urologist is helpful for children with NE, as long-term management may be needed for this stressful condition.

> ALERT: Medication should *NEVER* be first-line treatment for NE.

## INGUINAL HERNIA

An inguinal hernia is a protrusion of abdominal contents into the inguinal canal. Inguinal hernias are more common in males, with 1% to 5% of term newborns being affected, and 9% to 11% of preterm newborns affected (Ramsook, 2020). The right side is more often involved, in both sexes.

There are two types of inguinal hernias, indirect and direct. In males, during the prenatal period, the testes migrate into the scrotum via the *processus vaginalis*. Once a testis has migrated into the scrotum, the processus vaginalis closes or obliterates. Failure of this to occur results in an indirect inguinal hernia, which is the most common type in children (Ramsook, 2020). If the residual opening in the processus vaginalis is small, only peritoneal fluid can drain into the scrotum, resulting in a hydrocele (see section later in this chapter).

In females, this process is similar except the ovaries do not leave the abdominal cavity and the structure that fails to close is the *diverticulum of Nuck*, which extends into the labia majora (Ramsook, 2020). A direct inguinal hernia is a result of weakness in the floor of the inguinal canal and is rarely seen in pediatric patients.

### Subjective Findings

The health history may reveal groin swelling that increases during the day or worsens with crying, coughing, or sneezing.

### Risk Factors

The most common risk factors for inguinal hernias are:

- Prematurity
- Chronic lung disease (bronchopulmonary dysplasia, cystic fibrosis)
- Connective tissue disorder (such as Ehlers-Danlos Syndrome)

### Review of Systems

The most common manifestations revealed during the review of systems include:

- **Gastrointestinal:** abdominal pain, nausea and/or vomiting (particularly if hernia is incarcerated).
- **Genitourinary:** Groin swelling that increases with straining, such as when having a bowel movement, coughing, crying, or laughing. No change in voiding pattern.

### Objective Findings

The physical examination of the child with an inguinal hernia may reveal:

- A bulge in the inguinal area that may extend into the scrotum or labia.
- To assess for an inguinal hernia:
  - Find the internal ring. If the internal ring is empty, it is not a hernia.
  - If a "squish" is felt with bowel sliding under your fingers at the internal ring, the child has a hernia.
  - If a hernia is present, apply gentle pressure down and toward the scrotum or labia. The hernia should easily reduce.

> PRO TIP In children, an inguinal hernia can often be visualized when the infant or child is crying or laughing, or by having the child perform maneuvers such as blowing into a straw or putting their thumb in their mouth and blowing.

### Laboratory/Diagnostic Testing

The diagnosis of an inguinal hernia is typically based solely on clinical findings. However, if the diagnosis is uncertain, an ultrasound may be obtained and reveal the presence of peritoneal fluid or intestinal contents moving in and out of the peritoneal cavity through the hernia.

### Differential Diagnosis

The differential diagnosis for an inguinal hernia includes:

- Inguinal or femoral lymphadenopathy
- Hydrocele
- Soft tissue masses such as a lipoma or lymphoma
- Bartholin gland cyst
- Hematoma
- Sebaceous cyst

### Treatment/Management Plan

The management of inguinal hernias is manual or surgical reduction by a pediatric surgeon or pediatric urologist.

> ALERT: Inguinal hernias may become incarcerated, resulting in strangulation of the bowel. Findings include discoloration at hernia site, firm bulging, pain, nausea, or vomiting. Refer the child for an emergent reduction or surgical evaluation.

### Family Education

Teach the following:

- The hernia area should remain soft, painless, and the color of the child's skin.
- Keep the appointment with the pediatric surgeon or urologist.
- If the child experiences pain or discoloration at the site with nausea/vomiting, abdominal bloating, or loss of appetite, take the child to the emergency department.

### Referral

Any child with the finding of an inguinal hernia should be referred for an evaluation by a pediatric surgeon or pediatric urologist. If there is any concern for an incarcerated hernia, the child should be immediately referred to an emergency department.

# FEMALE GENITALIA ISSUES

Disorders of the female GU system include labial adhesions and vulvovaginitis.

## LABIAL ADHESIONS

Labial adhesions occur when the labia minora adhere together. This varies in severity from complete closure of the introitus to a partial fusion. Labial adhesions typically occur when estrogen levels are at their lowest, between 3 months and 6 years of age. Vulvovaginal inflammation may lead to labial adhesions.

### Subjective Findings

The health history may reveal:

- Inability to part labia

### Risk Factors

The most common risk factors for labial adhesions are:

- age under 5 years
- conditions leading to inflammation, such as poor hygiene, physical or chemical trauma, and infection

### Review of Systems

The most common manifestations revealed during the review of systems include:

- **Integumentary:** rash or redness to genitalia
- **Genitourinary:** urine dribbling
- **Psychologic:** history of trauma, abuse, or sexual abuse

### Objective Findings

The physical examination of the child with labial adhesions may reveal:

- Partial or complete closure of the introitus
- Erythema and/or swelling to the labia

### Laboratory/Diagnostic Testing

The diagnosis of labial adhesions is based upon the history and physical examination findings. Urinalysis and urine culture may be indicated, if the girl has urinary symptoms or pain with walking.

### Differential Diagnosis

The differential diagnosis for labial adhesions includes:

- Vaginitis
- Vulvovaginitis

### Treatment/Management Plan

Mild adhesions will typically resolve spontaneously at puberty. More severe adhesions that block urine flow, cause discomfort, or lead to UTIs should be treated. The first-line treatment is estrogen cream (0.1%), a small amount applied twice daily. Alternatively, betamethasone cream (0.05%) could also be used.

### Family Education

Teach the following:

- Use creams for separation sparingly, directly on the adherent area only.
- After adhesion release, use petroleum-based creams several times daily to prevent recurrence of adherence.
- Allow age-appropriate children to apply their own creams with guidance.
- Encourage parents to closely monitor the area, as the condition is known to recur (Laufer & Emans, 2020).

### Referral

For labial adhesions that do not respond to cream after an 8-week period, manual or surgical separation may be indicated, although this is rare. Refer to a pediatric urologist if labial adhesions do not resolve within 8 weeks, or if they recur.

> PRO TIP Labial adhesions will likely recur if parents are not properly taught after-separation care. The petroleum-based cream application is the most important treatment step.

## VULVOVAGINITIS

Vulvovaginitis, also known as vaginitis, is inflammation of the vulva and vagina. It can be caused by bacteria, yeast, parasites, exposure to environmental irritants or soaps and bubble baths, poor hygiene, chronic masturbation, restrictive clothing, and sexually transmitted infections (STIs). In children whose recurrent vulvovaginitis is thought to be secondary to the alkaline environment of the vagina, resolution is expected at puberty.

### Subjective Findings

The health history may reveal:

- Pruritus
- Dysuria
- Vaginal pain or soreness
- For older children and teens, one should inquire about sexual activity and possible exposure to STIs (Laufer & Emans, 2020)

### Risk Factors

The most common risk factors for vulvovaginitis are:

- Poor hygiene
- Exposure to environmental irritants, soaps, bubble baths
- Restrictive clothing such as leggings/tight jeans
- Chronic masturbation
- History of STIs

### Review of Systems

The most common manifestations revealed during the review of systems include:

- **Constitutional:** consumption of dietary irritants (typically acidic drinks, e.g., orange juice)
- **Genitourinary:** vaginal discharge, vaginal itching, reported discomfort or pain with vaginal cleaning or wiping
- **Lymphatic:** swollen lymph nodes
- **Dermatologic:** genitalia rash
- **Psychologic:** history of neglect, sexual abuse

### Objective Findings

The physical examination of the child with vulvovaginitis may reveal:

- Erythema to the vaginal area
- Vaginal discharge

### Laboratory/Diagnostic Testing

The diagnosis of vulvovaginitis is based upon the clinical findings. No laboratory or diagnostic testing is needed.

### Differential Diagnosis

The differential diagnosis for vulvovaginitis includes:

- Candidal vaginitis
- STI
- UTI

### Treatment/Management Plan

Treatment typically includes use of topical anti-yeast and/or steroid creams, applied together twice daily. Topical steroids should be used in small amounts and for no more than 7 days. If an allergic reaction is suspected, topical or oral antihistamines should be used. If parasite exposure is suspected, an antiparasitic should be used.

### Family Education

Teach the following:

- Encourage good hygiene, with regular bathing and proper rinsing with clean water after use of soap. Baby soaps or dye-free soaps are best; harsh soaps should be avoided. Avoid bubble baths or other bath additives. Dry the vaginal area well prior to dressing. Air drying is fine if towel drying is uncomfortable.
- Have the child wear cotton panties.
- Avoid wearing of tight or restrictive clothing. Gowns are preferred for night use and dresses for day use. These allow air circulation.
- In summer, remove wet bathing suit soon after swimming.
- Practice spread-leg voiding by abducting the legs during voiding to prevent vaginal pooling of urine.
- Discourage children from harsh wiping after toileting and from scratching the vaginal area.
- For recurrent irritations, such as seen in chronic day/night incontinence, instruct parents to use barrier creams to protect the skin.

Teens should be encouraged to avoid sexual activity. Educate parents to avoid use of perfumed detergents. (Laufer & Emans, 2020).

**PRO TIP** For comfort, children can be allowed to sit in a clean tub of warm water. Baking soda or vinegar can be added if parents desire. Cold compresses can also be used.

### Referral

The primary provider usually treats vulvovaginitis. In some cases, referral to a dermatologist, gynecologist, or pediatric urologist can be made for further management. Referral often depends on underlying causes of repeated irritation.

# MALE GENITALIA ISSUES

Common issues related to male genitalia include cryptorchidism, phimosis and paraphimosis, hydrocele, spermatocele, varicocele, epididymitis, hypospadias and chordee, testicular torsion, and meatal stenosis.

## CRYPTORCHIDISM

Cryptorchidism, also known as an undescended testicle, refers to one or both testicles not being located within the scrotum. It occurs in as many as 4% of full-term boys, and as many as 45% of preterm boys (Barthold & Hagerty, 2021). In embryologic development, the testes begin as germ cells developing within the posterior abdomen around the fifth week of gestation (Niederberger, 2016). In normal circumstances, the germ cells migrate from the posterior abdomen into the inguinal canal, and eventually the scrotum, and this is typically completed in the third trimester of pregnancy (Niederberger, 2016). Cryptorchidism occurs when there is an arrest in this descension.

Cryptorchidism is associated with decreased fertility. It was discovered that of the men who had undergone surgical correction for unilateral cryptorchidism as children, 96% of those men successfully fathered a child and of those men who had undergone surgical correction for bilateral cryptorchidism as children, only 70% had successfully fathered a child (Barthold & Hagerty, 2021). Cryptorchidism is also associated with germ cell tumors (Stephenson & Gilligan, 2021).

### Subjective Findings

The health history may reveal:

- Caregiver reports inability to locate testes even after a warm bath
- Seemingly underdeveloped scrotum

### Risk Factors

The most common risk factors for cryptorchidism are:

- Prematurity
- Low birth weight for gestational age

- Maternal diabetes
- Family history of cryptorchidism
- Maternal smoking
- Decreased androgen production
- Persistent Mullerian duct syndrome
- Chromosome abnormalities or other syndromes such as Klinefelter syndrome, Down syndrome, Eagle-Barrett (prune belly syndrome), or other congenital anomalies such as myelomeningocele, omphalocele, and gastroschisis (Barthold & Hagerty, 2021).

### Review of Systems

The most common manifestations revealed during the review of systems include:

- **Genitourinary:** empty scrotum, testis intermittently present in scrotum

### Objective Findings

The physical examination of the child with cryptorchidism may reveal:

- Empty scrotum
- Palpable testis within inguinal canal
- Ability to manipulate testis into superior aspect of scrotum, and once the testis is released, it immediately returns to its position within the inguinal canal
- Nonpalpable testis within scrotum or inguinal canal

**PRO TIP** Always perform a genitourinary examination during a well child visit.

### Laboratory/Diagnostic Testing

The diagnosis of cryptorchidism is based upon the clinical findings. It is not recommended to perform a scrotal/testicular ultrasound to identify the position of the testes, as ultrasound is not a sensitive test for positioning of the testes (Shields et al., 2019).

### Differential Diagnosis

The differential diagnosis for cryptorchidism includes:

- Retractile testis
- Ascended testis
- Intra-abdominal testis
- Vanishing/vanished testis
- Testicular agenesis (Barthold & Hagerty, 2021)

**PRO TIP** To differentiate between undescended testes and retractile testes, manipulate the testis into the scrotum, hold the testis in place for several seconds to fatigue the cremasteric muscle fibers, then release the testis.

- If the testis remains in the scrotum, then that is a retractile testis.
- If the testis immediately rebounds into its original position, then it is an undescended testis.

### Treatment/Management Plan

Spontaneous descension of undescended testes occurs in 34% to 43% of boys before 3 months of age (AUA, 2014). Even in premature infants, if the testes have not spontaneously descended by 6 months corrected age, then definitive repair with orchidopexy by a urologist is warranted (AUA, 2014). The rationale is that the likelihood of spontaneous descent at that point is low and the risks associated with general anesthesia are lower. Orchidopexy after puberty is associated with few positive effects on semen analysis, so the timing of definitive repair is important.

### Family Education

Teach the following:

- Due to the association between undescended testes and testicular cancer in the future, the child needs to perform monthly self-testicular examinations once puberty is entered.
- The average age for testicular cancer is young adulthood.

### Referral

If cryptorchidism is suspected, then referral to a pediatric urologist is warranted. If the patient has bilateral cryptorchidism with hypospadias or if the patient has bilateral cryptorchidism and ambiguous genitalia, then an evaluation for congenital adrenal hyperplasia and other disorders of sexual differentiation should be performed, as adrenal hyperplasia can be life-threatening. Such an evaluation should include genetics, endocrinology, and urology (AUA, 2014).

## PHIMOSIS AND PARAPHIMOSIS

Phimosis is a natural occurrence for infants and young boys. The prepuce, also known as the foreskin, naturally has a propensity to adhere to the glans of the phallus. These penile adhesions can lead to an inability to fully retract the foreskin. A preputial ring, a tight band of fibrinous tissue surrounding the glans, can also prevent full retraction of the foreskin. Both of these mechanisms of action can lead to phimosis.

Phimosis can be primary or secondary. Primary phimosis is what occurs naturally at birth (also termed *physiologic phimosis*). Secondary (pathologic) phimosis is due to other causes such as a postcircumcision circumferential scar, recurrent balanitis/balanoposthitis, forced retraction of the foreskin leading to the formation of fibrinous tissue, or phimosis that persists beyond 5 years of age (Palmer & Palmer, 2021).

The ability to retract the prepuce typically improves as the child ages. Therefore, as long as the patient has no complication due to being uncircumcised, it is no longer considered medically necessary to circumcise boys unless those complications arise. It is also natural for skin debris, called *smegma*, to accumulate on the glans of the phallus. At times, penile inclusion cysts can develop, which is the accumulation of smegma underneath the adhesion.

Paraphimosis is due to the prepuce becoming trapped proximal to the glans of the phallus. This can occur if the foreskin is retracted but not reduced afterward. The entrapped prepuce becomes edematous, forming a constrictive band around the glans that can lead to glanular gangrene.

### Subjective Findings

The health history may reveal:

- Inability to retract foreskin and/or to visualize the glans of the phallus
- Ballooning of the foreskin after voiding due to urine accumulating under the foreskin prior to draining out from the opening at the phimotic ring
- Inability to clean the glans of the phallus

#### Risk Factors

The most common risk factors for phimosis are:

- Congenital penile adhesions
- Recurrent inflammation
- Balanitis xerotica obliterans (Palmer & Palmer, 2021)

The most common risk factor for paraphimosis is:

- Failure to reduce foreskin

#### Review of Systems

The most common manifestations of phimosis revealed during the review of systems include:

- **Genitourinary:** inability to retract foreskin, visualize the glans of the phallus, and/or to clean the glans of the phallus; dysuria; redness of the prepuce; white milky drainage from phimotic opening (this is typically urine combined with smegma)

The most common manifestations of paraphimosis revealed during the review of systems include:

- **Genitourinary:** swelling just below the tip of the penis

### Objective Findings

The physical examination of the child with phimosis may reveal:

- A preputial ring, a tight band of fibrinous tissue surrounding the glans, preventing full retraction of foreskin

The physical examination of the child with paraphimosis may reveal:

- Edematous foreskin forming a constrictive band around the glans

#### Laboratory/Diagnostic Testing

The diagnoses of phimosis and paraphimosis are based upon the clinical findings. No laboratory or diagnostic testing is needed.

### Differential Diagnosis

The differential diagnosis for phimosis and paraphimosis includes:

- Phimosis
- Paraphimosis
- Balanitis

### Treatment/Management Plan

Physiologic phimosis simply requires GU hygiene. Low-potency topical corticosteroids can be applied twice daily to the phimotic ring for 6 to 8 weeks to assist in loosening the phimotic ring (Oettgen, 2017). If phimosis persists, it may be resolved with circumcision.

▶ ALERT: Paraphimosis is a medical emergency and requires immediate reduction of the edematous prepuce that has become entrapped proximal to the glans of the phallus.

### Family Education

Teach the following:

- Manipulate the foreskin by attempting to gently retract it with each diaper change, as well as at bath time, for diapered boys. For boys who are no longer in diapers, this should be performed a couple of times a day.
- Do not attempt to forcibly retract the foreskin. Once the foreskin is retractable, retract the foreskin at each diaper change and bath time, cleanse the phallus well, apply petroleum jelly, and reduce the foreskin upon completion to prevent recurrence of phimosis, and also to prevent paraphimosis.

### Referral

Refer infants or boys with pathologic phimosis to a pediatric urology specialist. If paraphimosis occurs, refer the child to the emergency room.

## HYDROCELE, SPERMATOCELE, AND VARICOCELE

Hydroceles, spermatoceles, and varicoceles are additional abnormalities that may be noted during assessment of the scrotum. A hydrocele is an accumulation of fluid in the scrotal sac. In a communicating hydrocele, the processus vaginalis has failed to close, leaving a small residual opening allowing only peritoneal fluid to pass through it. The swelling typically increases throughout the day when the child is more upright or standing, and then becomes smaller or even disappears when the child is recumbent. Fluid may also accumulate spontaneously around the testicle, which would be referred to as a reactive or noncommunicating hydrocele. Most commonly this is in response to a viral or bacterial infection or trauma. A smaller mobile mass present on palpation of the scrotal sac may represent a spermatocele (sperm-filled cyst; Brenner & Ojo, 2021).

When the structure that is responsible for the venous drainage of the testicle, known as pampiniform venous plexus, enlarges, a varicocele may develop. More commonly found on the left side, varicoceles may occur in 10% to 25% percent of teenage boys (Brenner & Ojo, 2021). They are not common in boys less than 10 years of age. The presence of a varicocele may lead to an increased risk of infertility because it can interfere with spermatogenesis. The grading system for varicocele is:

- *Grade I*—only palpable during Valsalva maneuvers
- *Grade II*—nonvisible, palpable without Valsalva maneuver
- *Grade III*—grossly visible (Brenner & Ojo, 2021).

### Subjective Findings

The health history may reveal:

- Painless scrotal swelling or mass noted in scrotum

### Risk Factors

The most common risk factors for a hydrocele are:

- Recent viral illness
- Epididymitis
- Onset of puberty
- History of prematurity

The most common risk factors for a varicocele are:

- Hyperthermia
- Hypoxia

There are no risk factors for the development of a spermatocele.

### Review of Systems

The most common manifestations revealed during the review of systems include:

- **Constitutional:** fever, myalgia
- **Gastrointestinal:** lower abdominal pain
- **Genitourinary:** scrotal swelling (particularly after prolonged standing or Valsalva maneuvers), palpable scrotal mass, scrotal pain

### Objective Findings

The physical examination of the child with a hydrocele may reveal:

- Unilateral or bilateral scrotal swelling that transilluminates (light held behind the scrotum shines through when the mass is cystic).
- Increased scrotal swelling with crying, straining, or other Valsalva maneuvers.
- Diffuse palpable mass within the scrotum. If this is a communicating hydrocele, the mass may be reducible.

The physical examination of a child with a varicocele may reveal:

- A mass, or "bag of worms," palpated superior to the testicle. Mass may enlarge with Valsalva maneuvers.

The physical examination of a child with a spermatocele may reveal:

- A small, mobile mass superior and posterior to the testicle, which also transilluminates

### Laboratory/Diagnostic Testing

The diagnosis of a hydrocele, spermatocele, or varicocele is based upon the clinical findings. No laboratory or diagnostic testing is needed.

### Differential Diagnosis

The differential diagnosis for hydrocele, spermatocele, and varicocele includes:

- Torsion of the appendix testis
- Orchitis
- Inguinal hernia
- Epididymitis
- Testicular tumor

### Treatment/Management Plan

In children, a noncommunicating hydrocele will typically resolve by age 2 years. If it does not, surgical evaluation may be warranted. If a communicating hydrocele is present, surgical intervention may be needed.

### Family Education

Teach the following:

- Hydroceles, spermatoceles, and varicoceles are typically benign and can be safely managed with observation.
- Boys with a history of spermatocele have an increased risk of infertility.

### Referral

Refer boys with a hydrocele, spermatocele, or varicocele to a pediatric urologist for evaluation and treatment.

## EPIDIDYMITIS

Epididymitis is inflammation of the epididymis with associated epididymal edema and pain. If the inflammation extends down to the testicle, it is considered epididymo-orchitis (Nickel, 2021). Acute epididymitis occurs when symptoms last less than 6 weeks, whereas with chronic epididymitis, symptoms last longer than 6 weeks. Epididymitis is usually caused by pathogens ascending into the urinary tract (Michel et al., 2015). UTIs may lead to epididymitis (particularly in younger boys) and STIs (most commonly chlamydia and gonorrhea) also cause epididymitis (Nickel, 2021). Some cases of epididymitis have noninfectious etiologies.

### Subjective Findings

The health history may reveal:

- Unilateral testicular pain that was gradual in onset
- Pain may radiate to abdomen or contralateral testicle occasionally
- Fever
- Urinary complaints such as urinary frequency, dysuria, urinary urgency

### Risk Factors

The most common risk factors for epididymitis are:

- STIs
- UTIs
- Activities predisposing boys and adolescents to epididymitis, include bicycle or motorcycle riding, sexual activity, and strenuous exercise (Brenner & Ojo, 2021)

### Review of Systems

The most common manifestations revealed during the review of systems include:

- **Constitutional:** unilateral testicular pain
- **Genitourinary:** symptoms of UTI or STI

### Objective Findings

The physical examination of the child with epididymitis may reveal:

- Unilateral epididymal tenderness and induration
- Normal cremasteric reflex
- positive Prehn sign (pain relief with lifting of scrotum on affected side)

### Laboratory/Diagnostic Testing

Epididymitis is suspected based on physical examination and history. It can be diagnosed by coupling clinical findings with scrotal/testicular ultrasound with Doppler (Wang et al., 2019). On testicular ultrasound, the epididymis will appear hyperemic. In an effort to treat the underlying cause, evaluate for chlamydia and gonorrhea (see chapter 31). Perform urine culture and sensitivity to rule out UTI.

### Differential Diagnosis

The differential diagnosis for epididymitis includes:

- Testicular torsion
- Torsion of testicular appendage
- Orchitis
- Idiopathic orchialgia

### Treatment/Management Plan

Management of epididymitis includes treatment of the underlying cause (Palmer & Palmer, 2021). If the underlying cause is an STI, then treatment of the STI is needed. If the underlying cause is a UTI, then culture-specific treatment of the UTI is needed. Nonsteroidal anti-inflammatory drugs (NSAIDs) are beneficial for pain management. Other supportive care options include the use of tight-fitted underwear, avoidance of strenuous activity, and elevation of the scrotum when possible.

### Family Education

Teach the following:

- When STI is the underlying cause:
  - Educate on safe sex practices.
  - Sexual partners within the 60 days prior to the symptoms should also be treated for the STI (Centers for Disease Control and Prevention, 2015).
- If the underlying cause is UTI and the patient is uncircumcised, then a discussion on the benefits of circumcision is warranted.

### Referral

Most cases of epididymitis can be managed by the primary care provider. However, referral to a pediatric urologist is necessary with chronic or recurrent epididymitis. If epididymitis is caused by a pathogen unrelated to an STI, then consider referral to a pediatric urologist to rule out other urinary tract abnormalities.

## HYPOSPADIAS AND CHORDEE

Hypospadias is characterized by the urethral meatus being positioned proximal to the orthotopic glanular location on the ventral aspect of the phallus. The diagnosis is further classified by the location of the urethral meatus as distal, midshaft, or proximal, with distal hypospadias comprising the majority of cases (van der Horst & de Wall, 2017). More specifically, the degree of hypospadias can also be described as glanular, coronal, midshaft, penoscrotal, scrotal, or perineal. The prevalence of hypospadias is 1 in 300 males (Snodgrass & Bush, 2021).

Hypospadias is commonly associated with ventral chordee and dorsal hooded foreskin (Snodgrass & Bush, 2021). Chordee is curvature of the penis, and it can be categorized as dorsal, ventral, lateral, or complex. It may occur with or without frank hypospadias, although ventral chordee is still technically considered on the spectrum of hypospadias (McCammon, 2021).

### Subjective Findings

The health history may reveal:

- Ectopic urethral meatus
- Asymmetric foreskin
- Curved penis
- Abnormal voiding stream

### Risk Factors

The most common risk factors for hypospadias are:

- First-degree relative with hypospadias
- Disorders of sex development (Snodgrass & Bush, 2021)
- Partial androgen insensitivity syndrome (Kosti et al., 2019)
- Pregestational diabetes and gestational diabetes (Yang et al., 2019)
- Prematurity
- Conceived by in vitro fertilization or intracytoplasmic sperm injection
- Lack of prenatal exposure to androgens
- Prenatal exposure to diethylstilbestrol (DES) or progestin (Ferri, 2020)

### Review of Systems

The most common manifestations revealed during the review of systems include:

- **Genitourinary:** Urethral meatus not in correct position, abnormal urinary stream, asymmetric foreskin

### Objective Findings

The physical examination of the child with hypospadias may reveal:

- Dorsal-hooded prepuce (foreskin) with a lack of ventral prepuce
- Ventral penile chordee
- Ectopic urethral meatus located proximal to the orthotopic glanular position on the ventral aspect of the phallus
- Glans of the phallus tilted downward (Snodgrass & Bush, 2021)

### Laboratory/Diagnostic Testing

The diagnoses of hypospadias and chordee are based upon the clinical findings. No laboratory or diagnostic testing is needed.

### Differential Diagnosis

The differential diagnosis for hypospadias and chordee includes:

- Chordee
- Megameatus
- Disorders of sexual differentiation
- Partial androgen insensitivity
- Micropenis

### Treatment/Management Plan

Surgical intervention may occur in one or multiple stages depending on the severity of the hypospadias and chordee (Snodgrass & Bush, 2021).

#### Family Education

Teach the following:

- Hypospadias can be familial
- Common complications of hypospadias repair include complete breakdown of the repair, development of a urethrocutaneous fistula, meatal stenosis, urethral stricture, urethral diverticulum (Ferri, 2020).
- The impact of hypospadias on fertility is related to the direction the semen exits from the phallus; it does not directly affect spermatogenesis.

#### Referral

If hypospadias and/or chordee is suspected, then refer the patient to a pediatric urologist.

## TESTICULAR TORSION

Testicular torsion occurs when the spermatic cord twists upon itself, causing an interruption of testicular blood flow (Palmer & Palmer, 2021). Several structures reside within the spermatic cord: the vas deferens, a vein, and an artery. These structures are covered by a layer of tunica vaginalis and that is covered by the cremasteric muscle. There are two types of testicular torsions, extravaginal and intravaginal. Extravaginal torsion is when the twisting occurs outside of the tunica vaginalis; this typically occurs perinatally. Intravaginal torsion is when the twisting occurs within the tunica vaginalis; this is the type that typically occurs in older children.

### Subjective Findings

The health history may reveal the following.

For older children:

- May have been of normal health and activity level prior to this
- May have reports of intermittent testicular discomfort that spontaneously resolved
- May have had a recent history of testicular trauma

For neonates:

- Reports of enlarged scrotum that was present at birth or developed shortly after birth
- Pain-free

#### Risk Factors

The most common risk factors for testicular torsion include:

- Family history.
- Age younger than 25 years.
- Bell clapper deformity (Palmer & Palmer, 2021).
  A bell-clapper deformity appears when the structure that secures the tunica vaginalis to the posterior scrotal wall is absent, allowing the testicle to move more freely within the scrotum.

#### Review of Systems

The most common manifestations revealed during the review of systems include the following.

For older children:

- **Constitutional:** pain causing awakening from sleep
- **Gastrointestinal:** referred abdominal or inguinal pain with/without vomiting
- **Genitourinary:** sudden onset of testicular pain, possible testicular trauma
- **Musculoskeletal:** altered gait due to pain

For neonates:

- **Constitutional:** pain-free
- **Genitourinary:** enlarged scrotum that was present at birth or developed shortly after birth

### Objective Findings

The physical examination of the older child with testicular torsion may reveal:

- Scrotal induration on affected side
- Testicular orientation may have a horizontal lie rather than a vertical one; affected side may appear higher than the contralateral side
- Absent cremasteric reflex on the affected side (highly sensitive for testicular torsion; Palmer & Palmer, 2021)
- Pain with palpation

The physical examination of the neonate with testicular torsion may reveal:

- Large, painless, scrotal mass

**PRO TIP** Perform testicular examination on all males with abdominal pain.

### Laboratory/Diagnostic Testing

The diagnosis of testicular torsion can be strongly suspected based upon the clinical findings; however, a scrotal/testicular ultrasound with Doppler is typically used to confirm the diagnosis (Wang et al., 2019). Ultrasound will demonstrate normal blood flow in the unaffected testicle, and no blood flow in the affected testicle.

The concept of intermittent testicular torsion is important to note. With intermittent testicular torsion, the testicle can become torsed, but then spontaneously detorse. In intermittent testicular torsion, if the testicle is not acutely torsed, then the ultrasound will in turn be normal. This coupled with a history of intermittent testicular pain with spontaneous resolution is suggestive of intermittent testicular torsion.

### Differential Diagnosis

The differential diagnosis for testicular torsion includes:

- Intermittent testicular torsion
- Epididymitis
- Gastroenteritis in patients who present with abdominal pain and vomiting
- Torsion of epididymal or testicular appendages
- Orchitis
- Incarcerated hernia

### Treatment/Management Plan

Testicular torsion is a medical emergency that requires immediate surgical intervention by a pediatric urologist. If testicular detorsion occurs within 4 to 8 hours of the first symptom, then the vast majority of the testicle can be salvaged. It is unlikely that a torsed testicle will be salvageable after 24 hours (Kolon & Canning, 2021).

### Family Education

Teach the following:

- Create an open line of communication so patients feel comfortable informing caregivers of testicular pain as soon as it is experienced.
- It is important to discuss this problem with young boys prior to its occurrence as a primary prevention measure in encounters such as well child office visits.

### Referral

Testicular torsion is a medical emergency that requires immediate surgical intervention by a urologist.

## MEATAL STENOSIS

Meatal stenosis refers to the narrowing of the urethral meatus. This is one of the most common complications of circumcision, but has also been seen as a complication of other penile surgeries such as hypospadias repair (Özen et al., 2019). Meatal stenosis can occur months after a penile surgery. The exact cause is unknown; however, several possible etiologies have been postulated. These etiologies include separation of the penile adhesion by way of lysis of penile adhesions or circumcision eliciting an inflammatory response, interruption of the penile frenular artery, chemical irritation by urine, or balanitis xerotica obliterans (Palmer & Palmer, 2021).

### Subjective Findings

Keep in mind that this condition may not be noticeable until toilet training (Özen et al., 2019). The health history may reveal:

- Abnormal urinary stream (spraying, deflection, deviation)
- Terminal hematuria (blood at the end of the urinary stream)
- Dysuria
- Urinary frequency or incontinence (Özen et al., 2019)
- Reports of "urine all over" the toilet or bathroom

### Risk Factors

The most common risk factors for meatal stenosis are history of circumcision or other penile surgery, little to no postoperative spreading of the urethral meatus, and balanitis xerotica obliterans.

### Review of Systems

The most common manifestations revealed during the review of systems include:

- **Genitourinary:** abnormal urinary stream, blood at the end of the urinary stream, dysuria, urinary frequency, urinary incontinence (Özen et al., 2019)

### Objective Findings

The physical examination of the child with meatal stenosis may reveal:

- Once the urethral meatus is spread, a small opening is noted due to scarring
- Palpable bladder
- If urinary stream is visualized, spraying, deflecting, or deviation (small caliber or high velocity; Özen et al., 2019)

**PRO TIP** In cases where the physical examination is borderline (not perfectly clear that meatus is of small size), visualizing the patient's urinary stream is helpful in the discernment of symptomatic meatal stenosis.

### Laboratory/Diagnostic Testing

The diagnosis of meatal stenosis is based upon the clinical findings. Incomplete bladder emptying may be noted on a post-void residual bladder scan, although no laboratory or diagnostic testing is needed.

### Differential Diagnosis

The differential diagnosis for meatal stenosis includes:

- Meatal stenosis
- Dysfunctional voiding
- UTI
- Hematuria

### Treatment/Management Plan

The definitive treatment for meatal stenosis is surgical intervention via meatoplasty or meatotomy by a pediatric urologist (Palmer & Palmer, 2021). It is important to counsel the caregivers on proper postoperative care, as recurrent meatal stenosis is possible. Diligent postoperative care can reduce the probability of recurrence.

### Family Education

Teach the following:

- Postoperative care is imperative to preventing recurrence of meatal stenosis

### Referral

If meatal stenosis is diagnosed or suspected, then a referral to a pediatric urologist for evaluation and/or definitive surgical repair is necessary.

## URINE SPECIMEN COLLECTION

Urine studies are most accurate when collected properly. Sterile specimen cups should be used as collection devices of choice for toilet-trained children. Collection devices used in the toilet bowl, often called "hats" because of their shape, should be avoided because these devices are not sterile.

Collection options include:

- Urine bag (adhesive bag placed around the perineum)
  - Used at the provider's discretion.
  - This is a noninvasive way to collect urine.
  - Often used in healthy-appearing older infants and children when a urine sample is requested, but caregivers are reluctant to allow catheterization.
  - A negative result avoids the need for catheterization.
  - Prior to application, the skin should be cleaned well, removing all oil, lotions, and creams.
  - After the area dries, the adhesive bag is placed starting in the bridge of skin between the genitals and rectum. It is then secured upward, making sure it adheres well.
  - Some caveats about use: These bags often leak and there are high contamination rates (Bajaj & Bothner, 2020).
- Urethral catheterization
  - Sterile intermittent catheterization should be used in non-toilet–trained children who are ill enough to warrant sterile urine collection.
  - Can be used in older ill children who cannot provide a voided sample.
- Suprapubic aspiration
  - Direct aspiration, using a needle placed through the skin above the pubis directly into the bladder.
  - Considered the gold standard for urine collection in young children acutely ill when a UTI is suspected.
  - Safe, rapid and little contamination risk.
  - Ultrasound guidance can be used.
  - Risks include bleeding, intestinal perforation, and infection.
- Voiding
  - Children can be assisted to collect a clean-catch midstream urine sample with the help of a parent.
  - Special care should be used to ensure that patient/parents are taught to clean well anteriorly to posteriorly with antiseptic wipes prior to collection.
  - The cup should remain closed and sterile until directly prior to collection.

- The urine should be initiated, then the specimen cup should be placed mid-stream to collect urine directly into the cup.
- The top should be replaced immediately.

## KEY POINTS

- To avoid UTI, teach proper hygiene.
- Urine culture is the gold standard for diagnosis of UTIs.
- In children with VUR, it is important to manage dysfunctional voiding habits and discourage voiding postponement.
- NE refers to bed wetting past the age of successful toilet training. Behavioral modification techniques are the first line of treatment, and bedwetting alarms are second-line; medications should be used only when behavioral modifications and bed-wetting alarms have been deemed unsuccessful.
- The infant or child with suspected incarcerated hernia should be referred to a pediatric surgeon or pediatric urologist for medical or surgical reduction.
- To avoid labial adhesions and vulvovaginitis, teach appropriate perineal hygiene.
- Paraphimosis is a medical emergency.
- Hypospadias is a diagnosis characterized by the urethral meatus being positioned proximal to the orthotopic glanular location on the ventral aspect of the phallus.
- Testicular torsion is a medical emergency. If treated within 4 to 8 hours of the first symptom, the likelihood of salvaging the testicle is increased.
- Cryptorchidism is one of the most common congenital genital anomalies. If the testis has not spontaneously descended by 6 months corrected age, the patient will most likely require definitive repair with an orchiopexy.
- Testicular torsion pain is typically sudden in onset, whereas epididymitis pain is typically gradual in onset.

## REFERENCES


American Academy of Pediatrics Subcommittee on Urinary Tract Infection, Steering Committee on Quality Improvement and Management. (2011). Urinary tract infection: Clinical practice guideline for the diagnosis and management of the initial UTI in febrile infants and children 2 to 24 months. *Pediatrics, 128*(3), 595–610. https://doi.org/10.1542/peds.2011-1330

American Urological Association. (2014). *Guideline statement: Evaluation and treatment of cryptorchidism.* https://www.auanet.org/guidelines/cryptorchidism-guideline

American Urological Association. (2017). *Guideline statement: Management and screening of primary vesicoureteral reflux in children.* https://www.auanet.org/guidelines/vesicoureteral-reflux-guideline#x3318

Bajaj, L., & Bothner, J. (2020). Urine collection techniques in infants and children with suspected urinary tract infections. *UpToDate.* https://www.uptodate.com/contents/urine-collection-techniques-in-infants-and-children-with-suspected-urinary-tract-infection

Barthold, J. S., & Hagerty, J. (2021). Etiology, diagnosis, and management of the undescended testis. In A. W. Partin, R. R. Dmochowski, L. R. Kavoussi, & C. A. Peters (Eds.), *Campbell-Walsh-Wein urology* (12th ed., Chapter 148). Elsevier.

Brenner, J. S., & Ojo, A. (2021). Causes of scrotal pain in children and adolescents. *UpToDate.* https://www.uptodate.com/contents/causes-of-scrotal-pain-in-children-and-adolescents

Centers for Disease Control and Prevention. (2015). Sexually transmitted diseases treatment guidelines 2015. *Morbidity and Mortality Weekly Report, 64*(3), 1–136. https://www.cdc.gov/mmwr/preview/mmwrhtml/rr6403a1.htm

Desmopressin: Pediatric drug information. (2021). *UpToDate.* https://www.uptodate.com/contents/desmopressin-pediatric-drug-information

Ferri, F. F. (2020). *Ferri's clinical advisor 2020.* Elsevier.

Khoury, A. E., & Bägli, D. J. (2021). Vesicoureteral reflux. In A. W. Partin, R. R. Dmochowski, L. R. Kavoussi, & C. A. Peters (Eds.), *Campbell-Walsh-Wein urology* (12th ed., Chapter 137). Elsevier.

Kolon, T. F., & Canning, D. A. (2021). Urologic evaluation of the child. In A. W. Partin, R. R. Dmochowski, L. R. Kavoussi, & C. A. Peters (Eds.), *Campbell-Walsh-Wein urology* (12th ed., Chapter 125). Elsevier.

Kosti, K., Athanasiadis, L., & Goulis, D. G. (2019). Long-term consequences of androgen insensitivity syndrome. *Maturitas, 127*, 51–54. https://doi.org/10.1016/j.maturitas.2019.06.004

Laufer, M., & Emans, S. (2020). Overview of vulvovaginal complaints in the prepubertal child. *UpToDate.* https://www.uptodate.com/contents/overview-of-vulvovaginal-complaints-in-the-prepubertal-child

McCammon, K. A. (2021). Surgery for benign disorders of the penis and urethra. In A. W. Partin, R. R. Dmochowski, L. R. Kavoussi, & C. A. Peters (Eds.), *Campbell-Walsh-Wein urology* (12th ed., Chapter 40). Elsevier.

Michel, V., Pilatz, A., Hedger, M. P., & Meinhardt, A. (2015). Epididymitis: Revelations at the convergence of clinical and basic sciences. *Asian Journal of Andrology, 17*(5), 756–763. https://doi.org/10.4103/1008-682X.155770

Nanda, G., Jahnukainen, T., & Vats, A. (2017). Urinary tract infections. In T. K. McInerny, H. M. Adam, D. E. Campbell, J. M. Foy, & D. M. Kamat (Eds.), *American Academy of Pediatrics textbook of pediatric care* (2nd ed., Chapter 344). American Academy of Pediatrics.

Neveus, T. (2019). The amount of urine voided in bed by children with enuresis. *Journal of Pediatric Urology, 15*(1), 31.e1–31.e5. https://doi.org/10.1016/j.jpurol.2018.08.006

Nickel, J. C. (2021). Inflammatory and pain conditions of the male genitourinary tract: Prostatitis and related pain conditions, orchitis, and epididymitis. In A. W. Partin, R. R. Dmochowski, L. R. Kavoussi, & C. A. Peters (Eds.), *Campbell-Walsh-Wein urology* (12th ed., Chapter 13). Elsevier.

Niederberger, C. S. (2016). Male infertility. In A. J. Wein, L. R. Kavoussi, A. W. Partin, & C. A. Peters (Eds.), *Campbell-Walsh urology* (11th ed., pp. 556–579). Elsevier.

Oettgen, A. B. (2017). Phimosis. In T. K. McInerny, H. M. Adam, D. E. Campbell, J. M. Foy, & D. M. Kamat (Eds.), *American Academy of Pediatrics textbook of pediatric care* (2nd ed., Chapter 312). American Academy of Pediatrics.

Oxybutynin: Drug information (2021). *UpToDate*. https://www.uptodate.com/contents/oxybutynin-pediatric-drug-information

Özen, M. A., Gündoğdu, G., Taşdemir, M., & Eroğlu, E. (2019). Are mechanical and chemical trauma the reason of meatal stenosis after newborn circumcision? *European Journal of Pediatrics, 178*(1), 77–80. https://doi.org/10.1007/s00431-018-3261-4

Palmer, L. S., & Palmer, J. S. (2021). Management of abnormalities of external genitalia in boys. In A. W. Partin, R. R. Dmochowski, L. R. Kavoussi, & C. A. Peters (Eds.), *Campbell-Walsh-Wein urology* (12th ed., Chapter 146). Elsevier.

Ramsook, C. (2020). Inguinal hernia in children. *UpToDate*. https://www.uptodate.com/contents/inguinal-hernia-in-children

Shaikh, N., & Hoberman, A. (2021). Urinary tract infections in infants older than one month and young children: Acute management, imaging, and prognosis. *UpToDate*. https://www.uptodate.com/contents/urinary-tract-infections-in-infants-older-than-one-month-and-young-children-acute-management-imaging-and-prognosis

Shields, L. B., White, J. T., Peppas, D. S., & Rosenberg, E. (2019). Scrotal ultrasound is not routinely indicated in the management of cryptorchidism, retractile testes, and hydrocele in children. *Global Pediatric Health, 6*. https://doi.org/10.1177/2333794X19890772

Snodgrass, W. T., & Bush, N. C. (2021). Hypospadias. In A. W. Partin, R. R. Dmochowski, L. R. Kavoussi, & C. A. Peters (Eds.), *Campbell-Walsh-Wein urology* (12th ed., Chapter 147). Elsevier.

Stephenson, A. J., & Gilligan, T. D. (2021). Neoplasms of the testis. In A. W. Partin, R. R. Dmochowski, L. R. Kavoussi, & C. A. Peters (Eds.), *Campbell-Walsh-Wein urology* (12th ed., Chapter 34). Elsevier.

Tu, N., & Baskin, L. S. (2020). Nocturnal enuresis in children: Management. *UpToDate*. https://www.uptodate.com/contents/nocturnal-enuresis-in-children-management

van der Horst, H. J., & de Wall, L. L. (2017). Hypospadias, all there is to know. *European Journal of Pediatrics, 176*(4), 435–441. https://doi.org/10.1007/s00431-017-2864-5

Wang, C. L., Aryal, B., Oto, A., Allen, B. C., Akin, O., Alexander, L. F., Bardo, D. M. E., Chong, J., Froemming, A. T., Gugham, P. F., Heller, M. T., Maranchie, J. K., Mody, R. N., Patel, B. N., Schieda, N., Turkbey, I. B., Venkatesan, A. M., Yoo, D. C., & Lockhart, M. E. (2019). ACR appropriateness criteria® acute onset of scrotal pain—without trauma, without antecedent mass. *Journal of the American College of Radiology*. https://doi.org/10.1016/j.jacr.2019.02.016

Williams, G., Hodson, E. M., & Craig, J. C. (2019). Interventions for primary vesicoureteric reflux. *Cochrane Database of Systemic Reviews*. https://doi.org/10.1002/14651858.CD001532.pub5

Yang, G. R., Dye, T. D., & Li, D. (2019). Effects of pre-gestational diabetes mellitus and gestational diabetes mellitus on macrosomia and birth defects in Upstate New York. *Diabetes Research and Clinical Practice, 155*, 107811. https://doi.org/10.1016/j.diabres.2019.107811

# Management of Reproductive Disorders

Nicole Lynne Audritsh

## Student Learning Outcomes

**Upon completion of this chapter the reader should be able to:**

1. Discuss pathophysiology and epidemiology of selected reproductive disorders in children or adolescents.
2. Differentiate subjective and objective findings for selected reproductive disorders in children or adolescents.
3. Choose appropriate laboratory or diagnostic tests for selected reproductive disorders in children or adolescents.
4. Utilize the differential diagnosis process to determine the diagnosis of reproductive disorders in children or adolescents.
5. Determine treatment plan, child/family education, and need for referral for children or adolescents with a reproductive system disorder.

## INTRODUCTION

Assessment, diagnosis, and management of adolescents with reproductive health disorders is a delicate balance between creating a trusting relationship with the child or adolescent, respecting parental wishes, providing informed consent, and participating in shared decision-making between the nurse practitioner and the adolescent. According to the federal Title X program, adolescents are legally able to obtain services related to family planning, contraception, and sexually transmitted infections (STIs) while protecting their confidentiality and allowing them to consent to treatment without a parent or guardian (Gudeman & Madge, n.d.). In a committee opinion released by the American College of Obstetricians (ACOG), it was suggested that best practice for care of the adolescent includes prioritizing the adolescent's control and choices, promoting empowerment, building trust, and ensuring that the adolescent feels physically and emotionally safe (2019).

According to the Centers for Disease Control and Prevention (CDC), one in seven children in the United States has experienced physical, emotional, or sexual abuse at some point in their lives (2020a). According to the Agency for Healthcare Research and Quality (AHRQ), one in five girls is sexually assaulted by age 13 (2016). Exposure to trauma is equal across all races, age groups, socioeconomic status, race, ethnicity, geography and sexual orientation (AHRQ, 2016). It is best for nurse practitioners to take a *trauma informed approach* to all gynecologic procedures in order to avoid triggers of painful memories in children who have experienced abuse. This is an approach aimed at engaging people with histories of trauma, which recognizes the presence of symptoms and acknowledges the role that it plays in the adolescent's life. Figure 29.1 shows the trauma-informed care (TIC) pyramid, which can direct practitioners in how to apply the principle to practice.

Patient-centered communication skills include screening every adolescent seen for intimate partner violence and then providing information about what safe relationships look like at adolescent well-checks. Additionally, modifying language when discussing gynecologic procedures, such as using "footrests" instead of stirrups and "table" instead of

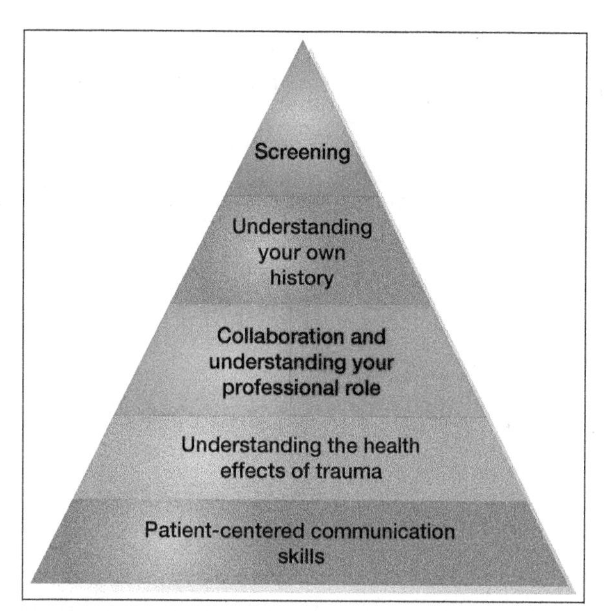


FIGURE 29.1 Trauma-informed care pyramid.

*Source*: From Raja, S., Hasnain, M., Hoersch, M., Gove-Yin, S., Rajagopalan, C., & Kruthoff, M. (2015). Trauma informed care in medicine: Current knowledge and future research directions. *Family and Community Health, 38*(3), 216–226. https://doi.org/10.1097/FCH.0000000000000071

bed, is important (AHRQ, 2016). If an adolescent is particularly uncomfortable about a necessary procedure, self-inserting the speculum and self-swabbing for STIs offers them an increased sense of control. While the nurse practitioner can encourage shared decision-making with the adolescent and the parent or guardian, it is important to remember that sexuality and reproductive health are new concepts to adolescents, so creation of a trusting environment over time will serve everyone involved.

Although the guidelines are continuously changing, the ACOG Foundation has published Women's Preventative Services guidelines at www.womenspreventivehealth.org/. Through the use of this web tool, the nurse practitioner can determine what gynecologic, reproductive, screening, and contraceptive methods are appropriate for adolescents/children based on age.

The content in this chapter maps to the following areas on the Pediatric Nursing Certification Board (PNCB) Pediatric Nurse Practitioner—Primary Care certification examination:

## CLINICAL PROBLEMS: REPRODUCTIVE DISORDERS

### CONTENT AREAS:

### II. Assessment and Diagnosis

**B. History and Physical Examination**

1. Obtain history of present illness
2. Obtain a comprehensive health history for new patients
3. Complete an interval history for established patients
4. Perform a review of systems
5. Perform a complete physical examination

**C. Diagnostic Testing and Screening**

1. Order and interpret office/clinic based screening tests
2. Order and interpret diagnostic laboratory tests
3. Order and interpret the results of diagnostic imaging tests

**D. Analyzing Information**

1. Integrate health history and physical examination findings into the plan of care
2. Assimilate findings from screening and diagnostic testing into plan of care

**E. Diagnosis**

1. Develop and prioritize differential diagnoses
2. Establish a diagnosis based on evaluation of patient data

### III. Management

**A. Child and Caregiver Counseling and Education**

1. Provide condition-specific counseling and education, including treatment options
2. Educate about benefits and potential adverse reactions of pharmacological interventions
3. Discuss non-pharmacological interventions
4. Counsel regarding the threshold for seeking follow-up care
5. Review the risks of non-adherence to recommended treatment

**B. Therapeutic Interventions**

1. Prescribe pharmacologic agents
2. Recommend the use of over-the-counter pharmacologic agents

3. Order or recommend non-pharmacologic treatments for the management of symptoms
4. Discuss use of complementary and alternative therapies as appropriate

**C. Procedures**

1. Perform procedures in accordance with diagnostic guidelines and plan of care (rapid tests)
2. Initiate life-saving techniques in response to urgent or emergent situations

**D. Collaboration and Referral**

2. Refer to specialists as indicated for evaluation, counseling, and/or treatment

**E. Care Coordination**

1. Facilitate patient and family-centered care for children of all ages with acute and chronic conditions

**F. Evaluation and Follow-up**

2. Establish a plan for follow-up care

### IV. Professional Role Responsibilities

**A. Leadership and Evidence-based Practice**

4. Develop, implement, and/or modify clinical practice guidelines

## ANATOMY AND PHYSIOLOGY

Adolescence is a time of transition between childhood and adulthood and is a time of surging hormones, rapid growth, cognitive maturation, and social changes.

### Biologic Development

Several terms are used to describe this period of rapid growth and biologic development. *Puberty* is the maturation and function of reproductive organs and the beginning of the development of secondary sex characteristics. There are three stages to the process of puberty: prepubescence, puberty, and postpubescence. *Prepubescence* is generally defined as the 2 years prior to the beginning of puberty when the child is developing minimal physical changes that reflect sexual maturity. *Puberty* is defined as the time when sexual maturity is complete; it is marked by the first menstrual period for girls and less obvious symptoms in boys. *Postpubescence* is the time by which skeletal growth is completed and reproductive function is established, generally occurring 1 to 2 years after the onset of puberty.

The physical changes of puberty are a result of chemical and hormonal activity that is controlled by the anterior pituitary gland after stimulus to the hypothalamus. The onset of puberty is a result of changing body accumulation of adipose tissue and changes in low amounts of estrogen that are released in order to stimulate long bone growth in girls. Primary sex characteristics are shown through the internal and external organs that carry out reproductive functions in each child. These include the ovaries, uterus, penis, testicles, and breasts. Secondary sex characteristics are the changes you can see on the outside of the body that signify hormonal changes, such as voice alterations, growth of facial and pubic hair, and changes in fat distribution, all of which have no roles in reproduction. Other significant physical changes occur as adolescents reach puberty, including achieving adult weight and height, formation of breast buds, and the closure of the epiphyseal in bones. It is believed that girls achieve the majority of their bone mass in early adolescence, creating a critical time for formation of long bones and thus preventing osteoporosis later in life.

Occurring simultaneously with the changes associated with puberty is the beginning of the menstrual cycle for adolescent girls. Estrogen is often referred to as the "feminizing" hormone and is often found in very low quantities in childhood. Early in prepubescence, the follicle stimulating hormone (FSH) begins to stimulate the ovaries to increase estrogen production. The positive feedback system of estrogen on the pituitary and hypothalamus glands stimulates a surge of luteinizing hormone (LH), thus stimulating ovulation (Schuiling & Lowe, 2017). The increase in estrogen causes an increase in density of the endometrial lining of the uterus, which eventually becomes the first menstruation. The pubertal changes that occur for girls most often occur in a predictable sequence, as shown in Table 29.1. These changes start with thelarche (breast bud development) around the age of 10 or 11, followed by adrenarche (pubic hair growth due to androgen stimulation), peak height velocity, and finally menarche around the age of 12 or 13 (Schuiling & Lowe, 2017). The timing of puberty in girls compared with the timing of puberty in boys is significantly earlier by approximately 2 years (Kritzler

**TABLE 29.1 Usual Sequence of Pubertal Changes by Gender**

| Girls | Boys |
|---|---|
| Breast changes | Enlargement of testicles |
| Rapid increase in height and weight | Growth of pubic hair, axillary hair, upper lip hair, hair on face |
| Growth of pubic hair | Rapid increase in height |
| Axillary hair appears | Changes in the larynx and penis size (usually concurrently) |
| Menstruation occurs (usually two years after first signs) | Nocturnal emission |

et al., 2017). Delayed puberty is defined as lack of thelarche by age 13 (Gibson et al., 2020).

The first menstrual cycle usually ranges from 2 to 7 days in length, and it is not uncommon for a young adolescent to have irregular cycles. Regular menstrual cycles are achieved within 24 months of menarche and include a menstrual cycle interval of 21 to 45 days, menses length of up to 7 days, and use of 3 to 6 pads or tampons per day. Menarche is often the most anticipated milestone event in an adolescent girl's life. While it is one that should be celebrated, it is often accompanied by trepidation, fear, and misinformation. This significant life event comes with physical, social, and emotional consequences that are important for clinicians to understand in order to provide holistic care.

The care of adolescents regarding reproductive concerns requires grace, creation of a trusting relationship, and the inclusion of their parent/guardian while allowing for adolescent privacy. Caring for adolescents in the area of gynecologic, sexual, and reproductive health allows an opportunity for the nurse practitioner to create trusting, lifelong relationships with adolescents. It is also an opportunity to educate and normalize topics that are intimidating for adolescents, such as sexual response, menstruation, and contraception. Providing care in a holistic, nurturing model will allow the adolescent to feel comfortable and thus provide more accurate information to the nurse practitioner.

## Sexual Maturation

Visible evidence of sexual maturation can be estimated by the clinician using the Tanner Scale (see Table 11.1). This is a reasonable tool to estimate how far the sexual maturation process has evolved in a certain adolescent, allowing the clinician to individualize education and anticipatory guidance during the appointment. Allowing time at each appointment for education and anticipatory guidance will encourage an open and trusting relationship with the adolescent and allow questions and concerns to be addressed, thus decreasing anxiety and trepidation.

## Psychosocial Development

The task of identity formation is to create a stable, understandable image of oneself that integrates not only one's past and current experiences, but also future experiences. Adolescence is an important time in regard to development of sexuality and sex-role identity. Adolescents are suddenly learning to adapt to intense hormonal changes, physiologic manifestations, and physical changes. The emergence of formal operational thinking begins during this time, and adolescents are likely to make decisions regarding sexuality and identity. During the latter part of adolescence, they are able to critically reason and think through the risks and benefits of sexual activity. In fact, one of the tasks of the adolescent period is to incorporate intimate relationships and sexuality by creating close relationships (Kansky & Allen, 2018). During this time in psychosocial development, adolescents will develop deep emotional and social identities separate from those of their families.

Additionally, this is the time when sexual identity forms. Adolescent focus will shift from relationships with same-sex peers to intimate, close relationships with opposite-sex or same-sex peers. A relationship between love and sexual expression is often seen around the middle adolescent period. Sexual identity is determined by incorporating sexual experiences, knowledge, and feelings within from previous relationships. Adolescents may be questioning their self-identity or may identify as straight, lesbian, gay, bisexual, or queer (refer to chapter __ for more information). Most often adolescents self-identify as heterosexual, but around 4% to 8% report same-sex attractions (Forcier & Olson-Kennedy, 2020).

Sexual orientation is a very important part of sexual identity. *Sexual orientation* is defined as the pattern of arousal or romantic attraction toward a person of the opposite gender (heterosexual or straight), the same gender (homosexual [lesbian or gay]), both genders (bisexual), all persons regardless of gender (pansexual), or having no attraction or desire at all (asexual). Adolescents who identify as anything other than heterosexual often have unique developmental issues and health challenges (Schuiling & Lowe, 2017).

# MENSTRUAL DISORDERS

A number of menstrual disorders may affect adolescent females. These include premenstrual syndrome, premenstrual dysphoric disorder, amenorrhea, and dysmenorrhea.

## PREMENSTRUAL SYNDROME

Throughout history there has been discussion in the fields of science and philosophy about the brain, menstruation, and behavioral connections that occur (Zielinksi & Lynne, 2017). In fact, many cultures still believe that premenstrual syndrome (PMS) is a cultural syndrome and not a physiological disorder. Some cultures believe that the uterus moves throughout the body, pulled by the moon during the premenstrual time, and that the discomforts occur based on where the uterus is located during its current travel (Zielinksi & Lynne, 2017). In other cultures, menstruation is a more positive experience for women and girls.

PMS is defined as a variety of symptoms such as irritability, food cravings, mood swings, irrational reactions and judgments, increased or decreased sex drive, migraines and headaches, unpredictable behavior and sometimes violence, along with dysmenorrhea, menorrhagia, and bloating (Zielinksi & Lynne, 2017). The following section focuses on menstrual-cycle pain and accompanying discomforts of the adolescent and the ways in which a nurse practitioner can offer solutions, validation, and hope to adolescents.

### Subjective Findings

The health history may reveal:

- Age of adolescent at first menstruation
- Last menstrual period
- Duration of cycles
- Quantity of bleeding
- Absence from school because of menstruation
- Increased arguments or disagreements with family and friends
- Effect of the symptoms on the adolescent's daily life, including self-image, relationships, school, extracurricular activities, and employment

### Risk Factors

The most common risk factors for PMS are:

- Family history of PMS
- Pre-existing anxiety or depression
- Lack of exercise
- High stress

### Review of Systems

The most common manifestations revealed during the review of systems include:

- **Constitutional:** lethargy, fatigue, food cravings or other alterations in appetite, weight gain with fluid retention, change in sleeping habits
- **Breasts:** increased breast size or other breast changes
- **Gastrointestinal:** abdominal bloating, constipation followed by diarrhea at the onset of menses, nausea/vomiting
- **Reproductive:** cramps
- **Neurologic:** irritability, headache or increase in migraines, irritability
- **Psychiatric:** crying, anger, change in affect, change in depression and/or anxiety, violent behavior, confusion, inability to concentrate

**PRO TIP** In the case of any topic surrounding reproductive health it is important to be vigilant and ask the parents to step out of the room in order to create a one-on-one trusting relationship with the adolescent. Ensure that the adolescent knows that the conversations between nurse practitioner and the adolescent are confidential, except in the case of suicidal or homicidal ideation. In some practices, a notice is sent to the parents before the adolescent's appointment notifying parents/guardians that they will be asked to leave the room for part of the interview. This fosters a trusting and open relationship with the adolescent to discuss menstruation, drug use, history of interpersonal violence and sexual assault, and sexual activity, all which are crucial to know before treatment of an adolescent.

### Objective Findings

There are no specific findings upon physical examination.

### Laboratory/Diagnostic Testing

The diagnosis of PMS is based upon the clinical findings (health history). No laboratory or diagnostic testing is needed. However, asking the adolescent to keep a diary of symptoms for 2 to 3 months will help with symptom evaluation and consistency with ovulation and menses.

## Differential Diagnosis

The differential diagnosis for PMS includes:

- A diagnosis of exclusion; all others must be ruled out
- Depression/anxiety
- Premenstrual dysphoric disorder
- Bipolar affective disorder
- Alcohol or substance abuse
- Personality disorder

## Treatment/Management Plan

The goal of management of PMS is to isolate the symptoms and treat symptomatically. There is very little evidence to support the use of dietary restrictions (including caffeine and salt). Nonpharmacologic management of PMS includes:

- Self-help strategies—Reassure the adolescent that this is a normal part of the menstruation process. Help them to understand why the symptoms are happening. Reassure them that they are in no grave danger.
- Vitamin B6 50 mg to 150 mg/day continuous use.
- Calcium carbonate supplementation: 1,200 to 1,600 mg/day.
- Chaste tree berry supplement.
- 30 to 60 minutes of exercise every day.
- Avoid known physical and emotional triggers.
- Cognitive behavioral therapy, group therapy, or relaxation therapy may improve psychologic issues.
- Mind-body techniques such as yoga, meditation, biofeedback, massage (Tharpe et al., 2017).

Pharmacologic management of PMS includes:

- Nonsteroidal anti-inflammatory drugs (NSAIDs; anti-prostaglandins such as Naprosyn) before and during menses may help reduce retention of fluid.
- Combined oral contraceptives or progesterone-only contraceptive pills may be helpful by suppressing ovulation and thus reducing physical symptoms, menstrual bleeding, and pain.
- Use of selective serotonin uptake reuptake inhibitors (SSRIs) has been shown to alleviate severe PMS (may take continuously or only during luteal phase each month).

### Family Education

Teach the following:

- Review the menstrual cycle and related hormonal changes.
- Suggest prospective menstrual charting or use of a reliable symptom tracker app.
- Reinforce the benefits of balanced diet and daily exercise.
- Encourage personal time for adolescent.
- Recommend stress-reducing techniques such as music, dance, yoga, meditation, or prayer (Tharpe et al., 2017).

### Referral

Premenstrual dysphoric disorder (PMDD) is a recognized psychiatric illness related to menstruation and encompasses cognitive, behavioral, emotional, and negative symptomatic changes that impair activities of daily living. If an adolescent demonstrates extreme severity in the symptoms related to PMS, they need a referral to psychiatry for evaluation for PMDD (Table 29.2).

# DYSMENORRHEA

Menstrual pain is one of the most common gynecologic complaints in the United States and one of the most feared issues associated with menses for adolescents (Zielinksi & Lynne, 2017). Menstrual pain that interrupts activities of daily living for adolescents, such as school, sports, work, and family life, is called *dysmenorrhea*. Dysmenorrhea causes physical and psychological distress during menstruation with prevalence rates ranging from 16% to 90% (Zielinksi & Lynne, 2017). This condition is the most commonly reported menstrual disorder, affecting up to 81% of girls and women (Zielinksi & Lynne, 2017). While dysmenorrhea is often accompanied by PMS and dysphoric disorders, it is often the most troublesome complaint experienced during menstruation.

The pain of dysmenorrhea is a result of intense uterine contractions during the menstrual phase of the cycle, which trigger endometrial prostaglandin production and release into the adolescent female's blood flow. Excessive amounts of prostaglandins cause the uterus to increase the intense contractions, which reduces uterine blood flow and causes ischemia and pain. The incidence of dysmenorrhea varies, with some studies showing up to 80% among adolescents and women in their early 20s, with more than half of these women experiencing a loss of days at school, interruption in sporting events, and interruption in work due to this condition (Zielinksi & Lynne, 2017).

Dysmenorrhea is classified into two categories: primary, with a lack of pelvic pathology; and secondary,

TABLE 29.2 **Symptoms of Premenstrual Disorder Versus Premenstrual Dysphoric Disorder**

| Criteria | PMS | PMDD |
|---|---|---|
| **Psychological Symptoms** | Depression<br>Anxiety<br>Anger/irritability<br>Confusion<br>Feelings of poor self-esteem and social withdrawal | Marked affective lability<br>Marked irritability or anger<br>Increased interpersonal conflicts<br>Markedly depressed mood, feelings of hopelessness, or self-depreciating thoughts<br>Marked anxiety, tension, feelings of being "on edge"<br>Decreased interest in usual activities<br>Insomnia or hypersomnia<br>Being overwhelmed or feeling out of control |
| **Physical Symptoms** | Nausea/vomiting<br>Food cravings<br>Constipation and then diarrhea at onset of menses<br>Headache/increase in migraines<br>Pelvic pain<br>Fatigue<br>Abdominal bloating<br>Mild weight gain | Same as PMS but more severe |
| **Diagnostic Criteria** | Symptoms:<br>begin up to 7 days prior to menses<br>end on menstrual cycle day 3–4<br>occur in at least two cycles<br>are not due to exacerbation of another disorder<br>impair activities of daily living | Five or more symptoms are associated with significant clinical distress and impairment of work, school, social activities, and interpersonal relationships<br>One or more of the following is present: marked anxiety, tension, marked depression, irritability, or affective lability<br>One or more of the following: decreased interest in usual activities, difficulty concentrating, fatigue, appetite changes, changes in sleep patterns, sense of feeling overwhelmed, physical symptoms such as breast tenderness, joint or muscle pain, bloating or weight gain<br>This is not an exacerbation of another disorder (e.g., major depressive disorder, bipolar syndrome)<br>Confirmed by prospective symptom charting for at least two cycles |

*Source*: Adapted from Zielinksi, R., & Lynne, S. (2017). Menstrual-cycle pain and premenstrual conditions. In K. D. Schuiling & F. E. Likis (Eds.), *Women's gynecologic health* (3rd ed., pp. 549–574). Jones & Bartlett Learning.

with identifiable organic pathology. Primary dysmenorrhea often begins 6 to 12 months after menarche. Symptoms are usually experienced with the onset of bleeding and continue for 8 to 72 hours into the cycle. Secondary dysmenorrhea is painful menstruation after years with no complaints. It usually begins in the early 20s to 30s and is characterized by pelvic organic pathology such as adenomyosis, leiomyomata (fibroid tumors), irritable bowel syndrome, endometriosis, or interstitial cystitis. Any process that can affect the pelvic viscera and cause acute or intermittent acute pain might be a source of secondary dysmenorrhea, including urinary tract infection, pelvic infection, STI, hernia, and pelvic relaxation or prolapse (Zielinksi & Lynne, 2017).

## Subjective Findings

The health history may reveal:

- Family history related to menstrual cycles
- Duration of the dysmenorrhea for the girl
- Girl's age at menarche
- Frequency and duration of menses
- Estimated menstrual flow (light, moderate, heavy)
- Absence from work or school
- Treatments used (both past and present)
- Abdominal cramps and pain, including location, onset, and duration, associated symptoms, and factors making the pain worse or better
- Age at first intercourse
- History of contraception

- STI
- Sexual abuse or trauma
- Obstetric history (if any)

## Risk Factors

The most common risk factors for dysmenorrhea are:

Primary:

- Early age at menarche (<12 years old)
- Body mass index (BMI) <20
- Smoking
- History of sexual abuse
- Premenstrual emotional symptoms (dysphoria)
- History of pelvic surgery
- Depression
- Nulliparity
- Heavy or prolonged menstrual flow
- Family history of dysmenorrhea
- Obesity

Secondary:

- Leiomyoma (fibroid)

## Review of Systems

The most common manifestations revealed during the review of systems include:

- **Constitutional:** pain (continuous abdominal, backache, abdominal cramps, general body aches)
- **Gastrointestinal:** nausea, vomiting, diarrhea
- **Neurologic:** dizziness

> **PRO TIP** When assessing the adolescent with dysmenorrhea, be sure you ask open-ended questions and remain aware for signs of depression and anxiety. When there are symptoms of depression or anxiety, it is important to assess whether the dysmenorrhea caused the symptoms or if they are underlying.

## Objective Findings

The physical examination of the child or adolescent with primary dysmenorrhea will typically reveal no abnormalities. Secondary dysmenorrhea may yield findings consistent with the pathologic condition causing it.

## Laboratory/Diagnostic Testing

The diagnosis of dysmenorrhea is based upon the clinical findings. No laboratory or diagnostic testing is needed in the case of primary dysmenorrhea. In the case of secondary dysmenorrhea, careful analysis of location and characteristics is the focus for the rest of the diagnostic testing. Testing may include urinalysis, quantitative human gonadotropin level (hCG), vaginal ultrasound and hysterosalpingogram to evaluate pelvic structures, laparoscopy to evaluate endometrial cavity, vaginal cultures and smears to evaluate for infectious process, and lower gastrointestinal evaluation.

## Differential Diagnosis

The differential diagnosis for dysmenorrhea includes:

- Imperforate hymen
- Lower vaginal agenesis
- Endometriosis
- Ovarian cysts
- Pelvic infection
- STI
- Urinary tract infection

## Treatment/Management Plan

Primary:

- Prostaglandin synthetase inhibitors and NSAIDs: Treatments of choice, most effective when started at beginning of menses and continued around the clock for 48 to 72 hours. Choices include:
  - Diclofenac potassium 50 mg PO q8h or 100 mg PO as loading dose followed by 50 mg q8 hours
  - Ibuprofen 400–800 mg PO q6h
  - Ketoprofen 25–50 mg PO q6–8h
  - Naproxen 500 mg PO, then 250 mg q6–8 h
- Combination hormonal contraception: A good choice, especially if concurrent contraception is needed or desired. The estrogen and progestin in the contraceptive act to suppress ovulation, which naturally reduces prostaglandin production and can relieve symptoms in adolescents with dysmenorrhea. Oral contraceptives suppress ovulation and endometrial growth, thereby decreasing menstrual volume and prostaglandin secretion (Zielinksi & Lynne, 2017).
- Depo medroxyprogesterone (DMPA): The choice to use DMPA is one that must be made carefully, knowing that the adolescent will need to return to the clinic every 12 weeks in order for the injection to be administered. Use of DMPA also promotes endometrial atrophy, decreased menstrual flow, and decreased secretion of prostaglandins (Zielinksi & Lynne, 2017).

An additional benefit of DMPA injections is amenorrhea in 55% to 60% of females by 12 months and 68% by 24 months (Zielinksi & Lynne, 2017).

- Progestin implant (Nexplanon/Implanon): Currently progestin implants are offered as a single rod inserted intradermally in the arm of the adolescent.
- Levonorgesterel-releasing intrauterine system (LNG-IUS): The intrauterine device (IUD) is a highly effective method in the treatment of dysmenorrhea with an additional benefit of 99% effective contraceptive control (Murphy et al., 2017). In adolescents with heavy or prolonged bleeding disorders, dysmenorrhea, leiomyomas, and pain due to endometriosis, the IUD can be life-changing.
- Self-help measures include regular exercise, warm heat compresses, yoga and relaxation exercises, acupuncture, and lifestyle changes including exercise and healthy food choices (King et al., 2019).
- Vitamin supplements
  - Vitamin E 200–400 IU PO BID 2 days prior to menses and 3 days after
  - Vitamins B1 and B6 daily
  - Magnesium: start daily during menses and continue until day 3 of menses (Tharpe et al., 2017)
- Herbal remedies
  - Vitex tea, tincture, or capsules
  - Evening primrose oil: 3–6 capsules/day
  - Crampbark and black haw tea (Tharpe et al., 2017)

Secondary:

- Treatment is consistent with the pathology

### Family Education

Teach the following:

- Starting NSAIDs at the beginning of menses and continuing around the clock for 48 to 72 hours is helpful to keep pain under control.
- Encourage the adolescent to maintain a healthy diet and exercise every day for 30 minutes each day.
- Understand that the adolescent may be feeling a loss of identity and control and validate her concerns and fears.

### Referral

When the cause for dysmenorrhea is suspected pelvic inflammatory disease (PID), hospital admission may be necessary if the adolescent does not improve within 48 hours after starting treatment.

## AMENORRHEA

Amenorrhea in an adolescent can be a sign of stress, pregnancy, over-exercise, malnutrition, or unexpected weight loss. It is important that the clinician complete a full reproductive, menstrual, obstetric, and comprehensive health history of the adolescent before continuing with the physical examination. Amenorrhea in an adolescent predisposes the child to infertility, increased risk of osteoporosis, scoliosis, stress fractures, and increased risk of breast and reproductive cancers (Gibson et al., 2020).

There are two subtypes of amenorrhea, primary and secondary. Primary amenorrhea is lack of a menstruation by the age of 15 in the presence of mature breast development or 3 years after thelarche (Gibson et al., 2020). Absence of menses for more than three cycles in a girl who has been having regular menstrual cycles, or longer than 6 months for a girl who was having cycles irregularly, is the definition of secondary amenorrhea (Gibson et al., 2020). In the case of secondary amenorrhea, polycystic ovary syndrome and functional hypothalamic amenorrhea are the most common causes (Tranoulis et al., 2020). Additionally, extreme athletes such as runners, gymnasts, and ballet dancers, and adolescents who suffer from anorexia nervosa and bulimia are among those with high rates of secondary amenorrhea. This condition is a symptom reflecting different etiologies and endocrine profiles.

The American Society for Colposcopy and Cervical Pathology (ASCCP) has recently updated guidelines regarding Papanicolaou testing in the adolescent population and does not recommend testing for any woman under the age of 21 years of age (Feldman et al., 2020). After careful interviewing and a thorough history are obtained, a pelvic examination on an adolescent child should only be performed if absolutely necessary in order to formulate a diagnosis. Most adolescents with anovulatory bleeding can be managed with nutritional counseling and medical therapy in the form of vitamin and mineral supplementation (Tharpe et al., 2017).

### Subjective Findings

Ascertain at what age the breast buds developed. The health history may reveal:

- Lack of menses

For girls who have previously menstruated, ascertain last menstrual period, age at first menarche, frequency and duration of menses, and estimated prior menstrual flow (light, moderate, heavy).

### Risk Factors

The most common risk factors for amenorrhea are:

- Eating disorders
- Participation in extreme sports

### Review of Systems

The most common manifestations revealed during the review of systems include:

- **Constitutional:** extreme weight loss, cyclic abdominal pain
- **Integumentary:** worsening acne, hirsutism

### Objective Findings

During the physical examination, determine the Tanner stage for breasts and pubic hair. The physical examination of the child or adolescent with amenorrhea may reveal:

- Low BMI
- Enlarged thyroid with possible nodularity
- Imperforate hymen, lower vaginal agenesis, female genital cutting, congenital labial fusion, cervical stenosis, ambiguous genitalia, or absence of the uterus, cervix, or vagina

### Laboratory/Diagnostic Testing

The diagnosis of amenorrhea is based upon the clinical and laboratory findings, including:

- Pelvic ultrasound
- Serum hCG (to rule out pregnancy)
- Serum $T_4$ and thyroid-stimulating hormone (TSH) may be low to normal
- FSH, LH, estradiol maybe low
- Prolactin should be normal
- Total testosterone to evaluate for polycystic ovary syndrome (PCOS) (Gibson et al., 2020; Tharpe et al., 2017)

### Differential Diagnosis

The differential diagnosis for amenorrhea includes:

- Pregnancy
- Hormonal contraception use
- Anorexia nervosa
- Bulimia
- Polycystic ovary syndrome
- Thyroid disease
- Primary ovarian insufficiency
- Adrenal mass
- Congenital adrenal hyperplasia
- Cushing syndrome
- Turner syndrome
- Intrauterine adhesions (Asherman syndrome)

### Treatment/Management Plan

Secondary amenorrhea (if hCG test is negative):

- Progestin challenge
  - Provera 10 mg PO for 10 days

    OR
  - Prometrium 400 mg at bedtime for 10 days
  - Expect withdrawal bleeding within 2 to 7 days after medication completion
  - If no withdrawal bleeding, refer to a gynecologist or a certified nurse-midwife (King et al., 2019)

### Family Education

Teach the following:

- Encourage the adolescent to maintain a healthy diet and exercise every day for 30 minutes each day.
- Counsel parents on need for balanced exercise and rest periods, especially in the cases of extreme athletes.

### Referral

If reproductive anomalies or abnormal laboratory results are present in the adolescent with primary amenorrhea, refer to a gynecologist. When the urine or blood test for hCG is positive, refer to a midwife or obstetrician for an initial pregnancy visit. For the adolescent displaying symptoms consistent with an eating disorder, refer for mental health services. Refer to social services any adolescent displaying evidence of food insecurity.

## INFECTIOUS DISORDERS OF THE FEMALE REPRODUCTIVE TRACT

Ordinarily, the vaginal pH of 3.5 to 4.0 promotes the growth of normal vaginal flora (mainly lactobacilli and acidogenic corynebacterial) with only a small quantity of candidal organisms present. When the pH is disrupted, overgrowth of other bacteria or *Candida* may occur, resulting in bacterial vaginosis or vulvovaginal candidiasis. Additionally, infection with particular sexually transmitted organisms may lead to PID in the adolescent.

· grey/white discharge
· ph > 4.5
clue cells
fishy smell

# BACTERIAL VAGINOSIS

Bacterial vaginosis (BV) is an alteration in the normal flora of the vagina with dominance of an anaerobic bacterium. It is the most common vaginal infection in women in the United States ages 15 to 44 (Jones, 2019). The occurrence of BV increases the risk for acquisition of STIs and human immunodeficiency virus (HIV); thus, it is important to identify its presence and treat the condition appropriately. Although not sexually transmitted, BV is more common in young women with multiple partners.

## Subjective Findings

The health history from the adolescent may reveal a grey, white, thin, malodorous discharge often with "fishy" smell.

## Risk Factors

Risk factors for developing bacterial vaginosis include:

- Douching (changes vaginal flora and pH)
- Sexual activity (especially unprotected intercourse)
- Increased number of sexual partners
- Females having sex with women
- Presence of intrauterine uterine device
- Being African American (Tharpe et al., 2017)

## Review of Systems

The review of systems for BV usually does not reveal other symptoms, although occasionally vaginal pruritus may be reported.

## Objective Findings

The physical examination of the child or adolescent with BV may reveal:

- Homogenous, adherent, whitish-gray discharge
- Presence of foul odor (fishy)

## Laboratory/Diagnostic Testing

Presence of three of the four Amsel criteria is diagnostic of BV:

- Vaginal pH >4.5
- Clue cells on saline wet mount
- Homogenous, white discharge
- Positive "whiff" test with addition of KOH to vaginal swab (results in an amine (fishy) odor)

## Differential Diagnosis

The differential diagnosis for BV includes:

- Trichomoniasis
- Candidiasis

## Treatment/Management Plan

Treatment is recommended for all adolescents with symptoms. Treatment options include:

- Metronidazole 500 mg orally, twice daily for 7 days
- Metronidazole gel 0.75%, one full applicator intravaginally at bedtime for 5 days
- Clindamycin cream 2%, intravaginally at bedtime for 7 days

For recurrent BV, prescribe metronidazole gel 0.75%, one full applicator intravaginally at bedtime, twice weekly for 4 to 6 months.

## Family Education

Teach the following:

- Avoid douching.
- Use condoms.
- Reduce the number of sexual partners.
- Adequately clean all sexual accessories between uses.
- If BV continues to recur, a long-term treatment may be prescribed.

# VULVOVAGINAL CANDIDIASIS

Vulvovaginal candidiasis occurs when there is inflammatory overgrowth of *Candida* invading the vulvovaginal epithelial cells. *Candida albicans* is the organism responsible for about 90% of cases. About 75% of women experience candidiasis at least once in their lives (Bornstein, 2019).

## Subjective Findings

Determine the health history from the adolescent, which may reveal vulval irritation and pruritus (possibly severe) with a white discharge.

## Risk Factors

Risk factors for the development of vulvovaginal candidiasis include:

- Diabetes mellitus
- Antibiotic, corticosteroid, oral contraceptive use
- HIV infection
- Obesity

### Review of Systems

The most common manifestations revealed during the review of systems include:

- **Genitourinary:** external dysuria
- **Reproductive:** vulvovaginal soreness

### Objective Findings

The physical examination of the child or adolescent with vulvovaginal candidiasis may reveal:

- Erythema of vulva and vagina
- White vaginal discharge (may be thick, curdy, and "cottage-cheese"-like)
- Discharge is usually adherent to vaginal walls

### Laboratory/Diagnostic Testing

To diagnose vaginal candidiasis, note that a vaginal pH will be normal (<4.5) and wet mount of vaginal secretions with 10% KOH will reveal pseudohyphae and budding yeast. A fungal culture confirms but is not necessary for diagnosis.

### Differential Diagnosis

The differential diagnosis for vulvovaginal candidiasis includes:

- Trichomoniasis
- Bacterial vaginosis
- Genital herpes
- Gonorrhea
- Chlamydia
- Localized provoked vulvodynia
- Vulvar dermatomes
- Allergic reaction

### Treatment/Management Plan

Treatment in the immunocompromised child or adolescent includes:

- Single dose of fluconazole 150 mg orally
- Over-the-counter miconazole or clotrimazole intravaginal cream or vaginal suppository for 7 days

### Family Education

Teach the following:

- Keep the vulva and vaginal area dry.
- Wear only nonabsorbent underwear and change if damp.
- Maintain a low-sugar diet.
- Keep diabetes mellitus under control.

## PELVIC INFLAMMATORY DISEASE

PID refers to a spectrum of acute and subacute infections of the upper female genital tract. The causative agent of the infection in 85% of cases is organisms causing an STI or bacterial vaginosis (Ross & Chacko, 2020; refer to chapter 31 for additional information on STIs). In PID, infection may occur in the uterus (endometritis), the fallopian tubes (salpingitis), and/or the ovaries (oophoritis). Perihepatitis, peritonitis, and/or tubo-ovarian abscess may also occur. Complications include ectopic pregnancy and scarring of the upper genital tract, resulting in infertility.

### Subjective Findings

Obtain a thorough reproductive and sexual history from the adolescent. The health history may reveal acute onset of abdominal pain.

### Risk Factors

The most common risk factors for PID include:

- Multiple sex partners
- Sexually active females younger than 25 years old
- Partner with an STI
- Previous episode of PID
- Lack of use of barrier contraception

### Review of Systems

The most common manifestations revealed during the review of systems include:

- **Constitutional:** lower abdominal pain (longer than 2 weeks' duration; may follow coitus, or happen with jarring movements or occur during or after menses), fever (more severe PID)
- **Genitourinary:** urinary frequency
- **Reproductive:** abnormal uterine bleeding, abnormal uterine discharge

### Objective Findings

The physical examination of the child or adolescent with PID may reveal:

- Abdominal tenderness with palpation, particularly in the lower quadrants

- Rebound tenderness or absent bowel sounds (with more severe PID)
- Purulent vaginal or endocervical discharge
- Adnexal, acute cervical motion or uterine tenderness with bimanual examination

### Laboratory/Diagnostic Testing

A presumptive diagnosis of PID may be made based on the subjective and physical examination findings. The following laboratory tests may be performed:

- Pregnancy test (rule out ectopic pregnancy)
- Saline microscopy of vaginal discharge (positive white blood cells sensitive for PID)
- Nucleic acid amplification tests (NAAT) for *Neisseria gonorrhoeae, Chlamydia trachomatis, Mycoplasma genitalum* (positive tests support PID diagnosis; negative tests do not rule out PID)
- Syphilis serology
- HIV testing

Pelvic imaging may be necessary in the acutely ill adolescent.

### Differential Diagnosis

The differential diagnosis for PID includes:

- Ectopic pregnancy
- Torsion of adnexal mass or ovarian cyst rupture
- Endometriosis
- Cystitis
- Appendicitis
- Irritable bowel syndrome
- Diverticulitis
- Functional pain

### Treatment/Management Plan

For sexually active adolescents presenting with lower abdominal pain, the nurse practitioner should have a low threshold for making the diagnosis of PID and prescribing treatment. Treat with ceftriaxone 250 mg intramuscularly as a single dose and doxycycline 100 mg orally twice a day for 14 days. The addition of metronidazole (500 mg twice daily) may also be considered.

### Family Education

Teach the following:

- The adolescent should abstain from sexual activity until treatment is completed and STI testing is negative.
- When sexual activity is resumed, practice safe sex methods.
- All sexual partners should be evaluated/treated for STIs.

### Referral

Refer for hospitalization any pregnant adolescent, or if severe clinical illness (high fever, nausea, vomiting, severe abdominal pain) is suspected.

## POLYCYSTIC OVARY SYNDROME

Polycystic ovary syndrome (PCOS) is associated with menstrual irregularities due to oligo-ovulation, or anovulation concurrently with clinical signs of hyperandrogenism. There is an increased LH:FSH ratio, increased androgen concentration, and decreased sex-hormone binding globulin, resulting in an increase in free testosterone. Metabolically, the outcome of PCOS is hyperinsulinemia and an increased risk for heart disease and diabetes.

Management of the adolescent with PCOS in a pediatric clinic focuses on symptom management, increasing regularity of menstrual cycles, contraceptive initiation, and cardiovascular disease health promotion. The pediatric nurse practitioner scope includes maintenance of PCOS and the pediatric nurse practitioner can use the opportunity to have conversations focused on reproductive and sexual health.

### Subjective Findings

The health history may reveal:

- Irregular menses (cycles 45–90 days apart)

### Risk Factors

There are no known risk factors for development of PCOS; however, once an individual has been diagnosed with PCOS she is at higher risk for endometrial cancers, heart disease, and diabetes, as obesity increases the risk of metabolic complications.

### Review of Systems

The most common manifestations revealed during the review of systems include:

- **Endocrine:** onset of hirsutism at puberty, signs of excess androgen production (acne, deep voice)

### Objective Findings

The physical examination of the child or adolescent with PCOS may reveal:

- Excessive hair growth on face, chest, buttocks
- Oily skin or acne
- Thinning hair or loss of hair on the head

### Laboratory/Diagnostic Testing

The diagnosis of PCOS is based upon the clinical findings. Additional testing may include:

- Pregnancy test (negative)
- Ultrasound assessment of ovaries may yield polycystic ovarian morphology in some adolescents, although it is not a required finding for diagnosis of PCOS in adolescents (Evans & Hoeger, 2020)

### Differential Diagnosis

The differential diagnosis for PCOS includes:

- Obesity
- Thyroid dysfunction
- Cushing disease
- Adrenal or ovarian tumors

### Treatment/Management Plan

The goal for a patient with PCOS is to lower the androgen levels, treat clinical manifestations, and decrease the long-term effects of hyperandrogenism. Encourage a healthy diet and increased physical activity. Combined oral contraceptive treatment may be used to manage hyperandrogenism and menstrual irregularity.

### Family Education

Teach the following:

- Because of the increased risk of heart disease, healthy diet and adequate exercise are especially important.
- Yearly monitoring of lipids and hemoglobin A1C.
- If the adolescent or child is obese, weight loss will be helpful for reduction of symptoms.

### Referral

Referral to a gynecologist is necessary for adolescents with PCOS if the symptoms cannot be managed in a primary care clinic or if the adolescent desires pregnancy.

## CONTRACEPTION

Contraceptive planning by an adolescent can be a very intimidating process. Therefore, it is important that the pediatric nurse practitioner feel comfortable discussing all of the options available to each young woman. A thorough menstrual history, sexual history including exposure to STIs and HIV and plans for sexual activity, along with a medical history are key to ensuring that the method chosen will be most effective with the least amount of side effects.

The adolescent population is still developing formal operational thinking, according to Piaget. Therefore, when prescribing contraceptive methods, it is important to remember that adolescents are predisposed to a lack of planning during this time of cognitive development. Discussions during contraceptive planning should be focused on ease of use, ability to remember daily dosing regimens, and cognitive abilities of the adolescent. Although the parent may be involved in helping the adolescent remember to take medications, beginning to use contraception is a good time to demonstrate personal responsibility and control over their own care. Ultimately, according to the Title X program, adolescents have legal authority for their own contraceptive planning, although some states' laws may conflict with those of Title X and require parental consent. The following section describes the appropriate contraceptive methods for an adolescent girl and family and patient education related to each.

### Subjective Findings

The health history may reveal:

- Regular or irregular menses

### Risk Factors

The most common risk factors for exclusions for using hormonal methods of contraception include:

- Migraines with aura
- Cardiovascular disease
- Hypertension
- Current/history of ischemic heart disease or stroke
  - Systemic lupus erythematosus
  - Rheumatoid arthritis
  - Unexplained vaginal bleeding

Refer to Exhibit 29.1 for additional information related to eligibility criteria for contraceptive use.

# Summary Chart of U.S. Medical Eligibility Criteria for Contraceptive Use

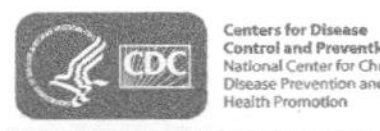


| Condition | Sub-Condition | Cu-IUD I | Cu-IUD C | LNG-IUD I | LNG-IUD C | Implant I | Implant C | DMPA I | DMPA C | POP I | POP C | CHC I | CHC C |
|---|---|---|---|---|---|---|---|---|---|---|---|---|---|
| Age | | Menarche to <20 yrs:2 | | Menarche to <20 yrs:2 | | Menarche to <18 yrs:1 | | Menarche to <18 yrs:2 | | Menarche to <18 yrs:1 | | Menarche to <40 yrs:1 | |
| | | ≥20 yrs:1 | | ≥20 yrs:1 | | 18-45 yrs:1 | | 18-45 yrs:1 | | 18-45 yrs:1 | | ≥40 yrs:2 | |
| | | | | | | >45 yrs:1 | | >45 yrs:2 | | >45 yrs:1 | | | |
| Anatomical abnormalities | a) Distorted uterine cavity | 4 | | 4 | | | | | | | | | |
| | b) Other abnormalities | 2 | | 2 | | | | | | | | | |
| Anemias | a) Thalassemia | 2 | | 1 | | 1 | | 1 | | 1 | | 1 | |
| | b) Sickle cell disease‡ | 2 | | 1 | | 1 | | 1 | | 1 | | 2 | |
| | c) Iron-deficiency anemia | 2 | | 1 | | 1 | | 1 | | 1 | | 1 | |
| Benign ovarian tumors | (including cysts) | 1 | | 1 | | 1 | | 1 | | 1 | | 1 | |
| Breast disease | a) Undiagnosed mass | 1 | | 2 | | 2* | | 2* | | 2* | | 2* | |
| | b) Benign breast disease | 1 | | 1 | | 1 | | 1 | | 1 | | 1 | |
| | c) Family history of cancer | 1 | | 1 | | 1 | | 1 | | 1 | | 1 | |
| | d) Breast cancer‡ | | | | | | | | | | | | |
| | i) Current | 1 | | 4 | | 4 | | 4 | | 4 | | 4 | |
| | ii) Past and no evidence of current disease for 5 years | 1 | | 3 | | 3 | | 3 | | 3 | | 3 | |
| Breastfeeding | a) <21 days postpartum | | | | | 2* | | 2* | | 2* | | 4* | |
| | b) 21 to <30 days postpartum | | | | | | | | | | | | |
| | i) With other risk factors for VTE | | | | | 2* | | 2* | | 2* | | 3* | |
| | ii) Without other risk factors for VTE | | | | | 2* | | 2* | | 2* | | 3* | |
| | c) 30-42 days postpartum | | | | | | | | | | | | |
| | i) With other risk factors for VTE | | | | | 1* | | 1* | | 1* | | 3* | |
| | ii) Without other risk factors for VTE | | | | | 1* | | 1* | | 1* | | 2* | |
| | d) >42 days postpartum | | | | | 1* | | 1* | | 1* | | 2* | |
| Cervical cancer | Awaiting treatment | 4 | 2 | 4 | 2 | 2 | | 2 | | 1 | | 2 | |
| Cervical ectropion | | 1 | | 1 | | 1 | | 1 | | 1 | | 1 | |
| Cervical intraepithelial neoplasia | | 1 | | 2 | | 2 | | 2 | | 1 | | 2 | |
| Cirrhosis | a) Mild (compensated) | 1 | | 1 | | 1 | | 1 | | 1 | | 1 | |
| | b) Severe‡ (decompensated) | 1 | | 3 | | 3 | | 3 | | 3 | | 4 | |
| Cystic fibrosis‡ | | 1* | | 1* | | 1* | | 2* | | 1* | | 1* | |
| Deep venous thrombosis (DVT)/Pulmonary embolism (PE) | a) History of DVT/PE, not receiving anticoagulant therapy | | | | | | | | | | | | |
| | i) Higher risk for recurrent DVT/PE | 1 | | 2 | | 2 | | 2 | | 2 | | 4 | |
| | ii) Lower risk for recurrent DVT/PE | 1 | | 2 | | 2 | | 2 | | 2 | | 3 | |
| | b) Acute DVT/PE | 2 | | 2 | | 2 | | 2 | | 2 | | 4 | |
| | c) DVT/PE and established anticoagulant therapy for at least 3 months | | | | | | | | | | | | |
| | i) Higher risk for recurrent DVT/PE | 2 | | 2 | | 2 | | 2 | | 2 | | 4* | |
| | ii) Lower risk for recurrent DVT/PE | 2 | | 2 | | 2 | | 2 | | 2 | | 3* | |
| | d) Family history (first-degree relatives) | 1 | | 1 | | 1 | | 1 | | 1 | | 2 | |
| | e) Major surgery | | | | | | | | | | | | |
| | i) With prolonged immobilization | 1 | | 2 | | 2 | | 2 | | 2 | | 4 | |
| | ii) Without prolonged immobilization | 1 | | 1 | | 1 | | 1 | | 1 | | 2 | |
| | f) Minor surgery without immobilization | 1 | | 1 | | 1 | | 1 | | 1 | | 1 | |
| Depressive disorders | | 1* | | 1* | | 1* | | 1* | | 1* | | 1* | |

| Condition | Sub-Condition | Cu-IUD I | Cu-IUD C | LNG-IUD I | LNG-IUD C | Implant I | Implant C | DMPA I | DMPA C | POP I | POP C | CHC I | CHC C |
|---|---|---|---|---|---|---|---|---|---|---|---|---|---|
| Diabetes | a) History of gestational disease | 1 | | 1 | | 1 | | 1 | | 1 | | 1 | |
| | b) Nonvascular disease | | | | | | | | | | | | |
| | i) Non-insulin dependent | 1 | | 2 | | 2 | | 2 | | 2 | | 2 | |
| | ii) Insulin dependent | 1 | | 2 | | 2 | | 2 | | 2 | | 2 | |
| | c) Nephropathy/retinopathy/neuropathy‡ | 1 | | 2 | | 2 | | 3 | | 2 | | 3/4* | |
| | d) Other vascular disease or diabetes of >20 years' duration‡ | 1 | | 2 | | 2 | | 3 | | 2 | | 3/4* | |
| Dysmenorrhea | Severe | 2 | | 1 | | 1 | | 1 | | 1 | | 1 | |
| Endometrial cancer‡ | | 4 | 2 | 4 | 2 | 1 | | 1 | | 1 | | 1 | |
| Endometrial hyperplasia | | 1 | | 1 | | 1 | | 1 | | 1 | | 1 | |
| Endometriosis | | 2 | | 1 | | 1 | | 1 | | 1 | | 1 | |
| Epilepsy‡ | (see also Drug Interactions) | 1 | | 1 | | 1* | | 1* | | 1* | | 1* | |
| Gallbladder disease | a) Symptomatic | | | | | | | | | | | | |
| | i) Treated by cholecystectomy | 1 | | 2 | | 2 | | 2 | | 2 | | 2 | |
| | ii) Medically treated | 1 | | 2 | | 2 | | 2 | | 2 | | 3 | |
| | iii) Current | 1 | | 2 | | 2 | | 2 | | 2 | | 3 | |
| | b) Asymptomatic | 1 | | 2 | | 2 | | 2 | | 2 | | 2 | |
| Gestational trophoblastic disease‡ | a) Suspected GTD (immediate postevacuation) | | | | | | | | | | | | |
| | i) Uterine size first trimester | 1* | | 1* | | 1* | | 1* | | 1* | | 1* | |
| | ii) Uterine size second trimester | 2* | | 2* | | 1* | | 1* | | 1* | | 1* | |
| | b) Confirmed GTD | | | | | | | | | | | | |
| | i) Undetectable/non-pregnant ß-hCG levels | 1* | 1* | 1* | 1* | 1* | | 1* | | 1* | | 1* | |
| | ii) Decreasing ß-hCG levels | 2* | 1* | 2* | 1* | 1* | | 1* | | 1* | | 1* | |
| | iii) Persistently elevated ß-hCG levels or malignant disease, with no evidence or suspicion of intrauterine disease | 2* | 1* | 2* | 1* | 1* | | 1* | | 1* | | 1* | |
| | iv) Persistently elevated ß-hCG levels or malignant disease, with evidence or suspicion of intrauterine disease | 4* | 2* | 4* | 2* | 1* | | 1* | | 1* | | 1* | |
| Headaches | a) Nonmigraine (mild or severe) | 1 | | 1 | | 1 | | 1 | | 1 | | 1* | |
| | b) Migraine | | | | | | | | | | | | |
| | i) Without aura (includes menstrual migraine) | 1 | | 1 | | 1 | | 1 | | 1 | | 2* | |
| | ii) With aura | 1 | | 1 | | 1 | | 1 | | 1 | | 4* | |
| History of bariatric surgery‡ | a) Restrictive procedures | 1 | | 1 | | 1 | | 1 | | 1 | | 1 | |
| | b) Malabsorptive procedures | 1 | | 1 | | 1 | | 1 | | 3 | | COCs: 3<br>P/R: 1 | |
| History of cholestasis | a) Pregnancy related | 1 | | 1 | | 1 | | 1 | | 1 | | 2 | |
| | b) Past COC related | 1 | | 2 | | 2 | | 2 | | 2 | | 3 | |
| History of high blood pressure during pregnancy | | 1 | | 1 | | 1 | | 1 | | 1 | | 2 | |
| History of Pelvic surgery | | 1 | | 1 | | 1 | | 1 | | 1 | | 1 | |
| HIV | a) High risk for HIV | 1* | 1* | 1* | 1* | 1 | | 1 | | 1 | | 1 | |
| | b) HIV infection | | | | | 1* | | 1* | | 1* | | 1* | |
| | i) Clinically well receiving ARV therapy | 1 | 1 | 1 | 1 | If on treatment, see Drug Interactions | | | | | | | |
| | ii) Not clinically well or not receiving ARV therapy‡ | 2 | 1 | 2 | 1 | If on treatment, see Drug Interactions | | | | | | | |

**Key:**

| | |
|---|---|
| 1 No restriction (method can be used) | 3 Theoretical or proven risks usually outweigh the advantages |
| 2 Advantages generally outweigh theoretical or proven risks | 4 Unacceptable health risk (method not to be used) |

**Abbreviations:** ARV = antiretroviral; C=continuation of contraceptive method; CHC=combined hormonal contraception (pill, patch, and, ring); COC=combined oral contraceptive; Cu-IUD=copper-containing intrauterine device; DMPA = depot medroxyprogesterone acetate; I=initiation of contraceptive method; LNG-IUD=levonorgestrel-releasing intrauterine device; NA=not applicable; POP=progestin-only pill; P/R=patch/ring; SSRI=selective serotonin reuptake inhibitor; ‡ Condition that exposes a woman to increased risk as a result of pregnancy. *Please see the complete guidance for a clarification to this classification: [illegible]

EXHIBIT 29.1 **Medical Eligibility Criteria (MEC) for Contraceptive Use**

*Source*: Centers for Disease Control and Prevention. (2020b). *Summary chart of U.S. medical eligibility criteria for contraceptive use.* https://www.cdc.gov/reproductivehealth/contraception/pdf/summary-chart-us-medical-eligibility-criteria_508tagged.pdf

## Summary Chart of U.S. Medical Eligibility Criteria for Contraceptive Use

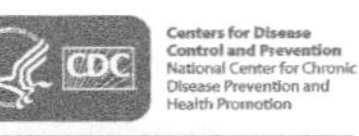


| Condition | Sub-Condition | Cu-IUD | | LNG-IUD | | Implant | | DMPA | | POP | | CHC | |
|---|---|---|---|---|---|---|---|---|---|---|---|---|---|
| | | I | C | I | C | I | C | I | C | I | C | I | C |
| Hypertension | a) Adequately controlled hypertension | 1* | | 1* | | 1* | | 2* | | 1* | | 3* | |
| | b) Elevated blood pressure levels (*properly taken measurements*) | | | | | | | | | | | | |
| | i) Systolic 140-159 or diastolic 90-99 | 1* | | 1* | | 1* | | 2* | | 1* | | 3* | |
| | ii) Systolic ≥160 or diastolic ≥100‡ | 1* | | 2* | | 2* | | 3* | | 2* | | 4* | |
| | c) Vascular disease | 1* | | 2* | | 2* | | 3* | | 2* | | 4* | |
| Inflammatory bowel disease | (*Ulcerative colitis, Crohn's disease*) | 1 | | 1 | | 1 | | 2 | | 2 | | 2/3* | |
| Ischemic heart disease‡ | Current and history of | 1 | | 2 | 3 | 2 | 3 | 3 | | 2 | 3 | 4 | |
| Known thrombogenic mutations‡ | | 1* | | 2* | | 2* | | 2* | | 2* | | 4* | |
| Liver tumors | a) Benign | | | | | | | | | | | | |
| | i) Focal nodular hyperplasia | 1 | | 2 | | 2 | | 2 | | 2 | | 2 | |
| | ii) Hepatocellular adenoma‡ | 1 | | 3 | | 3 | | 3 | | 3 | | 4 | |
| | b) Malignant‡ (hepatoma) | 1 | | 3 | | 3 | | 3 | | 3 | | 4 | |
| Malaria | | 1 | | 1 | | 1 | | 1 | | 1 | | 1 | |
| Multiple risk factors for atherosclerotic cardiovascular disease | (e.g., older age, smoking, diabetes, hypertension, low HDL, high LDL, or high triglyceride levels) | 1 | | 2 | | 2* | | 3* | | 2* | | 3/4* | |
| Multiple sclerosis | a) With prolonged immobility | 1 | | 1 | | 1 | | 2 | | 1 | | 3 | |
| | b) Without prolonged immobility | 1 | | 1 | | 1 | | 2 | | 1 | | 1 | |
| Obesity | a) Body mass index (BMI) ≥30 kg/m² | 1 | | 1 | | 1 | | 1 | | 1 | | 2 | |
| | b) Menarche to <18 years and BMI ≥ 30 kg/m² | 1 | | 1 | | 1 | | 2 | | 1 | | 2 | |
| Ovarian cancer‡ | | 1 | | 1 | | 1 | | 1 | | 1 | | 1 | |
| Parity | a) Nulliparous | 2 | | 2 | | 1 | | 1 | | 1 | | 1 | |
| | b) Parous | 1 | | 1 | | 1 | | 1 | | 1 | | 1 | |
| Past ectopic pregnancy | | 1 | | 1 | | 1 | | 1 | | 2 | | 1 | |
| Pelvic inflammatory disease | a) Past | | | | | | | | | | | | |
| | i) With subsequent pregnancy | 1 | 1 | 1 | 1 | 1 | | 1 | | 1 | | 1 | |
| | ii) Without subsequent pregnancy | 2 | 2 | 2 | 2 | 1 | | 1 | | 1 | | 1 | |
| | b) Current | 4 | 2* | 4 | 2* | 1 | | 1 | | 1 | | 1 | |
| Peripartum cardiomyopathy‡ | a) Normal or mildly impaired cardiac function | | | | | | | | | | | | |
| | i) <6 months | 2 | | 2 | | 1 | | 1 | | 1 | | 4 | |
| | ii) ≥6 months | 2 | | 2 | | 1 | | 1 | | 1 | | 3 | |
| | b) Moderately or severely impaired cardiac function | 2 | | 2 | | 2 | | 2 | | 2 | | 4 | |
| Postabortion | a) First trimester | 1* | | 1* | | 1* | | 1* | | 1* | | 1* | |
| | b) Second trimester | 2* | | 2* | | 1* | | 1* | | 1* | | 1* | |
| | c) Immediate postseptic abortion | 4 | | 4 | | 1* | | 1* | | 1* | | 1* | |
| Postpartum (*nonbreastfeeding women*) | a) <21 days | | | | | 1 | | 1 | | 1 | | 4 | |
| | b) 21 days to 42 days | | | | | | | | | | | | |
| | i) With other risk factors for VTE | | | | | 1 | | 1 | | 1 | | 3* | |
| | ii) Without other risk factors for VTE | | | | | 1 | | 1 | | 1 | | 2 | |
| | c) >42 days | | | | | 1 | | 1 | | 1 | | 1 | |
| Postpartum (*in breastfeeding or non-breastfeeding women, including cesarean delivery*) | a) <10 minutes after delivery of the placenta | | | | | | | | | | | | |
| | i) Breastfeeding | 1* | | 2* | | | | | | | | | |
| | ii) Nonbreastfeeding | 1* | | 1* | | | | | | | | | |
| | b) 10 minutes after delivery of the placenta to <4 weeks | 2* | | 2* | | | | | | | | | |
| | c) ≥4 weeks | 1* | | 1* | | | | | | | | | |
| | d) Postpartum sepsis | 4 | | 4 | | | | | | | | | |

| Condition | Sub-Condition | Cu-IUD | | LNG-IUD | | Implant | | DMPA | | POP | | CHC | |
|---|---|---|---|---|---|---|---|---|---|---|---|---|---|
| | | I | C | I | C | I | C | I | C | I | C | I | C |
| Pregnancy | | 4* | | 4* | | NA* | | NA* | | NA* | | NA* | |
| Rheumatoid arthritis | a) On immunosuppressive therapy | 2 | 1 | 2 | 1 | 1 | | 2/3* | | 1 | | 2 | |
| | b) Not on immunosuppressive therapy | 1 | | 1 | | 1 | | 2 | | 1 | | 2 | |
| Schistosomiasis | a) Uncomplicated | 1 | | 1 | | 1 | | 1 | | 1 | | 1 | |
| | b) Fibrosis of the liver‡ | 1 | | 1 | | 1 | | 1 | | 1 | | 1 | |
| Sexually transmitted diseases (STDs) | a) Current purulent cervicitis or chlamydial infection or gonococcal infection | 4 | 2* | 4 | 2* | 1 | | 1 | | 1 | | 1 | |
| | b) Vaginitis (*including trichomonas vaginalis and bacterial vaginosis*) | 2 | 2 | 2 | 2 | 1 | | 1 | | 1 | | 1 | |
| | c) Other factors relating to STDs | 2* | 2 | 2* | 2 | 1 | | 1 | | 1 | | 1 | |
| Smoking | a) Age <35 | 1 | | 1 | | 1 | | 1 | | 1 | | 2 | |
| | b) Age ≥35, <15 cigarettes/day | 1 | | 1 | | 1 | | 1 | | 1 | | 3 | |
| | c) Age ≥35, ≥15 cigarettes/day | 1 | | 1 | | 1 | | 1 | | 1 | | 4 | |
| Solid organ transplantation‡ | a) Complicated | 3 | 2 | 3 | 2 | 2 | | 2 | | 2 | | 4 | |
| | b) Uncomplicated | 2 | | 2 | | 2 | | 2 | | 2 | | 2* | |
| Stroke‡ | History of cerebrovascular accident | 1 | | 2 | | 2 | 3 | 3 | | 2 | 3 | 4 | |
| Superficial venous disorders | a) Varicose veins | 1 | | 1 | | 1 | | 1 | | 1 | | 1 | |
| | b) Superficial venous thrombosis (acute or history) | 1 | | 1 | | 1 | | 1 | | 1 | | 3* | |
| Systemic lupus erythematosus‡ | a) Positive (or unknown) antiphospholipid antibodies | 1* | 1* | 3* | | 3* | | 3* | 3* | 3* | | 4* | |
| | b) Severe thrombocytopenia | 3* | 2* | 2* | | 2* | | 3* | 2* | 2* | | 2* | |
| | c) Immunosuppressive therapy | 2* | 1* | 2* | | 2* | | 2* | 2* | 2* | | 2* | |
| | d) None of the above | 1* | 1* | 2* | | 2* | | 2* | 2* | 2* | | 2* | |
| Thyroid disorders | Simple goiter/ hyperthyroid/hypothyroid | 1 | | 1 | | 1 | | 1 | | 1 | | 1 | |
| Tuberculosis‡ (*see also Drug Interactions*) | a) Nonpelvic | 1 | 1 | 1 | 1 | 1* | | 1* | | 1* | | 1* | |
| | b) Pelvic | 4 | 3 | 4 | 3 | 1* | | 1* | | 1* | | 1* | |
| Unexplained vaginal bleeding | (suspicious for serious condition) before evaluation | 4* | 2* | 4* | 2* | 3* | | 3* | | 2* | | 2* | |
| Uterine fibroids | | 2 | | 2 | | 1 | | 1 | | 1 | | 1 | |
| Valvular heart disease | a) Uncomplicated | 1 | | 1 | | 1 | | 1 | | 1 | | 2 | |
| | b) Complicated‡ | 1 | | 1 | | 1 | | 1 | | 1 | | 4 | |
| Vaginal bleeding patterns | a) Irregular pattern without heavy bleeding | 1 | | 1 | 1 | 2 | | 2 | | 2 | | 1 | |
| | b) Heavy or prolonged bleeding | 2* | | 1* | 2* | 2* | | 2* | | 2* | | 1* | |
| Viral hepatitis | a) Acute or flare | 1 | | 1 | | 1 | | 1 | | 1 | | 3/4* | 2 |
| | b) Carrier/Chronic | 1 | | 1 | | 1 | | 1 | | 1 | | 1 | 1 |
| **Drug Interactions** | | | | | | | | | | | | | |
| Antiretrovirals used for prevention (PrEP) or treatment of HIV | Fosamprenavir (FPV)<br>All other ARVs are 1 or 2 for all methods. | 1/2* | 1* | 1/2* | 1* | 2* | | 2* | | 2* | | 3* | |
| Anticonvulsant therapy | a) Certain anticonvulsants (phenytoin, carbamazepine, barbiturates, primidone, topiramate, oxcarbazepine) | 1 | | 1 | | 2* | | 1* | | 3* | | 3* | |
| | b) Lamotrigine | 1 | | 1 | | 1 | | 1 | | 1 | | 3* | |
| Antimicrobial therapy | a) Broad spectrum antibiotics | 1 | | 1 | | 1 | | 1 | | 1 | | 1 | |
| | b) Antifungals | 1 | | 1 | | 1 | | 1 | | 1 | | 1 | |
| | c) Antiparasitics | 1 | | 1 | | 1 | | 1 | | 1 | | 1 | |
| | d) Rifampin or rifabutin therapy | 1 | | 1 | | 2* | | 1* | | 3* | | 3* | |
| SSRIs | | 1 | | 1 | | 1 | | 1 | | 1 | | 1 | |
| St. John's wort | | 1 | | 1 | | 2 | | 1 | | 2 | | 2 | |

**Updated in 2020.** This summary sheet only contains a subset of the recommendations from the U.S. MEC. For complete guidance, see: [illegible]. Most contraceptive methods do not protect against sexually transmitted diseases (STDs). Consistent and correct use of the male latex condom reduces the risk of STDs and HIV.

CS314239-A

**EXHIBIT 29.1 Medical Eligibility Criteria (MEC) for Contraceptive Use (*continued*)**

> **PRO TIP** A Medical Eligibility Criteria wheel from the CDC can be obtained for free at wwwn.cdc.gov/pubs/CDCInfoOnDemand.aspx?ProgramID=195

## Laboratory/Diagnostic Testing

No laboratory or diagnostic testing is needed, unless you are screening the adolescent for STIs.

## Prescribing Contraception

Table 29.3 provides effectiveness and first-year failure rate information, advantages and disadvantages, and management and follow-up for various contraceptives. Table 29.4 provides information related to timing with contraceptives.

## Family Education

Teach the following about the specific contraceptive prescribed (Table 29.5).

TABLE 29.3 **Information on Contraceptives**

| Contraceptive Method | Effectiveness/First Year Failure Rate | Advantages | Disadvantages or Side Effects | Management | Follow-Up |
|---|---|---|---|---|---|
| **Intrauterine Device (IUC)**<br>Levonorgestrel Intrauterine System (LNG-IUS): T-shaped plastic frame with levonorgestrel that is released. Methods last for 3 or 5 years. | Perfect use: 0.2%<br>Typical use: 0.2% | Ease of use.<br>Not dependent on action during intercourse.<br>Effective.<br>Reversible.<br>Can be used for adolescents with dysmenorrhea.<br>Effective for adolescents who don't want to use estrogen-based methods. | Altered menstrual bleeding patterns.<br>Risk of pelvic inflammatory disease.<br>Risk of spontaneous expulsion. | Thorough health history including STI exposure, sexual activity, and menstrual history.<br>Physical exam: speculum exam, STI cultures including gonorrhea and chlamydia.<br>Must have negative pregnancy test on file in office within 24 hours of placement.<br>See Table 29.4 for timing of placement. | Return to office as needed when desire change of contraceptive method.<br>No other routine follow-up is necessary. |
| Copper releasing IUC: T-shaped plastic device with copper wrapped around both vertical and horizontal stem. | Perfect use: 0.6%<br>Typical use: 0.2% | | | | |
| **Progestin-only Implant (Implanon/Nexplanon):**<br>Long-term contraceptive. Single rod-shaped implant placed subdermally in inner side of upper arm provides low-dose progestin to suppress LH, inhibiting ovulation in most users. | Perfect use: 0.05%<br>Typical use: 0.05% | Ease of use<br>Effective<br>Reversible—most users will ovulate within 6 weeks of removal<br>Contains no estrogen<br>Adolescents who suffer from dysmenorrhea may experience reduction in pain | Requires clinician insertion and removal by minor surgical procedure.<br>Pain, bruising, and risk for infection at insertion site.<br>Irregular, prolonged, more frequent uterine bleeding, especially in first few months.<br>No protection against STI/HIV.<br>Side effects include:<br>• Headaches<br>• Emotional lability<br>• Breast tenderness<br>• Acne | Thorough health history including past medical history, sexual history, menstrual history.<br>Elicit information from health history concerning any contraindications, risks, specific noncontraceptive benefits for use of progestin-only implant. | Return to office at any time to discuss side effects or to change contraceptive method.<br>No other follow-up necessary. |

*(continued)*

TABLE 29.3 **Information on Contraceptives** (*continued*)

| Contraceptive Method | Effectiveness/First Year Failure Rate | Advantages | Disadvantages or Side Effects | Management | Follow-Up |
|---|---|---|---|---|---|
| **Combined Oral Contraceptives (COC):**<br>Pill taken daily for contraception. Combination of estrogen and progestin. Must be taken at same time every day to suppress ovulation and prevent pregnancy. | Perfect use: 0.3%<br>Typical use: 9% | Ease of use<br>Reversible<br>Effective<br>May reduce incidence and severity of:<br>• Acne<br>• Dysmenorrhea<br>• Endometriosis<br>• Menstrual related migraine headaches<br>• Premenstrual syndrome | Does not protect against STI/HIV.<br>Requires daily compliance.<br>Possible side effects include:<br>• Breast tenderness<br>• Nausea<br>• Headaches<br>• Fatigue<br>• Weight gain<br>Potential for deep vein thrombosis and other clotting problems increases with estrogen use. | Thorough health history including past medical history, sexual history, menstrual history.<br>Elicit information from health history concerning any contraindications, risks, specific noncontraceptive benefits for use of COCs.<br>Ensure that adolescent is capable of daily dosing compliance. | Advise patient to return at any time to discuss side effects or to change contraceptive method.<br>No other routine follow-up necessary. |
| **Transdermal Contraceptive Patch System:**<br>Patch applied to skin: delivers continuous estrogen-progestin. New patch applied every week for three weeks. Fourth week without patch to induce withdrawal bleeding. | Perfect Use: 0.3%<br>Typical use: 9% | Ease of use<br>Reversible<br>Effective<br>Not a daily compliance issue | Does not offer STI/HIV protection.<br>Skin irritation at application site.<br>Side effects similar to those seen with COC. | Thorough health history including past medical history, sexual history, menstrual history.<br>Elicit information from health history concerning any contraindications, risks, specific noncontraceptive benefits for use of transdermal patch. | Advise patient to return at any time to discuss side effects or to change contraceptive method.<br>No other routine follow-up necessary. |
| **Contraceptive Vaginal Ring:**<br>Soft, clear plastic ring that delivers continuous estrogen and progestin. Worn in vagina for three weeks followed by one week without to induce withdrawal bleeding. | Perfect Use: 0.3%<br>Typical Use: 9% | Ease of use, no daily dosing<br>Reversible<br>Effective<br>Good menstrual cycle control | Does not protect against STI/HIV.<br>Side effects similar to those seen with COC.<br>Vaginal irritation. | Thorough health history including past medical history, sexual history, menstrual history.<br>Elicit information from health history concerning any contraindications, risks, specific noncontraceptive benefits for use of vaginal ring. | Advise patient to return at any time to discuss side effects or to change contraceptive method.<br>No other routine follow-up necessary. |

(*continued*)

TABLE 29.3 **Information on Contraceptives** (*continued*)

| Contraceptive Method | Effectiveness/First Year Failure Rate | Advantages | Disadvantages or Side Effects | Management | Follow-Up |
|---|---|---|---|---|---|
| **Progestin-Only Pills (POP):** Pill taken daily for contraceptive, composed of progestins in lower doses than COC. | Perfect Use: 0.3%<br>Typical use: 9% | Ease of use, no daily dosing<br>Reversible<br>Effective<br>Contains no estrogen, allowing adolescents who cannot have estrogen an option for daily dosing | Effectiveness can be compromised by drug interactions because of low-dose formulations.<br>STRICT daily dosing schedule (within 1 hour of same time every day).<br>Possible side effects:<br>• Increased menstrual irregularities<br>• Depression<br>• Breakthrough bleeding | Thorough health history including past medical history, sexual history, menstrual history.<br>Elicit information from health history concerning any contraindications, risks, specific noncontraceptive benefits for use of progestin-only pills. | Advise patient to return at any time to discuss side effects or to change contraceptive method.<br>No other routine follow-up necessary. |
| **Progestin-)nly Injectable Contraception (DMPA or "depo")** Intramuscular injection progestin administered in three-month intervals for contraception. | Perfect use: 0.2%<br>Typical Use: 6% | Ease of use<br>Effective<br>Long-term contraceptive option<br>Does not require compliance with daily dosing<br>Results in absence of menstrual bleeding in 50% of women by the end of the first year of use and 70% by end of second year<br>Contains no estrogen | Menstrual cycle abnormalities are very common.<br>Depression.<br>No protection against STI/ HIV.<br>Not immediately reversible.<br>Requires 3-month injection schedule.<br>Weight gain: average 5.4 lbs in first year.<br>Decreased bone density in long-term use (greater than 5 years). | Thorough health history including past medical history, sexual history, menstrual history.<br>Elicit information from health history concerning any contraindications, risks, specific noncontraceptive benefits for use of progestin injection. | Advise patient to return at any time to discuss side effects or to change contraceptive method.<br>MUST return to office in 12 weeks for injection. |

*Source*: Kelsey, B. M., & Nagtalon-Ramos, J. (2020). *Midwifery & woman's health nurse practitioner certification review guide* (5th ed.). Jones & Bartlett Learning.

## INITIAL PREGNANCY VISIT

In the United States in the past 20 years, we have seen a decrease in adolescent pregnancy rates (aged 15–19 years old) to a historic low at 22.3 per 1,000 females (Committee on Adolescent Health Care [CAHC], 2017). Despite the positive trends, the United States continues to have the highest adolescent pregnancy rates among developed countries with data (CAHC, 2017). The ACOG released a committee opinion in 2017 regarding the care of adolescents and reproductive health choices. That document outlines care of the teens and recommends that all adolescents should have access and counseling for all contraceptive methods without coercion from the clinician. The document also outlines the recommendation from ACOG and the American Academy of Pediatrics (AAP) for use of long-acting reversible contraception (LARK) in the

**TABLE 29.4 Timing of Contraceptive Methods**

| Intrauterine Device Placement | Progestin-Only Implant | Combined Oral Contraceptive (COC) & Progestin-Only Pills (POP) | Transdermal Contraceptive Patch (Xulane) | Contraceptive Vaginal Ring (Nuvaring) | Progestin-Only Injectable Contraception (DMPA or "depo") |
|---|---|---|---|---|---|
| Must be reasonably sure patient is not pregnant<br>• Within 7 days of start of menses<br>• No unprotected intercourse in the past 2 weeks<br>• Pregnancy test is negative in office no more than 24 hours from time of IUD placement | Insert within 1–5 days of menses; no backup method necessary<br>If adolescent has irregular menses, rule out pregnancy with negative pregnancy test within 24 hours of insertion | Reasonably certain patient is not pregnant: First pill of first day in office. Use back-up method for 7 days.<br>***OR***<br>Take first pill on first day of next menstrual period. No back-up method needed. | Reasonably certain patient is not pregnant: Apply patch on first day prescribed. Use back-up method for 7 days.<br>***OR***<br>Apply patch of first day of menses. No back up method needed. | Reasonably certain patient is not pregnant: Insert ring on first day prescribed. Use back-up method for 7 days.<br>***OR***<br>Insert ring on first day of menses. No back-up method needed. | Reasonably certain patient is not pregnant: Give injection in office. Use back-up method for 7 days.<br>***OR***<br>Administer injection on first day of menses. No back-up method needed. |

*Source*: Kelsey, B. M., & Nagtalon-Ramos, J. (2020). *Midwifery & woman's health nurse practitioner certification review guide* (5th ed.). Jones & Bartlett Learning.

**TABLE 29.5 Family Education About Contraceptive Methods**

| Intrauterine Device (IUD) | Progestin-Only Implant | Combined Oral Contraceptive (COC) & Progestin-Only Pills (POP) | Transdermal Contraceptive Patch (Xulane) | Contraceptive Vaginal Ring (Nuvaring) | Progestin-Only Injectable Contraception (DMPA or "depo") |
|---|---|---|---|---|---|
| **Signs of Infection**<br>• Pelvic pain<br>• Vaginal discharge<br>• Unexplained vaginal bleeding after the initial 60 days<br>**Warning Signs (PAINS)**<br>• (P) Period late or missed; abnormal spotting or bleeding<br>• (A) Abdominal pain<br>• (I) Infection—vaginal discharge<br>• (N) Not feeling well—fever, ache, chills<br>• (S) String missing, shorter or longer | **Warning signs**<br>• Abdominal pain (severe)<br>• Arm pain or signs of infection at site of insertion<br>• Heavy vaginal bleeding<br>• Missed menses after period of regularity<br>• Onset of severe headaches<br>Discuss use of condoms 100% of the time from start to finish to protect against STI/HIV.<br>Discuss possible bleeding changes and what is expected and not expected. | **Warning Signs (ACHES)—COC**<br>• Abdominal pain<br>• Chest pain<br>• Headaches<br>• Eye problems (blurry vision, blind spots)<br>• Severe leg pain<br>**Broad-Spectrum Antibiotics**<br>• Most broad-spectrum antibiotics (ampicillin, metronidazole, doxycycline, fluconazole) do NOT lower hormone levels or reduce effectiveness.<br>• A few do induce cytochrome P-450 enzyme activity and lower COC effectiveness (rifampin, rifapentine, griseofulvin).<br>• Some anticonvulsant medications reduce COC effectiveness.<br>Take pill at same time every day. If nausea occurs, take immediately before bed.<br>Use condoms 100% of the time from start to finish for protection against STI/HIV. | Apply patch to buttocks, shoulder, abdomen, upper torso excluding breasts, upper outer arm.<br>Apply new patch on same day each week for a total of three weeks.<br>Choose new site each week.<br>Discuss use of condoms 100% of the time from start to finish to protect against STI/HIV. | Wash hands before insertion.<br>Fold ring in half and gently insert into the vagina.<br>Leave ring in place for 3 weeks, then remove.<br>Insert new ring in 7 days. | **Warning Signs**<br>• Frequent intense headache<br>• Heavy bleeding<br>• Depression<br>• Severe abdominal pain<br>• Signs of infection at the injection site.<br>If late for injection, clinician will need to assess for pregnancy. If reasonably certain patient is not pregnant, injection can be given and a backup method should be used for 7 days. |

*Source*: Kelsey, B. M., & Nagtalon-Ramos, J. (2020). *Midwifery & woman's health nurse practitioner certification review guide* (5th ed.). Jones & Bartlett Learning.

form of intrauterine devices and implants for adolescents. Additionally, the AAP and ACOG recommend the discussion of dual-method use: pairing condoms with other forms of contraception in order to protect against pregnancy, STIs, and HIV as best practice for adolescents (CAHC, 2017). The pregnancy rate in the United States continues to decrease because clinicians are having open, honest, and safe conversations with adolescents about reproductive health care and their contraceptive choices.

## Subjective Findings

The health history may reveal:

- Lack of menses or abnormal vaginal bleeding
- Increased fatigue

### Risk Factors

The most common risk factors for adolescent pregnancy are:

- Hispanic and non-Hispanic black teens
- American Indian/Alaska native teens
- Teens who abuse substances such as drugs or alcohol
- Adolescents with a lack of knowledge about sex and/or contraception
- Adolescents with poor school performance, low self-esteem, and depression
- Any history of sexual, physical, or emotional abuse

### Review of Systems

The most common manifestations revealed during the review of systems include:

- **Constitutional:** increased weight
- **Gastrointestinal:** nausea or vomiting
- **Reproductive:** breast tenderness, absence of menses at expected time

## Objective Findings

The physical examination of the child or adolescent with suspected pregnancy may reveal:

- Enlarged uterus
- Chadwick's sign: Bluish cervix indicating increased blood flow

### Laboratory/Diagnostic Testing

The diagnosis of amenorrhea can be made with clinical signs and symptoms. However, the pediatric nurse practitioner needs to perform a urine hCG test in office to confirm or rule out pregnancy.

## Differential Diagnosis

The differential diagnosis for pregnancy includes other causes of amenorrhea such as anorexia nervosa or intensive physical activity or training.

## Treatment/Management Plan

Prescribe prenatal vitamins with folic acid (once daily). May try pyridoxine (vitamin B6) 10 to 25 mg orally every 6 to 8 hours to help with nausea until adolescent makes appointment with the certified nurse midwife (CNM) or obstetrician/gynecologist (OB/GYN).

### Family Education

Teach the following:

- Maintain a well-balanced, nutritious diet with plenty of fluid intake.
- Avoid use of alcohol and illicit drugs. Check with the provider about the safety of prescription medications.
- Get plenty of sleep and exercise regularly.
- Establish care with the CNM or OB/GYN immediately and maintain all visits for prenatal care.

### Referral

Any adolescent with a positive hCG, either urine or blood, should be referred to a CNM or OB/GYN immediately for prenatal care and planning for the pregnancy.

## KEY POINTS

- Pediatric nurse practitioners can work to make their clinic "teen friendly" by providing adolescents with confidential, private, respectful services with convenient office hours, and walk-in appointments. Create an open, trusting relationship with the adolescent that includes time to speak with the nurse practitioner without a parent or guardian present.
- All adolescents should have a reproductive health visit between ages 11 and 15 with regular reproductive health visits throughout their adolescent years. Nurse practitioners should have discussions including sexual history, STI and HIV screening, and private counseling with the adolescent patient.
- Studies show that the rate of adolescent pregnancy is lower in teens who have reproductive health visits with their clinician and are aware of the contraceptive management methods available to them.
- Be sure to assess each adolescent for a history of emotional, physical, and sexual assault.

- For PMS, have girls keep a symptom record for two or three cycles, then review with them and identify triggers and behavioral patterns that can be changed.
- Exercise and nutrition are key components of treatment plans for all reproductive disorders.
- Consider COC or IUD as first-line defense for dysmenorrhea.
- Primary dysmenorrhea often begins 6 to 12 months after menarche. Symptoms are usually experienced with the onset of bleeding and continue for 8 to 72 hours into the cycle.
- Thorough menstrual, obstetric, gynecologic, social, and nutritional history is a vital step in differential diagnosis for the adolescent with amenorrhea.
- ASCCP guidelines state that a pelvic examination of an adolescent should be completed **ONLY** when absolutely necessary and Papanicolaou testing in females under the age of 21 should not be done.
- If there is evidence of food insecurity, a referral to a mental health professional is recommended.
- Be sure to discuss all of the contraceptive options appropriate for each child or adolescent in depth at the initial contraceptive visit in order to document informed consent.
- The clinician needs to review CDC Medical Eligibility Criteria before prescribing any contraceptive method to the adolescent, to ensure safety of the method.
- Assess all physical and psychological symptoms when an adolescent presents with premenstrual symptoms to ensure that this is not a case of PMDD that needs to be referred to a mental health provider.
- Adolescents who are pregnant are considered emancipated minors and are able to make medical decisions for themselves. They should be seen by themselves if they present to a clinician's office without a parent for advice or care.

## REFERENCES

Agency for Healthcare Research and Quality. (2016). *Trauma-informed care.* https://www.ahrq.gov/ncepcr/tools/healthier-pregnancy/fact-sheets/trauma.html

American College of Obstetricians and Gynecologists. (2019). *Committee Opinion No. 777: Sexual assault.* https://www.acog.org/clinical/clinical-guidance/committee-opinion/articles/2019/04/sexual-assault

Bornstein, J. (2019). Benign disorders of the vulva & vagina. In A. H. DeCherney, L. Nathan, N. Laufer, & A. S. Roman (Eds.), *Current diagnosis & treatment: Obstetrics & gynecology* (12th ed., Chapter 40). McGraw-Hill Education.

Centers for Disease Control and Prevention. (2020a). *Child abuse and neglect prevention.* https://www.cdc.gov/violenceprevention/childabuseandneglect/index.html

Centers for Disease Control and Prevention. (2020b). *Summary chart of U.S. medical eligibility criteria for contraceptive use.* https://www.cdc.gov/reproductivehealth/contraception/pdf/summary-chart-us-medical-eligibility-criteria_508tagged.pdf

Committee on Adolescent Health Care. (2017). *Committee Opinion No. 699: Adolescent pregnancy, contraception, and sexual activity.* https://www.acog.org/-/media/project/acog/acogorg/clinical/files/committee-opinion/articles/2017/05/adolescent-pregnancy-contraception-and-sexual-activity.pdf

Evans, A., & Hoeger, K. M. (2020). Polycystic ovary syndrome and adolescents: Toward a better diagnosis and treatment. *Current Opinion in Endocrine and Metabolic Research, 12,* 105–111. https://doi.org/10.1016/j.coemr.2020.04.010

Feldman, S., Goodman, A., & Peipert, J. F. (2020). Screening for cervical cancer. *UpToDate.* https://www.uptodate.com/contents/screening-for-cervical-cancer#H41

Forcier, M., & Olson-Kennedy, J. (2020). Lesbian, gay, bisexual and other sexual minoritized youth: Epidemiology and health concerns. *UpToDate.* https://www.uptodate.com/contents/lesbian-gay-bisexual-and-other-sexual-minoritized-youth-epidemiology-and-health-concerns

Gibson, M. E. S., Fleming, N., Zuijdwijk, C., & Dumont, T. (2020). Where have all the periods gone? The evaluation and management of functional hypothalamic amenorrhea. *Journal of Clinical Research in Pediatric Endocrinology and Diabetes Society, 12*(Suppl. 1), 18–27. https://doi.org/10.4274/jcrpe.galenos.2019.2019.S0178

Gudeman, R., & Madge, S. (n.d.). *The federal Title X family planning program: Privacy and access rules for adolescents.* https://youthlaw.org/publication/the-federal-title-x-family-planning-program-privacy-and-access-rules-for-adolescents1

Jones, A. (2019). Bacterial vaginosis: A review of treatment, recurrence, and disparities. *The Journal for Nurse Practitioners, 15*(6), 420–423. https://doi.org/10.1016/j.nurpra.2019.03.010

Kansky, J., & Allen, J. P. (2018). Long-term risks and possible benefits associated with late adolescent romantic relationship quality. *Journal of Youth and Adolescents, 47*(7), 1531–1544. https://doi.org/10.1007/s10964-018-0813-x

Kelsey, B. M., & Nagtalon-Ramos, J. (2020). *Midwifery & woman's health nurse practitioner certification review guide* (5th ed.). Jones & Bartlett Learning.

King, T. L., Bruckner, M. C., Osborne, K., & Jevitt, C. M. (2019). *Varney's midwifery* (6th ed.). Jones & Bartlett Learning.

Kritzler, R. K., Long, D., & Plotnick, L. (2017). Puberty: Normal and abnormal. In T. K. McInerny, H. M. Adam, D. E. Campbell, J. M. Foy, & D. M. Kamat (Eds.), *American Academy of Pediatrics textbook of pediatric care* (2nd ed., Chapter 185). American Academy of Pediatrics.

Murphy, P. A., Hewitt, C. M., & Belew, C. (2017). Contraception. In K. D. Schuiling & F. E. Likis (Eds.), *Women's gynecologic health* (3rd ed., pp. 209–244). Jones & Bartlett Learning.

Ross, J., & Chacko, M. R. (2020). Pelvic inflammatory disease: Clinical manifestations and diagnosis. *UpToDate.* https://www.uptodate.com/contents/pelvic-inflammatory-disease-clinical-manifestations-and-diagnosis

Schuiling, K. D., & Lowe, L. K. (2017). Women's growth and development across the lifespan. In K. D. Schuiling & F. E. Likis (Eds.), *Women's gynecologic health* (3rd ed., pp. 17–35). Jones & Bartlett Learning.

Tharpe, N. J., Farley, C. L., & Jordan, R. G. (2017). *Clinical practice guidelines for midwifery & women's health* (5th ed.). Jones & Bartlett Learning.

Tranoulis, A., Soldatou, A., Georgiou, D., Mavrogianni, D., Loutradis, D. K., & Michala, L. (2020). Adolescents and young women with functional hypothalamic amenorrhea: Is it time to move beyond the hormonal profile? *Archives of Gynecology and Obstetrics, 301*(4), 1095–1101. https://doi.org/10.1007/s00404-020-05499-1

Zielinksi, R., & Lynne, S. (2017). Menstrual-cycle pain and premenstrual conditions. In K. D. Schuiling & F. E. Likis (Eds.), *Women's gynecologic health* (3rd ed., pp. 549–574). Jones & Bartlett Learning.

# Management of Hematologic and Oncologic Disorders

Sara Gerrie and Brandi M. Runnels

## Student Learning Outcomes

**Upon completion of this chapter the reader should be able to:**

1. Discuss pathophysiology and epidemiology of selected hematologic and oncologic disorders in children.
2. Differentiate subjective and objective findings for selected hematologic and oncologic disorders in children.
3. Choose appropriate laboratory or diagnostic tests for selected hematologic and oncologic disorders in children.
4. Utilize the differential diagnosis process to determine the diagnosis of hematologic and oncologic disorders in children.
5. Determine treatment plan, child/family education, and need for referral for children with a(n) hematologic and oncologic diagnosis.

## INTRODUCTION

Disorders of the blood are commonly encountered by the primary care provider. Symptomology can range from completely normal with only an abnormal laboratory value to life-threatening bleeding. While hematologic disorders may be followed by a hematologist, the primary care provider plays an important role in maintaining the overall health picture of the child. Signs and symptoms of oncologic disorders in children must be quickly identified for prompt treatment and, possibly, cure. Additionally, the primary care provider continues to follow the child undergoing cancer treatment for the purpose of promoting growth and development and otherwise maintaining health. Providers also have children in their care who are cancer survivors.

The content in this chapter maps to the following areas on the Pediatric Nursing Certification Board (PNCB) Pediatric Nurse Practitioner—Primary Care certification examination:

**CLINICAL PROBLEMS: HEMATOLOGY/ ONCOLOGY**

CONTENT AREAS:

**II. Assessment and Diagnosis**

**B. History and Physical Examination**

1. Obtain history of present illness
2. Obtain a comprehensive health history for new patients
3. Complete an interval history for established patients
4. Perform a review of systems
1. Perform a complete physical examination

**B. Diagnostic Testing and Screening**

1. Order and interpret office/clinic based screening tests
2. Order and interpret diagnostic laboratory tests
3. Order and interpret the results of diagnostic imaging tests

**C. Analyzing Information**

1. Integrate health history and physical examination findings into the plan of care
2. Assimilate findings from screening and diagnostic testing into plan of care

**B. Diagnosis**

1. Develop and prioritize differential diagnoses
2. Establish a diagnosis based on evaluation of patient data

## III. Management

**A. Child and Caregiver Counseling and Education**

1. Provide condition-specific counseling and education, including treatment options
2. Educate about benefits and potential adverse reactions of pharmacological interventions
3. Discuss non-pharmacological interventions
4. Counsel regarding the threshold for seeking follow-up care
5. Review the risks of non-adherence to recommended treatment

**A. Therapeutic Interventions**

1. Prescribe pharmacologic agents
2. Recommend the use of over-the-counter pharmacologic agents
3. Order or recommend non-pharmacologic treatments for the management of symptoms
4. Discuss use of complementary and alternative therapies as appropriate

**C. Collaboration and Referral**

2. Refer to specialists as indicated for evaluation, counseling, and/or treatment

**B. Care Coordination**

1. Facilitate patient and family-centered care for children of all ages with acute and chronic conditions

**C. Evaluation and Follow-up**

2. Establish a plan for follow-up care

## IV. Professional Role Responsibilities

**A. Leadership and Evidence-based Practice**

4. Develop, implement, and/or modify clinical practice guidelines

# HEMATOLOGIC DISORDERS: ANEMIA

*Anemia* is a reduction of the hemoglobin concentration in the blood. The normal range for hemoglobin is based primarily on age and sex. However, there is small differentiation among races noted on some charts. Hemoglobin and hematocrit are important levels to obtain and check against an acceptable reference, as differential will change based on age.

A phenomenon termed *physiologic anemia* exists where there is a decline in the hemoglobin within the first 2 to 3 months of life. This is the most common anemia in early life. The hemoglobin increases after nadir and reaches a more appropriate level by about the sixth month of life. This phenomenon is more pronounced in preterm infants.

## IRON-DEFICIENCY ANEMIA

Iron-deficiency anemia is a decreased hemoglobin concentration caused by a lack of sufficient iron. This can occur due to insufficient iron in the diet (less of a problem in developed countries), or a chronic mechanism of blood loss. In children, approximately 30% of daily iron needs for normal growth and development are obtained from dietary intake. Healthy full-term infants with no underlying disorder maintain enough iron storage for the first 5 to 6 months of life, making the diagnosis of iron-deficiency anemia unlikely before this age.

### Subjective Findings

The health history may reveal:

- Decreased energy
- Irritability
- Lack of iron in diet

The most common presentation of iron-deficiency anemia is an asymptomatic child found to have anemia with routine blood work. Severe and/or chronic disease can cause the symptoms noted earlier.

### Risk Factors

The most common risk factors for iron-deficiency anemia are:

- Lower socioeconomic status
- Prematurity
- Insufficient iron intake of solely breastfed infant
- Malabsorption disorder
- High cow milk intake in toddlers

### Review of Systems

The most common manifestations revealed during the review of systems include:

- **Constitutional:** decreased energy, poor feeding, pica

▶ ALERT: If pica is a presenting symptom, a blood lead level should be obtained to ensure that there is no lead poisoning (Leung & Hon, 2019).

### Objective Findings

The physical examination of the child with iron-deficiency anemia may reveal pallor.

### Laboratory/Diagnostic Testing

The diagnosis of iron-deficiency anemia is based on the laboratory findings of a microcytic (decreased mean corpuscular volume, or MCV) anemia in conjunction with a high total iron binding capacity, and a low serum ferritin level. Anemia thresholds are based upon age:

- Children 6 months to <5 years: hemoglobin <11 g/dL and ferritin <15 microgram/L
- Children 5 to <12 years: hemoglobin <11.5 g/dL and ferritin <15 micrograms/L

With the typical presentation for iron deficiency (<3 years of age and risk for low dietary iron), a complete blood count (CBC) will suffice, and successful treatment with iron supplementation will further confirm diagnosis. Low ferritin is always consistent with iron deficiency, but a higher ferritin level does not exclude a diagnosis of iron-deficiency anemia, as ferritin is an acute phase reactant.

PRO TIP The American Academy of Pediatrics (AAP) recommends routine screening for iron-deficiency anemia with a CBC at 1 year of age. Iron-deficiency anemia should be lower on differential in a child less than 6 months of age (term infant).

### Differential Diagnosis

The differential diagnosis for iron-deficiency anemia includes:

- Thalassemia trait
- Anemia of chronic disease
- Anemia of inflammation (following an infection or immunization)

### Treatment/Management Plan

Begin a trial therapy of iron (ferrous sulfate 3 mg/kg daily) for 4 weeks for those with mild anemia, and within 2 weeks if anemia is moderate to severe. The hemoglobin should demonstrate >1 g/dL increase. If the child is not reaching this threshold, the provider will need to evaluate for other causes. Iron supplementation should be continued until the child reaches a normal range of hemoglobin level for their age and a minimum of 3 months.

### Family Education

Teach the following:

- Iron supplementation starting at age 4 months for exclusively breastfed infants until receiving enough iron from solid foods or addition of formula. Start at age 2 weeks if infant was born prematurely.
- If utilizing formula to feed infant, a low-iron formula is *not* recommended.
- Limit cow's milk intake to less than 24 ounces per day (should not start cow's milk until 1 year of age).
- Provide diet with adequate intake of iron.

## LEAD POISONING

Children younger than 6 years of age are the most susceptible to lead poisoning due to their incomplete blood–brain barrier. This results in more severe symptoms involving the central nervous system (CNS). The majority of children will present asymptomatically, but symptomology is dependent on the amount and length of time of exposure to lead and the age of the child. Although paint manufactured now no longer contains lead, it was an ingredient in paint manufactured until the 1970s in the United States. Whether lead is ingested or inhaled, it is capable of distribution to the blood, soft tissues, and bone.

### Subjective Findings

The health history may reveal:

- Not meeting developmental milestones
- Neurobehavioral abnormalities
- Birth outside of United States or recent residence of another country

### Risk Factors

The most common risk factors for lead poisoning are:

- Younger than 6 years of age

- Lower socioeconomic status
- Residence in housing built before 1970s
- Exposure in countries still utilizing lead in gasoline, cookware, jewelry, toys, candy wrappers, and paint

### Review of Systems

The most common manifestations revealed during the review of systems include:

- **Constitutional:** weight loss
- **HEENT:** hearing loss
- **Gastrointestinal:** constipation, persistent vomiting
- **Neurologic:** speech difficulties, seizures, altered mental status

**PRO TIP** With lead poisoning, colic, abdominal pain, intermittent vomiting, and constipation occur.

### Objective Findings

The physical examination of the child with lead poisoning may reveal:

- Lethargy
- Language difficulty
- A lead line along gum line may be present with severe and prolonged lead exposure
- Diffuse abdominal tenderness
- Tremor

### Laboratory/Diagnostic Testing

Lead poisoning is diagnosed by venous sampling of blood to determine the lead level. The Centers for Disease Control and Prevention (CDC) specify a level of >5 mcg/dL as indicative of lead poisoning (CDC, 2020). Obtain abdominal radiograph for levels 15 to 44 mcg/dL with pica or >45 mcg/dL to rule out leaded foreign bodies or flecks that would indicate bowel decontamination procedures. Glycosuria may also be present.

### Differential Diagnosis

The differential diagnosis for lead poisoning includes:

- Anemia (acute or chronic, iron deficiency)
- Constipation
- Heavy metal toxicity

### Treatment/Management Plan

Treatment for lead poisoning is based on the severity and symptoms. Most children are asymptomatic and found to have lead poisoning through routine screening. Therefore, education and removal of lead from the child's environment are often sufficient. Chelation therapy will remove the lead from the body and should be performed in conjunction with a specialist for childhood lead poisoning. Often dimercaprol is utilized with the chelating agent of choice (succimer, calcium disodium edetate, or D-penicillamine). Chelation is only recommended for levels >45 mcg/dL. If encephalopathic, the child will likely require stabilization and airway protection by intubation and mechanical ventilation.

### Family Education

Teach the following:

- All sources of lead must be removed from the home.
- Avoid imported food, as the cans may contain lead.

▶ ALERT: While CDC guidelines set a reference level of >5 mcg/dL for lead poisoning, the AAP strongly states that there are no safe levels of lead. Even low-level poisoning can result in permanent neurologic damage. Public health authorities need to be notified of lead poisoning.

## HEMATOLOGIC DISORDERS: HEMOGLOBINOPATHIES

*Hemoglobinopathies* are genetic disorders resulting from a change in the structure of the hemoglobin molecule. These disorders result in inefficient oxygen transport to the tissues, as this is the main job of the red blood cell (RBC), where the protein hemoglobin is a component. These disorders are often chronic and lifelong and if symptomology is severe enough, it will require the inclusion of a hematologist as part of the care team.

## SICKLE CELL DISEASE

A standard RBC is round in shape, allowing for easy passage through the blood vessels. Children with sickle cell disease (SCD) have abnormally shaped RBCs in the shape of a sickle (crescent shape). These sickled RBCs do not always flow easily through the blood vessels due to their shape and can become stuck, leading to hemolytic anemia and vaso-occlusion, causing a sickle cell crisis.

SCD is inherited with hemoglobin S on the beta globin gene. One can also be a carrier (referred to as sickle cell trait) if they carry hemoglobin S on one beta globin gene but the other beta globin gene is normal. Children are screened at birth for SCDs on their newborn screening, as currently mandated testing in all 50 states (Pecker & Naik, 2018).

## Subjective Findings

The health history may reveal:

- Pain: in an infant this could manifest as less activity; younger children could lose interest in usual activities; teenagers may have difficulty concentrating in school
- Complaints of pain in fingers and toes

> **PRO TIP** Peripheral neuropathy can also be a finding in children with sickle cell anemia.

### Risk Factors

The most common risk factors for SCD are:

- African descent
- Both parents carrying sickle cell gene (carrier or have the disease)

### Review of Systems

The most common manifestations revealed during the review of systems include:

- **Constitutional:** pain
- **Respiratory:** history of asthma
- **Genitourinary:** priapism
- **Neurologic:** symptoms of stroke (severe headache, seizure activity, difficulty speaking, facial asymmetry, weakness in limbs)

## Objective Findings

The physical examination of the child with SCD may reveal:

- Swollen fingers and toes (dactylitis)
- Respiratory infection with wheezing
- Facial asymmetry
- Weakness in extremities

The symptoms presenting will likely be related to a complication of SCD or a manifestation of a pain crisis.

### Laboratory/Diagnostic Testing

All newborns are screened for SCD on their newborn screening with either hemoglobin electrophoresis, high performance liquid chromatography, or DNA testing. The preferred method of diagnosis is conducted by high performance liquid chromatography (HPLC). These studies can be ordered if the provider suspects sickle cell anemia and a newborn screen is unavailable.

> **PRO TIP** If a child has questionable laboratory findings for SCD at birth, repeating the tests at 6 months is appropriate. By this time all beta globin production should be complete and result in a more accurate finding.

## Differential Diagnosis

The differential diagnosis for SCD includes:

- Acute anemia
- Hemolytic anemia
- Sepsis
- Valvular heart disease
- Polycythemia vera
- Lupus erythematosus

## Treatment/Management Plan

The most common complication of SCD is a pain crisis that occurs from the sickled RBCs traveling through the bloodstream and causing damage and sequestration. Many children will start on an antineoplastic and antimetabolite medication called hydroxyurea. This medication works to reduce acute vaso-occlusive events (pain crises) by increasing the production of fetal hemoglobin (Rana et al., 2014). Children with more severe symptoms may require frequent blood transfusions as part of their treatment plan. Opioids are often prescribed to help children with pain crisis management.

As infection can be a trigger of a crisis, and streptococcus pneumoniae in particular may result in an overwhelming infection, most children with SCD will take penicillin prophylactically until age 5 years. Routine health maintenance, such as receiving timely immunizations, is important in this population. The mainstay of treatment is to prevent complications of SCD such as stroke and intracranial hemorrhage. Monitoring of blood pressure at all medical appointments and annual transcranial Doppler evaluation are necessary. Carefully monitor growth, as it can be delayed in children with SCD.

▶ ALERT: Asthma is a common comorbidity. Spirometry (once child is capable) is performed as routine health maintenance every 1 to 2 years.

### Family Education

Teach the following:

- Proper hydration is necessary to help prevent pain crises.
- Infections are serious in this population. Any signs of infection, such as fever, loss of appetite, fatigue, or decreased use of the restroom, should be evaluated promptly by a medical provider.
- Ensure that the influenza shot is administered every year and keep up with all immunizations.
- Before any surgeries, the child could need a blood transfusion.
- Genetic counseling should be provided for family planning of future children of the parents and any future children of the affected child.

### Referral

Refer to pediatric hematology, which will co-manage the care of the child with the primary care provider.

## THALASSEMIAS

The most common hemoglobinopathy is thalassemia. It is an inherited disorder in which the hemoglobin protein is altered and affects the production of RBCs. The type and severity of the disorder is determined by whether one or both genes of either the alpha or beta chain that make up the hemoglobin protein are affected. Children can have either alpha or beta thalassemia depending on which globin chain is reduced, and then are further subdivided into major, intermediate, and minor categories.

Alpha thalassemia major results in severe microcytic anemia with a condition called hydrops fetalis, and will typically result in a spontaneous abortion of the fetus in utero, as it is not compatible with life. Minor conditions of both alpha and beta thalassemia result from at least one normal chain gene and are typically asymptomatic in children showing a mild microcytic anemia. In beta thalassemia, a child may have beta thalassemia intermedia where they exhibit moderate microcytic thalassemia but are not transfusion-dependent. A child who is transfusion-dependent will have beta thalassemia major with severe microcytic anemia due to either one or both genes resulting in severe reduction or no production of the beta chain. In alpha thalassemia, the intermediate finding is known as hemoglobin H (HbH) disease (Taher et al., 2018).

### Subjective Findings

The health history may reveal:

- Fatigue, weakness, decreased activity
- Darker urine (hemolysis)
- Smaller child

Symptoms can range from asymptomatic (carrier) to severe anemia, growth deficit, and iron overload. The severity is dependent on the number of functional globin chains of the hemoglobin.

### Risk Factors

The most common risk factors for thalassemia are:

- Ancestry to areas of endemic malaria (sub-Saharan Africa, Southeast Asia, Mediterranean)
- Family history of thalassemia

### Review of Systems

The most common manifestations revealed during the review of systems include:

- **Constitutional:** fatigue

### Objective Findings

The physical examination of the child with thalassemia may reveal:

- Signs of hemolysis: jaundice, splenomegaly
- Signs of anemia: pallor
- Facial bone deformities
- Slow growth

### Laboratory/Diagnostic Testing

The standard workup includes a CBC, peripheral blood smear, and iron studies. A microcytic anemia will be noted on the CBC. For minor thalassemia, a mild microcytic anemia may be noted, or the CBC could be completely normal. Major and intermediate thalassemias can show an increased number of RBCs. Major thalassemia will have characteristic target or teardrop cells on smears. Iron studies should be performed to rule out iron deficiency and alert the provider to signs of iron overload. Definitive testing of thalassemia involves a hemoglobin analysis with globin gene testing.

### Differential Diagnosis

The differential diagnosis for thalassemia includes:

- Iron deficiency
- Anemia of chronic inflammation
- Liver disease

### Treatment/Management Plan

The only possible curative treatment for thalassemia is a bone marrow transplant, but due to the risk involved this is reserved for severe cases. Children with major beta thalassemia are transfusion-dependent and will require transfusions frequently to avoid hemolysis. Repeat transfusion results in iron overload and the necessity of chelation therapy. Gene therapy has been approved for use in Europe, but is not yet approved by the FDA for use in children in the United States.

### Family Education

Teach the following:

- Avoid taking iron supplementation.
- Take folic acid.
- Follow up with genetic counseling.

### Referral

Refer the child with thalassemia to pediatric hematology for co-management with the primary provider. Iron overload is the most important complication for children with thalassemia. This was previously attributed to transfusion frequency, but non-transfusion-dependent children with thalassemia were found to have higher iron stores than the average human due to increased absorption mechanisms. Providers should be careful to look for signs of iron overload at each visit.

## G6PD DEFICIENCY

Glucose-6-phosphate dehydrogenase (G6PD) is the enzyme responsible for protecting RBCs from oxidative injuries. Deficiency or defect of G6PD (also known as favism) is a rare X-linked inherited disorder with multiple variants. Variants cause symptomology from asymptomatic to severe deficiency-producing hemolytic anemia. Due to the X-linked characteristic of this disorder, males have more severe symptoms and females tend to be asymptomatic carriers.

### Subjective Findings

The health history may reveal:

- Neonatal jaundice
- Use of antimalarial medications
- Intake of fava beans
- Recent infection

▶ ALERT: The typical patient is asymptomatic with mild indication of hemolysis on laboratory findings found after an incident of oxidative stress. If the oxidative stress is related to a medication, there can be a sudden onset of jaundice, pallor, and dark urine about 2 to 4 days following the start of the medication.

### Risk Factors

The most common risk factors for G6PD deficiency are:

- Family history of inherited anemia
- Ancestry from geographic regions with high incidences of malaria
- African, Southern European, Middle Eastern, Chinese, or Southeast Asian heritage

### Review of Systems

The most common manifestations revealed during the review of systems include:

- **Constitutional:** abdominal or back pain
- **Integumentary:** yellow or pale skin color
- **Genitourinary:** darker urine

### Objective Findings

The physical examination of the child with G6PD deficiency may reveal:

- Jaundice
- Pallor
- Splenomegaly

### Laboratory/Diagnostic Testing

The diagnosis of G6PD deficiency is commonly found on routine specific screening (newborn or entrance into military service). Testing should be considered for any infant with unexplained neonatal jaundice. Peripheral blood smear may show bite and blister cells during an episode of hemolysis. In an acute episode of hemolysis, a decrease in hemoglobin concentration can be seen (3–4 g/dL from baseline) Luzzatto, L., & Arese, P. (2018).

ALERT: G6PD deficiency with an evidence of hemolytic anemia can falsely lower a HgbA1C level secondary to the increased RBC turnover. Infections can cause oxidative stress leading to hemolytic anemia. While some can be self-limiting and mild, others can be severe. It is important to treat infections promptly in these children with appropriate therapies.

## Differential Diagnosis

The differential diagnosis for G6PD deficiency includes:

- Autoimmune hemolytic anemia
- Bilirubin conjugation disorders
- Hemolytic disease of the newborn
- Sickle cell anemia
- Thalassemia

## Treatment/Management Plan

Treatment for this deficiency is to simply remove or resolve the trigger of oxidative stress. Treat the infection appropriately or stop the medication and find an alternative if necessary. If the child has severe anemia, they may need a blood transfusion. Luzzatto, L., & Arese, P. (2018). For neonates with jaundice, treatment (phototherapy) is focused on preventing kernicterus.

### Family Education

Teach the following:

- Avoid certain medications: nitrofurantoin, chlorpropamide, dabrafenib, dapsone, methylene blue, phenazopyridine, primaquine, rasburicase, and sulfa-containing medications (this is not an exhaustive list)
- Do not eat fava beans
- Avoid henna compounds (can also be found in hair dyes and inks for tattoos)
- Follow up with genetic counseling

### Referral

Refer to pediatric hematology for workup of hemolytic anemia. After a diagnosis of G6PD deficiency is made, children can easily be managed by their primary care provider and do not need to follow up with hematology unless they have severe symptomology.

PRO TIP Anemia and jaundice are the two characteristics commonly noted in the newborn period for infants with G6PD deficiency. These infants, if not already screened, should be tested as part of their workup and need close monitoring of bilirubin levels, as neurologic dysfunction can occur if left untreated. Those neonates with less severe G6PD deficiency will likely only show jaundice 2 to 3 days after birth.

# HEMATOLOGIC DISORDERS: BLEEDING DISORDERS

Bleeding disorders occur when there is a defect in the clotting mechanism, usually the lack of a specific clotting factor. These disorders are almost always inherited.

## HEMOPHILIA

Hemophilia A (factor VIII) and hemophilia B (factor IX) are bleeding disorders caused by coagulation factor deficiencies. These disorders are X-linked. While inheritance is most common, there are cases with no family history and presumed secondary to a new mutation. Hemophilia A is more common and more likely to be more severe than hemophilia B. Hemophilia C (factor XI) is autosomal recessive inheritance and common in Ashkenazi Jews.

### Subjective Findings

The health history may reveal:

- Spontaneous bleeding (epistaxis or nosebleed)
- Easy bruising
- Bleeding from gums during normal tooth brushing
- Delayed bleeding following trauma or minor surgical procedures (tooth extraction, circumcision)

### Risk Factors

The most common risk factors for hemophilia are:

- History of bleeding disorder in family, specifically bleeding symptoms in male family members

### Review of Systems

The most common manifestations revealed during the review of systems include:

- **Integumentary:** bruises easily
- **Hematologic:** abnormal bleeding

### Objective Findings

The physical examination of the child with hemophilia may reveal:

- Multiple bruises
- Hemarthrosis
- Forehead hematoma ("goose egg")

### Laboratory/Diagnostic Testing

Screening laboratory tests for hemostasis include platelet count, prothrombin time (PT), and activated partial thromboplastin time (aPTT). If the aPTT is prolonged, mixing studies are performed. If this corrects the aPTT, the diagnosis can be made of hemophilia A or B depending on which factor corrected the level. Factor activity levels are obtained following these studies. This measurement will reveal the degree of deficiency and severity. Severity based on factor level is as follows:

- Severe: less than 1%
- Moderate: 1%–5% level
- Mild: 6%–50% level

Of note, an aPTT can be normal in children with milder deficiencies.

ALERT: Factor VIII is an acute phase reactant. If the child is ill but mild hemophilia is suspected, a repeat factor activity level following recovery from illness is appropriate, as the level may have been falsely higher during the illness.

### Differential Diagnosis

The differential diagnosis for hemophilia includes:

- Von Willebrand disease
- Inherited platelet disorders
- Other factor deficiencies (more commonly factor XI and factor XIII deficiencies)
- Acquired factor inhibitors

### Treatment/Management Plan

Treatment with factor replacement can be done prophylactically or as an on-demand therapy. For children with severe hemophilia, a prophylactic factor administration may be ideal to help reduce risk of intracerebral hemorrhage and complications of long-term bleeding (Srivastava et al., 2020). The risk-to-benefit ratio will be considered with the child's hematologist, as prophylactic medications will require frequent venous access possibly necessitating a central line. An on-demand approach is standardly used for mild-to-moderately symptomatic children. Factor replacement is also given in the instance of acute bleeding or with surgery. Despite increased risk for bleeding, the child with hemophilia needs immunization as routinely recommended for all children. The primary care provider should consult with pediatric hematology to determine an individualized approach concerning whether the intramuscular or subcutaneous route should be used and timing of the injections based on factor replacement.

**PRO TIP** Utilize the smallest gauge needle possible for immunizations, do not rub the injection site, and apply ice for 3 to 5 minutes following injection. Allow the most experienced personnel to perform laboratory blood draws.

### Family Education

Teach the following:

- The child should wear a medical alert bracelet at all times.
- Avoid medications that increase the risk of bleeding, such as nonsteroidal anti-inflammatory drugs (NSAIDs).
- Inform all medical and dental providers of this disorder to ensure appropriate planning should the child need any type of surgery or procedures.
- Genetic counseling should be provided for parents and for the child's future offspring planning.
- Encourage exercise. Depending on the severity of disease, some restrictions may be put in place for contact sports. Make sure this is discussed with child's hematology provider.
- Consider emergency supply of factor replacement therapy when traveling, if appropriate.

### Referral

Refer to pediatric hematology. The child will be followed closely by a hematologist throughout the lifetime. The child should be referred to the closest designated hemophilia treatment center to allow for appropriate collaborative care.

## VON WILLEBRAND'S DISEASE

The most common inherited bleeding disorder is von Willebrand disease. von Willebrand factor, a protein, is used to help platelets to attach to the lining of blood vessels when there is an injury. Those with von Willebrand disease have either a deficiency or an abnormality. Most children have mild-to-moderate disease that manifests as bleeding that likely would not have occurred without use of an antiplatelet medication. There are three types (1–3), and classification is based on severity, with type 3 being the most severe and rarest. It has autosomal dominant inheritance patterns; therefore, both females and males are affected similarly (Sharma & Flood, 2017).

### Subjective Findings

The health history may reveal:

- Epistaxis for longer than 10 minutes
- Easy bruising
- Bleeding following surgery, especially dental procedures
- Heavy menstrual cycles

### Risk Factors

The most common risk factor for von Willebrand disease is family history of bleeding disorder.

### Review of Systems

The most common manifestations revealed during the review of systems include:

- **Integumentary:** easy bruising
- **Hematologic:** prolonged bleeding

### Objective Findings

The physical examination of the child with von Willebrand disease may reveal:

- Multiple bruises
- Cutaneous bleeding

### Laboratory/Diagnostic Testing

The majority of children will have completely normal CBCs and coagulation studies, but some cases may show a prolonged aPTT, thrombocytopenia, and/or microcytic anemia. High suspicion due to bleeding history warrants von Willebrand screening tests: VWF antigen, ristocetin cofactor, VWF functional assay, and factor VIII activity.

### Differential Diagnosis

The differential diagnosis for von Willebrand disease includes:

- Mild hemophilia A
- Inherited platelet disorders (such as Bernard-Soulier syndrome)
- Immune thrombocytopenia

### Treatment/Management Plan

The most important aspect in managing a child with von Willebrand disease is communication with all medical providers involved in any type of procedure or situation that could result in bleeding. The child's hematologist may trial DDAVP (in children >2 years old) to see if it will provide benefit to reduce bleeding for minor surgical procedures. Another option is to provide vWF concentrates. The purpose of either DDAVP or vWF concentrates is to increase von Willebrand factors and help the child clot more efficiently, more for a prophylactic effect. Antifibrinolytics, such as transexamic acid, are often used to treat bleeding symptoms following a procedure or for significant epistaxis. For females, it is prudent to discuss menstrual suppression if symptoms are significant. In severe cases of von Willebrand disease and following major surgeries with significant amounts of bleeding, platelet transfusions may be warranted (Sharma & Flood, 2017).

> **PRO TIP** For females, menstrual suppression can be extremely helpful and prevent significant anemia once a month.

### Family Education

Teach the following:

- The child should avoid NSAIDs and any other medications that may interfere with platelet function.
- For any surgeries, be sure to mention the child's von Willebrand disease, as they will require closer monitoring following surgery.
- Severe cases may require the need to avoid contact sports.

### Referral

Refer to pediatric hematology to co-manage this patient.

## IMMUNE THROMBOCYTOPENIA

Immune thrombocytopenia (ITP) is a diagnosis of exclusion for explanation of a platelet count less than 100,000 mcL with no other known cause. Though the cause is unknown, the condition is usually triggered by a viral infection. It can be primary or secondary with an underlying cause from an immune-mediated source such as systemic lupus erythematous or HIV. While most cases are resolved within 6 months, if it lasts longer than 12 months it is considered chronic. In immune thrombocytopenia, auto-antibodies attack platelet membrane antigens and inhibit platelet production and therefore lower the platelet count (Bussell, 2020).

### Subjective Findings

The health history may reveal:

- Recent viral illness (within about a month)
- Concern for new rash (might be described as dots on skin)

### Risk Factors

The most common risk factors for ITP are:

- Ages 2 to 5
- Recent viral infection

### Review of Systems

The most common manifestations revealed during the review of systems include:

- **Integumentary:** easy bruising
- **HEENT:** oral bleeding, epistaxis

### Objective Findings

The physical examination of the child with ITP may reveal:

- Petechiae, purpura, ecchymoses
- Mucocutaneous bleeding
- Absence of lymphadenopathy

These manifestations are found in an otherwise healthy child.

▶ ALERT: Although rare, the most concerning complication of ITP is intracranial hemorrhage. Any child with other symptomology concerning for intracranial hemorrhage should be evaluated immediately at an emergency department.

### Laboratory/Diagnostic Testing

Thrombocytopenia is the only outlier on the patient's complete blood count. The threshold for ITP diagnosis is a platelet count of <100,000/mcL. As ITP is a diagnosis of exclusion, the remainder of the CBC should be normal and any other abnormalities warrant further investigation for another cause of thrombocytopenia. Remember that white blood cell (WBC) count could be outside normal limits if there is evidence of a recent or ongoing infection. This infection could be the trigger for the episode of ITP.

### Differential Diagnosis

The differential diagnosis for ITP includes:

- Leukemia
- Active infections (e.g., Epstein-Barr virus, cytomegalovirus, hepatitis C)
- Bone marrow failure syndromes
- Autoimmune hemolytic anemia
- Hemolytic uremic syndrome
- Thrombotic thrombocytopenia (TTP)
- Disseminated intravascular coagulation (DIC)
- Drug exposure (much less common in children)

### Treatment/Management Plan

Typically, ITP will resolve itself without intervention within 6 months. Treatment will be to exercise watchful waiting and provide education for some restrictions for the child. A child with a platelet count <30,000 mcL is advised to avoid contact sports and reduce any activities where bleeding could easily occur. For example, if a child is prone to falling off their bike, this may be an activity to avoid until the platelet count improves.

No standard exists for how often to monitor the child's platelet count; frequency should be in accordance with the severity of symptoms. The healthcare provider may choose to obtain a platelet count once a week until evidence of recovery is shown and then space the platelet count checks further apart. Once the platelet count returns to normal, recheck again at 2, 4, and 6 months to ensure stability. Obviously, with any concerning symptoms the laboratory tests can be evaluated sooner. For any child showing signs of life-threatening bleeding, platelet transfusions, methylprednisolone, and intravenous immune globulin may be warranted (Bussell, 2020).

### Family Education

Teach the following:

- Avoid NSAIDs and antiplatelet/anticoagulant medications
- If emergency surgery is required for another problem, make diagnosis known to providers
- Postponement of elective surgeries may be warranted if the bleeding risk is too great

## Referral

Referral to pediatric hematology should be made if one cannot rule out other causes of thrombocytopenia or if concerned that the child may have a chronic case.

**PRO TIP** Platelet transfusions are not likely beneficial unless there is life-threatening bleeding.

# ONCOLOGIC DISORDERS

Childhood cancers constitute less than 1% of all cancers (American Cancer Society [ACS], 2020). The National Cancer Institute (NCI, 2021) estimated about 10,500 childhood cancer diagnoses in 2021. Cancer continues to be the leading cause of death from disease in children. Although the physiology of the disease is similar, cancers in children and adults are different. The most common adult cancers are prostate, breast, lung, and colon, whereas in pediatrics the most common are leukemias, lymphomas, brain tumors, and other various solid tumors. Unlike adult cancers, childhood cancers are not as likely to be caused by lifestyle and environmental factors. The exact causes of childhood cancers are unknown, but some genetic and parental exposure risks have been identified. Although the reasons may not be known, children with cancer seem to do much better than adults. This could be related to more aggressive treatments and multimodal approaches including combination therapy, e.g., chemotherapy and radiation. Childhood cancers have an overall 84% cure rate (ACS, 2020; Kline, 2014; NCI, 2021).

Leukemia is the most common malignancy in children, with acute lymphoblastic leukemia (ALL) being the most common type (ACS, 2020). CNS tumors are the most common solid tumors in children. Lymphomas, including non-Hodgkin's (NHL) and Hodgkin's lymphoma (HL), are seen in both children and adults. Other solid tumors mostly occurring in children include neuroblastoma, Wilms tumor, rhabdomyosarcoma, retinoblastoma, osteosarcoma (OGS), and Ewing sarcoma. The symptoms of childhood cancers can vary and can mimic many common disorders of childhood. Each cancer is unique, and prognosis can depend on many factors, including age, location, biology/histology of tumor, disease response to treatment, metastatic or nonmetastatic disease, and recurrence. Recurrence of cancer in children results in a worse prognosis (Kline, 2014). Table 30.1 shows peak ages of specific childhood cancers and overall prognosis at initial diagnosis.

**TABLE 30.1 Peak Ages of Childhood Cancers and Overall Prognosis at Initial Diagnosis**

| Cancer Type | Peak Age | 5-Year Event-Free Survival |
|---|---|---|
| Acute lymphoblastic leukemia (ALL)<br>Acute myelogenous leukemia (AML) | 2–5 years<br><2 years, then teens | Greater than 90%<br>60%–70% |
| NHL<br>HL | <10 years<br>>10 years | 85%–90% early detection<br>70%–90% advanced<br>90%–95% |
| CNS tumors | <15 years | Pilocytic astrocytoma 90%<br>Brain stem glioma <10%<br>Medulloblastoma 55%–76% |
| Neuroblastoma | <5 years with median age at 17 months | Very low risk: >85%<br>Low risk: 75%–85%<br>Intermediate risk: 50%–75%<br>High risk: <50% |
| OGS<br>Ewing's Sarcoma | 10–19 years (growth spurt)<br>10–19 years | No metastatic disease 65%–70%<br>Metastatic disease 20%–30%<br>No metastatic disease age <15 years: 76%<br>Age 15–19 years: 49%<br>Metastatic disease any age: 18%–30% |

*(continued)*

**TABLE 30.1 Peak Ages of Childhood Cancers and Overall Prognosis at Initial Diagnosis (*continued*)**

| Cancer Type | Peak Age | 5-Year Event-Free Survival |
|---|---|---|
| Wilms tumor | 2–3 years (<5 years) | 92% |
| Rhabdomyosarcoma | 2–6 years (embryonal)<br>10–18 years (alveolar) | >70% (with PAX7 gene)<br>10% (with PAX3 gene) |
| Retinoblastoma | Overall <4 years<br>Bilateral <7 months<br>Spontaneous 23 months | 96% |

ALL, acute lymphoblastic leukemia; AML, acute myelogenous leukemia; NHL, non-Hodgkin's lymphoma; HL, Hodgkin's lymphoma; CNS, central nervous system; OGS, osteogenic sarcoma.

*Sources*: Data from Dasgupta, R., Fuchs, J., & Rodeberg, D. (2016). Rhabdomyosarcoma. *Seminars in Pediatric Surgery, 25*, 276–283. https://doi.org/10.1053/j.sempedsurg.2016.09.011; Gamis, S., Alonzo, T. A., Perentesis, J. P., & Meshinchi, S. (2013). Children's Oncology Group's 2013 blueprint for research: Acute myeloid leukemia. *Pediatric Blood & Cancer, 60*(6), 964–971. https://doi.org/10.1002/pbc.24432; Kline, N. E. (2014). *Essentials of pediatric hematology/oncology nursing: A core curriculum* (4th ed.). Association of Pediatric Hematology Nursing; Lau, C., & Teo, W.-Y. (2020). Clinical manifestations and diagnosis of central nervous system tumors in children. *UpToDate.* Retrieved October 19, 2020, from https://www.uptodate.com/contents/clinical-manifestations-and-diagnosis-of-central-nervous-system-tumors-in-children; Mullassery, D., & Losty, P. (2016). Neuroblastoma. *Paediatrics and Child Health, 26*(2), 68–72. https://doi.org/10.1016/j.paed.2015.11.005; Ortiz, M. V., & Dunkel, I. J. (2016). Retinoblastoma. *Journal of Child Neurology, 31*(2), 227–236. https://doi.org/10.1177%2F0883073815587943; Pui, C.-H., Yang, J. J., Hunger, S. P., Pieters, R., Schrappe, M., Biondi, A., Vora, A., Baruchel, A., Silverman, L. B., Schmiegelow, K., Escherich, G., Horibe, K., Benoit, Y. C. M., Izraeli, S., Yeoh, A. E. J., Liang, D.-C., Downing, J. R., Evans, W. E., Relling, M. V., & Mullighan. (2015). Childhood acute lymphoblastic leukemia: progress through collaboration. *Journal of Clinical Oncology, 33*(27), 2938-2948. https://doi.org/10.1200/JCO.2014.59.1636; Starý, J., & Hrušák, O. (2016). Recent advances in the management of pediatric acute lymphoblastic leukemia. *F1000Research, 5*(F1000 Faculty Rev), 2635. https://doi.org/10.12688/f1000research.9548.1

## ANATOMY AND PHYSIOLOGY

Normal cells are part of the basic building blocks to maintain function of organ systems and tissue within the body. There are nearly 37 trillion cells in the human body. These cells have the ability to grow, divide, and stop when signaled; undergo cell apoptosis (death); secrete substances that make them stick together and not leave the part of the body in which they belong; have normal DNA and the normal number of chromosomes; and develop and function into mature working cells. Cancer cells, due to multiple factors and problems within the genes in a cell or group of cells, are not able to function like normal cells. These cells are not able to self-regulate and stop production or division, so they keep producing abnormal (immature) cells at a rapid pace. Injured cells that would normally be removed from the body stay due to problems within certain proteins. The adhesiveness of a normal cell is gone, so cancer cells can leave one part of the body and metastasize (spread) to other areas of the body. The DNA of cancer cells is atypical and usually has an abnormal number of chromosomes. Cancer cells are nonworking cells that take up space and accumulate rapidly in areas of the body. This in turn causes organ and blood dysfunction (Blaney et al., 2021; Mason, 2018).

## LEUKEMIA

Leukemia is the most common form of childhood cancer. This is cancer of the blood and blood-forming organs including the bone marrow, lymph nodes, and spleen. The blood is made up of nondifferentiated stem cells. Within the environment, signals are given to regulate proliferation and bring cells from an immature cell to a mature cell. When cells are malignant, they are unable to develop successfully and become mature working cells. These immature cells accumulate in the bone marrow, periphery, and organs. Normal cell division is then blocked as the bone marrow is filled with immature nonworking cells (leukemic or blast cells) in place of normal cells. These leukemic cells impair the normal function of the bone marrow (Hunger & Mulligan, 2015; Kline, 2014).

Abnormalities in the differentiation and cell division of the lymphoid cell lineage results in acute lymphocytic leukemia (ALL). ALL may also be called acute lymphoid leukemia, acute lymphoblastic leukemia, and precursor B and precursor T leukemia. ALL accounts for 75% to 80% of all leukemias, with a peak age for diagnosis of 2 to 5 years. AML is acute non-lymphoblastic or myeloid leukemia that accounts for about 15% to 20% of all leukemias, and chronic myeloid leukemia (CML) results from abnormal proliferation on myeloid cells and is associated with chromosomal translocations known as Philadelphia chromosome (Kline-Tilford & Haut, 2016).

## Subjective Findings

The health history may reveal:

- Infection symptoms
- Fever
- Bone pain (Horton & Steuber, 2019a)
- Bleeding (such as epistaxis)
- Swollen lymph nodes (Kline, 2014)

**PRO TIP** ALL should be suspected in a child with unexplained persistence of pallor, fever, bleeding/bruising, bone pain, hepatosplenomegaly, lymphadenopathy, or other uncommon findings (e.g., testicular swelling, neurologic findings, or evidence of tracheal obstruction or superior vena cava syndrome). A high degree of suspicion is required because the most common findings are nonspecific and may be difficult to distinguish from ordinary, self-limited diseases of childhood (Kline, 2014).

### Risk Factors

The most common risk factors for ALL are:

- Trisomy 21
- Schwachman-Diamond syndrome, neurofibromatosis
- Fanconi anemia, Bloom syndrome, ataxia telangiectasia
- Li-Fraumeni syndrome
- Acquired aplastic anemia
- Sibling of child with leukemia
- Twin with leukemia (risk decreases with age)
- Certain drugs and chemicals
- Ionizing radiation; prenatal maternal cigarette use, drug use, or alcohol consumption
- Petroleum product exposure (Kline, 2014)

### Review of Systems

The most common manifestations revealed during the review of systems include:

- **Constitutional:** fatigue, malaise, bone or abdominal pain, weight loss, anorexia
- **Integumentary:** pale color, bruising, petechiae
- **Genitourinary:** painless testicular swelling
- **Neurologic:** malaise, irritability
- **Lymphatic:** lymphadenopathy (Kleinman et al., 2021; Kline, 2014)

## Objective Findings

The physical examination of the child with leukemia may reveal:

- Lymphadenopathy
- Refusal to bear weight or walk, joint pain
- Bruising
- Pallor
- Hepatosplenomegaly
- Enlarged painless testis
- Swelling of face, neck, upper extremities
- Respiratory distress
- Neurologic findings (headache, vomiting, lethargy)
- Gingival hypertrophy (AML)
- Chloroma (AML; Kleinman et al., 2021; Kline, 2014)

### Laboratory/Diagnostic Testing

The CBC with differential may show blasts on peripheral smear. Additional laboratory tests performed by oncology include uric acid, lactate dehydrogenase (LDH), and bone marrow aspiration (Kline-Tilford & Haut, 2016).

▶ ALERT: If the CBC shows two or more cell lines (hemoglobin, platelets, neutrophils) as abnormal, there is a high suspicion for leukemia. The WBC count may present as high or low due to the number of immature blast cells. Hyperleukocytosis due to increased blood viscosity can present with a very high WBC count and is considered a medical emergency (Kline-Tilford & Haut, 2016).

## Differential Diagnosis

The differential diagnosis for leukemia includes:

- Other malignant disorders (e.g., Burkitt's lymphoma, aplastic anemia)
- Immune thrombocytopenia
- Infectious disease (e.g., mononucleosis, parvovirus, HIV, pertussis, osteomyelitis, tuberculosis)
- Autoimmune diseases (Silbert-Flagg & Sloand, 2017)

## Treatment/Management Plan

Treatment of leukemia may include chemotherapy, biotherapy, radiation, and possible bone marrow transplant (Kline, 2014).

### Referral

Refer the child with suspected leukemia to pediatric oncology.

## LYMPHOMA

Lymphoma is a malignancy involving the lymphoid cells and immune system. The etiology of lymphoma is not fully understood; however, it is believed that genetic, immunologic, and viral changes can influence cell development. NHL is derived from either mature or immature B or T cells. This type of lymphoma is fast-growing and systemic. The different classifications of NHL include lymphoblastic lymphoma, Burkitt lymphoma, diffuse large B cell lymphoma, and anaplastic large cell lymphoma. HL is slow growing and is diagnosed by the presence of malignant lymphoid Reed-Sternberg cells. These cells are characterized by their two nuclei and "owl eyes" appearance (Kline, 2014; Kline-Tilford & Haut, 2016).

### Subjective Findings

As with most childhood cancers, the health history may reveal symptoms similar to other diseases, so it can be difficult to differentiate among them. The health history may reveal:

*Non-Hodgkin's lymphoma*

- May be asymptomatic if not disseminated
- Difficulty swallowing or breathing
- Swelling in neck, face, upper extremities
- Symptoms of mediastinal mass (dysphagia, cough, wheezing, superior vena cava syndrome with jugular distention; Kline-Tilford & Haut, 2016) (Burkhardt & Hermesten, 2019)

*Hodgkin's Lymphoma*

- Painless swelling of lymph nodes
- Symptoms of mediastinal mass (Kleinman et al., 2021; Kline-Tilford & Haut, 2016)

▶ ALERT: Lymphadenopathy in supraclavicular region warrants high suspicion for HL.

### Risk Factors

The most common risk factors for lymphoma are:

- Genetic predisposition
- Environmental exposures
- Immunological diseases (Wiskott-Aldrich Syndrome, severe combined immunodeficiency, X-linked lymphoproliferative disease and ataxia telangiectasia; Silbert-Flagg & Sloand, 2017)
- EBV has been associated with Hodgkin's lymphoma (Diab et al., 2017)

### Review of Systems

The most common manifestations revealed during the review of systems include:

- **Constitutional:** fatigue (NHL), decreased appetite and weight loss (at least 10% body weight in 6 months—HL), fever (HL), night sweats (HL)
- **HEENT:** enlarged mass on neck (Kleinman et al., 2021)

### Objective Findings

The physical examination of the child with lymphoma may reveal:

- Lymphadenopathy
- Splenomegaly (Kleinman et al., 2021)

### Laboratory/Diagnostic Testing

Laboratory testing for lymphoma should include CBC with differential, reticulocyte count, erythrocyte sedimentation rate (ESR), and complete metabolic panel (CMP). A chest x-ray may reveal a mediastinal mass. A surgical biopsy of the involved site/lymph node may be performed. Pediatric oncology may order a positron emission tomography (PET) scan (Kline-Tilford & Haut, 2016).

### Differential Diagnosis

The differential diagnosis for lymphoma includes:

- Other malignant disorders, e.g., leukemias, aplastic anemia
- Infectious disease, e.g., mononucleosis, parvovirus, HIV, pertussis, osteomyelitis, tuberculosis
- Autoimmune diseases (Silbert-Flagg & Sloand, 2017)

### Treatment/Management Plan

Treatment of lymphoma includes chemotherapy, biotherapy, and radiation (Kline-Tilford & Haut, 2016).

### Referral

Refer the child with suspected lymphoma to pediatric oncology.

## CENTRAL NERVOUS SYSTEM TUMORS

CNS tumors include tumors of the brain and spinal cord. These tumors are the second most common childhood cancer and have the highest mortality rate of all pediatric cancers. Brain tumors can be malignant or benign and may develop quickly or over time

(Kline, 2014). The most common brain tumors are gliomas, and the peak age of diagnosis is 4 to 5 years (Kline-Tilford & Haut, 2016).

## Subjective Findings

Diagnosis can be difficult to establish, as symptoms often mimic other childhood illnesses and vary depending on location and growth of tumor. The health history may reveal:

- Headache
- Vomiting
- Visual changes
- Gait abnormalities (Kline, 2014)

**PRO TIP** Increased intercranial pressure (ICP) symptoms in children can present as a triad of symptoms: morning headaches, lethargy, nausea and vomiting. In infants, increased ICP is noted by such symptoms as irritability, increased head circumference, bulging fontanel, and the sun-setting sign (limited upward gaze and forced downward deviation of the eyes; Lau & Teo, 2020)

## Risk Factors

The most common risk factors for CNS tumors are:

- Genetic predisposition
- Neurocutaneous syndromes (tuberous sclerosis, neurofibromatosis)

## Review of Systems

The most common manifestations revealed during the review of systems include:

- **Constitutional:** persistent headaches
- **HEENT:** macrocephaly, diplopia
- **Gastrointestinal:** morning vomiting
- **Musculoskeletal:** ataxia
- **Neurologic:** seizure
- **Behavioral:** decline in school performance (Lau & Teo, 2020)

## Objective Findings

The physical examination of the child with a CNS tumor may reveal:

- Cranial nerve deficits
- Nystagmus
- Unequal pupillary reaction
- Altered mental status
- Unsteady gait
- Weakness

## Laboratory/Diagnostic Testing

Computed tomography (CT) scan of the brain or magnetic resonance imaging (MRI) of the brain (the preferred imaging test) may reveal the tumor (Kline, 2014).

**PRO TIP** When to image a child with headaches:

- Persistent headache (defined as a continuous or recurrent headache lasting for >4 weeks) with any of the following features: wakes from sleep, occurs upon waking, child <4 years of age, associated with disorientation or confusion, persistent vomiting upon waking)
- Visual findings, including any of the following: papilledema, optic nerve atrophy, new onset of nystagmus, reduced acuity not due to refractive error, visual field reduction, proptosis, new onset paralytic (noncomitant) squint
- Motor findings, including any of the following: regression in motor skills, focal motor weakness, abnormal gait and/or coordination, Bell's palsy with no improvement over 4 weeks, swallowing difficulties without an identifiable local cause (Lau & Teo, 2020)

## Differential Diagnosis

CNS tumors can be misdiagnosed as common childhood conditions (e.g., viral gastroenteritis, tension and migraine headaches). The differential diagnosis for CNS tumors includes:

- Brain abscess
- Intracranial hemorrhage
- Non-neoplastic hydrocephalus
- Arteriovenous malformations
- Aneurysms
- Indolent viral infections (Lau & Teo, 2020)

**PRO TIP** Children with CNS tumors generally present with more than one tumor-associated symptom or sign, which allows CNS tumors to be distinguished from other conditions.

### Treatment/Management Plan

Treatment of CNS tumors may include surgical resection, chemotherapy, biologic agents, and radiation.

### Referral

Refer the child with a suspected CNS tumor to pediatric oncology and pediatric neurosurgery.

## BONE TUMORS

Osteosarcoma (OGS) and Ewing's sarcoma are malignant tumors of the bone. Osteosarcoma is the most common bone tumor in children. It is formed by the overproduction of osteoid substance, which is formed prior to maturation of the bone. Classic Ewing's sarcoma occurs in the bone; however, Ewing's sarcoma can also present outside the bone and in this case is primarily neuroectodermal in nature (Kline, 2014).

### Subjective Findings

The health history may reveal:

- Symptoms similar to other musculoskeletal issues with a peak incidence in symptoms around growth spurts (Kline-Tilford & Haut, 2016).
- Dull aching pain, worse at night in bones, which commonly is associated with trauma
- May or may not have a soft tissue mass or swelling

### Risk Factors

The most common risk factors for a bone tumor are:

- Genetic predisposition
- Previous treatment for childhood cancers with radiation or chemotherapy
- Increased height
- Paternal occupation of farming

**PRO TIP** Genetic predisposition for OGS increases with hereditary retinoblastoma and Li-Fraumeni syndrome.

### Review of Systems

The most common manifestations revealed during the review of systems include:

- **Constitutional:** local pain worse at night and progressive over few months; with metastatic disease, fever, malaise, anorexia, or weight loss (Kline, 2014)

### Objective Findings

The physical examination of the child with a bone tumor may reveal:

- Swelling
- Mass at end of long bone
- Decreased range of motion
- Limp (Kleinman et al., 2021)

**PRO TIP** Ewing's sarcoma can present with pathological fractures.

### Laboratory/Diagnostic Testing

An x-ray of the affected extremity is warranted, and a CT scan or MRI of the extremity may also be needed. In OGS, radiographic findings can include starburst pattern, mixed regions of sclerosis, and lytic lesions of bones known as Codman's triangle (Kline-Tilford & Haut, 2016). A chest x-ray may be obtained to rule out metastatic disease. With Ewing's sarcoma, x-ray appearance is often associated with a lamellated or "onion skin" periosteal reaction. The ESR is usually elevated and LDH levels are used as a biomarker for prognosis. A biopsy of the tumor confirms the diagnosis (Kline, 2014).

### Differential Diagnosis

The differential diagnosis for a bone tumor includes:

- Osteomyelitis
- Osteochondroma
- Hemangiomas
- Histiocytosis (Silbert-Flagg & Sloand, 2017)

### Treatment/Management Plan

Treatment of bone tumors includes biopsy of the bone, chemotherapy, radiation (Ewing's only, as it is radiosensitive whereas OGS is not), and limb salvage procedure (Kline-Tilford & Haut, 2016).

### Referral

Refer the child with a suspected bone tumor to pediatric oncology and pediatric orthopedic surgery.

## NEUROBLASTOMA

Neuroblastoma is a spectrum of tumors that develop from the sympathetic nervous system and arise from primitive sympathetic ganglion cells. These tumors are often unpredictable in their ability to progress or spontaneously regress (Mullassery & Losty, 2016). They are able to secrete catecholamines. Neuroblastoma can develop anywhere in the sympathetic nervous system, and is most often found in the abdomen arising from the adrenal gland (two-thirds of cases; Kline-Tilford & Haut, 2016). These tumors are the most common extracranial solid tumors in children. Treatment and prognosis vary with age, histology, biology, and genetic factors. It is the most common tumor in infants, with overall prognosis being best for babies less than 1 year of age (Kline, 2014; Kline-Tilford & Haut, 2016).

### Subjective Findings

The health history may reveal symptoms similar to other pediatric illnesses, including:

- Poor feeding
- Abdominal mass or pain
- Pale color

#### Risk Factors

The most common risk factors for neuroblastoma are:

- Increased risk with NF type 1
- Hirschsprung disease
- Central hypoventilation (Ondine's curse)
- Genetics
- Family history (Silbert-Flagg & Sloand, 2017)

#### Review of Systems

The most common manifestations revealed during the review of systems include:

- **Constitutional:** weight loss
- **Musculoskeletal:** weakness
- **Neurologic:** listlessness, irritability (Kline, 2014)

▶ ALERT: Depending upon the location of the tumor, spinal cord compression may occur. Symptoms include paralysis, weakness, altered sensation in extremities, incontinence, and pain. It is considered an oncologic emergency and if not caught early can cause permanent paralysis (Kline, 2014).

### Objective Findings

The physical examination findings of the child with neuroblastoma is based on where the tumor is located and may reveal:

- Horner's syndrome (ptosis, miosis, anhidrosis)
- Paralysis or weakness if there is cord compression
- Hepatomegaly
- Abdominal mass
- Periorbital ecchymosis (raccoon eyes)
- Palpable subcutaneous nodules that are blue in color (referred to as blueberry muffin sign)
- Opsoclonus myoclonus ataxia syndrome (Kleinman et al., 2021; Kline-Tilford & Haut, 2016; Mullassery & Losty, 2016)

#### Laboratory/Diagnostic Testing

Ultrasound or CT with contrast may reveal the tumor. Urinary catecholamines (vanillylmandelic acid and homovannilic acid) are elevated in 90% to 95% of cases (Kline-Tilford & Haut, 2016; Mallasery & Losty, 2016). Pediatric oncology will continue further workup, including biopsy, bone marrow aspiration, bone scan, and metaiodobenzylguanidine imaging (Kline, 2014; Mullassery & Losty, 2016).

### Differential Diagnosis

The differential diagnosis for neuroblastoma includes:

- Trauma
- Lymphadenopathy
- Other malignancies such as leukemia and lymphoma
- Wilm's tumor (Silbert-Flagg & Sloand, 2017)

### Treatment/Management Plan

Treatment for these tumors is based on staging and risk factors. It may include observation or surgery alone, chemotherapy, radiation, or possible bone marrow transplant with stem cell rescue (Kline-Tilford & Haut, 2016).

#### Referral

Refer the child with a suspected neuroblastoma to pediatric oncology and pediatric surgery.

## RETINOBLASTOMA

Retinoblastoma is a congenital malignant intraocular tumor and the most common intraocular malignancy of childhood (Ortiz & Dunkel, 2016). It consists of a chalky white intraocular mass that commonly originates in the posterior eye and develops when tumor infiltrates through the optic nerve into the CNS. Prognosis is >95% if caught early and in infancy (Kline, 2014).

### Subjective Findings

The health history may reveal:

- Squinting
- Eye turning inward or outward
- Painful red eye (Kline, 2014)

### Risk Factors

The most common risk factors for retinoblastoma are:

- Mutation of RB1 gene (50% risk of passing gene on to family members)
- Familial history (Kline-Tilford & Haut, 2016)

**PRO TIP** Children who have had retinoblastoma are at an increased risk for osteosarcoma, as both disorders have the same gene mutation.

### Review of Systems

The most common manifestations revealed during the review of systems include a wandering eye (Kleinman et al., 2021).

### Objective Findings

The physical examination of the child with retinoblastoma may reveal:

- Leukoria (cat's eye reflex), which is a lack of red reflux (most common)
- Strabismus
- Esotropia
- Exotropia
- Decreased vision
- Hyphema (Kline, 2014; Ortiz & Dunkel, 2016)
- Irregular pupils (Kleinman et al., 2021)

**PRO TIP** Leukoria may be found inadvertently by a family member in photographs.

### Laboratory/Diagnostic Testing

Diagnostic testing includes an initial indirect and direct fundoscopic examination, an eye examination under anesthesia, and an ultrasound, CT scan, or MRI of the brain and orbits (Ortiz & Dunkel, 2016).

### Differential Diagnosis

The differential diagnosis for retinoblastoma includes:

- Primary retinal telangiectasia or Coats' disease
- Fetal vasculature
- Vitreous hemorrhage
- Cataract
- Retinal detachment
- Coloboma (Ortiz & Dunkel, 2016)

### Treatment/Management Plan

The goal of treatment for retinoblastoma is to preserve useful vision without compromising the child's chances for survival (Kline-Tilford & Haut, 2016). Treatment includes possible surgical enucleation of the eye, chemotherapy, radiation, or focal therapy (cryotherapy; Ortiz & Dunkel, 2016).

### Referral

Refer the child with a suspected retinoblastoma to pediatric oncology and pediatric ophthalmology.

## KIDNEY TUMORS

The most common kidney cancer in childhood is called Wilm's tumor (nephroblastoma). This is a large rapidly growing tumor that appears as an abdominal mass. It is mostly seen in children ages 2 to 5 years (Kleinman et al., 2021; Kline, 2014).

### Subjective Findings

The health history may reveal:

- Listlessness
- Poor feeding
- Pale
- Abdominal pain
- Weakness
- Irritability

### Risk Factors

The most common risk factors for a kidney tumor are:

- Genetics: Increased risk with aniridia, hemihypertrophy or genital or renal malformations, Beckwith-Weiderman syndrome, and other overgrowth syndromes
- Familial history
- Environmental (Kline, 2014)

### Review of Systems

The most common manifestations revealed during the review of systems include:

- **Constitutional:** pain, malaise, weight loss
- **Gastrointestinal:** asymptomatic abdominal mass
- **Genitourinary:** hematuria (Kleinman et al., 2021)

PRO TIP Many children with Wilm's tumor appear healthy without other symptoms. Many times the parent finds the mass (Kline, 2014).

### Objective Findings

The physical examination of the child with Wilm's tumor may reveal:

- Asymptomatic abdominal mass
- Hypertension (Kline, 2014)

PRO TIP If Wilm's tumor is suspected, palpate the abdomen gently, as Wilm's tumor can be fragile.

### Laboratory/Diagnostic Testing

Laboratory testing for Wilm's tumor includes CBC, urinalysis, and Comprehensive metabolic panel (including liver and renal function tests). Visualization of the tumor may occur with abdominal ultrasound or CT scan (Kline-Tilford & Haut, 2016).

### Differential Diagnosis

The differential diagnosis for Wilm's tumor includes:

- Hydronephrosis
- Polycystic kidney disease
- Neuroblastoma
- Rhabdomyosarcoma
- Lymphoma (Silbert-Flagg & Sloand, 2017)

### Treatment/Management Plan

Treatment for Wilm's tumor includes surgical excision (if unilateral, complete nephrectomy; if bilateral, partial nephrectomy, multiagent chemotherapy, and radiation therapy).

### Referral

Refer the child with a suspected Wilm's tumor to pediatric oncology and pediatric surgery or urology.

## RHABDOMYOSARCOMA

Rhabdomyosarcomas (RMSs) are malignant soft-tissue tumors that most often arise from cells of the skeletal muscles. Rhabdomyoblasts are the immature cells that are found in RMS. There are five main histological classifications of RMS; the two main types are embryonal and alveolar (Dasgupta et al., 2016). The most common type is embryonal, which is formed in the embryo and found most often in children (Ryan & Meyer, 2020).

### Subjective Findings

The health history may reveal:

- Symptoms similar to other illnesses
- Rhabdomyosarcoma can be in different locations of the body. The common symptoms are based on location:
  - Children <8 years most commonly have head and neck tumors
  - Adolescents: most likely to have extremity tumors
  - Infants: most likely are vaginal or bladder
  - Older children most likely nasopharynx (Kline, 2014)

### Risk Factors

The most common risk factors for rhabdomyosarcoma are:

- NF type 1, Hirschsprung disease, and central hypoventilation (Ondine's curse)
- Genetics: Li Fraumeni
- Family history (Ryan & Meyer, 2020)

PRO TIP Li Fraumeni is an autosomal dominant disorder usually associated with a germline mutation. Children with this syndrome have a genetically increased risk for certain cancers. Family cancer history is important (Evans, 2020).

### Review of Systems

The most common manifestation revealed during the review of systems is a painless mass.

### Objective Findings

The physical examination of the child with rhabdomyosarcoma is based on where the tumor is located and may reveal:

- A nontender mass with occasional overlying skin erythema at primary disease site
- The most common sites are head and neck, genitourinary, and extremities (Dasgupta et al., 2016)

### Laboratory/Diagnostic Testing

Diagnostic testing includes plain radiographs of the involved site and/or CT scan or MRI (Dasgupta et al., 2016; Kline, 2014).

### Differential Diagnosis

The differential diagnosis for rhabdomyosarcoma includes:

- Other malignancies
- Genetic syndromes: neurofibromatosis, Li Fraumeni syndrome, Beckwith Weideman (Kline-Tilford & Haut, 2016)

### Treatment/Management Plan

Treatment and management are based on staging and risk factors and may include surgical resection, chemotherapy, and radiation (Kline-Tilford & Haut, 2016).

### Referral

Refer the child with a suspected rhabdomyosarcoma to pediatric oncology and pediatric surgery.

## SUPPORTIVE CARE OF THE CHILD WITH CANCER

All children with cancer are managed at pediatric oncology centers by their specific oncology teams. Most of these specialized institutions are affiliated with the Children's Oncology Group (COG). COG is a large national organization that is committed to improving treatment and outcomes in childhood cancers by conducting disease-specific research. Treatment can vary from a few months to up to 3 years. Treatment may include surgery, chemotherapy, radiation, immunotherapy, targeted therapy, and/or stem cell transplant (National Cancer Institute, 2021). During therapy, children are encouraged to stay in contact with local primary care providers and continue to get routine physicals along with anticipatory guidance education. Scheduled vaccines are placed on hold until completion of therapy due to the variable response to vaccine when immunosuppressed (Horton & Steuber, 2019b). Once therapy is complete, the oncology team will work with primary care providers on immunization catch-up or revaccination.

Side effects of chemotherapy are addressed by the oncology team. Common side effects include neutropenia, anemia, thrombocytopenia (bleeding), mucositis, nausea and vomiting, and pain. The most common and problematic complication of children undergoing chemotherapy is infection. Fever may be the first indicator of an infection and in the setting of neutropenia should be treated as an oncologic emergency (Ahmed & Flynn, 2019). Psychologic and emotional support should be ongoing and can be provided within the community. Information related to caring for the childhood cancer survivor can be found in chapter 43.

▶ ALERT: The child undergoing chemotherapy who develops fever and neutropenia should have antibiotics administered within 60 minutes of presentation to the facility. Prompt initiation of antibiotics showed improved outcomes (Ahmed & Flynn, 2019).

## KEY POINTS

- The child with mild iron-deficiency anemia should be treated with ferrous sulfate 3 mg/kg/day and have labs rechecked in 4 weeks.
- Lead poisoning and its subsequent negative effects on childhood development may be prevented when screening recommendations are followed, allowing for early identification and treatment.
- The child with sickle cell disease may experience painful vaso-occlusive crises, demonstrate ongoing anemia, and is at increased risk for serious infection.
- With beta thalassemia major, chronic transfusion is necessary throughout life.
- To avoid oxidative stress leading to acute illness, the child with G6PD deficiency should avoid eating fava beans and using henna compounds, and not take medications such as nitrofurantoin or sulfa-containing drugs (among others).
- Hemophilia ranges from mild to severe, requires factor replacement to prevent serious bleeding, and may result in repeat joint pain from bleeding episodes.
- A milder bleeding disorder, von Willebrand's disease, may be treated with DDAVP or von Willebrand factor replacement.
- The child with immune thrombocytopenia has a platelet count less than 100,000 and may present with unusual bruising or bleeding.
- Leukemia is the most common form of cancer in children and is also the most treatable.
- The child with lymphoma may be asymptomatic or may present with painless lymph node swelling or swelling in the neck, face, or upper extremities, or may have a mediastinal mass.

- Central nervous system tumors, bone, and kidney tumors may be treated with surgery, chemotherapy, or radiation, or a combination of the three.
- Neuroblastoma most often presents as an abdominal mass.
- Symptoms of rhabdomyosarcoma vary depending upon their location.

## REFERENCES


Ahmed, N., & Flynn, P. (2019). Fever in children with chemotherapy-induced neutropenia. *UpToDate*. https://www.uptodate.com/contents/fever-in-children-with-chemotherapy-induced-neutropenia

American Cancer Society. (2020). *Cancer in children*. https://www.cancer.org/cancer/cancer-in-children.html

Blaney, S. M., Adamson, P. C., & Helaman, L. J. (2021). *Pizzo and Poplack's principles and practice of pediatric oncology* (8th ed.). Wolters Kluwer.

Bussell, J. B. (2020). Immune thrombocytopenia (ITP) in children: Clinical features and diagnosis. *UpToDate*. Retrieved October 19, 2020, from https://www.uptodate.com/contents/immune-thrombocytopenia-itp-in-children-clinical-features-and-diagnosis#H2035460624

Centers for Disease Control and Prevention. (2020). *Childhood lead poisoning prevention*. https://www.cdc.gov/nceh/lead/default.htm

Dasgupta, R., Fuchs, J., & Rodeberg, D. (2016). Rhabdomyosarcoma. *Seminars in Pediatric Surgery, 25*, 276–283. https://doi.org/10.1053/j.sempedsurg.2016.09.011

Diab, B., Sonia, Z., Hanene, S., Teheni, L., & Mounir, T. (2017). Prognostic significance of Epstein-Barr virus (EBV) infection in Hodgkin's lymphoma patients. *Journal of Infection and Chemotherapy, 23*(3), 121–130. https://doi.org/10.1016/j.jiac.2016.09.004

Evans, G. (2020). LiFraumeni syndrome. *UpToDate*. Retrieved October 19, 2020, from https://www.uptodate.com/contents/li-fraumeni-syndrome

Gamis, S., Alonzo, T. A., Perentesis, J. P., & Meshinchi, S. (2013). Children's Oncology Group's 2013 blueprint for research: Acute myeloid leukemia. *Pediatric Blood & Cancer, 60*(6), 964–971. https://doi.org/10.1002/pbc.24432

Hoffbrand, A. F., & Steensma, D. P. (2020). *Hoffbrand's essential haematology* (8th ed.). John Wiley & Sons.

Horton, T. M., & Steuber, C. P. (2019b). Overview of the treatment of acute lymphoblastic leukemia lymphoma in children and adolescents. *UpToDate*. Retrieved October 19, 2020, from https://www.uptodate.com/contents/overview-of-the-treatment-of-acute-lymphoblastic-leukemia-lymphoma-in-children-and-adolescents

Hunger, S., & Mulligan, C. (2015). Acute lymphoblastic leukemia in children. *New England Journal of Medicine, 373*(16), 1541–1552. https://doi.org/10.1056/NEJMra1400972

Kleinman, K., McDaniel, L., & Molloy, M. (Eds.). (2021). *The Harriet Lane handbook: A manual for pediatric house officers* (22nd ed.). Elsevier.

Kline, N. E. (2014). *Essentials of pediatric hematology/oncology nursing: A core curriculum* (4th ed.). Association of Pediatric Hematology Nursing.

Kline-Tilford, A. M., & Haut, C. (2016). *Lippincott certification review: Acute care pediatric nurse practitioner*. Wolters Kluwer.

Lau, C., & Teo, W.-Y. (2020). Clinical manifestations and diagnosis of central nervous system tumors in children. *UpToDate*. Retrieved October 19, 2020, from https://www.uptodate.com/contents/clinical-manifestations-and-diagnosis-of-central-nervous-system-tumors-in-children

Leung, A. K. C., & Hon, K. L. (2019). Pica: A common condition that is commonly missed—An update review. *Current Pediatric Reviews, 15*(3), 164–169. https://doi.org/10.2174/1573396315666190313163530

Luzzatto, L., & Arese, P. (2018). Favism and glucose-6-phosphate dehydrogenase deficiency. *New England Journal of Medicine, 378*(1), 60–71. https://doi.org/ 10.1056/NEJMra1708111

Mason, L. E. (2018). *Cancer cells vs. normal cells*. https://www.technologynetworks.com/cancer-research/articles/cancer-cells-vs-normal-cells-307366

Mullassery, D., & Losty, P. (2016). Neuroblastoma. *Paediatrics and Child Health, 26*(2), 68–72. https://doi.org/10.1016/j.paed.2015.11.005

National Cancer Institute. (2021). *Childhood cancers*. https://www.cancer.gov/types/childhood-cancers

Ortiz, M. V., & Dunkel, I. J. (2016). Retinoblastoma. *Journal of Child Neurology*, 31(2), 227–236. https://doi.org/10.1177%2F0883073815587943

Pecker, L. H., & Naik, R. P. (2018). The current state of sickle cell trait: Implications for reproductive and genetic counseling. *Blood, 132*(22), 2331–2338. https://doi.org/10.1182/blood-2018-06-848705

Pui, C.-H., Yang, J. J., Hunger, S. P., Pieters, R., Schrappe, M., Biondi, A., Vora, A., Baruchel, A., Silverman, L. B., Schmiegelow, K., Escherich, G., Horibe, K., Benoit, Y. C. M., Izraeli, S., Yeoh, A. E. J., Liang, D.-C., Downing, J. R., Evans, W. E., Relling, M. V., & Mullighan. (2015). Childhood acute lymphoblastic leukemia: progress through collaboration. *Journal of Clinical Oncology, 33*(27), 2938-2948. https://doi.org/10.1200/JCO.2014.59.1636

Rana, S., Houston, P. E., Wang, W. C., Iyer, R. V., Goldsmith, J., Casella, J. F., Reed, C. K., Rogers, Z. R., Waclawiw, M. A., & Thompson, B. (2014). Hydroxyurea and growth in young children with sickle cell disease. *Pediatrics, 134*(3), 465–472. https://doi.org/10.1542/peds.2014-0917

Ryan, C. W., & Meyer, J. (2020). Clinical presentation, histopathology, diagnostic evaluation, and staging of soft tissue sarcoma. *UpToDate*. Retrieved October 19, 2020, from https://www.uptodate.com/contents/clinical-presentation-histopathology-diagnostic-evaluation-and-staging-of-soft-tissue-sarcoma

Sharma, R., & Flood, V. H. (2017). Advances in the diagnosis and treatment of von Willebrand disease. *Blood, 130*(22), 2386–2391. https://doi.org/10.1182/blood-2017-05-782029

Silbert-Flagg, J., & Sloand, B. (2017). *Pediatric nurse practitioner certification review guide* (7th ed.). Jones and Bartlett Learning.

Srivastava, A., Santagostino, E., Dougall, A., Kitchen, S., Sutherland, M., Pipe, S. W., Carcao, M., Mahlangu, J., Rgani, M. V., Windya, J. L., Goddard, N. J., Mohan, R., Poonnoose, P. M., Felman, B. M., Lewis, S. Z., van den Berg, J. M., & Pierce, G. F. (2020). WFH guidelines for the management of hemophilia, 3rd edition. *Haemophilia, 26*(Suppl. 6), 1–158. https://doi.org/10.1111/hae.14046

Starý, J., & Hrušák, O. (2016). Recent advances in the management of pediatric acute lymphoblastic leukemia. *F1000Research, 5*(F1000 Faculty Rev), 2635. https://doi.org/10.12688/f1000research.9548.1

Stensvold, E., Krossnas, B. K., Lundar, T., Due-Tønnessen, B. J., Frič, R., Due-Tønnessen, P., Bechensteen, A. G., Myklebust, T. A., Johannesen, T. B., & Brandal, P. (2017). Outcome for children treated for medulloblastoma and supratentorial primitive neuroectodermal tumor (CNS-PNET)—A retrospective analysis spanning 40 years of treatment. *Acta Oncologica, 56*(5), 698–705. https://doi.org/10.1080/0284186X.2017.1301679

Taher, A. T., Weatherall, D. J., & Cappellini, M. D. (2018). Thalassemia. *Lancet, 391*(10116), 155–167. https://doi.org/10.1016/S0140-6736(17)31822-6

## FURTHER READING

Horton, T. M., & Steuber, C. P. (2019a). Overview of the clinical presentation and diagnosis of acute lymphoblastic leukemia/lymphoma in children. *UpToDate*. Retrieved October 19, 2020, from https://www.uptodate.com/contents/overview-of-the-clinical-presentation-and-diagnosis-of-acute-lymphoblastic-leukemia-lymphoma-in-children

# Management of Infectious Disorders

Laura Roettger

## Student Learning Outcomes

**Upon completion of this chapter the reader should be able to:**

1. Discuss pathophysiology and epidemiology of selected infectious disorders in children.
2. Differentiate subjective and objective findings of selected infectious disorders in children.
3. Choose appropriate laboratory or diagnostic tests for particular infectious disorders in children.
4. Utilize the differential diagnosis process to determine the diagnosis of particular infectious disorders in children.
5. Determine treatment plan, child/family education, and need for referral in children with particular infectious disorder diagnoses.

## INTRODUCTION

Pediatric infections are one of the most common reasons children are brought to see their healthcare provider, and the leading cause of mortality worldwide (Dadonaite, 2019). Pediatric infections are caused by pathogens, such as bacteria, viruses, parasites, or fungi. The chain of infection is the process by which any of these organisms is spread (Figure 31.1). Infants and young children demonstrate an increased promotion of the chain of infection as they place toys and their hands in the mouth, often drool, and at times experience leaking diapers. Poor hygiene, especially lack of handwashing, also increases a child's risk for infection. Complete immunization, proper handwashing and cleansing of surfaces, and avoidance of known sick contacts are methods for breaking the chain of infection.

Infections occur in four stages:

1. Incubation: Time from when the pathogen enters the body until the appearance of first symptoms; pathogens are growing and multiplying during this time.
2. Prodrome: Time from nonspecific symptom onset (fever, fatigue, malaise) until specific symptoms arise.
3. Illness: Time during which signs and symptoms specific to the disease are demonstrated in the child.
4. Convalescence: Time of recovery when symptoms of acute illness disappear.

The virulence of the infectious pathogen is dependent on both the organism's structure and its interaction with the host's defense mechanisms. The body's host-defense mechanisms prevent infections. These mechanisms include anatomic barriers such as the skin and mucociliary blanket of the airway; protective microbial flora normally found in the gastrointestinal tract; and lysozyme, interferon, and immunoglobin A found in body orifices. Additionally, gastric acid and bile have antimicrobial properties to rid the body of certain pathogens. Infections occur when the pathogens cause disruption or dysfunction of the body's host-defense mechanisms (Schwartz, 2019).

The content in this chapter maps to the following areas on the Pediatric Nursing Certification Board (PNCB) Pediatric Nurse Practitioner—Primary Care certification examination:

## CLINICAL PROBLEMS: INFECTIOUS DISEASE

### CONTENT AREAS:

### II. Assessment and Diagnosis

**B. History and Physical Examination**

1. Obtain history of present illness
2. Obtain a comprehensive health history for new patients
3. Complete an interval history for established patients
4. Perform a review of systems
5. Perform a complete physical examination

**C. Diagnostic Testing and Screening**

1. Order and interpret office/clinic based screening tests
2. Order and interpret diagnostic laboratory tests
3. Order and interpret the results of diagnostic imaging tests

**D. Analyzing Information**

1. Integrate health history and physical examination findings into the plan of care
2. Assimilate findings from screening and diagnostic testing into plan of care

**E. Diagnosis**

1. Develop and prioritize differential diagnoses
2. Establish a diagnosis based on evaluation of patient data

### III. Management

**A. Child and Caregiver Counseling and Education**

1. Provide condition-specific counseling and education, including treatment options
2. Educate about benefits and potential adverse reactions of pharmacological interventions
3. Discuss non-pharmacological interventions
4. Counsel regarding the threshold for seeking follow-up care
5. Review the risks of non-adherence to recommended treatment

**B. Therapeutic Interventions**

1. Prescribe pharmacologic agents
2. Recommend the use of over-the-counter pharmacologic agents
3. Order or recommend non-pharmacologic treatments for the management of symptoms
4. Discuss use of complementary and alternative therapies as appropriate

**C. Procedures**

1. Perform procedures in accordance with diagnostic guidelines and plan of care (rapid tests)
2. Initiate life-saving techniques in response to urgent or emergent situations

**D. Collaboration and Referral**

2. Refer to specialists as indicated for evaluation, counseling, and/or treatment

**E. Care Coordination**

1. Facilitate patient and family-centered care for children of all ages with acute and chronic conditions

**F. Evaluation and Follow-up**

2. Establish a plan for follow-up care

### IV. Professional Role Responsibilities

**A. Leadership and Evidence-based Practice**

4. Develop, implement, and/or modify clinical practice guidelines

## ANATOMY AND PHYSIOLOGY

The severity and outcome of the disease process may vary and in the pediatric population are influenced by age and impaired or lack of immunity. Certain pathogens manifest with more severe disease in utero than in children or adults. The fetus's protection against infectious disease is dependent on the transfer of maternal immunoglobulin G antibodies through the placenta. Further, in nonimmune pregnant mothers, the pathogen may cause mild disease in the mother, but malformations in or death of the fetus. Additionally, children younger than 3 years old with a diarrheal disease can quickly decompensate from a rapid fluid volume loss as compared with children or adolescents with diarrheal disease. A depletion or dysfunction of neutrophils observed in patients receiving chemotherapy or those with diabetes mellitus results in an increased risk for developing bacterial infections or invasive fungal infections. Disrupted integrity of epithelial surfaces caused by trauma or burns leads to an increased risk for bacterial or fungal infections. In addition, congenital absence of complement components C5, C6, C7, or C8 prevents the formation of a fully functioning membrane attack complex, which can lead to overwhelming infection and sepsis (Schwartz, 2019).

Infants and young children are more susceptible to infection due to immature responses of the immune system. Newborns are at increased risk for infection due to a decreased inflammatory response to invading pathogens. While cellular immunity is generally functional at birth, the body must encounter infectious agents and then develop immunity to new diseases for humoral immunity to occur. Infants are losing the passive immunity acquired from maternal antibodies, and have had limited disease exposure, placing them at higher risk. In young children, active immunity from vaccinations is not complete, placing them at an increased risk for communicable disorders. With current decreases in immunization rates, formerly infrequent childhood diseases such as measles are increasing in prevalence. The American Academy of Pediatrics (AAP, 2020a), the Centers for Disease Control and Prevention (CDC, 2020), and the National Association of Pediatric Nurse Practitioners (NAPNAP, 2015) advocate for the immunization of all children for whom a contraindication does not exist.

## GENERAL APPROACH TO CHILD WITH AN INFECTIOUS DISORDER

Infectious disease in children is diagnosed primarily through a collection of data gathered from a thorough history taking regarding the child, mother, and other family members, physical examination, and (on occasion) evaluation of laboratory testing or imaging results. Early diagnosis of an infectious illness and recognition of severe disease stages are important skills for the healthcare provider. Equally important is the healthcare provider's ability to effectively communicate care for the child during the course of the illness, as well as to provide preventative education regarding immunization and other protective measures.

When assessing a child with a potential infection, the health history provides a wealth of information that aids the provider in the diagnostic process. For all children with a potential infection, refer to Table 31.1 for suggested questions for various components of the health history.

# BACTERIAL INFECTIONS

Children often experience bacterial infections such as lymphadenitis, methicillin-resistant staph aureus (MRSA) infection, and cat scratch disease.

**TABLE 31.1 Questions for the Health History for a Potential Infection**

| Health History Component | Key Information | Questions to Ask |
|---|---|---|
| **History of Present Illness** | The timing of particular symptoms can provide important information for differentiating the diagnosis, particularly among the viral exanthems. | What symptoms are present? When did the symptoms start? Have the symptoms evolved since their appearance? Does anything relieve or worsen the symptoms? Has the child been around anyone else who is sick? |
| **Medical History** | Certain medical conditions can predispose a child or increase the risk for a child to contract an infectious disease. Immunosuppressed children are more susceptible to contracting illnesses and experiencing a severe case of the disease. Additionally, immunosuppressed children are at greater risk for experiencing recurrent infections. | Is the child immunocompromised or do they have an immunodeficiency?<br>Has the child taken chemotherapy or corticosteroids recently? |
| **Current and Recent Medications** | Recent antibiotic use is important for the provider to know when reviewing culture results for a resistant or recurrent bacterial infection. Antipyretic medications administered to the child may mask a fever. Accordingly, it is important for the provider to inquire about the dosing schedule of antipyretic medicines or preparations containing fever-reducing compounds. | What medications have you given your children? Has your child been on antibiotics recently? If so, obtain details. Have you given your child acetaminophen or ibuprofen? If so, ascertain dosing schedule. |
| **Immunizations** | Review of the immunization record is important especially when considering whether a child's presentation suggests a vaccine-preventable disease. | Ask about dates and specific immunizations, or review immunization record. |

(continued)

TABLE 31.1 **Questions for the Health History for a Potential Infection** (*continued*)

| Health History Component | Key Information | Questions to Ask |
|---|---|---|
| **Family Medical History** | Children are often exposed to infectious diseases within the family. For example, conjunctival drainage in the neonate following vaginal delivery from a mother who has a history of herpes simplex virus (HSV) raises suspicion of an ophthalmic herpes infection in the neonate. | Is anyone in the home ill? If so, what is the illness? Has the child been around anyone with similar symptoms? |
| **Social History** | Children who attend day care, school, or live in crowded conditions (e.g., shelters) are at increased risk of contracting illness. Recent travel or living in areas associated with an infectious disease outbreak can increase risk of contracting these diseases. Additionally, it is important to know whether the child lives in or has traveled to areas endemic to tick-borne diseases. Obtaining the adolescent's sexual history is important in determining their risk for sexually transmitted infections (STIs). | Does the child attend, school, day care, mother's morning out, or Sunday school? Has the child traveled recently inside or outside of the United States? If so, where and when? Is the adolescent sexually active? If sexually active, what type of protection is used? |
| **Exposure History** | Exposure to individuals with known illnesses or those who are at high risk for contracting illnesses, such as those with human immunodeficiency virus (HIV) or who have had contact with animals, can provide insight into the diagnosis of infections. For example, in a toddler refusing to eat, knowing the child has a sibling recently diagnosed with strep throat may assist in identifying this disease process that might not have been considered in a child unable to verbalize throat pain. | Is anyone in the home ill? Parents, siblings? Are there any known illnesses "going around" the school or day care? |
| **Nutrition/Elimination History** | Dehydration can impair the body's ability to function normally, and to an even greater degree when affected by an infectious disease. It is important to identify significant fluid loss due to insufficient fluid consumption that can complicate any infectious disease process. | What is your child's usual diet like? Has that changed in the past couple of days (or since the child became ill)? |
| **Complete Review of Systems** | Thorough questioning is central to identifying signs or symptoms characteristic of certain diseases that are absent from the guardian or patient report. | Perform a thorough review of systems. |

## LYMPHADENITIS

Lymphadenitis occurs when a lymph node becomes enlarged and tender (Figure 31.2). The diagnostic approach examines causes that require observation and reassurance because of an extensive diagnostic workup for children who appear ill. Infectious causes are most commonly associated with lymphadenitis (Healy, 2018).

### Subjective Findings

The health history may reveal lymph node enlargement with or without pain, and possibly fever. When obtaining the history, determine the duration and

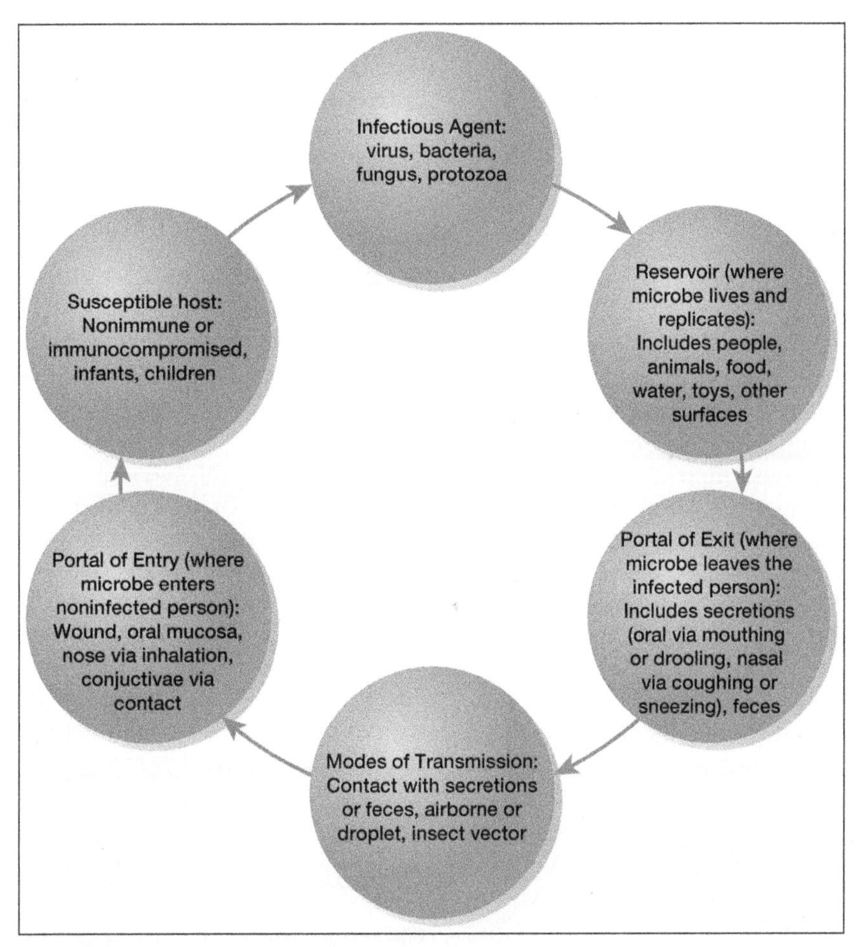


FIGURE 31.1 Chain of infection.

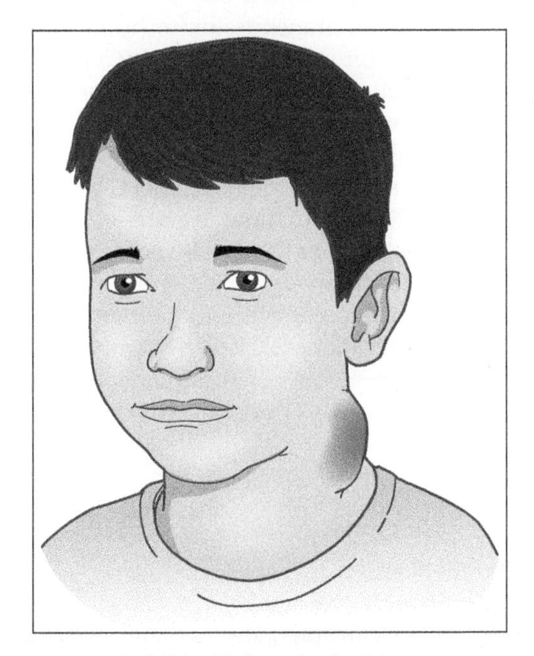

FIGURE 31.2 A child with lymphadenitis

change in size of the lymph node. Also ascertain the child's immunization status.

## Risk Factors

The most common risk factors for lymphadenitis are:

- Exposure to sick contacts
- History of tick bite
- Travel within and outside the United States (Healy, 2018)

## Review of Systems

The most common manifestations revealed during the review of systems include:

- **Constitutional:** fever, weight loss, fatigue
- **HEENT:** reddened eyes, sore throat, mouth sores
- **Respiratory:** cough
- **Musculoskeletal:** arthralgia, trauma

### Objective Findings

The physical examination of the child with lymphadenitis may reveal:

- Fever
- Irritability
- Lethargy
- Lymph node: a single erythematous, tender, and swollen lymph node. Lymph node alterations are differentiated as follow:
  - *Infected lymph nodes*: usually isolated, asymmetric, tender, warm, erythematous, and fluctuant.
  - *"Reactive/shotty" lymph nodes*: Small, soft, discrete, mobile, and minimally tender lymph nodes are considered reactive lymph nodes and occur frequently with many types of infections, particularly in young children. They are also termed "shotty" as they may feel like pieces of buckshot.
  - *Malignant lymph nodes*: tend to be nontender, hard, fixed, or matted.

### Laboratory/Diagnostic Testing

Children with bilateral lymphadenitis commonly have a viral upper respiratory infection, but group A *Streptococcus* must be ruled out. It is not recommended that children with bilateral lymphadenitis and mild illness (e.g., well-appearing, afebrile or low-grade fever, nonprogressive symptoms) undergo diagnostic workup (Healy, 2018).

The child with unilateral lymph node involvement and moderate illness (fever, tender node) should have diagnostic testing performed in order to guide medication treatment. This may include blood culture, culture from an open or draining wound if present, and/or needle aspiration of the node for organism identification (Healy, 2018).

### Differential Diagnosis

The differential diagnosis for lymphadenitis includes:

- Group A *Streptococcus* infection
- Epstein-Barr virus infection
- Cytomegalovirus (CMV)
- Cat scratch disease (CSD)
- Kawasaki disease
- Lymphoma
- Leukemia
- Tuberculosis

### Treatment/Management Plan

In children with acute, unilateral, cervical lymphadenitis and associated symptoms of fever, and adenitis without fluctuance, a 10- to 14-day course of antibiotic therapy is recommended. If no improvement occurs within 48 to 72 hours of initiation of treatment, cultures must be considered.

### Family Education

Teach the family:

- Complete the entire course of antibiotic therapy.
- Contact the nurse practitioner (NP) if there is no improvement within 48 to 72 hours of treatment initiation or if new symptoms arise.

### Referral

Refer a child for intravenous antibiotic therapy if, after incision and drainage, the child with acute unilateral cervical lymphadenitis has associated symptoms of fever and adenitis with fluctuance.

Refer to a pediatric infectious disease specialist the child who is ill-appearing, continues to be febrile, or has progressing symptoms and persistent lymphadenopathy (6–8 weeks with no decrease in size) for further evaluation and treatment. Refer the child with fixed nontender nodes to a pediatric hematologist/oncologist for further workup and evaluation.

## CAT SCRATCH DISEASE

CSD is a zoonosis caused by *Bartonella henselae*, a hemotropic gram-negative bacterium. *B. henselae* is harbored and spread among cats and about half of all cats are infected. Transmission to humans occurs via scratches and bites from a cat, or by a cat licking a human wound. Although rare, dogs also carry *B. hensalae*. The incidence rate of CSD is highest in children ages 5 to 9 years (9.4 cases/100,000 population), and in southern areas of the United States (6.5 cases/100,000 population; Nelson et al., 2016). Primary manifestation of the disease is lymphadenopathy proximal to the wound site, with most patients recovering spontaneously without intervention or experiencing complications. However, immunocompromised patients are at risk for suffering complications of the disease.

### Subjective Findings

The health history may reveal:

- Low-grade fever
- Papule or pustule at wound site
- Enlarged, tender lymph node proximal to wound site
- History of playing with cats (particularly kittens)

### Risk Factors

The most common risk factor for CSD is playing with kittens or cats.

### Review of Systems

The most common manifestations revealed during the review of systems include:

- **Constitutional:** low-grade fever
- **Integumentary:** kitten or cat scratch
- **Lymphatic:** tender lymph node

### Objective Findings

The physical examination of the child with CSD may reveal:

- Papule or pustule at wound site, which may be painful, warm, or open
- Enlarged, erythematous, tender lymph node proximal to wound site

### Laboratory/Diagnostic Testing

The diagnosis of CSD is based upon the clinical findings and positive exposure history. If the test is available, a polymerase chain reaction (PCR) result will be positive (CDC, 2020).

### Differential Diagnosis

The differential diagnosis for CSD includes:

- Local lymphadenopathy
- Lymphadenitis
- Methicillin-resistant *Staphylococcus aureus* (MRSA)

### Treatment/Management Plan

The treatment plan is focused on supportive care and possibly antibiotic treatment. Nonsteroidal anti-inflammatory drugs (NSAIDs), such as acetaminophen or ibuprofen, may be used to reduce fever and treat. Warm compresses may also be applied to the area of lymphadenopathy to decrease pain. Most cases of CSD resolve without treatment, although disseminated disease is prevented with azithromycin. The recommended dosing for azithromycin is:

- For children >45.5 kg: 500 mg on day 1, followed by 250 mg for 4 days
- For children ≤45.5 kg: 10 mg/kg on day 1, followed by 5 mg/kg for 4 days

### Family Education

Teach the family:

- Refrain from owning a house cat younger than 1 year of age in households with immunocompromised individuals.
- Wash hands immediately after handling cats.
- Use flea collars on house cats and dogs.
- Treat house cats and dogs for fleas (CDC, 2020).

# VIRAL INFECTIONS

Children, particularly young children, are exposed to and contract a large number of viral infections. Infections discussed in this section include hand, foot, and mouth disease (HFMD), adenovirus, mumps, and HIV.

## HAND, FOOT, AND MOUTH DISEASE

HFMD is most frequently caused by Coxsackievirus A16 and Enterovirus A71 (EV-A71), and occurs worldwide with outbreaks concentrating in day cares, schools, camps, and military communities (Figure 31.3). The majority of cases occur in children younger than 7 years old in the summer and early fall seasons. Transmission of the virus occurs via respiratory or fecal-oral routes, and the incubation period is 2 to 7 days (Romero, 2020).

### Subjective Findings

The health history may reveal:

- Fever, fussiness, and anorexia
- Mouth and throat pain
- Rash on the hands and/or feet

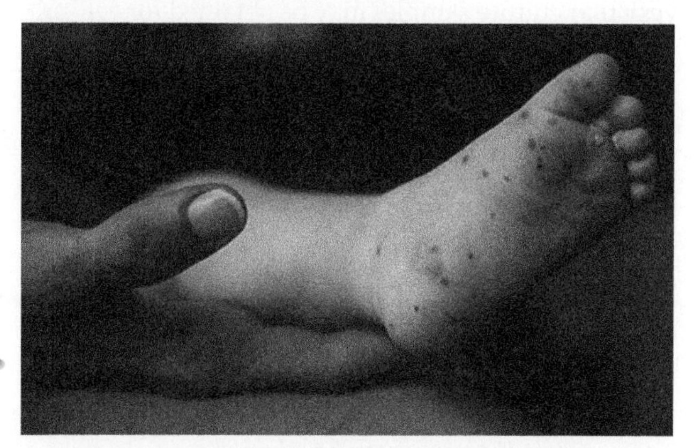

**FIGURE 31.3** Spots on feet as a symptom of HFM.

*Source*: Centers for Disease Control and Prevention. (2021). Hand, foot, and mouth disease. https://www.cdc.gov/hand-foot-mouth/index.html.

### Risk Factors

The most common risk factors for HFMD are:

- Age younger than 5 to 7 years
- Day care, school, or summer camp attendance

### Review of Systems

The most common manifestations revealed during the review of systems include:

- **Constitutional:** fever, refusal to eat or drink (preverbal child)
- **HEENT:** sores in mouth, mouth or throat pain (verbal child)
- **Gastrointestinal:** abdominal pain, emesis, diarrhea
- **Integumentary:** spots on hands and/or feet

### Objective Findings

The physical examination of the child with HFMD may reveal:

- Rash on tongue, buccal mucosa, hands, and feet typically, although it may also involve soft/hard palates, lips, tonsils, buttocks, legs, and arms
- Rash changes over time, so findings may include erythematous macules (1–5 mm) that progress to vesicles surrounded by an erythematous halo, then rupture of vesicles with grayish-yellow base with erythematous rim
- Nail dystrophy/Beau lines (transverse ridges of nail plate), or onychomadesis (occurring 1 to 2 months after HFMD); occurs with the more severe disease caused by novel Coxsackie A6

### Laboratory/Diagnostic Testing

Diagnosis of HFMD is made based upon the clinical presentation. If diagnosis is uncertain, throat, stool, or vesicular culture samples may be obtained for cell culture or nucleic acid amplification.

### Differential Diagnosis

The differential diagnosis for HFMD includes:

- Aphthous ulcers
- Herpes simplex gingivostomatitis
- Eczema herpeticum
- Erythema multiforme major
- Contact dermatitis
- Varicella

### Treatment/Management Plan

Management for HFMD is supportive in nature, with fever resolution occurring within 4 days and throat lesions resolving within 3 to 10 days. Manage pain and fever with an antipyretic such as acetaminophen or an NSAID such as ibuprofen (Romero, 2020).

### Family Education

Teach the family:

- Discuss infection prevention measures.
- Stress the importance of good hand hygiene.
- Exclude from day care and school while the child is febrile, has open blisters, or has extensive drooling from mouth lesions (Romero, 2020).

### Referral

Refer for hospitalization when the child is dehydrated or if encephalitis, meningitis, flaccid paralysis, or myocarditis is a concern.

## ADENOVIRUS INFECTION

Adenovirus is a family of more than 60 DNA viruses that causes about 5% to 10% of febrile illnesses in infants and young children (Flomenberg & Kojaoghlanian, 2021). Adenoviruses cause infection in children throughout the year, and disease transmission occurs via aerosol droplets, fecal-oral route, and contaminated fomites. In the neonate, disease can spread transvaginally. The most common system affected is the respiratory system, with symptoms commonly lasting 3 to 5 days (and up to 2 weeks). In infants and young children, adenovirus predominantly manifests as an illness of the respiratory, cardiac, gastrointestinal, or genitourinary system.

### Subjective Findings

The health history may reveal:

- Fever
- Rhinorrhea
- Cough
- Watery or itchy eyes
- Diarrhea (Flomenberg & Kojaoghlanian, 2021)

### Risk Factors

The most common risk factors for adenovirus infection are:

- Day-care attendance
- Exposure to an infected individual

### Review of Systems

The most common manifestations revealed during the review of systems include:

- **Constitutional:** fever, malaise
- **HEENT:** watery, itchy, and/or red eyes, rhinorrhea, sneezing, sore throat, hoarseness

- **Respiratory:** cough
- **Gastrointestinal:** diarrhea, abdominal pain
- **Neurologic:** headache

### Objective Findings

The physical examination of the child with adenovirus infection may reveal:

- Cervical lymphadenopathy
- Conjunctivitis
- Otitis media
- Exudative tonsillitis
- Wheezes or crackles in lung fields

### Laboratory/Diagnostic Testing

Diagnostic testing to confirm adenovirus is important in differentiating the infection from other illnesses that require specific treatment. A chest radiograph reveals diffuse bilateral pulmonary infiltrates in a child with adenoviral pneumonia. Nasopharyngeal swabs or aspirates, throat swabs or washes, sputum, tracheal aspirates, bronchoalveolar lavage, conjunctival swabs or scrapings, stool or rectal swabs, urine, blood, cerebrospinal fluid (CSF), and tissue samples may be collected in the early phases of the illness and demonstrate persistence of adenovirus for weeks in children. In immunocompromised children, adenovirus may be shed in the urine or stool for months without symptoms; therefore, it is important to interpret culture results based on current symptoms (Flomenberg & Kojaoghlanian, 2021).

### Differential Diagnosis

The differential diagnosis for adenovirus includes:

- Rhinovirus (common cold)
- Influenza
- Respiratory syncytial virus (RSV)
- Parainfluenza
- Human metapneumovirus
- Norovirus

### Treatment/Management Plan

Most adenovirus infections are self-limiting and treatment is mainly supportive. However, immunocompromised children may experience severe illness and antiviral medication may be recommended due to the risk of severe disease and complications (Munoz & Flomenberg, 2020).

### Family Education

Teach the family:

- Careful and diligent handwashing is important to prevent transmission of the virus through fomites, fecal matter, or contact with conjunctival secretions.
- Use respiratory hygiene/cough etiquette practices such as covering the mouth and nose when coughing or sneezing, using nearest waste receptacle to dispose of used tissues, and proper handwashing after contact with respiratory secretions (Munoz & Flomenberg, 2020).

### Referral

Refer neonates, immunocompromised children, or those with severe disease to a pediatric infectious disease specialist (Munoz & Flomenberg, 2020).

## MUMPS

Mumps is a highly contagious viral illness resulting in parotitis and is spread via respiratory droplet, direct contact, and fomites. The incubation period ranges from 12 to 25 days, and infectivity begins prior to onset of parotitis, continuing for at least 5 days following that onset (Albrecht, 2020c). The illness is self-limited, with treatment focused on symptomatic amelioration, and is preventable via vaccination. Since vaccination for mumps began, cases of mumps in the United States have decreased by 99% (Albrecht, 2020c).

### Subjective Findings

The health history may reveal:

- Fever
- Neck swelling

### Risk Factors

The most common risk factors for mumps are children who are not immunized against mumps and children who are immunocompromised.

### Review of Systems

The most common manifestations revealed during the review of systems include:

- **Constitutional:** fever, fatigue, anorexia
- **HEENT:** neck swelling, tenderness near the parotid area, possible earache
- **Musculoskeletal:** myalgia
- **Neurologic:** headache

### Objective Findings

The physical examination of the child with mumps may reveal:

- Parotid gland swelling
- Erythematous and enlarged orifice of Stensen's duct

### Laboratory/Diagnostic Testing

Laboratory confirmation may be established with detection of mumps virus RNA with reverse-transcriptase polymerase chain reaction (RT-PCR) or serum mumps IgM antibody (Albrecht, 2020c).

### Differential Diagnosis

The differential diagnosis for mumps includes:

- Bacterial parotitis
- Epstein-Barr virus infection
- CSD
- HIV infection

### Treatment/Management Plan

Treatment of mumps is symptomatic. Monitor for complications such as orchitis, oophoritis, meningitis, encephalitis, deafness, and rarely arthritis, pancreatitis, and myocarditis (Albrecht, 2020c).

### Family Education

Teach the family:

- Use an antipyretic such as acetaminophen to reduce fever and pain from parotid swelling.
- The child must stay home from school and other outside activities, preferably in a separate room, until at least 5 days after the onset of symptoms.
- Ensure that all other family members are immunized against mumps (Albrecht, 2020c).

## HUMAN IMMUNODEFICIENCY VIRUS INFECTION

Transmission of HIV to children occurs through vertical transmission (mother to fetus or newborn), and horizontal modes (risky behaviors such as infected needle use or unprotected sexual activity). Clinical manifestations of pediatric HIV infection are variable and nonspecific. With early diagnosis and prompt initiation of highly effective, combination antiretroviral therapy (ART), infection with opportunistic illnesses, incidence of comorbidities, and mortality can be greatly reduced. Comorbidities associated with HIV infection include developmental delay, mental health disorders (e.g., anxiety, mood disorders, and substance abuse disorders), dyslipidemia, cardiomyopathy, accelerated atherosclerosis, insulin resistance, diabetes mellitus, decreased bone mineral density, and chronic kidney disease (Gillespie, 2021).

### Subjective Findings

The health history may reveal:

- Anorexia
- Diarrhea
- Recurrent fevers or infections

### Risk Factors

Children and adolescents at high risk of contracting HIV infection are those who:

- Experience perinatal exposure to HIV-positive mother
- Use injectable drugs
- Have sex with HIV-infected partners or those whose HIV status is unknown
- Exchange sex for money or drugs
- Are males who have sex with other males, including sexual abuse

### Review of Systems

The most common manifestations revealed during the review of systems include:

- **Constitutional:** anorexia, fever
- **Respiratory:** fast breathing, nonproductive cough, progressive shortness of breath
- **Gastrointestinal:** diarrhea
- **Immune:** recurrent bacterial infections

### Objective Findings

The physical examination of the child with HIV infection may reveal:

- Oral candidiasis (early sign in children with history of perinatal exposure)
- Lymphadenopathy (early sign)
- Hepatosplenomegaly (early sign)
- Delayed milestone attainment, loss of milestones, loss of cognitive ability (early sign in children with history of perinatal exposure)
- *Pneumocystis jirovecii* pneumonia—formerly known as pneumocystis carinii pneumonia (PCP) presents with tachypnea and nonproductive cough, with rales

and rhonchi as a late sign, in 50% of untreated children presenting during the first year of life
- Wasting syndrome—persistent weight loss greater than 10% of baseline, crossing downward 2 or more percentiles on pediatric weight-for-age chart, less than fifth percentile on weight-for-height chart over two consecutive measurements separated by 30 days with a history of diarrhea or fever
- HIV encephalopathy
- Microcephaly
- Acquired symmetric motor deficits

### Laboratory/Diagnostic Testing

Screening for HIV infection is dependent on the age of presentation in the child. Maternal HIV antibodies persist in infants until the age of 18 months. Therefore, serologic testing for the presence of HIV DNA and RNA confirms HIV diagnosis in children younger than 18 months of age. Further, it is recommended that a follow-up antibody test be performed between 12 and 18 months old to confirm HIV infection (Gillespie, 2019).

For the identification of HIV infection in children older than 18 months, a testing algorithm is recommended. Fourth-generation combination HIV-1/HIV-2 immunoassay is obtained initially. If the fourth-generation combination assay is positive, HIV-1/HIV-2 antibody differentiation immunoassay is performed. A plasma HIV RNA level is recommended if the fourth-generation test is positive and the confirmatory HIV-1/HIV-2 antibody differentiation immunoassay is negative or uncertain (Sax, 2020).

For patients with suspected *Pneumocystis jirovecii* pneumonia, a chest radiograph will show bilateral perihilar interstitial infiltrates that become homogenous and diffuse later in the disease process (Gillespie, 2019).

### Differential Diagnosis

The differential diagnosis for HIV infection includes:

- Primary immunodeficiency
- Mononucleosis
- Lymphadenopathy
- Malnutrition or failure to thrive
- Constitutional growth delay

### Treatment/Management Plan

With the introduction of combination ART, there has been a sharp decline in morbidity and mortality rates associated with HIV. Early identification and treatment is key to preventing the incidence rate of opportunistic infections in children. Studies evaluating ART regimens have shown improved virologic, immunologic, and overall health of children and adolescents infected with HIV (Gillespie, 2021). A brief overview of drug therapy is described for the primary care provider, as the child and adolescent with HIV infection is primarily managed by the immunologist or infectious disease specialist.

ART therapy acts on preventing HIV replication through the different stages that comprise the HIV life cycle: entry, reverse transcription, integration, replication, assembly, and budding and maturation. Chemokine coreceptor (CCR5) antagonists and fusion inhibitors act on blocking HIV during the entry stage. Nucleoside/nucleotide reverse transcriptase inhibitors (NRTIs) and non-nucleoside reverse transcriptase inhibitors (NNRTIs) inhibit the process of reverse transcription. Integrase strand transfer inhibitors (INSTIs) inhibit the process of integration. Protease inhibitors inhibit budding and maturation of new viral proteins that emerge (Fletcher, 2021).

### Family Education

Teach the family:

- Always administer all doses of anti-HIV medications.
- Adolescents 15 to 18 years old should be screened once for HIV based on risk assessment (sexually active adolescents, and those who possess other risk factors for transmission of HIV such as intravenous drug users; Committee on Pediatric AIDS, 2011).

### Referral

Children and adolescents diagnosed with HIV infection should be referred to a pediatric infection disease specialist or immunologist for management of the disease process (Committee on Pediatric AIDS, 2011).

## VIRAL EXANTHEMS

The classic childhood diseases (excluding mumps) are viral infections resulting in exanthems of the skin. A rash or skin eruption is also referred to as an *exanthem*. The viral exanthems of childhood each demonstrate a particular pattern of fever presentation and a distinct rash pattern. Childhood immunizations have resulted in a significant decrease in the incidence of certain viral exanthems, such as varicella (chickenpox), rubella (German measles), and measles.

## VARICELLA

Varicella zoster virus (chickenpox) is a DNA virus in the herpes virus family (Figure 31.4). Since the introduction of the varicella vaccine in 1995, incidence

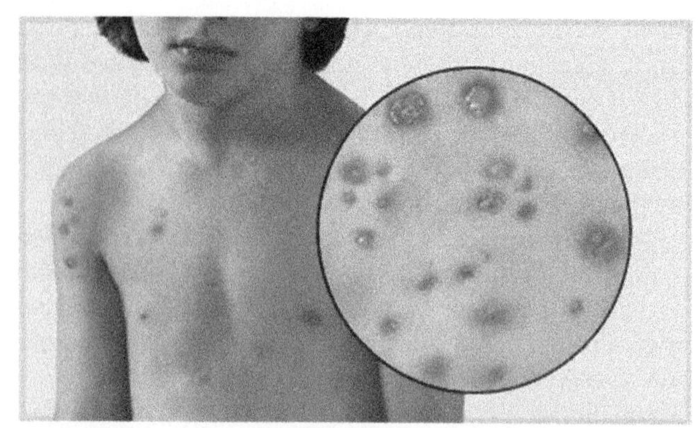

FIGURE 31.4 All three stages of the chickenpox rash (red bumps, blisters, and scabs) appear on the body at the same time.

*Source*: © 1995–2020. The Nemours Foundation/KidsHealth®. Reprinted with permission. https://kidshealth.org/en/parents/chicken-pox.html

rates have declined to 3.9 per 100,000 population in states reporting to the National Notifiable Diseases Surveillance System, with the greatest reduction observed in children ages 5 to 14 years old (Albrecht, 2019b). Transmission of the virus occurs via the following modes: droplet, direct cutaneous contact, and airborne. The incubation period ranges from 10 to 21 days, and infectivity begins 48 hours prior to the onset of the rash until crusting of lesions (Albrecht, 2019a).

## Subjective Findings

The health history may reveal:

- Fever
- Rash (usually beginning on the trunk, then extending to the entire body)

### Risk Factors

The most common risk factors for varicella infection are:

- Children who are unimmunized and are exposed to the virus
- Children who are immunocompromised

### Review of Symptoms

The most common manifestations revealed during the review of systems include:

- **Constitutional:** fever, malaise, anorexia (these precede the rash)
- **Integumentary:** extremely pruritic rash
- **HEENT:** sore throat (precedes the rash)

## Objective Findings

The physical examination of the child with varicella may reveal:

- A classic rash in varying stages
  - Findings may include macules (early), papules, vesicles, pustules, and crusted lesions on the trunk, face, and extremities
- Temporary hypopigmentation (arising 1–2 weeks after crusts fall off)

### Laboratory/Diagnostic Testing

Varicella is diagnosed based upon the clinical presentation. Infection may be confirmed with serologic testing for the presence of IgG antibodies to varicella, and real-time PCR assays obtained from skin lesions, cerebral spinal fluid, or bronchoalveolar lavage (Albrecht, 2020a).

## Differential Diagnosis

The differential diagnosis of varicella includes:

- Herpes zoster (shingles)
- Herpes simplex virus (HSV)
- HFMD
- Impetigo

## Treatment/Management Plan

In healthy individuals, varicella is a self-limited illness. Symptom management and supportive care are used for previously healthy children. However, in children with a history of malignancy, corticosteroid use, or immunosuppressive therapy, HIV infection, or solid organ transplantation, the impaired immunity increases the risk of complications and death (Albrecht, 2019a).

### Family Education

Teach the family:

- Give oral antihistamines and/or use topical antipruritis agents (such as calamine lotion or pramoxine cream) to relieve pruritus.
- Oatmeal baths may also relieve pruritus.
- Administer weight-appropriate doses of acetaminophen or ibuprofen to reduce fever.
- Ensure adequate hydration, as fever may lead to dehydration in children.
- Symptomatic management includes the use of antihistamines to reduce pruritis, and acetaminophen and NSAIDs (e.g., ibuprofen) to treat fever.

- Children must avoid day-care and school settings until all lesions are crusted (usually about 6 days following initial appearance), when children are no longer contagious.
- Immunization is recommended for all children in two doses; first dose administered between 12 and 18 months old and the second dose administered between 4 and 6 years old (Albrecht, 2019b).

### Referral

Refer children who are immunocompromised or unvaccinated adolescents for hospitalization to receive intravenous treatment with valacyclovir or acyclovir for 7 to 10 days as recommended to reduce the risk of complications and death (Albrecht, 2020d).

## ROSEOLA INFANTUM (EXANTHEMA SUBITUM)

Roseola is caused by human herpesvirus 6 (HHV-6), HHV-7, enteroviruses (coxsackieviruses A and B, and echoviruses), adenovirus, and parainfluenza virus (type 1). Ninety percent of roseola cases are in children younger than 2 years of age. The classic disease pattern is characterized by a 3- to 5-day period of fever (possibly exceeding 40 °C/104 °F) followed by a blanching macular or maculopapular rash starting on the neck and trunk and spreading to the face and extremities and disappearing within a few hours to 2 days (Tremblay & Brady, 2019). See Figure 31.5.

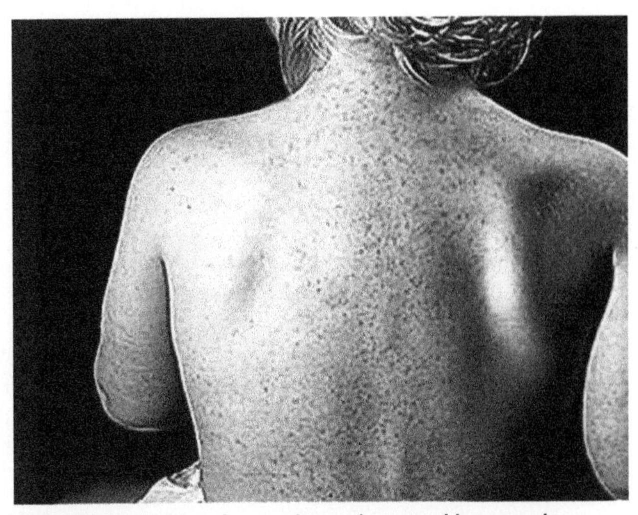

**FIGURE 31.5** Maculopapular rash caused by roseola infantum.

*Source*: Used with permission of Mayo Foundation for Medical Education and Research, all rights reserved. https://www.mayoclinic.org/diseases-conditions/roseola/symptoms-causes/syc-20377283

### Subjective Findings

The health history may reveal:

- Fever for 3 to 5 days
- Nonpruritic rash

### Risk Factors

The most common risk factor for roseola is being a child under 2 years of age.

### Review of Systems

The most common manifestations revealed during the review of systems include:

- **Constitutional:** fever
- **HEENT:** eye redness, eyelid swelling, runny nose
- **Respiratory**: cough
- **Gastrointestinal:** diarrhea, vomiting
- **Neurologic:** possible irritability (most children are active and alert)

### Objective Findings

The physical examination of the child with roseola may reveal:

- Otherwise healthy appearance
- Erythematous macular/maculopapular rash on neck, trunk, face, or extremities (blanches)
- Palpebral conjunctivitis
- Eyelid edema
- Rhinorrhea
- Macules or ulcers at the uvulopalatoglossal junction
- Cervical (most common), postauricular, and/or occipital lymphadenopathy

### Laboratory/Diagnostic Testing

Roseola is diagnosed by clinical presentation. If diagnosis must be confirmed, virologic studies of suspected pathogens should be obtained. Serologic testing for the common causative organisms includes HHV-6, HHV-7, enterovirus, adenovirus, or parainfluenza virus type 1 (Tremblay & Brady, 2019).

### Differential Diagnosis

The differential diagnosis of roseola includes:

- Rubella
- Rubeola
- Enteroviral infections
- Erythema infectiosum
- Scarlet fever
- Drug rash

### Treatment/Management Plan

Most children with roseola recover spontaneously. Treatment is supportive (Tremblay & Brady, 2019).

### Family Education

Teach the family:

- Administer acetaminophen or ibuprofen in weight-appropriate dosing for fever management.
- Ensure adequate hydration.
- Practice good hygiene to prevent spread of the disease (Tremblay & Brady, 2019).

## MEASLES

Measles is a highly contagious infection resulting from the measles virus. It occurs worldwide and about 90% of nonimmune persons will develop measles after exposure to the virus (Gans & Maldonado, 2019). Person-to-person contact is not required, and it may be transmitted in public places. Individuals infected with the measles virus are contagious from about 5 days before the onset of the rash until 4 days after its appearance (Figure 31.6).

### Subjective Findings

The health history may reveal:

- Fever
- Cold symptoms
- Rash

### Risk Factors

The most common risk factors for measles are children who are not immunized against it and those who are immunocompromised.

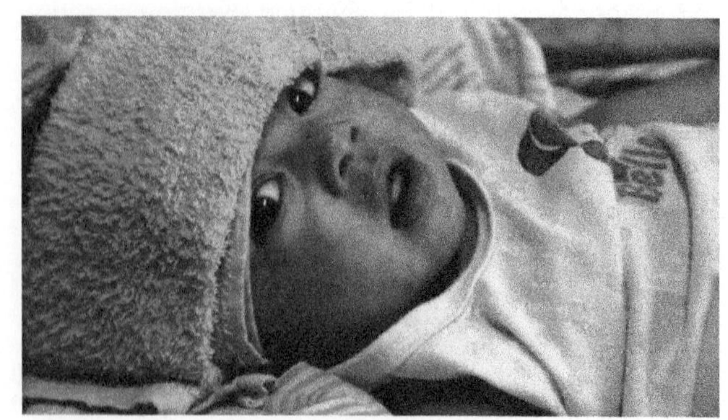

FIGURE 31.6 Exanthem stage shows blanching rash.

*Source*: CDC. https://www.cdc.gov/measles/index.html

### Review of Systems

The most common manifestations revealed during the review of systems include:

- **Constitutional:** fever, malaise, anorexia (prodromal stage)
- **Integumentary:** rash (begins after fever and cold symptoms)
- **HEENT:** red eyes, runny nose, congestion
- **Respiratory:** cough

### Objective Findings

The physical examination of the child with measles reveals different findings depending upon the stage of the illness.

- *Incubation stage* (lasting 6–21 days), the child is usually asymptomatic.
- *Prodromal stage* (lasting 2–8 days), note fever (40 °C, 104 °F), conjunctivitis, coryza, Koplik spots (1–3 mm whitish, bluish, grayish elevations with an erythematous base observed in buccal and labial mucosa, lasting about 12 to 72 hours, and disappearing prior to the exanthem phase).
- *Exanthem stage* shows erythematous, maculopapular, blanching rash appearing first on the face and spreading cephalocaudally and centrifugally (lasts 6–7 days, darkening first to a brownish color and disappearing in the order it appeared). Also occurring during the exanthem phase are high fever (peaks 2–3 days after appearance of the rash), pharyngitis, nonpurulent conjunctivitis, and lymphadenopathy.

### Laboratory/Diagnostic Testing

Diagnosis of measles is made with serologic testing for serum IgM antibody, measles IgG antibody, viral culture, or detection of measles virus RNA by RT-PCR (Gans & Maldonado, 2019).

### Differential Diagnosis

The differential diagnosis of measles includes:

- Common viral respiratory illnesses (rhinovirus, parainfluenza, influenza, adenovirus, RSV)
- Varicella
- Roseola
- Erythema infectiosum
- Rubella
- HFMD
- Group A *Streptococcus* infection
- Drug rash
- Infectious mononucleosis

- Kawasaki disease
- *Mycoplasma pneumoniae* infection
- Rocky Mountain spotted fever (RMSF)

### Treatment/Management Plan

Measles is a self-limiting illness with treatment focusing on fever reduction, hydration maintenance, and treatment of secondary infections (i.e., bacterial pneumonia or otitis media; Gans & Maldonado, 2019).

### Family Education

Teach the family:

- Give weight-appropriate doses of acetaminophen as needed for fever reduction.
- Encourage the child to consume adequate fluids.
- The cough may persist for 2 to 3 weeks after the rash disappears.
- If antibiotics are prescribed for a secondary bacterial infection, complete the entire course of medication.
- Prevent measles infection by immunization. The vaccine is a 2-dose series with the first dose administered at 12 to 18 months old, and the second dose being given at 4 to 6 years of age (Gans & Maldonado, 2019).

## RUBELLA

Rubella is a member of the Togaviridae family. With introduction of the vaccination in 1969, annual cases rapidly declined, and in 2004, rubella and congenital rubella syndrome were declared eliminated in the United States (Edwards, 2020). Globally, rubella outbreaks continue to occur in some countries. Rubella is acquired via inhalation of infectious large-particle aerosols and is amplified by close or prolonged contact with infected persons. The incubation period ranges from 12 to 23 days and many individuals remain asymptomatic, although infected. Rubella infection acquired during pregnancy may result in congenital rubella syndrome in the newborn and imay results in birth defects such as cataracts.

### Subjective Findings

The health history may reveal:

- Low-grade fever
- Rash

### Risk Factors

Children at high risk of contracting rubella are those who are unimmunized and are exposed to infected individuals (via international travel).

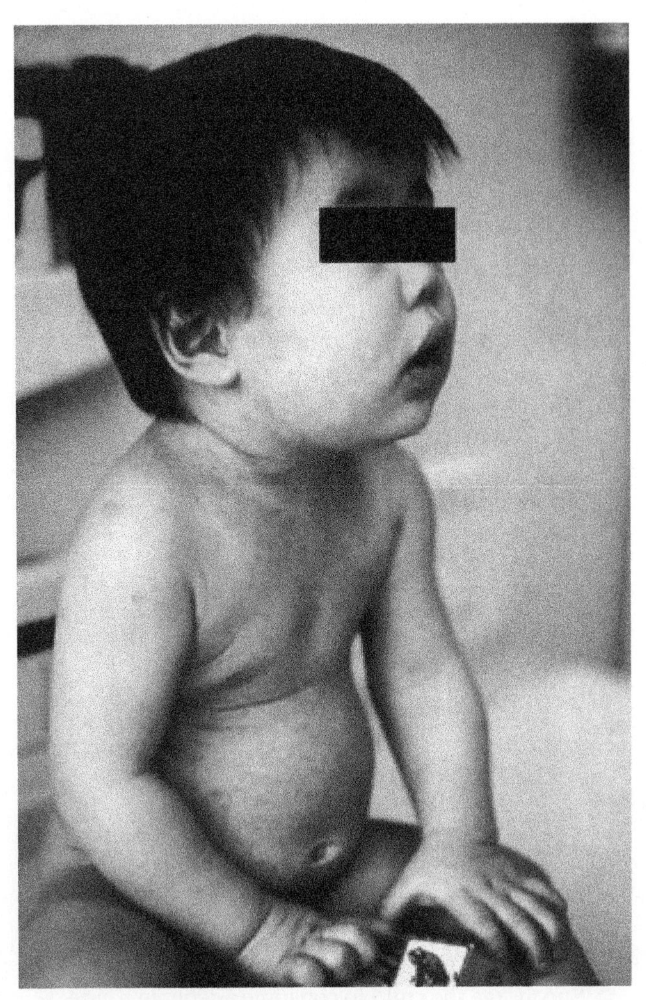

FIGURE 31.7 This baby has a mild rash with pink and red spots caused by rubella.

*Source*: CDC. https://www.cdc.gov/rubella/about/photos.html

### Review of Systems

The most common manifestations revealed during the review of systems include:

- **Constitutional:** low-grade fever
- **Integumentary:** rash (Figure 31.7)
- **HEENT:** reddened eyes
- **Musculoskeletal:** Arthritis/arthralgia, particularly of the knees, wrists, and fingers (common in adolescents)

### Objective Findings

The physical examination of the child with rubella may reveal:

- Lymphadenopathy (posterior cervical, posterior auricular, and suboccipital)

- Pinpoint, pink maculopapular rash first appearing on face and spreading to trunk, then extremities (becoming generalized within 24 hours of onset), lasting 1 to 8 days
- Mild nonexudative conjunctivitis
- Forchheimer spots (small red spots) on soft palate

### Laboratory/Diagnostic Testing

Rubella infection is diagnosed via enzyme immunoassay (EIA) to detect IgM antibodies to rubella.

### Differential Diagnosis

The differential diagnosis of rubella includes:

- Group A *Streptococcus*
- Parvovirus
- Infectious mononucleosis
- Measles
- Drug rash

### Treatment/Management Plan

Treatment is supportive and includes controlling fever reduction and pain management (Edwards, 2020).

### Family Education

Teach the family:

- Give weight-appropriate doses of acetaminophen as needed for fever reduction.
- Encourage the child to consume adequate fluids.
- Exclude from day care and school for 7 days after rash onset.
- Use NSAIDs (e.g., ibuprofen) to reduce the pain of arthralgia or arthritis.
- Prevent rubella infection by immunization. The vaccine is a 2-dose series with the first dose administered at 12 to 18 months old, and the second dose given at 4 to 6 years of age (Edwards, 2020).

## FIFTH DISEASE (ERYTHEMA INFECTIOSUM)

Fifth disease (erythema infectiosum) is caused by parvovirus B19 (a single-stranded DNA virus in the *Parvoviridae* family) and spreads via the respiratory and contact routes, as well as vertically. The incubation period of parvovirus B19 ranges from 4 to 21 days, with some children appearing asymptomatic or presenting with nonspecific flu-like symptoms (Jordan, 2021a). In addition to causing fever and rash with fifth disease, parvovirus B19 destroys erythrocyte progenitor cells, which causes a decrease in hematocrit. In healthy children, red blood cell production recovers within 10–14 days (Jordan, 2020). Children with a history of sickle cell disease, thalassemia, hereditary spherocytosis, or iron deficiency anemia are at particular risk for suffering an aplastic crisis with severe anemia (Jordan, 2021a).

### Subjective Findings

The health history may reveal:

- Fever
- Flu-like symptoms
- Rash (following the first two symptoms)

### Risk Factors

The most common risk factors for fifth disease are:

- Exposure to other young children
- Day-care attendance
- Living in crowded environments

### Review of Systems

The most common manifestations revealed during the review of systems include:

- **Constitutional:** fever
- **Integumentary:** rash (2–5 days following the other symptoms)
- **HEENT:** coryza
- **Gastrointestinal:** nausea, diarrhea
- **Musculoskeletal:** arthralgia
- **Neurologic:** headache

### Objective Findings

The physical examination of the child with fifth disease may reveal:

- Circumoral pallor
- Erythematous malar rash (slapped-cheek appearance; see Figure 31.8)
- Reticulated (lace-like) rash on trunk and extremities as facial rash fades

### Laboratory/Diagnostic Testing

In the presence of classic clinical symptoms, no laboratory diagnosis is necessary. However, if the presentation is atypical or unclear, diagnosis can be confirmed with serologic parvovirus B19-specific IgM antibody (Jordan, 2021a).

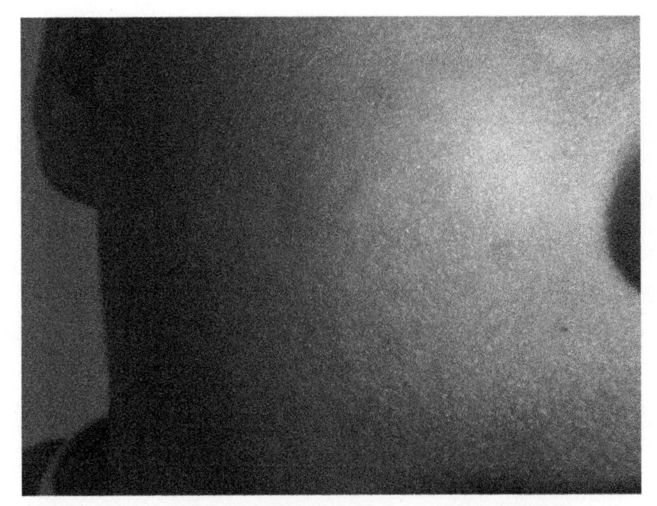

FIGURE 31.8 Slapped-cheek rash from fifth disease.

*Source*: Kostolansky, S., & Waymack, J. R. (2020). *Erythema infectiosum*. https://www.ncbi.nlm.nih.gov/books/NBK513309

### Differential Diagnosis

The differential diagnosis for fifth disease includes:

- Roseola
- Rubella
- Measles
- Enterovirus
- Group A Streptococcus
- Drug rash

### Treatment/Management Plan

Fifth disease is a self-limited, mild illness that is primarily managed with symptomatic care (fever reduction and pain management; Jordan, 2021b).

### Family Education

Teach the family:

- To prevent transmission of the disease, practice good hygiene such as covering the face with a tissue when coughing or sneezing or doing so into the elbow, and limiting exposure to sick contacts.
- Use acetaminophen in weight-appropriate doses to reduce fever.
- Encourage adequate fluid consumption.
- In the adolescent, use NSAIDs such as ibuprofen to manage pain of arthritis/arthralgia.
- Provide pregnant adolescents with education on the risk of infection if exposed to parvovirus B19 (risk of fetal anemia and hydrops; Jordan, 2021b).

# SEXUALLY TRANSMITTED INFECTIONS

Newborns may be affected by sexually transmitted infections (STIs) from exposure in utero or via the birth process. Children and adolescents may become infected via sexual activity. The AAP recommends that adolescents 11 to 21 years old should be screened for STIs based on risk assessment (AAP, 2020b; U.S. Preventive Services Task Force, 2019). STIs include chlamydia, gonorrhea, genital herpes, syphilis, and trichomoniasis (Tables 31.2 and 31.3).

## CHLAMYDIA

*Chlamydia trachomatis* is a sexually transmitted gram-negative bacterium that is commonly asymptomatic and is observed to have the highest prevalence of infection in younger males and females age 15 to 24 years old (Hsu, 2019b). Pregnant mothers who are infected with chlamydia place their newborns at risk for acquiring the infection, presenting with conjunctivitis (15%–50% risk) or pneumonia (5%–20% risk) 5 to 14 days following delivery (Hammerschlag, 2018). Co-infection with *Neisseria gonorrhea* has been documented to be as high as 50%, providing sufficient evidence to support the screening of STIs in adolescents with chlamydial infection (Hsu, 2019b).

Complications of chlamydial infection include pelvic inflammatory disease (PID); scarring of the fallopian tubes, ovaries, endometrial lining, and perineum; and increased risk for ectopic pregnancy and tubal infertility (Hsu, 2019b). Studies have also identified that chlamydial infection during pregnancy can cause premature rupture of membranes, preterm delivery, and low-birth-weight infants. Further, co-infection increases the transmission of HIV vertically to the neonate (Hsu, 2019b).

## GONORRHEA

Gonorrhea infection is caused by the gram-negative coccus *Neisseria gonorrhoeae*. Gonorrhea presenting in adolescents predominates as an asymptomatic illness but is associated with serious comorbidities such as PID, epididymitis, infertility, ectopic pregnancy, chronic pelvic pain, endocarditis, and meningitis. Additional perinatal complications include chorioamnionitis, premature rupture of membranes, preterm birth, low birth weight, small for gestational age infants, and spontaneous abortion. The untreated pregnant adolescent has a 30% to 50% increased risk

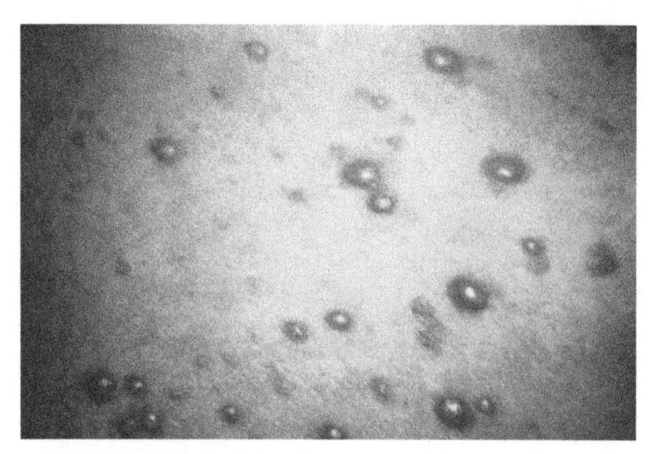

FIGURE 31.9 Herpes simplex virus type 2.

*Source*: Centers for Disease Control and Prevention/Dr. K.L. Herman. *Public health image library*. https://phil.cdc.gov/Details.aspx?pid=5407

of transmission of infection to the fetus, manifesting as ophthalmia neonatorum, pharyngitis, arthritis, and gonococcemia (Ghanem, 2020). Without early diagnosis and treatment in the neonate, infection can cause corneal ulceration, perforation, and blindness. Epidemiologic patterns indicate growing concern for widespread drug resistance, highlighting the significance of being familiar with surveillance data in the healthcare provider's practice region (Ghanem, 2020).

## GENITAL HERPES

Genital herpes is a common, recurrent, viral infection (Figure 31.9). Transmitted by skin-to-skin contact, genital herpes is most often a result of HSV-2 infection, though HSV-1 infection is increasing in genital herpes especially in younger females and males having sex with males (Albrecht, 2020b). Genital herpes occurs as a result of oral, anal, or vaginal sex. For information on the pathogenesis of HSVs, refer to chapter 19. Pregnant adolescent females may transmit the infection to their newborns via vaginal delivery. Complications of genital herpes infections include meningitis, proctitis, and sacral radiculitis (severe primary infection).

## TRICHOMONIASIS

Trichomoniasis infection (or "trich") is caused by the anaerobic, flagellated protozoan parasite *Trichomoniasis vaginalis*. It is transmitted via vaginal-penile intercourse or vulva-to-vulva contact. Trichomoniasis infection during pregnancy places the adolescent at risk for premature rupture of membranes, preterm labor, and delivery of a low birth weight infant. HIV transmission rates are increased in the presence of trichomoniasis infection.

## SYPHILIS

Syphilis is a chronic STI caused by infection with *Treponema pallidum*. The spirochete enters the skin through microscopic breaks in the skin during sexual intercourse, though infection may also occur with kissing, biting, or oral-genital sex (Fantasia, 2017). Syphilis infection consists of four stages: primary, secondary, latent, and tertiary. Complications include meningitis, paresis, tabes dorsalis, and meningovascular syphilis. The spirochete crosses the placenta, so newborns of mothers infected with syphilis may experience congenital syphilis infection or neurosyphilis.

### Subjective Findings

The health history may reveal the symptoms listed in Table 31.2.

**TABLE 31.2 Common STI Symptoms**

| Chlamydia | Gonorrhea | Herpes | Syphilis | Trichomoniasis |
|---|---|---|---|---|
| Dysuria<br>Urinary frequency<br>Eye drainage (newborn) | Vaginal pruritis<br>Mucopurulent vaginal or penile discharge | Painful urination<br>Painful, burning rash or paresthesia in and around the genital region | Chancre at point of entry | Most are asymptomatic<br>Vaginal or penile discharge<br>Dysuria, urgency and frequency of urination |

STI, sexually transmitted infection

*Sources*: Data from Albrecht, M. A. (2020b). Epidemiology, clinical manifestations, and diagnosis of genital herpes simplex viral infection. *UpToDate*. https://www.uptodate.com/contents/epidemiology-clinical-manifestations-and-diagnosis-of-genital-herpes-simplex-virus-infection; Fantasia, H. C. (2017). Sexually transmitted infections. In K. D. Schuiling & F. E. Likis (Eds.), *Women's gynecologic health* (3rd ed., pp. 17–35). Jones & Bartlett Learning; Ghanem, K. G. (2020). Clinical manifestations and diagnosis of Neisseria gonorrheae in adults and adolescents. *UpToDate*. https://www.uptodate.com/contents/clinical-manifestations-and-diagnosis-of-neisseria-gonorrhoeae-infection-in-adults-and-adolescents; Hammerschlag, M. R. (2018). Chlamydia trachomatis infections in the newborn. *UpToDate*. https://www.uptodate.com/contents/chlamydia-trachomatis-infections-in-the-newborn; Hsu, K. (2019a). Clinical manifestations and diagnosis of chlamydia trachomatis infections. *UpToDate*. https://www.uptodate.com/contents/clinical-manifestations-and-diagnosis-of-chlamydia-trachomatis-infections.

## Risk Factors

The most common risk factors for STIs in children and adolescents are:

- Perinatal exposure to a mother with a history of *Chlamydia, Gonorrhea,* genital herpes, or syphilis
- Having a new sex partner
- Having more than one sex partner, a sex partner who has multiple partners, or a partner with a history of STIs
- Inconsistent use of condoms with nonmonogamous partners
- Having a previous or current history of STI
- Exchanging sex for money or drugs
- Being a male having sex with other males (including sexual abuse)

## Review of Systems

The most common manifestations revealed during the review of systems include:

*Chlamydia*

- **Constitutional:** absence of or low-grade fever (newborn), pain (if abdominal or pelvic, suspect PID in females)
- **HEENT:** eye drainage or thick nasal secretions (newborn)
- **Respiratory:** cough (newborn)
- **Genitourinary:** unilateral testicular tenderness or pain with ejaculation in males

*Gonorrhea*

- **Constitutional:** abdominal pain (increased suspicion for PID)
- **HEENT:** eyelid edema (newborn), sore throat
- **Gastrointestinal:** symptoms of proctitis (cramping rectal pain [tenesmus]), anorectal pain, rectal fullness, constipation, anorectal bleeding, mucopurulent anal discharge
- **Genitourinary:** dysuria, urinary frequency or hesitancy, unilateral testicular pain or swelling
- **Reproductive:** intermenstrual bleeding, menorrhagia, pain with sexual intercourse (increased suspicion for PID)

*Herpes*

- **Constitutional:** fever, malaise

*Syphilis*

- Primary
  - **Integumentary:** chancre
- Secondary
  - **Integumentary:** lesions on palms of hands and soles of feet
- Tertiary
  - **Constitutional:** weakness
  - **Musculoskeletal:** weakness

*Trichomoniasis*

- **Integumentary:** vulvar pruritus
- **Genitourinary:** vaginal or penile discharge

## Objective Findings

The physical examination of the child with chlamydia, gonorrhea, genital herpes, syphilis, and trichomoniasis may reveal symptoms shown in Table 31.3.

**TABLE 31.3 Symptoms of Common STI Exams**

| Chlamydia | Gonorrhea | Herpes | Syphilis | Trichomoniasis |
|---|---|---|---|---|
| *In the newborn:*<br>■ Mild to severe swelling of eyelids with a watery or mucopurulent discharge<br>■ Staccato cough, paroxysms, tachypnea, crackles, mild to moderate hypoxemia<br>In the older child or adolescent:<br>■ Cervical motion tenderness<br>■ Adnexal tenderness | *In the newborn:*<br>■ Conjunctivitis with eyelid edema and discharge<br>*In the older child or adolescent:*<br>■ Cervical discharge<br>■ Friable cervical mucosa<br>■ Abdominal, uterine, adnexal, or cervical motion tenderness with palpation (high suspicion for PID) | *In the older child or adolescent:*<br>■ 2–3 mm clusters of vesicles with surrounding erythema and edema on the shaft of the penis, prepuce, or glans penis (male) and labia minora, labia majora, or mons (female)<br>■ Inguinal lymphadenopathy | *Primary:*<br>■ Chancre on vulva, vagina, cervix, penis, or at any site of entry<br>*Secondary:*<br>■ Lymphadenopathy<br>■ Localized or diffuse mucocutaneous lesions on palms of hands and soles of feet.<br>*Tertiary:*<br>■ Neuromuscular development issues | ■ Erythema, edema, excoriation of vulva<br>■ Red speckles (strawberry spots) on vagina or cervix<br>■ Homogenous, watery, yellowish-green discharge<br>■ Vaginal pH >5.0<br>■ Cervix may bleed when touched |

STI, sexually transmitted infection

*Sources*: Data from Albrecht, M. A. (2020b). Epidemiology, clinical manifestations, and diagnosis of genital herpes simplex viral infection. *UpToDate*. https://www.uptodate.com/contents/epidemiology-clinical-manifestations-and-diagnosis-of-genital-herpes-simplex-virus-infection; Fantasia, H. C. (2017). Sexually transmitted infections. In K. D. Schuiling & F. E. Likis (Eds.), *Women's gynecologic health* (3rd ed., pp. 17–35). Jones & Bartlett Learning; Ghanem, K. G. (2020). Clinical manifestations and diagnosis of *Neisseria gonorrheae* in adults and adolescents. *UpToDate*. https://www.uptodate.com/contents/clinical-manifestations-and-diagnosis-of-neisseria-gonorrhoeae-infection-in-adults-and-adolescents; Hammerschlag, M. R. (2018). Chlamydia trachomatis infections in the newborn. *UpToDate*. https://www.uptodate.com/contents/chlamydia-trachomatis-infections-in-the-newborn; Hsu, K. (2019a). Clinical manifestations and diagnosis of chlamydia trachomatis infections. *UpToDate*. https://www.uptodate.com/contents/clinical-manifestations-and-diagnosis-of-chlamydia-trachomatis-infections.

Adolescent females who are experiencing symptoms of PID (see chapter 29) should have a complete cervical evaluation to determine upper vaginal tract involvement.

## Laboratory/Diagnostic Testing

With chlamydia infection, the urinalysis may demonstrate pyuria and a leukocyte esterase test may be positive. Nucleic acid amplification testing, via vaginal swab in adolescent females and a first-catch urine specimen in male adolescents, is the diagnostic method of choice for identifying *C. trachomatis* or *N. gonorrhea* infection (Ghanem, 2020; Hsu, 2019a). In a neonate with *Chlamydia pneumoniae*, hyperinflation with bilateral, symmetrical interstitial infiltrates will be observed on chest x-ray.

Herpes infection may be confirmed with a positive viral culture of vesicular fluid obtained from the base of the vesicle or ulcer. PCR assay for HSV is the most sensitive test (Albrecht, 2020b).

For suspected syphilis, serologic testing with the highly sensitive venereal disease research laboratory test is used for screening. If positive, the fluorescent treponemal antibody absorption test can determine the presence of antibodies to *Treponema palladium.*

In the female with suspected trichomoniasis, a pelvic examination or self-swab may be used. Testing will yield a vaginal pH of >5.0 with trichomonads seen on a wet prep. A urethral swab is used in males. The definitive test is positive culture for *Trichomoniasis vaginalis.*

**PRO TIP** Having an adolescent woman swab her own vagina can be empowering and much less intimidating. Educate the patient to place nucleic acid amplification test (NAAT) swabs inside the vagina and make a "figure 8" motion to collect the specimen. If the individual is uncomfortable, a speculum examination can be done and the NP can collect the specimen.

## Differential Diagnosis

The differential diagnosis for chlamydia and/or gonorrhea includes:

- Trichomonas vaginalis
- Mycoplasma dentalium
- HSV
- Syphilis
- Testicular torsion (*Gonorrhea*)

For gonorrhea, the differential diagnosis may include chlamydial infection; for *Chlamydia trachomatis* infection, the differential diagnosis may include gonorrhea.

The differential diagnosis for genital herpes includes:

- Behçet syndrome
- Chancroid
- Fungal infection
- Granuloma inguinale
- Lymphogranuloma venereum
- Neoplasm
- Sexual trauma
- Syphilis

The differential diagnosis for trichomoniasis includes:

- Bacterial vaginosis
- Candidiasis
- Trauma from foreign body

The differential diagnosis for syphilis includes:

- Genital carcinoma
- Trauma (skin wound)

## Treatment/Management Plan

All cases of chlamydia, gonorrhea, and syphilis must be reported to the local health department. For all STIs, all partners should be evaluated and treated.

### Medications to Treat STIs

Medications for the treatment of STIs are listed in Table 31.4.

**TABLE 31.4 Pharmacological Treatment of STIs**

| Chlamydia | Gonorrhea | Genital Herpes | Syphilis | Trichomoniasis |
|---|---|---|---|---|
| Azithromycin 1 gm orally as a one-time dose<br>OR<br>Doxycycline (avoid in second and third trimesters of pregnancy)<br>OR<br>Amoxicillin<br>OR<br>Erythromycin | Ceftriaxone 250 mg IM<br>AND<br>Azithromycin 1 gm orally as a one-time dose | Acyclovir 400 mg orally three times a day for 7–10 days (first clinical episode) | Benthazine penicillin G 2.4 million units IM as a single dose | Metronidazole 2 gm orally as a one-time dose<br>STIs, sexually transmitted infections. |

STIs, sexually transmitted infections. (Workowski & Bolan, 2015)

Workowski, K. A., & Bolan, G. A. (2015). Sexually transmitted diseases treatment guidelines, 2015. *Morbidity and Mortality Weekly Report—Recommendations and Reports, 64*(RR3), 1–137. https://www.ncbi.nlm.nih.gov/pmc/articles/PMC5885289

Oral erythromycin or azithromycin is the recommended treatment for neonatal Chlamydia pneumonia and conjunctivitis (Hammerschlag, 2018). The CDC recommends treatment for both chlamydia and gonorrhea when gonorrhea testing is positive, and chlamydia infection has not been ruled out (St. Cyr et al., 2020).

## Family Education

Teach the family:

- Adolescents and pregnant patients should adhere to the treatment plan and abstain from sexual activity until 7 days after starting treatment, and once sexual partners have been treated.
- Inform adolescent females with Chlamydia infection they should be screened for pregnancy, especially considering doxycycline toxicity to a fetus.
- Offer testing for other STIs, as they are at increased risk for contracting other diseases.
- Teach safe sex practices.
- Counsel adolescents and pregnant clients about the importance of adhering to the treatment plan and abstaining from sexual activity until 7 days after starting treatment, and once sexual partners have been treated.
- Patients should notify all sexual contacts within the past 60 days, and it is recommended that these partners also receive evaluation and treatment for gonorrhea infection (Seña & Cohen, 2021)
- Educate that there is no cure for genital herpes, but that treatment may suppress the ulcer.

## Referral

Refer all females with genital herpes, PID, or syphilis to a women's health specialist. All pregnant adolescents with PID must be hospitalized for intravenous therapy.

# TICK-BORNE INFECTIONS

Tick-borne infections are diseases caused by infectious agents that are transmitted directly from ticks (as vectors) to humans. Young children are at particular risk for contracting tick-borne diseases, as they are unaware of the health risks around them. The immature immune system of the younger child results in a decreased capacity to resist tick-borne diseases. Many times the child with Lyme disease or RMSF may initially present with nonspecific symptoms.

## LYME DISEASE

Lyme disease is a tick-borne illness caused primarily in the United States by *Borrelia burgdorferi*, transmitted through a tick bite. The illness presents differently depending on the stage of the disease process. The disease process is categorized in three stages: early localized, early disseminated, and late disease (Shapiro, 2021).

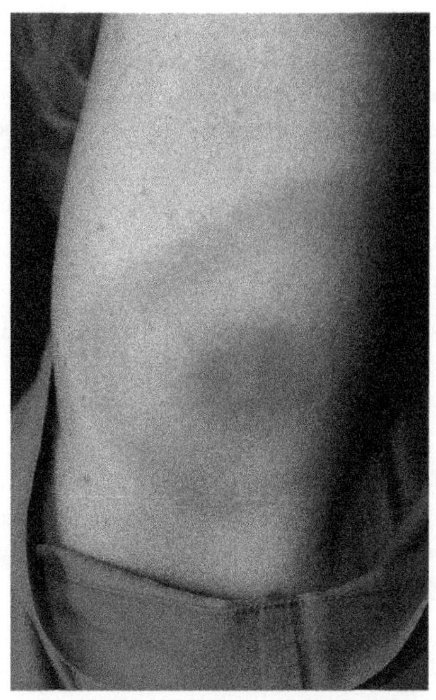

**FIGURE 31.10 Erythema migrans. Distinct bull's-eye appearance denotes stage 1 of Lyme disease.**

*Source*: Centers for Disease Control and Prevention/James Gathany.

The classical presentation of the disease is heralded with the appearance of erythema migrans (termed a bull's-eye rash due to a central clearance) in 89% of patients within 3 to 30 days after a tick bite during the early localized stage (Figure 31.10). Lyme disease most commonly presents as a homogenous erythematous rash, which begins as a red macule at the site of the tick bite, but may be found elsewhere on the body, and can be pruritic or burning but is seldom painful. The rash may progress with a vesicular or necrotic center due to an accelerated inflammatory response (Shapiro, 2021).

The early disseminated stage usually occurs weeks to several months after the tick bite. In this stage the organism has entered the bloodstream and disseminated into the tissues commonly affected: the central nervous system and heart. Extracutaneous systems are involved, and patients manifest with facial palsy, meningitis, and carditis.

Late disease presents months to years after the tick bite. Typically the disease during this stage manifests with intermittent or persistent arthritis in large joints, particularly in the knee (occurs in greater than 90% of patients; Shapiro, 2021).

Early diagnosis and treatment during the early localized phase is critical in preventing complications of the central nervous system and heart. Complications of the heart include carditis presenting with complete heart block (Shapiro, 2021).

## Subjective Findings

The health history may reveal:

- History of playing in or camping in the woods
- Rash
- Vague complaints of head or neck pain

### Risk Factors

The most common risk factor for Lyme disease is residing or playing in areas that are wooded or have high grass.

### Review of Systems

The most common manifestations revealed during the review of systems include:

- **Constitutional:** fever, fatigue, pain (headache or neck pain with early disseminated disease)
- **HEENT:** facial drooping (early disseminated)
- **Musculoskeletal:** arthralgia (late), myalgia (late), swollen and tender joint(s) (late)

## Objective Findings

The physical examination of the child with Lyme disease may reveal:

- Erythematous rash with central clearing
- Facial nerve palsy (unilateral or bilateral)

### Laboratory/Diagnostic Testing

Diagnosis of Lyme disease can be challenging to healthcare providers, as there is variability with the timing and characteristics of clinical manifestations. The healthcare provider's interpretation of cases suspected of Lyme disease must consider the regions that are endemic to Lyme disease, and seasonal implications; Lyme disease is more prevalent in the summer and fall months. Diagnosis of Lyme disease may be made on clinical presentation alone, especially in the case of a child who lives in or has traveled to an area that is endemic for Lyme disease, and is presenting with the characteristic erythema migrans rash. Serology is not required or recommended in the preceding case description, as the mounting of the antibody response may be delayed. A special circumstance when Lyme disease is strongly considered arises for the child presenting with multiple erythema migrans. There are a few specific cases when the diagnostic process is more involved. For example, for a child presenting with facial nerve involvement without a history of erythema migrans, serology may not be positive until several weeks after the onset of palsy. Therefore, it becomes extremely important for the healthcare provider to assess for the presence of symptoms related to meningitis, such as nuchal rigidity, papilledema, or severe headache. If the child presents with facial palsy and signs of meningitis with a diagnosis of Lyme disease, a lumbar puncture is warranted (Shapiro, 2021).

The testing algorithm employed in a child suspected of Lyme disease is two-pronged. A whole cell-based enzyme-linked immunosorbent assay (ELISA) or immunofluorescent assay (IFA) followed by a Western Blot test is recommended to confirm diagnosis. If the ELISA or IFA is negative, no further testing is warranted. Patients with a positive ELISA or IFA must have a positive Western Blot to confirm diagnosis. Alternatively, if the Western Blot is negative and the ELISA or IFA is positive, Lyme disease is not confirmed. It is important to keep in mind that antibodies may persist for years after Lyme disease is treated and cured; therefore, testing for Lyme disease is not recommended in the absence of clinical disease (Hu, 2019).

## Differential Diagnosis

The differential diagnosis for Lyme disease includes:

- Erythema multiforme
- Nummular eczema
- Tinea corporis
- Cellulitis
- Granuloma annulare
- Spider bite

## Treatment/Management Plan

In children 8 years and older, prescribe doxycycline for a 14- to 21-day course of therapy. Pregnant adolescents and children under 8 years of age should receive amoxicillin (Meissner, 2017).

### Family Education

Teach the family:

- Complete the entire course of drug therapy to prevent disseminated disease.
- Symptoms largely improve within 20 days following the initiation of treatment, although some symptoms

may persist for months and usually resolve within 6 months.

- Testing of the tick is not required.
- Check children for ticks following outdoor activities in wooded areas, especially in areas endemic to Lyme disease.
- Apply DEET (N, N-diethyl-m-toluamide), which contains tick repellent, on children older than 2 months old.
- Oil of lemon eucalyptus, also known as P-menthane diol (PMD) is a plant-based repellent that gives protection time similar to low concentrations of DEET-containing products. It is not recommended for children less than 3 years old (Hu, 2019).
- Doxycycline is associated with photosensitivity; use sun protection measures such as sunscreen, hats, and long-sleeved shirts (Sexton & McClain, 2021).

## ROCKY MOUNTAIN SPOTTED FEVER

RMSF is caused by an aerobic gram-negative bacterium, *Rickettsia rickettsii*, transmitted through a tick bite (usually a wood tick or dog tick). RMSF occurs throughout the United States, most concentrated in the southeastern and south-central states, and during the spring and early summer months. RMSF presents with symptoms within 2 to 14 days in an infected child. Symptoms are usually abrupt and may range from mild to disseminated disease; therefore, prompt diagnosis and early treatment are critical to reducing risk of mortality and morbidity. Rash occurs in approximately 88% to 90% of patients (Sexton & McClain, 2021).

### Subjective Findings

The health history may reveal a history of fever or rash (Figure 31.11).

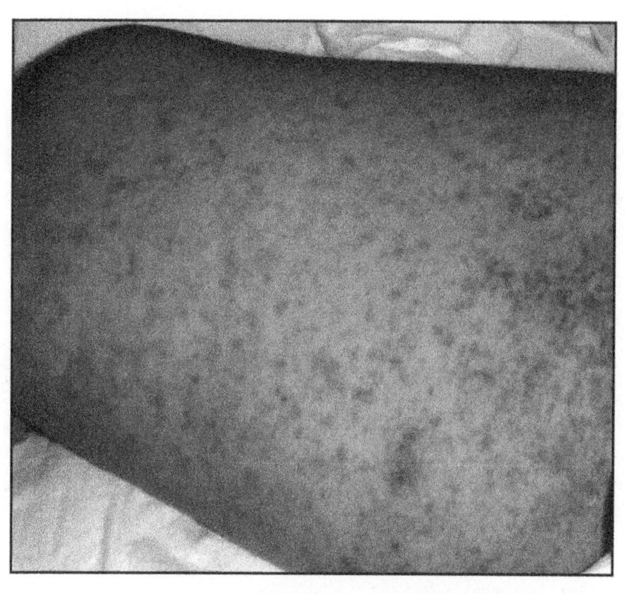

FIGURE 31.11 Maculopapular rash with central petechiae associated with Rocky Mountain spotted fever.

*Source*: CDC. https://www.cdc.gov/mmwr/volumes/65/rr/rr6502a1.htm#F20_down

### Risk Factors

The most common risk factors for RMSF are:

- Residing or playing in areas that are wooded or have high grass
- Exposure to dogs
- American Indian ethnicity

### Review of Systems

The most common manifestations revealed during the review of systems include:

- **Constitutional:** fever, malaise, abdominal pain
- **Integumentary:** rash
- **Gastrointestinal:** nausea with or without emesis
- **Musculoskeletal:** myalgia, arthralgia
- **Neurologic:** severe headache

### Objective Findings

The physical examination of the child with RMSF may reveal:

- Conjunctival erythema
- Blanching erythematous rash with macules (1 to 4 mm) progressing to petechiae beginning on the ankles and wrists, spreading to trunk
- Pedal edema
- Abnormal mentation
- Seizures (late)
- Cranial nerve palsies (late)
- Transient deafness (late)

### Laboratory/Diagnostic Testing

The diagnosis of RMSF is based upon the clinical findings. No laboratory or diagnostic testing is needed.

### Differential Diagnosis

The differential diagnosis for RMSF includes:

- Drug rash
- Meningococcal meningitis

### Treatment/Management Plan

Antimicrobial therapy should be initiated early, ideally within 5 days of symptom onset. Doxycycline is the preferred treatment and has been endorsed by the AAP for treatment in children and pregnant adolescents. It should be administered for 3 days after the patient has become afebrile. Doxycycline can cause teeth staining in children younger than 8 years old; however, studies have shown that dental staining did not occur in permanent teeth when short courses of antibiotic therapy were administered. Children with mild illness will show improvement 48 to 72 hours after initiation of treatment. Children with severe illness will show improvement 5 days after initiation of treatment (Sexton & McClain, 2019).

### Family Education

Teach the family:

- Complete the entire course of drug therapy.
- Symptoms largely improve within 3 days following the initiation of treatment.
- Testing of the tick is not required.
- Check children for ticks following outdoor activities in wooded areas, especially in areas endemic to Lyme disease.
- Apply DEET (N, N-diethyl-m-toluamide), which contains tick repellent, on children older than 2 months old.
- Oil of lemon eucalyptus, also known as PMD, is a plant-based repellent that gives protection time similar to low concentrations of DEET-containing products. It is not recommended for children under 3 years old (Hu, 2019).
- Doxycycline is associated with photosensitivity; use sun protection measures such as sunscreen, hats, and long sleeve shirts (Sexton & McClain, 2019).

### Referral

Children with mild illness may be treated safely as outpatients; however, children with severe disease must be hospitalized.

## FEVER

Fever is a common reason for children to visit the primary care provider. *Fever* is defined as a rectal temperature of 38 degrees Celsius (100 °F) or greater in children younger than 3 months old. The etiology of the fever can be a viral infection, bacterial infection, or related to an immunodeficiency. Human rhinovirus, RSV, influenza, and parainfluenza are among the common viral pathogens that affect young children. *Escherichia coli* and group B *Streptococcus* are the most common bacterial pathogens affecting infants younger than 3 months old. Other bacterial pathogens to consider include *S. aureus*, *Streptococcus pneumoniae*, *Salmonella* species, *Enterococcus faecalis*, *Enterobacter cloacae*, *Moraxella catarrhalis*, *Klebsiella* species, and *Citrobacter* species.

Neonates, infants 28 days and younger, have a greater risk for invasive bacterial disease. Invasive bacterial disease includes bacteremia/sepsis, bacterial meningitis, bacterial pneumonia, skin and soft tissue infections, osteomyelitis, bacterial gastroenteritis, septic arthritis, or urinary tract infection (UTI; Smitherman & Macias, 2021).

## FEVER WITHOUT A SOURCE (IN THE CHILD YOUNGER THAN 3 MONTHS)

Management of infants with fever is dependent on appearance, clinical symptoms, and evidence of risk factors. Neonates 28 days old and younger need a full evaluation for sepsis, as they are particularly at risk for HSV, meningitis, bacteremia/sepsis, or UTI. UTI is the predominant illness caused by bacterial infection in infants younger than 3 months of age (Smitherman & Macias, 2021).

### Subjective Findings

The health history may reveal presence of fever, lack of other symptoms, and lack of known exposure to sick individuals. Ascertain the immunization status. The healthcare provider must also ask about exposure to sick contacts and symptoms such as rhinorrhea, cough, wheeze, vomiting, diarrhea, blood or mucus in the stool, or rash (Smitherman & Macias, 2021). These additional symptoms may lead the provider to an alternative diagnosis and reason for the fever.

### Review of Systems

It is important for the healthcare provider to obtain medical history about the infant, household contacts, and mother to determine the source of infection. The most common manifestations revealed during the review of systems include:

- **Constitutional:** poor feeding, increased sleepiness
- **Neurologic:** lethargy, irritability

## Risk Factors

The most common risk factors for invasive bacterial disease are:

- Infants younger than 28 days old
- Ill appearance
- Rectal temperature greater than 38.6 °C (101.5 °F)
- Unimmunized against pneumococcal and *Haemophilus influenzae* type B infections
- Prematurity
- Infants who require respiratory or parenteral nutritional support
- Maternal history of group B streptococcus, genital herpes chlamydia, or gonorrhea
- Maternal prolonged rupture of membranes or intrapartal fever
- Chromosomal or congenital anomaly

## Objective Findings

The physical examination of the child with fever and possible invasive bacterial disease may reveal clinical findings associated with acute suppurative otitis media, pneumonia, omphalitis, bacterial arthritis, osteomyelitis, cutaneous cellulitis or abscess, meningitis, HSV, or bronchiolitis (Smitherman & Macias, 2021).

## Laboratory/Diagnostic Testing

A full sepsis laboratory workup is warranted for all infants:

- Who are ill-appearing
- Younger than 28 days old
- Who are highly suspicious for herpes infection (i.e., mucocutaneous vesicles, seizures, focal neurologic findings, history of maternal herpes infection)
- Infants 29 to 60 days old:
  - With a rectal temperature greater than 38.6 °C
  - History of congenital or chromosomal abnormalities
  - Who require respiratory or parenteral nutritional support
  - Who have received antibiotic therapy in the past 3 to 7 days
- Infants 29 to 90 days old with a focal infection and abnormal white blood cell count, absolute band count, inflammatory markers, or urinalysis

A full sepsis laboratory workup includes the following diagnostic tests:

- Complete blood count (CBC) with differential
- Blood or serum glucose (to permit comparison with CSF glucose)
- Inflammatory markers (e.g., PCT and C-reactive protein [CRP], if rapidly available [i.e., within 60 minutes])
- Blood culture
- Urinalysis
- Urine culture (by bladder catheterization or suprapubic aspiration)
- Chest radiograph
- Stool culture in infants with diarrhea or stool containing blood or mucus
- CSF cell count with differential, glucose and protein, bacterial culture and gram stain, PCR as indicated based upon clinical risk:
  - Enterovirus studies during time of high prevalence or in patients with CSF pleocytosis
  - HSV in infants with clinical findings or increased risk of maternal HSV transmission
  - CSF for viral culture if there is pleocytosis; if there is a limited CSF sample, prioritize PCR over viral culture.
- Additional studies are often obtained for patients with signs of septic shock:
  - Prothrombin time (PT), partial thromboplastin time (aPTT), international normalized ratio (INR)
  - Fibrinogen and D-dimer
  - Serum lactate
  - Serum total bilirubin and alanine aminotransferase
  - Ionized calcium

Well-appearing infants 29 to 60 days old who do not have a focal bacterial infection, HSV symptoms, and other risk factors for invasive bacterial disease and a rectal temperature less than 38.6 °C (101.5 °F) should have the following diagnostic testing:

- CBC with differential
- PCT (only if results are rapidly available [i.e., within 60 minutes])
- CRP (only if results are rapidly available [i.e., within 60 minutes])
- Blood culture
- Urinalysis
- Urine culture (by transurethral bladder catheterization or suprapubic aspiration)
- Chest radiograph in patients with signs of respiratory illness (e.g., cough, tachypnea, or abnormal breath sounds)

Well-appearing infants 61 to 90 days old with a rectal temperature less than 38.6 °C (101.5 °F) should have a urinalysis with urine culture completed unless immunizations have not been administered; in the latter case a CBC with blood culture is also recommended (Smitherman & Macias, 2021).

### Family Education

Teach the family:

- In the infant younger than 90 days of age, a rectal temperature > 100.4 °F is considered a fever.
- If the infant has a fever, the infant should be seen by the healthcare provider.
- Do not give fever-reducing medications to infants less than 90 days of age unless instructed to do so by a healthcare provider.

## KEY POINTS

- The severity and outcome of infectious disease processes can vary, and are dependent on the host's defense mechanisms, age, population, and medical history (e.g., diabetes mellitus, diarrhea, or chemotherapy).
- Conducting a comprehensive health history is important in generating and prioritizing differential diagnoses for the child based on their presentation of symptoms and history. Information that the healthcare provider must obtain includes: history of present illness, medical history, current and recent medications, immunization history, family medical history, exposure history, nutrition/elimination history, and complete review of systems.
- Management of infants and children younger than 36 months old with fever is dependent on age, appearance, clinical symptoms, and evidence of risk factors. Neonates 28 days old and younger need a full evaluation for sepsis, as they are particularly at risk for HSV, meningitis, bacteremia/sepsis, or UTI.

## REFERENCES


Albrecht, M. A. (2019a). Clinical features of varicella-zoster virus infection: Chickenpox. *UpToDate*. https://www.uptodate.com/contents/clinical-features-of-varicella-zoster-virus-infection-chickenpox

Albrecht, M. A. (2019b). Epidemiology of varicella-zoster virus infection: Chickenpox. *UpToDate*. https://www.uptodate.com/contents/epidemiology-of-varicella-zoster-virus-infection-chickenpox

Albrecht, M. A. (2020a). Diagnosis of varicella zoster virus infection. *UpToDate*. https://www.uptodate.com/contents/diagnosis-of-varicella-zoster-virus-infection

Albrecht, M. A. (2020b). Epidemiology, clinical manifestations, and diagnosis of genital herpes simplex viral infection. *UpToDate*. https://www.uptodate.com/contents/epidemiology-clinical-manifestations-and-diagnosis-of-genital-herpes-simplex-virus-infection

Albrecht, M. A. (2020c). Mumps. UpToDate. https://www. *UpToDate*.com/contents/mumps

Albrecht, M. A. (2020d). Treatment of varicella (chickenpox) infection. *UpToDate*. https://www.uptodate.com/contents/treatment-of-varicella-chickenpox-infection

American Academy of Pediatrics. (2020a). *Immunizations*. https://www.aap.org/en-us/about-the-aap/aap-press-room/campaigns/immunizations/Pages/default.aspx

American Academy of Pediatrics. (2020b). *Recommendations for preventive pediatric healthcare*. https://downloads.aap.org/AAP/PDF/periodicity_schedule.pdf

Centers for Disease Control and Prevention. (2020). *Bartonella infection (cat scratch disease, trench fever, Carrion's disease): For healthcare providers*. https://www.cdc.gov/bartonella/clinicians/index.html

Centers for Disease Control and Prevention. (2020, April 2). *Vaccines and preventable diseases*. https://www.cdc.gov/vaccines/vpd/should-not-vacc.html.

Committee on Pediatric AIDS. (2011). Adolescents and HIV infection: The pediatrician's role in promoting routine testing. *Pediatrics, 128*(5), 1023–1029. https://doi.org/10.1542/peds.2011-1761

Dadonaite, B. (2019). *What are children dying from and what can we do about it?* https://ourworldindata.org/what-are-children-dying-from-and-what-can-we-do-about-it

Edwards, M. S. (2020). Rubella. *UpToDate*. https://www.uptodate.com/contents/rubella

Fantasia, H. C. (2017). Sexually transmitted infections. In K. D. Schuiling & F. E. Likis (Eds.), *Women's gynecologic health* (3rd ed., pp. 17–35). Jones & Bartlett Learning.

Fletcher, C. V. (2021). Overview of antiretroviral agents used to treat HIV. *UpToDate*. https://www.uptodate.com/contents/overview-of-antiretroviral-agents-used-to-treat-hiv

Flomenberg, P., & Kojaoghlanian, T. (2021). Pathogenesis, epidemiology, and clinical manifestations of adenovirus infection. *UpToDate*. https://www.uptodate.com/contents/pathogenesis-epidemiology-and-clinical-manifestations-of-adenovirus-infection

Gans, H., & Maldonado, Y. A. (2019). Measles: Clinical manifestations, diagnosis, treatment, and prevention. *UpToDate*. https://www.uptodate.com/contents/measles-clinical-manifestations-diagnosis-treatment-and-prevention

Ghanem, K. G. (2020). Clinical manifestations and diagnosis of Neisseria gonorrheae in adults and adolescents. *UpToDate*. https://www.uptodate.com/contents/clinical-manifestations-and-diagnosis-of-neisseria-gonorrhoeae-infection-in-adults-and-adolescents

Gillespie, S. L. (2019). Diagnostic testing for sax infection in infants and children younger than 18 months. *UpToDate*. https://www.uptodate.com/contents/diagnostic-testing-for-hiv-infection-in-infants-and-children-younger-than-18-months

Gillespie, S. L. (2021). Pediatric sax infection: Classification, clinical manifestations, and outcome. *UpToDate*. https://www.uptodate.com/contents/pediatric-hiv-infection-classification-clinical-manifestations-and-outcome

Hammerschlag, M. R. (2018). Chlamydia trachomatis infections in the newborn. *UpToDate*. https://www.uptodate.com/contents/chlamydia-trachomatis-infections-in-the-newborn

Healy, C. M. (2018). Cervical lymphadenitis in children: Diagnostic approach and initial management. *UpToDate.* https://www.uptodate.com/contents/cervical-lymphadenitis-in-children-diagnostic-approach-and-initial-management

Hsu, K. (2019a). Clinical manifestations and diagnosis of chlamydia trachomatis infections. *UpToDate.* https://www.uptodate.com/contents/clinical-manifestations-and-diagnosis-of-chlamydia-trachomatis-infections

Hsu, K. (2019b). Epidemiology of chlamydia trachomatis infections. *UpToDate.* https://www.uptodate.com/contents/epidemiology-of-chlamydia-trachomatis-infections

Hu, L. (2019). Diagnosis of Lyme disease. *UpToDate.* https://www.uptodate.com/contents/diagnosis-of-lyme-disease

Jordan, J. A. (2020). Microbiology, epidemiology, and pathogenesis of parvovirus B19 infection. *UpToDate.* https://www.uptodate.com/contents/microbiology-epidemiology-and-pathogenesis-of-parvovirus-b19-infection

Jordan, J. A. (2021a). Clinical manifestations and diagnosis of parvovirus B19 infection. *UpToDate.* https://www.uptodate.com/contents/clinical-manifestations-and-diagnosis-of-parvovirus-b19-infection

Jordan, J. A. (2021b). Treatment and prevention of parvovirusB19 infection. *UpToDate.* https://www.uptodate.com/contents/treatment-and-prevention-of-parvovirus-b19-infection

Meissner, H. C. (2017). Lyme disease. In T. K. McInerny, H. M. Adam, D. E. Campbell, J. M. Foy, & D. M. Kamat (Eds.), *American Academy of Pediatrics textbook of pediatric care* (2nd ed., Chapter 287). American Academy of Pediatrics.

Munoz, F. M., & Flomenberg, P. (2020). Diagnosis, treatment, and prevention of adenovirus infection. *UpToDate.* https://www.uptodate.com/contents/diagnosis-treatment-and-prevention-of-adenovirus-infection

National Association of Pediatric Nurse Practitioners. (2015). NAPNAP position statement on immunizations. *Journal of Pediatric Health Care, 29,* A11–A12. https://doi.org/10.1016/j.pedhc.2014.12.001

Nelson, C. A., Saha, S., & Mead, P. S. (2016). Cat-scratch disease in the United States, 2005–2013. *Emerging Infectious Diseases, 22*(10), 1741–1746. https://dx.doi.org/10.3201/eid2210.160115

Romero, J. R. (2020). Hand, foot, and mouth disease and herpangina. *UpToDate.* https://www.uptodate.com/contents/hand-foot-and-mouth-disease-and-herpangina

Sax, P. E. (2020). Screening and diagnostic testing for HIV infection. *UpToDate.* https://www.uptodate.com/contents/screening-and-diagnostic-testing-for-hiv-infection

Schwartz, D. A. (2019). Infectious and parasitic diseases. In E. Rubin & H. M. Reisner (Eds.), *Essentials of Rubin's pathology* (7th ed., pp. 175–217). Wolters Kluwer.

Seña, A. C., & Cohen, M. S. (2021). Treatment of uncomplicated Neisseria gonorrheae infections. *UpToDate.* https://www.uptodate.com/contents/treatment-of-uncomplicated-neisseria-gonorrhoeae-infections

Sexton, D. J., & McClain, M. T. (2019). Treatment of Rocky Mountain spotted fever. *UpToDate.* https://www.uptodate.com/contents/treatment-of-rocky-mountain-spotted-fever

Sexton, D. J., & McClain, M. T. (2021). Clinical manifestations and diagnosis of Rocky Mountain spotted fever. *UpToDate.* https://www.uptodate.com/contents/clinical-manifestations-and-diagnosis-of-rocky-mountain-spotted-fever

Shapiro, E. D. (2021). Lyme disease: Clinical manifestations in children. *UpToDate.* https://www.uptodate.com/contents/lyme-disease-clinical-manifestations-in-children

Smitherman, H. F., & Macias, C. G. (2021). Febrile infant (younger than 90 days of age): Outpatient evaluation. *UpToDate.* https://www.uptodate.com/contents/febrile-infant-younger-than-90-days-of-age-outpatient-evaluation

St. Cyr, S., Barbee, L., Workowski, K.A., Bachmann, L. H., Pham, C., Schlanger, K., Torrone, E., Weinstock, H., Kersh, E. N., & Thorpe, P. (2020). Update to CDC's treatment guidelines for gonococcal infection, 2020. *MMWR Morbidity and Mortality Weekly Report,* 69(50), 1911–1916. https://www.cdc.gov/mmwr/volumes/69/wr/mm6950a6.htm?s_cid=mm6950a6_w

Tremblay, C., & Brady, M. T. (2019). Roseola infantum (exanthem subitem). *UpToDate.* https://www.uptodate.com/contents/roseola-infantum-exanthem-subitum

U.S. Preventive Services Task Force. (2019). *Final recommendation statement Chlamydia and Gonorrhea: Screening.* https://www.uspreventiveservicestaskforce.org/Page/Document/RecommendationStatementFinal/chlamydia-and-gonorrhea-screening

# Management of Immune and Rheumatic Disorders

Paula Barbel and Danielle R. Stratton

## Student Learning Objectives

Upon completion of this chapter the reader should be able to:

1. Discuss pathophysiology and epidemiology of selected immune and rheumatic disorders in children.
2. Differentiate subjective and objective findings of selected immune and rheumatic disorders in children.
3. Choose appropriate laboratory or diagnostic tests for particular immune and rheumatic disorders in children.
4. Utilize the differential diagnosis process to determine diagnosis of immune or rheumatic disorders in children.
5. Determine treatment plan, child/family education, and need for referral in children with a(n) immune and rheumatic disorder.

## INTRODUCTION

Immune and rheumatic diseases do not occur frequently in children, but have a significant effect on the child's quality of life. They are generally expressed as the collection of symptoms and objective findings that mark the disease. Many immune and rheumatic disorders share similar results for laboratory testing, making the clinical findings even more important in the diagnostic process, although defined diagnostic criteria do exist for some of the disorders. The immune and rheumatic disorders discussed in this chapter include allergy, primary immunodeficiencies, autoimmune disease, and inflammatory disorders.

The content in this chapter maps to the following areas on the Pediatric Nursing Certification Board (PNCB) Pediatric Nurse Practitioner—Primary Care certification examination:

### CLINICAL PROBLEMS: IMMUNOLOGY/RHEUMATOLOGY

CONTENT AREAS:

**II. Assessment and Diagnosis**

**B. History and Physical Examination**

1. Obtain history of present illness
2. Obtain a comprehensive health history for new patients
3. Complete an interval history for established patients
4. Perform a review of systems
5. Perform a complete physical examination

**C. Diagnostic Testing and Screening**

1. Order and interpret office/clinic based screening tests
2. Order and interpret diagnostic laboratory tests
3. Order and interpret the results of diagnostic imaging tests

**D. Analyzing Information**

1. Integrate health history and physical examination findings into the plan of care
2. Assimilate findings from screening and diagnostic testing into plan of care

**E. Diagnosis**

1. Develop and prioritize differential diagnoses
2. Establish a diagnosis based on evaluation of patient data

## III. Management

### A. Child and Caregiver Counseling and Education

1. Provide condition-specific counseling and education, including treatment options
2. Educate about benefits and potential adverse reactions of pharmacological interventions
3. Discuss non-pharmacological interventions
4. Counsel regarding the threshold for seeking follow-up care
5. Review the risks of non-adherence to recommended treatment

### B. Therapeutic Interventions

1. Prescribe pharmacologic agents
2. Recommend the use of over-the-counter pharmacologic agents
3. Order or recommend non-pharmacologic treatments for the management of symptoms
4. Discuss use of complementary and alternative therapies as appropriate

### C. Procedures

1. Perform procedures in accordance with diagnostic guidelines and plan of care (rapid tests)
2. Initiate life-saving techniques in response to urgent or emergent situations

### D. Collaboration and Referral

2. Refer to specialists as indicated for evaluation, counseling, and/or treatment

### E. Care Coordination

1. Facilitate patient and family-centered care for children of all ages with acute and chronic conditions

### F. Evaluation and Follow-up

2. Establish a plan for follow-up care

## IV. Professional Role Responsibilities

### A. Leadership and Evidence-based Practice

4. Develop, implement, and/or modify clinical practice guidelines

# ANATOMY AND PHYSIOLOGY

In children, the spleen is functional at birth and the thymus is quite enlarged at birth, remaining so until about 10 years of age, then involuting slowly throughout later childhood and adulthood. As maternal T cells do not cross the placenta, the fetal thymus begins production of T cells early in gestation, and cellular immunity does not cross the placenta. Delayed hypersensitivity reactions are mediated by T cells rather than antibodies, and skin test responses are diminished until about 1 year of age, as the infant demonstrates a decreased ability to mount an inflammatory response. Because the fetus is normally in an antigen-free environment, only trace amounts of immunoglobulins (specifically immunoglobulin M [IgM]) are produced. The newborn acquires immunoglobulin G (IgG) transplacentally from the mother. Over the first months of life, as the transplacental IgG is catabolized, these levels wane over time and result in a physiologic hypogammaglobulinemia between 2 and 6 months of age until self-production of IgG reaches higher levels. Immunoglobulins A, D, E, and M do not cross the placenta, requiring an antigenic challenge for production.

# ALLERGY

An immune-mediated response to a foreign substance resulting in an adverse physiologic reaction, allergy is a common reason for primary care visits in pediatrics, and affects up to 25% of the population in developed countries (Covar et al., 2020). The most frequent etiologic factors include medications, infections, food, immunizations, and malignancies (Paller & Mancini, 2016). The skin is a common organ of involvement, especially in medication and infectious hypersensitivity reactions.

The extent of an allergic response is determined by environmental and host factors as well as the duration, rate, and amount of exposure to the allergen. In IgE-mediated allergy, the allergic response involves antigen-specific IgE antibodies. When the antibody encounters the antigen (allergen), rapid cell activation occurs, with cytokines and potent mediators being released. The atopic disorders (asthma, allergic rhinitis, and atopic dermatitis) are discussed in chapter 33. Food and sting allergy, as well as erythema multiforme (EM), drug eruptions, and urticaria, are further discussed in this chapter.

## FOOD ALLERGY

Food allergy can lead to significant medical complications and affects about 8% of children (Covar et al., 2020). For younger children, the most common food allergens are milk, soy, eggs, wheat, peanuts and tree nuts, fish and shellfish. Older children and adults may have lifelong allergy, most often to peanuts/tree nuts, fish, and shellfish (Volkman & Chiu, 2019). Usually occurring within minutes of exposure, reactions may

BOX 32.1 **Latex Allergy**

An IgE-mediated response to exposure to latex that is common in gloves in healthcare settings occurs in some children. These children must avoid exposure to latex due to the risk of anaphylaxis. Screen all children for latex allergy. Foods with cross-reactivity to latex include apple, apricot, avocado, banana, carrot, celery, cherry, chestnut, fig, grape, kiwi, melon, nectarine, papaya, passion fruit, pear, peach, plum, pineapple, potato, and tomato. Instruct the family of a child with latex allergy to avoid those foods. The CDC's latex allergy prevention guide is available at www.cdc.gov/niosh/docs/98-113/pdfs/98-113.pdf?id=10.26616/NIOSH-PUB98113

also occur up to 2 hours after ingestion. There is also cross-reactivity of certain foods and latex, which can cause allergy in some children, as shown in Box 32.1.

## Subjective Findings

The health history may reveal:

- Ingestion of a known or unknown allergen
- Hives
- Itching

### Risk Factors

The most common risk factor for food allergy is personal or family history of atopic disease.

### Review of Systems

The most common manifestations revealed during the review of systems include:

- **Integumentary:** flushing, hives
- **HEENT:** facial swelling, throat or mouth itching, runny nose
- **Gastrointestinal:** abdominal pain, vomiting, diarrhea

## Objective Findings

The physical examination of the child with food allergy may reveal:

- Erythema and/or edema of the lips, oral cavity, and face
- Hives
- Nasal congestion

▶ ALERT: Swelling of the tongue, uvula, or pharynx may indicate upper airway swelling not visible on examination. Wheezing may be an ominous sign and anaphylaxis should be considered.

### Laboratory/Diagnostic Testing

Prick skin testing may reveal the food allergen. Additional testing should be determined by the pediatric allergist.

## Treatment/Management Plan

Avoidance of the food allergen has long been the mainstay of treatment for food allergy. Reintroduction of the food should occur at a time determined by the specialist. Some children and adolescents may need to carry an epinephrine auto-injector for avoidance of prophylaxis. Prescribe epinephrine to be administered intramuscularly, at the following doses:

- 7.5 kg to <15 kg: 0.1 mg
- 15 kg to <30 kg: 0.15 mg
- ≥30 kg: 0.3 mg (Lexicomp, 2020)

The dose may be repeated once if anaphylactic symptoms persist. Implement an anaphylaxis action plan with the child and family (Exhibit 32.1).

New guidelines related to peanut introduction were introduced recently by the National Institute of Allergy and Infectious Diseases and have been endorsed by the American Academy of Pediatrics. Rather than avoiding peanut introduction in the first year of life, with research demonstrating decreased incidence of peanut allergy development, it is now recommended that peanuts be introduced during the first year (Sicherer, 2017). Introduce peanut-containing foods in a developmentally appropriate manner (powdered food additive, pureed in smoothie, etc.) according to these guidelines:

- Infants without eczema or any food allergy: age-appropriate introduction and cultural preference
- Infants with mild to moderate eczema: around 6 months
- Infants with severe eczema, egg allergy, or both: around 4 to 6 months depending upon results of peanut-specific IgE or skin prick test (Sicherer, 2017)

### Family Education

Teach the following:

- The majority of childhood food allergies are lost over time, although the precise time cannot be predicted.

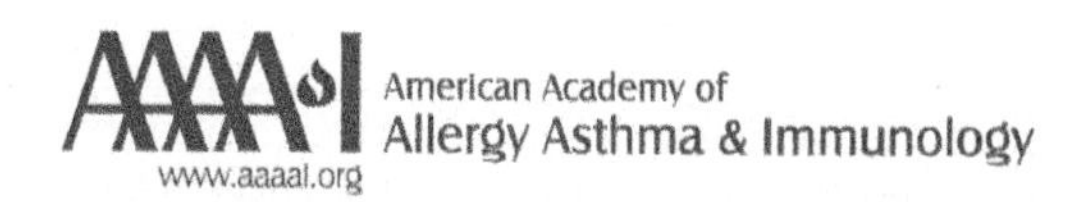


# Anaphylaxis Emergency Action Plan

**Patient Name:** ______________________________ **Age:** __________

**Allergies:** ______________________________

**Asthma** ☐ **Yes *(high risk for severe reaction)*** ☐ **No**

**Additional health problems besides anaphylaxis:** ______________________________

______________________________

**Concurrent medications:** ______________________________

______________________________

**Symptoms of Anaphylaxis**

| | |
|---|---|
| MOUTH | itching, swelling of lips and/or tongue |
| THROAT* | itching, tightness/closure, hoarseness |
| SKIN | itching, hives, redness, swelling |
| GUT | vomiting, diarrhea, cramps |
| LUNGS* | shortness of breath, cough, wheeze |
| HEART* | weak pulse, dizziness, passing out |

***Only a few symptoms may be present. Severity of symptoms can change quickly.***
****Some symptoms can be life-threatening. ACT FAST!***

## Emergency Action Steps - DO NOT HESITATE TO GIVE EPINEPHRINE!

1. **Inject epinephrine in thigh using (check one):**

☐ **0.1 mg (16.5 lbs to less than 33 lbs) Specify brand:** ______________________

☐ **0.15 mg (33 lbs to less than 66 lbs) Specify brand:** ______________________

☐ **0.3 mg (66 lbs or more) Specify brand:** ______________________

**IMPORTANT: ASTHMA INHALERS AND/OR ANTIHISTAMINES CAN'T BE DEPENDED ON IN ANAPHYLAXIS.**

**2. Call 911 or emergency medical services (before calling contact)**

**3. Emergency contact #1: home**__________ **work**__________ **cell**__________

**Emergency contact #2: home**__________ **work**__________ **cell**__________

**Emergency contact #3: home**__________ **work**__________ **cell**__________

**Comments:** ______________________________

______________________________

______________________________
**Doctor's Signature/Date/Phone Number**

______________________________
**Parent's Signature (for individuals under age 18 yrs)/Date**

This information is for general purposes and is not intended to replace the advice of a qualified health professional. For more information, visit www.aaaai.org.  9/2020

EXHIBIT 32.1 **Anaphylaxis Emergency Action Plan.**

*Source*: Reproduced with permission from the American Academy of Allergy, Asthma & Immunology, © 2020.

- Be vigilant when caring for the child with a food allergy.
- Read food labels to ensure that you know what the food contains, to avoid accidental ingestion.
- Have the child wear a medical alert bracelet for severe allergy.
- Make sure the child, the childcare center, and the school are aware of foods that should be avoided.
- Connect with food allergy networks for additional support:
  - Food Allergy & Anaphylaxis Connection Team: www.foodallergyawareness.org
  - Food Allergy Research & Education: www.foodallergy.org

### Referral

When there is concern about identification of the allergen, refer to the child to pediatric allergy/immunology for additional testing if needed. It may be helpful for the family to consult with a dietician experienced with food allergy.

## INSECT STING ALLERGY

Children and adolescents may also demonstrate an IgE-mediated response to insect stings, especially those from the Hymenoptera class (bees, wasps, ants, yellow jackets, hornets). A sting will usually result in a local reaction, but a systemic or anaphylactic reaction may also occur. In response to the insect's venom, a hypersensitivity response is triggered. Other insect bites are discussed in chapter 19.

### Subjective Findings

The health history will reveal a recent sting, of which the child is acutely aware.

#### Risk Factors

The risk factor for insect sting allergy is familial history of insect sting allergy.

#### Review of Systems

The most common manifestations revealed during the review of systems include:

- **Constitutional:** pain at the sting site
- **Integumentary:** edema at the sting site (possible erythema), pruritus
- **Respiratory:** difficulty breathing, chest tightness, (systemic reaction or anaphylaxis)

### Objective Findings

Note if the stinger remains. The physical examination of the child with allergy from an insect sting may reveal:

- Urticarial wheal
- Papular reaction
- Cellulitis appearance (large local reaction)
- With mild systemic reactions: flushing
- With severe systemic reactions: dyspnea, wheeze, hoarseness, hypotension, loss of consciousness

#### Laboratory/Diagnostic Testing

Skin testing is indicated for children with systemic reactions to insect stings.

### Differential Diagnosis

The differential diagnosis for insect sting includes insect bite.

### Treatment/Management Plan

Antihistamines may be useful for decreasing itching, and corticosteroids are helpful with larger reactions to decrease edema and inflammation. Any child with a previous anaphylactic reaction to a Hymenoptera sting should wear a medical alert bracelet and be prescribed an epinephrine autoinjector (see instructions in the preceding "Food Allergy" section).

#### Family Education

Teach the following:

- When a child is stung on an extremity, remove jewelry or constrictive clothing.
- Scrape away the stinger with a credit card or your fingernail (do not pull it out).
- Elevate the extremity and apply pressure intermittently.
- With future stings, to minimize the reaction, administer diphenhydramine as soon as possible.
- Teach children never to disturb an ant hill nor a bee or wasp nest.
- Prevent insect stings by wearing protective clothing and shoes when outdoors.
- Use insect repellents (with a maximum concentration of 30% n,n-diethyl-meta-toluamide [DEET] in infants and children older than 2 months; Stein & Barnett, 2017).

#### Referral

Children who experience severe systemic reactions and have a positive skin test should receive venom immunotherapy.

# ERYTHEMA MULTIFORME

EM is an uncommon, self-limited hypersensitivity reaction characterized by erythematous targetoid cutaneous lesions with or without mucosal ulcerations. Only 20% of cases occur in the pediatric population (Paller & Mancini, 2016). In children, the most common precipitating factors include infections and medications. Herpes simplex virus (HSV) and *Mycoplasma pneumoniae* are the most frequently encountered infectious etiologies, while antibiotics (especially penicillins) are the most frequently implicated medications (Zoghaib et al., 2019). There are two forms of EM: major (involving both skin and mucosal surfaces) and minor (sparing mucosal surfaces). The diagnosis is typically based on clinical findings and the mainstay of management is supportive care.

## Subjective Findings

The health history may reveal:

- Recent HSV infection (e.g., herpes labialis, or "cold sore") or other preceding illness
- Recent medication change (e.g., treatment with antibiotic such as penicillin)
- Erythematous targetoid rash involving palms/soles and spreading centripetally
- Discomfort with eating/drinking (in children with mucosal involvement)

## Risk Factors

The most common risk factors for EM are:

- Recent infection (HSV or *M. pneumoniae*)
- Recent medication change

## Review of Systems

The most common manifestations revealed during the review of systems include:

- **Constitutional:** low-grade fever and/or malaise (not required for diagnosis)
- **Integumentary:** acute onset rash with or without pruritus
- **HEENT:** oral discomfort (if mucosal involvement present)

## Objective Findings

The physical examination of the child with EM may reveal:

- Erythematous to violaceous fixed macular or papular targetoid lesions
- Targetoid lesions are comprised of three distinct zones: central dusky region with or without bulla or necrosis, paler edematous area, and rim of erythema
- Symmetric distribution—beginning on acral sites/extremities and spreading to involve trunk, face, and neck
- If mucosal involvement:
  - Erosions of buccal mucosa and/or tongue
  - Erosions, crusting, and swelling of the lips

## Laboratory/Diagnostic Testing

The diagnosis of EM is based upon the clinical findings. No laboratory or diagnostic testing is needed. If the diagnosis is unclear, skin biopsy may be considered.

## Differential Diagnosis

The differential diagnosis for EM includes:

- Stevens-Johnson syndrome/toxic epidermal necrolysis
- *M. pneumoniae*-induced rash and mucositis
- Generalized fixed drug eruption
- Urticaria
- Leukocytoclastic vasculitis
- Viral exanthem

## Treatment/Management Plan

The management of EM is supportive, as the reaction is self-limited and will resolve over 2 to 3 weeks (Paller & Mancini, 2016; Zoghaib et al., 2019). Supportive care can include oral antihistamines for relief of pruritus and topical analgesic mouth washes if there is mucosal involvement. Although less common in the pediatric population, recurrences of the eruption can occur. If the eruption is found to be secondary to HSV, consideration can be given to prophylactic antiviral therapy for 6 to 12 months to prevent recurrence (Paller & Mancini, 2016; Zoghaib et al., 2019).

## Family Education

Teach the following:

- EM is a hypersensitivity reaction to an infection or medication.
- It is a self-limited disease that should resolve in 2 to 3 weeks without complication.
- Recurrence is possible, although not common, in children who have HSV-associated EM.

### Referral

In children with severe mucositis, which is impairing adequate hydration or nutrition, consideration should be given to inpatient supportive care.

## DRUG ERUPTIONS

Drug eruptions are hypersensitivity reactions to medications. Many present with cutaneous findings; in the outpatient setting, cutaneous eruptions account for 1.5% of drug reactions. The most common drug eruption is exanthematous (morbilliform; Perez & Dyer, 2020). In the pediatric population, another frequently encountered cutaneous drug eruption is serum sickness-like reaction. Although rare, Stevens-Johnson syndrome/toxic epidermal necrolysis and drug reaction with eosinophilia and systemic symptoms (DRESS) are medical emergencies.

The common denominator in all cutaneous drug eruptions is the recent initiation of or change in a medication. The most frequently implicated medications are antibiotics, anticonvulsants, and nonsteroidal anti-inflammatory drugs (NSAIDs). Each drug eruption is unique in its presentation and management.

### Subjective Findings

The health history may reveal:

- Initiation of new medication or change in dose of current medication
- History of prior known medication allergies
- New-onset pruritic rash

### Risk Factors

The most common risk factors for drug eruptions are:

- Initiation of a new medication or change in dose of a chronic medication.
- For exanthematous drug eruptions, the most common culprit medications include anticonvulsants, penicillins, and sulfonamides (Perez & Dyer, 2020).
- For serum sickness-like reaction, the most common culprit medications are cephalosporins (cefaclor most commonly associated historically), penicillins, sulfonamides, minocycline, and bupropion (Perez & Dyer, 2020).

### Review of Systems

The most common manifestations revealed during the review of systems include:

*Exanthematous/morbilliform drug eruption:*

- **Constitutional:** low-grade fever
- **Integumentary:** erythematous macular and papular rash, pruritus

*Serum Sickness-Like Reaction:*

- **Constitutional:** low-grade fever, malaise
- **Integumentary:** urticarial rash
- **Musculoskeletal:** arthralgias
- **Gastrointestinal:** gastrointestinal (GI) upset
- **Neurologic:** headache

### Objective Findings

The physical examination of the child with an exanthematous drug eruption may reveal:

- Erythematous macules and papules coalescing into patches and plaques; most commonly begins on the trunk, spreading symmetrically to become generalized
- Involvement of palms/soles is common
- Eruption does not involve mucous membranes

The physical examination of the child with serum sickness-like reaction may reveal:

- Erythematous fixed urticarial and polycyclic papules and plaques, often generalized
- Lesions may become violaceous to ecchymotic centrally
- Periarticular swelling of joints such as metacarpophalangeals, knees, etc.

### Laboratory/Diagnostic Testing

The diagnosis of both exanthematous drug eruptions and serum sickness-like reaction are based upon the clinical findings. No laboratory or diagnostic testing is needed. In both, eosinophilia is often present, but not required for diagnosis.

### Differential Diagnosis

The differential diagnosis for exanthematous drug eruption includes:

- Viral exanthem
- Mononucleosis
- Bacterial infection (such as staphylococcal scalded skin syndrome or scarlet fever)
- Early stages of other drug eruptions (such as EM, drug reaction with eosinophilia and systemic symptoms)
- Kawasaki disease (KD)

The differential diagnosis for serum sickness-like reaction includes:

- Urticaria
- Urticarial vasculitis
- EM

### Treatment/Management Plan

The management of both exanthematous drug eruption and serum sickness-like reaction is supportive care and removal of the culprit medication. Oral antihistamines can be given to relieve pruritus in both eruptions. In serum sickness-like reaction, NSAIDs can be used to alleviate arthralgias. Exanthematous drug eruptions typically occur 7 to 14 days after initiation of the culprit medication; however, if it is a repeat exposure, the eruption can occur within hours of administration (Perez & Dyer, 2020). It is expected to evolve over 7 to 14 days, first turning red/brown, followed by superficial desquamation (Perez & Dyer, 2020). Serum sickness-like reaction is a self-limiting eruption that is expected to resolve in 2 to 3 weeks after discontinuation of the culprit medication (Paller & Mancini, 2016; Zoghaib et al., 2019).

### Family Education

Teach the following:

- Drug eruptions are hypersensitivity reactions to certain medications, often new antibiotics or antiepileptics.
- Exanthematous drug eruptions and serum sickness-like reaction are both self-limited conditions that are expected to resolve within 2 to 3 weeks after discontinuation of the culprit medication.
- The mainstay of treatment is discontinuation of suspected medication and supportive care.

### Referral

The preceding drug eruptions are more common in the pediatric population and are self-limiting conditions. Severe drug eruptions such as drug reaction with eosinophilia and systemic symptoms, and Stevens-Johnson syndrome/toxic epidermal necrolysis are rare in this population but are important to recognize. These occurrences are medical emergencies and should be referred for inpatient care.

Drug reaction with eosinophilia and systemic symptoms can present similarly to exanthematous drug eruption. The eruption is similar in morphology; however, it starts on the face and spreads caudally. A hallmark feature is the presence of facial edema, which occurs in approximately 70% of affected children (Perez & Dyer, 2020). Children with drug reaction with eosinophilia and systemic symptoms typically appear unwell and have associated fever. As stated in the name, this eruption can have systemic involvement (liver is the most common extracutaneous site); therefore, prompt determination of culprit medication, laboratory evaluation, and treatment are required (Perez & Dyer, 2020).

Stevens-Johnson syndrome/toxic epidermal necrolysis is quite rare; it is estimated to affect approximately 3 individuals in 4 million annually (Perez & Dyer, 2020). Children typically present with a prodrome of flu-like symptoms (fever, headache, malaise, arthralgias). There is eventual painful eruption that often presents as targetoid macules that progress to bullae and desquamation (Paller & Mancini, 2016). Mucosal surfaces are almost always involved (can involve ocular, oral, and genital mucosa). The severity of disease is based on total body surface area (TBSA) involved; less than 10% TBSA is classified as Stevens-Johnson syndrome, while greater than 30% TBSA is classified as toxic epidermal necrolysis. With increased TBSA involvement comes increased risk of electrolyte imbalances, thermal dysregulation, and infection risk. Children with suspected Stevens-Johnson syndrome/toxic epidermal necrolysis should be promptly referred for multidisciplinary inpatient care involving a burn team and dermatology.

## PRIMARY IMMUNODEFICIENCIES

Although rare, primary immunodeficiencies may be hereditary or congenital. They may be related to cellular immunity deficiencies or humoral deficiencies (or a combination of the two), complement deficiencies, or phagocytic system defects (Chinn, 2019). Primary immunodeficiencies include agammaglobulinemia, common variable immunodeficiency disease, hyper IgM, selective IgA deficiency, and antibody subclass deficiency, among others. Children with primary immunodeficiencies often experience a significant number of milder infections, though some of them may be more severe. Their quality of life is also negatively affected by the amount of sick days, and they may fail to thrive or have developmental delay (Abbott & Hauk, 2020). Appropriate treatment of primary immunodeficiency decreases the number of infections experienced and helps the child to experience a more normal life.

### Subjective Findings

The health history may reveal:

- Recurrent infection
- Recurrent fever
- Delayed growth

BOX 32.2 **Warning Signs of Primary Immunodeficiency**

Warning signs of primary immunodeficiency include:

- Six or more respiratory tract infections or four or more episodes of acute otitis media in 1 year
- Two or more episodes of severe sinusitis or pneumonia in 1 year
- Infant failing to grow normally or gain weight
- Treatment with antibiotics for 2 months or longer with little effect
- Recurrent abscesses involving an organ or deep skin
- Persistent or recurrent oral candidiasis or integumentary fungal infection
- Infections requiring intravenous antibiotics to clear
- Two or more serious infections in a lifetime (such as meningitis or sepsis)
- Family history of primary immunodeficiency or unexplained early death (before age 30 years)
- Complications from a live vaccine
- Chronic diarrhea, nonhealing wounds, extensive skin lesions, or unexplained fevers

*Source*: Data from Butte, M. J., & Stiehm, E. R. (2020). Approach to the child with recurrent infections. *UpToDate*. Retrieved October 25, 2020, from https://www.uptodate.com/contents/approach-to-the-child-with-recurrent-infections; Jeffrey Modell Foundation. (2016). *10 warning signs*. http://www.info4pi.org/library/educational-materials/10-warning-signs

## Risk Factors

The most common risk factors for primary immunodeficiency are:

- Age over 4 months (waning of maternal immunity)
- Family history of immunodeficiency

## Review of Systems

The most common manifestations revealed during the review of systems include (Box 32.2):

- **Constitutional:** recurrent fever (often without explanation), poor growth or failure to gain weight, malaise
- **Integumentary:** fungal infection, skin lesions
- **HEENT:** recurrent runny nose or ear pain, persistent thrush
- **Gastrointestinal:** diarrhea

## Objective Findings

The physical examination of the child with a primary immunodeficiency may be completely normal or may reveal:

- Low weight, length/stature, or body mass index for gender and age
- Thrush
- Lymphadenopathy (hyper IgM)
- Splenomegaly (hyper IgM)
- Fungal skin infection or other skin lesions

▶ ALERT: Severe combined immunodeficiency (SCID) is a rare disorder of severe deficiency in T-cell number or function and is fatal in the first year of life if untreated. Despite being universally screened for in all 50 states at birth, an unidentified infant with SCID may present with persistent, recurrent, opportunistic infection, chronic diarrhea, failure to thrive, or unexplained severe respiratory illness. SCID constitutes an emergency and the infant should be immediately referred to pediatric immunology.

## Laboratory/Diagnostic Testing

Primary immunodeficiency is diagnosed based upon immunoglobulin and subclass levels. Order IgA, IgG (with subclasses), IgM, and IgE levels. T-cell number and function should also be measured. Additionally, assess antibody function with measurement of antibody response to natural infection or immunization. The complete blood count (CBC) may reveal lymphopenia.

## Differential Diagnosis

The differential diagnosis for primary immunodeficiency includes:

- Autoimmune disorder
- Secondary immunodeficiency
- Malnutrition
- Protein-losing disorder (gastroenteropathy or kidney disease)
- Drug-induced hypogammaglobulinemia (corticosteroids, immune modulators, certain anti-epileptic drugs)
- Transient hypogammaglobulinemia of infancy

### Treatment/Management Plan

The usual treatment for primary immunodeficiency is intravenous (IV) gammaglobulin therapy prescribed by a pediatric immunologist or infective disease specialist and administered at a specialty clinic.

### Family Education

Teach the following:

- Treatment is focused on preventing recurrent infection, thereby permitting adequate growth and development.
- Obtain support through the Immune Deficiency Foundation network—https://primaryimmune.org/living-pi/programs

### Referral

Refer children with suspected primary immunodeficiency or SCID to a clinic specializing in primary immunodeficiency in children. These clinics offer a multidisciplinary approach, utilizing a team consisting of pediatric allergy/immunology and pediatric infectious disease specialists.

# AUTOIMMUNE DISEASES

## SYSTEMIC LUPUS ERYTHEMATOSUS

Systemic lupus erythematosus (SLE) is a disease found worldwide. It is an autoimmune disease that has an unclear etiology, in which the level of severity can range from very mild to life-threatening. SLE is characterized by abnormalities and multiorgan involvement, in which the immune system attacks its own tissues, in turn causing widespread inflammation throughout the body. This can lead to tissue damage in the affected organ(s). Childhood-onset SLE is relatively rare, usually seen between the ages of 10 and 15; however, it can occur at any age, and is more prominent in minority females. When symptoms present, they manifest more aggressively than in adult-onset SLE. SLE is a chronic, noncurable disease, but medications in combination with leading a healthy lifestyle can help to maintain and control it (Centers for Disease Control and Prevention [CDC], 2018b; Wong et al., 2019).

The cause of SLE is unknown; however, it is believed that one or a combination of reasons are linked, such as hormonal and environmental factors. Genetic factors have also been found to play a role. A child in a family with a history of SLE is at high risk of developing the disease (CDC, 2018b; Wong et al., 2019).

### Subjective Findings

The health history may reveal:

- Frequent infections
- Fever
- Rash on face, eyelashes and/or body
- Recurring ulcers in the nose, mouth, and/or throat (CDC, 2018b; Klein-Gitelman, 2019).

### Risk Factors

The most common risk factors for SLE are:

- Female gender
- Age 15 years and older
- Minority racial groups
- Immediate family member with SLE (CDC, 2018b)

### Review of Systems

The most common manifestations revealed during the review of systems include:

- **Constitutional:** fever, malaise, nonspecific fatigue, appetite change, weight change, abdominal pain
- **Integumentary:** photosensitivity, hair loss
- **HEENT:** swollen neck glands, neck stiffness
- **Respiratory:** cough, shortness of breath or difficulty breathing
- **Cardiovascular:** chest pain, extremity edema
- **Gastrointestinal:** constipation, diarrhea
- **Genitourinary:** dysuria, difficulty urinating
- **Musculoskeletal:** joint discomfort/pain/swelling/stiffness, decreased range of motion, weakness, loss of muscle size, muscle spasm
- **Neurologic:** tremor, involuntary movement, incoordination, numbness, feeling of "pins and needles" or tingling, memory problems
- **Hematologic:** anemia, easy bruising or bleeding
- **Psychiatric:** having disruptive thoughts or perceptions about reality or what is not real (psychosis)

### Objective Findings

The physical examination of the child with SLE may reveal:

- Lymphadenopathy
- Nose, mouth, or throat ulcers
- Malar rash on face (one of the most recognizable signs of SLE)
- Nailfold capillary changes
- Possibly flat affect, withdrawn, quiet, anxious, sad (CDC, 2018b; Klein-Gitelman, 2019; Wong et al., 2019)

### Laboratory/Diagnostic Testing

Diagnosing SLE in both children and adults can be difficult because of the multitude of symptoms that can present and mimic other diseases. Although not diagnostic of SLE, an antinuclear antibody (ANA) test, if positive, is indicative of an autoimmune process (more likely to make autoantibodies of SLE). Complement levels, specifically C3 and C4, will be low, while C-reactive protein (CRP) and erythrocyte sedimentation rate (ESR) will be high. Particular antibody testing in SLE may reveal:

- Antibodies to double-stranded DNA (anti-dsDNA) are usually elevated in SLE.
- Phospholipids (aPLs) such as lupus anticoagulant (LA) and anticardiolipin antibodies may also be positive, placing the child at risk for a stroke because they can result in the narrowing of the blood vessels, leading to a thrombus.
- Anti-Smith antibody (Sm) and ribonucleoproteins (RNPs) may be be present.
- A screening urinalysis may raise questions concerning renal function.

### Differential Diagnosis

The differential diagnosis for SLE includes:

- Contact dermatitis
- Seborrheic dermatitis
- Tinea faciei
- Pityriasis rubra pilaris
- Phototoxic (also known as photo allergic) drug eruptions
- Polymorphous light eruption (PMLE)
- Drug-induced SLE
- Stevens-Johnson syndrome
- Infectious causes—viral infections can give a false positive ANA test
- Antiphospholipid antibody syndrome
- Malignancies (acute lymphoblastic leukemia can sometimes show a positive ANA result)
- Dermatomyositis
- Polymyositis
- Erythropoietic protoporphyria
- Scleroderma
- Chilblains, also known as perniosis (CDC, 2018b; Klein-Gitelman, 2019).

### Treatment/Management Plan

The main goal of treatment for individuals with SLE, especially in childhood, is to achieve the lowest possible disease progression and activity in the body, to help promote long-term survival. Preventing organ damage, minimizing drug toxicities when they are prescribed, and improving quality of health and life are key components. Other important factors are support of and education for children and families about the disease, plan of care and treatment, promotion of healthy habits and lifestyle, and what role all these factors play in the management of this disease.

Treatment for SLE is individualized based on the child, their comorbidities, disease severity, disease activity, and the child and family's plan of care preferences. Pharmacologic and nonpharmacologic interventions are assessed to determine the best plan of individualized care. The first-line treatment is glucocorticoids with hydroxychloroquine. They have been found to be safe and efficacious treatments for SLE and necessary to attain adequate control of the disease in children with mild SLE. Hydroxychloroquine or chloroquine are key maintenance medications and help to lower risk of kidney involvement. However, with disease progression, multiorgan and/or severe end-organ involvement, treatment with additional disease-modifying medications is necessary. In children with mild SLE who do not have renal involvement, NSAIDs are used if the child is having musculoskeletal symptoms. Once these symptoms resolve, then the NSAIDs should be discontinued, because children with SLE are at higher risk of developing aseptic meningitis from NSAIDs.

Depending on the disease severity, progression and organ involvement are how the second line of therapy is chosen. Children and adolescents with progressive or severe SLE will require a more aggressive treatment course with immunosuppressants such as rituximab, cyclophosphamide, or mycophenolate. These have been found to have the best long-term success rates in children with severe SLE. These disease-modifying agents are taken into careful consideration for each child or adolescent, especially when considering cyclophosphamide, because of potential gonadotoxic and nephrotoxic effects (Klein-Gitelman, 2019; Wong et al., 2019). Belimumab may also be considered.

### Family Education

Teach the following:

- Ask questions. Knowledge is power, and the family knows the child best.
- Maintain and keep the child's daily activities to encourage the child to have a normal lifestyle to promote social and emotional development.

- Promote lifelong healthy habits, including good nutrition and exercise (must keep moving their muscles and joints to prevent stiffness) with weight-bearing exercise being particularly important for healthy bones.
- When on corticosteroids it is important to limit sugar to avoid weight gain. Guide the child, parents, and their family to learn about SLE and what support is available to them
- SLE is a chronic disease, but proper treatment and close follow-up decrease the risk of flare-ups.
- Strongly encourage the child to go to all healthcare team visits scheduled, and follow the developed individualized care plan.
- Learn the child's triggers and what symptoms present that may mean a flare-up is developing, to catch it early, possibly stop it, or make it less severe.
- Call the healthcare team to advocate early, to start any treatment regimen immediately.
- Encourage talking with the child's school to help them understand the child's health, their needs, and support systems they may require.
- Encourage the family to seek support groups, such as The Lupus Foundation of America (CDC, 2018b; Klein-Gitelman, 2019; Lupus Foundation of America, 2020).

### Referral

Refer the child or adolescent with SLE to a pediatric rheumatologist who specializes in childhood SLE. If the child develops issues with organs because of the SLE (such as kidney failure), refer to the corresponding pediatric specialist.

## ACUTE RHEUMATIC FEVER

Acute rheumatic fever (ARF) is a multisystem autoimmune inflammatory response to an untreated or partially treated pharyngeal group A Streptococcus infection. The mechanisms of how ARF develops are not fully understood; however, genetic susceptibility and molecular mimicry are considered to play a role in the autoimmune response that results in immunoglobulins attacking the heart, central nervous system (CNS), cutaneous tissue, and joints (Sika-Paotonu et al., 2017). Symptoms typically appear 2 to 3 weeks after a group A Streptococcus infection. The most clinically significant sequela of ARF is damage to the mitral and aortic valves, which can lead to rheumatic heart disease (Munteanu et al., 2018).

### Subjective Findings

The health history may reveal:

- Fever (occurs in approximately 70% to 75% of children)
- History of recent sore throat and/or upper respiratory infection (URI)
- Swollen, tender, red joints, most common in the knees, ankles, elbows, and wrists

### Risk Factors

The most common risk factors for ARF are:

- Family history of ARF

ARF is rare in the United States, but continues to be a cause of cardiovascular morbidity and mortality in children globally, particularly in developing countries (Gewitz et al., 2015).

- Low socioeconomic status, including large households and poor access to health care
- Child between 5 and 15 years of age

### Review of Systems

The most common manifestations revealed during the review of systems include:

- **Constitutional:** fever, fatigue, abdominal pain
- **Integumentary:** nonpruritic macular or papular rash
- **Cardiovascular:** chest pain
- **Musculoskeletal:** swollen, painful, red, hot joints
- **Neurologic:** uncontrollable jerky movements of the hands, face, and feet that cease when asleep

### Objective Findings

The diagnosis of ARF is based upon the Revised Jones Criteria for Rheumatic Fever and must have evidence of preceding streptococcal infection. The child must have two major manifestations or one major and two minor manifestations. The criteria are stratified into two risk categories: (1) Low risk (ARF incidence ≤2 per 100,000 school-age children or all-age rheumatic heart disease prevalence ≤1 per 1,000) and (2) moderate to high risk (Sika-Paotonu et al., 2017). The physical examination of the child with ARF may reveal:

*Major Criteria (low-risk populations):*

- Carditis (clinical and subclinical): occurs in 50% to 70% of initial cases, most often due to valvulitis leading to mitral valve regurgitation and (less often) aortic valve regurgitation. A holosystolic murmur is heard at the aortic or mitral area. Tachycardia (out of proportion to the fever) and a pericardial rub may be found on examination. A pansystolic murmur with mitral valve regurgitation and a diastolic murmur can be heard if severe (CDC, 2018a).

- Polyarthritis and migratory arthritis: In 75% of cases, joint inflammation, redness, and tenderness. This can involve multiple joints with onset at different times or simultaneously (known as migratory polyarthritis), most commonly in the knees, ankles, elbows, and wrists. However, arthritis is also common in several other rheumatologic disorders, and therefore is nonspecific. Joint pains can last for days up to a week and resolve without treatment in a month (Sika-Paotonu et al., 2017).
- Sydenham's chorea (also known as St. Vitus's dance): In 10% to 30% of cases, this is a neurologic disorder characterized by uncontrollable jerky movements of the hands, face, and feet; muscle weakness; and behavioral changes such as restlessness or crying. These symptoms cease while asleep and increase with purposeful movement.
- Erythema marginatum (also known as erythema annulare): In < 6% of cases, this is a bright pink, nonpruritic macular or papular rash seen on the trunk and occasionally limbs.
- Subcutaneous nodules: In up to 10% of cases, painless, firm nodules over bony prominences that range from millimeters to 2 centimeters. These typically resolve within a month (Steer & Gibofsky, 2020).

*Minor Criteria (low-risk populations):*

- Fever: (In >90% of children) ≥38.5 °C or 101.3 °F. Low-grade fevers are more common in high-risk groups.
- Polyarthralgia.
- ESR ≥60 mm/hour and CRP ≥3 mg/dL (Steer & Gibofsky, 2020).
- Prolonged PR interval on ECG: These will vary by age. First degree is commonly seen in children with ARF, if severe, can lead to junctional rhythm and complete heart block.

*Major Criteria (moderate- to high-risk population):*

- Carditis (clinical and/or subclinical)
- Monoarthritis, polyarthritis, and/or polyarthralgia
- Chorea
- Erythema marginatium
- Subcutaneous nodules

*Minor Criteria (moderate- to high-risk population):*

- Fever ≥38 °C
- Monoarthralgia
- Prolonged PR interval
- ESR ≥30 mm/hr and/or CRP ≥3.0 mg/dL (Sika-Paotonu et al., 2017; Szczygielska et al., 2018)

## Laboratory/Diagnostic Testing

Laboratory and diagnostic testing includes ESR (elevated), CRP (elevated), CBC with differential (will show leukocytosis, normocytic anemia), and rapid strep test, throat culture, or elevated serology (anti-streptolysin O titer (ASO) titer and anti-deoxyribonuclease B titer). A chest x-ray, electrocardiogram, and echocardiogram evaluate the heart and its rhythm.

## Differential Diagnosis

The differential diagnosis for ARF includes:

- Congenital heart disease
- Congenital mitral and aortic valve abnormalities
- Infective endocarditis
- Myocarditis
- Cardiomyopathy
- Avascular necrosis
- Leukemia
- Idiopathic pain syndromes
- KD
- SLE
- Juvenile idiopathic arthritis (JIA)
- Reactive arthritis
- Subcutaneous granuloma annulare
- Fibromas
- Xanthomas

## Treatment/Management Plan

Any child with suspected ARF should be hospitalized for close monitoring and treatment. Treatment for ARF includes:

- Antibiotic treatment with benzathine penicillin G (BPG) intramuscular within 10 days of onset is the recommended first-line therapy. If allergic to penicillin, erythromycin can be used to treat. For secondary prophylaxis to prevent recurrent rheumatic fever, BPG is given once every 4 weeks.
- NSAIDs for relief of symptoms of joint pain. Joint pain is very responsive to treatment with NSAIDs. If joint pain fails to respond to NSAIDs or corticosteroids, the diagnosis of ARF should be re-examined. Aspirin should be avoided in children due to the risk of Reye syndrome. Treatment duration is typically 1 to 2 weeks, although some children will require a longer duration (Sika-Paotonu et al., 2017).
- Corticosteroids can be used for children with severe carditis. Children and adolescents with severe carditis, heart block, or congestive heart failure will be managed and treated by a pediatric cardiologist.

- Chorea is usually self-limiting and resolves within a week to months. If the chorea is significantly affecting the child or places them at risk for injury, valproic acid and carbamazepine can be used as first-line treatment.
- Ensure that they receive an annual influenza vaccination.

### Family Education

Teach the following:

- Primary prevention: It is important to treat strep throat infections and complete the course of antibiotics as prescribed.
- Secondary prevention: Children and caregivers need to know about ARF, rheumatic heart disease, and the importance of completing the course of secondary prophylaxis which lasts until age 21, or 10 years after symptom onset (Sika-Paotonu et al., 2017).

### Referral

The child with ARF should be referred to pediatric cardiology. Additional specialty consultations may include a pediatric infectious disease specialist and pediatric rheumatologist.

▶ ALERT: Any child presenting with symptoms of ARF needs to be hospitalized. Subclinical carditis may be present without any findings on auscultation.

# INFLAMMATORY DISORDERS

## IMMUNOGLOBULIN A VASCULITIS

Immunoglobulin A vasculitis, also known as Henoch-Schönlein purpura (HSP), is the most common acute vasculitis in children. Ig A vasculitis is characterized by IgA1 immune deposits in the small vessels, with complement and neutrophil infiltration leading to vascular inflammation involving the skin, GI tract, joints, and kidneys (Heineke et al., 2017). Most cases of Ig A vasculitis are seen in the fall and winter, with approximately 50% of cases preceded by an upper respiratory tract infection. Most cases resolve without treatment; however, rarely, a small subset of children with Ig A vasculitis can develop nephritis/glomerulonephritis (leading cause of morbidity), GI bleeding, intussusception, bowel necrosis or perforation, and CNS involvement.

### Subjective Findings

The health history may reveal:

- Recent viral illness
- Joint pain and swelling
- Rash

### Risk Factors

The most common risk factors for IgA vasculitis are:

- Having a preceding viral illness or streptococcal infection
- Gender—Higher incidence in males (1.5:1 male: female ratio)
- Age—most cases occurring in children less than 10 years old, with a peak age of 6 years old
- Genetic predisposition—more common in Asians

### Review of Systems

The most common manifestations revealed during the review of systems include:

- **Constitutional:** abdominal pain
- **Integumentary:** rash, edema of the eyes, hands, or scrotum (if nephrotic syndrome occurs)
- **Gastrointestinal:** nausea, vomiting, bloody stools
- **Genitourinary:** bloody or tea-colored, or frothy urine
- **Musculoskeletal:** joint pain and swelling (arthralgia occurs in approximately 75% of children, mostly in the knees and ankles, and is typically migratory without warmth or erythema).

### Objective Findings

The physical examination of the child with IgA vasculitis may reveal:

- Palpable purpura without thrombocytopenia and coagulopathy (typically the first sign to appear), commonly on the lower extremities and buttocks. The rash may also have erythematous wheals that may turn into ecchymosis or necrotic lesions.
- Joint edema and decreased range of motion.
- Abdominal pain—colicky pain that may be accompanied by nausea and vomiting.
- Hematuria or proteinuria occurs in 20% to 55% of children with IgA vasculitis; onset is 1–3 months after the appearance of the rash.

Diagnosis is based on clinical findings and the diagnostic criteria outlined by the European League Against Rheumatism (EULAR) and the Paediatric Rheumatology European Society (PRES) in conjunction with

Paediatric Rheumatology International Trials Organization (PRINTO):

- Mandatory criterion—Purpura or petechiae with lower limb predominance (without thrombocytopenia and coagulopathy)
- Minimum of one of the following symptoms:
  - Diffuse abdominal pain with acute onset
  - Histopathology showing leukocytoclastic vasculitis or proliferative glomerulonephritis, with predominant immunoglobulin A deposits
  - Arthritis or arthralgia of acute onset
  - Renal involvement—proteinuria or hematuria (Hetland et al., 2017)

### Laboratory/Diagnostic Testing

Laboratory and diagnostic testing includes:

- CBC with differential—normochromic anemia, leukocytosis, normal platelet count
- Elevated ESR, CRP, serum IgA levels
- PT, PTT, and bleeding time—usually normal
- Complete metabolic panel (CMP; elevated blood urea nitrogen and creatinine, hypoalbuminemia)
- Urinalysis may demonstrate red blood cell casts, hematuria, proteinuria
- Skin punch biopsy may reveal leukocytoclastic vasculitis

▶ ALERT: Any child presenting with palpable purpura, joint pain, and edema should receive a workup for renal involvement.

### Differential Diagnosis

The differential diagnosis for IgA vasculitis includes:

- Purpura
- Hypersensitivity vasculitis
- SLE
- JIA
- Rheumatic fever
- Septic arthritis
- Toxic synovitis
- Churg-Strauss syndrome
- Acute hemorrhagic edema of infancy
- Infectious disease
- Appendicitis
- Irritable bowel disease (Dedeoglu & Kim, 2019)

### Treatment/Management Plan

Symptomatic management is indicated for cases without renal involvement. This includes pain management, hydration, bed rest, and wound care if skin necrosis is present. The use of prednisone for treatment of renal involvement is controversial, as several studies have shown no benefit in terms of disease course and resolution; however, prednisone has been used in cases of severe abdominal pain. Immunosuppressive and immunomodulatory medications such as mycophenolate mofetil, dapsone, and rituximab have been used with positive effects; however, these should be reserved for children with chronic, persistent, or complicated courses (Hetland et al., 2017).

**PRO TIP** Urinalysis and blood pressure should be measured at all subsequent well child visits to screen for development of late renal involvement.

### Family Education

Teach the following:

- Course of the illness and signs/symptoms of complications such as glomerulonephritis, CNS involvement, intussusception, GI bleeding.
- Educate families/caregivers on the use of NSAIDs and keeping the child hydrated.

### Referral

Refer the child with renal involvement to pediatric nephrology. If a skin punch biopsy is needed, consultation with pediatric dermatology is appropriate.

## JUVENILE IDIOPATHIC ARTHRITIS

JIA, considered to be an autoinflammatory disorder, occurs in children under the age of 16 years. Although the pathogenesis is not completely understood, it appears that a combination of genetic predisposition and a triggering factor such as an antecedent viral illness cause immune dysregulation. The result is inflammation of the synovial membrane and sometimes other body systems with waxing and waning of symptoms. At times the symptoms appear to be in remission, and at other times, when the disease flares, they are worse.

It is unclear how JIA will affect a child. Some children may experience symptoms for a short time, lasting only a few months. When symptoms last at least 6 weeks, the condition is considered chronic and some children encounter the challenge of facing symptoms for the rest of their lives. About 1 child in every 1,000 will develop arthritis (American College of Rheumatology [ACR], 2020).

Several types of juvenile arthritis exist, each presenting differently. Oligoarticular arthritis involves five or fewer joints and accounts for about half of the cases of JIA (ACR, 2020). Systemic juvenile arthritis (sJIA) occurs in about 10% of cases (ACR, 2020). Polyarticular JIA (involving more than five joints) occurs in 20% to 35% of children with JIA, while psoriatic arthritis and enthesitis-related arthritis account for another 5% to 10% of cases (Wu & Rabinovich, 2020). Although a particular cause for JIA has not been identified, its development may follow a viral illness in genetically susceptible individuals.

### Subjective Findings

The health history may reveal:

- Joint pain, stiffness or swelling
- Difficulty with daily living activities (such as playing, walking, running, dressing, etc.)
- Limping with ambulation (Wu & Rabinovich, 2020)

### Risk Factors

The most common risk factors for JIA are:

- Genetic susceptibility (human leukocyte antigen markers, vary by type of JIA)
- Female gender (polyarticular, oligoarticular)
- Age 2 to 4 years (polyarticular, oligoarticular)
- Age 10 to 14 years (polyarticular)
- Age 1 to 5 years (systemic; Wu & Rabinovich, 2020).

### Review of Systems

The most common manifestations revealed during the review of systems include:

- **Constitutional:** appetite loss, fatigue, poor sleep quality, quotidian fever (daily fever spike ≥38.5 °C (≥101.3 °F) with normothermia in between [systemic JIA])
- **Integumentary:** rash (systemic JIA)
- **HEENT:** conjunctival inflammation
- **Respiratory:** chest pain or cough (systemic JIA)
- **Musculoskeletal:** decreased joint range of motion, weakness (Haumann & Merola, 2019; Kimura, 2020; Wu & Rabinovich, 2020).

### Objective Findings

The physical examination of the child with JIA may reveal:

- Macular, salmon-pink rash that can be evanescent (systemic JIA)
- Uveitis
- Joint edema, warmth, tenderness, decreased range of motion; any number of joints may be involved
- Lymphadenopathy
- Hepatosplenomegaly (Haumann & Merola, 2019; Kimura, 2020; Wu & Rabinovich, 2020).

▶ ALERT: Macrophage activation syndrome (MAS) is a severe complication that could occur in the initial stage of systemic JIA disease and should be treated as a life-threatening emergency. MAS is characterized by an atypical rash (if present at the time), persistent fever, a decrease in white blood cells, decrease in red blood cells, decrease in platelets, coagulopathy, hyperferritinemia, and hepatitis. This can occur in the first few days to weeks of the onset of systemic JIA (Kimura, 2020).

### Laboratory/Diagnostic Testing

There are currently no specific laboratory or diagnostic tests specific to JIA. ESR and CRP are either elevated or significantly elevated depending upon the type of JIA. The antinucleic antibody (ANA) may be positive in some cases of oligoarticular, polyarticular, or psoriatic arthritis. ANA does not assist with diagnosis; rather, it is used to determine risk of uveitis. Rheumatoid factor will be positive in only a small percentage of cases of polyarthritis. In the child with sJIA, the CBC may reveal anemia, and elevated white blood cell and platelet counts.

### Differential Diagnosis

The differential diagnosis for JIA includes:

- Osteomyelitis
- Septic arthritis
- Reactive arthritis
- Transient synovitis
- Hypermobility syndrome
- Lyme disease
- Serum sickness
- Immunoglobulin A vasculitis
- KD
- SLE
- Sarcoidosis
- Inflammatory bowel disease
- Malignancy
- Trauma

### Treatment/Management Plan

The main goals of treatment are to relieve the child's discomfort, delay or prevent joint degeneration, and maintain/restore range of motion, muscle strength, and joint function. Additionally, it is important to promote optimal growth and development, and physical activity, along with social and emotional development.

Management in most cases of JIA is a combination approach. Medication, physical therapy, and encouragement to exercise at home are first-line treatment. Occasionally, NSAIDs alone are effective for children with JIA. Some cases of JIA require corticosteroid joint injections. When JIA is not responsive to treatment with NSAIDs or corticosteroids, the specialist may recommend disease-modifying antirheumatic drugs (DMARDs) (Haumann & Merola, 2019; Wu & Rabinovich, 2020).

### Family Education

Teach the following:

- Ask questions. Knowledge is power, and the family knows the child best.
- Maintain and keep the child's daily activities to encourage a normal lifestyle to promote social and emotional development.
- Promote lifelong healthy habits. Make sure the child eats a well-balanced diet with plenty of calcium and vitamin D (and daily folate supplement if taking DMARDs, specifically methotrexate) and encourage daily exercise to prevent joint stiffness.
- A warm bath in the morning may ease overnight stiffness.
- Support groups may be beneficial to the family and child—the Arthritis Foundation (arthritis.org) has many resources.
- Talk with the child's school to help them understand the child's health, their needs, and support systems they may require.

**PRO TIP** For children on DMARDs:

- Avoid live vaccines
- Avoid trimethoprim-containing medications (with methotrexate)
- Hold DMARDs for acute viral illnesses until child is fever-free
- Ensure that child continues to receive annual flu vaccination

### Referral

Refer children with JIA to a pediatric rheumatologist. A team comprised of the child's primary care provider, rheumatologist, and physical therapist will all work together to develop the best plan of care and method of treatment for the child.

## KAWASAKI DISEASE

KD, also known as mucocutaneous lymph node syndrome, is a self-limiting disease of acute vascular inflammation. However, the cardiac sequelae of KD can be very serious. The most common complication of KD is coronary artery aneurysm; however, other cardiac complications include myocardial dysfunction, myocardial infarction, and arrhythmias. After treatment, children will require frequent follow-up to monitor for the development of arrhythmias, heart failure, coronary artery dilation, aneurysm, and valvular insufficiency (Newburger et al., 2016).

### Subjective Findings

The health history may reveal:

- High fever >101 °F, lasting 5 or more days, likely refractory to antipyretics
- Antecedent nonspecific respiratory or GI symptoms (prodrome)

### Risk Factors

Risk factors for the development of KD include:

- Familial history of KD, particularly siblings and parents
- Asian ancestry
- Male gender
- 6 months to 5 years of age (Lin & Wu, 2017)

### Review of Systems

The most common manifestations revealed during the review of systems include

- **Constitutional:** fever; prolonged fever lasting 5 or more days
- **Integumentary:** rash
- **HEENT:** eye redness

### Objective Findings

The physical examination of the child with KD may reveal:

- Bilateral bulbar conjunctival injection
- Oral mucous membrane changes: erythema of lips and oral mucosa, "strawberry tongue," cracked lips
- Desquamation of fingers
- Cervical lymphadenopathy
- Polymorphous rash
- Peripheral extremity changes: erythema of palms and soles, indurated edema and erythema of hands and feet (Newburger et al., 2016)

**PRO TIP** The objective findings of KD often may not present at the same time. Therefore, it may be important to repeat the assessment and examination multiple times in order to make a diagnosis of KD.

### Laboratory/Diagnostic Testing

The diagnosis of KD requires the presence of fever for at least 5 days, in addition to four of the five revealing symptoms of mucocutaneous inflammation, as listed earlier. If a child exhibits more than four of the symptoms, an early diagnosis of KD can be made on the fourth day of illness. While not included in the diagnostic criteria, the following laboratory and imaging results are supportive of the diagnosis, and may even be used in diagnosing atypical or incomplete KD in children with fewer than four of the presenting symptoms:

- elevated CRP, ESR, ferritin
- CBC: thrombocytopenia, lymphocytosis, normocytic normochromic anemia
- CMP: elevated transaminases, hyponatremia, elevated triglycerides
- Urinalysis: pyuria
- Echocardiogram to rule out coronary artery aneurysm (repeat at 2 weeks and 6 weeks later)

▶ ALERT: Echocardiogram should be obtained as soon as the diagnosis of KD is made in order to establish a baseline of coronary artery measurements for comparison with subsequent imaging.

### Differential Diagnosis

The differential diagnosis of KD includes:

- Systemic JIA
- Stevens-Johnson syndrome
- Rocky Mountain spotted fever
- Staphylococcal toxic shock syndrome
- Rheumatic fever
- Adenovirus
- Epstein-Barr virus
- Measles

### Treatment and Management

Treat KD with aspirin and IV immunoglobulin (IVIG) therapy. Giving both medications is associated with decreased incidence of the development of coronary artery aneurysm. Prescribe aspirin 30–100 mg/kg per day in four divided doses. While the specific mechanism is unknown, IVIG is most effective if given within 7 to 10 days of the onset of fever (Newburger et al., 2016). Administer a dose of IVIG as:

- 2 g/kg in one dose

  or

- 400 mg/kg daily for 4 days

▶ ALERT: Live-virus immunizations should be postponed for at least 11 months after a child has received IVIG therapy, due to decreased immunogenicity.

### Family Education

Teach the following:

- Check the child's temperature every 6 hours until 48 hours after the last time a fever was noted.
- Later, if the child feels warm or symptoms of KD are present, take the child's temperature.
- Make sure to keep the follow-up appointment at 7 to 10 days after diagnosis.
- Limit activity as determined by the pediatric cardiologist (Sundel, 2020).

### Referral

Refer to pediatric cardiology for echocardiogram reading and follow-up regarding development of coronary artery aneurysm. If the diagnosis is unclear, refer to pediatric infectious disease.

## JUVENILE FIBROMYALGIA SYNDROME

Initially fibromyalgia was only diagnosed in adults; however, this disorder is increasingly being seen in children and adolescents, although rarely occurring in children younger than 4 years old. Juvenile fibromyalgia syndrome (JFMS) is characterized by widespread musculoskeletal pain that has been present for more than 3 months. This is in combination with a number of other presenting symptoms that may vary from child to child; however, sleep disturbances and fatigue are typically reported. It can affect people of all ages. The etiology and emergence of this disorder is unknown. One commonality that is indicated is a central sensitization component that is at the origin of the syndrome. It has also been found that there is a genetic predisposition in children leading them to be more susceptible of developing fibromyalgia, and triggers play a role in activating the inflammatory response and symptoms, such as viral illnesses or infections, traumatic injuries, and events that cause emotional or physical stress (CDC, 2020; Kimura & Walco, 2021).

### Subjective Findings

The symptoms of JFMS may not be the same from one child to another, with the report of symptoms ranging from very mild to severe, with different parts of the body being affected, and varying over time. However, one commonality in all children who suffer from fibromyalgia is chronic pain and discomfort. The symptoms may be reported to come and go over time, and must be present for at least 3 months before diagnosis.

The health history of the child or adolescent may reveal:

- Tiredness, fatigue
- Pain
- Sleep disturbances
- Sensitivity to temperature (cold and/or heat; CDC, 2020; Kimura & Walco, 2021)

### Risk Factors

The most common risk factors for JFMS include:

- Family history of fibromyalgia or other autoimmune or autoinflammatory diseases
- Age between 10 and 15 years
- Past history of frequent illnesses, especially viral infections
- Childhood diagnosis of SLE or JIA
- Repetitive injuries, overuse or repetitive stress on joint(s)
- Past history of traumatic or stressful events, such as motor vehicle accidents, post-traumatic stress disorder (PTSD)
- Female gender
- Poor sleeping habits
- Physical or psychological stress
- Lack of physical activity (CDC, 2020; Kimura & Walco, 2021)

### Review of Systems

The most common manifestations revealed during the review of systems include:

- **Constitutional:** headache, widespread pain, discomfort, and stiffness occurring bilaterally, above and below the waist, tiring easily or quickly (even with light activity or exercise), lingering exhaustion, difficulty sleeping through the night, waking up feeling tired, change in appetite or weight
- **Gastrointestinal:** abdominal pain, constipation, irritable bowel syndrome (IBS), bloating, diarrhea
- **Musculoskeletal:** history of restless leg syndrome
- **Neurologic:** history of migraines; tingling or numbness in hands and feet; issues with concentration, thinking, and memory; feeling of "pins and needles" or "tingles"
- **Psychiatric/Behavioral:** depression, anxiety, behavioral changes (CDC, 2020; Kimura & Walco, 2021)

### Objective Findings

The physical examination of the child or adolescent with JFMS may be normal, or it may reveal:

- Tired appearance
- Tender points, allodynia and/or hyperalgesia in the following areas: occiput, low cervical, trapezius, supraspinatus, second ribs, lateral epicondyles, gluteal, greater trochanter, knees
- Joint hypermobility
- Flat affect (CDC, 2020; Kimura & Walco, 2021)

### Laboratory/Diagnostic Testing

There are no specific laboratory, diagnostic, or imaging tests for JFMS. Diagnosis is based on the presentation of typical symptoms, clinical characteristics, history of present illness, family history, and physical examination (CDC, 2020; Kimura & Walco, 2021).

### Differential Diagnosis

The differential diagnosis for JFMS includes:

- Growing pains
- Other pain syndromes
- Chronic fatigue syndrome (CFS), which is rare to see and diagnose in children
- JIA
- SLE
- Complex regional pain syndrome type 1 (CRPS), previously referred to as reflex sympathetic dystrophy, post-traumatic sympathetic dystrophy, and Sudeck's atrophy
- Other autoimmune or auto-inflammatory diseases (Kimura & Walco, 2021)

### Treatment/Management Plan

The main goals of treatment are pain relief; maintenance of range of motion, muscle strength, and function of joints; and promotion of optimal growth and development, physical activity, and social and emotional development.

Over-the-counter (OTC) pain relievers such as acetaminophen and NSAIDs are not usually effective in treating the pain associated with JFMS. Anti-epileptic drugs such as gabapentin and pregabalin may be effective at reducing pain in some children. Selective serotonin reuptake inhibitors (SSRIs) such as fluoxetine may be helpful, but children and adolescents should be carefully monitored while on SSRIs. Tricyclic antidepressants such as amitriptyline, particularly at bedtime, help in relief of a combination of symptoms and may assist with initiating sleep when this is a concern (Kimura & Walco, 2020).

### Family Education

Teach the following:

- Parents will become experts on the child's needs.
- Encourage them and the child, if developmentally appropriate, to learn what fibromyalgia is and how best to manage it daily (learning to decrease the triggers that exacerbate the symptoms).
- Low-impact, aerobic exercises as well as muscle strengthening exercises (even if they hurt) will help maintain range of motion, muscle strength, and joint function.
- Good sleep hygiene and routine will help improve the child's quality of sleep.
- Maintain and keep the child's daily low-impact activities, to encourage the child to have a normal lifestyle to promote social and emotional development.
- Use relaxation techniques to learn to reduce stress and minimize triggers (meditation, yoga, massage therapy, acupressure, or acupuncture).
- Support groups can be very helpful, either parent-to-parent connections, or child/adolescent support groups.
- Teach children coping and psychological mechanisms to help identify stressful triggers that may make the pain or discomfort worse, as well as to help through painful days.
- Talk with the child's school to help them understand the child's health, their needs, and support systems they may require. Children should attend school, using graduated return to school as needed (Kimura & Walco, 2020).

### Referral

A multidisciplinary approach is needed for children with fibromyalgia. Refer to pediatric psychology for the institution of cognitive behavioral therapy (CBT). CBT will enhance self-regulation of pain as well as coping strategies. Refer to pediatric physical therapy as needed for assistance with graduated exercise training.

## KEY POINTS

- Those diagnosed with SLE who receive proper preventative care, education, guidance, and medical care significantly improve their quality and function of life.
- It is important for the maintenance and treatment to refer children with SLE to a pediatric rheumatologist and any multidisciplinary specialists as organ systems are affected.
- In ARF, Sydenham's chorea erythema marginatum, and subcutaneous nodules are self-limiting.
- Prompt recognition of signs/symptoms of ARF is necessary to prevent further valvular damage.
- Education on the importance of adherence to secondary prophylaxis for ARF is essential.
- IgA vasculitis will be self-limiting in the vast majority of individuals, requiring only symptomatic care, although children should be monitored closely for renal involvement and complications.
- Reassure family/caregivers regarding the course of IgA vasculitis and educate them regarding complications.
- JIA is often not apparent in early stages of the disease and can be difficult to diagnose because there are no diagnostic tests, but early recognition, diagnosis, and treatment can help in the prevention of long-term damage of joints as well as help maintain function and prevent severe pain.
- Refer the child with JIA to a pediatric rheumatologist for guidance, maintenance, and treatment of the disease.
- KD is a self-limiting disease that requires a timely diagnosis of exclusion to decrease the potential for serious cardiac sequelae, such as coronary artery aneurysm.
- All children diagnosed with KD require an echocardiogram as soon as possible.
- Fibromyalgia is not harming the child or adolescent's body systems; therefore, treatment is not about healing, but rather about maintaining and controlling symptoms so the child may live a happy, healthy life.
- Medications may not be necessary for fibromyalgia; however, they may have to be used on a short-term basis to manage those children or adolescents affected more severely by their symptoms, especially with sleep disturbances, mood changes, and/or significant discomfort or pain.

## REFERENCES


Abbott, J. K., & Hauk, P. J. (2020). Immunodeficiency. In W. W. Hay, M. J. Levin, M. J. Abzug, & M. Bunik (Eds.), *Current diagnosis & treatment: Pediatrics* (25th ed., Chapter 33). McGraw-Hill Education.

American College of Rheumatology. (2020). *Juvenile arthritis.* https://www.rheumatology.org/I-Am-A/Patient-Caregiver/Diseases-Conditions/Juvenile-Arthritis

Butte, M. J., & Stiehm, E. R. (2020). Approach to the child with recurrent infections. *UpToDate.* https://www.uptodate.com/contents/approach-to-the-child-with-recurrent-infections

Centers for Disease Control and Prevention. (2018a). *Acute rheumatic fever.* https://www.cdc.gov/groupastrep/diseases-public/rheumatic-fever.html

Centers for Disease Control and Prevention. (2018b). *Systemic lupus erythematosus (SLE).* https://www.cdc.gov/lupus/facts/detailed.html

Centers for Disease Control and Prevention. (2020). *Fibromyalgia.* https://www.cdc.gov/arthritis/basics/fibromyalgia.htm

Chinn, I. K. (2019). Primary humoral immunodeficiencies: An overview. *UpToDate.* https://www.uptodate.com/contents/primary-humoral-immunodeficiencies-an-overview

Covar, R. A., Fleischer, D. M., Cho, C., & Boguniewicz, M. (2020). Allergic disorders. In W. W. Hay, M. J. Levin, M. J. Abzug, & M. Bunik (Eds.), *Current diagnosis & treatment: Pediatrics* (25th ed., Chapter 38). McGraw-Hill Education.

Dedeoglu, F., & Kim, S. (2019). IgA vasculitis (Henoch-Schönlein purpura): Clinical manifestations and diagnosis. *UpToDate.* https://www.uptodate.com/contents/iga-vasculitis-henoch-schonlein-purpura-clinical-manifestations-and-diagnosis

Gewitz, M. H., Baltimore, R. S., Tani, L. Y., Sable, C. A., Shulman, S. T., Carapetis, J., Remenyi, B., Taubert, K. A., Bolger, A. F., Beerman, L., Mayosi, B. M., Beaton, A., Pandian, N. G., & Kaplan, E. L. (2015). Revision of the Jones criteria for the diagnosis of acute rheumatic fever in the era of doppler echocardiography. *Circulation, 131,* 1806–1818. https://doi.org/10.1161/CIR.0000000000000205

Haumann, J. S., & Merola, J. F. (2019). *Juvenile idiopathic arthritis in child.* https://www.visualdx.com/visualdx/diagnosis/juvenile+idiopathic+arthritis?moduleId=102&diagnosisId=52268

Heineke, M. H., Ballering, A. V., Jamin, A., Ben Mkaddem, S., Monteiro, R. C., & Van Egmond, M. (2017). New insights in the pathogenesis of immunoglobulin A vasculitis (Henoch-Schönlein purpura). *Autoimmunity Reviews, 16*(12), 1246–1253. https://doi.org/10.1016/j.autrev.2017.10.009

Hetland, L. E., Sursrud, K. S., Lindahl, K. H., & Bygum, A. (2017). Henoch-Schönlein purpura: A literature review. *Acta Dermato Venereologica, 97*(10), 1160–1166. https://doi.org/10.2340/00015555-2733

Jeffrey Modell Foundation. (2016). *10 warning signs.* http://www.info4pi.org/library/educational-materials/10-warning-signs

Kimura, Y. (2020). Systemic juvenile idiopathic arthritis: Clinical manifestations and diagnosis. *UpToDate.* Retrieved October 20, 2020, from https://www.uptodate.com/contents/systemic-juvenile-idiopathic-arthritis-clinical-manifestations-and-diagnosis

Kimura, Y., & Walco, G. A. (2020). Fibromyalgia in children and adolescents: Treatment and prognosis overview. *UpToDate.* https://www.uptodate.com/contents/fibromyalgia-in-children-and-adolescents-treatment-and-prognosis-overview

Kimura, Y., & Walco, G. A. (2021). Fibromyalgia in children and adolescents: Clinical manifestations and diagnosis. *UpToDate.* https:// www.uptodate.com/contents/fibromyalgia-in-children-and-adolescents-clinical-manifestations-and-diagnosis

Klein-Gitelman, M. (2019). Systemic lupus erythematosus (SLE) in children: Treatment, complications, and prognosis. *UpToDate.* https://www.uptodate.com/contents/systemic-lupus-erythematosus-sle-in-children-treatment-complications-and-prognosis

Lexicomp. (2020). *Lexicomp clinical drug information* (version 5.7.1) [Mobile app]. App store. https://apps.apple.com/us/app/lexicomp/id313401238

Lin, M.-T., & Wu, M.-H. (2017). The global epidemiology of Kawasaki disease: Review and future perspectives. *Global Cardiology Science and Practice, 2017*(20). https://doi.org/10.21542/gcsp.2017.20

Lupus Foundation of America. (2020). *Understanding lupus.* https://www.lupus.org/resources/what-is-lupus

Munteanu, V., Petaccia, A., Contecaru, N., Amodio, E., & Agostoni, C. V. (2018). Paediatric acute rheumatic fever in developed countries: Neglected or negligible disease? Results from an observational study in Lombardy (Italy). *AIMS Public Health, 5*(2), 135–143. https://doi.org/10.3934/publichealth.2018.2.135

Newburger, J. W., Takahashi, M., & Burns, J. C. (2016). Kawasaki disease. *Journal of the American College of Cardiology, 67*(14), 1738–1749. https://doi.org/10.1016/j.jacc.2015.12.073

Paller, A. S., & Mancini, A. J. (2016). *Hurwitz clinical pediatric dermatology: A textbook of skin disorders of childhood and adolescence* (5th ed.). Elsevier.

Perez, C. E., & Dyer, J. A. (2020). Cutaneous drug eruptions in pediatrics: A primer. *Pediatric Annals, 49*(3), e132–e139. https://doi.org/10.3928/19382359-20200224-01

Sicherer, S. H. (2017). *How to implement new peanut allergy prevention guidelines.* https://www.aappublications.org/news/2017/05/09/Peanut050917

Sika-Paotonu, D., Beaton, A., Raghu, A., Steer, A., & Carapetis, J. (2017). Acute rheumatic fever and rheumatic heart disease. In J. J. Ferretti, D. L. Stevens, & V. A. Fischetti (Eds.), *Streptococcus pyogenes: Basic biology to clinical manifestations.* University of Oklahoma Health Sciences Center. https://www.ncbi.nlm.nih.gov/books/NBK425394/

Steer, A., & Gibofsky, A. (2020). Acute rheumatic fever: Clinical manifestations and diagnosis. *UpToDate.* https://www.uptodate.com/contents/acute-rheumatic-fever-clinical-manifestations-and-diagnosis

Stein, D. H., & Barnett, N. K. (2017). Insect bites and infestations. In T. K. McInerny, H. M. Adam, D. E. Campbell, J. M. Foy, & D. M. Kamat (Eds.), *American Academy of Pediatrics textbook of pediatric care* (2nd ed., Chapter 277). American Academy of Pediatrics.

Sundel, R. (2020). Kawasaki disease: Initial treatment and prognosis. *UpToDate.* https://www.uptodate.com/contents/kawasaki-disease-initial-treatment-and-prognosis

Szczygielska, I., Hernik, E., Kotodziejczyk, B., Gazda, A., Maślińska, M., & Gietka, P. (2018). Rheumatic fever—New diagnostic criteria. *Reumatologia, 56*(1), 37–41. https://doi.org/10.5114/reum.2018.74748

Volkman, K. K., & Chiu, A. M. (2019). Allergy. In K. J. Marcdante & R. M. Kliegman (Eds.), *Nelson's essentials of pediatrics* (8th ed., Section 14). Elsevier.

Wong, V., Winter, M. W., Tan, B., Burgin, S., & Prasad, P. (2019). *Systemic lupus erythematosus in child.* https://www.visualdx

.com/visualdx/diagnosis/systemic+lupus+erythematosus?moduleId=102&diagnosisId=51886

Wu, E. Y., & Rabinovich, C. E. (2020). Juvenile idiopathic arthritis. In R. M. Kliegman, J. St. Geme, N. J. Blum, S. S. Shah, R. C. Tasker, K. M. Wilson, & R. E. Behrman (Eds.), *Nelson textbook of pediatrics* (21st ed., Chapter 180). Elsevier.

Zoghaib, S., Kechichian, E., Souaid, K., Soutou, B., Helou, J., & Tomb, R. (2019). Triggers, clinical manifestations, and management of pediatric erythema multiforme: A systematic review. *Journal of the American Academy of Dermatology, 81*(3), 813–822. https://doi.org/10.1016/j.jaad.2019.02.057

CHAPTER **33**

UNIT IV

# Management of Atopic Disorders

Stacy B. Buchanan, Kathleen P. Thompson, and Elizabeth Neptune

## Student Learning Outcomes

**Upon completion of this chapter the reader should be able to:**

1. Discuss pathophysiology and epidemiology of selected atopic disorders in children.
2. Differentiate subjective and objective findings of selected atopic disorders in children.
3. Choose appropriate laboratory or diagnostic tests for particular atopic disorders in children.
4. Utilize the differential diagnosis process to determine atopic dermatitis, asthma, or allergic rhinitis diagnosis in children.
5. Determine treatment plan, child/family education, and need for referral in children with a(n) atopic dermatitis, allergic rhinitis, or asthma diagnosis.

## INTRODUCTION

**Atopic disorders** are common disorders of the pediatric population. Atopic disorders include atopic dermatitis (AD), asthma, and allergic rhinitis. These three conditions are commonly referred to as the *atopic triad* and are also grouped with other allergic disorders which in total affect about 25% of the population (Covar et al., 2020). The worldwide prevalence for allergic rhinitis is close to 13%, asthma 12%, and AD 8% (Pols et al., 2015). This chapter explores each of these disorders and reviews treatment modalities for use in the outpatient setting.

The content in this chapter maps to the following areas on the Pediatric Nursing Certification Board (PNCB) Pediatric Nurse Practitioner—Primary Care certification examination:

**CLINICAL PROBLEMS: HEENT, DERMATOLOGY, PULMONOLOGY**

CONTENT AREAS:

**II. Assessment and Diagnosis**

**B. History and Physical Examination**

1. Obtain history of present illness
2. Obtain a comprehensive health history for new patients
3. Complete an interval history for established patients
4. Perform a review of systems
5. Perform a complete physical examination

**C. Diagnostic Testing and Screening**

1. Order and interpret office/clinic based screening tests
2. Order and interpret diagnostic laboratory tests
3. Order and interpret the results of diagnostic imaging tests

**D. Analyzing Information**

1. Integrate health history and physical examination findings into the plan of care
2. Assimilate findings from screening and diagnostic testing into plan of care

**E. Diagnosis**

1. Develop and prioritize differential diagnoses
2. Establish a diagnosis based on evaluation of patient data

### III. Management

**A. Child and Caregiver Counseling and Education**

1. Provide condition-specific counseling and education, including treatment options
2. Educate about benefits and potential adverse reactions of pharmacological interventions
3. Discuss non-pharmacological interventions
4. Counsel regarding the threshold for seeking follow-up care
5. Review the risks of non-adherence to recommended treatment

**B. Therapeutic Interventions**

1. Prescribe pharmacologic agents
2. Recommend the use of over-the-counter pharmacologic agents
3. Order or recommend non-pharmacologic treatments for the management of symptoms
4. Discuss use of complementary and alternative therapies as appropriate

**C. Procedures**

1. Perform procedures in accordance with diagnostic guidelines and plan of care (rapid tests)
2. Initiate life-saving techniques in response to urgent or emergent situations

**D. Collaboration and Referral**

2. Refer to specialists as indicated for evaluation, counseling, and/or treatment

**E. Care Coordination**

1. Facilitate patient and family-centered care for children of all ages with acute and chronic conditions

**F. Evaluation and Follow-up**

2. Establish a plan for follow-up care

### IV. Professional Role Responsibilities

**A. Leadership and Evidence-based Practice**

4. Develop, implement, and/or modify clinical practice guidelines

## ATOPIC DERMATITIS

The skin is the largest organ of the body and its primary function is to protect the body. AD is an inflammatory condition resulting in pruritis and rash. AD appears in infancy or childhood, can be ongoing through adulthood, and carries a prevalence risk of 15% to 20% in industrialized nations (Simpson et al., 2019). Often, children of color are more affected more often than Caucasians (Geria & Alexis, 2016). AD is a common condition that can be debilitating. The cause of AD is multifactorial, including genetic predisposition, environmental factors, and socioeconomic factors (Bager et al., 2016).

Genetics play a role as a determinant in the development of AD, particularly when an atopic disorders affects a first-degree relative (Bager et al., 2016; Prok & Torres-Zegarra, 2020). The **filaggrin** protein is found in cells that make up the outermost, protective layer of skin (epidermis) and if disrupted may allow the skin to become compromised (Bager et al., 2016). Skin barrier disruption permits irritant exposure, resultant inflammation, and the development of AD (Simpson et al., 2019).

A lack of moisture in the skin results in cutaneous hyperreactivity and pruritis, the hallmark symptom of AD. Scratching occurs after allergen and irritant exposure, humidity changes, and excessive sweating. Redness of the skin is further exacerbated with the itch-scratch cycle (Bager et al., 2016). In chronic cases, lichenification and pigmentation changes occur.

The exact etiology of AD has yet to be determined. As mentioned previously, those who have a defect in the filaggrin protein are more likely to manifest symptoms of AD. Triggers such as stress, climate changes, exposure to allergens, and environmental irritants can exacerbate AD (Simpson et al., 2019). Infection with *Staphylococcus* bacteria triggers an IgE-mediated response in some children and can lead to an outbreak of AD symptoms (Bager et al., 2016).

### Subjective Findings

The health history may reveal:

- Recurrent pruritis
- Rash

### Risk Factors

The most common risk factors for atopic dermatitis are:

- Genetic predisposition
- Exposure to environmental triggers.

### Review of Systems

The most common manifestations revealed during the review of systems include:

- **Constitutional:** sleep disruption from itching
- **Integumentary:** recurrent, itchy rash

### Objective Findings

The physical examination of the child with atopic dermatitis may reveal:

- Dry skin
- Patches of erythematous skin, crusting, scaling, scabbing, or lichenification
  - Usually on cheeks, torso extensor surface in infants
  - Typically, in flexural creases on children 2 years and older
  - Sparing of the groin area

ALERT: Be sure to recognize whether the lesions are secondarily infected!

### Laboratory/Diagnostic Testing

The diagnosis of AD is based upon the clinical findings. No laboratory or diagnostic testing is needed. Identification of food allergy through allergy testing can be beneficial if a food allergy is a suspected trigger for AD.

### Differential Diagnosis

The differential diagnosis for AD includes:

- Psoriasis
- Contact dermatitis
- Tinea corporis
- Scabies

### Treatment/Management Plan

The primary mode of prevention and treatment includes the use of emollient moisturizers. The skin is dry and adding moisture is always a part of the care of children with AD (Prok & Torres-Zegarra, 2020). Moisturizers should always be fragrance- and dye-free to avoid further irritation of the skin. Lotions are generally unacceptable as emollients in AD, as they may contain alcohol or other irritants and are composed of a large percentage of water, which evaporates quickly. A cream, gel, balm, oil, or ointment would serve to treat xerosis and prevent water loss. Choose an emollient with the family's input, considering preference, safety, effectiveness, and cost. Many emollients are readily available for purchase over the counter.

Some families may be interested in using a natural or alternative emollient product rather than a commercial moisturizer. Petroleum jelly is inexpensive, an excellent emollient, and generally does not result in adverse effects. In contrast, vegetable shortening can be more expensive and, in some cases, result in additional inflammation. Currently, few studies support the use of other alternative products. Olive oil should probably not be used, as it may induce an inflammatory reaction or irritant contact dermatitis. Virgin coconut oil works well to prevent water loss, has an anti-inflammatory effect, and presents low risk for contact dermatitis. Sunflower seed oil decreases inflammation, treats skin dysfunction, and carries no risk for allergic dermatitis (Karagounis et al., 2019).

In addition to emollients, there are several options to consider depending upon the severity of symptoms once moisturizing becomes insufficient in treating a child with AD. Pharmacologic treatments include topical corticosteroids, calcineurin inhibitor topical creams, phosphodiesterase inhibitor ointments, a monoclonal antibody, and cyclosporine. Children with severe AD may benefit from wet wrap therapy (National Eczema Foundation, 2020).

### Medical Treatment

#### *Topical Corticosteroids*

Topical corticosteroids vary in potency and are formulated in creams and ointments. Generally, ointments are more potent than creams. The potency of topical corticosteroids ranges from VII (least potent) to I (super potent). Utilizing a steroid potency chart (such as Table 33.1) will assist with choosing a mild or moderate potency topical steroid. Adverse effects include atrophy, striae, and telangiectasia.

#### *Calcineurin Inhibitor Topical Creams*

Considering topical steroid use to be the second line in the defense against AD, the third-line treatment modalities include calcineurin inhibitor topical creams (pimecrolimus, tacrolimus). Tacrolimus has been used with caution in the treatment of AD in children, considering the potential for lymphoma development, but recent evidence refutes that thinking (Ohtsuki et al., 2018). However, complaints of pain and/or burning at the application sites may limit the use of this medication (Kimler et al., 2019).

**TABLE 33.1 Topical Corticosteroid Potency**

| Potency | Corticosteroid (Vehicle) |
|---|---|
| Least Potent—VII | Hydrocortisone hydrochloride 1% (C, O)<br>Hydrocortisone hydrochloride 2.5% (C, L, O)<br>Hydrocortisone acetate 1% (C, O)<br>Hydrocortisone acetate 2.5% (C, L, O)<br>Pramoxine hydrochloride 1.0% (C, L, O)<br>Pramoxine hydrochloride 2.5% (C, L, O) |
| Low Potency—VI | Betamethasone valerate 0.05% (L)<br>Desonide 0.05% (C)<br>Flucinolone acetonide 0.01% (C, S, Oil)<br>Triamcinolone acetonide 0.1% (C) |
| Low-Mid Strength—V | Betamethasone dipropionate 0.05% (L)<br>Betamethasone valerate 0.1% (C)<br>Fluticasone acetonide 0.025% (C)<br>Fluticasone propionate 0.05% (C)<br>Hydrocortisone valerate 0.2% (C) |
| Mid Strength—IV | Hydrocortisone valerate 0.2% (O)<br>Fluocinolone acetonide 0.025% (O)<br>Mometasone furoate 0.1% (C)<br>Triamcinolone acetonide 0.1% (C) |
| High-Mid Strength—III | Betamethasone dipropionate 0.05% (C)<br>Betamethasone valerate 0.1% (O)<br>Fluocinonide 0.05% (C)<br>Fluticasone propionate 0.005% (O)<br>Triamcinolone acetonide 0.1% (O) |
| High Potency—II | Betamethasone dipropionate 0.05% (C, O)<br>Fluocinonide 0.05% (C, O, G, S)<br>Mometasone furoate 0.1% (O) |
| Super Potency—I | Betamethasone dipropionate 0.05% (C, O)<br>Clobetasol propionate 0.05% (C, O)<br>Halobetasol propionate 0.05% (C, O) |

C, cream; O, ointment; L, lotion; G, gel; S, Solution

*Source*: Adapted from Kimler, K. A., McDonald, D., & Shah, P. B. (2019). Treatment of atopic dermatitis in pediatric patients: Nursing implications. *Pediatric Nursing, 45*(5), 215–223, 230.

### *Phosphodiesterase-4 Inhibitors*

A newer alternative in topical therapy would be a phosphodiesterase-4 (PDE-4) inhibitor called crisaborole ointment. PDE-4 inhibitors are effective because they suppress the release of cytokines and limit pruritis (Kimler et al., 2019). The most common adverse effect of crisaborole is pain at the application site, though otherwise adverse effects are rare.

### *Systemic Therapies*

In uncontrolled moderate to severe AD, systemic therapy may be considered. Systemic medications for AD include monoclonal antibodies and cyclosporin.

### *Monoclonal Antibody Therapy*

The first monoclonal antibody therapy, dupilumab, is approved for children and adolescents 11 years of age and older with uncontrolled moderate to severe AD. Dupilumab targets the interleukin-4 alpha receptor, a key mediator in AD (Kimler et al., 2019). It is given via subcutaneous injection with doses based on weight and age:

- 6 years to 17 years
  - 15 to less than 30 kg: 600 mg (as two 300 mg injections) initially, with maintenance dose of 300 mg every 4 weeks
  - 30 kg to less than 60 kg: 400 mg (as two 200 mg injections) initially, with maintenance dose of 200 mg every 2 weeks
  - Over 60 kg: 600 mg (as two 300 mg injections) initially, with maintenance dose of 300 mg every 2 weeks
  - Age 18 years and older: 600 mg (as two 300 mg injections) initially, with maintenance dose of 300 mg every 2 weeks

### *Cyclosporine*

Cyclosporine may be considered as an adjunct therapy for those children with refractory AD that has been difficult to manage. Cyclosporine works as an immune modulator that suppresses cytokine release in T-cells (Kimler et al., 2019). Prescribe 3 to 5 mg/kg/day in two divided doses for 2 to 4 months, with a gradual tapering over several months (Spergel & Lio, 2020). Adverse reactions to be considered with the use of cyclosporine include hypertension, edema, headache, and increased susceptibility to infection, each of which must be considered prior to the initiation of therapy (Kimler et al., 2019).

### *Treatment Decision Making*

All children with AD require the use of emollients at least twice daily. Refer to Table 33.2 for medication guidance in relation to the severity of AD and its state of control. For more severe disease, use a taper-down approach (as severity lessens or disease improves, change medication and/or frequency).

### *Wet Wrap Therapy*

Wet wrap therapy may benefit some children with severe AD who experience a generalized exacerbation. Topical corticosteroids are applied to the affected areas, which are then wrapped with either wet cotton gauze or a wet garment. Dry wraps or a dry garment is then applied, taking care not to dislodge the wet

**TABLE 33.2 Medications for Atopic Dermatitis Based on Severity**

| Severity | Medication | Frequency/Duration |
|---|---|---|
| Maintenance | TCI or PDI to areas usually involved | Twice weekly |
| Controlled | TCI or PDI to areas usually involved | Twice daily/2 weeks |
| Mild | Low-potency CS *and* TCI or PDI | Twice daily/3–5 days |
| Moderate | Medium-potency CS *and* TCI or PDI | Twice daily/3–5 days |
| Severe | High-potency CS *and* TCI or PDI | Twice daily/3–5 days |
| Uncontrolled | Dupilumab | Initial dose, then every 2 to 4 weeks |
| Refractory | Cyclosporin | Twice daily/2–4 months, then tapered |

CS, corticosteroid; TCI, topical calcineurin inhibitor; PDI, phosphodiesterase-4 (PDE-4) inhibitor

*Sources*: Adapted from Kimler, K. A., McDonald, D., & Shah, P. B. (2019). Treatment of atopic dermatitis in pediatric patients: Nursing implications. *Pediatric Nursing, 45*(5), 215–223, 230; Oberlin, K. E., & Nanda, S. (2019). Atopic dermatitis made easy: The Schachner Ladder. *Pediatric Dermatology, 36*, 1017–1018. https://doi.org/10.1111/pde.13862; Spergel, J. M., & Lio, P. A. (2020). Management of severe atopic dermatitis (eczema) in children. *UpToDate*. Retrieved June 18, 2020, from https://www.uptodate.com/contents/management-of-severe-atopic-dermatitis-eczema-in-children

wrap. The wrap may be worn for 2 hours or overnight (Spergel & Lio, 2020).

### Family Education

Teach the following:

- Moisturization is the number-one treatment choice.
- Reduce bathing frequency and use warm, rather than hot, water.
- All laundry detergent, bath soap, and topical products should be fragrance-free.
- Pat dry (rather than rub) after bathing or showering and immediately apply moisturizer while skin is damp.
- Bleach baths may reduce severity (use ¼ cup bleach in a full bath, 1/8 cup bleach in a half bath; Chopra et al., 2017).
- Use medications as instructed by provider.
- Teach families how to use wet wraps if needed (https://nationaleczema.org/eczema/treatment/wet-wrap-therapy).
- Information about commercially available wet-dry pajamas may be found at www.soothems.com/blogs/news/how-to-wet-wrap-using-soothems-eczema-therapy-pajamas (Soothems, 2020).

### Referral

If management of AD through traditional means does not result in control of symptoms, then referral should be considered. A dermatologist and/or allergist may be appropriate for children with refractory AD. Some children may require allergy testing to determine if food allergies trigger the AD exacerbations.

## ALLERGIC RHINITIS

Affecting a significant number of children, allergic rhinitis is a common chronic condition having multiple environmental causes. Inhalants trigger the immune (IgE-mediated) response, resulting in increased nasal secretions, turbinate swelling, and pruritis of the nasal mucosa. Occurring seasonally or perennially, common triggers include pollen, mold, dust mites, cockroaches, and pet dander (de Shazo & Kemp, 2020). About 10% to 14% of children with allergic rhinitis also have asthma (Covar et al., 2020). Resulting in significant childhood morbidity, allergic rhinitis occurring in isolation does not affect childhood mortality. Sleep-disordered breathing may occur as a result of allergic rhinitis and is linked to poor school performance, as are attention difficulties experienced by seasonal sufferers during pollen season (de Shazo & Kemp, 2020).

### Subjective Findings

The health history may reveal:

- Persistent rhinorrhea (seasonally or perennially)
- Chronic nasal congestion
- Sneezing
- Frequent upper respiratory infections including sinusitis and otitis media
- Snoring
- Headaches

### Risk Factors

The most common risk factors for allergic rhinitis are:

- Family or personal history of atopy
- Exposure to environmental factors
- Maternal smoking in the first year of life

## Review of Systems

The most common manifestations revealed during the review of systems include:

- **Constitutional:** snoring, night awakening
- **HEENT:** itchy, watery eyes, sneezing
- **Neurologic:** headache

## Objective Findings

The physical examination of the child with allergic rhinitis may reveal:

- Clear rhinorrhea
- Allergic shiners (i.e., periorbital hyperpigmentation, dark circles under the eyes caused by nasal and sinus congestion)
- Pale, boggy, enlarged turbinates
- Allergic "salute" (transverse white line or crease across nose from habit of rubbing the nose in a typically upward movement)

## Laboratory/Diagnostic Testing

The diagnosis of allergic rhinitis is based upon the clinical findings. No laboratory or diagnostic testing is needed, though a nasal smear may be positive for eosinophilia, though this is not diagnostic. To identify specific allergens, skin testing or a radioallergosorbent test (RAST) may be used (Covar et al., 2020).

## Differential Diagnosis

The differential diagnosis for allergic rhinitis includes:

- Viral upper respiratory infection
- Acute or chronic bacterial rhinosinusitis
- Significantly deviated septum
- Nasal polyps
- Adenoidal hypertrophy
- Rhinitis medicamentosa (rebound congestion from overuse of nasal decongestants)

## Treatment/Management Plan

Treatment of allergic rhinitis consists of trigger avoidance, saline washes, antihistamines, intranasal corticosteroids, and (in older children) possibly decongestants. First-generation antihistamines such as diphenhydramine and hydroxyzine may cause excess sedation or a paradoxical excitatory response in young children, so they are not routinely used. Second-generation antihistamines are generally well tolerated, and most are available without prescription. Table 33.3 provides dosage recommendations.

**TABLE 33.3 Antihistamines for Allergic Rhinitis**

| Medication | Age | Dosage |
|---|---|---|
| **Cetirizine** (tablet, chewable tablet, dispersible tablet, liquid) | | |
| | 6–23 months | 2.5 mg daily |
| | 2–5 years | 2.5–5 mg daily |
| | 6 years or older | 5–10 mg daily, or 2.5 mg twice a day |
| **Loratadine** (tablet, rapidly disintegrating tablet, liquid) | | |
| | 2–5 years | 5 mg daily |
| | 6 years or older | 10 mg daily |
| **Desloratadine** (tablet, orally-dissolving tablet, liquid) | | |
| | 6–11 months | 1 mg daily |
| | 1–5 years | 1.25 mg daily |
| | 6–11 years | 2.5 mg daily |
| | 12 years or older | 5 mg daily |
| **Fexofenadine** (tablet, orally disintegrating tablet, liquid) | | |
| | 6–23 months | 15 mg twice a day |
| | 2–11 years | 30 mg twice a day |
| | 12 years or older | 60 mg twice a day, or 180 mg (extended release) once daily |
| **Levocetirizine** (prescription only, available as tablet, liquid) | | |
| | 6 months–5 years | 1.25 mg daily |
| | 6–11 years | 2.5 mg daily |
| | 12 years or older | 5 mg daily |

Intranasal corticosteroid therapy reduces swelling of nasal mucosa and provides symptomatic relief of nasal congestion. Prescribe intranasal corticosteroids as follows:

- Mometasone, fluticasone furoate—one spray in each nostril once daily (2–11 years), two sprays in each nostril once daily (12 years and older)
- Fluticasone propionate—one to two sprays/nostril once daily (4 years and older)
- Budesonide, triamcinolone—one to two sprays/nostril once daily (6 years and older)
- Flunisolide—one spray/nostril three times a day or two sprays/nostril twice a day (6–14 years)
- Ciclesonide—two sprays/nostril once daily (6 years and older for seasonal allergic rhinitis, and 12 years and older for perennial allergic rhinitis)

Adjunct therapies that may also help include:

- For mast cell stabilization: cromolyn sodium intranasal spray, 1 spray/nostril 3–4 times daily (2 years and older; or ipratropium bromide intranasal solution

(0.03%), 2 sprays/nostril 2–3 times daily (6 years and older)
- Antihistamine ophthalmic preparations such as naphazoline
- In older children, nasal decongestants and ophthalmic vasoconstrictors may relieve congestion and redness but should not be used for longer than 4 days, as rebound rhinorrhea or conjunctival redness may occur

ALERT: Nosebleeds can occur as a side effect of intranasal steroid use.

### Family Education

Teach the following:

- Eliminate pet dander and dust mites by keeping all pets out of child's bedroom, avoiding stuffed animals, removing carpets and rugs from the child's bedroom, washing all linens weekly in very hot water
- Avoid all exposure to cigarette smoke (no parental smoking in the home or car)
- Keep windows closed during pollen season
- Routinely clean all surfaces in the home
- Utilize commercially prepared normal saline nasal spray or make at home with 1 cup distilled water, ½ teaspoon salt, and ¼ teaspoon baking soda; use a bulb syringe to instill in the nose
- Treatment with nasal sprays can be difficult in younger children; think of a fun game or treat as a reward for receiving a nasal spray
- Caution families about intranasal corticosteroid side effects of nasal irritation or soreness, and epistaxis (which may commonly occur with chronic use)

**PRO TIP** Instruct parents and children to tilt the head forward and aim the tip of the nasal spray toward the ear to avoid injuring the nasal septum and decrease the likelihood of swallowing the medication.

### Referral

For children who are unresponsive to treatment, refer to a pediatric allergy specialist for identification of exact triggers and consideration for immunotherapy. Refer children suspected of having further anatomy issues such as nasal polyps to a pediatric otolaryngologist (Seidman et al., 2015).

## ASTHMA

Asthma is the most common chronic respiratory disease in children and adults (Fuchs et al., 2017). It is a heterogeneous, chronic inflammatory disorder of the airways that causes recurrent episodes of wheezing, cough, shortness of breath, and chest tightness. The inflammation is thought to be caused by many cellular elements including mast cells, eosinophils, T lymphocytes, macrophages, neutrophils, and epithelial cells (Wingrove, 2016). These cellular elements are the targets of treatments. The clinical triad of asthma refers to tissue edema, excess mucus production, and bronchial constriction (Figure 33.1). This bronchoconstriction is often reversible with treatments (Wingrove, 2016). The cause of childhood asthma is not fully understood; however, there are indications that both environmental exposures (such as allergens, infections, microbes, and pollutants), and stress and genetic susceptibilities play a role. There is no cure for asthma, so the goal of treatment is to adequately control symptoms and prevent serious asthma exacerbations, which can often be achieved by avoiding triggers (Appendix A).

With asthma being one of the most common chronic diseases in childhood, it is not unexpected that the prevalence continues to increase rapidly worldwide. Asthma affects an estimated 300 million people of all ethnicities worldwide across all ages (Fuchs et al., 2017). It affects an estimated 6.1 million children under the age of 18 years old and accounts for more than 10 million lost school days per year (American Lung Association [ALA], 2020). When comparing prevalence of children with asthma, there is a lower prevalence in children under 5 years of age, which likely is due to difficulty diagnosing asthma in this age group. Data from the Centers for Disease Control and Prevention (CDC) regarding children shows that males have a higher prevalence than females (2018). Prevalence is also higher among children of color as compared with White children (CDC, 2018). Asthma is responsible for 3,388 deaths a year (across all ages), and Black Americans are two to three times more likely to die from asthma than any other group is (CDC, 2018). Asthma exacerbations are the third leading cause of hospitalization among children (CDC, 2018).

### Subjective Findings

The health history may reveal:

- Wheezing with upper respiratory infections

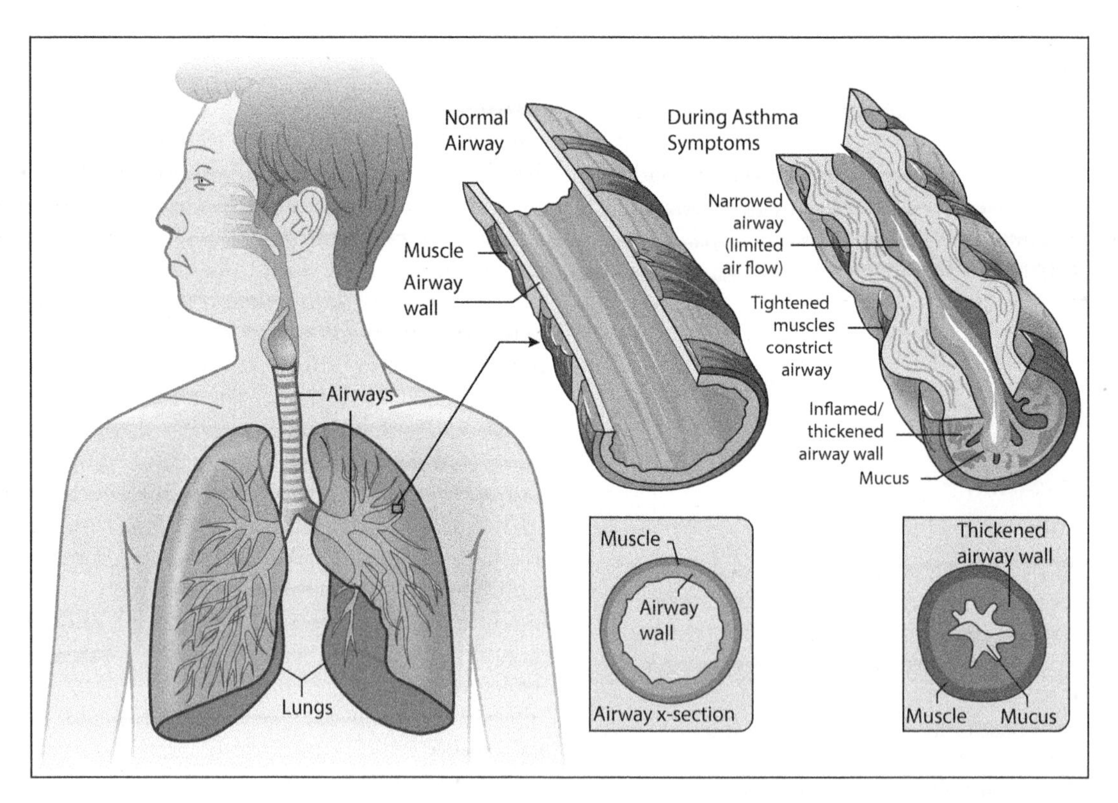


FIGURE 33.1 The pathophysiology of asthma.

- Increased coughing or wheezing with exposure to environmental triggers such as smoking and pet dander, with exercise or stressful situations
- Nighttime cough and/or wheezing (Figure 33.2)

## Risk Factors

The most common risk factors for asthma are:

- Family or personal history of atopic or allergic disease (e.g., allergic rhinitis, AD, food allergies)
- Lower socioeconomic status
- Infections early in life, especially common viral respiratory infections such as rhinovirus, respiratory syncytial virus, adenovirus, human metapneumovirus, and influenza
- Environmental exposure to tobacco smoke
- Low birth weight and decreased lung function at birth (CDC, 2018; Fuchs et al., 2017)

## Review of Systems

The most common manifestations revealed during the review of systems include:

- **Constitutional:** difficulty keeping up with peers during physical activity

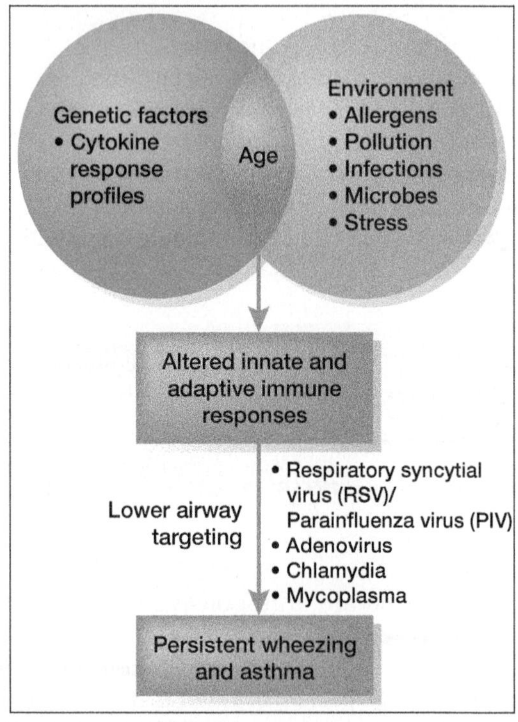


FIGURE 33.2 Host factors and environmental exposures that cause asthma.

- **Respiratory:** chest tightness, wheezing, nighttime cough and/or wheezing

## Objective Findings

The physical examination of the child with asthma may reveal:

- Transverse nasal crease (allergic salute)
- Rhinitis
- Frequent cough
- Tachypnea and accessory muscle usage
- Expiratory wheeze on auscultation
- Diminished aeration on auscultation
- Forced, prolonged expiratory phase
- Changes in oxygenation saturation as noted by pulse oximetry
- Rash consistent with AD

## Laboratory/Diagnostic Testing

In children 5 years and younger, the diagnosis of asthma is challenging. This is due to periodic episodes of respiratory symptoms like wheezing and cough that often are caused by viral respiratory infections, which is common in pediatrics, especially for children less than 2 years of age (Global Initiative for Asthma [GINA], 2020a). Additionally, it is not possible to routinely assess airflow limitation or bronchodilator responsiveness in children less than 5 years of age (GINA, 2020a). There are no specific tests to definitively diagnose asthma with certainty in children 5 years and younger; however, there are several useful adjuncts worth discussing.

A therapeutic trial of treatment with a short acting beta-2 agonist (SABA) and regular low-dose inhaled corticosteroids (ICS) may provide some insight about a possible diagnosis of asthma (GINA, 2020a). The trial should be evaluated by daytime/nighttime symptom control, frequency of wheezing episodes, and number of exacerbations. A diagnosis of asthma is supported if there is clinical improvement during the trial and deterioration when the trial is stopped. The therapeutic trial may have to be repeated in order to be certain of the diagnosis (GINA, 2020a).

Radiographic imaging is rarely indicated to confirm a diagnosis of asthma. Nevertheless, if there is doubt of the diagnosis, a chest x-ray may be beneficial to exclude structural abnormalities such as congenital lobar emphysema, vascular ring, inhaled foreign body, or chronic infectious process (GINA, 2020a).

Allergy testing via skin-prick testing or allergen-specific immunoglobulin E may be helpful in aiding the diagnosis of asthma. The presence of allergic sensitization is found in the majority of children with asthma once they are over the age of 3 (GINA, 2020a). It is important to note that the absence of sensitization to common aeroallergens does not exclude the diagnosis of asthma. Allergic sensitization has proven to be a good predictor for the development of persistent asthma (GINA, 2020b).

There are several pediatric risk profile tools that have been developed to identify children 5 years and younger who have a high risk of developing persistent asthma symptoms. The Tucson Children's Respiratory Study developed the Asthma Predictive Index (API) for children who have had four or more wheezing episodes in a year (GINA, 2020a). Although additional research is needed to further validate the risk profile, one study found that a positive API had a four- to tenfold greater chance of developing asthma between the ages of 6 to 13 years than those with a negative API (GINA, 2020a). Approximately 95% of children with a negative API remained asthma free (GINA, 2020a).

In children younger than 5 years of age, the ability to obtain reproducible expiratory maneuvers is limited. Subsequently, lung function testing, bronchial provocation testing, and other physiological tests do not have a major role in diagnosing asthma at such a young age. However, by 5 years of age, many children are able to perform reproducible spirometry if taught by experienced technicians (GINA, 2020a).

Pulmonary function testing of forced vital capacity (FVC) and forced expiratory volume in 1 second (FEV1) are useful tools for assessing airway obstruction, especially if there is a positive response after bronchodilator administration. Spirometry, which is an objective measurement of asthma control, aids with identifying obstruction in children with low symptom awareness, allows for disease progression tracking, and measures response to therapy (Wingrove, 2016). Spirometry is obtained by having a child inhale deeply, close to total lung capacity, and then forcefully exhale into the spirometer as hard and fast as possible to reach residual volume (Stickle, 2018). Additionally, the child must completely seal their lips on a mouthpiece and have a nasal clip to prevent air from escaping through the nares (Wingrove, 2016). Visual cues, such as blowing out candles, are helpful to aid the child on focusing throughout the test to improve result validity (GINA, 2020a; Wingrove, 2016). Spirometry testing is repeated three times to prove reproducibility. Computer programs measure the volume and rate of exhaled air into the device and calculate percentages based on predicted values; these are based on gender, height, and ethnicity. Ability to reach 80% of predicted value is considered normal. Below 80% is obstruction, especially if there is a disproportionate reduction in the FEV1 to FVC ratio (Table 33.4; Wingrove, 2016). Then, a bronchodilator is administered, and the test is repeated. A bronchodilator response is considered positive when there is 12% or more change in FVC, FEV1, and the FEV1/FVC ratio. A positive response is highly suggestive of a reversible airway obstruction that is seen in asthma (GINA, 2020a; Wingrove, 2016).

In children age 5 and older, fractional exhaled nitric oxide (FeNO) testing may be used. FeNO measures the amount of nitric oxide (an inflammation byproduct) exhaled, in parts per billion (ppb). In children 5 to 12 years of age, levels of > 35 ppb support a diagnosis of asthma, while levels of 50 ppb indicate asthma in children older than 12 years. Though it should not be used alone to determine either asthma control or for clinical course prediction, it may be useful when the diagnosis or therapeutic approach is uncertain (National Heart, Lung, and Blood Institute [NHLBI], 2020).

## Differential Diagnosis

A definitive diagnosis of asthma in pediatrics is challenging, since many disorders have similar signs and symptoms. This is especially true in children younger than 5 years of age. It is imperative to consider and exclude alternative causes that have symptoms of wheeze, cough, and breathlessness prior to confirming the diagnosis of asthma, because the differential has important clinical consequences (GINA, 2020b). Refer to Table 33.5 for common differential diagnoses of asthma in children 5 years or younger and their key clinical features.

**TABLE 33.4 Pulmonary Function Test to Assess Severity of Asthma**

| | Persistent | | |
|---|---|---|---|
| **Intermittent** | **Mild** | **Moderate** | **Severe** |
| Normal FEV1 between exacerbations<br>FEV1 >80% predicted<br>FEV1/FVC >85% | FEV1 ≥80% predicted<br>FEV1/FVC >80% | FEV1 = 60%–80% predicted<br>FEV1/FVC = 75%–80% | FEV1 <60%<br>FEV1/FVC <75% |

FEV1, forced expiratory volume in one second; FVC, forced vital capacity

*Sources*: Adapted from Global Initiative for Asthma. (2020). *Pocket guide for asthma management and prevention*. https://ginasthma.org/pocket-guide-for-asthma-management-and-prevention; Liu, A. H., Spahn, J. D., & Sichere, S. H. (2020). Childhood asthma. In R. M. Kliegman, J. St. Geme, N. J. Blum, S. S. Shah, R. C. Tasker, K. M. Wilson, & R. E. Behrman (Eds.), *Nelson textbook of pediatrics* (21st ed., Chapter 169). Elsevier; National Heart, Lung, and Blood Institute. (2020). *Asthma*. https://www.nhlbi.nih.gov/health-topics/asthma 2019; Wingrove, B. R. (2016). An overview of pediatric asthma. *Physician Assistant Clinics*, 1(4), 563–582. https://doi.org/10.1016/j.cpha.2016.05.005

Typical features of asthma increase the likelihood of an accurate asthma diagnosis; these include cough, wheeze, shortness of breath, and/or chest tightness, which vary in intensity and over time. Cough is often worse at night or early in the morning. The symptoms may start following a trigger such as viral upper respiratory infection, weather changes, exposure to an allergen or irritant, exercise, laughing, and irritants such as car exhaust fumes, smoke, or strong smells. Features decreasing the likelihood of asthma include chronic sputum production, isolated cough, chest pain, shortness of breath resulting in lightheadedness or dizziness, and noisy inspiration when having breathing difficulty during exercise (GINA, 2020a). Refer to the algorithm in Figure 33.3.

## Treatment/Management Plan

The goal of asthma management is to relieve and control symptoms and prevent exacerbation and asthma-related deaths (GINA, 2020a). Successful management requires a partnership between child and their family and the healthcare provider. It is important to assess the child's goals and have shared decision-making in treatment options. GINA has established an asthma management cycle of assess, adjust treatment, and review response (Figure 33.3).

Once the diagnosis of asthma has been made, it is recommended to start treatment right away with daily low-dose ICS and SABA as needed (GINA, 2020a). Even children with mild intermittent asthma can have severe exacerbations and should be started on low-dose ICS. Treatment should be increased in a stepwise approach based on NHLBI guidelines (see Figure 33.4a–c). If the child has asthma symptoms or is waking from asthma once or more per week, the healthcare provider should initiate therapy at step 3 or 4 with medium-dose ICS –long-acting beta-agonist (LABA) and refer to a specialist. If the initial asthma presentation is with severely uncontrolled asthma or an acute exacerbation, then a short course of oral systemic steroids should be given as well as starting a regular controller treatment at step 3 or 4 with medium-dose ICS-LABA and refer to a specialist (see Figure 33.4a–c).

When stepping up treatment, reassess the child's response in 4 to 6 weeks if age 4 or younger, or in 2 to 6 weeks if over 5 years of age. Assessing control is based on a report of the child's symptoms and objective data with pulmonary function tests. Each clinic visit, the child/family should answer questions regarding frequency of symptoms over the past 4 weeks. A record of how often the symptoms are present will indicate if the child's asthma is well controlled, partially controlled, or uncontrolled (GINA, 2020a; NHLBI, 2020).

**TABLE 33.5 Asthma Differential Diagnoses in Children Less Than 6 Years Old, with Typical Clinical Features**

| Diagnosis | Typical Clinical Features |
|---|---|
| Recurrent viral respiratory tract Infections | Usually cough, rhinorrhea <10 days; no symptoms between infections |
| Gastroesophageal reflux | Cough when feeding; recurrent chest infections; poor response to asthma medications; episodes of emesis after a large feed |
| Foreign body aspiration | Abrupt, severe cough and/or stridor during eating or play; recurrent chest infections & cough; focal vesicular sounds |
| Persistent bacterial bronchitis | Persistent productive cough; poor response to asthma medications |
| Tracheomalacia | Noisy breathing with rigorous activity like eating, crying, or with upper airway infections (noisy inspiration if extrathoracic or expiration if intrathoracic); harsh cough; inspiratory or expiratory retractions; symptoms typically present since birth; poor response to asthma medications |
| Tuberculosis | Persistent noisy respirations and cough; fever unresponsive to normal antibiotics; lymphadenopathy; poor response to bronchodilators or inhaled corticosteroids; known contact with tuberculosis |
| Congenital heart disease | Cardiac murmur; cyanosis when eating; failure to thrive; tachycardia; tachypnea or hepatomegaly; poor response to asthma medications |
| Cystic fibrosis | Cough starts shortly after birth; recurrent chest infections; failure to thrive (malabsorption); loose, greasy, bulky stools |
| Primary ciliary dyskinesia (PCD) | Cough and recurrent chest infections; neonatal respiratory distress, chronic ear infections and persistent nasal discharge from birth; poor response to asthma medications; approximately 50% of children with PCD have situs inversus (congenital anomaly where visceral organs are reversed from correct positioning) |
| Vascular ring | Persistently noisy breathing; poor response to asthma medications |
| Bronchopulmonary dysplasia | Prematurity; very low birth weight; need for prolonged mechanical ventilation or supplemental oxygen; difficulty with breathing since birth |
| Immune deficiency | Failure to thrive; persistent febrile episodes and infections (including nonrespiratory) |

*Source*: Adapted from: Global Initiative for Asthma. (2020). *Global strategy for asthma management and prevention*. https://ginasthma.org/reports

When asthma symptoms have been well controlled for 3 months, consider stepping down therapy. However, ICS should not be completely stopped in adolescents (GINA, 2020a; NHLBI, 2020). The timing of stepping down treatment should be when the child's triggers are low and it is not peak viral respiratory season. The summer is usually a good time for families to step down treatment.

**PRO TIP** The NHLBI (2020) does not recommend the use of cromolyn, montelukast, or theophylline for the treatment of asthma, as these drugs have been demonstrated to be of limited use, have undesirable adverse effects, or require additional monitoring.

Pharmacotherapy is crucial to management; however, it is important to avoid medications that can cause severe exacerbations, such as nonsteroidal anti-inflammatory drugs (NSAIDs) and aspirin. With each clinic appointment and/or medication change, a new asthma action plan should be completed as part of the treatment plan. School-age children should have asthma action plans for home and school as well as controller medications for both home and school.

Treatment for children <5 years old is a challenge due to difficulty with diagnosis in this age group. Step 1 treatment should be an inhaled SABA administered as needed. Step 2 treatment should be daily low-dose ICS plus SABA as needed. If 3 months of Step 2 treatment does not achieve symptom control, then refer to a specialist (GINA, 2020a; NHLBI, 2020).

**PRO TIP** The NHLBI recommends initiating inhaled corticosteroids in children less than 4 years of age, who experience recurrent wheezing, at the start of a respiratory infection (NHLBI, 2020).

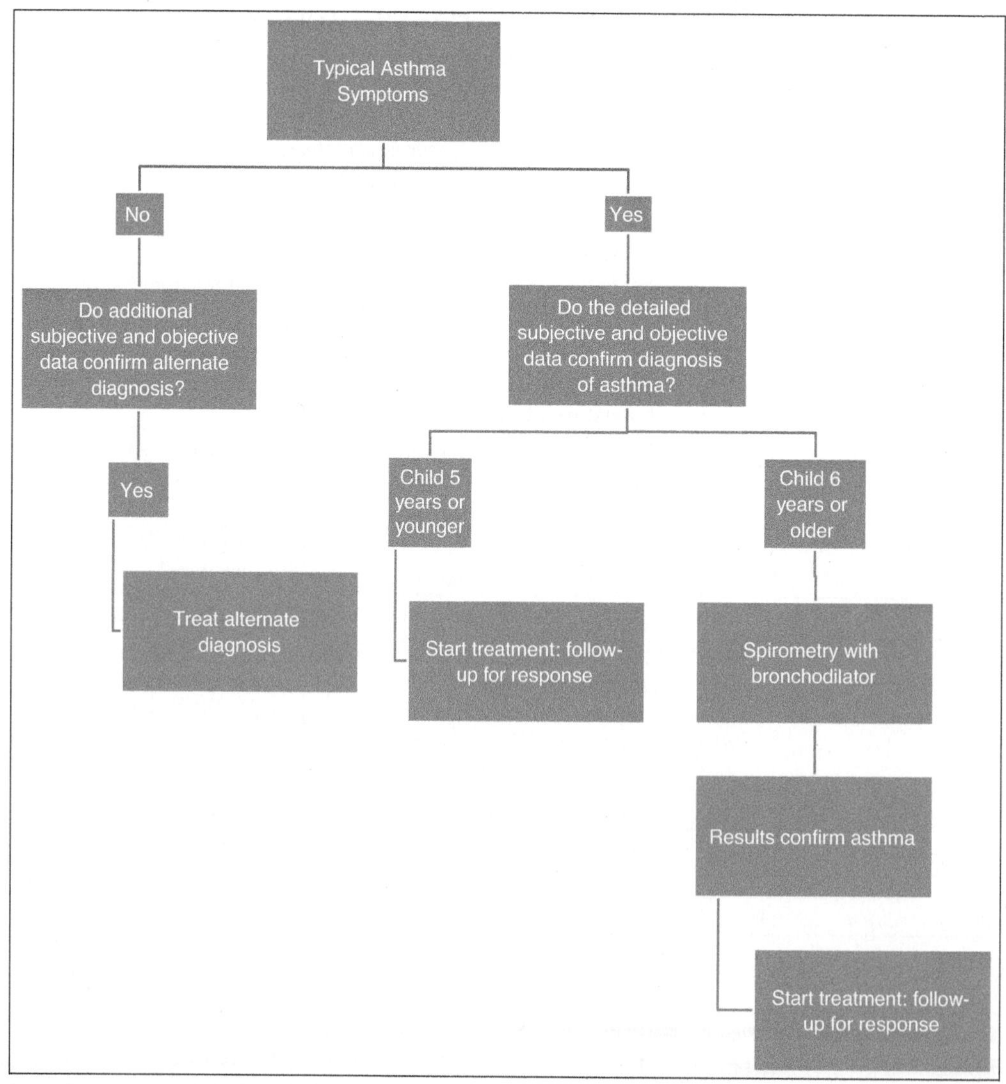


FIGURE 33.3 Asthma treatment decision tree.

The type of inhaler device is crucial to sufficient medication delivery and must be considered based on the child's age and developmental stage. A metered-dose inhaler (MDI) with a valved spacer—with or without face mask, depending on child's age and developmental stage—is the preferred delivery system (GINA, 2020a). In order to optimally deliver medication, the child should take five to 10 breaths to empty the spacer. For children ages 0 to 3, an MDI with spacer and face mask or nebulizer with face mask can be used to deliver medication. In children 4 years old or older, an MDI with spacer and mouthpiece or face mask can be used. Children and families should be trained in clinic and observed using the inhaler to ensure adequate delivery of medication.

Pharmacologic treatment is not the only component of asthma management. Treatment success depends on a trusted medical home, partnership between child/family and healthcare provider, skills training for inhaler devices, nonpharmacologic strategies to avoid triggers, and ensuring environmental control when possible (GINA, 2020a).

**PRO TIP** Administration of nebulized medications can be difficult for toddlers. Recommend redirection with alternative activity during therapy. Demonstrate use of all inhaled medications in the office and allow parents and school-aged children to demonstrate use to ensure understanding.

## Family Education

Asthma education is key to the successful management of pediatric asthma and should be reviewed at every follow-up appointment. Adherence to the medical

**(A)**

| Treatment | Intermittent Asthma | Management of Persistent Asthma In Individuals Ages 0-4 Years | | | | |
|---|---|---|---|---|---|---|
| | STEP 1 | STEP 2 | STEP 3 | STEP 4 | STEP 5 | STEP 6 |
| **Preferred** | PRN SABA and At the start of RT1: Add short course daily ICS^ | Daily low-dose ICS and PRN SABA | Daily low-dose ICS-LABA and PRN SABA^ or Daily low-dose ICS + montelukast,* or daily medium-dose ICS, and PRN SABA | Daily medium-dose ICS-LABA and PRN SABA | Daily high-dose ICS-LABA and PRN SABA | Daily high-dose ICS-LABA + oral systemic corticosteroid and PRN SABA |
| **Alternative** | | Daily montelukast* or Cromolyn,*and PRN SABA | | Daily medium-dose ICS + montelukast* and PRN SABA | Daily high-dose ICS + montelukast* and PRN SABA | Daily high-dose ICS + montelukast*+ oral systemic corticostroid old and PRN SABA |
| | | | For children age 4 years only and Step 3 and Step 4 on Management of Persistent Asthma in Individuals in individuals Age 5-11 years diagram | | | |

**Assess Control**

- First check adherence, inhaler technique, environmental factors,^ and comorbid conditions.
- **Step up** if needed; reassess n 4-6 weeks
- **Step down** if possible (if asthma is well controlled for at least 3 consecutive months)

Consult with asthma specialist if Step 3 or higher is required, Consider consultation at Step 2.

Control assessment is a key element of asthma care. This involves both impairment and risk. Use of objective measures, self-reported control, and health care utilization are complementary and should be employed on an ongoing basis, depending on the individual's clinical situation.

**(B)**

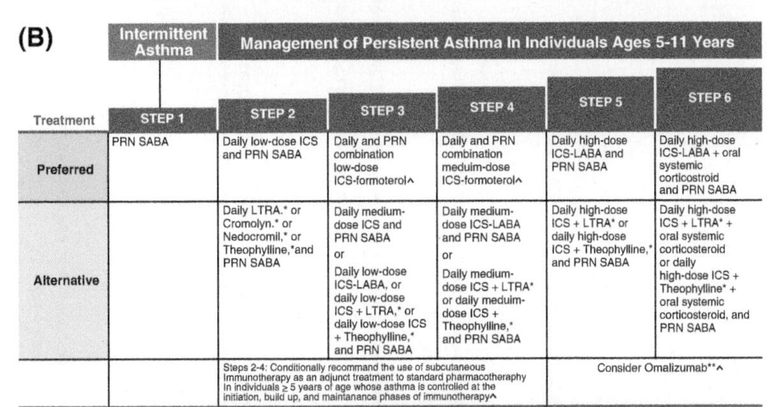

| Treatment | Intermittent Asthma | Management of Persistent Asthma In Individuals Ages 5-11 Years | | | | |
|---|---|---|---|---|---|---|
| | STEP 1 | STEP 2 | STEP 3 | STEP 4 | STEP 5 | STEP 6 |
| **Preferred** | PRN SABA | Daily low-dose ICS and PRN SABA | Daily and PRN combination low-dose ICS-formoterol^ | Daily and PRN combination meduim-dose ICS-formoterol^ | Daily high-dose ICS-LABA and PRN SABA | Daily high-dose ICS-LABA + oral systemic corticostroid and PRN SABA |
| **Alternative** | | Daily LTRA.* or Cromolyn.* or Nedocromil,* or Theophylline,*and PRN SABA | Daily medium-dose ICS and PRN SABA or Daily low-dose ICS-LABA, or daily low-dose ICS + LTRA,* or daily low-dose ICS + Theophylline,* and PRN SABA | Daily medium-dose ICS-LABA and PRN SABA or Daily medium-dose ICS + LTRA* or daily meduim-dose ICS + Theophylline,* and PRN SABA | Daily high-dose ICS + LTRA* or daily high-dose ICS + Theophylline,* and PRN SABA | Daily high-dose ICS + LTRA* + oral systemic corticosteroid or daily high-dose ICS + Theophylline* + oral systemic corticosteroid, and PRN SABA |
| | | Steps 2-4: Conditionally recommand the use of subcutaneous Immunotherapy as an adjunct treatment to standard pharmacotheraphy In individuals ≥ 5 years of age whose asthma is controlled at the initiation, build up, and maintanance phases of immunotherapy^ | | | Consider Omalizumab**^ | |

**Assess Control**

- First check adherence, inhaler technique, environmental factors,^ and comorbid conditions.
- **Step up** if needed; reassess in 2-6 weeks
- **Step down** if possible (if asthma is well controlled for at least 3 consecutive months)

Consult with asthma specialist if Step 4 or higher is required, Consider consultation at Step 3.

Control assessment is a key element of asthma care. This involves both impairment and risk. Use of objective measures, self-reported control, and health care utilization are complementary and should be employed on an ongoing basis, depending on the individual's clinical situation.

**(C)**

| Treatment | Intermittent Asthma | Management of Persistent Asthma In Individuals Ages 12+ Years | | | | |
|---|---|---|---|---|---|---|
| | STEP 1 | STEP 2 | STEP 3 | STEP 4 | STEP 5 | STEP 6■ |
| **Preferred** | PRN SABA | Daily low-dose ICS and PRN SABA or PRN concomitant ICS and SABA^ | Daily and PRN combination low-dose ICS-formoterol^ | Daily and PRN combination medium-dose ICS-formoterol^ | Daily medium-high dose ICS-LABA + LAMA and PRN SABA^ | Daily high-dose ICS-LABA + oral systemic corticosteroids + PRN SABA |
| **Alternative** | | Daily LTRA* and PRN SABA or Cromolyn,*or Nedocromil,* or Zileuton,* or Theophylline,* and PRN SABA | Daily medium-dose ICS and PRN SABA or Daily low-dose ICS-LABA, or daily low-dose ICS + LAMA,^or daily low-dose ICS + LTRA,* and PRN SABA or Daily low-dose ICS + Theophylline* or Zileuton,* and PRN SABA | Daily medium-dose ICS-LABA or daily medium-dose ICS + LAMA, and PRN SABA^ or Daily medium-dose ICS + LTRA,* or daily medium-dose ICS + Theophylline,* or daily medium-dose ICS + Zileuton,* and PRN SABA | Daily medium-high dose ICS-LABA or daily high-dose ICS + LTRA,* and PRN SABA | |
| | | Steps 2-4: Conditionally recommand the use of subcutaneous Immunotherapy as an adjunct treatment to standard pharmacotheraphy In individuals ≥ 5 years of age whose asthma is controlled at the initiation, build up, and maintenance phases of immunotherapy^ | | | Consider adding Asthma Biologics (e.g. anti-IgE, anti-IL5,and-IL5R anti-IL4/IL13)** | |

**Assess Control**

- First check adherence, inhaler technique, environmental factors,^and comorbid conditions.
- **Step up** if needed; reassess n 2-6 weeks
- **Step down** if possible (if asthma is well controlled for at least 3 consecutive months)

Consult with asthma specialist if Step 4 or higher is required, Consider consultation at Step 3.

Control assessment is a key element of asthma care. This involves both impairment and risk. Use of objective measures, self-reported control, and health care utilization are complementary and should be employed on an ongoing basis, depending on the individual's clinical situation.

FIGURE 33.4 (**A**) Stepwise approach for management of asthma in individuals ages 0–4 years. (**B**) Stepwise approach for management of asthma in individuals ages 5–11 years. (**C**) Stepwise approach for management of asthma in individuals ages 12 years and older.

*Source*: National Heart, Lung, and Blood Institute. (2020). *2020 focused updates to the asthma management guidelines.* https://www.nhlbi.nih.gov/health-topics/asthma-management-guidelines-2020-updates

# ASTHMA ACTION PLAN

For: ____________ Doctor: ____________ Date: ____________

Doctor's Phone Number: ____________ Hospital/Emergency Department Phone Number: ____________

**GREEN ZONE**

DOING WELL

- No cough, wheeze, chest tightness, or shortness of breath during the day or night
- Can do usual activities

**And, if a peak flow meter is used,**

**Peak flow:** more than ____________
(80 percent or more of my best peak flow)

My best peak flow is: ____________

**Daily Medications**

| Medicine | How much to take | When to take it |
|---|---|---|
| | | |
| | | |
| | | |
| | | |
| | | |

| **Before exercise** | ☐ ____________ | ☐2 or ☐4 puffs ______ | 5 minutes before exercise |
|---|---|---|---|

**YELLOW ZONE**

ASTHMA IS GETTING WORSE

- Cough, wheeze, chest tightness, or shortness of breath, or
- Waking at night due to asthma, or
- Can do some, but not all, usual activities

-Or-

**Peak flow:** ______ to ______
(50 to 79 percent of my best peak flow)

1st **Add: quick-relief medicine—and keep taking your GREEN ZONE medicine.**

____________ (quick-relief medicine) ______ Number of puffs **or** ☐Nebulizer, once — Can repeat every ______ minutes up to maximum of ______ doses

2nd **If your symptoms (and peak flow, if used) return to GREEN ZONE after 1 hour of above treatment:**

☐Continue monitoring to be sure you stay in the green zone.

-Or-

**If your symptoms (and peak flow, if used) do not return to GREEN ZONE after 1 hour of above treatment:**

☐Take: ____________ (quick-relief medicine) ______ Number of puffs **or** ☐Nebulizer

☐Add: ____________ (oral steroid) mg per day For ______ (3-10) days

☐Call the doctor ☐before/ ☐within______ hours after taking the oral steroid.

**RED ZONE**

MEDICAL ALERT!

- Very short of breath, or
- Quick-relief medicines have not helped,
- Cannot do usual activities, or
- Symptoms are same or get worse after 24 hours in Yellow Zone

-Or-

**Peak flow:** less than ____________
(50 percent of my best peak flow)

**Take this medicine:**

☐ ____________ (quick-relief medicine) ______ Number of puffs **or** ☐Nebulizer

☐ ____________ (oral steroid) mg

**Then call your doctor NOW.** Go to the hospital or call an ambulance if:

- You are still in the red zone after 15 minutes AND
- You have not reached your doctor.

DANGER SIGNS

- **Trouble walking and talking due to shortness of breath**
- **Lips or fingernails are blue**

- **Take ______ puffs of ____________ (quick relief medicine) AND**
- **Go to the hospital or call for an ambulance ____________ (phone) NOW!**

See the reverse side for things you can do to avoid your asthma triggers.

EXHIBIT 33.1 **Asthma Action Plan for Home and School**

*Source*: National Heart, Lung, and Blood Institute. (2020). *2020 focused updates to the asthma management guidelines.*

management plan affects the child's outcome and overall quality of life. Follow-up appointments are needed to assess disease control, and to revise daily and exacerbation management plans, and are important teaching opportunities for the child and family. Education should focus on basic asthma understanding, individual risk factors, proper technique of inhalation devices, and written asthma action plans (GINA, 2020a).

Asthma action plans have two components (Exhibit 33.1). The first is a daily routine management plan that details regular asthma medication use and other factors to avoid, in an effort to keep asthma in good control. The second component of asthma action plans is a chart to manage and recognize worsening asthma symptoms, describe indicators of impending exacerbations, identify what medications to take, and specify when and how to contact the primary care provider and/or proceed to urgent/emergent medical care (Liu et al., 2020; National Heart, Lung, and Blood Institute, 2020).

▶ ALERT: Multiple episodes of wheezing requiring oral steroid use indicate poorly controlled asthma. Underutilization of asthma medications can lead to frequent exacerbations. Be sure parents know what respiratory distress looks like and when to call 911 for help.

In addition to the asthma action plan, teach families:

- Wash spacers regularly (at least monthly) to ensure proper medication delivery.
- Children should rinse the mouth with water and spit the water out after using the inhaler.
- Have young children drink water after using their inhaler if they are unable to rinse and spit. Then follow by brushing their teeth to prevent ICS-related thrush.
- Refer to the allergic rhinitis section in this chapter for information on allergy avoidance if the child's asthma is triggered by allergies.

## Referral

Primary care providers are very capable of treating mild to moderate asthma when utilizing the stepwise therapy guide from the Global Initiative for Asthma. There are some children, however, who will benefit from referral to either a pediatric allergist or a pulmonologist for further care. A general rule to follow is to refer children younger than 4 years of age with moderate persistent asthma to a pediatric asthma specialist. For children 5 years and older, a specialist is recommended if they require step 4 or above of asthma therapy and to be strongly considered when they require step 3 (GINA, 2020a; Liu et al., 2020). Additionally, if allergen immunotherapy or anti-immunoglobulin (Ig) E therapy is being considered, the child should be under the care of a pediatric allergy/immunology specialist to guide this therapy. Early referral for sub-specialty care is recommended for children 5 years and younger with the following clinical signs and symptoms that are suggestive of an alternative diagnosis:

- Failure to thrive
- Neonatal or very early onset of symptoms (especially if associated with failure to thrive)
- Emesis associated with respiratory symptoms
- Continuous wheezing
- Failure to respond to asthma medications (inhaled ICS, oral steroids, or SABA)
- No association of symptoms with typical triggers, such as viral upper respiratory tract infection
- Focal lung or cardiovascular signs, or finger clubbing
- Hypoxemia out of proportion for a viral illness (GINA, 2020a)

## KEY POINTS

- AD is a chronic, yet treatable condition.
- Moisturization is an important treatment plan at any stage of AD.
- Proper application of medications to areas affected by AD is key.
- Involve parents by teaching them about AD, what to expect, and when to call for help.
- Allergic rhinitis is a clinical diagnosis usually not requiring any type of laboratory or diagnostic testing.
- Symptom control is the goal of therapy for allergic rhinitis.
- Asthma is a chronic condition requiring proper use of medications to reach symptom control.
- Asthma action planning is critical to caring for children with asthma.

## REFERENCES

American Lung Association. (2020). *The impact of asthma.* https://www.lung.org/lung-health-diseases/lung-disease-lookup/asthma/learn-about-asthma/impact-of-asthma

Bager, P., Wohlfahrt, J., Thyssen, J. P., & Melbye, M. (2016). Filaggrin genotype and skin diseases independent of atopic dermatitis in childhood. *Pediatric Allergy and Immunology, 27*(2), 162–168. https://doi.org/10.1111/pai.12511

Centers for Disease Control and Prevention. (2018). *Asthma: Reports and publications*. https://www.cdc.gov/asthma/reports_publications.htm

Chopra, R., Vakharia, P., Sacotte, R., & Silverberg, J. (2017). Efficacy of bleach baths in reducing severity of atopic dermatitis: A systematic review and meta-analysis. *American College of Allergy, Asthma, and Immunology, 119*, 435–440. https://doi.org/10.1016/j.anai.2017.08.289

Covar, R. A., Fleischer, D. M., Cho, C., & Boguniewicz, M. (2020). Allergic disorders. In W. W. Hay Jr., M. J. Levin, M. J. Abzug, & M. Bunik (Eds.), *Current diagnosis & treatment: Pediatrics* (25th ed., Chapter 38). McGraw-Hill.

deShazo, R. D., & Kemp, S. F. (2020). Allergic rhinitis: Clinical manifestations, epidemiology, and diagnosis. *UpToDate*. https://www.uptodate.com/contents/allergic-rhinitis-clinical-manifestations-epidemiology-and-diagnosis

Fuchs, O., Bahmer, T., Rabe, K. F., & von Mutius, E. (2017). Asthma transition from childhood into adulthood. *The Lancet Respiratory Medicine, 5*(3), 224–234. https://doi.org/10.1016/S2213-2600(16)30187-4

Geria, A. N., & Alexis, A. F. (2016). Atopic dermatitis and other eczemas. In A. P. Kelly, S. C. Taylor, H. W. Lim, & A. M. Anido Serrano (Eds.), *Taylor and Kelly's dermatology for skin of color* (2nd ed., Chapter 27). McGraw-Hill Education.

Global Initiative for Asthma. (2020a). *Global strategy for asthma management and prevention*. https://ginasthma.org/reports

Global Initiative for Asthma. (2020b). *Pocket guide for asthma management and prevention*. https://ginasthma.org/pocket-guide-for-asthma-management-and-prevention

Karagounis, T., Gittler, J., Rotemberg, V., & Morel, K. (2019). Use of "natural" oils for moisturization: Review of olive, coconut, and sunflower seed oil. *Pediatric Dermatology, 36*(1), 9–15. https://doi.org/10.1111/pde.13621

Kimler, K. A., McDonald, D., & Shah, P. B. (2019). Treatment of atopic dermatitis in pediatric patients: Nursing implications. *Pediatric Nursing, 45*(5), 215–223, 230.

Liu, A. H., Spahn, J. D., & Sichere, S. H. (2020). Childhood asthma. In R. M. Kliegman, J. St. Geme, N. J. Blum, S. S. Shah, R. C. Tasker, K. M. Wilson, & R. E. Behrman (Eds.), *Nelson textbook of pediatrics* (21st ed., Chapter 169). Elsevier.

National Eczema Foundation. (2020). *Wet wrap therapy*. https://nationaleczema.org/eczema/treatment/wet-wrap-therapy

National Heart, Lung, and Blood Institute. (2020). *2020 focused updates to the asthma management guidelines*. https://www.nhlbi.nih.gov/health-topics/asthma-management-guidelines-2020-updates

Oberlin, K. E., & Nanda, S. (2019). Atopic dermatitis made easy: The Schachner Ladder. *Pediatric Dermatology, 36*, 1017–1018. https://doi.org/10.1111/pde.13862

Ohtsuki, M., Morimoto, H., & Nakagawa, H. (2018). Tacrolimus ointment for the treatment of adult and pediatric atopic dermatitis: Review on safety and benefits. *The Journal of Dermatology, 45*, 936–942. https://doi.org/10.1111/1346-8138.14501

Pols, D. H. J., Wartna, J. B., van Alphen, E. I., Moed, H., Rasenberg, N., Bindels, P. J. E., & Bohnen, A. M. (2015). Interrelationships between atopic disorders in children: A meta-analysis based on ISAAC questionnaires. *PLoS ONE, 10*(7), e0131869. https://doi.org/10.1371/journal.pone.0131869

Prok, L. D., & Torres-Zegarra, C. X. (2020). Skin. In W. W. Hay Jr., M. J. Levin, M. J. Abzug, & M. Bunik (Eds.), *Current diagnosis & treatment: Pediatrics* (25th ed., Chapter 15). McGraw-Hill.

Seidman, M. D., Gurgel, R. K., Lin, S. Y., Schwartz, S. R., Baroody, F. M., Bonner, J. R., Dawson, D. E., Dykewicz, M. S., Hackell, J. M., Han, J. K., Ishman, S. L., Krouse, H. J., Malekzadeh, S., Mims, J. W., Omole, F. S., Reddy, W. D., Wallace, D. V., Walsh, S. A., Warren, B. E., . . . Nnacheta, L. C. (2015). Clinical practice guideline: Allergic rhinitis executive summary. *Otolaryngology—Head and Neck Surgery, 152*(2), 197–206. https://doi.org/10.1177/0194599814562166

Simpson, E. L., Leung, D. Y. M., Eichenfield, L. F., & Boguniewicz, M. (2019). Atopic dermatitis. In S. Kang, M. Amagai, A. L. Bruckner, A. H. Enk, D. J. Margolis, A. J. McMichael, & J. S. Orringer (Eds.), *Fitzpatrick's dermatology* (9th ed., Chapter 22). McGraw-Hill Education

Soothems. (2020). *How to wet wrap using Soothems eczema therapy pajamas*. https://www.soothems.com/blogs/news/how-to-wet-wrap-using-soothems-eczema-therapy-pajamas

Spergel, J. M., & Lio, P. A. (2020). Management of severe atopic dermatitis (eczema) in children. *UpToDate*. Retrieved June 18, 2020, from https://www.uptodate.com/contents/management-of-severe-atopic-dermatitis-eczema-in-children

Stickle, D. (Ed.). (2018). Spirometry: An Integral integral tool for diagnosing and managing pediatric asthma. *RT: The Journal for Respiratory Care Practitioners, 31*(2), 12–16.

Wingrove, B. R. (2016). An overview of pediatric asthma. *Physician Assistant Clinics, 1*(4), 563–582. https://doi.org/10.1016/j.cpha.2016.05.005

## FURTHER READING

Host factors and environmental exposures that cause asthma. From Section 2, Definition, Pathophysiology and Pathogenesis of Asthma, and Natural History of Asthma https://www.nhlbi.nih.gov/files/docs/guidelines/03_sec2_def.pdf

Expert Panel Report 3: Guidelines for the Diagnosis and Management of Asthma.

National Asthma Education and Prevention Program, Third Expert Panel on the Diagnosis and Management of Asthma. National Heart, Lung, and Blood Institute, August 2007.

# Management of Musculoskeletal Disorders

Lindsey Locke and Leslie N. Rhodes

## Student Learning Outcomes

**Upon completion of this chapter, the reader should be able to:**

1. Discuss pathophysiology and epidemiology of musculoskeletal disorders in children.
2. Differentiate subjective and objective findings of musculoskeletal disorders in children.
3. Choose appropriate laboratory or diagnostic tests for musculoskeletal disorders in children.
4. Utilize the differential diagnosis process to identify the most accurate diagnosis of musculoskeletal disorders in children.
5. Determine treatment plan, child/family education, and need for referral in children with a musculoskeletal disorder.

## INTRODUCTION

The musculoskeletal system is a vital part of the human body. It provides postural support, protects vital organs, and allows for movement. Many causes of musculoskeletal pain are benign in nature and resolve on their own. However, assuring the family as to the benign nature of injury and typical resolution pattern is a large part of caring for musculoskeletal injuries in children.

Children are at increased risk for musculoskeletal disorders, particularly injuries due to their development stage and activity level. Many of the musculoskeletal disorders result in pain. During the health history, use the mnemonic OLD CARTS (**O**nset, **L**ocation, **D**uration, **C**haracteristics, **A**ggravating factors, **R**elieving factors, **T**iming, and **S**everity) to inquire about the pain. Also, if an injury has occurred, always ask about the mechanism of injury (how it occurred and position of the injured body part).

The content in this chapter maps to the following areas on the Pediatric Nursing Certification Board (PNCB) Pediatric Nurse Practitioner—Primary Care certification examination:

**CLINICAL PROBLEMS: MUSCULOSKELETAL DISORDERS**

CONTENT AREAS:

**II. Assessment and Diagnosis**

**B. History and Physical Examination**

1. Obtain history of present illness
2. Obtain a comprehensive health history for new patients
3. Complete an interval history for established patients
4. Perform a review of systems
5. Perform a complete physical examination

**C. Diagnostic Testing and Screening**

1. Order and interpret office/clinic based screening tests
2. Order and interpret diagnostic laboratory tests
3. Order and interpret the results of diagnostic imaging tests

**D. Analyzing Information**

1. Integrate health history and physical examination findings into the plan of care

2. Assimilate findings from screening and diagnostic testing into plan of care

**E. Diagnosis**

1. Develop and prioritize differential diagnoses
2. Establish a diagnosis based on evaluation of patient data

## III. Management

**A. Child and Caregiver Counseling and Education**

1. Provide condition-specific counseling and education, including treatment options
2. Educate about benefits and potential adverse reactions of pharmacological interventions
3. Discuss non-pharmacological interventions
4. Counsel regarding the threshold for seeking follow-up care
5. Review the risks of non-adherence to recommended treatment

**B. Therapeutic Interventions**

1. Prescribe pharmacologic agents
2. Recommend the use of over-the-counter pharmacologic agents
3. Order or recommend non-pharmacologic treatments for the management of symptoms
4. Discuss use of complementary and alternative therapies as appropriate

**C. Procedures**

1. Perform procedures in accordance with diagnostic guidelines and plan of care (rapid tests)
2. Initiate life-saving techniques in response to urgent or emergent situations

**D. Collaboration and Referral**

2. Refer to specialists as indicated for evaluation, counseling, and/or treatment

**E. Care Coordination**

1. Facilitate patient and family-centered care for children of all ages with acute and chronic conditions

**F. Evaluation and Follow-up**

2. Establish a plan for follow-up care

## IV. Professional Role Responsibilities

**A. Leadership and Evidence-based Practice**

4. Develop, implement, and/or modify clinical practice guidelines

# ANATOMY AND PHYSIOLOGY

The musculoskeletal system is composed of 206 bones and is divided into the axial and appendicular skeleton (Figure 34.1). Other structures include muscles, fascia, ligaments, cartilage, tendons, and joints. In children, each long bone contains a growth plate, known as the physis. The physis separates the epiphysis (the end of a long bone) from the diaphysis (the central part of a long bone) and varies in thickness depending on the age of the child and location of the physis. Damage to the physis can disrupt normal bone growth and potentially lead to long-term deformities. The bones of children are more porous than those of adults, causing them to bow or bend before fracturing. However, because of the abundant blood supply, children's bones tend heal more quickly than adults' bones.

# PACKAGING DEFORMITIES

There are many deformities classified as packaging disorders. These disorders are the result of restricted space for the developing fetus in utero, resulting in

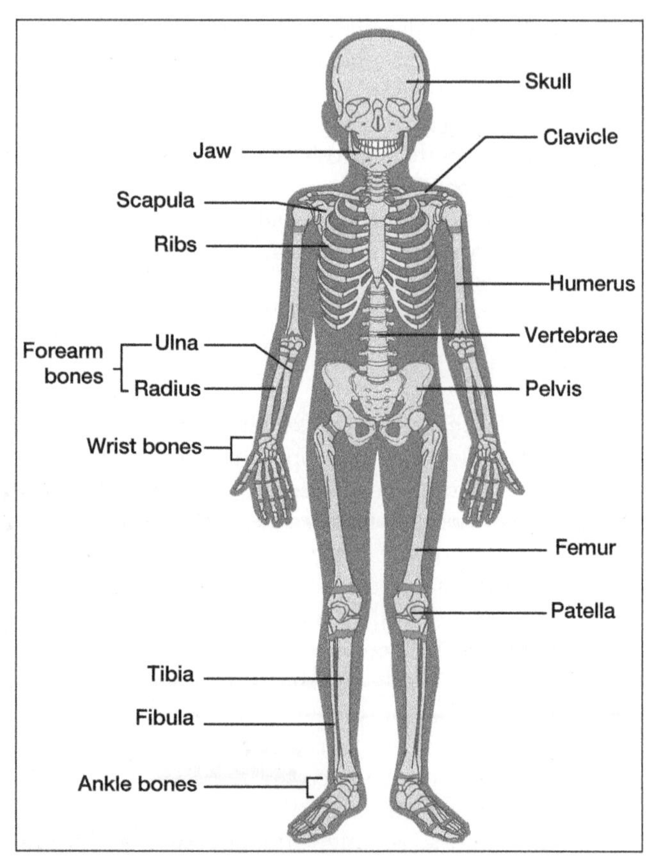


FIGURE 34.1 Musculoskeletal system.

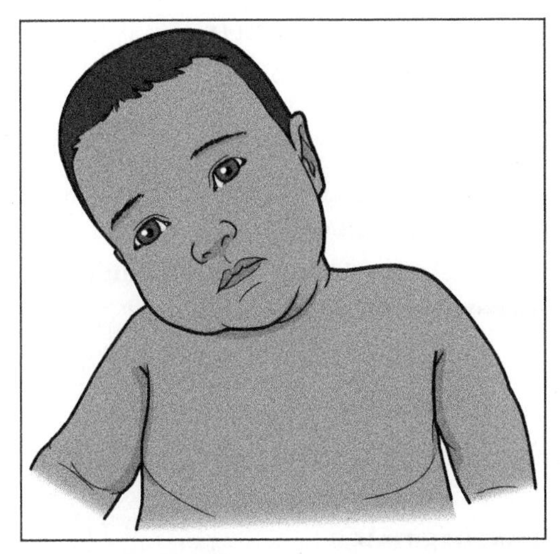

FIGURE 34.2 Tortocollis.

*Source*: Chiocca, E. M. (2019). *Advanced pediatric assessment* (3rd ed.). Springer Publishing Company.

abnormal bending of the arms and legs. The conditions include, but are not limited to, congenital torticollis, developmental dysplasia of the hip (DDH), clubfoot deformity, and metatarsus adductus (MA).

## CONGENITAL TORTICOLLIS

Torticollis is associated with head tilt and rotation contralateral to the sternocleidomastoid muscle of the affected side (Figure 34.2). Torticollis can be a congenital or acquired condition, with congenital being the most common cause and presenting soon after birth (Ozuah & Skae, 2017).

### Subjective Findings

Determine the history of present illness from the parent and child (as age allows). Ask about the birth history, developmental milestones achieved, and history of recent illness.

The health history may reveal:

- Head tilt
- Head rotation
- Feeding difficulties

### Risk Factors

The most common risk factor for congenital torticollis is intrauterine positioning.

### Review of Systems

The most common manifestations revealed during the review of systems include:

- **Constitutional:** fever or absence of it, difficulty feeding
- **Musculoskeletal:** associated conditions (DDH, MA)
- **Neurologic:** irritability

### Objective Findings

The physical examination of the child with torticollis may reveal:

- Head tilt and rotation
- Limited passive range of motion (ROM)
- Palpable, painless mass

### Laboratory/Diagnostic Testing

The diagnosis of torticollis is based upon the clinical findings. No laboratory or diagnostic testing is needed. An ultrasound, magnetic resonance imaging (MRI), or computerized tomography (CT) may be warranted if the condition persists (Ozuah & Skae, 2017).

### Differential Diagnosis

The differential diagnosis for torticollis includes:

- Vertebral anomalies
- Ocular torticollis
- Clavicle fracture
- Neck mass
- Plagiocephaly (flattening of an infant's head in one area)
- Lesions of central and peripheral nervous system (Macias & Gan, 2019a)

### Treatment/Management Plan

The first-line treatment includes a variety of home stretching exercises and/or physical therapy. This can be managed by the primary care provider with follow-up every 2 to 4 weeks, and rarely requires surgical intervention (Macias & Gan, 2019b).

### Family Education

Teach the following:

- Environmental changes may be beneficial in the treatment of torticollis. This includes modifying the environment to encourage the child to stretch the sternocleidomastoid muscle (i.e., with diaper changes).

- During feeding, position the child so the child is encouraged to actively rotate the chin toward the affected side.
- Encourage adult-observed tummy time (prone positioning) to encourage head lifting.
- Passive stretching is used to lengthen the shortened sternocleidomastoid muscle. There is no research to support the exact technique for stretching exercises; however, multiple studies have shown that more intense stretching exercises have a positive correlation with faster healing (Macias & Gan, 2019b).

### Referral

Refer to specialists as follows:

- Physical therapy if home stretching is unsuccessful after 4 weeks.
- Pediatric orthopedic surgeon if greater than 6 months of age with unresolved sign and symptoms and limited ROM (Macias & Gan, 2019b).

## DEVELOPMENTAL DYSPLASIA OF THE HIP

Developmental dysplasia of the hip (DDH or hip dysplasia) is abnormal development of the hip joint of an infant. Hip dysplasia can result in dislocation and/or subluxation. The severity of the disorder varies with each child (International Hip Dysplasia Institute [IHDI], 2018).

### Subjective Findings

The health history may reveal:

- Leg length discrepancy (LLD)
- Leg turning outward on the side with DDH
- Uneven skin folds of the gluteals and/or thighs
- Limited abduction

### Risk Factors

The most common risk factors for DDH are:

- Birth history, especially first-born females who are breech in utero
- Twins or multiples
- Positive family history of DDH
- History of other packaging deformities

### Review of Systems

The most common manifestations revealed during the review of systems include:

- **Musculoskeletal:** other associated conditions such as torticollis, clubfoot, and/or MA

### Objective Findings

The physical examination of the child with DDH may reveal:

- + Galeazzi sign (LLD)
- + Barlow sign (hip dislocation; Figure 34.3A)
- + Ortolani maneuver (reduction of a dislocated hip; examine hips one at a time; Figure 34.3B)
- Limited hip abduction
- + Trendelenburg sign (if patient is of walking age; Figure 34.4)
- Uneven skin folds of the gluteals and/or thighs (Rosenfeld, 2019b; Figure 34.5)

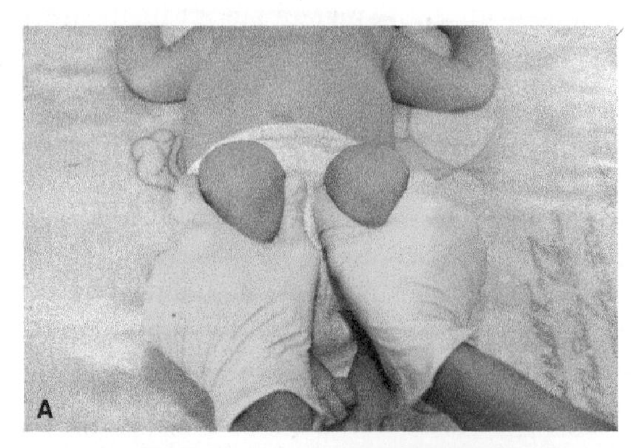


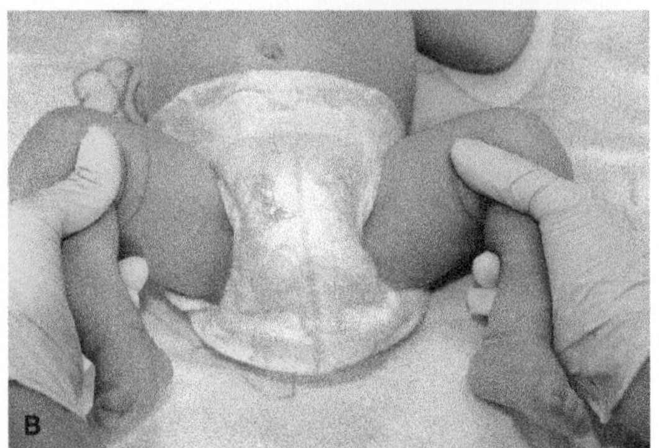


FIGURE 34.3 (A) Barlow sign. (B) Ortolani maneuver.

*Source*: Chiocca, E. M. (2019). *Advanced pediatric assessment* (3rd ed.). Springer Publishing Company.

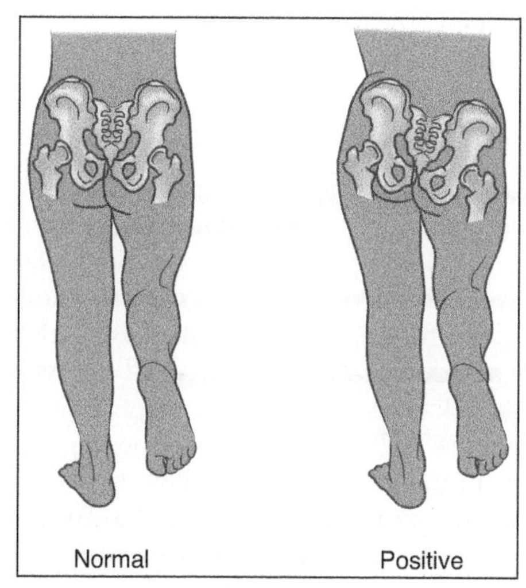


FIGURE 34.4 Trendelenburg sign.

*Source*: Chiocca, E. M. (2019). *Advanced pediatric assessment* (3rd ed.). Springer Publishing Company.

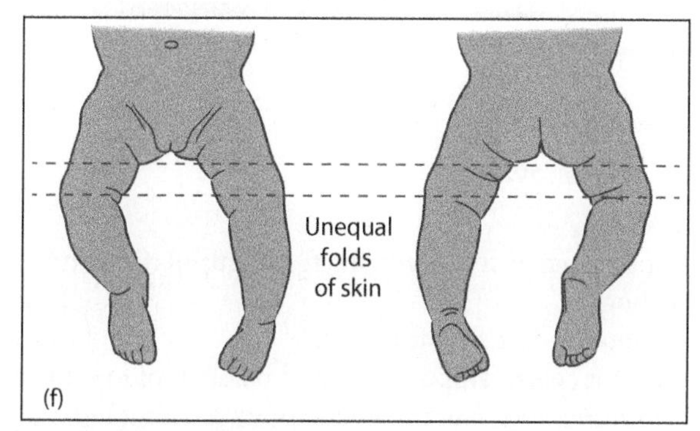


FIGURE 34.5 Asymmetrical thigh and gluteal folds.

*Source*: Chiocca, E. M. (2019). *Advanced pediatric assessment* (3rd ed.). Springer Publishing Company.

**PRO TIP** Always examine one hip at a time using gentle pressure when performing the Barlow and Ortolani maneuvers independent of each other.

## Laboratory/Diagnostic Testing

The diagnosis of DDH is based upon the examination findings during a well child visit. A hip ultrasound is the diagnostic test most commonly ordered in an infant who is 4 to 6 weeks of age with suspected DDH. Additionally, the American Academy of Pediatrics (AAP) recommends a hip ultrasound for any infant 6 weeks of age or younger with other risk factors associated with DDH. Radiographs (x-rays) are used when the femoral head begins to ossify at around 6 months of age.

## Differential Diagnosis

The differential diagnosis for DDH includes:

- Proximal femoral focal deficiency (PFFD)
- Coxa vara
- Hemihypertrophy or hemihyperplasia
- Sacral agenesis with limb deformity (Rosenfeld, 2019b)

## Treatment/Management Plan

Treatment for DDH is dependent on the age of the child at diagnosis and the severity of the disorder. Infants who are less than 6 months of age with DDH can be treated nonoperatively with braces, which allow the hips to be held in the correct position for hip joint development. These braces include Pavlik harnesses and hip abduction braces. After the age of 6 months, or if the infant has failed conservative treatment, surgical intervention may be needed. This can include a variety of procedures, such as a closed reduction and casting of the affected hip or an open reduction with or without osteotomies.

## Family Education

Teach the following:

- How to put on and take off a Pavlik harness and/or hip abduction brace.
- Educate parents on how to remove the brace daily to check for femoral nerve palsy.
- Healthy hip positioning—hips should naturally fall to the side, with the hips and knees flexed, while supporting the thighs (IHDI, 2018).
- Safe swaddling—avoid swaddling baby too tight with the legs extended (IHDI, 2018).
- Cast care if needed.
- Car safety in cast if needed.
- Inform families of the need for regular follow-up with the pediatric orthopedic surgeon until skeletal maturity.

## Referral

Any infant with a positive examination, inconclusive examination, or positive risk factors should be referred to a pediatric orthopedic surgeon who specializes in the treatment of DDH (Rosenfeld, 2021).

# CONGENITAL TALIPES EQUINOVARUS

Congenital talipes equinovarus, also known as clubfoot, is a deformity of the foot at birth that is characterized by midfoot cavus, forefoot adductus, hindfoot varus, and hindfoot equinus. The cause can be idiopathic or neurogenic and affects nearly one in 1,000 live births per year (Clunie, 2017).

## Subjective Findings

The health history may reveal:

- Turning in of one or both feet
- History of torticollis or DDH

## Risk Factors

The most common risk factors for congenital talipes equinovarus are:

- Intrauterine positioning
- Positive family history of clubfoot
- Male gender

## Review of Systems

The most common manifestations revealed during the review of systems include:

- **Musculoskeletal:** other associated conditions such as torticollis or DDH

## Objective Findings

The physical examination of the child with congenital talipes equinovarus may reveal:

- Midfoot cavus
- Forefoot adductus
- Hindfoot varus
- Hindfoot equinus
- Calf atrophy on the affected side
- Shorter and wider foot on the affected side
- Medial and posterior creases in skin

## Laboratory/Diagnostic Testing

The diagnosis of congenital talipes equinovarus is based upon examination findings. No laboratory or diagnostic testing is needed.

## Differential Diagnosis

The differential diagnosis for congenital talipes equinovarus includes:

- MA
- Calcaneovalgus foot deformity
- Congenital vertical talus
- Tibial torsion

## Treatment/Management Plan

The treatment for congenital talipes equinovarus is serial casting known as the Ponsetti method. This should begin immediately upon diagnosis. Serial casting, with long leg casts, involves weekly manipulation of the foot deformity. The total amount of time in casts is dependent upon the severity of the deformity and the response to treatment. Following serial casting, most patients require a percutaneous Achilles tendon lengthening to prevent recurrence of the deformity and allow for proper brace wear. Once the patient is healed from the TAL, typically 3 weeks, he or she is transitioned to braces with bars and shoes to maintain correction. Braces are to be worn 23 out of 24 hours per day for the first 3 months. After this, the patient is transitioned to nighttime/naptime brace wear up until they reach 3 years of age. If the deformity recurs, repeat serial casting and/or surgical correction may be indicated (Rhodes et al., 2018).

## Family Education

Teach the following:

- Cast care
- Importance of weekly visits for manipulation and casting
- Adherence to using the brace
- Monitor color, temperature, and position of toes in cast
- Immunizations can be given above the long leg cast
- Developmental milestones such as crawling and walking may be reached despite casting

## Referral

Any patient with a known or suspected congenital talipes equinovarus foot deformity should be referred to a pediatric orthopedic surgeon to begin treatment as soon as possible for the most favorable outcomes.

# METATARSUS ADDUCTUS

MA is defined as medial deviation (adduction) of the forefoot while the hindfoot remains in a neutral position, unlike congenital talipes equinus (McKee-Garrett, 2020).

## Subjective Findings

The health history may reveal:

- "Bean-shaped" foot
- History of other packaging deformities

### Risk Factors

The most common risk factors for MA are:

- Intrauterine positioning
- First pregnancies
- Twin pregnancies
- Positive family history
- More common in girls (McKee-Garrett, 2020)

### Review of Systems

The most common manifestations revealed during the review of systems include:

- **Musculoskeletal:** complaints of in-toeing if patient is of walking age, other associated packaging deformities

### Objective Findings

The physical examination of the child with MA may reveal:

- Forefoot adduction
- Hindfoot in neutral position
- "C"-shaped foot
- Deep medial crease
- Lateral convex border
- Widened space between first and second toes

### Laboratory/Diagnostic Testing

The diagnosis of MA is based upon the clinical findings. No laboratory or diagnostic testing is needed.

### Differential Diagnosis

The differential diagnosis for MA includes:

- Congenital talipes equinovarus
- Internal tibial torsion
- Femoral anteversion

### Treatment/Management Plan

Up to 90% of cases of MA resolve on their own (McKee-Garrett, 2020). If spontaneous resolution does not occur, serial casting with manipulation and/or surgery may be indicated, though this is rare. Serial casting and manipulation in children who are less than 8 months of age have more favorable outcomes.

### Family Education

Teach the following:

- Condition usually resolves spontaneously by the age of 4
- Home stretching program (laterally directed pressure on the head of the first metatarsal, held for 10 seconds; perform five times per affected foot with diaper changes)

### Referral

Referral to a pediatric orthopedic surgeon for evaluation of whether serial casting and manipulation and/or surgical intervention is warranted if no improvement with home stretching exercises is seen after 4 to 6 weeks of beginning treatment (Rosenfeld, 2020).

# INJURIES

Musculoskeletal injuries are one of the most common reasons for seeking care in the pediatric population. These include sprains, strains, fractures, overuse injuries, and dislocations. Each of these injuries is a result of trauma to varying degrees.

## SPRAINS AND STRAINS

Sprains and strains are often a result of sports injuries, though they may result simply from running, playing, or falling. A sprain occurs when a ligament is forced, resulting in a stretch or sometimes even rupture. Sprains most often occur as a result of an outside force. The most common sprain occurs in the ankle (Kim & Shoval, 2019). A strain occurs when a muscle has been injured as a result of a muscle contraction. Strains are most often caused by a dynamic injury.

### Subjective Findings

The health history may reveal:

- Traumatic event leading to the injury
- Pain
- Swelling
- Bruising

### Risk Factors

The most common risk factor for sprains and strains is participation in sports, running, throwing, or jumping, not warming up properly, and anabolic steroid use.

### Review of Systems

The most common manifestations revealed during the review of systems include:

- **Musculoskeletal:** immediate sharp pain, hearing or feeling a "pop" or "snap," pain with weight-bearing, limited ROM

### Objective Findings

The physical examination of the child with a *sprain* may reveal:

- Tenderness and bruising over the injured ligament
- Swelling
- Joint instability (in severe sprains)

The physical examination of the child with a *strain* may reveal:

- Pain
- Swelling
- Bruising with or without an associated muscle injury

### Laboratory/Diagnostic Testing

The diagnoses of ligamentous sprains and muscular strains are based upon the clinical findings. No laboratory or diagnostic testing is needed. X-rays (plain radiographs) may be ordered to rule out fracture or dislocation.

### Differential Diagnosis

The differential diagnosis for sprains and strains includes:

- Contusion
- Fracture
- Dislocation
- Infection
- Rheumatologic disorders
- Hematologic disorders
- Neoplastic abnormalities

### Treatment/Management Plan

Management of sprains and strains includes rest, ice, compression, and elevation (RICE). Treatment should begin immediately to minimize the amount of swelling. Relative rest helps prevent reinjury while allowing motion to help with recovery. Ice minimizes swelling and decreases pain by constricting the blood vessels and dulling pain receptors. Ice should be applied to the injured site for 20 minutes at a time, and be applied every 2 hours to avoid thermal injuries to the skin. Compression using an elastic wrap or bandage limits swelling and should also be applied above and below the injury. Elevation above the level of the heart decreases the amount of swelling and increases lymphatic and venous return.

**PRO TIP** Be sure to check pulses and capillary refill after applying an elastic wrap or bandage to ensure that the wrap is not too constricting.

### Family Education

Teach the following:

- RICE is the treatment for both sprains and strains.
- Adherence to treatment is vital for attaining a good outcome.
- Relative rest is very important to decrease the risk of further injury.

### Referral

Refer to orthopedics if a fracture is suspected or if a sprain does not appear to be healing properly.

## FRACTURES AND DISLOCATIONS

Direct impact to bone and joints can result in fractures and/or dislocations. A fracture is a disruption in the bone tissue resulting in deformation or a break. Pediatric fractures are unique in that they may involve the physis (growth plate) and may not be obvious on radiographs. Damage to the growth plate may result in a limb-length discrepancy after healing. In general, ligaments in children are functionally stronger than bone; thus, a higher percentage of injuries that result in sprains and/or strains in adults end up causing fractures in children (Egol et al., 2020). Due to differences in structure, pediatric fractures occur with less force than those of adults and are typically caused by a bending, compression, or torsion mechanism. In children, a variety of fracture patterns occur, including complete, buckle, bowing, greenstick, comminuted, transverse, avulsed, oblique, and spiral. Figure 34.6 shows illustrations of some common pediatric fractures.

Dislocation includes displacement of a bone from the original position in a joint and may vary in degree of displacement. A common dislocation seen by primary care providers is a radial head subluxation, also known as a nursemaid elbow, most common in children ages 1 to 5. A subluxation of the radial head occurs anteriorly, away from the capitellum, when a sudden upward motion of the extended arm causes excessive traction. More than 50% of patients experience pain and one-third of patients have had a previous nursemaid's elbow (Crowther-Radulewicz, 2019).

### Subjective Findings

From the parent and child (as age allows), determine how the injury occurred. Ask specifically about the mechanism of injury and the direction of force. Determine the level of pain and if there is a history of previous injuries.

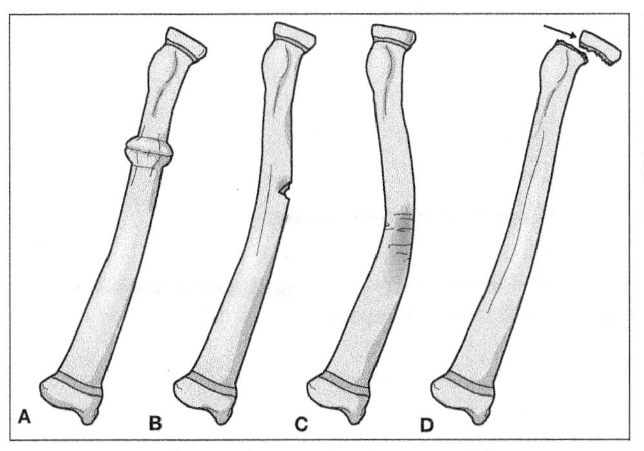


FIGURE 34.6 Common pediatric fractures. (**A**) Buckle (**B**) greenstick (**C**) bowing (**D**) Salter-Harris I (separated growth plate with displaced epiphysis [arrow]).

**PRO TIPS** A history that is vague or an injury that is inconsistent with the history should lead the practitioner to consider nonaccidental trauma (abuse).

## Risk Factors

The most common risk factors for fractures are:

- Male sex
- Lack of proper nutrition
- Lack of weight-bearing activities
- Obesity
- High levels of activity (Allison et al., 2020)

## Review of Systems

The most common manifestations revealed during the review of systems include:

- **Musculoskeletal:** pain, hearing or feeling a "pop" or "snap", limited ROM, inability to bear weight on affected extremity, protection of affected extremity

## Objective Findings

The physical examination of the child with fractures and dislocations may reveal:

- Obvious deformity
- Tenderness with palpation over injury site
- Swelling and discoloration
- Laceration of skin if fracture is open
- Fracture blisters
- Decreased capillary refill time
- Weak or absent pulses
- Paresthesias

**PRO TIP** Signs and symptoms of compartment syndrome can be remembered using the 5 Ps: pain, pallor, parasthesias, pulselessness, and paralysis. The 3 As are also helpful: increasing agitation and anxiety and the increased need for anesthetic medications.

## Laboratory/Diagnostic Testing

The diagnosis of fractures and dislocations is based upon the clinical and radiographic findings. Anterioposterior and lateral X-rays, to include above and below the affected joint, may be obtained. The Salter-Harris fracture classification system is unique to pediatric fractures and differentiates fractures based on epiphyseal involvement (Figure 34.7). Depending on the site of the injury, other views and/or tests, such as CT or MRI, may be warranted. For suspected radial head subluxation, confirm absence of fracture via x-ray prior to attempting reduction.

## Differential Diagnosis

The differential diagnosis for fractures and dislocations includes:

- Genetic disorders
- Metabolic bone disease
- Benign bone tumors
- Endocrine disorders
- Malignancy
- Nonaccidental trauma

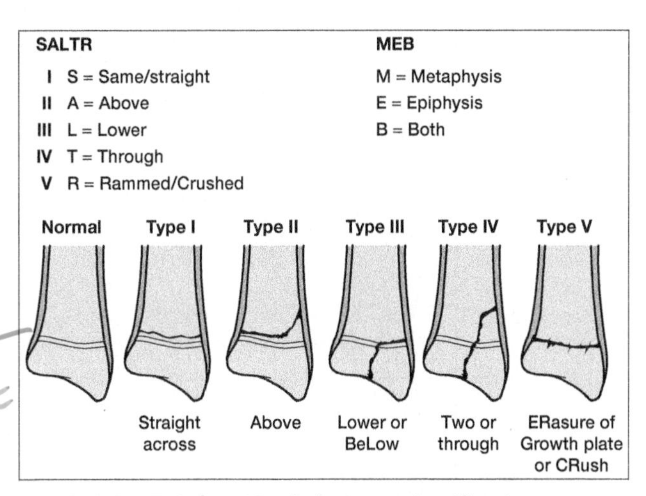


FIGURE 34.7 Salter-Harris fracture classification system.

*Source:* Shea, S. S., & Hoyt, K. (2016). *Family Emergent/urgent and ambulatory care: The pocket NP.* Springer Publishing Company.

### Treatment/Management Plan

Stabilize the suspected injury. This could include casting, surgical intervention, and/or reduction of the injury. If a fracture and/or dislocation is suspected, refer the child to a pediatric orthopedic surgeon to ensure prompt treatment of the injury. If the growth plate is damaged, a limb-length discrepancy may occur after healing and the patient should be followed by a pediatric orthopedic surgeon.

### Procedure: Reduction of Radial Head Subluxation (Figure 34.8)

1. Educate patient and family that the elbow is not in the proper place and needs to be put back into place.
2. Warn patient and family that the patient will experience temporary pain during the procedure but that the pain should subside once the elbow is in the proper place.
3. Position the patient in a family member's lap prior to the procedure.
4. Place your thumb on the radial head, while supporting the affected elbow.
5. In one swift motion, press down on the radial head while fully supinating the forearm and extending the elbow. Then, fully flex the elbow while keeping the forearm supinated and your thumb on the radial head.

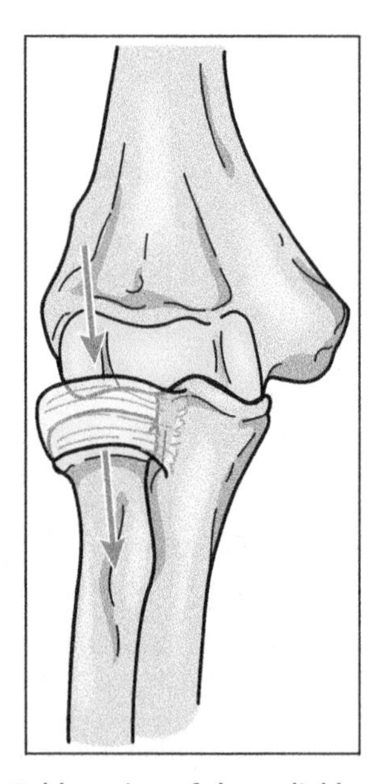

FIGURE 34.8 Subluxation of the radial head.

*Source*: Reproduced from Cuccurullo, S. J. (2020). *Physical medicine and rehabilitation board review* (4th ed.). Springer Publishing Company.

6. Once the reduction has taken place, a click will be felt and/or heard (Crowther-Radulewicz, 2019).

### Family Education

Teach the following:

- Cast/splint and dressing care
- RICE
- Signs and symptoms of compartment syndrome
- Weight-bearing status of affected extremity after treatment
- Importance of follow-up visits to ensure proper healing
- Post-reduction radial head subluxation: Child should regain full use of the arm within 30 minutes of the procedure. Restraining the affected extremity is not needed. *Avoid upward pulling motion to child's arms.* Educate family members to watch for signs and symptoms of repeated radial head subluxation or decreased use of affected arm post-procedure. Instruct family members to seek medical attention if the patient develops fever, redness, or swelling around the elbow (Crowther-Radulewicz, 2019)

### Referral

Refer children with confirmed or suspected fractures to a pediatric orthopedic surgeon to ensure prompt treatment of the injury.

▶ ALERT: Emergent referral and immediate orthopedic consultation is indicated for open fractures, injuries with vascular and/or nerve compromise, signs/symptoms of compartment syndrome, and deep lacerations over an affected joint.

## OVERUSE SYNDROMES

Overuse injuries occur from repetitive stress that causes microdamage to a bone, muscle or tendon. Hard and soft tissue breakdown is a normal, daily occurrence, and the body continually remodels these tissues so that they recuperate fully. In overuse syndromes, the normal reparative process is not allowed sufficient recovery time, thus injury occurs.

Overuse injuries include Osgood-Schlatter Disease (OSD), Little League elbow, Little League shoulder, patellofemoral pain syndrome, shin splints, Sever's Disease and stress fractures. Children are at increased risk for overuse injuries due to having immature bones that are unable to handle much stress.

## Subjective Findings

The health history may reveal:

- Pain in affected area following physical activity
- Pain at the time of activity with or without limiting performance
- Chronic pain that does not subside even with rest
- Activities that are performed in a repetitive manner (e.g., sport, position played, number of games, other sports or activities that may stress the same tissue)

### Risk Factors

The most common risk factors for overuse injuries are:

- Participation in some form of organized sports
- Overuse of the affected extremity without properly allowing the healing process to occur

### Review of Systems

The most common manifestations revealed during the review of systems include:

- **Integumentary**: swelling, bruising
- **Musculoskeletal**: pain, limp, guarding of affected extremity, decreased ROM, deformity

## Objective Findings

The physical examination of the child with overuse injuries may reveal tenderness and swelling. Refer to Table 34.1 for particular history and physical examination findings associated with each overuse syndrome.

### Laboratory/Diagnostic Testing

The diagnosis of overuse injuries is typically based upon the clinical findings. Plain radiographs (x-rays) and/or CT/MRI may be necessary to rule out other injuries.

## Differential Diagnosis

The differential diagnosis for overuse injuries includes:

- Sprain
- Strain
- Fracture
- Infection

## Treatment/Management Plan

The treatment for overuse injuries includes relative rest of the affected extremity for an adequate amount of time to ensure healing. Nonsteroidal anti-inflammatory drugs (NSAIDs) and ice will help with pain and inflammation. Immobilization may be needed for certain conditions; methods include braces, casts, and/or splints. Gradual reintroduction to sports or activities is imperative to prevent further injury and is usually achieved with specific stretching and strengthening exercises.

**TABLE 34.1 Clinical Findings With Overuse Syndromes**

| History and Physical Examination Findings | Overuse Syndrome |
|---|---|
| Swelling, pain, and tenderness directly over the tibial tubercle | Osgood-Schlatter disease (OSD) |
| Anterior knee pain | Patella-femoral pain syndrome |
| Gradual onset of shoulder pain that is increased with throwing, especially a curve ball | Little League shoulder |
| Tenderness to palpation over medial elbow, elbow pain with activity, decreased ROM and locking of elbow | Little League elbow |
| Pain with palpation to the tibia in a child with a history of repetitive running | Shin splints |
| Pain with jumping activities and/or repetitive running and positive calcaneal squeeze test | Sever disease |

### Family Education

Teach the following:

- With proper rest, most overuse injuries have complete resolution without any surgical intervention.
- With overuse syndromes, growth may be affected if adequate healing is not achieved.

### Referral

If the patient experiences persistent signs and symptoms despite conservative management, consider referral to physical therapy for sport-specific training and or a referral to a pediatric orthopedic surgeon if the patient does not achieve positive outcomes with physical therapy.

# ADOLESCENT IDIOPATHIC SCOLIOSIS

Adolescent idiopathic scoliosis (AIS) is the most common disorder of the pediatric spine and is often diagnosed during well child visits. The etiology of AIS is unknown; however, it is often familial in nature and affects approximately 3% of the general population (Scherl, 2020).

## ADOLESCENT IDIOPATHIC SCOLIOSIS

**AIS** is a three-dimensional, side-to-side "S" shaped curvature with rotation of the spine greater than 10 degrees. It can affect the cervical, thoracic, or lumbar spine or a combination of these. Although there are other types of scoliosis, AIS is the type most commonly seen in primary care. Other types of scoliosis include infantile, juvenile, congenital, and neuromuscular. AIS occurs during adolescence, is most often diagnosed around age 11, and the cause is unknown (Scherl, 2020). Lateral curvature of the spine progresses most rapidly during the adolescent's period of peak height velocity (PHV).

> **PRO TIP** Curves tend to progress more during times of rapid growth. In girls, this typically occurs during the first 18 months after their first menses.

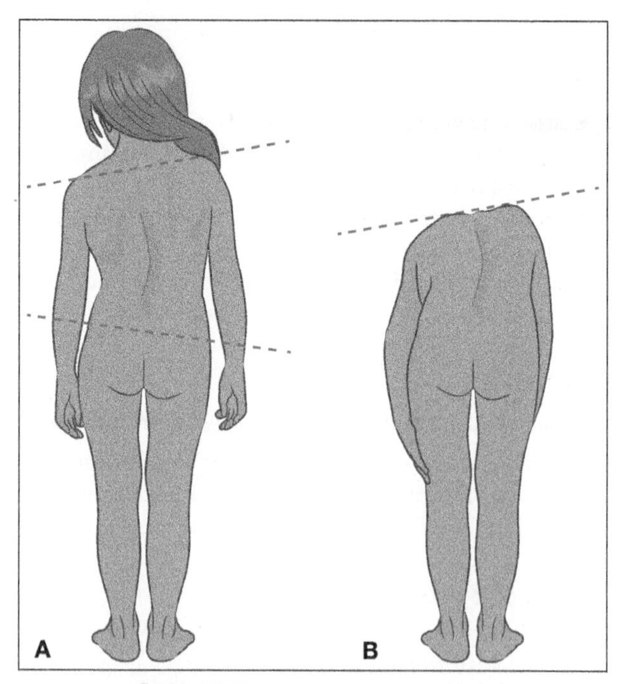


FIGURE 34.9 Adams forward-bend test. (**A**) Lateral curvature of spine is visible: right shoulder is elevated. (**B**) In Adams forward bend test, note the right scapula appears higher and reveal a rib hump.

*Source*: Chiocca, E. M. (2019). *Advanced pediatric assessment* (3rd ed.). Springer Publishing Company.

### Subjective Findings

The health history may reveal:

- Positive family history of AIS
- A gradual onset of uneven shoulders, one hip higher than the other, one shoulder sticking out farther than the other, or humpback
- Lack of pain
- Recent growth spurt

### Risk Factors

The most common risk factors for AIS are:

- Positive family history
- Female gender
- Premenarchal status

### Review of Systems

The most common manifestations revealed during the review of systems include:

- **Genitourinary:** bowel and/or bladder incontinence
- **Musculoskeletal:** noticeable rib hump, one leg shorter than other, numbness or pain in lower extremities, weakness in either upper or lower extremities

### Objective Findings

Observe the child from behind with the child's feet together and arms hanging by the sides. Then observe the child from behind with the Adams forward bend test (Figure 34.9). When available, use a scoliometer to measure the angle of trunk rotation (ATR). The physical examination of the child with AIS may reveal:

- Shoulder and/or waistline asymmetry
- Unilateral prominent shoulder blade or difference in the level of the shoulders or scapulae
- Obvious curvature of spine, or head shifted to one side (trunk shift)
- Excessive lordosis
- Tenderness to palpation of the spine
- Thoracic or lumbar spine prominence on one side with the Adams forward bend test
- ATR via scoliometer of 7° (5° in the obese child) or greater (Scherl, 2020)

> **PRO TIP** If the patient complains of back pain on examination, it is not likely caused from the scoliosis, but from participation in daily activities without proper conditioning. If this is the case, physical therapy may be indicated for core strengthening and hamstring stretching.

### Laboratory/Diagnostic Testing

The diagnosis of AIS is based upon the clinical and radiographic findings. Standing posterior-anterior and lateral radiographs of the entire spine are the gold standard for diagnosis. Curvature of greater than 10 degrees via the Cobb angle measurement on radiographs indicates the presence of AIS (Scherl, 2020).

If the curve is abnormal in presentation (left thoracic, double thoracic, high thoracic, or isolated left lumbar curve), an MRI may be indicated. An MRI may also be warranted if the patient has an abnormal physical exam, such as pain to palpation of spine, numbness and/or tingling of lower extremities, altered gait pattern or decreased muscle strength (Bosch & Rab, 2021).

**PRO TIP** A 7-degree curve with the scoliometer generally correlates with a 20-degree curve on radiograph.

### Differential Diagnosis

The differential diagnosis for AIS includes:

- Neuromuscular scoliosis
- Congenital scoliosis
- Schumann's kyphosis
- Sprengel deformity
- Limb length discrepancy
- Neurofibromatosis
- Malignancy

### Treatment/Management Plan

The treatment for AIS is dependent on the degree of curvature, the patient's age, and the patient's PHV. The Cobb angle is used to measure the degree of curvature on radiographs. Treatment consists of observation, bracing, or surgery. Treatment is based on the degree of curvature and the level of skeletal maturity (Table 34.2).

**ALERT:** Changes in the neuromuscular examination (such as pain, weakness, and/or bowel or bladder incontinence) require immediate evaluation and diagnostic testing.

**TABLE 34.2 Treatment for AIS Based on Degree of Curve and Skeletal Maturity**

| Degree of Curve | Skeletally Immature | Skeletally Mature |
|---|---|---|
| 10°–20° | Observation; follow up every 4–6 months with repeat radiographs | Observation |
| 25°–40° | Brace worn until skeletally mature | Observation |
| >40° | Surgical intervention | Observation until curve reaches 50° |

### Family Education

Teach the following:

- Adherence to instructions for brace wear is vital in preventing further progression of the curve.
- Patient needs to return to the clinic if they begin experiencing pain, bowel and/or bladder incontinence, muscle weakness, or the development of an altered gait pattern.
- Physical therapy is generally not indicated for AIS.

### Referral

Refer to a pediatric orthopedic surgeon if the ATR is 5 to 7 degrees, or the Cobb angle on x-ray is measured as 10 degrees or greater.

# LOWER EXTREMITY CONDITIONS

Many lower extremity conditions are seen in primary care. Most of these conditions are benign and self-limiting. The most commonly seen lower extremity conditions are genu varum, genu valgum, in-toeing, and idiopathic toe walking.

## GENU VARUM AND GENU VALGUM

Genu varum, also known as physiologic bowed legs, is a variation of normal and most often presents in children up to the age of 3 years old. Natural progression of growth begins with the appearance of genu varum at birth. This is thought to occur due to tight intrauterine packaging. Genu varum typically resolves around age 3 when the child returns to neutral. As the child grows, around the age of 4, the child transitions into genu valgum, or knock-knees. Genu valgum is typically seen in children up to 7 years of age. After the age of 7, a slightly valgus or neutral position remains throughout adulthood.

**PRO TIP** You can easily remember the difference between genu valgum and genu varum by thinking about "gum" that makes the knees stick together for genu valgum and a truck fitting through the varus deformity sounding like "vrmmm" for genu varum.

### Subjective Findings

The health history of a patient with physiologic genu varum may reveal:

- Painless "bowed legs"

- Excessive falling
- In-toeing
- Early ambulator

The health history of a patient with genu valgum may reveal:

- Painless "knock-knees"
- Cosmetic concerns

### Risk Factors

The most common risk factors for physiologic genu varum and genu valgum are:

- Family history
- Birth history

### Review of Systems

The most common manifestations revealed during the review of systems include:

- **Musculoskeletal:** misalignment of lower extremities or obvious deformity, gait disturbances

### Objective Findings

The physical examination of the child with *physiologic genu varum* may reveal:

- Bowed legs
- Associated internal tibial torsion (Weintraub, 2017)

The physical examination of the child with *genu valgum* may reveal:

- Knock-knees
- Awkward gait (Weintraub, 2017)
  Refer to Figure 34.10.

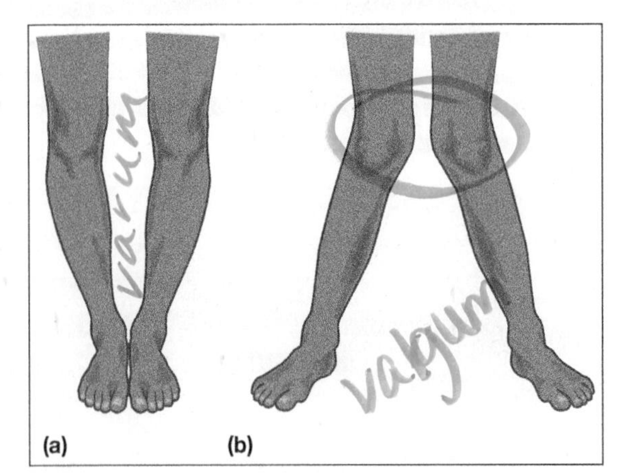


FIGURE 34.10 Genu varum; genu valgum.

*Source*: Chiocca, E. M. (2019). *Advanced pediatric assessment* (3rd ed.). Springer Publishing Company.

### Laboratory/Diagnostic Testing

The diagnosis of physiologic genu varum and genu valgum is based upon the clinical findings. No laboratory or diagnostic testing is needed unless pathologic or metabolic causes are suspected.

### Differential Diagnosis

The differential diagnosis for genu varum and genu valgum includes:

- Rickets
- Blount disease
- Chondroplasia or neuromuscular disorder
- Osteogenesis imperfecta
- Infection
- Trauma
- Tumor (Weintraub, 2017)

▶ ALERT: If a child presents to clinic with genu varum between the ages of 2 and 4, is overweight, and is an early ambulator (walker), be aware that this could be Blount disease (pathologic tibia vara) and will need close monitoring and likely a referral to a pediatric orthopedist.

### Treatment/Management Plan

No treatment is indicated for physiologic genu varum, as it often spontaneously resolves with time. Blount disease does require early intervention before the age of 4. If the patient does not begin showing improvement after the age of 2, a referral is indicated for an evaluation for possible Blount disease.

No treatment is indicated for genu valgum prior to the age of 7. After age 7, surgery may be indicated to correct the deformity. Referral to a pediatric orthopedist is indicated if the patient is not showing any improvement by the age of 7.

### Family Education

Teach the following:

- Most cases of physiologic genu varum resolve by age 3.
- Most cases of genu valgum resolve by age 7.
- No restriction of activities is indicated in either genu varum or genu valgum.
- No treatment is indicated in genu varum as long as it is physiologic and not pathologic.
- Genu valgum that persists beyond age 7 may require operative intervention (Rosenfeld, 2019a).

### Referral

Referral to pediatric orthopedics is necessary when the patient is at risk for a pathologic condition. A referral is also indicated if the genu varum or genu valgum appear to be worsening on repeat examination. If genu valgum persists beyond 7 years of age, referral is indicated for possible operative intervention.

## IN-TOEING

In-toeing is often caused by internal tibial torsion and femoral anteversion. Tibial torsion is described as a rotational abnormality of the tibia and is most often found around the age of 6 to 12 months. This is commonly physiologic and results from intrauterine packaging. Tibial torsion frequently spontaneously resolves around age 6. Femoral anteversion is an excessive rotational abnormality of the femur, with the general population having some degree of rotation. In-toeing caused by femoral anteversion tends to increase up to the age of 5, with complete resolution by age 8 (Weintraub, 2017).

### Subjective Findings

The health history may reveal:

- Pigeon-toeing
- Awkward run
- May trip or fall more often than other children
- "W" sits (sits on floor with both knees forward, legs bent at knees, with heels pointing toward the buttocks—the legs form a 'W')
- Positive family history

### Risk Factors

The most common risk factors for in-toeing are:

- Positive family history
- Intrauterine positioning

### Review of Systems

The most common manifestations revealed during the review of systems include:

- **Musculoskeletal:** misalignment or obvious deformity, gait disturbances

### Objective Findings

The physical examination of the child with in-toeing (tibial torsion) may reveal:

- Increased thigh-foot angle on prone examination
- Increased foot progression angle when ambulating
- Increased internal tibial rotation with the patella facing forward

The physical examination of the child with in-toeing (femoral anteversion) may reveal:

- "Kissing" patella when ambulating
- Increased thigh-foot angle on prone examination
- Increased foot progression angle when ambulating
- Limited external rotation of the hips

### Laboratory/Diagnostic Testing

The diagnosis of in-toeing is based upon the clinical findings. No laboratory or diagnostic testing is needed.

### Differential Diagnosis

The differential diagnosis for in-toeing includes:

- Associated hip disorders such as DDH
- Neuromuscular disorders such as cerebral palsy
- MA

### Treatment/Management Plan

Treatment for in-toeing includes reassurance and observation. Internal tibial torsion and femoral anteversion are both self-limiting and resolve on their own with time.

### Family Education

Teach the following:

- Reassure that braces and therapy are not indicated, as they have not been shown to be effective.

**PRO TIP** Sitting in the "W" position does not increase the deformity and does not have to be avoided.

### Referral

If tibial torsion and femoral anteversion have not completely resolved by the age of 8, referral to a pediatric orthopedist is indicated.

## IDIOPATHIC TOE-WALKING

Idiopathic toe-walking is commonly seen in young children around walking age who have yet to develop a heel-toe walking pattern. The most common cause is a tight Achilles tendon. Some children adopt normal walking patterns with time. Persistent toe-walking beyond the age of 2 years may be idiopathic or habitual in nature, but warrants further investigation as it may result from a neuromuscular disorder (Weintraub, 2017).

### Subjective Findings

The health history may reveal:

- Walks on toes

### Risk Factors

The most common risk factor for idiopathic toe-walking is:

- Positive family history

### Review of Systems

The most common manifestations revealed during the review of systems include:

- **Musculoskeletal:** toe-walking gait

### Objective Findings

Perform a complete neurologic examination to rule out other underlying disorders that may cause in-toeing. Assess ROM of the hips, knees, and ankles. The physical examination of the child with idiopathic toe-walking may reveal tight Achilles tendon, but also the ability to place the foot flat.

### Laboratory/Diagnostic Testing

The diagnosis of idiopathic toe-walking is based upon the clinical findings. No laboratory or diagnostic testing is needed.

### Differential Diagnosis

The differential diagnosis for toe-walking includes:

- Cerebral palsy
- Arthrogryposis
- Muscular dystrophy (MD)
- Leg length discrepancy
- Spinal cord abnormalities
- Charcot-Marie-Tooth disease (Weintraub, 2017)

### Treatment/Management Plan

Observation of idiopathic toe-walking until the age of 3 is acceptable, or passive range-of-motion/stretching exercises may be helpful. For the older child with persistent toe-walking, serial casting may be prescribed by the orthopedic surgeon. (Weintraub, 2017).

### Family Education

Teach the following:

- Children do not acquire their adult gait pattern until 7 years of age (Weintraub, 2017).
- Instruct the patient and family on proper heel cord stretching exercises.

### Referral

Consider physical therapy referral for tight Achilles tendon. If an Achilles tendon contracture occurs, refer to a pediatric orthopedist.

# PEDIATRIC HIP DISORDERS

Patients often present to their primary care provider with knee or groin pain that likely originates from the hip. The two most commonly seen pediatric hip disorders are slipped capital femoral epiphysis (SCFE) and Legg-Calve-Perthes disease (LCPD).

## SLIPPED CAPITAL FEMORAL EPIPHYSIS (SCFE)

A SCFE is a pediatric hip disorder that commonly occurs in adolescents between the ages of 11 and 16 years (Boutis, 2020). A SCFE is described as the displacement of the femoral head from the femoral neck through the physis. It is classified as acute, chronic, or acute on chronic (acute worsening of the chronic condition) and is considered stable or unstable based on the patient's weight-bearing ability. Avascular necrosis is the most serious complication and is caused by disruption of the blood supply to the epiphysis (Boutis, 2020).

### Subjective Findings

The health history may reveal:

- Hip pain
- Groin pain
- Knee pain
- Thigh pain
- Vague history of recent trauma
- Pain with ambulation
- Inability to bear weight on the affected leg
- Altered gait pattern

### Risk Factors

The most common risk factors for SCFE are:

- African American or Polynesian descent
- Obesity
- Male gender
- This is not a risk factor for SCFE
- Certain underlying conditions, including juvenile arthritis, renal failure, endocrinopathies, and certain human leukocyte antigen types
- History of previous radiation or chemotherapy (Boutis, 2020)

### Review of Systems

The most common manifestations revealed during the review of systems include:

- **Constitutional:** pain in hip or referred to thigh or knee
- **Musculoskeletal:** inability to bear weight, or a change in gait pattern, recent trauma

### Objective Findings

The physical examination of the child with SCFE may reveal:

- Walking with an externally rotated leg
- Decreased internal rotation
- Decreased abduction and extension
- Antalgic gait pattern (a gait that develops as a way to avoid pain) with associated limp
- Hip, groin, thigh, and/or knee pain

**PRO TIP** Always examine the patient's hips if the child is having knee pain. Many patients present to the office with only knee pain complaints, which may cause a delay in diagnosis.

### Laboratory/Diagnostic Testing

The diagnosis of SCFE is based upon the clinical and radiographic findings. Common findings on anteroposterior and lateral x-rays include widening of the growth plate and/or femoral head displacement, often resembling a "scoop of ice cream falling off the cone." An endocrine workup is often warranted in patients with SCFE to rule out any underlying endocrinopathies.

### Differential Diagnosis

The differential diagnosis for SCFE includes:

- LCPD
- Fracture
- Avascular necrosis
- Septic hip
- Osteoarthritis (Kienstra & Macias, 2021)

### Treatment/Management Plan

Treatment for a SCFE is dependent on the severity of the slip. The goal of treatment is to prevent further slippage and is achieved through surgical intervention by a pediatric orthopedic surgeon (Kienstra & Macias, 2021).

### Family Education

Teach the following:

- Surgery is often performed within 24 hours of diagnosis
- Adherence to non-weight-bearing is vital to prevent further slippage until evaluated by an orthopedic surgeon
- Postoperative care
- There is an increased risk of the patient developing degenerative joint disease even with fixation, and the patient may require a total hip replacement later in life (Kienstra & Macias, 2021)

### Referral

Referral to a pediatric orthopedic surgeon is imperative to produce the most favorable outcome for the patient.

## LEGG-CALVE-PERTHES DISEASE

LCPD is a pediatric hip disorder that causes deficient blood flow to the femoral head. It most often affects children 4 to 9 years of age, affecting both hips in only 10% of cases (Boutis, 2020). The four stages of LCPD are necrosis, fragmentation, reossification, and healing.

### Subjective Findings

The health history may reveal:

- Gradual onset of a limp
- Possible pain
- Pain that is relieved by rest and exacerbated by activity
- Intermittent hip, knee, thigh, or groin pain

### Risk Factors

The most common risk factors for LCPD are:

- Age between 4 and 9 )'ears
- Male gender
- Caucasian
- Positive family history
- Delayed skeletal maturation
- Being small for age (Boutis, 2020)

### Review of Systems

The most common manifestations revealed during the review of systems include:

- **Constitutional:** mild or intermittent pain of thigh, groin, hip, or knee
- **Musculoskeletal:** gradual onset of a limp, with decreased ROM of affected leg

### Objective Findings

The physical examination of the child with LCPD may reveal:

- Trendelenburg gait (see Figure 34.5)
- Decreased internal rotation

- Decreased abduction
- Muscle atrophy
- LLD (Walter & Tassone, 2019)

**PRO TIP** Always examine the patient's hips if the child is having thigh or knee pain, as many patients with LCPD present to the office not complaining of hip pain—thereby causing a delay in diagnosis.

### Laboratory/Diagnostic Testing

The diagnosis of LCPD is based upon the clinical and radiographic findings. Anteroposterior and frog-leg views may show a flattened femoral head depending on the phase of disease (Boutis, 2020).

### Differential Diagnosis

The differential diagnosis for LCPD includes:

- Limp
- Fracture
- Juvenile idiopathic arthritis
- Rheumatoid arthritis
- Septic arthritis
- Transient synovitis
- SCFE
- Sickle cell disease
- Endocrinopathies such as hypothyroidism
- Skeletal dysplasia (Hernandez & Li, 2018)

### Treatment/Management Plan

Treatment for LCPD is dependent on the severity of the disease and the age of the child. The goal of treatment is to maintain flexibility and ROM of the hip, control pain, and maintain proper position of the femoral head. Nonoperative interventions include NSAIDs to help with pain management, casts and/or braces, and activity restriction. Surgical interventions include arthrogram, closed reduction and casting, tendon release and/or osteotomies. Surgery is not recommended in children who are under 6 years of age (International Perthes Study Group, 2020).

### Family Education

Teach the following:

- Educate the family that the disease process often takes years to resolve
- Maintaining hip ROM is crucial

### Referral

Referral to a pediatric orthopedic surgeon is imperative to produce the most favorable outcome for the patient. Referral to a physical therapist is needed to help maintain flexibility and ROM of the hip. If other conditions are suspected, referral to the appropriate specialist is warranted.

# INFECTIOUS/INFLAMMATORY DISORDERS

Many childhood illnesses can result in infectious and/or inflammatory disorders of the musculoskeletal system. The infection usually involves a joint, mainly of the hips and knees. Osteomyelitis and septic arthritis are two diagnoses that are infectious in nature; transient synovitis is caused by an inflammatory reaction.

## OSTEOMYELITIS

Osteomyelitis is an infection of the bone that affects children of all ages. Osteomyelitis is more common in children than adults. Most cases are diagnosed in the later summer and early fall months and following a viral illness or upper respiratory infection (URI). The most common organism to cause osteomyelitis is *Staphylococcus aureus* (Rhodes et al., 2018).

### Subjective Findings

The health history may reveal:

- Recent viral illness or URI
- Fever
- Gradual onset of pain
- Inability to bear weight on the affected extremity
- Decreased ROM
- Limping

### Risk Factors

The most common risk factor for osteomyelitis is a recentl diagnosis of a URI or viral illness. A history of a traumatic event also increases a child's risk for developing osteomyelitis.

### Review of Systems

The most common manifestations revealed during the review of systems include:

- **Constitutional:** pain, fever, fatigue; in infants, poor feeding

- **Musculoskeletal:** limp, refusal or inability to bear weight, decreased ROM
- **Neurologic:** irritability in infants

### Objective Findings

The physical examination of the child with osteomyelitis may reveal:

- Irritability with being examined
- Lethargy
- Tenderness to palpation over affected joint
- Warmth, erythema, edema of affected area

### Laboratory/Diagnostic Testing

Laboratory findings indicative of osteomyelitis include elevated white blood cell (WBC) count, elevated C-reactive protein (CRP), and increased erythrocyte sedimentation rate (ESR). Blood cultures may also be positive. Radiographic images may reveal soft tissue swelling, with bony changes noted later in the illness. MRI with contrast is the gold standard for diagnosis (Rhodes et al., 2018).

### Differential Diagnosis

The differential diagnosis for osteomyelitis includes:

- Septicemia
- Cellulitis
- Septic arthritis
- Malignancy
- Bone infarction (Krogstad, 2020b)

▶ ALERT: It is important to rule out Ewing sarcoma, leukemia, and lymphoma when considering a diagnosis of osteomyelitis.

### Treatment/Management Plan

Antibiotic therapy is essential in the treatment of osteomyelitis. Once a causative organism has been identified, the appropriate antibiotic should be started to target the infection. The duration of treatment is dependent on the organism and the antibiotic chosen, most often requiring 6 weeks of treatment (may begin with intravenous and transition to oral medication when tenderness, fever, WBC count, and CRP are all either resolved or decreasing).

### Family Education

Teach the following:

- Children typically respond well to the treatment of osteomyelitis and do not suffer any long-term effects.
- Adherence to antibiotic therapy, duration, and frequency is vital in resolving the infection.

### Referral

If osteomyelitis is suspected, refer the patient to the emergency department or for direct hospitalization to ensure timely and appropriate treatment.

## SEPTIC ARTHRITIS

Septic arthritis is an infection involving the joint. Septic arthritis affects children of all ages and can present in any joint; however, children who are less than 5 years of age are most likely to present with septic arthritis. The most common causative organism is *Staphylococcus aureus* (Yee-Guardino & Goldfarb, 2017).

### Subjective Findings

The health history may reveal acute onset of illness and pain with motion of the involved joint. Determine recent use of antibiotics and the child's vaccination status.

### Risk Factors

The most common risk factor for septic arthritis is being a hospitalized neonate with multiple possible sources of infection. Other risk factors include joint trauma, skin lesions, underlying rheumatologic and hematologic conditions, prosthetic joints, and immunocompromise (Krogstad, 2020a).

### Review of Systems

The most common manifestations revealed during the review of systems include:

- **Constitutional:** fever, pain, fatigue
- **Respiratory:** symptoms of a URI
- **Musculoskeletal:** limp, decreased ROM, inability to bear weight on affected extremity

### Objective Findings

The physical examination of the child with septic arthritis may reveal:

- Current fever
- Lethargy
- Irritability with being examined
- Holding affected extremity in a flexed, abducted, slightly externally rotated position
- Warmth
- Edema

- Severe pain with ROM of the affected joint (Krogstad, 2020a)

### Laboratory/Diagnostic Testing

The diagnosis of septic arthritis is based upon the clinical and laboratory findings. After referral has been made, a joint aspirate will be obtained. Fluid will be tested for a cell count and culture as well as a gram stain. A CBC with differential, CRP, ESR, and blood cultures should also be ordered. Radiographic images may reveal soft tissue swelling; however, they are not diagnostic. Ultrasound of the affected area is helpful in identifying a subperiosteal fluid collection and may be used to guide aspiration of the affected joint. MRI is highly sensitive in diagnosing septic arthritis (Krogstad, 2020a).

▶ ALERT: Early diagnosis and treatment of septic arthritis is key for producing the most favorable long-term outcomes and avoidance of joint damage and disability.

### Differential Diagnosis

The differential diagnosis for septic arthritis includes:

- Osteomyelitis
- Rheumatologic disorders
- Transient synovitis
- LCPD
- SCFE
- Fracture (Krogstad, 2020a)

### Treatment/Management Plan

Septic arthritis is an orthopedic emergency requiring immediate hospitalization for surgical drainage and intravenous antibiotic therapy. The mainstay of treatment includes appropriate antibiotic therapy and surgical intervention. Before initiating antibiotic therapy, cultures should be obtained.

#### Family Education

Teach the following:

- Adherence to antibiotic therapy is vital to the long-term outcome of septic arthritis.
- The patient may require a prolonged hospitalization until the infection is cleared, and often may require multiple operations.

#### Referral

Refer as follows:

- It is critical to refer to the emergency room for suspected septic arthritis.
- Consultation with a pediatric orthopedic surgeon or pediatric interventional radiologist is required for aspiration of joint fluid and determination of the causative organism.
- An infectious disease specialist is often consulted during the hospitalization for antibiotic regimen and recommended duration of treatment.
- A pediatric orthopedic surgeon is also consulted for surgical incision and drainage of the affected joint.

▶ ALERT: Septic arthritis is an orthopedic emergency.

## TRANSIENT SYNOVITIS

Transient synovitis is an inflammatory condition that must be distinguished from septic arthritis. Transient synovitis is a diagnosis of exclusion and most often affects children ages 3 to 8. It is the most common cause of hip pain in children and occurs more often in males. The cause of transient synovitis is unknown, but may be linked to viral illness (Walter & Tassone, 2019).

### Subjective Findings

The health history may reveal:

- Recent URI
- Acute onset of pain in the hip, groin, thigh, or knee

#### Risk Factors

The most common risk factors for transient synovitis are:

- Male gender
- Age 3 to 8 years
- Recent upper respiratory or other viral infection (Walter & Tassone, 2019)

#### Review of Systems

The most common manifestations revealed during the review of systems include:

- **Constitutional:** pain, possible fever
- **Musculoskeletal:** limp

### Objective Findings

The physical examination of the child with transient synovitis may reveal:

- Painful limp
- Holds hip in a normal position

**PRO TIP** Patients with transient synovitis are more likely to allow ROM of the affected joint, as this condition is not as painful as septic arthritis.

### Laboratory/Diagnostic Testing

The diagnosis of transient synovitis is based upon the clinical and laboratory findings. Because transient synovitis is a diagnosis of exclusion, laboratory testing is beneficial in ruling out other possible diagnoses. Typically, WBC count, CRP, and ESR are normal. There is no indication for radiographic evaluation of transient synovitis.

### Differential Diagnosis

The differential diagnosis for transient synovitis includes:

- Septic arthritis
- Trauma
- Juvenile idiopathic arthritis
- Rheumatologic disorder
- Malignancy (Walter & Tassone, 2019)

### Treatment/Management Plan

Once septic arthritis has been ruled out, transient synovitis is treated with rest and NSAIDs. The condition is self-limiting and typically resolves within 1 to 2 weeks.

### Family Education

Teach the following:

- Transient synovitis is self-limiting and resolves with time.
- Monitor the patient for signs of septic arthritis (fever, inability to bear weight, and extreme pain with ROM of the joint). If any of these changes occur, medical care should be sought immediately.
- NSAIDs decrease inflammation as well as help with pain management and should be utilized regularly until the condition resolves.

### Referral

If the patient has persistent pain that worsens, or develops signs and symptoms of septic arthritis, the child must be referred to the emergency room for evaluation by a pediatric orthopedic surgeon.

## KEY POINTS

- Congenital torticollis usually resolves with stretching exercises and/or physical therapy; follow up every 2 to 4 weeks until the condition is resolved.
- The AAP suggests that all infants with risk factors for DDH receive a hip ultrasound at the age of 6 weeks, despite a normal physical exam.
- Clubfoot casting will not keep the child from reaching developmental milestones such as crawling and walking.
- Reassure parents of children with MA that the condition will most likely resolve on its own over time without any treatment.
- Monitor the child with a sprain or strain every 2 to 3 weeks to assess for improvement. Patients may return to activity once they have regained full ROM, have complete return of both strength and proprioception, and minimal pain.
- Close follow-up of fractures is indicated to ensure proper healing and position of the bone.
- Complete resolution of overuse injury may take weeks to years depending on the type of overuse injury.
- AIS does not cause back pain and is more common in females.
- Stretching and/or braces are not indicated in physiologic genu varum or genu valgum, as they have not been shown to be effective.
- Reassure the patient's family that in-toeing most often resolves on its own with time and that braces are not necessary.
- If SCFE is suspected or diagnosed on x-ray, keep the patient non-weight–bearing until an evaluation by an orthopedic surgeon.
- Many patients with LCPD do not complain of hip pain, but do complain of thigh and knee pain, delaying a proper diagnosis. *Always* check the hips if a patient is complaining of thigh or knee pain.
- If osteomyelitis is suspected, refer the patient to the emergency department for further workup.
- Septic arthritis is an orthopedic emergency.
- Children with transient synovitis should be reexamined in 1 to 2 weeks to ensure that the transient synovitis has resolved and the patient has regained full, painless ROM of the joint.

## REFERENCES

Allison, R. M., Birken, C. S., Lebovic, G., Howard, A. W., L'Aabbe, M. R., Morency, M.-E., Maquire, J. L., & the TARGet Kids! Collaboration. (2020). Consumption of cow's milk in early childhood and fracture risk: A prospective cohort study. *American Journal of Epidemiology, 189*(2), 146–155. https://doi.org/10.1093/aje/kwz216

Bosch, P., & Rab, G. T. (2021). Chapter 12: Pediatric orthopedic surgery. In P. J. McMahon, & H. B. Skinner (Eds.), *Current diagnosis & treatment in orthopedics* (6th ed.). McGraw-Hill.

Boutis, K. (2020). Pediatric orthopedic emergencies. In J. E. Tintinalli, O. J. Ma, D. M. Yealy, G. D. Meckler, S. Stapczynski,

D. M. Cline, & S. H. Thomas (Eds.), *Tintinalli's emergency medicine: A comprehensive study guide* (9th ed., Chapter 141). McGraw-Hill Education.

Clunie, G. (2017). Prenatal diagnosis. In T. K. McInerny, H. M. Adam, D. E. Campbell, J. M. Foy, & D. M. Kamat (Eds.), *American Academy of Pediatrics textbook of pediatric care* (2nd ed., Chapter 82). American Academy of Pediatrics.

Crowther-Radulewicz, C. (2019). *Orthopedic procedures* [Online module]. http://www.pncb.org

Egol, K., Koval, J. K., & Zuckerman, J. D. (2020). *Handbook of fractures* (6th ed.). Wolters Kluwer.

Hernandez, J., & Li, C. D. (2018). Legg-Calve-Perthes disease in emergency medicine. *eMedicine.* https://emedicine.medscape.com/article/826935-overview

International Hip Dysplasia Institute. (2018). *Infant and child hip dysplasia.* http://www.hipdysplasia.org.

International Perthes Study Group. (2020). *Treatment by age.* https://perthesdisease.org/treatment-by-age

Kienstra, A. J., & Macias, C. G. (2021). Evaluation and management of slipped capital femoral epiphysis (SCFE). *UpToDate.* https://www.uptodate.com/contents/evaluation-and-management-of-slipped-capital-femoral-epiphysis-scfe

Kim, H., & Shoval, H. A. (2019). Pediatric musculoskeletal medicine. In R. Mitra (Ed.), *Principles of rehabilitation medicine* (pp. 1046–1067). McGraw-Hill.

Krogstad, P. (2020a). Bacterial arthritis: Clinical features and diagnosis in infants and children. *UpToDate.* https://www.uptodate.com/contents/bacterial-arthritis-treatment-and-outcome-in-infants-and-children

Krogstad, P. (2020b). Hematogenous osteomyelitis in children: Evaluation and diagnosis. *UpToDate.* https://www.uptodate.com/contents/hematogenous-osteomyelitis-in-children-evaluation-and-diagnosis

Macias, C. G., & Gan, V. (2019a). Congenital muscular torticollis: Clinical features and diagnosis. *UpToDate.* https://www.uptodate.com/contents/congenital-muscular-torticollis-clinical-features-and-diagnosis

Macias, C. G., & Gan, V. (2019b). Congenital muscular torticollis: Management and prognosis. *UpToDate.* https://www.uptodate.com/contents/congenital-muscular-torticollis-management-and-prognosis/

McKee-Garrett, T. M. (2020). Lower extremity positional deformations. *UpToDate.* https://www.uptodate.com/contents/lower-extremity-positional-deformations

Ozuah, P. O., & Skae, C. C. (2017). Torticollis. In T. K. McInerny, H. M. Adam, D. E. Campbell, J. M. Foy, & D. M. Kamat (Eds.), *American Academy of Pediatrics textbook of pediatric care* (2nd ed., Chapter 203). American Academy of Pediatrics.

Rhodes, J., Erickson, M. A., Tagawa, A., & Niswander, C. (2018). Orthopedics. In W. W. Hay, M. J. Levin, R. R. Deterding, M. J. Abzug, & J. M. Sondheimer (Eds.), *Current diagnosis and treatment: Pediatrics* (24th ed., Chapter 26). McGraw-Hill Education.

Rosenfeld, S. B. (2019a). Approach to the child with knock-knees. *UpToDate.* https://www.uptodate.com/contents/approach-to-the-child-with-knock-knees

Rosenfeld, S. B. (2019b). Developmental dysplasia of the hip: Clinical features and diagnosis. *UpToDate.* https://www.uptodate.com/contents/developmental-dysplasia-of-the-hip-clinical-features-and-diagnosis

Rosenfeld, S. B. (2020). Approach to the child with in-toeing. *UpToDate.* https://www.uptodate.com/contents/approach-to-the-child-with-in-toeing

Rosenfeld, S. B. (2021c). Developmental dysplasia of the hip: Treatment and outcome. *UpToDate.* https://www.uptodate.com/contents/developmental-dysplasia-of-the-hip-clinical-features-and-diagnosis

Scherl, S. A. (2020). Adolescent idiopathic scoliosis: Clinical features, evaluation, and diagnosis. *UpToDate.* https://www.uptodate.com/contents/adolescent-idiopathic-scoliosis-clinical-features-evaluation-and-diagnosis

Walter, K. D., & Tassone, J. C. (2019). Orthopedics. In K. J. Marcdante & R. M. Kliegman (Eds.), *Nelson's essentials of pediatrics* (8th ed., Section 26). Elsevier.

Weintraub, B. (2017). Foot and leg problems. In T. K. McInerny, H. M. Adam, D. E. Campbell, J. M. Foy, & D. M. Kamat (Eds.), *American Academy of Pediatrics textbook of pediatric care* (2nd ed., Chapter 156). American Academy of Pediatrics.

Yee-Guardino, S., & Goldfarb, J. (2017). Septic arthritis. In T. K. McInerny, H. M. Adam, D. E. Campbell, J. M. Foy, & D. M. Kamat (Eds.), *American Academy of Pediatrics textbook of pediatric care* (2nd ed., Chapter 328). American Academy of Pediatrics.

# Management of Neuromuscular Disorders

Leslie N. Rhodes and Brittany Williams

## Student Learning Outcomes

**Upon completion of this chapter the reader should be able to:**

1. Discuss pathophysiology and epidemiology of selected neuromuscular disorders in children.
2. Differentiate subjective and objective findings of selected neuromuscular disorders in children.
3. Choose appropriate laboratory or diagnostic tests for particular neuromuscular disorders in children.
4. Utilize the differential diagnosis process to determine neuromuscular diagnosis in children.
5. Determine treatment plan, child/family education, and need for referral in children with a neuromuscular diagnosis.

## INTRODUCTION

A variety of neuromuscular disorders may affect children, with each resulting in some degree of temporary or permanent muscular dysfunction. These disorders may be a congenital anomaly (neural tube defects), genetic in nature (muscular dystrophy [MD], spinal muscular atrophy [SMA]), or acquired (cerebral palsy [CP], Bell palsy). Bell palsy is a temporary condition, but the others result in significant motor dysfunction that is lifelong in nature. They affect the child's development and acquisition of motor skills, often resulting in handicaps. The primary care provider plays an important role by maintaining a high index of suspicion in identification of the disorder early and as the coordinator of many specialists or interventions.

The content in this chapter maps to the following areas on the Pediatric Nursing Certification Board (PNCB) Pediatric Nurse Practitioner—Primary Care certification examination:

**CLINICAL PROBLEMS: NEUROLOGY**

CONTENT AREAS:

**II. Assessment and Diagnosis**

**B. History and Physical Examination**

1. Obtain history of present illness
2. Obtain a comprehensive health history for new patients
3. Complete an interval history for established patients
4. Perform a review of systems
5. Perform a complete physical examination

**C. Diagnostic Testing and Screening**

1. Order and interpret office/clinic based screening tests
2. Order and interpret diagnostic laboratory tests
3. Order and interpret the results of diagnostic imaging tests

**D. Analyzing Information**

1. Integrate health history and physical examination findings into the plan of care
2. Assimilate findings from screening and diagnostic testing into plan of care

**E. Diagnosis**

1. Develop and prioritize differential diagnoses
2. Establish a diagnosis based on evaluation of patient data

## III. Management

**A. Child and Caregiver Counseling and Education**

1. Provide condition-specific counseling and education, including treatment options
2. Educate about benefits and potential adverse reactions of pharmacological interventions
3. Discuss non-pharmacological interventions
4. Counsel regarding the threshold for seeking follow-up care
5. Review the risks of non-adherence to recommended treatment

**B. Therapeutic Interventions**

1. Prescribe pharmacologic agents
3. Order or recommend non-pharmacologic treatments for the management of symptoms

**D. Collaboration and Referral**

2. Refer to specialists as indicated for evaluation, counseling, and/or treatment

**E. Care Coordination**

1. Facilitate patient and family-centered care for children of all ages with acute and chronic conditions

**C. Evaluation and Follow-up**

2. Establish a plan for follow-up care

## IV. Professional Role Responsibilities

**A. Leadership and Evidence-based Practice**

4. Develop, implement, and/or modify clinical practice guidelines

# BELL PALSY

Bell palsy is a sudden or acute, unilateral weakening or paralysis of the facial nerve (cranial nerve [CN] VII) without sensory involvement. This results from venous congestion in the nerve canal and edema of the facial nerve, further contributing to compression of the nerve. The most common cause is a postinfectious viral illness. The palsy involves both the upper and lower face on one side, which distinguishes it from a stroke. Onset occurs quickly and can progress to the peak of severity within hours. The symptoms of Bell palsy may last from 1 to 9 weeks (Ryan, 2020).

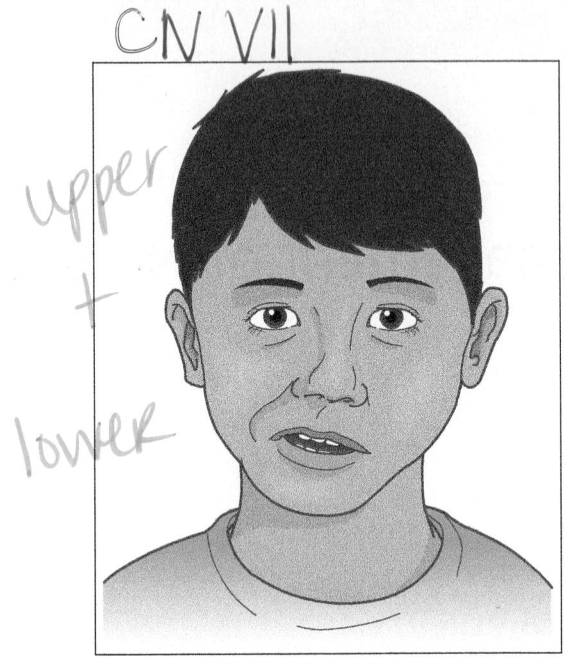

FIGURE 35.1 Facial symptoms of Bell palsy.

There are many potential causes for facial nerve palsies, including congenital, infectious, inflammatory, neoplastic, traumatic, and idiopathic (Zaidman, 2020). The incidence of Bell palsy in children is 3:100,000 in those under 10 years of age (Falchek, 2019). Commonly associated conditions include rubella, herpes simplex, Lyme disease, Epstein-Barr virus, cytomegalovirus, mumps, human immunodeficiency virus, *Mycoplasma pneumoniae*, and sarcoidosis. A preceding illness is often identified, but is not a requirement for diagnosis (Figure 35.1).

**PRO TIP** Acute otitis media is the number-one cause of Bell palsy in children (Patterson, 2019).

## Subjective Findings

The health history may reveal:

- Difficulty moving forehead
- Droopy eyebrows or drooping of the mouth corner
- Unable to close the eye
- Trauma (Falchek, 2019; Patterson, 2019)

## Risk Factors

The most common risk factors for Bell palsy are:

- Previous viral infection
- Exposure to Lyme disease and tick bites

### Review of Systems

The most common manifestations revealed during the review of systems include:

- **HEENT:** decreased tears on the affected side, itchy and/or burning eyes, ear pain, isophonia
- **Neurologic:** facial paralysis, headache, hyperacusis (sensitivity to sound on the affected side), difficulty eating food and drinking (may have dribbling on the weak side), difficulty keeping the mouth closed, dysgeusia (foods don't taste the same)

### Objective Findings

The physical examination of the child with Bell palsy reveals:

- Motor changes of the upper and lower facial muscles on one side
- Disappearance of the nasolabial fold
- Unilateral smooth forehead
- Full, equal strength in bilateral upper and lower extremities (Falchek, 2019; Patterson, 2019)

Other findings may include:

- Absence of complete blinking on the affected side
- Decreased or absent corneal reflex on the affected side but not the unaffected side
- Drawing of the mouth to the unaffected side

**PRO TIP** An examination of the ear canal is important to evaluate for a herpetic lesion in addition to otitis media (Flemming & Jones, 2015).

### Laboratory/Diagnostic Testing

The diagnosis of Bell palsy is based upon the clinical findings. No laboratory or diagnostic testing is needed unless the child's symptoms do not resolve over a 6-week period or other neurologic symptoms develop (Flemming & Jones, 2015). If there is possibility of exposure to Lyme disease, serologic testing may be recommended (Patterson, 2019).

### Differential Diagnosis

The differential diagnosis for Bell palsy includes:

- Trauma
- Infection (otitis media, Lyme disease, Epstein-Barr virus, herpes simplex virus)
- Inflammatory conditions
- Tumor
- Metabolic conditions
- Congenital/genetic disorders (such as Moebius syndrome; Falchek, 2019)

### Treatment/Management Plan

The underlying cause as well as severity of the facial nerve palsy will dictate the treatment plan. The goals of treatment are to restore facial muscle function and avoid corneal damage. If the child is unable to fully close the eye, prescribe ocular lubricant to be used multiple times a day in order to prevent corneal abrasion. Protect the eye by using a patch or tape. Prescribe prednisone 1 to 2 mg/kg/day up to 60 to 80 mg in a 24-hour period for 5 days. This should be initiated within the first 48 hours of symptoms for the best results. The addition of antiviral therapy to corticosteroid therapy has not been shown to improve outcomes. However, in children who have severe symptoms and/or if there is a possibility of herpes, valacyclovir 20 mg/kg/dose three times a day with a maximum of 1,000 mg per dose for 1 week should also be prescribed (Falchek, 2019; Patterson, 2019).

### Family Education

Teach the following:

- Children and adolescents who experience an isolated palsy of CN VII have a 60% to 70% chance of full recovery.
- Typically, 3 weeks after the initial onset, children begin showing signs of recovering function, most often improving control of mimetic facial movements.

### Referral

A referral to a pediatric neurologist is indicated if the child does not have resolution of symptoms within 3 to 6 weeks, if there is a relapsing pattern, or if new neurologic symptoms develop.

▶ ALERT: If a child has bilateral facial palsy, Guillain-Barré or other infectious, inflammatory, or metabolic disease should be considered. These conditions warrant more immediate treatment (Falchek, 2019).

## CEREBRAL PALSY

CP is a permanent, static, nonprogressive condition resulting from an injury to the brain during fetal or infant development. Common causes are stroke, hypoxic ischemic event, malformations of the brain, early traumatic brain injury, infection, and prematurity. Associated symptoms can include impaired cognition and communication, epilepsy, musculoskeletal problems, and visual or hearing impairment. These children can range from mildly affected to severely affected based on the extent and location of the injury. Although CP is not a progressive condition, the clinical presentation may change with time as the child grows (Barkoudah & Glader, 2019a).

CP is classified based on the types of movement and distribution. The types of movement include spastic, athetoid, ataxic, and mixed. *Spastic* is defined as being unable to completely relax a muscle, causing increased tone. *Athetoid* is defined as slow movements that are involuntary or uncontrolled. *Ataxic* is defined as lack of coordination of movements and balance. Mixed indicates a combination of two types, with the most common types being spastic and athetoid. The distribution may be hemiplegic, diplegic, triplegic, and quadriplegic. Hemiplegic is defined as affecting one side of the body, while diplegic affects both lower extremities. Triplegic typically affects both lower extremities and one upper extremity, whereas quadriplegic affects both upper and both lower extremities (Glader & Barkoudah, 2019a).

## Subjective Findings

Gather a detailed birth history. The health history may reveal:

- Delayed milestones
- Abnormal gait
- Poor balance
- Abnormal posture
- Muscles that are too tight or too loose

## Risk Factors

The most common risk factors for CP are:

- Difficult delivery
- Prematurity
- Postmaturity
- Postnatal central nervous system injury
- APGAR score less than 3 at 10 minutes
- Microcephaly
- Exposure to maternal infection
- Maternal hypothyroidism, intracranial hemorrhage, toxemia, preeclampsia, antepartal hemorrhage, and maternal stroke
- Fetal distress
- Coagulation in the fetus or newborn
- Neonatal seizures (Barkoudah & Glader, 2019b)

## Review of Systems

The most common manifestations revealed during the review of systems include:

- **Constitutional:** poor growth
- **Cognitive:** intellectual disability, language and learning disability
- **HEENT:** hearing loss, impaired visual acuity, difficulty speaking
- **Gastrointestinal:** constipation
- **Genitourinary:** neurogenic bladder
- **Musculoskeletal:** spasticity, difficulty with movement, neglecting an extremity
- **Neurologic:** seizures

## Objective Findings

The physical examination of the child with CP may reveal:

- Developmental delay with varying degrees of impairment
- Preferred handedness; unilateral weakness
- Impaired vision
- Impaired hearing
- Absent or delayed speech development
- Uncoordinated suck and swallow
- Brisk deep tendon reflexes
- Persistent primitive reflexes
- Joint contractures, most often hamstrings and abductors
- Scoliosis
- Hip subluxation
- Usually increased tone
- Occasionally decreased tone
- Asymmetric movements

## Laboratory/Diagnostic Testing

The diagnosis of CP is one of exclusion. Imaging can be used to guide the diagnosis. A referral to a pediatric neurologist for appropriate magnetic resonance imaging (MRI) of the brain is warranted if CP is suspected or has not yet been confirmed.

**PRO TIP** It is important to remember that CP is a central condition and not a peripheral condition.

## Differential Diagnosis

The differential diagnosis for CP includes:

- Motor syndromes
- Connective tissue disorders

- Inborn errors of metabolism
- Fetal alcohol syndrome
- Tumor
- Brain malformation
- Neurodegenerative disorders
- Developmental or traumatic lesions of the brain or spinal cord (Glader & Barkoudah, 2019b)

### Treatment/Management Plan

Family-centered care is imperative for promotion of good outcomes for children with CP. Including the child in the plan of care is a very important part of the treatment. Family-centered care can best be found through a multidisciplinary clinic where multiple needs are addressed at one time, avoiding various appointments at different locations, which often results in fractured care.

Health maintenance visits should occur more frequently in order to address the multiple chronic conditions associated with CP. Some children will have increased caloric needs related to degree of spasticity, whereas others require fewer calories based on activity levels. Appropriate intake for adequate growth and development should be monitored and managed by a registered dietitian in conjunction with the primary care provider. Gastroesophageal reflux disease (GERD) frequently occurs in children with CP; monitor for symptoms of GERD. Some children are less able to manage their oral secretions and may experience frequent respiratory infections.

It is important to manage and assess every aspect of activity. These activities include dressing, bathing, sitting, standing, positioning, transporting, and mobilizing. Families require assistance with innovative ways to incorporate these activities into their everyday lives. Occupational and physical therapists should be actively involved in these activities, with the ultimate goal being to maximize independence and decrease limitations. The sooner early intervention programs are incorporated into the child's care, the better the outcome. Assistive devices can help children navigate their world more efficiently. Although by definition, CP is static encephalopathy, other deformities can develop as the child grows, especially if the child maintains poor positioning for long periods of time. Range-of-motion exercises are also necessary to assist with contracture prevention. Prevention of osteopenia may be achieved with vitamin D and calcium supplementation, daily exercise, and the use of equipment such as a vertical, supine, or prone stander. The American Academy for Cerebral Palsy and Developmental Medicine has published a care pathway for osteoporosis, available at www.aacpdm.org/publications/care-pathways/osteoporosis. Physical therapy, occupational therapy, and speech therapy can be provided in the home, school, or outpatient setting as the child grows in order to improve mobility and communication throughout their lifespan (Barkoudah & Glader, 2019b).

### Family Education

Teach the following:

- Help families to understand that just because their child has motor impairments that are sometimes severe, the child often does not have cognitive impairment.
- Families should treat every child the same, involving them in conversations and including them as part of the family unit.
- Initiating physical, speech, occupational, and developmental therapies at a young age is vital to growth and development of children with CP.
- It is important to be optimistic about the child's communication ability. Even though the child may not appear to communicate effectively, assistive devices are available to help the child communicate in ways that they otherwise may not be able to communicate.

### Referral

Treatment for spasticity (botulinum toxin, baclofen, or diazepam) is selected by a CP specialist. Seizures are monitored and treated by a pediatric neurologist. Musculoskeletal conditions such as contractures, scoliosis, and hip subluxation should be managed by a pediatric orthopedic surgeon.

Depending upon the child's individual assessment, additional referrals to subspecialists may also include a developmental pediatric specialist, pediatric ophthalmologist, pulmonologist, endocrinologist, cardiologist, urologist, gastroenterologist, geneticist, otolaryngologist, audiologist, and dentist.

## MYELOMENINGOCELE

Spina bifida is the most common neural tube defect, resulting in abnormal formation of the spine or spinal cord during early embryonic development (Bowman, 2020). Spina bifida includes three different types: spina bifida occulta, myelomeningocele, and meningocele. This section focuses solely on myelomeningocele because spina bifida occulta is mild and usually asymptomatic (commonly seen as an asymptomatic finding), and meningocele is extremely rare. The prevalence of spina bifida is around 1:1,000 pregnancies around the world; due to the recommendation of prenatal folic acid supplementation, the rate is 0.64 per 1,000 (Levey & Korth, 2019).

**PRO TIP** It is recommended that all women of childbearing age take at least 400 mcg of folic acid daily in order to prevent neural tube defects if pregnancy were to occur.

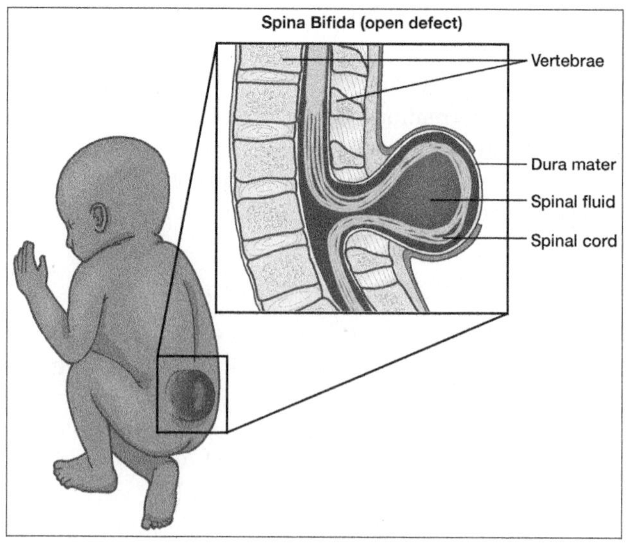


FIGURE 35.2 Myelomeningocele.

## Subjective Findings

The health history may reveal:

- Increased head size
- Decreased sensation in the lower extremities
- Decreased movement of the lower extremities

## Risk Factors

The most common risk factor for spina bifida is maternal folic acid deficiency and nutritional deficiencies. Other risk factors include maternal diabetes, obesity, use of valproic acid or carbamazepine, alcohol consumption during pregnancy, and maternal hypothermia during early pregnancy (Levey & Korth, 2019).

## Review of Systems

The most common manifestations revealed during the review of systems include:

- **Cognitive:** learning disabilities
- **Integumentary:** patch of hair on the back
- **Gastrointestinal:** chronic constipation, inability to control bowel movements
- **Genitourinary:** urinary incontinence, inability to void, frequent urinary tract infections
- **Musculoskeletal:** lower extremity weakness, decreased sensation in lower extremities

## Objective Findings

The physical examination of the child with myelomeningocele may reveal (Figure 35.2):

- A protruding sac of meninges and spinal cord at the level of the defect at birth
- A tuft of hair at the level of the defect
- A sacral dimple at the level of the defect
- Absence of anal wink, indicating impaired sphincter control
- Dysplastic overlying muscle and skin at the site of the defect
- Macrocephaly due to hydrocephalus
- Skin breakdown
- Clubfoot
- Scoliosis
- Hip dysplasia
- Joint contractures
- Other congenital abnormalities

*Thoracic-level lesion may reveal:*

- Flaccid paralysis of the lower extremities
- Loss of sensation to dermatome distribution below the defect
- Variable core weakness
- Respiratory compromise (likely in high thoracic lesions)
- Palpable fecal mass
- Distended bladder secondary to urinary retention

*High lumbar-level lesion may reveal:*

- Voluntary hip flexion and adduction
- Flaccid paralysis of the knees, ankles, and feet
- Loss of sensation to dermatome distribution below the defect
- May ambulate using braces and crutches
- Palpable fecal mass
- Distended bladder

*Midlumbar-level lesion may reveal:*

- Strong hip flexion and adduction
- Fair knee extension
- Flaccid paralysis of ankles and feet
- Loss of sensation to dermatome distribution below the defect
- Palpable fecal mass
- Distended bladder

*Low lumbar-level lesion may reveal:*

- Strong hip flexion, extension, and adduction as well as knee extension
- Weak ankle and toe range of motion
- Loss of sensation to dermatome distribution below the defect
- Palpable fecal mass
- Distended bladder

*Sacral-level lesion may reveal:*

- Lower extremities function normally
- Sensation may be impaired in distal lower extremities
- Palpable fecal mass
- Distended bladder (Bowman, 2020)

### Laboratory/Diagnostic Testing

Myelomeningocele can be diagnosed based on prenatal ultrasound. Elevated maternal serum alpha-fetoprotein at 16 to 18 weeks' gestation should prompt referral for further evaluation. A chromosomal microarray (CMA) can help determine if there is a genetic cause. Postnatal diagnosis is confirmed based on clinical findings. Imaging is indicated in children who are found to have hydrocephalus (Levey & Korth, 2019).

### Differential Diagnosis

The differential diagnosis for myelomeningocele includes:

- Other neural tube defects

### Treatment/Management Plan

Myelomeningocele is often diagnosed prenatally based on ultrasound. Once diagnosed, it is important for the mother to seek care at a high-risk maternal fetal center, as the birth will require planning with specialists. The delivery via cesarean section results in an immediate transfer to a neonatal intensive care unit for appropriate care prior to surgical intervention by a pediatric neurosurgeon. It is important to use latex-free gloves during the delivery process and subsequent care, as these children are at risk for developing a fatal latex allergy (Bowman, 2020).

Myelomeningocele requires early surgical closure of the defect in order to prevent infection as well as damage to the exposed neural sac. Further diagnostic testing can identify the specific tissue malformation and level of involvement. This can include ultrasound, computed tomography (CT) scan, and/or MRI. Determining the level of involvement by careful assessment of the newborn before and during the closure is important for long-term planning. Monitor head circumference in the evaluation of hydrocephalus.

Multidisciplinary clinics are vital for the management of these children with complex multisystem involvement. The healthcare team may include neurosurgeons, urologists, orthopedists, neurologists, pediatric primary care providers, physical therapists, and occupational therapists. Pediatric primary care providers are vital in coordinating the care of all of the specialists, particularly if a multidisciplinary clinic is not available. Pediatric primary care providers are also needed for well child visits and anticipatory guidance, along with providing management for acute care needs. Children with myelomeningocele may routinely need more frequent evaluation by their pediatric primary care provider secondary to potential challenges with coexisting conditions. Urinary tract infection or constipation may commonly occur, as urinary and bowel elimination is often impaired depending upon the level of the lesion. It is imperative to check the child thoroughly for skin breakdown. As a child ages, potential psychosocial needs increase. Primary care providers assist with acquisition of community resources in order to allow the child the opportunity to function at their highest level.

### Family Education

Teach the following:

- Proper urinary catheterization technique as well as a bowel program in order to prevent skin breakdown and constipation.
- Support groups are available for children with myelomeningocele and their families to help with the chronic grief for the loss of normalcy.
- The signs and symptoms of Chiari II malformation (posterior brain bulging through foramen ovale) as well as shunt malfunctions, as these can both lead to emergent complications.

▶ ALERT: Increased injuries may occur due to decreased sensation. Parents should be educated on temperature control and frequent position changes.

## Referral

A pediatric neurosurgeon is involved from the beginning for repair of the defect, and often continued follow-up for hydrocephalus and shunt management is required. Consult a pediatric urologist to assist with the management of bowel and bladder function, as well as prevention and management of urinary tract infections. Refer to a pediatric orthopedist for management of scoliosis, hip dysplasia, clubfoot, and joint contractures. If seizures occur, consult a pediatric neurologist for evaluation and management. Physical therapists and occupational therapists work with the child to assist with gaining and maintaining function, mobility, and independence throughout all stages of life. When available, children should frequently be evaluated by a multidisciplinary team to achieve best outcomes. Additionally, support with transition to adult providers will be needed.

# MUSCULAR DYSTROPHY

The most common type of MD is Duchenne dystrophy with an X-linked inheritance pattern. The incidence of Duchenne MD (DMD) is 1:3,500 male live births (Nance, 2019). It results in progressive weakness due to degeneration of muscle fibers. Boys typically demonstrate symptoms by the age of 5 years.

Children with DMD initially appear to be developing normally. There may be delayed gross motor milestones, including delayed walking up to age 18 months. As the child grows, they become clumsier than their peers and further progress to having trouble keeping up with their peers during activities. The child has difficulty getting up from the floor, may be unable to jump, and may experience more frequent falls. Muscle involvement typically begins with proximal muscles prior to moving distally. Calf hypertrophy is a common sign of DMD. Prognosis is poor, as most individuals die due to respiratory and/or cardiac causes by age 30 (Nance, 2019).

PRO TIP Refer mothers of males with DMD for genetic counseling about their carrier status and for future pregnancies.

## Subjective Findings

The health history may reveal:

- Slow acquisition of milestones
- Poor head control
- Growth delays
- Increased clumsiness
- Unable to run by age 3
- Struggles to go up stairs
- Difficulty going from floor sitting to standing
- Abnormal gait
- Walks on toes
- Muscle pain or cramps (Darras, 2020)

## Risk Factors

The most common risk factor for DMD is family history of muscular dystrophies.

## Review of Systems

The most common manifestations revealed during the review of systems include:

- **HEENT:** dysphagia
- **Respiratory:** increased respiratory infections, sleep apnea
- **Cardiovascular:** cardiomyopathy
- **Gastrointestinal:** constipation, reflux, gastroparesis
- **Musculoskeletal:** muscle weakness/fatigue, muscle cramps, gait abnormalities, contractures, pseudohypertrophy of the gastrocnemius, lordosis, scoliosis
- **Developmental:** loss of motor skills, developmental delay (Muscular Dystrophy Association, 2021)

## Objective Findings

The physical examination of the child with DMD may reveal:

- Toe walking
- Enlarged calves
- Fibrotic-feeling muscles
- Positive Gower's sign (using hands to walk up the legs when standing from floor)
- Waddling gait
- Lordosis
- Respiratory weakness
- Hypotonia
- Hyporeflexia or areflexia
- Proximal weakness (Darras, 2020)

▶ ALERT: Be concerned that a child may have DMD if they have a positive Gower's sign, calf hypertrophy, and inability to keep up with peers. Appropriate referrals for diagnosis should be made as soon as the diagnosis is suspected.

## Laboratory/Diagnostic Testing

The diagnosis of DMD is based upon the clinical findings, genetic testing, muscle biopsy, and electromyography (EMG). Given the availability of genetic testing, EMG testing is less commonly used now. Genetic testing confirms the mutation in the dystrophin gene. DMD exonic duplication or deletion is noted in 70% of cases, and new mutations of the dystrophin gene are continuing to develop (Nance, 2019). A creatine kinase greater than 10 times the normal level can be an early identifier of the disease. Liver function tests may also show elevated results. Muscle biopsy will reveal an absence of dystrophin. EMG may show increased insertional activity and small myopathic motor unit.

### Differential Diagnosis

The differential diagnosis for DMD includes:

- Liver disease
- SMA
- Other muscular dystrophies (Darras, 2020)

### Treatment/Management Plan

Supportive care is instrumental in the treatment of DMD. There is currently no cure for the disease. A multidisciplinary team is ideal in managing the complex care of these children. Braces may be necessary to help prevent extremity contractures. Surgical tendon releases may be indicated to improve range of motion of extremities. Posterior spinal fusion may be indicated for scoliotic curves to prevent further pulmonary decline.

Children are likely to become wheelchair-dependent by early adolescence. Annual influenza vaccinations are recommended for the child as well as everyone in the household due to the child's increased risk for respiratory compromise. Weight management is important for prolonging the onset of comorbidities associated with this condition. Treatment with corticosteroids and deflazacorts remains controversial. If these medications are being used, the immunization schedule may require adjusting. A specialist in DMD will prescribe medications as indicated.

## Family Education

Teach the following:

- Safety measures related to increased risk of falls, potential need for increased trunk support, adjustments to car seats for additional support as needed.
- Increased visits to a primary care provider are indicated to manage the multiple comorbidities associated with DMD.
- Family counseling is indicated for future pregnancies.
- Support groups can help caregivers and children deal with the diagnosis.

## Referral

Refer to a pediatric neurologist for monitoring of the neurodegenerative disease process. A dietitian consult will be helpful if weight management is needed. If or when lung function becomes affected, refer to a pediatric pulmonologist, as the child may eventually require positive pressure ventilation. Consult a pediatric cardiologist for monitoring of cardiomyopathy. Pediatric orthopedic surgeons should be consulted as needed for bracing or surgical intervention. Physical therapy, occupational therapy, and speech therapy are indicated for promotion of increased quality of life and independence.

# SPINAL MUSCULAR ATROPHY

SMA is a progressive, autosomal recessive disorder of the neuromuscular system caused by degeneration of the anterior horn cells of the spinal cord and motor nuclei in the lower brain stem. There are four different types of SMA, defined based on the age of onset and progression rate. The incidence of SMA is 4 to 10 per 100,000 live births (Bodamer, 2020).

SMA type 1, also known as Werdnig-Hoffman disease, is the most fatal and severe form. It may present with mild weakness at birth; however, by 6 months of age the child will have hypotonia, weakness, and areflexia. Children with type 1 are never able to sit. Progression of SMA type 1 eventually leads to respiratory failure by 2 years of age. SMA type 2 is typically diagnosed between 6 and 18 months and characterized by symmetric, proximal weakness affecting lower extremities more than upper extremities. These children are never able to stand or walk independently. SMA type 3, also known as Kugelberg-Welander disease, typically has proximal weakness also affecting the lower extremities more than upper extremities. However, these children typically gain the ability to walk later but may lose that ability as the disease progresses. SMA type 4 accounts for only 5% of cases, is late in onset (possibly into adulthood), and the child achieves all milestones and has a normal life span (Bodamer, 2020).

## Subjective Findings

The health history may reveal:

*SMA type 1:*

- Alert and happy appearance
- Floppy limbs and core
- Decreased activity
- Delayed motor milestone
- Increased secretions
- Weak cry
- Abnormal tongue movements
- Feeding problems
- Failure to thrive
- History of decreased fetal movements

*SMA type 2:*

- Unable to stand
- Unable to walk
- Delayed gross motor skills
- Dysphasia
- Abnormal tongue size
- Abnormal tongue movements
- Weakness, particularly in the lower extremities

*SMA type 3:*

- Weakness
- Increased falls
- Difficulty climbing stairs (Bodamer, 2020)

## Risk Factors

SMA is transmitted in an autosomal recessive pattern. Genetics is the only risk factor.

## Review of Systems

The most common manifestations revealed during the review of systems include:

- **Constitutional:** difficulty feeding
- **Respiratory:** breathing difficulties
- **Musculoskeletal:** decreased activity, weakness in core muscles and extremities

## Objective Findings

The physical examination of the child with SMA may reveal:

*SMA Type 1:*

- Tongue fasciculation
- Axial and appendicular hypotonia
- Absent reflexes
- Paradoxical breathing
- Frog-leg posture at rest

*SMA Types 2 and 3:*

- Weakness
- Tongue atrophy
- Tongue fasciculation
- Absent reflexes
- Scoliosis
- Joint contractures

**PRO TIP** Tongue fasciculations in a young child are highly suggestive of SMA.

## Laboratory/Diagnostic Testing

The diagnosis of SMA is based upon the clinical findings and genetic testing. Most children have deletions or abnormalities in SMN (survival motor neuron; Bodamer, 2020).

## Differential Diagnosis

The differential diagnosis for SMA includes:

- Other genetic neuromuscular disorders
- Hypoxic-ischemic myelopathy
- Guillain-Barré syndrome
- Arthrogryposis
- Muscular dystrophy
- Myasthenia gravis

## Treatment/Management Plan

A multidisciplinary team is vital in the management of children who have SMA. This team should include a physical therapist, occupational therapist, speech therapist, dietitian, orthopedist, neurologist, and pulmonologist. The primary care provider may facilitate interventions or orders as prescribed by the pediatric subspecialist.

**PRO TIP** The specialist may prescribe a disease-modifying therapy such as nusinersen (intrathecal, 4 loading doses, then once every 4 months), onasemnogene abeparvovec (intravenous infusion given once only), or risdiplam (only daily oral therapy). If prescribed for a child the primary care provider is caring for, it will be important to understand the adverse effects and precautions needed in relation to these medications.

### Family Education

Teach the following:

- Genetic counseling is necessary for future pregnancies.
- Survival in SMA Types 1, 2, and 3 has been improving with the advancement of the medical field.
- Routine vaccination is important, especially for respiratory illnesses such as influenza and respiratory syncytial virus.
- It is important to discuss end-of-life goals with children and families early, as respiratory failure can ensue quickly and be fatal.
- Intelligence is preserved in these children, so it is important to include them in decision-making as well as everyday life.

ALERT: Minor respiratory infections in these children may quickly lead to respiratory failure.

### Referral

Refer to pediatric physical, occupational, and speech therapists for assistance with mobility, activities of daily living, and feeding. The goal of physical therapy is to increase range of motion and prevent contractures. The use of a wheelchair for mobility will be required at some point in most children with any of type of SMA. A custom seating system is helpful to further prevent progression of scoliosis. Consult a registered dietitian for appropriate management of the child's nutrition to avoid a catabolic state. Pediatric orthopedic consultation is needed for management of any contractures and scoliosis that develop. These can be managed with nonoperative or operative interventions. Pediatric neurology may be needed to manage the progressive nature of the disease. Refer to pediatric pulmonology for management of the child's respiratory status, including chest physiotherapy, cough assist, and secretion management (Bodamer, 2020).

## KEY POINTS

- It is important to rule out other infectious, inflammatory, or metabolic conditions prior to making the diagnosis of Bell palsy.
- Testing the CNs by having the child wrinkle their forehead or raise their eyebrows, tightly close their eyes, show their teeth and/or smile and puff out their cheeks test the most commonly affected muscles in Bell palsy.
- The goal of treatment of CP is to maximize the child's independence as well as their functional abilities while reducing the extent of disability.
- Care of the child with myelomeningocele requires a multidisciplinary approach.
- The pediatric primary care provider is instrumental in ensuring that the child with myelomeningocele receives adequate care and referrals.
- Children with DMD appear to be developing normally until around age 3, when they are unable to keep up with their peers, and continue to progressively worsen.

## REFERENCES


Barkoudah, E., & Glader, L. (2019a). Cerebral palsy: Epidemiology, etiology, and prevention. *UpToDate*. Retrieved October 28, 2020, from https://www.uptodate.com/contents/cerebral-palsy-epidemiology-etiology-and-prevention

Barkoudah, E., & Glader, L. (2019b). Cerebral palsy: Overview of management and prognosis. *UpToDate*. Retrieved October 28, 2020, from https://www.uptodate.com/contents/cerebral-palsy-overview-of-management-and-prognosis

Bodamer, O. A. (2020). Spinal muscular atrophy. *UpToDate*. Retrieved October 28, 2020, from https://www.uptodate.com/contents/spinal-muscular-atrophy

Bowman, R. M. (2020). Overview of the management of myelomeningocele (spina bifida). *UpToDate*. Retrieved October 28, 2020, from https://www.uptodate.com/contents/overview-of-the-management-of-myelomeningocele-spina-bifida

Darras, B. T. (2020). Duchenne and Becker muscular dystrophy: Clinical features and diagnosis. *UpToDate*. Retrieved October 28, 2020, from https://www.uptodate.com/contents/duchenne-and-becker-muscular-dystrophy-clinical-features-and-diagnosis

Falchek, S. J. (2019). Bell palsy. In M. D. Cabana (Ed., pp. 106–107), *The 5-minute pediatric consult* (8th ed.). Wolters Kluwer.

Flemming, K. D., & Jones, L. K. (Eds.). (2015). *Mayo Clinic neurology board review: Clinical neurology for initial certification and MOC*. Oxford University Press.

Glader, L., & Barkoudah, E. (2019a). Cerebral palsy: Clinical features and classifications. *UpToDate*. Retrieved October 28, 2020, 2020, from https://www.uptodate.com/contents/cerebral-palsy-clinical-features-and-classification

Glader, L., & Barkoudah, E. (2019b). Cerebral palsy: Evaluation and diagnosis. *UpToDate*. Retrieved October 28, 2020, from https://www.uptodate.com/contents/cerebral-palsy-evaluation-and-diagnosis

Levey, E. B., & Korth, S. A. (2019). Neural tube defects. In M. D. Cabana (Ed.), *The 5-minute pediatric consult* (8th ed., pp. 624–625). Wolters Kluwer.

Muscular Dystrophy Association. (2021). *Duchenne muscular dystrophy*. https://www.mda.org/disease/duchenne-muscular-dystrophy

Nance, J. R. (2019). Muscular dystrophies. In M. D. Cabana (Ed.), *The 5-minute pediatric consult* (8th ed., pp. 602–603). Wolters Kluwer.

Patterson, M.C. (2019). Facial nerve palsy in children. *UpToDate*. https://www.uptodate.com/contents/facial-nerve-palsy-in-children.

Ryan, M. M. (2020). Bell palsy. In R. M. Kliegman, J. St. Geme, N. J. Blum, S. S. Shah, R. C. Tasker, K. M. Wilson, & R. E. Behrman (Eds.), *Nelson textbook of pediatrics* (21st ed., Chapter 635). Elsevier.

Zaidman, C. (2020). Facial nerve palsy in children. *UpToDate*. Retrieved October 28, 2020, from https://www.uptodate.com/contents/facial-nerve-palsy-in-children

# Management of Neurologic Disorders

Lai Brooks, Beth Heuer, and Mariah Morris

## Student Learning Outcomes

**Upon completion of this chapter the reader should be able to:**

1. Discuss pathophysiology and epidemiology of selected neurologic disorders in children.
2. Differentiate subjective and objective findings of selected neurologic disorders in children.
3. Choose appropriate laboratory or diagnostic tests for particular neurologic disorders in children.
4. Utilize the differential diagnosis process to determine neurologic diagnoses in children.
5. Determine treatment plan, child/family education, and need for referral in children with a neurologic diagnosis.

## INTRODUCTION

Neurologic disorders in the pediatric population can include congenital, infectious, and genetic etiologies. Understanding the source of the specific neurologic condition will allow the practitioner to assess and manage the child efficiently. This chapter discusses common pediatric neurologic disorders by focusing on important subjective and objective findings, along with appropriate diagnosis, management, education, and referral for each specific disorder identified.

The content in this chapter maps to the following areas on the Pediatric Nursing Certification Board (PNCB) Pediatric Nurse Practitioner—Primary Care certification examination:

**CLINICAL PROBLEMS: NEUROLOGY**

CONTENT AREAS:

**II. Assessment and Diagnosis**

**B. History and Physical Examination**

1. Obtain history of present illness
2. Obtain a comprehensive health history for new patients
3. Complete an interval history for established patients
4. Perform a review of systems
5. Perform a complete physical examination

**C. Diagnostic Testing and Screening**

1. Order and interpret office/clinic based screening tests
2. Order and interpret diagnostic laboratory tests
3. Order and interpret the results of diagnostic imaging tests

**D. Analyzing Information**

1. Integrate health history and physical examination findings into the plan of care
2. Assimilate findings from screening and diagnostic testing into plan of care

**E. Diagnosis**

1. Develop and prioritize differential diagnoses
2. Establish a diagnosis based on evaluation of patient data

## III. Management

### A. Child and Caregiver Counseling and Education

1. Provide condition-specific counseling and education, including treatment options
2. Educate about benefits and potential adverse reactions of pharmacological interventions
3. Discuss non-pharmacological interventions
4. Counsel regarding the threshold for seeking follow-up care
5. Review the risks of non-adherence to recommended treatment

### B. Therapeutic Interventions

1. Prescribe pharmacologic agents
2. Recommend the use of over-the-counter pharmacologic agents
3. Order or recommend non-pharmacologic treatments for the management of symptoms
4. Discuss use of complementary and alternative therapies as appropriate

### C. Procedures

1. Perform procedures in accordance with diagnostic guidelines and plan of care (rapid tests)
2. Initiate life-saving techniques in response to urgent or emergent situations

### D. Collaboration and Referral

2. Refer to specialists as indicated for evaluation, counseling, and/or treatment

### E. Care Coordination

1. Facilitate patient and family-centered care for children of all ages with acute and chronic conditions

### F. Evaluation and Follow-up

2. Establish a plan for follow-up care

## IV. Professional Role Responsibilities

### A. Leadership and Evidence-based Practice

4. Develop, implement, and/or modify clinical practice guidelines

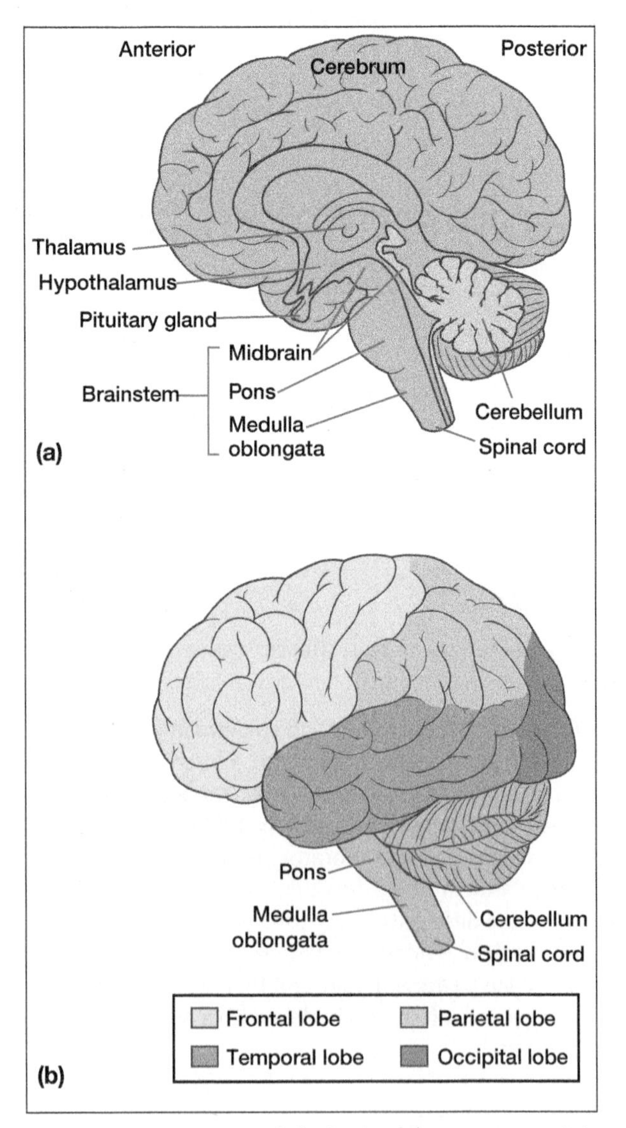


FIGURE 36.1 Anatomy of the brain. (a) Structures of the brain. (b) Lobes of the brain.

*Source*: Chiocca, E. M. (2019). *Advanced pediatric assessment* (3rd ed.). Wolters Kluwer.

# ANATOMY AND PHYSIOLOGY

Compared with adults, there are anatomic differences in the brain and spinal cord of children (Figure 36.1). The heads of infants and children <8 years of age are larger and disproportionate in size to the rest of their body. The larger head and weaker neck muscles make them more susceptible to head injury. The pediatric brain continues to grow and develop rapidly as the child grows. For example, children begin life with fontanels and sutures that eventually close, the cranium becomes thicker, the brain and spinal cord undergo myelination, and cervical ligaments and muscles become stronger (Figaji, 2017). Rapid neurodevelopmental processes also occur, and the pediatric brain will be close to adult size by age 5. The pediatric spinal cord is also immature and does not begin to resemble an adult spine until 8 to 9 years of age (Figaji, 2017).

In addition, the pediatric brain is not as developed as the adult brain and is more pliable. Having plasticity can be an asset, as children who suffer from stroke have better outcomes than adults with history of stroke. However, the brain of infants is less myelinated, the cranium is thinner, and the presence of open sutures and larger subarachnoid spaces makes infants more susceptible to hematoma in the event of trauma (Lee & Fleisher, 2019).

# GENERAL APPROACH TO THE CHILD WITH A NEUROLOGIC DISORDER

When a child presents with a potential neurologic disorder, it is important to obtain a comprehensive history and complete a thorough physical examination. Based on these clinical findings, with the differential diagnosis in mind, laboratory and diagnostic testing may then be ordered. The general approach to assessment of the child with a potential neurologic disorder is as follows.

## Subjective Findings

For the child with a suspected neurologic disorder, obtain a complete health history including:

- History of present illness—for all symptoms, note the onset, location, duration, character, aggravating or relieving factors, timing, and severity (OLDCARTS).
- Medications, including dose, route, and frequency (current and past as applicable).
- Allergies—medications, food, environmental. If there is an allergy, also document the child's reaction.
- Pregnancy and birth history—include prenatal history such as mother's age, previous pregnancies and miscarriages, maternal exposure to illness or infections that could affect brain development (Zika, toxoplasmosis, rubella, cytomegalovirus, herpes [TORCH] infections), and any abnormal prenatal testing (laboratory and ultrasound). Birth history should include age of gestation at time of delivery, route of delivery, and any complications during the birth process. Also discuss Apgar scores and whether there was any neonatal intensive care unit (NICU) stay. Review results of newborn screening along with the newborn hearing test.
- Past medical history—any previous surgeries or hospitalizations, any chronic conditions.
- Family history—any pertinent family history of neurologic or developmental issues.
- Social history—discuss where and with whom child lives, any day-care attendance.
- Developmental history—review when child met developmental milestones.
- Academic history—discuss if child is at appropriate grade level for age and if there are any cognitive difficulties at school.

## Risk Factors

The most common risk factors for neurologic disorders include:

- Prematurity
- Diagnosed genetic condition
- Family history of neurologic disorder
- Trauma/injury

## Review of Systems

The most common manifestations revealed during the review of systems include:

- **Constitutional:** sleep difficulties
- **HEENT:** dysphagia, strabismus, headache, head pain
- **Respiratory:** respiratory difficulties
- **Gastrointestinal:** gastroesophageal reflux
- **Neurologic:** delayed milestones, cognitive difficulties, dizziness, balance disturbances
- **Musculoskeletal:** low muscle tone, abnormal or involuntary movements (Kotagal, 2019)

## Objective Findings

The physical examination of the child with a neurologic disorder may reveal:

- Observe the child and how they interact with the parent/caregiver prior to examining the child. Watching how the child plays and interacts helps the practitioner to assess fine and gross motor skills along with attention span and developmental level (Kotagal, 2019).
- Depending on the age of the child, the examination may differ. For a newborn, you would elicit newborn reflexes. A toddler may feel most comfortable sitting on the parent's lap during the examination. The teenage child may want to discuss things privately with the practitioner without the parent in the room, so it is important to assess the age and developmental level of the child during your examination.
- Assess fontanels, sutures, and head circumference in the infant.
- Test each cranial nerve (I–XII) as appropriate and applicable, observing any abnormalities (Figure 36.2).
- Assess motor function and strength in upper and lower extremities. Observe for any weakness, stiffness, or involuntary movements. Grade the level of strength out of five.
- Assess coordination by performing rapid alternating hand movements, finger-to-nose-finger testing. Observe gait and ask the child to perform tandem walk as appropriate.

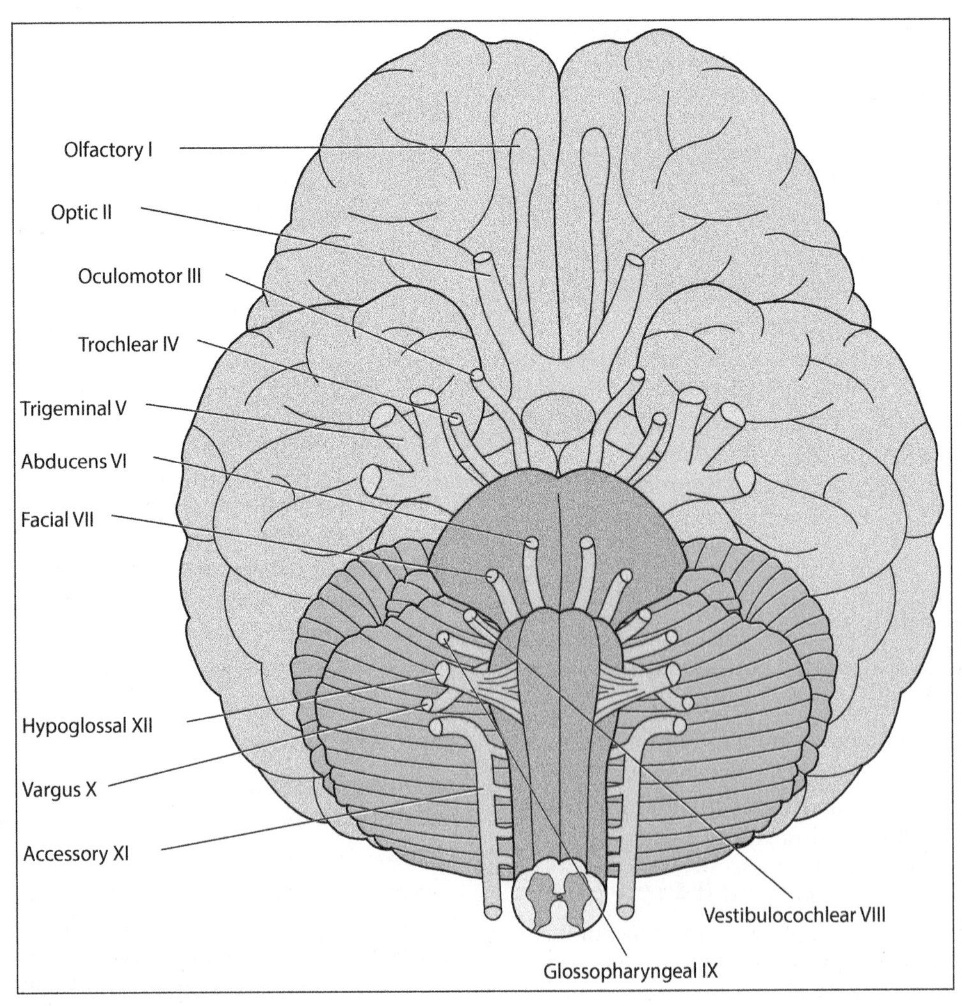


FIGURE 36.2 The cranial nerves.

*Source*: From Myrick, K. M., & Karosas, L. M. (2020). *Advanced health assessment and differential diagnosis*. Wolters Kluwer.

- Assess sensory function using dull and pin-prick sensations.
- Elicit deep tendon reflexes in the older child.
- Assess for any abnormalities noted in the spine and/or head.

# INFECTIOUS DISORDERS

Two common pediatric infectious neurologic disorders are meningitis and encephalitis.

## MENINGITIS

*Meningitis* is inflammation of the meninges or tissue that surrounds the brain and spinal cord and can be either bacterial or viral in origin. Meningitis will vary in severity, origin, and outcome based on the cause, the child's age and health status, and immunization history.

Bacterial meningitis can be caused by several strains of bacteria and is most likely to occur during the first month of life (Edwards & Baker, 2018). In the United States, *Streptococcus pneumoniae* (streptococcus) and *Neisseria meningitidis* (meningococcus) are the two most common bacterial strains to cause bacterial meningitis (Kaplan & Di Pentima, 2019). *Escherichia coli* and *Listeria monocytogenes* can also cause bacterial meningitis (Kronman et al., 2019a). Bacterial meningitis is more dangerous than viral meningitis because it can cause long-term neurologic damage.

There are several viruses that can cause viral meningitis. Enterovirus is one of the most common causes of viral meningitis (Kaplan & Di Pentima, 2019). Viral meningitis is more common and less severe than bacterial meningitis and typically occurs in late summer or early fall. Transmission of viral meningitis is via airborne droplets and/or direct contact with a person with viral meningitis, during the birthing process, or through animal bites (Kaplan & Di Pentima, 2019).

## Subjective Findings

The health history will vary depending on the age of the child. Ask about recent infection (ear, upper respiratory, sinus), fever, lethargy, change in oral intake, change in sleeping habits, recent exposure to ill contacts, and any recent travel to an endemic area (e.g., Sub-Saharan Africa for bacterial meningitis). Also determine recent antibiotic use, as this may alter results of cultures obtained.

### Risk Factors

The most common risk factors for bacterial meningitis in the neonate are:

- Positive maternal group B streptococci (GBS) status during delivery
- Prematurity
- Low birth weight
- Premature rupture of membranes
- Traumatic delivery
- Maternal prenatal infection
- Abnormalities of the urinary tract (Edwards & Baker, 2018)

The most common risk factors for bacterial meningitis in the child older than 1 month are:

- Being underimmunized (Hib, pneumococcus)
- Recent travel to endemic area
- Recent bacterial infection
- Recent head trauma or surgery
- Cochlear implants
- Other congenital anatomic defects (i.e., urinary tract anomaly; Kaplan, 2018)

The most common risk factors for viral meningitis are:

- Recent viral infection (e.g., influenza, enterovirus, arbovirus, or mumps; Di Pentima & Kaplan, 2018).

### Review of Systems

The most common manifestations revealed during the review of systems include:

- **Constitutional:** fever or difficulty regulating temperature, decreased oral intake, difficulty nursing in the infant
- **HEENT:** headache, recent ear or upper respiratory infection; in the older child, photophobia
- **Gastrointestinal:** vomiting/diarrhea
- **Neurologic:** Increased fussiness or irritability of newborn; older child: confusion, seizure
- **Musculoskeletal:** nuchal rigidity
- **Dermatologic:** skin rash, recent insect or tick bite for possible viral origin (Kaplan, 2018)

## Objective Findings

The physical examination of the child with meningitis may reveal:

- Ill appearance
- Vital sign abnormalities: Positive fever, tachycardia, tachypnea, possible enlargement of head circumference
- Bulging fontanel
- Positive Kernig and Brudzinski signs
- Change in mental status
- Papilledema
- Seizures
- Petechiae or purpura on extremities following maculopapular rash (common with *N. meningitidis*)
- May see mouth ulcers (herpangina), hand-foot-mouth disease, conjunctivitis, lymphadenopathy with viral meningitis (Kaplan, 2018)

**PRO TIP** Suspect possible meningitis in a newborn or infant that presents with fever, seizure-like events, poor feeding, and lethargy. Do not delay diagnosis or treatment, as bacterial meningitis is a medical emergency. Send infant to the emergency department immediately if you suspect meningitis.

### Laboratory/Diagnostic Testing

The diagnosis of meningitis is based upon the clinical findings, laboratory results, and the specimen results from a lumbar puncture (LP). Cerebrospinal fluid (CSF) should be evaluated for gram stain and culture, cell count, protein, and glucose as well as viral polymerase chain reaction (PCR) if viral origin is suspected. CSF will reveal elevated white blood cell count (WBC) and protein, and decreased glucose in the presence of bacteria (Edwards & Baker, 2018). Platelet count may be low. CSF and blood for culture should be obtained to identify causative bacterial organism or to rule out bacterial causes (Edwards & Baker, 2018). With viral meningitis, a viral pathogen may be identified in the CSF or other specimens such as throat, blood, rectal, urine, or stool (Di Pentima &

Kaplan, 2018). Consider obtaining a head computerized tomography (CT) scan prior to LP in infants or children with signs of increased intracranial pressure (Di Pentima & Kaplan, 2018).

Consider ordering prothrombin time/partial thromboplastin times (PT/PTT) in children presenting with purpura or petechiae. Additionally, if herpes simplex virus (HSV) or Epstein-Barr virus (EBV) infection is suspected, consider ordering HSV PCR and/or EBV titers to rule out or confirm that source of viral meningitis.

### Differential Diagnosis

The differential diagnosis for meningitis includes:

- Bacterial versus viral meningitis
- Lyme disease
- Other viral/bacterial illness
- Encephalitis
- Brain tumor
- Brain abscess (Di Pentima & Kaplan, 2018; Kaplan, 2018)

▶ ALERT: Bacterial meningitis is a medical emergency, so diagnosis and treatment must be prompt.

### Treatment/Management Plan

Empiric antibiotic therapy known to achieve significant levels in the CSF should begin immediately after LP. Third-generation cephalosporins and vancomycin are commonly used (Kaplan, 2018). Once cultures identify the causative organism, antibiotics can be tailored and changed accordingly. Treatment for viral meningitis is supportive care: intravenous (IV) fluids, rest, and acetaminophen or ibuprofen for pain and fever. Antiviral drugs may be used if HSV or varicella are cause of meningitis.

### Family Education

Teach the following:

- If a parent suspects their child may have meningitis, they should seek help immediately and go to the emergency department.
- Families should report any fever greater than 38.0 °C (100.4 °F) in the neonate and greater than 38.3 °C (101 °F) in an infant to their child's primary care provider.
- Parents should report nuchal rigidity, altered level of consciousness, seizure, or unrelenting, severe headache.
- The child will most likely be admitted to hospital for IV antibiotics if bacterial meningitis is diagnosed.
- Avoid exposure to insect bites.
- Provide supportive care to the child at home if viral meningitis is diagnosed.
- Proper handwashing should be used to prevent transmission or spread.

### Referral

Depending on clinical manifestations such as the presence of seizures or suspected long-term deficits, a pediatric neurologist may be consulted.

## ENCEPHALITIS

Encephalitis is inflammation of the brain parenchyma with associated altered neurologic function such as change in mental status/behavior/personality, seizures, and/or speech or motor deficits (Hardarson, 2018). Viruses are the main cause of pediatric encephalitis, although encephalitis can be from a bacterial cause or from a parasite such as Toxoplasma gondii, which causes toxoplasmosis.

### Subjective Findings

The health history may be nonspecific with encephalitis and may reveal:

- Fever
- Headache
- Lethargy or irritability
- Poor feeding/nursing
- Decreased oral intake in an older child
- Seizures
- Behavioral changes in older child
- Exposure to virus via ill contact or insect bite

Ask about recent immunization status and any recent travel (Hardarson, 2018; Messacar et al., 2018).

### Risk Factors

The most common risk factors for encephalitis are:

- Exposure to specific viruses via respiratory droplets or contaminated food/drink.
- Exposure from insect bites can lead to arboviruses and enteroviruses, which are the most common viruses to cause encephalitis.
- Exposure to equine West Nile virus may also be a risk factor (Kronman et al., 2019b).
- HSV is also known to cause encephalitis.

- Other viruses such as varicella or exposure to mumps or Lyme disease are risk factors for encephalitis (Messacar et al., 2018).

### Review of Systems

The most common manifestations revealed during the review of systems include:

- **Constitutional:** fever, decreased oral intake or decreased nursing in the infant
- **HEENT:** headache
- **Neurologic:** lethargy, irritability, or fussiness in infant; mood or behavioral changes, altered mental status in older child
- **Musculoskeletal:** joint pain or stiffness (Hardarson, 2018; Kronman et al., 2019b)

### Objective Findings

The physical examination of the child with encephalitis may reveal:

- Altered mental status in older child
- Fussiness/irritability in infant
- Fever
- Bulging fontanel
- Positive Kernig or Brudzinski sign
- Diminished reflexes
- Weakness of extremities
- Abnormality of cranial nerve exam
- Presence of rash—this will vary depending on causative agent. Vesicular rash is common with HSV, whereas maculopapular rash is seen with West Nile virus. Other causes for rash include hand, foot, and mouth disease and Rocky Mountain Spotted fever (Hardarson, 2018)

### Laboratory/Diagnostic Testing

The diagnosis of encephalitis is based upon the clinical findings along with laboratory testing, neuroimaging, and an LP. Brain magnetic resonance imaging (MRI) shows areas of edema and inflammation. Children with HSV encephalitis may have hemorrhagic findings on brain MRI (Hardarson, 2018). CSF should be analyzed for cell count and differential (elevated WBC), protein (may be elevated), and glucose (usually normal). CSF should also be sent for culture to identify causative organism. Also obtain a serum complete blood count (CBC) with differential and platelets to look for elevated WBC. Blood cultures and a toxicology screen will also be performed. An electroencephalogram (EEG) should also be ordered if seizure-like activity is demonstrated by the child.

**PRO TIP** Suspect possible HSV encephalitis in a newborn or infant who presents with fever, seizure-like events, poor feeding, lethargy. Do not delay diagnosis or treatment, as HSV meningitis is a medical emergency. Send the child to the emergency department immediately if you suspect encephalitis.

### Differential Diagnosis

The differential diagnosis for encephalitis includes:

- Meningitis
- Head trauma/injury
- Brain tumor
- Drug intoxication
- Seizures
- Systemic lupus erythematosus (Hardarson, 2018; Kronman et al., 2019b)

### Treatment/Management Plan

Begin empirical treatment for suspected encephalitis with acyclovir, as HSV encephalitis is a devastating condition. Empiric antibiotics may also be warranted if a bacterium is suspected as the cause. Supportive treatment is also indicated and includes antipyretics, rest, and an increase in fluids. In the presence of seizures, or abnormal EEG, antiepileptic drugs (AEDs) may be started (Hardarson, 2018).

▶ ALERT: Encephalitis can be a dangerous situation, so diagnosis and treatment must be prompt.

### Family Education

Teach the following:

- Stay up to date on immunizations, especially measles, mumps, rubella (MMR), varicella, and meningococcal vaccines.
- Children should wear insect repellent and long-sleeved clothing when outside, especially at dusk.
- Avoid exposure to ticks.
- Wash fruits and vegetables and cook meat thoroughly.
- Report any fever greater than 37 °C (100.4 °F) in the neonate and greater than 38.3 °C (101 °F) in an infant to the primary care provider.

- Report signs of altered mental status or behavioral changes.
- Hearing will have to be evaluated following diagnosis of encephalitis and developmental follow-up is needed for at least 1 year after diagnosis (Kronman et al., 2019b; Messacar et al., 2018).

### Referral

Depending on clinical manifestations (presence of seizures or suspected long-term deficits), a neurologist may be consulted.

## NONINFECTIOUS DISORDERS

A number of noninfectious disorders of the neurologic system also affect children and adolescents. Children may experience chronic headaches or have breath-holding spells (BHSs). Tics and Tourette syndrome may occur in children. A genetic mutation causes Rett syndrome (RS) in girls.

## HEADACHES

Headaches are a common reason children may require primary care treatment. The complaint of headache increases with the child's age and is most times nonpathologic (Gladstein, 2017). Headaches are classified as either primary or secondary. Secondary headaches occur less frequently and result from a pathologic origin. Acute headaches may be associated with a febrile illness (White, 2019). In children chronic headaches are more often migraines, or tension-type, rather than cluster headaches.

Migraine headaches are recurrent headaches that are moderate to severe in intensity and are described as throbbing pain in the bitemporal or bifrontal regions that worsens with activity/exercise. Migraine headaches can also be hereditary and can last from a few hours to 1 or 2 days. Tension headaches are characterized by nonthrobbing, diffuse pain that is mild to moderate in severity and does not worsen with activity/exercise. They may last from 30 minutes to several days. Cluster headaches are characterized by severe pain, usually unilateral in the frontal or periorbital region, last less than 3 hours, occur in clusters, and rarely present in a child less than 10 years of age (Bonthius & Hershey, 2020).

### Subjective Findings

Ask about onset, location, duration, characteristics, associated symptoms, aggravating and alleviating factors, timing, and severity of the headaches. Refer to Table 36.1 for a comparison of pain and associated symptoms for migraine, tension, and cluster headaches.

During the health history, ask questions about family history of headaches, any known triggers (such as certain foods), and frequency of headaches. Obtaining a headache diary will help aid diagnosis of the type of headache the child may be having (Bonthius & Hershey, 2020).

> ALERT: Occipital headaches, headaches that wake a child up from sleep at night or that occur first thing in the morning, require further investigation, as they can be a sign of a serious underlying condition (White, 2019).

### Risk Factors

The most common risk factors for headaches are:

- Family history of headaches
- Known triggers (allergies or specific foods such as pizza, chocolate, caffeine)
- Concurrent upper respiratory infection or other febrile illness

**TABLE 36.1 Characteristics of Chronic Headaches**

| Characteristics | Migraine | Tension | Cluster |
|---|---|---|---|
| Pain | Throbbing, bilateral moderate-intensity pain, increases with exertion | Non-throbbing, mild to moderate pain, does not increase with exertion | Severe unilateral pain |
| Associated symptoms | Aura, photophobia, phonophobia, nausea, vomiting | photophobia OR phonophobia (not both), no associated nausea/vomiting | Several episodes occur within the timeframe of a few hours |

*Sources*: Data from Bonthius, D. J., & Hershey, A. D. (2020). Headache in children: Approach to evaluation and general management strategies. *UpToDate*. Retrieved July 25, 2020, from https://www.uptodate.com/contents/headache-in-children-approach-to-evaluation-and-general-management-strategies; White, C. P. (2019). Headache in children and young people. *Paediatrics and Child Health, 29*(11), 476–480. https://doi.org/10.1016/j.paed.2019.07.011

- Dehydration
- Poor sleeping habits
- Vision problems
- Hormonal changes (female)
- Excess video game or tablet use

### Review of Systems

The most common manifestations revealed during the review of systems include:

- **Constitutional:** poor eating and sleeping habits
- **Respiratory:** upper respiratory infection symptoms (acute headache)
- **Neurologic:** head pain (see Table 36.1)

▶ ALERT: Reports of dizziness, confusion, gait abnormalities, or seizure indicate the possibility of secondary headache (a pathologic cause).

## Objective Findings

The physical examination of the child with headaches is typically normal unless the child is experiencing a headache during examination or a suspected secondary headache occurs. Pain may be noted upon palpation of face/head/sinuses. When an infectious process is responsible for an acute headache, fever and tachycardia may occur. Perform a complete neurologic examination. Papilledema, abnormal cranial nerve testing, involuntary movements, or gait abnormalities suggest a possible secondary headache (Bonthius & Hershey, 2020).

### Laboratory/Diagnostic Testing

The diagnosis of headache is most often based upon a thorough history and clinical findings. Obtaining a thorough history is the most important aspect for diagnosing the type of headache. Most children who present to primary care with headaches have primary headaches; therefore, neuroimaging is not warranted. If the neurologic examination is abnormal, papilledema is present, or the practitioner suspects increased intracranial pressure, brain MRI is the recommended first line for testing (Bonthius & Hershey, 2019). Consider neuroimaging also if there has been a recent change or sudden onset of headaches (Gladstein, 2017). In most cases laboratory testing is not necessary. Potential headache causes may be ruled out with a CBC, erythrocyte sedimentation rate (ESR), and thyroid function testing. If there is a history of seizure-like events, consider an EEG. When increased intracranial pressure is suspected (such as with pseudotumor cerebri), an LP to measure opening pressure may be useful (Bonthius & Hershey, 2020).

## Differential Diagnosis

The differential diagnosis for headache includes:

- Acute headache related to an infectious process (upper respiratory infection, meningitis, encephalitis, sinusitis)
- Migraine vs. tension vs. cluster headache
- Brain tumor (other secondary pathology)
- Intracranial hemorrhage
- Cerebrovascular infarction (stroke)
- Drug intoxication
- Head trauma/injury
- Temporomandibular joint syndrome

## Treatment/Management Plan

Treatment is based on the underlying condition causing the headaches. For primary (nonpathological) headaches, nonsteroidal anti-inflammatory drugs (NSAIDs) are the first pharmacologic choice, followed by acetaminophen. Nonpharmacologic interventions include stress management, increased hydration, avoidance of dietary triggers and other allergens, adequate sleep, and avoidance of prolonged use of video games and tablets. The first-line pharmacologic intervention for chronic headache is a triptan medication. Preventive medications used for chronic headache include amitriptyline, propranolol, and topiramate, among others.

PRO TIP Rizatriptan and zolmitriptan are available as a melting tablet, which may be better tolerated in younger children (and easier to administer).

### Family Education

Teach the following:

- Keep a headache diary to accurately document occurrence, location, severity, triggers, and alleviating and aggravating symptoms.
- Practice stress management techniques, ensure adequate sleep, avoid prolonged use of video games/tablets.
- Avoid known and common headache triggers.
- Limit use of over-the-counter NSAIDs and acetaminophen to avoid rebound headaches.
- Take prescription medication as prescribed if applicable.

- Report any sudden onset or recent change in headaches, a headache that wakes the child up at night, or one that occurs upon awakening (Bonthius & Hershey, 2020; Gladstein, 2017).

### Referral

Refer to a pediatric neurologist for treatment and management when the headaches are refractory to treatment, or when a pathologic process is suspected. Headaches associated with behavioral or mood changes also warrant a neurology referral (Bonthius & Hershey, 2020; Gladstein, 2017).

## BREATH-HOLDING SPELLS

BHSs are a type of benign paroxysmal episode in which a child briefly stops breathing and loses consciousness after an upsetting or painful triggering event. BHS is an involuntary phenomenon in which the child experiences crying or emotional upset that leads to a prolonged period of soundless expiration accompanied by a color change (pallor or cyanosis). Most episodes subside with deep inspiration, but some are more severe. There is no postictal period involving sleep or excessive lethargy. The incidence of BHS is approximately 5% in otherwise healthy children ages 6 months to 5 years (Leung et al., 2019). Spells are very rare in children younger than 6 months of age, and typically resolve spontaneously by school age. About 20% to 30% of children have a family history of BHS with an autosomal dominant trait (Bidabadi et al., 2019). Caregivers often find these events to be extremely frightening despite their benign nature, as the child is unconscious and appears lifeless, although usually for no more than a few seconds.

Autonomic nervous system dysregulation, vagally mediated cardiac inhibition, and delayed myelination of the brain stem contribute to BHS. There is also a notable association between BHSs and iron-deficiency anemia (Ahmed, 2016). Children may experience cyanotic BHS, pallid BHS, or mixed types. The cyanotic type accounts for more than 70% of cases (Leung et al., 2019). A cyanotic spell is typically precipitated by anger or frustration. The child typically emits a short cry, followed by involuntary breath-holding during expiration, becomes either limp or rigid, and cyanotic with a brief loss of consciousness. Some children experience momentary twitching or clonic movements. As the child inhales, consciousness is restored. With the pallid type, episodes are usually precipitated by fear or pain. In these spells, a crying response may be absent, or is often brief or "silent." The apneic episode may consist of a single deep gasp before the loss of consciousness, with either limp or rigid posturing. The heart rate slows and the child becomes pale and possibly diaphoretic. As with cyanotic spells, generalized twitching or clonic movements may occur. The child will exhibit significant pallor until the episode spontaneously resolves. The events last for less than 1 minute. Severe types may have associated changes in consciousness and loss of muscle tone or tonic-clonic activity similar to that seen in seizures occur in combination with the events.

### Subjective Findings

The health history may reveal brief unconscious periods with color change.

### Risk Factors

The most common risk factors for BHSs are:

- Family history (first-degree relative)
- Male gender
- RS
- 16p11.2 microdeletion syndrome

Research has suggested that certain temperamental characteristics may predispose children to have BHSs (Leung et al., 2019). Children noted to have a low threshold of responsiveness, who are easily frustrated, and who are slow to recover from negative emotional states were found to be more prone to these spells.

### Review of Systems

The most common manifestations revealed during the review of systems include:

- **Constitutional:** rapid development of cyanosis or pallor during spells
- **Respiratory:** caregiver report that child emits a short, loud cry, leading to a sudden involuntary holding of the breath in forced expiration during episode
- **Neurologic:** loss of consciousness, seizure (rare, and if the apneic spell is prolonged)
- **Musculoskeletal:** stiffness or generalized clonic movements

### Objective Findings

The physical examination of the child with BHSs is typically normal, unless the child experiences a spell during the examination due to anger or fear (e.g., anticipation of receiving immunizations).

### Laboratory/Diagnostic Testing

If the history and physical examination are normal, laboratory evaluation is usually not necessary in children with cyanotic BHSs. Because there is an association between BHS and iron-deficiency anemia, an anemia workup is appropriate, including a CBC and ferritin level. If the history is suspicious for seizure, then an EEG can be obtained (EEG is normal in BHS). An echocardiogram should be considered in children with frequent, severe pallid BHSs to rule out prolonged QT syndrome. Neuroimaging such as MRI is not indicated, as studies suggest that although BHS can be prolonged, there is no permanent neuronal damage (Dai & Demiryürek, 2019).

### Differential Diagnosis

The differential diagnosis for BHS includes:

- Prolonged QT syndrome
- Congenital heart disease
- Hyperekplexia (startle syndrome)
- Laryngospasm
- Seizures, epilepsy
- Sepsis
- Shuddering spells
- Vasovagal syncope

### Treatment/Management Plan

Treatment for both cyanotic and pallid types of BHS involves providing education to the caregivers. They will require reassurance that the child will outgrow these episodes and that BHS does not cause delays in the child's subsequent development. If iron-deficiency anemia is present, it should be treated with iron supplementation (refer to chapter 30 for additional information). For children with prolonged bradycardia and asystole associated with BHS, a cardiac pacemaker may be considered.

### Family Education

Teach the following:

- BHS is involuntary, benign, self-limiting, usually does not require treatment, and the child will outgrow these episodes
- During an episode, remain calm
- Apply appropriate firm limits in parenting, without the concern that the child will get upset and have a BHS
- Follow through with cardiopulmonary resuscitation (CPR) training
- Report to the practitioner if there are prolonged episodes or if the event has characteristics that are different from previous BHSs
- Call 911 if the child is not breathing for longer than 1 minute or if they are not waking up after the episode has ended

### Referral

BHS should be observed by an experienced practitioner for a diagnosis to be determined. If the practitioner cannot distinguish if the child is having BHS versus another medical condition, then the child should be referred to a pediatric cardiologist or neurologist for further workup. Refer to a pediatric cardiologist for evaluation if there are concerns about an underlying cardiac disorder. Refer to a pediatric neurologist if the event description or the child's medical history makes a compelling argument for seizures.

## TIC DISORDERS

Simple motor or vocal tics are benign, nonpathological occurrences and are common among children, yet may cause anxiety for the parents and the child. Most often tics are noticed around the ages of 6 to 7 years, with peaks occurring around 10 to 13 years of age and diminishing throughout adolescence (King, 2017). Simple motor tics may include eye blinking, sudden head or shoulder jerks, or extremity jerks. Complex motor tics involve multiple muscle groups and can manifest as hitting, jumping, or punching. Simple vocal tics may include humming, throat clearing, sniffing, and grunting, whereas complex vocal tics will include words or phrases. Tics occur in up to 2% of children, with Tourette syndrome occurring at a rate of 0.2% to 0.9% of the school-age population and males being affected four times more often than females (Hirschtritt et al., 2016).

Tourette syndrome is a neuropsychiatric disorder that is diagnosed when a child has had both motor and vocal tics present for at least 1 year. The tics do not have to be concurrent and may come and go. Complex motor tics associated with Tourette syndrome include repeating another person's words (echolalia), repeating their own words (palilalia), or yelling obscenities (coprolalia; Hirschtritt et al., 2016). The etiology of Tourette syndrome is likely multifactorial in nature, including genetic vulnerability (King, 2017). Tourette syndrome is also exacerbated by stressful situations, anxiety, fear, and excitement.

## Subjective Findings

The health history may reveal:

- Simple motor and/or vocal tics
- Complex vocal and/or motor tics
- Occurrence of vocal and motor tics that have occurred simultaneously or independently for at least one year (Tourette syndrome)

### Risk Factors

The most common risk factors for tics are:

- Male gender
- Being school age

Additional risk factors for Tourette syndrome are:

- Family history
- Having a diagnosis of attention deficit hyperactivity disorder (ADHD), or obsessive-compulsive disorder (OCD; King, 2017)

### Review of Systems

The most common manifestations revealed during the review of systems include:

- **Constitutional:** sleep disturbances, poor school performance
- **Musculoskeletal:** possible muscle pain from motor tics
- **Neurologic:** presence of motor and/or vocal tics
- **Psychiatric:** possible depression related to bullying or anxiety related to tics (Hirschtritt et al., 2016; Jankovic, 2019b; King, 2017)

## Objective Findings

The physical examination of the child with tics or Tourette syndrome will be normal, unless the child is having tics during the examination. The child may be able to suppress tics for a short amount of time; however, the urge will still be present (Jankovic, 2019b; King, 2017). Ask to see a video of tics, if possible, for classification purposes.

### Laboratory/Diagnostic Testing

The diagnosis of tics or Tourette syndrome is based mainly upon the history. The child may display motor or vocal tics during the examination, but that is not a requirement for diagnosis. No laboratory or diagnostic testing is needed.

## Differential Diagnosis

The diagnosis of tics is made based on the history and by ruling out any other underlying condition or medication side effect explanation for the tics. Tourette syndrome diagnosis requires the age of onset of the tics to be before age 18 years and for both motor and vocal tics being present simultaneously or independently for at least 1 year (Jankovic, 2019b). The differential diagnosis for Tourette syndrome includes:

- Seizures
- Dystonia
- Chorea
- Autism
- Pediatric autoimmune neuropsychiatric disorder associated with streptococcus (PANDAS)
- ADHD (Jankovic, 2019b; King, 2017)

## Treatment/Management Plan

No pharmacological treatment is necessary if tics are not bothersome. Discuss relaxation methods to decrease anxiety and ensure adequate sleep habits. Comprehensive behavioral intervention for tics has been shown to be effective in the reduction of tics. If tics continue to be bothersome, consider pharmacologic measures such as guanfacine, clonidine, or atypical antipsychotic drugs for Tourette syndrome (Jankovic, 2019a; King, 2017). Treating comorbidities such as ADHD, OCD, and anxiety may also help to reduce the frequency of tics demonstrated.

Note: Psychostimulant medications used to treat ADHD can increase the frequency and severity of tics, and it is important to work with the child and family on managing both sets of symptoms. For example, the family may prefer to continue use of a stimulant and add in a second medication to treat the tics. Conversely, the family may wish to trial a nonstimulant ADHD medication to see if the ADHD symptoms can be adequately controlled and if the tics will lessen in severity.

**PRO TIP** Focus on coping strategies and nonpharmacologic interventions and reserve pharmacologic treatment for tics that are bothersome to the child (not the parent).

## Family Education

Teach the following:

- Do not criticize or draw attention to tics. Reaffirm with the family that tics are involuntary acts and that the child will most likely outgrow the tics (this is comforting to the family)

- Continue to monitor for progression or worsening of tics
- Counseling and behavioral therapy are recommended for tics, and comprehensive behavioral intervention for Tourette syndrome
- If pharmacologic treatment is prescribed, discuss potential side effects of medication

### Referral

Refer to a pediatric neurologist to help confirm the diagnosis if needed, if psychiatric conditions are suspected or confirmed, and for psychiatric pharmacologic treatment when necessary.

▶ ALERT: There is no need to pharmacologically treat tics unless the tics are bothering the child.

## SEIZURES

A seizure is the clinical manifestation of an abnormal and excessive synchronization of an area of cortical neurons. Seizures are a consequence of neurologic or systemic disorders with structural, genetic, immune, metabolic, or infectious etiologies. The incidence of unprovoked seizures in children ranges from 63 to 134 per 100,000 children per year, with the highest rates occurring in the first year of life, and 65% to 70% have no apparent cause (Auvin, 2016). A first seizure does not necessarily mean that the child will develop epilepsy.

During a seizure, a group of neurons generate abnormal electrical firing, possibly due to an imbalance of inhibitory (gamma-aminobutyric acid [GABA]) and excitatory cells (glutamate). Seizure discharge transmission depends on excitatory synapses. The immature central nervous system is more susceptible to being converted from a normal neuronal network to a hyperexcitable one; which causes abnormal firing of neurons. Seizure phenomena may consist of altered consciousness, sensory, motor, autonomic, or behavioral events. Clinical seizures usually last <3 minutes and stop spontaneously. If seizures last longer, they are less likely to stop spontaneously. Delay in treatment is associated with a higher likelihood of poor response to abortive therapy.

Seizures are classified into two groups: focal and generalized. Focal (or partial) seizures only arise from one area of the brain and can be either simple or complex. A simple focal seizure may be characterized by jerking of one or more parts of the body, or sensory changes such as smelling specific odors or experiencing tingling sensations. This type of seizure lasts <1 minute. Complex focal seizures typically arise from the temporal lobe, and last between 1 and 2 minutes. Complex partial seizures involve impairment of consciousness, and often have a postictal period, during which the child is lethargic/sleepy. A secondary generalized seizure starts as a focal seizure but then spreads to both sides of the brain, causing loss of consciousness and tonic-clonic movements.

Generalized seizures are caused by widespread, excessive, electrical discharge in both brain hemispheres. Seizure movements can be described as *tonic* (muscles stiffening), *atonic* (loss of tone, also referred to as "drop seizures"), *clonic* (rhythmic jerking), *myoclonic* (sudden brief jerking or twitching), *absence* (staring spells, with possible automatisms such as lip smacking or eye blinking), and *tonic-clonic*. In generalized seizures, there is loss of consciousness and children experience a postictal period.

## FEBRILE SEIZURE

Febrile seizures are single, brief convulsions that occur in young children and are triggered by fever (typically >101 °F/38.3 °C), usually during rise or fall of the fever (National Institute of Neurological Disorders and Stroke [NINDS], 2020). They typically occur in young children between the ages of 6 months and 5 years. Febrile seizure is the most common neurologic condition in children (DiSano et al., 2020). Most children experiencing febrile seizures are neurologically normal and do not develop epilepsy. There is a 33% chance that febrile seizures will recur (Smith et al., 2019). The risk of recurrence is increased with age younger than 18 month, body temperature less than 40 °C, fever less than 1 hour prior to seizure onset, family history of febrile seizure and developmental abnormalities (Saguil & Servey, 2020). Febrile seizures typically present as generalized tonic-clonic convulsions that only last a few minutes. Less common presentations include eye rolling, rigid (stiff) limbs, or focal motor movements.

### Subjective Findings

Caregivers will typically describe that the child has had a sudden high fever. It is important to get a thorough description of the seizure, if known. Ask about whether it was generalized or if there were specific focal findings. Determine if the child lost consciousness, the duration of the episode, and if the child had postictal confusion or sleepiness.

## Risk Factors

The most common risk factors for febrile seizure are:

- Past medical history of seizure, either afebrile or febrile
- Children at highest risk for recurrence are those who have their first febrile seizure prior to age 18 months, have the seizure as their *first* sign of illness, have a relatively low temperature with their first febrile seizure, or have a family history of febrile seizures (NINDS, 2020)
- Familial seizure disorder

## Review of Systems

The review of systems may reveal a recent viral illness or exposure to sick contacts. The most common manifestations revealed during the review of systems include those associated with a febrile illness:

- **Constitutional:** fever, ear pain, recent onset of headache
- **Integumentary:** rash
- **HEENT:** drainage from the ear, runny nose, sore throat
- **Respiratory:** cough, cold, or congestion
- **Gastrointestinal:** nausea, vomiting, diarrhea
- **Genitourinary:** dysuria, urinary frequency
- **Neurologic:** seizures (provoked/unprovoked), lethargy, change in balance or coordination
- **Lymphatic:** swollen lymph nodes

## Objective Findings

The physical examination of the child with febrile seizure may reveal:

- Well-appearing child
- Elevated temperature
- Fontanel soft and flat
- Irritable but easily consoled
- Nasal or upper airway congestion
- Neurologically normal

▶ ALERT: Be aware of signs of increased intracranial pressure which may indicate meningitis: increased blood pressure, decreased/increased pulse rate, decreased respirations, bulging anterior fontanel, and sunset eyes.

## Laboratory/Diagnostic Testing

EEG is not routinely indicated for neurologically intact children presenting with a single febrile seizure. MRI is reserved for children with focal abnormality on EEG, presence of complex (focal or prolonged) seizure, and any focal neurologic deficits, however brief, following the seizure. An LP is suggested for all infants under 6 months of age, but otherwise only if meningitis is suspected. Draw a blood glucose; other blood studies are usually not indicated (Mikaty & Tchapyjnikov, 2020).

## Differential Diagnosis

The differential diagnosis for febrile seizure includes:

- Epileptic condition
- Central nervous system infection, including meningitis
- Metabolic or toxic encephalopathy
- BHSs
- Anoxia
- Central nervous system tumor
- Hypoglycemia
- Febrile shivering, shaking rigor
- Syncope

## Treatment and Management

The goal of treatment should be to identify the source of the febrile illness. Reducing the fever with antipyretics reduces discomfort during the child's illness, but has not been shown to prevent the onset of a febrile seizure or prevent subsequent seizures from occurring. Children who have experienced a brief febrile seizure are typically not prescribed prophylactic antiepileptic medications to prevent future seizures, as side effects outweigh any benefits. However, prolonged febrile seizures are associated with the potential for injury and an increased risk of developing epilepsy, so some neurologists may consider prescribing medication, such as rectal diazepam, to be administered in the event of recurrent lengthy seizures.

## Family Education

Teach the following:

- Basic emergency measures, including positioning child to prevent aspiration and not putting anything in the child's mouth.
- Time the seizure and note whether it is generalized or focal in nature.
- Use antipyretics to relieve the child's discomfort when a fever is present; however, studies have indicated that this does not reduce the child's risk of having another febrile seizure.

- In those children who have had a prolonged previous seizure, instruct on the use of rectal diazepam if warranted.
- No current evidence links occasional febrile seizures with permanent neurologic damage or learning issues.

### Referral

Hospitalization for febrile seizure is usually not indicated unless the seizure is either very prolonged or is accompanied by a serious infection, or if the child is <6 months of age (NINDS, 2020). Referral should be made to a pediatric neurologist for management of febrile seizures if the child has developmental and neurologic abnormalities or develops seizures without fever. These children have an increased risk of developing epilepsy.

## EPILEPSY

Epilepsy is a brain disorder resulting in a long-term predisposition to generate seizures. Epilepsy may be defined by any of the following conditions:

- At least two unprovoked seizures occurring greater than 24 hours apart
- One unprovoked seizure along with sufficient EEG clinical information to credibly establish an ongoing tendency to develop recurrent seizures
- Diagnosis of an epilepsy syndrome

One in 26 people will develop epilepsy in their lifetime. It is estimated that one in 150 children is diagnosed with epilepsy by age 10, with highest incidence of diagnosis during infancy (Aaberg et al., 2017). Epilepsy is not necessarily a lifelong diagnosis. It is considered to be resolved if:

- the individual has been seizure free for 10 consecutive years (at least 5 years off antiepileptic medication)
- when the person has passed the age of an age-dependent epilepsy syndrome

Causes of epilepsy include genetic variations, congenital or acquired structural brain changes, autoimmune or metabolic disorders, or chronic infection (such as human immunodeficiency syndrome or tuberculosis). Finding the root cause of a child's epilepsy can help determine the child's prognosis. Triggers for seizures may include illness, hyperventilation, flashing or strobe lights, menses, exercise, poor sleep, certain medications (e.g., diphenhydramine can lower seizure threshold), missed doses of medication or prescribed medication weans, use of alcohol or recreational drugs, and stress.

Epileptic syndromes include:

- Self-limited epilepsy with centrotemporal spikes (most common, accounts for 15% to 25% of all childhood epilepsies). Peak age of onset is between the ages of 7 and 8 years, usually resolving by age 16.
- Infantile spasms are characterized by a specific EEG pattern (hypsarrhythmia). The child experiences flexion/extension spasms in arms, legs, and head; the spasms are unpredictable and vary in duration.
- Lennox-Gastaut syndrome is characterized by the child having multiple seizure types. Children typically have an underlying brain malformation or injury.
- Dravet syndrome or severe myoclonic epilepsy of infancy is an intractable epilepsy syndrome which usually presents in the first year of life.
- Juvenile myoclonic epilepsy presents with multiple seizure types (tonic-clonic seizures, myoclonic jerks, and absence seizures), occurring most frequently in the morning, and including generalized tonic-clonic seizures, myoclonic jerks, and absence seizures.
- Child absence epilepsy most commonly occurs in children ages 4 to 10 years, is characterized by behavioral arrest and impaired consciousness, with spells typically lasting only a few seconds; spells can occur hundreds of times per day and can be mistaken by parents and teachers for inattention.

### Subjective Findings

In the child who has not had a witnessed tonic-clonic seizure episode, the health history may reveal:

- Lack of response when child is called or touched
- Decline in grades and concerns for inattention
- Child reports seeing flashing lights or smelling certain odors
- Findings such as blood on the child's pillow (from tongue-biting) or new-onset nocturnal enuresis associated with nighttime seizures
- Yelling, thrashing, unexplained laughter or running
- Episodes of blinking, lip smacking, eye deviation, or twitching

### Risk Factors

The most common risk factors for epilepsy are:

- Brain malformations (congenital or acquired, such as after brain injury or stroke)
- Genetic or metabolic syndromes (may include neurofibromatosis, tuberous sclerosis, RS)
- Family history of epilepsy or febrile seizures

- Central nervous system infections such as encephalitis or meningitis
- Conditions causing intellectual and developmental disabilities
- Anoxic events

## Review of Systems

The most common manifestations revealed during the review of systems include:

- **HEENT:** microcephaly or macrocephaly, dysmorphic features
- **Integumentary:** neurocutaneous findings (e.g., café-au-lait spots with neurofibromatosis type I, facial hemangioma with Sturge Weber syndrome, adenoma sebaceum or ash leaf spots with tuberous sclerosis)
- **Neurologic:** alteration in mental status, changes in balance or coordination, focal or lateralizing weakness, presence of seizure during the evaluation

▶ ALERT: A Todd's paralysis can occur acutely following a seizure. The child may experience temporary limb weakness or hemiplegia, without long-term consequences (Xu et al., 2020).

## Objective Findings

The physical examination of a child with epilepsy may reveal:

- Dysmorphic features
- Indications of developmental delay
- Neurocutaneous lesions
- Diaphoresis or clamminess (possibly related to hypoglycemia)
- Microcephaly or macrocephaly
- Early closing of fontanels or sutures (infants)
- Signs of head trauma
- Focal or lateralizing weakness or deficits
- Signs of increased intracranial pressure

PRO TIP Hyperventilation (such as having the child blow on a pinwheel) may elicit an absence seizure.

## Laboratory/Diagnostic Testing

Recent advances in genetic, metabolic, and neuroimaging techniques have improved accuracy of the comprehensive diagnosis of epilepsy. EEG is the most important neurophysiologic study for the diagnosis, prognosis, and treatment of epilepsy. An EEG should be performed for 45 minutes to 1 hour. In children with new-onset seizures, a complete laboratory evaluation includes CBC, comprehensive metabolic panel, and blood or urine toxicology screening. Metabolic testing is critical in infants with epilepsy. Epilepsy genetic panels and autoimmune markers in blood and CSF may also be tested. LP with CSF studies is not done routinely unless there is suspicion of infection or a metabolic or autoimmune component to the seizure presentation. Neuroimaging is imperative for children with developmental abnormalities, focal abnormalities on EEG, and focal seizures. Brain lesions or areas of congenital malformations can be the focus of seizures. Identifying these areas is pertinent in determining if they can be surgically removed and give the child an opportunity to have decreased seizures or become seizure-free. For the child on an antiepileptic medication, it is essential to monitor drug levels, typically drawn as a trough level before the morning dose. The side-effect profile of the medication also determines other monitoring parameters, including blood counts and renal and hepatic function.

## Differential Diagnosis

The differential diagnosis for epilepsy in children includes:

- BHSs
- Central nervous system tumor or infection
- Fainting (syncope)/vasovagal syncope
- Hypoglycemia (low blood sugar)
- Inattention (possibly ADHD)
- Migraine with confusion
- Movement disorders: tics, tremors, dystonia
- Panic attacks
- Parasomnias, such as night terrors
- Psychogenic nonepileptic seizures ( also referred to as pseudoseizures)
- Sandifer syndrome (infants experiencing arching/stiffening associated with gastrointestinal reflux disease)

## Treatment/Management

The standard of treatment for epilepsy is the use of AEDs. AEDs enhance inhibitory processes or oppose excitatory processes. Although they do not treat the underlying cause, the mechanism of action prevents seizures from occurring. Determining the appropriate medication largely depends on the child's age and the seizure type. An important concept is that the neurologist should treat the seizures, not the EEG. Many children will have a persistently abnormal EEG, especially if there is an underlying issue such as a structural brain difference or a genetic or metabolic disorder. In a number of epilepsy syndromes, such as absence seizures or self-limited epilepsy with centro-temporal spikes, neurologists often consider weaning the child from antiepileptic medications if the child has been seizure free for 2 to 3 (up to 5) years and the EEG has normalized.

In children with intractable seizures, there are other management options, especially when AEDs have been ineffective or caused excessive side effects. The ketogenic diet can be used successfully in some children who have not had success with AEDs. The diet is comprised a very large percentage of fats, a small amount of protein, and very low amounts of carbohydrates. While effective in reducing seizure frequency in approximately one-third of children, this diet can be difficult for some children and families to maintain. Another treatment option is surgical implantation of a vagal nerve stimulator, and other neuromodulation therapies are on the horizon. Finally, surgical resection of the seizure locus, ranging from lesionectomy to hemispherectomy, can provide relief to children for whom other treatments have failed.

## Family Education

Teach the following:

- Obtain training in seizure first aid. Both the Epilepsy Foundation (www.epilepsy.com/learn/seizure-first-aid-and-safety/first-aid-seizures-stay-safe-side) and the Centers for Disease Control and Prevention (CDC; www.cdc.gov/epilepsy/about/first-aid.htm) have information available on managing seizures.
- Medication dosing, side effects, and the importance of not missing doses.
- Children may have excessive daytime tiredness when medications are started or doses are changed, but this is generally short-term.
- Behavioral changes may be seen with medications such as levetiracetam. Supplementing with Vitamin B-6 (pyridoxine) may be beneficial.
- Work with the school to institute a seizure action plan (www.epilepsy.com/learn/managing-your-epilepsy/seizure-action-plans), which includes the protocol for seizures if they should occur at school. First aid, rescue seizure medication instructions, family notification, and when to call 911 are all essential components of the plan.
- Keeping a seizure diary or using a seizure tracking app may assist the specialist with evaluating therapy response and determining seizure management.
- Find out about the state's driver's license law (in most states an individual is not permitted to drive until seizure-free for 6 months to 1 year).
- Pregnancy should be avoided while taking antiepileptic medications, which potentially may be teratogenic.

▶ ALERT: Abrupt withdrawal of antiepileptic medications can provoke a seizure in a child who has remained seizure-free on medication. Families must be cautioned to never stop medications abruptly or without the guidance of their neurologist.

## Referral

When a child is suspected of having seizures, refer to a pediatric neurologist for accurate diagnosis and treatment. The practitioner and neurologist will become partners in the care of the child with seizures.

▶ ALERT: *Status epilepticus* refers to more than 30 minutes of either continuous seizure activity OR more than two sequential seizures without full recovery of consciousness between seizures.

To reduce associated morbidity and mortality, current guidelines recommend rapidly stopping both clinical and electrical seizure activity. To stabilize the child, intramuscular midazolam or intravenous (IV) lorazepam or diazepam is used to stop seizures lasting at least 5 minutes. If the seizure continues past the 20-minute mark, the second phase of treatment involves single-dose IV administration of fosphenytoin, valproic acid, or levetiracetam (Glauser et al., 2016).

# RETT SYNDROME

RS is a neurodevelopmental disorder that is the most common cause of profound intellectual disability in females. The incidence of RS in the United States is ~1 in 10,000 girls by age 12 (National Organization for Rare Disorders [NORD], 2015). Most cases of RS are caused by mutations in the MECP2 gene on the X-chromosome, with a wide phenotypic presentation of MECP2, depending on the location, type, and severity of the mutation. RS is characterized by early presentation of hypotonia but otherwise apparently normal development, followed by psychomotor regression and the emergence of midline hand stereotypies (Tarquinio et al., 2017). The most common phenotype is severe, with early-onset encephalopathy, infantile spasms, global developmental delay, and intellectual disability. There are cases involving much milder symptoms as well. Survival of children with RS is often into adulthood, with the 35-year survival rate at 70% (Bernstein & Glaze, 2020). Originally, RS was considered lethal in males, as it has an X-linked dominant inheritance. Although this syndrome has a higher incidence in females, rare cases are also documented in males (NORD, 2015).

RS presentations can be categorized as either classic or variant/atypical; most girls with RS have a classic form. The natural history of classic RS can be divided into four stages with significant clinical features:

- *Stage I*—developmental arrest (6–18 months): normal early development, then significant neurodevelopmental deterioration between 6 and 18 months of age; head growth decelerates and eye contact and interactive play may diminish. Seizures commonly occur in children with RS, and may have their onset prior to or during this stage, or later.
- *Stage II*—rapid deterioration or developmental regression (1–4 years): regression in previously acquired skills, including spoken language and the ability to make purposeful hand/finger movements. Stereotypical hand movements begin, including hand wringing, squeezing, or clapping, or hand-to-mouth movements emerge. Children can exhibit screaming, inconsolable crying, or panic attacks. May demonstrate autism-like features, bruxism, tremors, apraxia, and seizures.
- *Stage III*—pseudostationary (2–10 years): during this stage a plateau is reached that can last for decades. Some children show small improvements in communication skills, eye contact, and social interactions. Persistent issues include bruxism, stereotypical hand movements, and breathing irregularities.
- *Stage IV*—late motor deterioration (>10 years): Though some children with classic RS never learn to walk, it is during this stage that those who could previously ambulate lose this ability. Motor symptoms include muscle wasting, spasticity, dystonia, and quadriparesis. Scoliosis or kyphoscoliosis and joint contractures develop. Breathing issues continue, as do seizures. Hyperventilation episodes occur only when the child is awake and can worsen with stress. Sleep problems are another common finding and include sleep disordered breathing, insomnia, and parasomnias (Bernstein & Glaze, 2020).

In variant (or atypical) RS, not all of the classic symptoms may be present. In one variant, the infant displays severe hypotonia and developmental delays during the first few months of life. In other variants, the child may not develop microcephaly, and may have more aggression and significant autism features (NORD, 2015).

## Subjective Findings

The health history may reveal:

- Examine developmental milestones, particularly identifying decline in motor functioning, language regression, and cognitive abilities.
- Identify the onset of symptoms (typically between 5 and 12 months of age).
- Determine if there has been regression followed by a period of stabilization and some recovery in the four main categories of purposeful hand movements, spoken language, gait, and hand stereotypies.

## Risk Factors

About 99% of the time, the genetic mutation causing RS in a child is sporadic (NORD, 2015).

## Review of Systems

The most common manifestations revealed during the review of systems include:

- **Constitutional:** impaired sleep
- **HEENT:** bruxism, intermittent esotropia
- **Respiratory:** hyper- or hypoventilation episodes
- **Cardiovascular:** cold, discolored hands and feet (autonomic instability can occur)
- **Gastrointestinal:** feeding issues (chewing and swallowing difficulty), regurgitation, dysphagia, constipation
- **Neurologic:** BHPs, ataxia, seizures
- **Musculoskeletal:** scoliosis, joint contractures
- **Neurodevelopment:** social withdrawal, significant communication impairment, tantrums, screaming, agitation, stereotypical hand movements; girls with RS almost always prefer people to objects and enjoy affection, whereas males with RS often have more significant autism features.

## Objective Findings

The physical examination of the child with RS may reveal:

- Declines on all growth curves
- Tooth damage from bruxism

- Positive eye contact, communication with intense eye pointing
- Electrocardiogram abnormality (prolonged QT syndrome)
- Hypo- or hyperventilation, apneic pauses
- Ataxia or inability to walk
- Irritability
- Scoliosis
- Hypertonia, spasticity, joint contractures
- Hypotonia
- Stereotypic hand movements (hand wringing/ squeezing, clapping/tapping, mouthing or washing/ rubbing)

## Laboratory/Diagnostic Testing

The diagnosis of RS is based on initial clinical features and can be confirmed by molecular genetic testing. A Rett/Angelman syndrome panel, MECP2 gene sequencing, epilepsy panel, and X-linked disorders panels can all pick up RS mutations. To rule out metabolic disorders, testing of plasma amino acids, acylcarnitine profile, ammonia, serum lactate and pyruvate, and urine organic acids is warranted. Genetic testing will most commonly reveal a mutation of the MECP2 gene (but may also show a mutation in CKDL5 or FOXG1). As a component of diagnostic testing for developmental plateau or if seizures are suspected, an EEG may be ordered. EEG patterns seen in children with RS can vary from normal to mild background slowing initially. As developmental regression occurs, the EEG will become moderately slower and the appearance of multifocal epileptiform abnormalities can be identified. After age 3, EEG is almost universally abnormal in children with RS (Tarquinio et al., 2017). An echocardiogram should be performed by age 5 due to concerns for prolonged QT syndrome; if normal, it is repeatedly typically every other year. Polysomnography may be necessary for children with significant sleep disruption, snoring, and apnea. A swallow study may be indicated for children with dysphagia.

## Differential Diagnosis

The differential diagnosis for RS includes:

- Acquired epileptic aphasia
- Angelman syndrome
- Autism spectrum disorder
- Benign congenital hypotonia
- Cerebral palsy
- CDKL5 deficiency disorder
- Encephalitis
- Epileptic encephalopathy
- Fetal alcohol syndrome
- Metabolic disorders, including lysosomal or peroxisomal storage diseases , and inborn errors of metabolism such as phenylketonuria
- Other neurodegenerative disorders including mitochondrial disorders or spinocerebellar degeneration
- Prader-Willi syndrome
- Tuberous sclerosis

## Treatment/Management Plan

Treatment planning for children with RS is highly individualized, with early developmental therapies focused on maximizing each child's potential (NORD, 2015). Multiple medical specialists may be involved, and coordination of care is essential. The inability to communicate verbally can be stressful for both the child and family. Some children with RS exhibit hearing loss, especially as they get older, and hearing aids may be necessary. Augmentative and alternative communication devices can be utilized to facilitate the child's ability to communicate their thoughts and needs.

Management of sleep problems may include use of weighted blankets and relaxation techniques, supplements such as melatonin, and off-label use of antidepressants or other psychotropic medications. Antireflux medications may be indicated in the presence of gastroesophageal reflux disease, and some children may require fundoplication to reduce severe discomfort. Adequate nutrition is essential, and children may require gastrostomy tube feeding to enhance their caloric intake. Experts typically do not prescribe antiseizure medications for children without clear epileptic seizures, even if the child has an abnormal EEG. As the child gets older, osteopenia is a risk, and management of bone health becomes an important focus.

## Family Education

Teach the following:

- The child will require high levels of care due to their multiple disabilities.
- Plan for special education.
- Many resources are available at www.rettsyndrome.org.

## Referral

Refer the child with RS to:

- Developmental behavioral pediatrics
- Early intervention (birth to 3) services to help with all developmental therapies (may be provided at home, in special needs day care, or in the home)

- Physical, occupational, and speech therapy
- Genetics
- Pediatric neurology
- Augmentative and assistive communication evaluation (to determine appropriate communication technology depending on the child's abilities and needs)
- Pediatric pulmonary, orthopedics, gastroenterology, cardiology, psychiatry as symptoms present

# NEUROLOGIC INJURIES

Neurologic injuries occurring in children and adolescents (i.e., fractures, contusions, and concussions) can arise from various causes. Injuries can be incidental or accidental. In the following section, subjective and objective findings for neurologic injuries are discussed. Pertinent diagnostic testing, potential differential diagnoses, and appropriate management and education for head injuries and concussion are presented.

## CLOSED HEAD INJURY

Head injuries are any type of trauma that results in injury to the scalp, skull, or brain (Schutzman, 2020). Head injuries or trauma can occur from various incidents in a child's life. Most head injuries are minor and occur in males (Schutzman, 2020). Head injury in a newborn or infant who is not yet mobile is concerning for abuse. Other common accidental head injuries include accidental falls while at school or home, sports-related injuries, motor vehicle accidents, or a physical assault.

### Subjective Findings

The health history may reveal:

- Reported fall off bed or couch by an infant or an accidental fall at school, home, or extracurricular activities of older child during play/physical activity (including sports-related injury)
- Physical assault by another person (child or adult)
- History of motor vehicle accident

**PRO TIP** Suspect possible child abuse for reports of fall in a not-yet-mobile infant. Also perform skeletal survey to rule out any other injuries/fractures in an infant you suspect of being abused (younger than age 1, do a skeletal survey if there is a skull fracture).

### Risk Factors

The most common risk factors for head injuries in children are:

- Accidental falls
- Playing sports
- Motor vehicle accidents
- Abuse

### Review of Systems

The most common manifestations revealed during the review of systems include:

Infant:

- **Constitutional:** poor nursing, parent reports child is not acting normally
- **Neurologic:** lethargy, fussiness, seizure-like events

Older child:

- **HEENT:** headache, photophobia, phonophobia
- **Gastrointestinal:** vomiting
- **Neurologic:** dizziness, difficulty with concentration or memory, depression or anxiety, change in mental status, possible loss of consciousness after injury, seizure-like activity
- **Dermatologic:** scalp laceration, bruising, or hematoma (goose-egg; Korn & Babl, 2020; Schutzman, 2020)

### Objective Findings

The physical examination of the child with a minor closed head injury may reveal a normal physical examination except for the possibility of scalp laceration or hematoma.

▶ ALERT: Findings indicating a more serious head injury include altered mental status, bulging anterior fontanelle in an infant, periorbital ecchymosis, unequal pupil size, unilateral weakness, or limited range of motion (Korn & Babl, 2020; Schutzman, 2020).

### Laboratory/Diagnostic Testing

The diagnosis of minor closed head injury is based upon the history, clinical findings, and neuroimaging. A head computed tomography (CT) scan is used to identify contusion, hematoma, swelling, or hemorrhage. A skull x-ray may identify fractures.

### Differential Diagnosis

The differential diagnosis for minor closed head injury includes:

- Headaches
- Meningitis

- Abuse
- Poisoning or overdose

## Treatment/Management Plan

For minor head injury, treatment may occur at home with close monitoring. The child should rest. Apply ice to the area of injury. Use acetaminophen as needed for pain (avoid the use of aspirin and ibuprofen).

### Family Education

Teach the following:

- Seek care if child has worsening of symptoms (persistent vomiting, difficult to arouse, confusion, weakness, or seizure-like activity).
- Continue to follow up with provider for weekly visits to monitor for further sequalae.
- Avoid accidents by baby-proofing home, providing constant supervision of infants and young children, and having the child wear protective sports gear.
- Wear seatbelts in cars and helmets for bicycles and scooters. Infants and young children need to be in car seats (Schutzman, 2019).

### Referral

Refer to a pediatric neurologist if there is continued worsening of symptoms or seizure-like events occur.

# MILD TRAUMATIC BRAIN INJURY

Mild traumatic brain injury (mTBI), formerly termed *concussion*, is defined as an acute brain injury resulting from external mechanical force to the head, neck, or face. mTBI is indicated when both of the following occur:

1. **One** of the following:

- Confusion or disorientation
- Loss of consciousness for 30 minutes or less,
- Posttraumatic amnesia for less than 24 hours,
- Other transient neurologic abnormalities (focal signs/symptoms or seizure)

2. Glasgow Coma Scale score is 13 to 15, 30 minutes following the injury or upon presentation to healthcare facility (Lumba-Brown et al., 2018)

The highest incidence of mTBI occurs in boys who are active in collision sports, although any head injury in any sport can result in mTBI (Meehan & O'Brien, 2020a).

## Subjective Findings

The health history may reveal:

- Direct force to head, neck, or face
- Report of immediate confusion and/or amnesia after injury that lasts for several minutes
- Report of loss of consciousness immediately following injury
- Nausea, vomiting, vertigo, dizziness, headache, neck pain
- In days to weeks following injury: persistent headache, difficulty staying on task and focusing at school, photophobia, phonophobia, changes in attitude/behavior (Meehan & O'Brien, 2020a)

The CDC guidelines recommend using a validated rating tool such as the Post-Concussion Symptom Inventory or the Health and Behavior Inventory in order to distinguish subtle symptoms associated with mTBI (CDC, 2021).

### Risk Factors

The most common risk factors for concussion are:

- A previously sustained concussion
- Any participation in a contact sport such as football, soccer, or hockey

### Review of Systems

The most common manifestations revealed during the review of systems include:

- **Constitutional:** pain (headache)
- **HEENT:** photophobia, phonophobia
- **Gastrointestinal:** nausea, vomiting
- **Neurologic:** confusion, amnesia, loss of consciousness following injury, dizziness, vertigo
- **Psychiatric:** behavioral or emotional changes, difficulty concentrating in school (Korn & Babl, 2020; Meehan & O'Brien, 2020a)

## Objective Findings

Perform a complete physical examination of the child or adolescent with suspected mTBI. Pay particular attention to the neck and neurologic examination. Examination of the neck may reveal muscle strain or ligament sprain. Perform a detailed neurologic examination including balance, gait, mental status, and cognition. It is helpful to use a validated assessment tool such as:

- Balance Error Scoring System—available at https://theconcussionblog.files.wordpress.com/2011/02/bessprotocolnata09.pdf)

- Standardized Assessment of Concussion—available at https://cbirt.org/sites/cbirt.org/files/resources/sac_informational_kit_001.pdf)
- Sports Concussion Assessment Tool 5th edition (SCAT5, for adolescents 13 years or older)—available at http://scat5.cattonline.com
- Child-Sports Concussion Assessment Tool 5th edition (Child SCAT5, for children ages 5 to 12 years)—available at http://childscat5.cattonline.com (Korn & Babl, 2020; Meehan & O'Brien, 2020a)

Children and adolescents with mTBI generally exhibit normal cranial nerve, sensory, and motor findings.

▶ ALERT: If focal deficits or abnormalities (such as confusion, difficulty with memory, light sensitivity, uneven pupils, slurred speech, blank stare, or difficulties with balance, coordination, and gait) are noted, prompt evaluation for intracranial or spinal cord injury is warranted.

## Laboratory/Diagnostic Testing

Head CT does not reveal mTBI and should only be considered if child has seizure-like activity, focal neurologic deficits, or there is concern of intracranial injury (Meehan & O'Brien, 2020a). Skull x-ray may be done to rule out skull fracture.

## Differential Diagnosis

The differential diagnosis for mTBI includes:

- Migraine
- Transient ischemic attack
- Drug intoxication
- Syncope
- Hypoglycemia
- Intracranial injury

**PRO TIP** Use the Acute Concussion Evaluation (ACE) tool for assessment and decision-making for mTBI (available atwww.cdc.gov/headsup/pdfs/providers/ace_v2-a.pdf)

## Treatment/Management Plan

Neurocognitive and physical rest is essential, so remove the child from school and sports. The timing for return to school (cognitive activity) and to sports varies depending upon the particular child. Treat associated neurologic symptoms as appropriate. Manage headaches with acetaminophen or ibuprofen, nausea with ondansetron, and sleep difficulties with melatonin (Meehan & O'Brien, 2020b).

▶ ALERT: Worsening of neurologic symptoms post-mTBI is concerning and requires immediate referral to a pediatric neurologist.

Preventing a second injury is critical. Gradually increase the intensity and length of school activities as the child is able, without exacerbation of symptoms. If the child continues with difficulty focusing and staying on task, academic accommodations may be needed (Lumba-Brown et al., 2018). If the child wants to return to sports, the child must be fully asymptomatic at rest and with exertion prior to being cleared to return to play. After 48 hours of rest, the child may participate in light aerobic exercise (5–10 minutes of walking, exercise bike, or light jogging) at home, but never to the point of exertion. Physical activity is increased gradually, based on the absence of symptoms. Moderate activity includes brief running, and moderate-intensity stationary bicycling and weight-lifting (less repetition, less weight). Heavy activity includes sprinting/running, high-intensity stationary biking, regular weightlifting program, or noncontact-specific drills. The next step is return to controlled practice, followed eventually by return to competition. If at any point any neurologic symptoms return, the child should not participate in sport/exercise and should revisit the healthcare provider (CDC, 2021). Periodic retesting with the SCAT5 or Child-SCAT5 may be useful if it was performed at baseline.

**PRO TIP** The Acute Concussion Evaluation (ACE) Care Plan is a useful tool for communicating return to school and return to play (available atwww.cdc.gov/headsup/pdfs/providers/ACE_care_plan_school_version_a.pdf).

## Family Education

Teach the following:

- Educate the parents and child about the signs and symptoms of mTBI.
- Report any worsening neurologic issues: persistent headache, continued nausea/vomiting/dizziness, behavioral/mood changes, academic difficulties.
- Ensure that the child does not return to school or sports without being asymptomatic and without prior medical clearance from a healthcare professional.

- Be sure the child wears protective equipment while playing sports.

## Referral

If neurologic symptoms persist, or a seizure-like event occurs, refer the child to a pediatric neurologist.

## KEY POINTS

- When considering meningitis or encephalitis, obtain a thorough history and complete physical exam to rule out other potential causes of illness.
- Remember to review maternal GBS status at time of delivery in the newborn with suspected meningitis and maternal HSV status at time of delivery in the newborn with suspected encephalitis.
- Urge families to take measures to avoid exposure to mosquito and tick bites, for protection from certain organisms causing meningitis or encephalitis.
- Make sure children are up to date on vaccines, to avoid certain types of meningitis or encephalitis.
- For the child with suspected encephalitis or bacterial meningitis, send them to the emergency department quickly, as diagnosis and treatment should be prompt!
- Obtaining a thorough history and utilizing a headache diary is essential for accurate diagnosis of headaches.
- The majority of headaches in children are nonpathologic, and management of headaches focuses on avoidance of triggers and proper medication for pain relief.
- Refer to a pediatric neurologist when headache treatment is not working or a suspected secondary headache occurs.
- BHSs are benign and typically outgrown by children by age 6. Parents benefit from education and reassurance.
- Tics are benign and do not have pathologic origin.
- Tourette's syndrome is involuntary, can be hereditary, and can be diagnosed when the child has had vocal and motor tics either simultaneously or independently for at least 1 year and the onset was prior to age 18.
- Nonpharmacologic strategies for the treatment of tics are promotion of coping mechanisms and stress reduction. Pharmacologic treatment is not necessary unless the tics are bothersome to the child.
- A single febrile seizure does not require imaging or EEG. Laboratory evaluation should focus on finding a source for the fever if the child remains ill.
- Families must be cautioned never to stop antiepileptic medications abruptly and without the guidance of their neurologist.
- Girls with a regression in development occurring after 6 months of age should be evaluated for RS.
- Treatment strategies for RS involve active physical, occupational, and speech therapies; augmentative communication; management of seizures; and coordination of care for the child's complex needs.
- Close monitoring is crucial following head injury.
- Remember to baby-proof the home, have children wear protective sports gear, and use other protective equipment to avoid head injuries.
- Neurocognitive and physical rest is essential following concussion.
- Child *must* be asymptomatic at rest and exertion and have medical clearance prior to return to sports and recreational activities after mTBI.

## REFERENCES

Aaberg, K. M., Gunnes, N., Bakken, I. J., Søraas, C. L., Berntsen, A., Magnus, P., Lossius, M. I., Stoltenberg, C., Chin, R., & Surén, P. (2017). Incidence and prevalence of childhood epilepsy: A nationwide cohort study. *Pediatrics, 139*(5), e20163908. https://doi.org/10.1542/peds.2016-3908

Ahmed, B. (2016). Iron status in children with severe breath-holding spells. *International Journal of Medicine and Pharmaceutical Science, 6*, 31–36.

Auvin, S. (2016). Pathophysiology of seizures in the developing brain. In J. M. Pellock, D. R. Nordli, R. Sankar, & J. W. Wheless (Eds.), *Pellock's pediatric epilepsy: Diagnosis and therapy* (4th ed., pp. 3–20). Springer Publishing Company.

Bernstein, B., & Glaze, D. G. (2020). Rett syndrome. *eMedicine.* Retrieved July 25, 2020, from https://emedicine.medscape.com/article/916377-overview#a1

Bidabadi, E., Poornabi Dazi, S., Mashouf, P., & Shahraki, T. (2019). Effectiveness of iron therapy on breath holding spells in children. *Iranian Journal of Child Neurology, 13*(4), 155–161.

Bonthius, D. J., & Hershey, A. D. (2020). Headache in children: Approach to evaluation and general management strategies. *UpToDate.* Retrieved July 25, 2020, from https://www.uptodate.com/contents/headache-in-children-approach-to-evaluation-and-general-management-strategies

Centers for Disease Control and Prevention. (2021). *Heads up.* https://www.cdc.gov/headsup/index.html

Chiocca, E. M. (2019). *Advanced pediatric assessment* (3rd ed.). Wolters Kluwer.

Dai, A. I., & Demiryürek, A. T. (2019). Effectiveness oral theophylline, piracetam, and iron treatments in children with simple breath-holding spells. *Journal of Child Neurology, 35*(1), 25–30. https://doi.org/10.1177/0883073819871854

Di Pentima, C., & Kaplan, S. L. (2018). Viral meningitis: Clinical features and diagnosis in children. *UpToDate.* Retrieved July 25, 2020, from https://www.uptodate.com/contents/viral-meningitis-clinical-features-and-diagnosis-in-children

DiSano, M., Pestanta-Knight, E., & Gupta, A. (2020). Seizures not diagnosed as epilepsy. In V. Wasade & M.

Spanaki (Eds.), *Understanding epilepsy: A study guide for the boards* (pp. 165–175). Cambridge University Press.

Edwards, M. S., & Baker, C. J. (2018). Bacterial meningitis in the neonate: Clinical features and diagnosis. *UpToDate*. Retrieved July 25, 2020, from https://www.uptodate.com/contents/bacterial-meningitis-in-the-neonate-clinical-features-and-diagnosis

Figaji, A. A. (2017). Anatomical physiological differences between children and adults relevant to traumatic brain injury and the implications for clinical assessment and care. *Frontiers in Neurology, 8*(685). https://doi.org/10.3389/fneur.2017.00685

Gladstein, J. (2017). Headache. In T. K. McInerny, H. M. Adam, D. E. Campbell, J. M. Foy, & D. M. Kamat (Eds.), *American Academy of Pediatrics textbook of pediatric care* (2nd ed., Chapter 157). American Academy of Pediatrics.

Glauser, T., Shinnar, S., Gloss, D., Alldredge, B., Arya, R., Bainbridge, J., Bare, M., Bleck, T., Dodson, W. E., Garrity, L., Jagoda, A., Lowenstein, D., Pellock, J., Riviello, J., Sloan, E., & Treiman, D. M. (2016). Evidence-based guideline: Treatment of convulsive status epilepticus in children and adults: Report of the Guideline Committee of the American Epilepsy Society. *Epilepsy Currents, 16*(1), 48–61. https://doi.org/10.5698%2F1535-7597-16.1.48

Hardarson, H. S. (2018). Acute viral encephalitis in children: Clinical manifestations and diagnosis. *UpToDate*. Retrieved July 25, 2020, from https://www.uptodate.com/contents/acute-viral-encephalitis-in-children-clinical-manifestations-and-diagnosis

Hirschtritt, M. E., Dy, M. E., Yang, K. G., & Scharf, J. M. (2016). Child neurology: Diagnosis and treatment of Tourette syndrome. *Neurology, 87*, e65–e67. https://doi.org/10.1212/WNL.0000000000002977

Jankovic, J. (2019a). Tourette syndrome: Management. *UpToDate*. Retrieved July 25, 2020, from https://www.uptodate.com/contents/tourette-syndrome-management

Jankovic, J. (2019b). Tourette syndrome: Pathogenesis, clinical features, and diagnosis. *UpToDate*. Retrieved July 25, 2020, from https://www.uptodate.com/contents/tourette-syndrome-pathogenesis-clinical-features-and-diagnosis

Kaplan, S. L. (2018). Bacterial meningitis in children older than one month: Clinical features and diagnosis. *UpToDate*. Retrieved July 25, 2020, from https://www.uptodate.com/contents/bacterial-meningitis-in-children-older-than-one-month-clinical-features-and-diagnosis

Kaplan, S. L., & Di Pentima, C. (2019). Patient education: Meningitis in children: Beyond the basics. *UpToDate*. Retrieved July 25, 2020, from https://www.uptodate.com/contents/meningitis-in-children-beyond-the-basics

King, R. A. (2017). Tics. In T. K. McInerny, H. M. Adam, D. E. Campbell, J. M. Foy, & D. M. Kamat (Eds.), *American Academy of Pediatrics textbook of pediatric care* (2nd ed., Chapter 202). American Academy of Pediatrics.

Korn, P. A., & Babl, F. (2020). Minor head injury and concussion in children. In J. E. Tintinalli, O. Ma, D. M. Yealy, G. D. Meckler, J. Stapczynski, D. M. Cline, & S. H. Thomas (Eds.), *Tintinalli's emergency medicine: A comprehensive study guide* (9th ed., Chapter 111). McGraw-Hill.

Kotagal, S. (2019). Detailed neurologic assessment of infants and children. *UpToDate*. Retrieved July 25, 2020, from https://www.uptodate.com/contents/detailed-neurologic-assessment-of-infants-and-children

Kronman, M. P., Crowell, C. S., & Vora, S. B. (2019a). Meningitis. In: K. J. Marcdante & R. M. Kliegman (Eds.), *Nelson's essentials of pediatrics* (8th ed., pp. 386–388). Elsevier.

Kronman, M. P., Crowell, C. S., & Vora, S. B. (2019b). Encephalitis. In: K. J. Marcdante & R. M. Kliegman (Eds.), *Nelson's essentials of pediatrics* (8th ed., pp. 389–390). Elsevier.

Lee, L. K., & Fleisher, G. R. (2019). Trauma management: Unique pediatric considerations. *UpToDate*. Retrieved July 25, 2020, from https://www.uptodate.com/contents/trauma-management-unique-pediatric-considerations

Leung, A. K., Leung, A. A., Wong, A. H., & Hon, K. L. (2019). Breath-holding spells in pediatrics: A narrative review of the current evidence. *Current Pediatric Reviews, 15*(1), 22–29. https://doi.org/10.2174/1573396314666181113094047

Lumba-Brown, A., Yeates, K. O., Sarmiento, K., Breiding, M. J., Haegerich, T. M., Gioia, G. A., Turner, M., Benzel, E. C., Suskauer, S. J., Giza, C. C., Joseph, M., Broom, C., Weissman, B., Gordon, W., Wright, D. W., Moser, R. S., McAvoy, K., Ewing-Cobbs, L., Duhaime, A.-C., . . . Timmons, S. D. (2018). Centers for Disease Control and Prevention guideline on the diagnosis and management of mild traumatic brain injury among children. *JAMA Pediatrics, 172*(11), e182853. https://doi.org/10.1001/jamapediatrics.2018.2853

Meehan, W. P., & O'Brien, M. J. (2020a). Concussion in children and adolescents: Clinical manifestations and diagnosis. *UpToDate*. Retrieved July 25, 2020 from https://www.uptodate.com/contents/concussion-in-children-and-adolescents-clinical-manifestations-and-diagnosis

Meehan, W. P., & O'Brien, M. J. (2020b). Concussion in children and adolescents: Management. *UpToDate*. Retrieved July 25, 2020, from https://www.uptodate.com/contents/concussion-in-children-and-adolescents-management

Messacar, K., Fischer, M., Dominguez, S. R., Tyler, K. L., & Azburg, M. J. (2018). Encephalitis in U.S. children. *Infectious Disease Clinics of North America, 32*(1), 145–162. https://doi.org/10.1016/j.idc.2017.10.007

Mikaty, M. A., & Tchapyjnikov, D. (2020). Seizures in childhood. In R. M. Kliegman, J. St. Geme, N. J. Blum, S. S. Shah, R. C. Tasker, K. M. Wilson, & R. E. Behrman (Eds.), *Nelson textbook of pediatrics* (21st ed.). Elsevier.

Myrick, K. M., & Karosas, L. M. (2020). *Advanced health assessment and differential diagnosis*. Wolters Kluwer.

National Institute of Neurologic Disorders and Stroke. (2020). *Febrile seizures fact sheet*. https://www.ninds.nih.gov/Disorders/Patient-Caregiver-Education/Fact-Sheets/Febrile-Seizures-Fact-Sheet

National Organization for Rare Disorders. (2015). *Rett syndrome*. https://rarediseases.org/rare-diseases/rett-syndrome

Saguil, A., & Servey, J. (2020). Predicting the likelihood of a recurrent febrile seizure. *American Family Physician, 101*(8), 497–498. https://www.aafp.org/afp/2020/0415/p497.html

Schutzman, S. (2019). Minor head trauma in infants and children: Management. *UpToDate*. Retrieved July 25, 2020, from https://www.uptodate.com/contents/minor-head-trauma-in-infants-and-children-management

Schutzman, S. (2020). Minor head trauma in infants and children: Clinical features and evaluation. *UpToDate*. Retrieved July 25, 2020, from https://www.uptodate.com/contents/minor-blunt-head-trauma-in-infants-and-young-children-less-than2-years-clinical-features-and-evaluation

Smith, D. K., Sadler, K. P., & Benedum, M. (2019). Febrile seizures: Risks, evaluation, and prognosis. *American Family Physician, 99*(7), 445–450. https://www.aafp.org/afp/2019/0401/p445.html

Tarquinio, D. C., Hou, W., Berg, A., Kaufmann, W., Lane, J., Skinner, S. A., Motil, K. J., Neul, J. L., Percy, A. K., & Glaze, D. (2017). Longitudinal course of epilepsy in Rett

syndrome and related disorders. *Brain, 140*(2), 306–318. https://doi.org/10.1093/brain/aww302
White, C. P. (2019). Headache in children and young people. *Paediatrics and Child Health, 29*(11), 476–480. https://doi.org/10.1016/j.paed.2019.07.011
Xu, S.-Y., Li, Z.-X., Wu, X.-W., Li, L., & Li, C.-X. (2020). Frequency and pathophysiology of post-seizure Todd's paralysis. *Medical Science Monitor, 26*, e920751-1–e920751-4. https://dx.doi.org/10.12659%2FMSM.920751

## FURTHER READING

Abdel-Mannan, O., Taylor, H., Donner, E. J., & Sutcliffe, A. G. (2019). A systematic review of sudden unexpected death in epilepsy (SUDEP) in childhood. *Epilepsy and Behavior, 90*, 99–106. https://doi.org/10.1016/j.yebeh.2018.11.006
Akpinar, M., Ocal, M., & Irdem, A. (2019). Ventricular repolarization changes in children with breath holding spells. *Journal of Electrocardiology, 55*, 116–119. https://doi.org/10.1016/j.jelectrocard.2019.05.01
Choi, Y. J., Jung, J. Y., Kim, J. H., Kwon, H., Park, J. W., Kwak, Y. H., Kim, D. K., & Lee, J. H. (2019). Febrile seizures: Are and future risk of afebrile epileptic seizure based on the national sample cohort in South Korea, 2002-2013. *Seizure: European Journal of Epilepsy, 64*, 77–83. https://doi.org/10.1016/j.seizure.2018.12.004
Cosentino, L., Vigli, D., Franchi, F., Laviola, G., & Filippis, B. (2019). Rett syndrome before regression: A time window of overlooked opportunities for diagnosis and intervention. *Neuroscience and Biobehavioral Reviews, 107*, 115–135. https://doi.org/10.1016/j.neubiorev.2019.05.013
Mehta, C. E., Brady, P., & Gaddam, S. (2020). Status epilepticus. In V. Wasade & M. Spanaki (Eds.), *Understanding epilepsy. A study guide for the boards* (pp. 189–202). Cambridge University Press.
Olson, H., Rudloe, T., Loddenkemper, T., Harper, M. B., & Kimia, A. A. (2018). Should patients with complex febrile seizure be admitted for further management? *American Journal of Emergency Medicine, 36*(8), 1386–1390. https://doi.org/10.1016/j.ajem.2017.12.059
Rubenstein, S., & Levy, A. (2019). Seizures in childhood: Aetiology, diagnosis, treatment, and what the future may hold. *European Medical Journal Neurology, 7*(1), 62–70. https://www.emjreviews.com/neurology/article/seizures-in-childhood-aetiology-diagnosis-treatment-and-what-the-future-may-hold

# Management of Endocrine Disorders

Mandi Cafasso, Brandi Guyton, and Exie Meredith

## Student Learning Outcomes

**Upon completion of this chapter the reader should be able to:**

1. Discuss pathophysiology and epidemiology of selected endocrine disorders in children.
2. Differentiate subjective and objective findings of selected endocrine disorders in children.
3. Choose appropriate laboratory or diagnostic tests for particular endocrine disorders in children.
4. Utilize the differential diagnosis process to determine endocrine diagnosis in children.
5. Determine treatment plan, child/family education, and need for referral in children with a an endocrine disorder.

## INTRODUCTION

The primary care provider has the challenge of being knowledgeable about the actions of all body systems and differentiating symptoms among those systems, while considering the most common etiologies first. This skill becomes even more crucial when caring for children who may be unable to verbalize symptoms. As pediatric healthcare providers, we rely on parents and caregivers to provide details of a child's feelings, including the intensity, frequency, and duration of symptoms. While this may be feasible in the acutely ill child, for a child who is suffering from a chronic ailment(s), the details in the history may be less specific and, therefore, differential diagnoses may be harder to determine. The ability to identify endocrine disorders relies significantly on an adequate history and physical examination. However, there are additional details that can assist the primary care provider to recognize endocrine disorders. In this chapter we discuss a myriad of endocrine disorders, many with generalizable signs and symptoms at presentation to the primary care office. As a pediatric primary care provider, you will be able to feel confident in your ability to recognize the child who needs further evaluation by an endocrine specialist.

The content in this chapter maps to the following areas on the Pediatric Nursing Certification Board (PNCB) Pediatric Nurse Practitioner—Primary Care certification examination:

### CLINICAL PROBLEMS: ENDOCRINOLOGY

CONTENT AREAS:

**II. Assessment and Diagnosis**

**B. History and Physical Examination**

1. Obtain history of present illness
2. Obtain a comprehensive health history for new patients
3. Complete an interval history for established patients
4. Perform a review of systems
5. Perform a complete physical examination

**C. Diagnostic Testing and Screening**

1. Order and interpret office/clinic based screening tests
2. Order and interpret diagnostic laboratory tests
3. Order and interpret the results of diagnostic imaging tests

**D. Analyzing Information**

1. Integrate health history and physical examination findings into the plan of care
2. Assimilate findings from screening and diagnostic testing into plan of care

**E. Diagnosis**

1. Develop and prioritize differential diagnoses
2. Establish a diagnosis based on evaluation of patient data

## III. Management

**A. Child and Caregiver Counseling and Education**

1. Provide condition-specific counseling and education, including treatment options
2. Educate about benefits and potential adverse reactions of pharmacological interventions
3. Discuss non-pharmacological interventions
4. Counsel regarding the threshold for seeking follow-up care
5. Review the risks of non-adherence to recommended treatment

**B. Therapeutic Interventions**

1. Prescribe pharmacologic agents
2. Recommend the use of over-the-counter pharmacologic agents
3. Order or recommend non-pharmacologic treatments for the management of symptoms
4. Discuss use of complementary and alternative therapies as appropriate

**D. Collaboration and Referral**

2. Refer to specialists as indicated for evaluation, counseling, and/or treatment

**E. Care Coordination**

1. Facilitate patient and family-centered care for children of all ages with acute and chronic conditions

**F. Evaluation and Follow-up**

2. Establish a plan for follow-up care

## IV. Professional Role Responsibilities

**A. Leadership and Evidence-based Practice**

4. Develop, implement, and/or modify clinical practice guidelines

## ANATOMY AND PHYSIOLOGY

The endocrine system is comprised of nine main hormone-producing, miniature organs called *glands* (Figure 37.1). Each of the glands produces various chemicals and hormones that affect nearly every cell in the body. The main hormone-producing glands in the body are the hypothalamus, pituitary, parathyroid, pancreas, thyroid, adrenal, pineal, and gonads (ovaries and testes). The key to appropriate hormone release or inhibition is communication within the system and the environment.

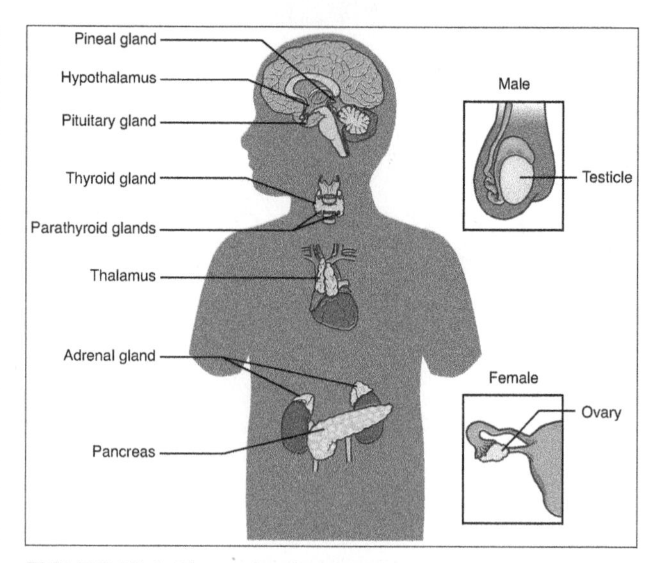


FIGURE 37.1 The endocrine system.

Communication within the endocrine system occurs via feedback loop. This happens when the hypothalamus communicates with the pituitary gland or "master gland" to either stimulate production or halt production of hormones in the end target gland. Continuous and ongoing feedback to the hypothalamus and the pituitary from the target glands controls the cascade of hormone release and production. For instance, production of thyroid hormone is the result of the hypothalamic release of thyrotropin-releasing hormone (TRH), which triggers the release of thyroid-stimulating hormone (TSH) or thyrotropin from the pituitary gland, which in turn causes the release of thyrotropin (T4) from the thyroid gland.

## GENERAL APPROACH TO CHILD WITH AN ENDOCRINE DISORDER

### Subjective Findings

The health history may reveal:

- Delays in development
- Abnormal growth
- Changes in energy levels
- Abnormal changes in weight
- Changes in stool patterns

### Risk Factors

The most common risk factors for an endocrine disorder are:

- Family history of endocrine disorders
- Genetic mutations

### Review of Systems

As previously mentioned, the hormones produced in the endocrine system affect nearly every cell in the body. Because of this, a thorough and complete review of systems can aid in appropriate diagnosis, but also can assist in ruling out certain endocrinopathies. The most common manifestations revealed during the review of systems include:

- **Constitutional:** abnormal growth, sleep problems
- **Integumentary:** dry skin, change in hair or nails
- **HEENT:** exophthalmos, vision changes, goiter
- **Respiratory:** shortness of breath
- **Cardiovascular:** palpitations, night sweats, changes in blood pressure
- **Breasts:** nipple discharge, breast buds, gynecomastia
- **Gastrointestinal:** change in weight or appetite, constipation, diarrhea
- **Genitourinary:** increased urination, urination at night
- **Musculoskeletal:** pain, swelling, stiffness
- **Neurologic:** headache, tremor, fainting, brain anomaly
- **Endocrine:** temperature intolerance, sweating, increased thirst
- **Psychiatric:** anxiety, depression, change in mood

### Objective Findings

The physical examination of the child with an endocrine disorder is nonspecific in many cases and may reveal:

- Goiter
- Abnormal weight changes or other growth parameters
- Alterations in development
- Abnormal vital signs
- Changes in mood

## THYROID DISORDERS

The thyroid gland is a butterfly-shaped gland in the lower portion of the neck that sits over the top of the tracheal rings. The thyroid gland is responsible for production the thyroxine (T4) which is critical in the control of metabolism, growth, and development as well as cardiac and bone health. Thyroid diseases occur when the body produces too little (hypothyroid) or too much (hyperthyroid) thyroid hormone. In this section, we discuss hypo- and hyperthyroidism, and assessment, diagnosis, and management of these disorders.

## CONGENITAL HYPOTHYROIDISM

Congenital hypothyroidism (CH) is a treatable condition that has been screened in neonates in nearly all developed countries since the 1970s (Deladoëy Van Vliet & Giguère, 2015). If left untreated, it is one of the most common causes of mental retardation and growth delay in children. The typical screening of the newborn occurs within the first 24 to 48 hours of life and positive screening results occur in one in 2,500 babies.

The most common form of CH results from abnormal thyroid gland development (dysgenesis) in 85% of infants. Errors occurring in thyroid hormone biosynthesis (dyshormonogenesis) account for about 15% of primary hypothyroidism (Bona et al., 2015). CH should also be further identified as transient or permanent. Permanent CH should be considered in infants with TSH over 40 mIU/mL. Caregivers of children with permanent CH should be educated on the importance of medication adherence and the necessity of lifelong treatment (Wassner, 2018).

Transient CH is often diagnosed in infants with a TSH value between 20 to 39 mIU/mL. These babies have a temporary decrease in thyroid hormone production that usually resolves around 3 years of age (Wassner, 2018). Caregivers of children with transient CH should be educated on the importance of medication adherence and the necessity of treatment for the protection of critical brain development through the age of 3 years.

### Subjective Findings

The health history may reveal:

- Decreased activity
- Increased sleepiness
- Feeding difficulties
- Prolonged jaundice
- Constipation (Wassner, 2018)

### Risk Factors

Most instances of congential hypothyroidism are thought to be sporadic. The most common risk factors for congenital hypothyroidism are:

- Infantile gestation greater than 42 weeks
- Infants born to mothers with autoimmune thyroid disease

- Infants with increased iodine exposure or decreased maternal iodine exposure
- Infants with liver hemangiomas (Bona et al., 2015)
- Preterm infants
- Very low birth weight infants
- Twins (Olivieri, 2015)

## Review of Systems

The most common manifestations revealed during the review of systems include:

- **Constitutional:** feeding problems, sleepiness, poor linear growth
- **Integumentary:** dry skin
- **Respiratory:** respiratory distress
- **Cardiovascular:** palpitations, night sweats, changes in blood pressure
- **Gastrointestinal:** constipation
- **Neurologic:** brain anomaly, hoarse cry
- **Endocrine:** temperature intolerance, hypothermia, sweating, goiter

## Objective Findings

The physical examination of the child with CH may reveal:

- Swollen facies
- Large fontanels
- Macroglossia (large tongue)
- Umbilical hernia
- Lethargy
- Mottled skin
- Hypothermia
- Bradycardia (Kamat & Adam, 2018)

## Laboratory/Diagnostic Testing

The diagnosis of CH is rarely based upon the clinical findings. A newborn screening resulting in a TSH over 40 mIU/mL is justification for immediate treatment and referral to a pediatric endocrine specialist. If TSH result is less than 40 mIU/mL, the clinician may choose to delay treatment until serum results are obtained in 24 to 48 hours. If the resultant serum TSH at 3 to 5 days is greater than 20 mIU/mL, treatment should be started and continued through age 3 years to protect neurocognitive development (Wassner, 2018). Children with primary hypothyroidism can have hyperlipidemia noted on the laboratory evaluation.

## Differential Diagnosis

Because most industrialized countries have a newborn screening modality for the disease, differential diagnoses may not have to be considered. However, in those children with clinical manifestations that develop after birth or in the absence of newborn screening, the differential diagnosis for CH includes:

- Constitutional growth delay
- Short stature
- Malabsorption syndrome
- Growth hormone deficiency (GHD)
- Constipation
- Depression (Sinha & Bauer, 2016)

## Treatment/Management Plan

Families should be notified immediately of abnormal newborn screening results by the primary care provider, and advised about the necessity of a referral to a pediatric endocrine specialist. Due to the notable and rapid effects on neurocognitive development, replacement of thyroxine should be started once abnormal testing is confirmed. Babies are generally started on levothyroxine for replacement at a dose of 10 to 15 mcg/kg/day. The American Academy of Pediatrics (AAP and Pediatric Endocrine Society [PES], 2018) recommend an office follow-up with a pediatric endocrine specialist 1 to 2 weeks after starting levothyroxine and at intervals of 2 weeks until TSH has normalized. Once the TSH has normalized, repeat free T4 and thyrotropin levels should be obtained every 1 to 2 months until 6 months of age; every 3 to 4 months until 3 years of age; and then every 6 to 12 months until completion of growth. According to the AAP, a thyroid scan is optional, but will distinguish sporadic disease from familial goitrous thyroid dyshormonogenesis (Kamat & Adam, 2018).

## Family Education

Teach the following:

- Importance of medication adherence
  - Medication should be crushed and mixed in formula, breast milk, or water.
  - Providers should be notified if the infant is on a soy-based formula, as it may interfere with absorption.
- Anticipatory guidance regarding normal development with proper management and monitoring.

## Referral

Infants with CH should be referred within the first 1 to 2 weeks of life to a pediatric endocrine specialist for management.

## ACQUIRED HYPOTHYROIDISM

The most common cause of acquired hypothyroidism in children and adolescents is Hashimoto's thyroiditis. Hashimoto's thyroiditis is an autoimmune disorder that causes inflammation of the thyroid gland and over time ultimately leads to decreased production of thyroid hormone. Hypothyroidism occurs in one in 1,250 children and is usually permanent, requiring lifelong treatment with thyroxine replacement (AAP & PES, 2018).

Other causes of primary acquired hypothyroidism include surgery, radiation, or medication. Acquired hypothyroidism that results from pituitary anomaly is called secondary or central-acquired hypothyroidism. In this section, we discuss autoimmune-acquired hypothyroidism.

### Subjective Findings

The health history may reveal:

- Decreased activity/energy
- Fatigue
- Weight gain
- Constipation
- Dry skin

### Risk Factors

The most common risk factors for acquired hypothyroidism are:

- Genetic conditions such as Down, Noonan, DiGeorge, Williams, or Turner syndrome
- Additional autoimmune diseases, such as celiac disease and type 1 diabetes mellitus (DM)
- Positive family history
- Female gender
- Adolescent age (Vigone et al., 2018)

### Review of Systems

The most common manifestations revealed during the review of systems include:

- **Constitutional:** altered growth (particularly declining stature velocity), appetite changes, sleep problems
- **Integumentary:** hair loss
- **HEENT:** swelling in face or neck
- **Musculoskeletal:** pain, swelling, stiffness
- **Neurologic:** fainting
- **Endocrine:** cold intolerance
- **Psychiatric:** anxiety, depression, change in mood

### Objective Findings

The physical examination of the child with autoimmune acquired hypothyroidism may reveal:

- Goiter (pebbly or rubbery consistency)
- Weight gain related to fluid retention
- Poor growth
- Dry skin
- Swollen facies, coarse features
- Altered pubertal development for age
- Bradycardia
- Hypotension

### Laboratory/Diagnostic Testing

The diagnosis of autoimmune-acquired hypothyroidism is based upon clinical findings and laboratory evaluation. Upon seeing a child with suspicion for acquired hypothyroidism, the provider should evaluate biochemical markers including TSH and free T4. Thyrotropin levels will be elevated and free T4 levels will be low in those with overt hypothyroidism requiring treatment. In order to differentiate autoimmune-acquired hypothyroidism from other causes, a thyroid peroxidase antibody and/or thyroglobulin level can be assessed. A positive level is confirmatory of Hashimoto's thyroiditis (LaFranchi, 2020a).

### Differential Diagnosis

The differential diagnosis for autoimmune-acquired hypothyroidism includes:

- Sick euthyroidism
- Iodine deficiency
- Medication-induced hypothyroidism
- Radiation to thyroid
- Thyroid surgery

### Treatment/Management Plan

Thyroxine replacement is the first choice for treatment of autoimmune-acquired hypothyroidism. Recommendations for dosing vary with age and are also weight-dependent. Children with hypothyroidism should be managed by an endocrine specialist for close monitoring of growth and development. Initial doses for children with TSH over 10 mIU/mL can be administered in consultation with a pediatric endocrine specialist.

▶ ALERT: Extremely elevated TSH values (>50 mIU/mL) require modified dosing to avoid fluid retention. Rapid correction of thyrotropin values in the child who is severely hypothyroid can cause heart failure (Udovcic et al., 2017).

## Family Education

Teach the following:

- Importance of medication adherence
- Treatment may cause temporary behavior symptoms
- Full growth potential may not be restored in the child with short stature and marked bone age delay (LaFranchi, 2020a)

## Referral

Children with a TSH value over 50 mIU/mL should be referred urgently to a pediatric endocrine specialist. Children with TSH above the reference range and/or free T4 below reference range should be referred to a pediatric endocrine specialist. In cases of mild hypothyroidism, TSH 5–10 mIU/mL and no symptoms, consider repeat testing at 2 to 3 months before referring to a specialist.

**PRO TIP** In the obese child, mild elevations are seen in the TSH and typically do not require treatment if free T4 is normal.

# HYPERTHYROIDISM (GRAVES DISEASE)

Hyperthyroidism (Graves disease) is an overproduction of thyroxine from the thyroid gland. In most cases, hyperthyroidism is caused by an autoimmune process whereby the thyroid gland produces excess thyroid hormone as a result of the body's production of thyroid-stimulating antibodies. These antibodies also cause growth of the gland, resulting in a goiter. Hyperthyroidism results in many clinical manifestations that may be very subtle and cause symptoms for months or even years before diagnosis.

A distinguishing characteristic of Graves disease seen in 50% to 75% of individuals with hyperthyroidism is exophthalmos. This ophthalmopathy is not caused by high thyroxine levels, but rather by an inflammation of the extraocular muscles caused by the autoimmune process (LaFranchi, 2020b).

## Subjective Findings

The health history may reveal:

- Weight loss or failure to gain weight
- Stare (eyes appear widely open)
- Lid lag (sclera seen above iris when child looks down)
- Diarrhea
- Sweating
- Decreased attention
- Decreased school performance

## Risk Factors

The most common risk factors for hyperthyroidism are:

- Family history of autoimmune thyroid disease.
- Family history of autoimmune hypothyroidism
- Female gender (5:1)
- Older than 11 years
- Down syndrome
- Turner syndrome (LaFranchi, 2020b)

## Review of Systems

The most common manifestations revealed during the review of systems include:

- **Constitutional:** fatigue, poor sleep, increased appetite
- **Integumentary:** hair and nail changes
- **HEENT:** change in eye appearance, neck swelling
- **Cardiovascular:** fast heartbeat
- **Gastrointestinal:** increased stooling
- **Musculoskeletal:** weakness
- **Neurologic:** tremor, ataxia
- **Psychiatric:** anxiety, restlessness, mood swings

## Objective Findings

According to the PES guidelines, the physical examination of the child with hyperthyroidism may reveal:

- Warm or clammy skin
- Soft nails
- Thin hair
- Exophthalmos
- Lid lag
- Goiter (firm consistency)
- Tachycardia
- Widened pulse pressure
- Decreased muscle mass
- Tremors
- Tongue fasciculations (small contractions of muscle fibers)
- Hyperactive deep tendon reflexes (PES, 2019b)

## Laboratory/Diagnostic Testing

The diagnosis of hyperthyroidism is based upon laboratory testing that should include TSH, free T4, and T3. The typical laboratory pattern seen with hyperthyroidism is a significant elevation of the free T4 and T3 with suppression of the TSH. After confirming that a child is biochemically hyperthyroid, the clinician should investigate the possible cause of the condition.

If clinical manifestations do not include goiter and ophthalmopathy suggestive of Graves disease, the healthcare provider should order tests of serum antithyroid peroxidase antibody, thyroid-stimulating immunoglobulin (TSI), and antithyroglobulin antibodies. TSIs are measurable in at least 60% of individuals with Graves disease. Antithyroid antibodies are present in Graves disease, but are typically much more elevated in the thyrotoxic phase of autoimmune thyroiditis (LaFranchi, 2020b).

Another diagnostic test that can be utilized if the TSI is negative is the radioactive iodine uptake test and scan. Children with biochemical markers consistent with hyperthyroidism and negative antibodies should be referred to a pediatric endocrine specialist for ordering of this test.

## Differential Diagnosis

The differential diagnosis for hyperthyroidism includes:

- Thyroid storm

▶ ALERT: Fever and altered mental status seen with thyroid storm indicate a medical emergency.

- Thyrotoxic phase of autoimmune acquired hypothyroidism
- Toxic goiter
- Toxic nodule
- Tumor
- Thyroid hormone resistance
- Thyroid injury
- Medication-induced hyperthyroidism

## Treatment/Management Plan

There are several choices of treatment for the child with hyperthyroidism. Antithyroid medication, radioactive iodine therapy, and thyroidectomy are all considerations for treatment of hyperthyroidism. In most cases a child is started on antithyroid drug therapy in the hope that the child will achieve remission of the disease. The treatment of choice is methimazole, due to the severity of the side effects associated with propylthiouracil. Dosing recommendations range between 0.25 to 1 mg/kg/day. Daily dose is divided into two to three doses initially and is dependent upon the severity of the elevation of free T4 and size of the goiter. Treatment in children is suggested for at least 18 months to 2 years, with increased chance of remission in those who are treated for longer periods of time. Prior to initiating therapy the clinician should check serum white blood cells, alanine aminotransferase, aspartate aminotransferase, and gamma-glutamyl transpeptidase. Mild elevation of these values is not uncommon in the child with hyperthyroidism, and they provide a baseline for monitoring of medication-induced agranulocytosis and neutropenia, as well as hepatitis.

Radioactive iodine therapy is not recommended for children less than 10 years of age due to low risk of malignancies. Thyroidectomy, however, should be considered in children under the age of 5 years. Rates of remission are decreased in children of younger age (Ross et al., 2016).

**PRO TIP** Children with palpitations and tremors can be treated with beta-blockers for symptom management until thyroid hormone levels normalize. Atenolol is the drug of choice for symptom management and is typically dosed at 1 to 2 mg/kg/day.

### Family Education

Teach the following:

- Lifelong monitoring in children and adolescents with Graves disease is required.
- The recurrence of Graves hyperthyroidism is in children is variable.
- Most relapses will occur within 1 year of discontinuing antithyroid drugs.

### Referral

A provider who suspects that a child has hyperthyroidism should urgently refer the child to a pediatric endocrine specialist for evaluation and management.

# DIABETES MELLITUS

DM is one of the most commonly diagnosed chronic conditions in the pediatric population. DM is irregular metabolism of carbohydrates in the body, which results in hyperglycemia. DM results from abnormal secretion or utilization of insulin by the beta cells of the pancreas. DM is a comorbid condition associated with a number of different diseases, including cystic fibrosis, pancreatitis, Cushing disease, growth hormone excess, and glucagon-secreting tumors. Medications that can also cause diabetes include glucocorticoids, cyclosporine, tacrolimus, and atypical antipsychotic drugs (Levitsky & Misra, 2020).

The most common forms of diabetes are type 1 DM and type 2 DM. A total destruction of the beta cells through an autoimmune process defines the physiology of type 1 DM. Type 2 DM results in hyperglycemia due to resistance to insulin in addition to a deficiency in insulin production. Characteristics of the child and symptoms at presentation aid in distinguishing the two forms of DM.

## TYPE 1 DIABETES MELLITUS

Type 1 DM results in genetically susceptible individuals after one or more possible environmental factors initiates an autoimmune response resulting in pancreatic beta cell destruction (Pietropaolo, 2020). The destruction of these cells results in an absolute insulin deficiency, leading to hyperglycemia and requiring insulin administration. Environmental factors include viruses, perinatal factors, receipt of monoclonal antibodies, and dietary factors such as cow's milk and cereal consumption. The beta cell destruction occurs over a lengthy period (years), so children are asymptomatic for quite a while. Approximately 67% of children under the age of 19 years diagnosed with diabetes in the United States are diagnosed with type 1 DM. Annually, nearly 96,000 are estimated to develop type 1 DM worldwide (Mayer-Davis et al., 2018). About 30% of children with type 1 DM will have diabetic ketoacidosis at presentation (Glaser, 2020).

### Subjective Findings

Symptoms of type 1 DM are generally quite rapid in onset. The health history may reveal:

- Increased thirst
- Increased urination
- Increased appetite
- Weight loss
- Fatigue
- Nausea and/or vomiting

▶ ALERT: Children with symptoms of DM require urgent referral to a pediatric endocrine specialist.

### Risk Factors

The most common risk factors for the development of type 1 DM are:

- Having a first-degree relative with diabetes
- Non-Hispanic white ethnicity
- 4 to 6 years of age
- 10 to 14 years of age (Levitsky & Misra, 2020)

PRO TIP ★ In addition to the subjective findings listed previously, the following characteristics might assist the clinician in considering a diagnosis of type 1 DM:

- Acute, rapid presentation of symptoms
- Presenting with ketosis
- Lack of acanthosis nigricans
- Prepubertal

### Review of Systems

The most common manifestations revealed during the review of systems include:

- **Constitutional:** increased appetite, weight loss, fatigue
- **HEENT:** vision changes, fruity-smelling breath (diabetic ketoacidosis)
- **Respiratory:** shortness of breath (diabetic ketoacidosis)
- **Gastrointestinal:** abdominal pain
- **Genitourinary**: increased urination, nocturia, enuresis
- **Musculoskeletal:** weakness
- **Neurologic:** headache

PRO TIP ★ Children with type 1 DM often present with increased thirst and increased urination, including nocturia.

### Objective Findings

According to the PES guidelines, the physical examination of the child with type 1 DM may reveal:

- Tachypnea
- Tachycardia
- Dehydration
- Fruity breath smell
- Weight loss (PES, 2019a)

▶ ALERT: Children with signs and symptoms of ketosis (nausea, vomiting, abdominal pain, mental status change) should be immediately referred to the emergency room.

## Laboratory/Diagnostic Testing

The diagnosis of type 1 DM is based upon laboratory testing, including random blood glucose over 200 mg/dL or fasting blood glucose over 126 mg/dL. Urine ketones and glucose will be seen on a urinalysis in most children presenting with symptoms of type 1 DM. About 30% of the children and adolescents with new-onset type 1 DM will present with diabetic ketoacidosis (Levitsky & Misra, 2020). After conferring with a pediatric endocrine specialist, additional testing may be considered to assist in confirming a diagnosis of type 1 DM. Additional testing may include:

- Complete metabolic panel
- Hemoglobin (Hgb) A1c (>6.5%)
- Complete blood count
- C-peptide (low)
- Islet cell antibody profile (GAD-65, IA2, IAA, ZnT8)
- Oral glucose tolerance test (OGTT)

**PRO TIP** While Hgb A1c over 6.5% is consistent with a diagnosis of DM, the International Society of Pediatric and Adolescent Diabetes cautions against making a diagnosis of type 1 DM based on Hgb A1c alone (Mayer-Davis et al., 2018).

## Differential Diagnosis

The differential diagnosis for type 1 DM includes:

- Type 2 DM
- Medication-induced DM
- Stress-induced hyperglycemia
- Monogenic onset of DM of young (MODY)

## Treatment/Management Plan

For children with type 1 DM, insulin replacement is life-sustaining. Children who present with ketonuria should begin insulin therapy within 6 hours of testing in order to avoid metabolic decompensation and ketoacidosis (Danne et al., 2018). There are a number of insulin management regimens that should be considered for the child with type 1 DM. Considerations for treatment choice should include insulin needs, age of child, diet, exercise/sports schedule, and duration of diabetes.

One option for insulin administration is a regimen of basal-bolus therapy (BBT) or multiple daily injection therapy. BBT involves a combination of long-acting insulin or basal insulin and short-acting insulin or bolus insulin in a subcutaneous injection. Another method to achieve the basal-bolus regimen is via an insulin pump, which provides children with a continuous infusion of short-acting insulin (basal). The pump is also utilized for boluses of insulin with meals and hyperglycemia. BBT is intended to mimic the physiological insulin profile, as doses are adjusted for carbohydrate intake (Danne et al., 2018). Consultation with a pediatric endocrine specialist at diagnosis will accelerate appropriate care and dosing of insulin for the child. The goals of insulin treatment are normalization of blood sugar to achieve euglycemia when fasting.

In addition to insulin therapy, blood glucose monitoring is a key component of diabetes management. Improved glycemic control is associated with increased frequency of blood glucose monitoring. Recommendations for blood glucose testing is four or more times a day, usually before meals and snacks, before bedtime, prior to exercising, or any time the blood glucose may be low (Riddle et al., 2020). Another option for self-monitoring of blood glucose is continuous glucose monitoring.

## Family Education

Teach the following:

- Type 1 DM is an autoimmune disease that requires insulin administration for regulation of blood sugar and prevention of ketoacidosis.
- Children with type 1 DM should be seen by a pediatric endocrine specialist for management and evaluation of Hgb A1c every 3 months.
- Children with type 1 DM are recommended to test blood sugar at least four times a day.
- Parents must have an active role in the management of type 1 DM throughout childhood and as the child gets older, until the child can become independent in self-care.
- Children in school will need a DM plan discussed with the school nurse and teacher.
- Children who have type 1 DM can live normal lives, participate in sports, grow and develop normally.

## Referral

Primary care providers are often the first to see children with symptoms of diabetes, most commonly polyuria, polyphagia, and polydipsia. Children with suspicion for type 1 diabetes should be referred to a pediatric endocrine specialist. Children with fingerstick blood glucose levels of 200 or greater should be immediately referred to a local diabetes specialist, preferably with direct provider communication so as not to delay treatment. If ketones are present or the child is extremely dehydrated or appears ill, they should be referred to the ER immediately (Dayton & Silverstein, 2016).

## TYPE 2 DIABETES MELLITUS

Type 2 DM is a condition in which the body develops a resistance to insulin and an overall decrease in insulin production. This decrease in the efficacy of insulin results in hyperglycemia. The pathogenesis of type 2 DM is complicated, as there are a number of risk factors, such as genetics, environment, and possible beta-cell destruction. We know that type 2 DM is more commonly associated with the obese child. However, obesity is not a distinct characteristic that differentiates between type 1 DM and type 2 DM, as type 1 diabetics can be obese. Moreover, the child with type 2 DM is more likely to have acanthosis nigricans, which is an indicator of insulin resistance, than the obese child with type 1 DM. The evidence does suggest that type 2 DM in children has different features than in adults: i.e., in children it seems to have more rapidly progressive decline in beta cell function and accelerated complications of DM (Riddle et al., 2020).

Although the incidence of childhood obesity seems to have stabilized, there continues to be a rise in incidence of type 2 DM. The SEARCH for Diabetes in Youth study showed that in children 10 to 19 years of age, the incidence of DM increased between 2002 and 2012 from nine per 100,000 to 12.5 per 100,000, respectively (Mayer-Davis et al., 2017). Almost 80% of children diagnosed with type 2 diabetes are obese, and 10% are overweight (Laffel & Svoren, 2020).

### Subjective Findings

While nearly half of children and adolescents with type 2 DM have no symptoms, the health history may reveal:

- Increased thirst
- Increased urination
- Night-time urination
- Weight gain or weight loss
- Darkening of the skin
- Vaginal discharge or vulvovaginitis, in adolescent girls

### Risk Factors

The most common risk factors for type 2 DM are:

- Obesity
- Positive family history
- Female gender
- ethnicity; children of Native American, African American, Hispanic, Asian American, and Pacific island descent are at increased risk for the development of type 2 DM
- Children born to mothers with diabetes or gestational diabetes and females with polycystic ovarian syndrome are also at increased risk

### Review of Systems

The most common manifestations revealed during the review of systems include:

- **Constitutional:** fatigue, overweight or obese
- **Integumentary:** skin darkening (acanthosis nigricans)
- **HEENT:** blurry vision
- **Breasts:** gynecomastia in males and prepubertal girls
- **Gastrointestinal**: abdominal pain
- **Genitourinary:** increased urination, urination at night
- **Neurologic:** headache
- **Psychiatric:** behavior problems, mood changes

### Objective Findings

The physical examination of the child with type 2 DM may reveal:

- Overweight/obese
- Acanthosis nigricans
- Females: vaginal discharge or vulvovaginitis

PRO TIP Only 5% to 12% of children with diabetic ketoacidosis on presentation have type 2 DM.

### Laboratory/Diagnostic Testing

The diagnosis of type 2 DM is based upon the clinical findings and laboratory or diagnostic testing. Children over age 10 years or with onset of puberty (whichever occurs earlier), with a body mass index (BMI) ≥85% *and* risk factors (as listed previously; Laffel & Svoren, 2020; Riddle et al., 2020) should be screened. If results are normal, these children should be retested a minimum of every 3 years or more often if BMI is increasing (Laffel & Svoren, 2020; Riddle et al., 2020). Diagnosis of type 2 DM may be made based on any of the following:

- Hgb A1c greater than or equal to 6.5% (48 mmol/mol; should be certified by the National Glycohemoglobin Standardization Program)
- Random plasma blood glucose greater than or equal to 200 mg/dL

- Fasting plasma blood glucose >126 mg/dL
- Oral glucose tolerance test >200 mg/dL at 2 hours (Laffel & Svoren, 2020)

In the obese child or adolescent, evaluate for comorbidities with these additional laboratory tests:

- Liver function test with gamma-glutamyl transpeptidase
- 25-OH Vitamin D
- TSH with reflex free T4
- Fasting lipid profile

**PRO TIP** Hgb A1c less than 6.5% in a child with signs/symptoms of DM does not exclude the diagnosis. A second test should be done to confirm the diagnosis.

## Differential Diagnosis

The differential diagnosis for type 2 DM includes:

- Type 1 DM
- Medication-induced DM
- Stress-induced hyperglycemia
- MODY
- Pre-DM
    - Hgb A1c 5.7 to 6.4%
- Impaired fasting glucose
    - Fasting blood glucose between 100 and 125 mg/dL
- Impaired glucose tolerance
    - Plasma blood glucose ≥140 to 199 mg/dL on an OGTT

## Treatment/Management Plan

As mentioned previously, almost all children with type 2 DM are overweight or obese. Excess weight contributes to insulin resistance. Weight reduction of 7% to 10% has been associated with an improvement in insulin sensitivity and secretion (American Diabetes Association [ADA], 2019). Weight management and lifestyle modification are the first steps in treatment of the child with type 2 DM. While the ideal treatment team for a child with this diagnosis is multidisciplinary, including an endocrine specialist, nurse educator, dietitian, and mental health professional, primary care clinicians should begin providing anticipatory guidance on weight management at the time of referral to an endocrinologist.

Consultation with a registered dietitian who specializes in pediatrics is recommended to assist in developing goals for weight management. Most children with type 2 DM should have goals set to achieve a reduction in weight. Although the BMI will decrease with weight maintenance as children grow, most children with type 2 DM are severely obese, warranting an intense approach to weight management. In addition to dietary management, the primary care provider should encourage increasing physical activity to at least 1 hour daily and decreasing screen time to less than 2 hours a day.

Metformin is the first-line medication in treatment of children and adolescents with type 2 DM. According to the ADA, the TODAY study found that nearly half of the children who were prescribed metformin for management of type 2 DM achieved glycemic control (2019).

Due to the high incidence of complication and/or comorbidities associated with type 2 DM, the primary care provider should evaluate children with diabetes for signs and symptoms of nephropathy, neuropathy, retinopathy, nonalcoholic fatty liver disease, obstructive sleep apnea, and cardiovascular disease. Identification of polycystic ovarian syndrome in the female adolescent should also be considered.

## Family Education

Teach the following:

- Children with BMI >85% and at least one other risk factor will be screened for type 2 DM at minimum every 3 years.
- Lifestyle modification should be a priority. Providers should screen families for psychosocial barriers to implementation of lifestyle changes, such as food insecurity, stable housing, and access to safe areas for physical activity.
- Additional testing for complications associated with type 2 DM is warranted.
- Depressive symptoms and disordering eating are not uncommon in children and adolescents with type 2 DM. Mental health concerns should be addressed immediately if observed by the family (ADA, 2019).

## Referral

All children with type 2 DM should be referred to a pediatric endocrine specialist for management and evaluation. Children with an identified comorbid condition should be referred to the appropriate specialist.

# GROWTH DISORDERS

The most common causes of short stature and inappropriate puberty in children are familial or constitutional growth delay. In order to know which children should be evaluated for a growth disorder, it is important to have a good understanding of normal growth expectations. Linear growth velocity and mid parental height are reliable indicators for determination of inappropriate growth in children. There are a number of medical concerns that should be in the differential diagnosis list for the child with short stature and inappropriate puberty.

Height predictions are based upon genetic potential and can be calculated using the following equations:

- *For girls*: [father's height in inches –5 + mother's height]/2
- *For boys*: [mother's height in inches +5 + father's height]/2

Most children between the age of 3 and pubertal entry will grow about an inch every 6 months, or 2 inches a year (Richmond & Rogol, 2020b). This is a normal growth rate that should allow the child to maintain a growth percentile. In this section we discuss causes of poor growth, including constitutional delay of growth and puberty (CDGP), GHD, and precocious puberty.

## GROWTH HORMONE DEFICIENCY

GHD is a rare condition that results in inadequate production and secretion of growth hormone. Children with GHD have a slowed growth velocity leading to growth failure. GHD can be congenital, acquired, or idiopathic in nature (a disorder that arises from an unknown cause; Levy & Head, 2016). A child may have a history of neonatal hypoglycemia or prolonged neonatal jaundice. In general, GHD is caused by genetic mutations or processes within the body that affect hypothalamic or pituitary function (Richmond & Rogol, 2020c).

### Subjective Findings

The health history may reveal:

- Poor growth
- Short stature
- Small penis
- Decreased energy levels

### Risk Factors

The most common risk factors for GHD are:

- Family history and history of brain surgery
- Brain anomaly
- Brain injury
- Brain radiation

### Review of Systems

The most common manifestations revealed during the review of systems include:

- **Constitutional:** decreased energy levels
- **Integumentary:** abnormal fat distribution for age with increase in abdominal fat
- **HEENT:** immature look of facies
- **Psychiatric:** anxiety, mood changes

### Objective Findings

The physical examination of the child with GHD may reveal:

- Growth failure
- Severely short stature
- Delayed bone age
- Immature facies
- Immature voice
- Underdeveloped nasal bridge
- Frontal bossing (prominent, protrusion) of skull
- Abnormal distribution of fat described as "infantile" or "orange peel"
- Delayed puberty
- Sparse or thin hair

### Laboratory/Diagnostic Testing

The diagnosis of GHD is based upon clinical findings with confirmation through a growth hormone stimulation test ordered by a pediatric endocrine specialist. Insulin-like growth factor-1 (IGF-1) and insulin-like growth factor binding protein-3 (IGFBP-3) may be low. Children with severe growth failure should undergo a bone-age x-ray for confirmation of delay. Additional laboratory testing can be ordered, but should be done in consultation with an endocrine specialist. Confirmation of GHD is done via provocative testing (any test that is done to trigger or cause a suspected disorder), but initial evaluation will include investigation of potential underlying organic causes of poor growth and short stature (Levy & Head, 2016).

**PRO TIP** Growth hormone (GH) is secreted in a pulsatile fashion; therefore, random sampling of blood for GH level is inadequate to aid in diagnosis.

### Differential Diagnoses

The differential diagnoses for GHD include:

- Insufficiency nutrition leading to growth delay
- Prolonged glucocorticoid treatment leading to growth failure

- Gastrointestinal disease
- Rheumatologic disease
- Chronic kidney disease
- Severe heart disease
- Type 1 DM
- Hypothyroidism
- CDGP
- Genetic syndromes (Turner syndrome, SHOX mutations, Noonan, Russell-Silver, skeletal dysplasia)
- Idiopathic short stature
- Familial short stature
- History of small height for gestational age
- Growth hormone insensitivity

### Treatment/Management Plan

Children with a diagnosis of GHD should be prescribed recombinant growth hormone under the supervision of a pediatric endocrine specialist. Doses of growth hormone are determined based on weight, growth response, and laboratory test evaluation. Frequent follow-up, every 3 to 6 months, with an endocrine specialist is necessary for appropriate dosing.

#### Family Education

Teach the following:

- GHD is a medical indication for growth hormone treatment/replacement.
- Growth hormone assists in achieving normal growth, but also has a number of metabolic effects that are important throughout the life span, including support of metabolism, bone health, and heart health. Children with complete GHD may require lifelong hormone replacement.

#### Referral

Children with concerns for poor growth and clinical characteristics of GHD should be referred to a pediatric endocrine specialist.

## CONSTITUTIONAL DELAY OF GROWTH AND PUBERTY

CDGP is a variation of normal growth. These children are also known as "late bloomers." Children with this condition usually have a family history positive for CDGP and may also have a low normal growth velocity until puberty begins. The typical age of entry into puberty or breast development for girls with CDGP is 12 years of age and menarche by 16 years. Boys with CDGP generally do not have testicular enlargement, the hallmark sign of puberty, until 14 years of age and can have continued growth beyond age 16 years.

> **PRO TIP** Tanner staging of secondary sex characteristics, such as pubic hair, is not indicative of pubertal entry.

### Subjective Findings

The health history may reveal:

- Short stature
- Reported poor growth
- Poor appetite

#### Risk Factors

The most common risk factors for CDGP are positive family history of "late bloomers."

#### Review of Systems

The most common manifestations revealed during the review of systems include:

- **Constitutional:** abnormal growth with poor weight gain
- **Psychiatric:** anxiety, depression

### Objective Findings

The physical examination of the child with CDGP may reveal:

- Height below the third percentile
- Low normal growth velocity
- Underweight/low BMI
- Immature appearance
- Delayed dental development

#### Laboratory/Diagnostic Testing

The diagnosis of CDGP is based upon the clinical findings of short stature, pubertal delay, and positive family history. A bone-age x-ray can be obtained to confirm suspicion for CDGP. A bone age delayed more than 1 year from the chronological age supports the diagnosis.

### Differential Diagnosis

The differential diagnosis for CDGP includes:

- Insufficiency of nutrition leading to growth delay
- Prolonged glucocorticoid treatment leading to growth failure

- Gastrointestinal disease
- Rheumatologic disease
- Chronic kidney disease
- Severe heart disease
- Type 1 DM
- Hypothyroidism
- GHD
- Genetic syndromes (Turner syndrome, SHOX mutations, Noonan, Russell-Silver, skeletal dysplasia)
- Primary hypogonadotropic hypogonadism (Richmond & Rogol, 2020a)

### Treatment/Management Plan

The child with CDGP should be reassured that their development is normal. Observation of the child with serial measurements of height and pubertal progression over 1 to 2 years is a reasonable approach and can assist in clarifying the diagnosis (Crowley & Pitteloud, 2020). Treatment for the child with CDGP should be reserved for those with significant pubertal delay or those with psychosocial detriment due to the delay. For girls over the age of 12 years, pubertal initiation can be achieved with estradiol therapy. Administration of testosterone via intramuscular injection, for a period of 6 months at low doses, will often provide a pubertal "jump start" in boys older than 14 years.

Deficiencies in nutrition should be addressed with referral to a registered pediatric dietitian for further education on healthy ways to increase calories in the growing child. Nutrition is important in timing of puberty. Some studies have shown that increased adipose tissue correlates to earlier puberty in girls, just as low levels of adiposity, such as seen in children with low BMIs or intense athletes, can delay puberty (Villamoor & Jansen, 2016).

### Family Education

Teach the following:

- Children with a family history of "late bloomers" will generally follow genetics.
- Children with CDGP can develop normally and grow to a normal adult height without intervention.
- Psychosocial detriment related to delayed puberty and short stature is a reason to consider initiation of puberty with a pediatric endocrine specialist.
- Adequate caloric intake is necessary for normal growth and development.

### Referral

A referral to a pediatric endocrine specialist is warranted in children who desire pubertal initiation with hormone therapy.

**PRO TIP** From start to finish, puberty takes about 4 years to complete. Children without progression of puberty over a 2-year span should be referred to a pediatric endocrine specialist for evaluation.

## PRECOCIOUS PUBERTY

The development of secondary sexual characteristics in children younger than the mean for sex is considered precocious. In general, girls with breast development prior to age 8 years and testicular enlargement in boys prior to age 9 define precocious puberty. However, variations in the mean age of pubertal entry seem to exist across race/ethnicity and body mass index (BMI) (Harrington & Palmert, 2020).

Precocious puberty is most commonly central in nature (CPP) with early activation of the hypothalamic pituitary axis. However, peripheral precocious puberty can occur from excess secretion of sex hormones from the gonads or adrenal glands, or exogenous exposure to hormones. Nearly 90% of CPP in girls and 60% in boys is idiopathic in nature; other cases may result from lesions in the central nervous system.

Early onset of puberty can lead to short stature, as increased production of sex hormones results in advancement of the bone age and decreases the overall duration of growth in a child (Guaraldi et al., 2016). Psychosocial issues can also arise, including difficulty in school and with peers due to uncontrollable emotional lability. However, there are no studies that show a correlation between CPP and long-term psychological or behavioral problems.

### Subjective Findings

The health history may reveal:

- Rapid growth
- Acne
- Pubic hair
- Underarm hair
- Body odor
- Breast development

## Risk Factors

The most common risk factors for central precocious puberty are:

- Positive family history
- Female gender
- African-American ethnicity

## Review of Systems

The most common manifestations revealed during the review of systems include:

- **Constitutional:** rapid growth, increased sleep, change in weight or appetite
- **Integumentary:** oily skin, acne
- **Breasts:** breast buds, gynecomastia
- **Neurologic:** headache
- **Psychiatric:** change in mood, emotional lability

## Objective Findings

The physical examination of the child with precocious puberty may reveal:

- Tall for age
- Body odor
- Axillary hair
- Pubic hair
- Tanner stage II breasts (boys may also have breast buds)
- Estrogenized vaginal mucosa
- Phallic enlargement
- Testicular volume ≥4 mL

## Laboratory/Diagnostic Testing

The diagnosis of precocious puberty is based upon the clinical findings. Confirmation of precocious puberty can be accomplished with a bone-age x-ray that is 2 or more years advanced. However, children with benign premature adrenarche (early development of pubic and/or underarm hair) can also have an advanced bone age. Progressive adrenarche or bone age above two standard deviations beyond chronological age should undergo laboratory testing. Laboratory testing should be completed in the morning and consist of a luteinizing hormone, follicle-stimulating hormone, and estradiol or testosterone test. This evaluation allows for determination of the activity of the hypothalamic-pituitary axis.

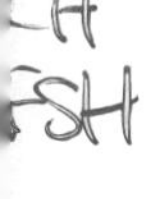

A brain magnetic resonance imaging scan with contrast should be obtained on all boys with CPP and girls with signs of puberty prior to age 6 years, since higher rates of central nervous system anomalies are seen in these groups. A pelvic ultrasound can be helpful in distinguishing central precocious puberty from premature thelarche (breast development) in girls without clear biochemical and physical evidence of puberty.

**PRO TIP** For children whose physical examination is not consistent with laboratory test results, a gonadotropin-releasing hormone stimulation test can be performed by a pediatric endocrine specialist.

## Differential Diagnoses

The differential diagnoses for central precocious puberty include:

- Premature thelarche—isolated breast development, normal height velocity, normal bone age, absence of other characteristics of puberty
- Premature adrenarche—appearance of axillary and/or pubic hair, body odor, acne
- Peripheral precocious puberty

## Treatment/Management Plan

Puberty can be halted using a gonadotropin-releasing hormone agonist (GnRHa) to preserve final adult height if treatment is initiated at the appropriate time (Eugster, 2019). Treatment should be reserved for girls younger than age 6 years to get the most benefit for adult height. All boys with a compromised height should be considered for treatment. Generally, girls who are treated with GnRHa remain on treatment until bone age is approximately 12 years or height is near 60 inches. Boys are treated until bone age of 13 years is reached or height is near 64 inches (Eugster, 2019).

Parental anxiety regarding menarche often leads to request for administration of GnRHa to delay menses. Reassurance should be provided to parents experiencing anxiety and discussion of options for menstrual management should be considered.

## Family Education

Teach the following:

- Precocious puberty is defined by breast development in girls prior to age 8 years and testicular enlargement in boys prior to age 9 years.
- Preservation of adult height is the most common reason to consider treatment for early puberty, because children with precocious development stop growing.
- Psychosocial issues and parental anxiety alone are not indications for treatment.

**PRO TIP** Children with developmental delay and signs of early puberty may be candidates for treatment with GnRHa and should be referred to a pediatric endocrine specialist.

### Referral

Referral should be made to a pediatric endocrine specialist for the girl with breast development prior to age 8 years and for the boy with testicular enlargement prior to age 9 years.

## ADRENAL INSUFFICIENCY

Inadequate production and release of adrenocortical hormones defines adrenal insufficiency. Adrenocortical hormones are produced in the adrenal cortex and include glucocorticoids, mineralocorticoids, and adrenal androgens. These hormones play a critical role in maintaining whole-body homeostasis, especially during times of stress. For example, one role of glucocorticoids (i.e., cortisol) is to convert protein to carbohydrates for regulation of blood sugar. Additionally, mineralocorticoids, such as aldosterone, assist in regulation of electrolyte balance, which aids in blood pressure maintenance (Donohoue, 2018).

## PRIMARY ADRENAL INSUFFICIENCY

Primary adrenal insufficiency is manifested by problems with production of glucocorticoids, mineralocorticoids, and adrenal androgens within the adrenal cortex. The most common cause of primary adrenal insufficiency in infants is congenital adrenal hyperplasia (CAH), but older children could have adrenal insufficiency as a result of autoimmune disease caused by antiadrenal antibodies. Other possible causes of adrenal insufficiency in children and adolescents are tuberculosis, adrenoleukodystrophy, adrenomyeloneuropathy, or late-onset adrenal hyperplasia (Donohoue, 2018).

▶ ALERT: Babies are screened for CAH on the newborn screen, as many are asymptomatic at birth. However, salt-wasting CAH can precipitate adrenal crisis and is more commonly missed in boys. Infant girls may present with ambiguous genitalia and no other overt symptoms of adrenal insufficiency.

## CENTRAL ADRENAL INSUFFICIENCY

Central adrenal insufficiency can result from a decrease in release of adrenocorticotropic hormone (ACTH) from the pituitary or decrease in production of corticotropin-releasing hormone (CRH) from the hypothalamus. The inadequate production of these hormones results in glucocorticoid deficiency, but not mineralocorticoid deficiency; therefore, symptoms may vary slightly from primary adrenal insufficiency (Donohoue, 2019).

### Subjective Findings

The health history may reveal:

- Salt craving (primary)
- Weight loss (primary)
- Fatigue
- Nausea and vomiting
- Morning headaches
- Dizziness (primary)

### Risk Factors

The specific causes of adrenal insufficiency seem to vary by population; thus the incidence of overall primary adrenal insufficiency is unknown. Risk factors seem to be associated with genetic mutations and prior diagnosis of autoimmune disease, although children with prolonged endogenous exposure to corticosteroids are also at risk (Bornstein et al., 2016).

### Review of Systems

The most common manifestations revealed during the review of systems include:

- **Constitutional:** anorexia
- **Integumentary:** hyperpigmentation of the skin (chronic adrenal insufficiency)
- **Gastrointestinal:** nausea, vomiting
- **Genitourinary:** decreased urination, ambiguous genitalia (infant)
- **Musculoskeletal:** weakness

### Objective Findings

The physical examination of the child with adrenal insufficiency may reveal:

- Failure to thrive
- Lethargy
- Hypotension

- Dehydration
- Tachycardia
- Precocious puberty (late-onset CAH)

▶ ALERT: Clinical and laboratory findings of adrenal crisis are dehydration, hypotension, shock, acute abdominal pain, fever, lethargy, mental status change, hyponatremia, hyperkalemia, and hypoglycemia. Children displaying these symptoms should be seen for care in the emergency department.

## Laboratory/Diagnostic Testing

The diagnosis of adrenal insufficiency is based upon the clinical findings of fatigue, nausea and vomiting, morning headaches, low blood sugar, low blood pressure, and failure to thrive. Diagnosis of primary adrenal insufficiency can be made with a laboratory test result of low *morning* serum cortisol and elevated ACTH. Confirmation of suspicions for primary adrenal insufficiency occurs with failure of a corticotropin stimulation test, which is considered the gold standard test for the diagnosis and is done upon consultation of a pediatric endocrine specialist (Bornstein et al., 2016).

Secondary or central adrenal insufficiency will be confirmed with low cortisol and low ACTH levels on serum testing.

## Differential Diagnosis

The differential diagnosis for adrenal insufficiency includes:

- Chronic fatigue syndrome
- Depression
- GHD

## Treatment/Management Plan

Treatment of adrenal insufficiency involves hormone replacement. Glucocorticoid replacement is life-sustaining in children with deficiency. Children will be prescribed hydrocortisone three times a day at doses equivalent to physiologic replacement (7–10 mg/m$^2$). Children with confirmed mineralocorticoid deficiency should be treated with fludrocortisone and infants with mineralocorticoid deficiency should receive sodium chloride supplementation for the first year of life.

Frequent follow-up, every 3 to 6 months (depending on age) with a pediatric endocrine specialist for assessment of growth, blood pressure, and general health is recommended.

▶ ALERT: Children and adolescents who are subjected to physiologic stress will require additional doses of glucocorticoids, up to 50 mg/m$^2$. Children who are unable to tolerate oral medication should be given the glucocorticoid as an injection (Donohoue, 2019).

## Family Education

Teach the following:

- Replacement of glucocorticoids and in some cases mineralocorticoids is life-sustaining in children with adrenal insufficiency.
- Children who are stressed with illness or injury will require additional doses of glucocorticoid and should receive an injection if unable to tolerate oral medication.
- Frequent follow-up with a pediatric endocrine specialist is necessary for long-term management of the condition.
- Genetic counseling may be warranted upon receiving diagnosis for identification of risks to other family members.

## Referral

Children who may have adrenal insufficiency should be referred immediately to a pediatric endocrine specialist.

## KEY POINTS

- Newborns with suspicion for hypothyroidism should have a serum blood test for TSH and free T4, and it is urgent that they be referred to a pediatric endocrine specialist.
- The best laboratory evaluation for determination of hypothyroidism after the newborn period includes TSH, free T4, and thyroid antibodies tests.
- Type 1 DM is an autoimmune condition that causes destruction of the insulin-producing beta cells in the pancreas, resulting in an absolute deficiency in insulin production, which requires insulin administration via injection or insulin pump.
- Type 2 DM is caused by the body's resistance to insulin effects in addition to a decrease in insulin secretion. Most children who have type 2 DM are overweight or obese.

- GHD is a medical condition that requires treatment for adequate growth, metabolism, bone health, and heart health.
- With constitutional delay, optimizing nutrition and caloric intake is a necessary step in promoting growth in children.
- Precocious puberty refers to girls with breast development prior to age 8 years and testicular enlargement in boys prior to age 9.
- All newborns are screened for CAH on the newborn screen. Girls may present with ambiguous genitalia, but boys will likely be asymptomatic at birth.

## REFERENCES


American Academy of Pediatrics and Pediatric Endocrine Society. (2018). *Pediatric endocrinology fact sheet: Acquired hypothyroidism in children: A guide for families*. https://downloads.aap.org/dosp/acquired_hypothyroidism.pdf

American Diabetes Association. (2019). 13. Children and adolescents: Standards of medical care in diabetes—2019. *Diabetes Care, 42*(S1), S148–S164. https://doi.org/10.2337/dc19-S013

Bona, G., Bellone, S., Prodam, F., & Monzani, A. (2015). Etiology of congenital hypothyroidism. In G. Bona, F. De Luca, & A. Monzani (Eds.), *Thyroid diseases in childhood: Recent advances from basic science to clinical practice* (pp. 27–32). Springer.

Bornstein, S., Allolio, B., Arlt, W., Barthel, A., Don-Wauchope, A., Hammer, G., Husebye, E., Merke, D., Murat, M. H., Stratakis, C., & Torpy, D. (2016). Diagnosis and treatment of primary adrenal insufficiency: An Endocrine Society clinical practice guideline. *Journal of Clinical Endocrinology and Metabolism, 101*(2), 364–389. https://doi.org/10.1210/jc.2015-1710

Crowley, W., & Pitteloud, N. (2020). Approach to the patient with delayed puberty. *UpToDate*. Retrieved October 24, 2020, from https://www.uptodate.com/contents/approach-to-the-patient-with-delayed-puberty

Danne, T., Phillip, M., Buckingham, B., Jarosz-Chbot, P., Saboo, B., Urakami, T., Battelino, T., Hanas, R., & Codner, E. (2018). ISPAD Clinical Practice Consensus Guidelines 2018: Insulin treatment in children and adolescents with diabetes. *Pediatric Diabetes, 19* (27), 115–135. https://doi.org/10.1111/PEDI.12718

Dayton, K., & Silverstein, J. (2016). What the primary care provider needs to know to diagnose and care for adolescents with type 1 diabetes. *The Journal of Pediatrics, 179*, 249–256. http://doi.org/10.1016/j.jpeds.2016.08.077

Deladoëy Van Vliet, G., & Giguère, Y. (2015). Neonatal screening for congenital hypothyroidism: What it has taught us about thyroid and brain development. In G. Bona, F. De Luca, & A. Monzani (Eds.), *Thyroid diseases in childhood: Recent advances from basic science to clinical practice* (2015, pp. 33–42). Springer Publishing Company.

Donohoue, P. (2018). Diagnosis of adrenal insufficiency in children. *UpToDate*. Retrieved October 24, 2020, from https://www.uptodate.com/contents/diagnosis-of-adrenal-insufficiency-causes-in-children

Donohoue, P. (2019). Causes and clinical manifestations of primary adrenal insufficiency in children. *UpToDate*. Retrieved October 24, 2020, from https://www.uptodate.com/contents/causes-and-clinic-manifestations-of-primary-adrenal-insufficiency-in-children

Endocrine Society. (2020). *The endocrine system*. https://www.hormone.org/what-is-endocrinology/the-endocrine-system

Eugster, E. (2019). Treatment of central precocious puberty. *Journal of the Endocrine Society, 3*(5), 965–972. https://doi.org/10.1210/js.2019-00036

Glaser, N. (2020). Clinical features and diagnosis of diabetic ketoacidosis in children and adolescents. *UpToDate*. Retrieved October 23, 2020, from https://www.uptodate.com/contents/clinical-features-and-diagnosis-of-diabetic-ketoacidosis-in-children-and-adolescents

Guaraldi, F., Guglielmo, G., Gori, D., & Ghizzoni, L. (2016). Management of endocrine disease: Long-term outcomes of the treatment of central precocious puberty. *European Journal of Endocrinology, 174*(3), R79–R87. https://doi.org/10.1530/EJE-15-0590

Harrington, J., & Palmert, M. (2020). Definition, etiology and evaluation of precocious puberty. *UpToDate*. Retrieved October 23, 2020, from https://www.uptodate.com/contents/definition-etiology-and-evaluation-of-precocious-puberty

Kamat, D., & Adam, H. (2018). *Quick reference guide to pediatric care* (2nd ed.). American Academy of Pediatrics.

Laffel, L., & Svoren, B. (2020). Epidemiology, presentation and diagnosis of type 2 diabetes mellitus in children and adolescents. *UpToDate*. Retrieved October 23, 2020, from https://www.uptodate.com/contents/epidemiology-presentation-and-diagnosis-of-type-2-diabetes-mellitus-in-children-and-adolescents

LaFranchi, S. (2019). Approach to acquired goiter in children and adolescents. *UpToDate*. Retrieved October 23, 2020, from https://www.uptodate.com/contents/approach-to-acquired-goiter-in-children-and-adolescents

LaFranchi, S. (2020a). Acquired hypothyroidism in childhood and adolescence. *UpToDate*. Retrieved October 23, 2020, from https://www.uptodate.com/contents/acquired-hypothyroidism-in-childhood-and-adolescence

LaFranchi, S. (2020b). Clinical manifestations and diagnosis of Graves disease in children and adolescents. *UpToDate*. Retrieved October 23, 2020, from https://www.uptodate.com/contents/clinical-manifestations-and-diagnosis-of-graves-disease-in-children-and-adolescents

Levitsky, L. L., & Misra, M. (2020). Epidemiology, presentation, and diagnosis of type 1 diabetes mellitus in children and adolescents. *UpToDate*. Retrieved October 23, 2020, from https://www.uptodate.com/contents/epidemiology-presentation-and-diagnosis-of-type-1-diabetes-mellitus-in-children-and-adolescents

Levy, R., & Head, J. (2016). *Growth hormone deficiency*. https://rarediseases.org/rare-diseases/growth-hormone-deficiency

Mayer-Davis, E., Kahkosa, A., Jefferies, C., Dabelea, D., Balde, N., Gong, C., Aschner, P., & Craig, M. (2018). ISPAD Clinical Practice Consensus Guidelines 2018: Definition, epidemiology and classification of diabetes in children and adolescents. *Pediatric Diabetes, 19*(Suppl. 27), 7–19. https://doi.org/10.1111/PEDI.12773

Mayer-Davis, E., Lawrence, J., Dabelea, D., Divers, J., Isom, S., Dolan, L., Imperatore, G., Linder, B., Marcovina, S., Pettit, D., Pihoker, C., Saydah, S., & Wagernknecht, L. (2017). Incidence trends of type 1 and type 2 diabetes among youths, 2002–2012. *New England Journal of*

*Medicine, 376*(15), 1419–1429. https://doi.org/10.1056/NEJMoa1610187

Olivieri, A. (2015). Epidemiology of congenital hypothyroidism. In G. Bona, F. De Luca, & A. Monzani (Eds.), *Thyroid diseases in childhood: Recent advances from basic science to clinical practice* (pp. 53–63). Springer.

Pediatric Endocrine Society. (2019a). *Child with suspected hyperglycemia.* https://mk0pesendoklgy8upp97.kinstacdn.com/wp-content/uploads/2020/09/Child-with-suspected-hyperglycemia-final-1.pdf

Pediatric Endocrine Society. (2019b). *Child with suspected hyperthyroidism.* https://pedsendo.org/clinical-resource/child-with-suspected-hyperthyroidism

Pietropaolo, M. (2020). Pathogenesis of type 1 diabetes mellitus. *UpToDate.* Retrieved October 24, 2020, from https://www.uptodate.com/contents/pathogenesis-of-type-1-diabetes-mellitus

Richmond, E. J., & Rogol, A. D. (2020a). Causes of short stature. *UpToDate.* Retrieved October 23, 2020, from https://www.uptodate.com/contents/causes-of-short-stature

Richmond, E. J., & Rogol, A. D. (2020b). Diagnostic approach to children and adolescents with short stature. *UpToDate.* Retrieved March 22, 2020, from https://www.uptodate.com/contents/diagnostic-approach-to-children-and-adolescents-with-short-stature

Richmond, E. J., & Rogol, A. D. (2020c). Diagnosis of growth hormone deficiency in children. *UpToDate.* Retrieved October 23, 2020, from https://www.uptodate.com/contents/diagnosis-of-growth-hormone-deficiency-in-children

Riddle, M., Bakris, G., Blonde, L., Boulton, A., D'Alessio, D., DiMeglio, L., Gonder-Frederick, L., Hood, K., Hu, F., Kahn, S., Kaul, S., Leiter, L., Moses, R., Rich, S., Rosentstock, J., & Wylie-Rossett, J. (Eds.). (2020). Diabetes technology: Standards of medical care in diabetes—2020. *Diabetes Care, The Journal of Clinical and Applied Research and Education, 43*(Suppl. 1), 577–588. https://doi.org/10.2337/dc20-S007

Ross, D., Burch, H., Cooper, D., Greenlee, C., Laurberg, P., Maia, A., Rivkees, S., Samuels, M., Sosa, J., Stan, M., & Walter, M. (2016). 2016 American Thyroid Association guidelines for diagnosis and management of hyperthyroidism and other causes of thyrotoxicosis. *Thyroid, 26*(10), 1343–1421. https://doi.org/10.1089/thy.2016.0229

Sinha, S. K., & Bauer, A. J. (2016). *Pediatric hypothyroidism.* https://reference.medscape.com/article/922777-overview

Udovcic, M., Pena, R., Patham, B., Tabatabai, L., & Kansara, A. (2017). Hypothyroidism and the heart. *Methodist Debakey Cardiovascular Journal, 13*(2), 55–59. https://doi.org/10.14797/mdcj-13-2-55

Vigone, M., Capalbo, D., Weber, G., & Salerno, M. (2018). Mild hypothyroidism in childhood: Who, when, and how should be treated. *Journal of the Endocrine Society, 2*(9), 1024–1039. https://doi.org/10.1210/js.2017-00471

Villamoor, E., & Jansen, E. (2016). Nutritional determinants of the timing of puberty. *Annual Review of Public Health, 37*, 33–36. https://doi.org/10.1146/annurev-publhealth-031914-122606

Wassner, A. (2018). Congenital hypothyroidism. *Clinics in Perinatology, 45*(1), 1–18. https://doi.org/10.1016/j.clp.2017.10.004

# Management of Genetic Disorders

Holly Lydigsen

## Student Learning Outcomes

**Upon completion of this chapter the reader should be able to:**

1. Discuss pathophysiology and epidemiology of selected genetic disorders in children.
2. Differentiate subjective and objective findings of selected genetic disorders in children.
3. Choose appropriate laboratory or diagnostic tests for particular genetic disorders in children.
4. Utilize the differential diagnosis process to determine genetic diagnosis in children.
5. Determine treatment plan, child/family education, and need for referral in children with a genetic diagnosis.

## INTRODUCTION

In general, genetic disorders are rare; however, it is estimated that approximately 10,000 different genetic conditions exist and affect millions of people worldwide (World Health Organization [WHO], 2020). A genetic disorder occurs when there is a pathogenic change or a biological change (such as imprinting) to the DNA structure. Genetic disorders are complex and diverse. Some of the pathogenic and biological changes that result in genetic disorders include chromosomal; mitochondrial; Mendelian (autosomal recessive, autosomal dominant, and X-linked); inborn errors of metabolism; and alterations to the DNA due to mechanisms such as deletion, duplication, imprinting, and methylation (Nussbaum et al., 2016).

Children and adolescents with genetic disorders often require the help of a primary care clinician as well as a multidisciplinary team. Advanced practice nurses need to be aware of signs and symptoms of a possible genetic disorder, when to refer to a pediatric geneticist, and how to find resources on disorders. This chapter covers only a few different disorders, including a few types of chromosomal anomalies, Mendelian disorders, inborn errors of metabolism, and one disorder of nonclassical inheritance.

The content in this chapter maps to the following areas on the Pediatric Nursing Certification Board (PNCB) Pediatric Nurse Practitioner—Primary Care certification examination:

**CLINICAL PROBLEMS: GENETICS**

CONTENT AREAS:

**II. Assessment and Diagnosis**

**B. History and Physical Examination**

1. Obtain history of present illness
2. Obtain a comprehensive health history for new patients
3. Complete an interval history for established patients

The author would like to thank the following experts who offered advice for this chapter:
Eniko K. Pivnick, MD, Medical Genetics, Le Bonheur Children's Hospital, Memphis, TN; and
Nora A. Urraca, MD, PhD, Medical Genetics, Le Bonheur Children's Hospital, Memphis, TN.

4. Perform a review of systems
5. Perform a complete physical examination

**C. Diagnostic Testing and Screening**

1. Order and interpret office/clinic based screening tests
2. Order and interpret diagnostic laboratory tests
3. Order and interpret the results of diagnostic imaging tests

**D. Analyzing Information**

1. Integrate health history and physical examination findings into the plan of care
2. Assimilate findings from screening and diagnostic testing into plan of care

**E. Diagnosis**

1. Develop and prioritize differential diagnoses
2. Establish a diagnosis based on evaluation of patient data

### III. Management

**A. Child and Caregiver Counseling and Education**

1. Provide condition-specific counseling and education, including treatment options
2. Educate about benefits and potential adverse reactions of pharmacological interventions
3. Discuss non-pharmacological interventions
4. Counsel regarding the threshold for seeking follow-up care
5. Review the risks of non-adherence to recommended treatment

**B. Therapeutic Interventions**

1. Prescribe pharmacologic agents
2. Recommend the use of over-the-counter pharmacologic agents
3. Order or recommend non-pharmacologic treatments for the management of symptoms
4. Discuss use of complementary and alternative therapies as appropriate

**C. Procedures**

1. Perform procedures in accordance with diagnostic guidelines and plan of care (rapid tests)
2. Initiate life-saving techniques in response to urgent or emergent situations

**D. Collaboration and Referral**

2. Refer to specialists as indicated for evaluation, counseling, and/or treatment

**E. Care Coordination**

1. Facilitate patient and family-centered care for children of all ages with acute and chronic conditions

**F. Evaluation and Follow-up**

2. Establish a plan for follow-up care

### IV. Professional Role Responsibilities

**A. Leadership and Evidence-based Practice**

4. Develop, implement, and/or modify clinical practice guidelines

## GENERAL APPROACH TO CHILD WITH A GENETIC DISORDER

A pediatric genetic examination usually includes a head-to-toe assessment with special attention to any unusual (dysmorphic) physical features and changes to growth and development. When assessing for syndromic features, it is important to consider ethnicity and family traits. Whenever a child has a birth defect, physical abnormality, delayed growth or development, or an acute illness without explanation, referral to a pediatric geneticist should be considered (Seibert et al., 2016).

### Subjective Findings

The health history may reveal:

- Prenatal history
- Gestational age
- Difficulties during pregnancy (including any miscarriages and/or stillbirths), any medications or illnesses during pregnancy
- Birth growth parameters (height, weight, and head circumference)
- Past history of illnesses and hospitalizations
- Developmental history (including delays or regression)
- Food avoidances
- History of seizures or birth defects
- Family history of any birth defect, developmental delay, developmental regression, learning problems, or cognitive impairment, early age of onset for a disease, reproductive problems (multiple miscarriages and stillbirths)

Also, create a three-generation family pedigree (Seibert et al., 2016; Figure 38.1).

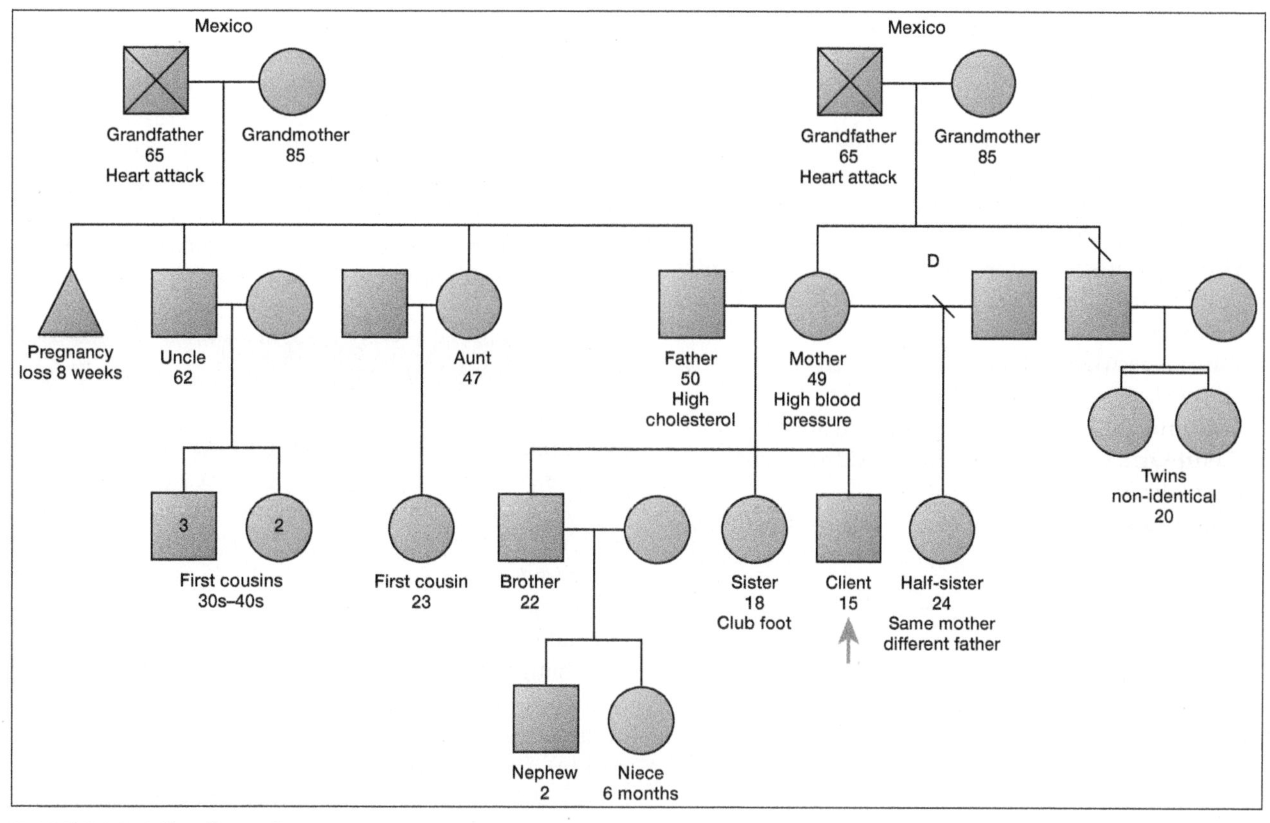


FIGURE 38.1 Family pedigree.

*Source*: Reproduced with permission from *Understanding genetics: A New York, Mid-Atlantic guide for patients and health professionals*. http://ncbi.nlm.nih.gov/books/NBK115557

## Recurrence Risk

An estimated recurrence risk of a genetic disorder is dependent on the child's diagnosis and the family pedigree. When a disorder is caused by a single gene defect, recurrence risk can be predicted based on Mendel's principle of segregation and the mode of inheritance.

Briefly, for autosomal dominant disorders with one affected heterozygous parent, there is a 50% chance of having an affected offspring for each pregnancy; notably, some autosomal dominant disorders are lethal with two copies of the mutated gene, meaning that for these disorders affecting childbearing, individuals have only a single mutated allele (i.e., are heterozygous) and each parent is heterozygous for the same mutated allele. With autosomal recessive disorders with a carrier mother and father, there is a 25% chance of having an affected child, a 50% chance of having a carrier, and a 25% chance of having an unaffected noncarrier child. For X-linked inheritance with a carrier mother, there is a 50% chance of having an affected male and 50% chance of having a female carrier for each pregnancy. For fathers with an X-linked condition, 100% of daughters will be carriers and no sons will be carriers or affected. Females may be affected due to skewed X-linked inactivation. When predicting recurrence risk of Mendelian disorders, it is important to consider the risk *for each pregnancy*; thus, while two carriers have a 25% chance of conceiving a child with an autosomal recessive disorder, it is possible that four out of four children in a family could be affected. For chromosomal disorders, recurrence risk will vary based on the specific diagnosis. For disorders with complex inheritance (heart defects, neural tube defects, cleft lip/palate), an estimated recurrence risk is given based on the family history and empirical risks for the disorder (Firth & Hurst, 2017). To locate genetic services, see the American College of Medical Genetics site: https://clinics.acmg.net.

### Review of Systems

The most common manifestations revealed during the review of systems include:

- **Constitutional**: abnormal growth and/or development, congenital abnormality
- **Integumentary:** history of rashes, poor wound healing, birth marks
- **HEENT:** unusual features not consistent with family or ethnicity, vision and/or hearing problems, feeding problems
- **Cardiovascular:** history of heart defect
- **Respiratory:** unexplained lung disease
- **Gastrointestinal:** history of structural abnormalities
- **Genitourinary:** history of urinary, kidney, genital anomalies
- **Musculoskeletal:** history of unexplained fractures, weakness, missing/extra digits, or missing all or a segment of an extremity
- **Neurologic:** seizures, developmental delay or regression, learning problems, unusual cry, behavioral problems or changes
- **Psychiatric:** mental health problems (Seibert et al., 2016)

### Objective Findings

The physical examination of the child with a genetic disorder may reveal:

- Short/tall stature, failure to thrive (FTT)/obesity, changes in growth velocity, looks different from family
- Hypotonia/hypertonia, abnormal reflexes, poor coordination
- Macro/microcephaly, abnormal head and/or face shape, frontal bossing, asymmetrical facial features, highly arched eyebrows, synophrys (unibrow), abnormal hair line, long eyelashes, different eye shape/size/spacing, coloboma, nystagmus, ptosis, epicanthal folds, abnormal nose shape, abnormal ear shape/appearance/position, ear pits or creases, smaller or more prominent features (eyes, ears, jaw), abnormal or high palate, bifid uvula, unusually shaped teeth, crowded teeth, abnormal dentition pattern, short/webbed neck
- Abnormally spaced nipples, pectus abnormalities, other breast abnormalities (e.g., underdeveloped breasts in pubescent female, gynecomastia in males)
- Hernia, protruding/distended abdomen, hepatomegaly, splenomegaly
- Inguinal hernia, small or large genitals, ambiguous genitalia, hypospadias, undescended testes, abnormal hair development, imperforate anus
- Hypermobile joints, contractures of joints, skeletal disproportion, pes planus (flat feet), syndactyly, polydactyly, ectrodactyly, clinodactyly (curved pinkie finger), single transverse crease, deep creases on palmar or plantar surfaces, scoliosis, kyphosis
- Extra skin folds, hyperelastic skin, axial freckling, six or more café-au-lait spots, hypopigmented and hyperpigmented skin areas, neurofibromas, sparse hair, hirsutism, abnormal nails (Seibert et al., 2016)

# CHROMOSOMAL DISORDERS

Humans have 46 chromosomes. Chromosome pairs one through 22 are autosomal (non-sex chromosomes) and the 23rd pair is made up of the sex chromosomes (Clarke, 2020). Therefore, a "normal" male karyotype is 46, XY (22 pairs of autosomes, 1 X chromosome, and 1 Y chromosomes) and females with 46, XX (22 pairs of autosomes and 2 X chromosomes). Chromosomal abnormalities include genetic disorders that are a result of a change in the expected number of chromosomes or in their structure. Numerical abnormalities can result in an extra set of 23 chromosomes (triploidy or tetraploidy), but most commonly are the result of an addition or deletion of an entire chromosome (aneuploidy) or just part of a chromosome. Some common chromosomal anomalies include: trisomy 21 (Down syndrome [DS]), trisomy 18 (Edwards' syndrome), trisomy 13 (Patau syndrome), monosomy X (Turner syndrome [TS]), 47XXY* (*among other chromosomal variants, Klinefelter syndrome [KS]), and XXX syndrome (Jones et al., 2014).

## DOWN SYNDROME

DS is a chromosomal disorder that occurs in 1 in 800 newborns and affects males and females, racial and ethnic groups equally. DS is the most common genetic cause of intellectual disability and results in characteristic facial features, cognitive impairment, hypotonia, and other birth defects due to the additional genetic material from an extra copy of chromosome 21 (Genetics Home Reference [GHR], 2020a). Ninety-five percent of DS cases occur because all cells have three copies of chromosome 21 (trisomy 21), due to nondisjunction (failure of the chromosomes to separate) during meiosis. Translocation of chromosome 21 (extra chromosome 21 is attached to another chromosome) occurs in 3% to 4% of cases, and mosaicism (in which some cells have a third copy of chromosome 21, and some cells have the expected two copies due to nondisjunction that occurs during mitosis) occurs in 1% to 2% of cases (Bull & Committee on Genetics [COG], 2011). The features of DS are similar for trisomy 21, translocation DS, and mosaic DS; therefore, chromosome analysis is recommended for all children with DS to provide genetic counseling and determine recurrence risk.

Children with DS have a higher incidence of ear infections and sinusitis, and experience an increased incidence of morbidity due to respiratory infections. Despite an increased incidence of leukemia, children with DS respond well to treatment. Polycythemia may be noted if the child has chronic sleep apnea. High altitude pulmonary edema is more common is children with DS. They also demonstrate an increased response to psychoactive medications (Bull & COG, 2011).

## Subjective Findings

The family health history may reveal:

- History of miscarriages (translocation 21, also known as "familial Down syndrome")
- Decreased fetal movement in utero due to hypotonia
- Abnormalities on prenatal screening or ultrasound result
- Delayed developmental milestones (Bull & COG, 2011)

### Recurrence Risk

Recurrence risk depends on the mother's age, the child's karyotype, and the parental karyotypes if the child has a translocation form of DS. For a mother who is 30 years of age or older, the risk of having a child with trisomy 21 increases with her age (Samson-Fang & Goldman-Luthy, 2019). The reason for this is that during oogenesis, the process of meiosis halts during Prophase 1 and the homologous chromosomes remain paired until oogenesis resumes at the time of maturing an individual egg. For older mothers, the homologous chromosomes have been paired longer and are more difficult to separate, and thus are more prone to nondisjunction.

ALERT: Approximately 4% of children have DS due to a translocation of chromosome 21. In this case, parental karyotypes are recommended to provide recurrence risk counseling. Accurate diagnosis by karyotype and genetic counseling is essential.

## Review of Systems

The most common manifestations revealed during the review of systems include:

- **Constitutional:** smaller size/growth difficulties, sleep problems, feeding difficulties
- **HEENT:** vision problems (60%), hearing problems (75%), frequent ear infections and respiratory infections, delayed dental eruption, and hypodontia (23%)
- **Cardiovascular:** heart defect (50% risk)
- **Endocrine:** hypothyroidism (4% to 18%, risk increases with age)
- **Gastrointestinal:** gastroesophageal reflux disease, constipation, Hirschsprung's syndrome, celiac disease, gastrointestinal atresia
- **Neurologic:** hypotonia, developmental delay, autism spectrum disorder, behavioral problems, seizures
- **Hematological:** leukemia, polycythemia, transient myeloproliferative disorder, anemia, iron deficiency (Bull & COG, 2011)

## Objective Findings

The physical examination of the child with DS may reveal:

- Smaller for growth parameter (plot all growth on special growth charts for DS (Centers for Disease Control and Prevention, 2019)
- Microcephaly or brachycephaly
- Up-slanting palpebral fissures, epicanthal folds
- Nystagmus
- Midface hypoplasia, depressed nasal bridge
- Smaller mouth, protruding tongue
- Dental abnormalities such as delayed eruption of teeth, small and missing teeth
- Low-set ears/posteriorly rotated ears
- Excessive skin at nape of neck
- Noisy breathing/referred upper airway sounds
- Heart murmur
- Single palmar creases on hands, sandal gap on feet, acquired hip dysplasia, hypotonia (Bull & COG, 2011; Figure 38.2)

PRO TIP Narrow ear canals can make visualization of tympanic membranes challenging; therefore, a smaller speculum may be required.

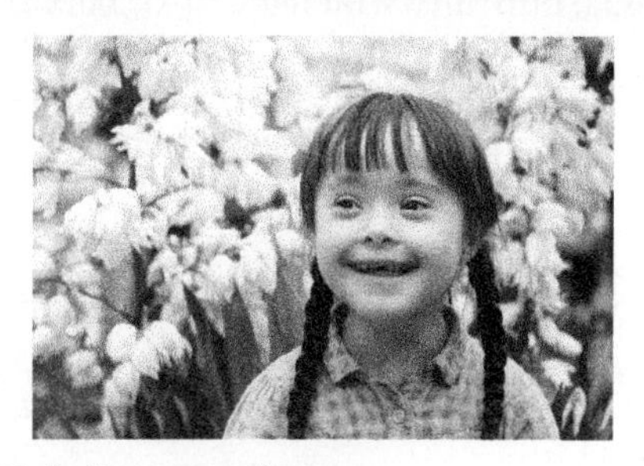

FIGURE 38.2 Down syndrome.

## Laboratory/Diagnostic Testing

The diagnosis of DS may be based upon clinical findings; however, it is important to confirm by a karyotype an organized picture of all the chromosomes. A karyotype will confirm diagnosis of DS and distinguish between trisomy 21, translocations, and mosaicism (by comparing chromosome counts in different cells) and is essential for providing parents with accurate counseling on recurrence risk (Firth & Hurst, 2017). If only thyroxine (T4) is completed through the state newborn screening program, obtain a thyroid-stimulating hormone (TSH) concentration to evaluate for congenital hypothyroidism (Bull & COG, 2011).

**PRO TIP** Use a karyotype; do not complete a chromosomal microarray (CMA) for diagnosis of DS, as CMA cannot detect balanced chromosomal rearrangements.

### Differential Diagnosis

The differential diagnosis for DS includes:

- Microdeletion or microduplication disorder
- Physical features (such as upward-slanting eyes) may be a familial trait

### Treatment/Management Plan

Guided by the American Academy of Pediatrics (AAP), recommendations for children from prenatal to 21 years of age include:

- Electrocardiogram (ECG) and echocardiogram (ECHO) completed by a pediatric cardiologist prior to discharge after birth
- If the child has a congenital heart defect, monitor for signs and symptoms of congestive heart failure at all visits
- Obtain a swallow assessment if the child has marked hypotonia, difficulty with feeding, or failure to thrive (FTT)
- Eye examination at birth, annually from 1 to 5 years, every 2 years from 5 to 13 years, then every 3 years from 13 to 21 years of age
- Hearing assessment at birth
- Audiology and otolaryngology assessment at 6 months, 12 months, and annually
- History and examination for duodenal or anorectal atresia at birth
- At every visit, ask about constipation and evaluate dietary intake; consider hypotonia, hypothyroidism, gastrointestinal anomalies, Hirschsprung's disease
- Screen for hypothyroidism at birth, 6 months, 12 months, and annually
- Hemoglobin annually
- Discuss atlantoaxial instability with parents and monitor for evidence of myopathy at every visit; cervical x-rays for preparticipation (sports) examination
- Assess for symptoms of obstructive sleep apnea at every visit; consider polysomnography
- Screen for celiac disease annually starting at 1 year of age
- Assess for developmental progress and refer to local early childhood interventions services at birth
- Assess for behavioral issues from age 1 year and throughout childhood
- Establish optimal dietary and physical exercise patterns throughout childhood
- Discuss physical and psychosocial changes through puberty, need for gynecologic care in pubescent female, sexual development, and sexual behavior during adolescence and after
- Facilitate transition: guardianship, financial planning, behavioral problems, school placement, vocational training, independence with self-care from 13 years and older (Bull & COG, 2011)

## Family Education

Teach the following:

- Counsel on diagnosis and recurrence risk (or refer to genetics).
- Provide information on common health considerations and treatment and management recommendations as described by the AAP.
- Discuss the importance of early intervention services (physical, occupational, and speech therapies).
- Provide routine childhood vaccinations, including influenza.
- Consider prophylaxis for respiratory syncytial virus (dependent upon comorbidities).
- Stress the importance of cervical spine support and positioning due to possibility of atlantoaxial instability (Bull & COG, 2011).
- Refer family to support groups, such as:
  - National Association for Down Syndrome—www.nads.org
  - National Down Syndrome Congress: www.ndsccenter.org
  - National Down Syndrome Society: www.ndss.org

▶ ALERT: Parent should contact pediatrician if neck pain, changes in bladder or bowel habits, change in gait, or other symptoms of spinal cord compression occur, due to the possibility of atlantoaxial instability. Prompt referral to an pediatric orthopedic surgeon or pediatric neurosurgeon is recommended.

### Referral

Refer to a pediatric geneticist for appropriate testing and counseling as needed and early intervention services at birth and/or diagnosis. Also, refer to cardiology, audiology, ophthalmology, otolaryngology, endocrinology, neurology, gastroenterology, nutrition, orthopedics, and hematology for baseline studies as appropriate based on the child's history and findings on physical examination.

## TURNER SYNDROME

Turner syndrome (TS) is a chromosomal anomaly that occurs only in females. TS occurs in about 1 in 2,000 to 2,500 liveborn girls worldwide and is a result of partial or complete loss (monosomy) of one copy of the X chromosome. Clinical presentation is widely variable due to mosaicism. Common characteristics include short stature; cardiac, skeletal, and kidney abnormalities; lymphedema; and reproductive problems (early loss of ovarian function and infertility). Most females have normal intelligence; however, developmental delay, learning disabilities, and behavioral problems may occur. About one-third of affected children are diagnosed in the neonatal period, one-third in childhood, and one-third in adolescence (GHR, 2020f). TS is usually not inherited and has a population frequency of 0.4 in 1,000 live births (Clarke, 2020).

### Subjective Findings

The health history may reveal:

- Developmental delay and/or learning problems
- Abnormal tooth eruption
- Delayed puberty, absence of menarche, infertility (GHR, 2020g)

### Review of Systems

The most common manifestations revealed during the review of systems include:

- **HEENT:** vision problems (amblyopia, strabismus, ptosis, refractive errors), recurrent ear infections, sensorineural hearing loss
- **Cardiovascular:** cardiac abnormalities (congenital heart defects, aortic root dilatation/dissection, ischemic heart disease and cerebrovascular disease)
- **Gastrointestinal:** gastroesophageal reflux disease, celiac disease, transaminitis
- **Genitourinary:** renal abnormalities (horseshoe kidney, hypoplasia, renal ectopia), ambiguous genitalia
- **Musculoskeletal:** vitamin D deficiency, osteoporosis, history of fractures
- **Neurologic:** neurocognitive issues (intellectual disability in about 10%, learning disabilities)
- **Endocrine:** hypothyroidism, autoimmune thyroiditis, metabolic syndrome (obesity, glucose intolerance), pubertal delay/ovarian insufficiency (Shankar & Backeljauw, 2017).

▶ ALERT: Cardiac abnormalities are the cause of early mortality.

### Objective Findings

The physical examination of the child with TS may reveal:

- Short stature (most common finding in TS)
- Down-slanted palpebral fissures, epicanthal folds
- Short, broad, webbed neck
- Narrow palate, micrognathia
- Low-set ears
- Heart murmur
- Lymphedema of hands/feet
- Delayed puberty, decreased breast and body hair development
- Scoliosis, kyphosis, pes planus, pectus excavatum (Shankar & Backeljauw, 2017)

### Laboratory/Diagnostic Testing

The diagnosis of TS is based upon result of karyotype analysis of (45, X) or in mosaicism (45, X/46, XX) (Firth & Hurst, 2017). For karyotype results: 45, X or 45,X/46,XY, additional genetic testing for presence of the sex-determining region Y protein (SRY) should be completed.

### Differential Diagnosis

The differential diagnosis for TS includes:

- Familial short stature
- Madelung deformity (abnormal growth of the wrist)
- SHOX gene mutation (resulting in short stature)
- Noonan syndrome (NS)
- Mayer-Rokitansky-Kuster-Hauser syndrome (genetic disorder resulting in absence of the uterus and vagina)
- Congenital adrenal hyperplasia (Firth & Hurst, 2017)

### Treatment/Management Plan

Treatment of TS requires a multidisciplinary approach. Initial evaluations are recommended at diagnosis with surveillance ongoing. These include:

- Pediatric genetics evaluation.
- Cardiology evaluation and diagnosis and ongoing screening/management (ECHO, cardiac magnetic resonance imaging [MRI], ECG).
- Otolaryngology/audiology evaluation starting at 9 to 12 months of age, treatment of middle ear infections, placement of myringotomy tubes if needed, and audiology follow-up every 5 years.
- Pediatric ophthalmology evaluation by 12 to 18 months, and minimum annual follow-up.
- Dental evaluation for abnormal tooth eruption and crown abnormalities at diagnosis, and then at least annually.
- Pediatric endocrinology referral for evaluation of thyroid function, glucose intolerance, and growth hormone treatment (recommended at 4–6 years or sooner). Monitoring of gonadotropins (yearly at about 11 years of age prior to induction of puberty) and estrogen/progestin replacement therapy. Counseling on fertility preservation options and induction of puberty.
- Gastroenterology evaluation for signs/symptoms of inflammatory bowel disease (abdominal pain, weight loss, diarrhea, or gastrointestinal bleed). Screening for celiac disease at 2 to 3 years and at least every 2 years after that. Monitoring of liver function starting at 10 years of age, then annually.
- Kidney ultrasound at diagnosis to assess for horseshoe kidney, hypoplasia, and renal ectopia.
- Orthopedic evaluation for scoliosis (annual examination for scoliosis or every 6 months if on growth hormone therapy), kyphosis, vertebral wedging, pes planus, cubitus valgus, pectus excavatum, patellar laxity (assess for skeletal abnormalities at 5–6 years of age and at 12–14 years of age), vitamin D deficiency (screen at 9–11 years and every 2–3 years after that), osteoporosis, and increased fracture risk (DEXA scans after adult hormone replacement has been initiated and every 5 years after that).
- Dermatology for evaluation of changes in melanocytic nevi (Shankar & Backeljauw, 2017).
- Low self-esteem, depression, and anxiety should be addressed early on.

### Family Education

Teach the following:

- Provide counseling on recurrence risk and associated health problems.
- Inform that most women with TS lead independent lives.
- Educate that the majority of women with TS are infertile (Firth & Hurst, 2017).
- Refer family to support groups:
  - Turner Syndrome Foundation: https://turnersyndromefoundation.org
  - Turner Syndrome Society of the United States: www.turnersyndrome.org
  - Turner Syndrome Support Society: www.tss.org.uk

### Referral

Refer all girls with suspected TS to clinical genetics and pediatric endocrinology. Additional referrals (as warranted by the clinical manifestations the girl is experiencing) may include pediatric, cardiology, orthopedics, ophthalmology, otolaryngology, gastroenterology, dentist, and dermatology. The girl with TS may also be referred to a gynecologist.

## KLINEFELTER SYNDROME

KS is a chromosomal condition that affects approximately 1 in 650 males of all racial and ethnic groups and can affect both physical and intellectual development (GHR, 2020c). At least one additional X chromosome is always present; boys with KS most commonly have the karyotype 47,XXY but other variants exist (48,XXXY; 48,XXYY). KS is not inherited. It is thought that the extra X chromosome occurs early in embryogenesis as a result of a nondisjunction error. The extra copy of multiple genes on the X chromosome is thought to be responsible for the clinical manifestations seen with KS (GHR, 2020c). Many individuals with KS have mild features and are never diagnosed.

### Subjective Findings

The health history may reveal:

- Difficulty with coordination and motor skills
- Difficulty with learning, language delay
- Delayed/incomplete puberty
- Gynecomastia (GHR, 2020c)

### Risk Factors

Advanced parental age has been linked to increased risk of KS, and postfertilization nondisjunction occurs in approximately 10% of individuals (Radicioni et al., 2010).

### Review of Systems

The most common manifestations revealed during the review of systems include:

- **Musculoskeletal:** difficulty with coordination and motor skills, hypotonia
- **Neurologic:** developmental delay, learning difficulties, dyslexia, attention deficit, autistic behaviors
- **Endocrine:** delayed-onset or incomplete puberty, breast development, smaller testes after puberty
- **Immunological:** autoimmune disorders
- **Psychiatric:** low self-esteem, mood disorders, anxiety, behavioral problems (GHR, 2020c)

### Objective Findings

The physical examination of the child with KS may reveal:

- Tall stature
- Broad lips
- Sparse body hair
- Gynecomastia
- Small testes, small penis, bifid scrotum, cryptorchidism, inguinal hernia, hypospadias
- Fifth finger clinodactyly (curved pinky finger)
- Reduced upper to lower segment ratio
- Pes planus (flat feet)
- Hypotonia
- Speech and language difficulties/neurodevelopmental disorders (Radicioni et al., 2010)

▶ ALERT: Further evaluate the boy with cryptorchidism and a mild developmental disorder for the presence of KS.

### Laboratory/Diagnostic Testing

The diagnosis of KS is based upon karyotype result of 47,XXY or in mosaicism (47, XXY/46, XY) (GHR, 2020c).

### Differential Diagnosis

The differential diagnosis for KS includes:

- Familial tall stature
- Another chromosomal anomaly
- Other disorder causing hypogonadism, such as Kallman syndrome (Defendi, 2020)

### Treatment/Management Plan

*Infancy and Childhood:*

- Physical examination and assessment of growth parameters and testes.
- Development and learning evaluation and support.

*Adolescence and Adulthood:*

- Annual physical examination and assessment of growth parameters, blood pressure, testes, gynecomastia, varicose veins.
- Neuropsychology evaluation.
- Dual-energy x-ray absorptiometry DEXA) scan (a bone mineral density test), vitamin D, serum calcium phosphate levels initially, then every 2 years. Provide treatment for osteoporosis, if needed.
- Monitor for the development of metabolic syndrome, type 2 diabetes, hypertension, and/or autoimmune disorders.

### Family Education

Teach the following:

- Support groups can be very helpful:
  - Association for X and Y Chromosome Variations: https://genetic.org/variations/about-47xxy
  - The Focus Foundation: https://thefocusfoundation.org/x-y-chromosomal-variations/xxy
- Counsel about genetic etiology, recurrence risk, and recommended management

### Referral

Refer to clinical genetics/pediatric endocrinology for measurement of sex hormone levels, ultrasound of testes, and initiation of testosterone replacement therapy (TRT) as needed.

Refer to developmental pediatrics and early intervention (if under age 3). Refer to urology for scrotal and penile anomalies.

## MENDELIAN SYNDROMES

Mendelian syndromes are single-gene (monogenic) disorders that usually follow a pattern of inheritance in families but can also be a result of new (*de novo*) changes in an individual, such as those due to errors in normal cellular processes (e.g., replication error) or exposure to mutagens in the environment.

Autosomal dominant and recessive conditions are due to a change on an autosome (chromosomes 1–22), whereas X-linked disorders are due to a change on the X chromosome. *Autosomal dominant* conditions require only one copy of a gene with a pathogenic change. *Autosomal recessive* conditions are due to two pathogenic changes (mutations) in a gene; affected individuals are usually children of parents who are both carriers of the disorder. Autosomal recessive conditions are more common in people who are consanguineous (biologically related). X-linked disorders have a more severe effect on males, since they have only a single X chromosome. This results in a single X-linked recessive mutation that causes disease in males who are hemizygous for the X chromosome. Likewise, X-linked dominant disorders are more likely to be lethal in males than in females. The effects of X-linked dominant disorders vary in females due to skewed X-linked inactivation; some females have a disproportionate percentage of activated X chromosomes with the pathogenic change (Nussbaum et al., 2016).

## NOONAN SYNDROME

NS is an inherited disorder that occurs in 1 in 1,000 to 2,500 individuals (GHR, 2020e). There is no gender, racial, or ethnic predisposition and symptoms are widely variable among affected individuals, even within the same family. NS is a multisystem disorder that results in heart defects, bleeding problems, distinctive facial features, short stature, skeletal malformations, developmental delay, and an increased risk for leukemia or other cancers.

### Subjective Findings

The health history may reveal:

- Distinctive facial and musculoskeletal features that are more obvious in infancy and become less obvious during childhood
- Developmental delay, learning problems, intellectual disability (25%; Allanson & Roberts, 2019)

### Risk Factors

NS is inherited in an autosomal dominant manner, although individuals with NS may have a *de novo* or new mutation. NS in a parent results in a 50% chance of NS for each pregnancy due to autosomal dominant inheritance. Less commonly, NS is caused by a change in the LZTR1 gene, which can be inherited in an autosomal dominant or recessive pattern. With a recessive pattern, carrier parents have a 25% chance of having a child affected with NS for each pregnancy (Allanson & Roberts, 2019).

### Review of Systems

The most common manifestations revealed during the review of systems include:

- **Constitutional:** feeding difficulties as an infant
- **HEENT:** hearing loss
- **Cardiovascular:** heart defect (pulmonary valve stenosis in 20%–50%), heart disease (hypertrophic cardiomyopathy in 20%–30%) lymphedema
- **Musculoskeletal:** short stature, skeletal anomalies, swelling of lower extremities
- **Endocrine:** delayed puberty
- **Hematological:** bleeding problems, mild bruising, nose bleeds to severe bleeding (Allanson & Roberts, 2019)

### Objective Findings

The physical examination of the child with NS may reveal:

*Newborn:*

- Head: macrocephaly, small face, narrow temples, tall forehead
- Eyes: widely spaced, epicanthal folds, ptosis, horizontal or downward-slanting eyelids (95%)
- Nose: broad, short, depressed nasal root and full tip
- Ears: low-set, posteriorly rotated, oval shaped, thick helix
- Lips: upper with deeply grooved philtrum, full
- Neck: short with excess skin and low hairline (55%)

*Toddler:*

- Hair: may be wispy

*Middle-Late Childhood:*

- Hair: curly or wooly
- Face: less expressive (myopathic-like in appearance)

*Adolescence:*

- Face: wide at forehead with pointed chin (inverted triangle), features are sharper in appearance
- Eyes: less prominent
- Nose: narrow nasal root, thin nasal bridge
- Neck: longer, webbing of skin more pronounced

*In General:*

- Skeletal: chest deformity (superior: pectus carinatum, inferior: pectus excavatum); widely spaced nipples; low-set, rounded shoulders; scoliosis (10%–15%); vertebral and rib anomalies; joint contractures; abnormal forearm carrying angles; hyperextensibility
- Skin: abnormal pigmentation, including multiple pigmented nevi, café-au-lait spots, lentigines, keratosis pilaris (upper arms, face; Romano et al., 2010)

### Laboratory/Diagnostic Testing

The diagnosis of NS is based upon the clinical findings and confirmed by molecular testing (DNA sequencing of a panel of the eight genes related to NS). Approximately 50% of cases of NS are due to sequence changes in the PTPN11 gene. NS is most often inherited in an autosomal dominant pattern, but can also be due to a new (*de novo*) mutation, autosomal recessive inheritance, or gonadal mosaicism of a parent (Allanson & Roberts, 2019). Knowing the specific mutation guides genetic counseling regarding the risk of having subsequent children with the disorder.

### Differential Diagnosis

The differential diagnosis for NS includes:

- Neurofibromatosis type 1 (NF1)
- TS
- Watson syndrome
- NS with multiple lentigines (NSML)
- Cardiofaciocutaneous (CFC) syndrome
- Noonan-like syndrome with loose anagen hair
- Costello syndrome (Tafazoli et al., 2017)

### Treatment/Management Plan

The treatment/management plan includes the following:

- Monitor growth parameters three times a year for the first 3 years, then annually.
- Complete developmental screening annually.
- Complete regular oral examination and recommend dental evaluation at 1 to 2 years of age and then annually.
- Ophthalmology examination at diagnosis and follow-up at least every 2 years.
- Hearing evaluation at diagnosis, then annually throughout childhood; treat ear infections promptly.
- Laboratory work at diagnosis and every 6 to 12 months: complete blood count with differential, prothrombin time, activated partial thromboplastin.
- Evaluate for cryptorchidism by 1 year of age, kidney ultrasound at diagnosis.
- Examine chest and back for skeletal abnormalities and complete radiographs for abnormal findings.
- Monitor for problems with balance, weakness, paresthesia; obtain brain MRI if present.
- Monitor for signs and symptoms of hypothyroidism (goiter, fatigue, constipation, poor growth); obtain thyroid function tests and antibodies if present (Romano et al., 2010).

### Family Education

Teach the following:

- Counsel on genetic etiology, recurrence risk, and recommended health maintenance
- Refer family to support groups:
  - National Organization for Rare Disorders (NORD): https://rarediseases.org/rare-diseases/noonan-syndrome
  - Noonan Syndrome Foundation: www.teamnoonan.org

### Referral

Refer as follows:

- Clinical genetics at diagnosis
- Early intervention (up to 3 years of age), developmental pediatrics
- Pediatric cardiology for evaluation at diagnosis
- Pediatric endocrinology for growth pattern deceleration, delayed puberty (girls with no breast development at 13 years/boys with no testicular enlargement at 14 years)
- Pediatric nephrology if abnormalities on kidney ultrasound
- Pediatric urology for orchiopexy if cryptorchidism present
- Pediatric hematology if bleeding symptoms occur or as determined by abnormal bloodwork
- Pediatric neurology if seizures are suspected (Romano et al., 2010)

## MARFAN SYNDROME

Marfan syndrome is an inherited disorder that occurs in 1 in 5,000 births worldwide (GHR, 2020d). There is no gender, racial, or ethnic predisposition and symptoms vary from mild to severe. Marfan syndrome is a multisystem connective-tissue disorder that affects the cardiovascular, ocular, and skeletal systems due to mutations or changes in the FBN1 gene and the resulting abnormal fibrillin protein.

### Subjective Findings

The health history may reveal (Figure 38.3):

- Family history of Marfan syndrome (first-degree relative)
- Tall and thin stature, scoliosis, pectus excavatum or carinatum
- Vision problems

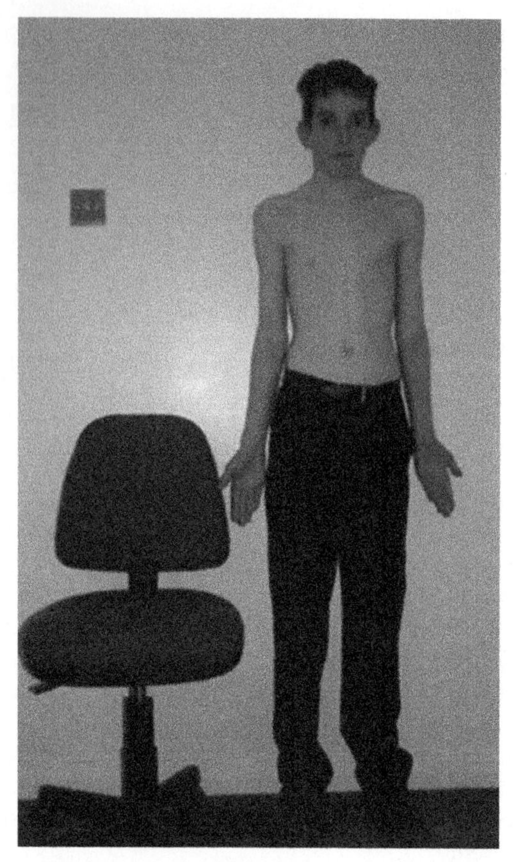

FIGURE 38.3 Marfan syndrome.

*Source*: Reproduced with permission from Dean, J. C. S. (2007). Marfan syndrome: Clinical diagnosis and management. *European Journal of Human Genetics, 15*(7), 724–733. https://doi.org/10.1038/sj.ejhg.5201851

- Abnormal ECHO result (Wright & Connolly, 2021)
- Flexible joints
- Chronic pain in bones and joints

## Risk Factors

Marfan syndrome is inherited in an autosomal dominant manner. For an affected parent, there is a 50% chance of having a child with Marfan syndrome for each pregnancy. Twenty-five percent of cases of Marfan syndrome are due to a *de novo* mutation (Dietz, 2017).

## Review of Systems

The most common manifestations revealed during the review of systems include:

- **HEENT:** vision problems, cataracts, myopia
- **Cardiovascular:** abnormal echocardiogram result, thoracic, abdominal, or another aortic aneurysm, valvular disease
- **Respiratory:** pneumothorax
- **Gastrointestinal:** hernia
- **Musculoskeletal:** skeletal abnormalities, long arms, legs
- **Integumentary:** Poor wound healing, abnormal scars, striae (Wright & Connolly, 2021)

## Objective Findings

The physical examination of the child with Marfan syndrome may reveal:

- Three of five facial features: dolichocephaly, malar hypoplasia, enophthalmos, retrognathia, down-slanting palpebral fissures
- Ectopia lentis, retinal detachment
- Chest asymmetry or pectus carinatum or excavatum
- Reduced upper segment/lower segment and increased arm span/height without severe scoliosis
- Scoliosis >20 degrees or thoracolumbar kyphosis
- Positive wrist/thumb sign (confirms arachnodactyly)
- Reduced elbow extension
- Hindfoot deformity
- Pes planus
- Skin striae (Wright & Connolly, 2021)

## Laboratory/Diagnostic Testing

The diagnosis of Marfan syndrome is based upon the clinical findings and confirmed with molecular testing of the FBN1 gene. Additional diagnostics assisting with the diagnosis include:

- Myopia (–3 diopters on ophthalmology evaluation)
- Mitral valve prolapse (on echocardiogram)
- Dilated aortic root (Z-score of ≥3 for <20-year-old or ≥2 for ≥20 years old) from echocardiogram result
- Dural ectasia on MRI of spine
- Protrusio acetabulae on radiographs (Wright & Connolly, 2021)

## Differential Diagnosis

The differential diagnosis for Marfan syndrome includes:

- Loeys-Dietz syndrome
- Congenital contractural arachnodactyly
- Heritable thoracic aortic disease
- Ehlers-Danlos syndrome
- Homocystinuria
- Stickler syndrome
- Fragile X syndrome (FXS; Dietz, 2017)

### Treatment/Management Plan

The treatment/management plan includes the following:

- *Vision:* annual examination, eyeglass prescription for refractive errors, surgical treatment of dislocated lens
- *Dental:* antibiotic prophylaxis may be recommended by cardiologist when mitral or aortic valve regurgitation is present
- *Cardiology:* annual ECHO
- *Skeletal:* scoliosis surgery, pectus surgery, orthotics for pes planus (Dietz, 2017)

▶ ALERT: Avoid prescribing fluoroquinolones due to increased risk of aortic aneurysm or dissection (U.S. Food and Drug Administration, 2018).

### Family Education

Teach the following:

- Counsel on genetic etiology, recurrence risk, and health surveillance recommendations.
- Refer family to support groups:
  - The Marfan Foundation: www.marfan.org
  - NORD: https://rarediseases.org/rare-diseases/marfan-syndrome
- Advise to avoid contact and competitive sports, isometric exercises, carrying heavy backpack at school, and activities that cause joint injury/pain.
- Recommend evaluation of family members.
- Recommend that family and school nurse have emergency letter or emergency alert card (see www.marfan.org).

▶ ALERT: Teach to avoid use of cardiovascular stimulants (decongestants, caffeine, vasoconstrictive agents) and LASIK procedures (Dietz, 2017).

### Referral

Refer to the following:

- Clinical genetics
- Pediatric cardiology for annual ECHO, possible medications to decrease stress on the aorta, CT or MRA scans of entire aorta (may need pediatric cardiothoracic surgery referral for repair of aortic root)
- Pediatric ophthalmology
- Pediatric orthopedist (for skeletal anomaly, scoliosis, or pes planus)

## NEUROFIBROMATOSIS

NF1 is an inherited disorder that occurs in 1 in 3,000 individuals (Gutmann et al., 2017). There is no sex, racial, or ethnic predisposition, and symptoms are widely variable, even within a family. NF1 is a multisystem disorder characterized by the following: multiple birthmarks (café-au-lait spots); freckling in the axillary and inguinal areas; iris Lisch nodules; plexiform neurofibromas; optic pathway and other gliomas of the central nervous system; scoliosis; sphenoid wing dysplasia; vasculopathy; and learning disabilities. NF1 may be inherited in an autosomal dominant fashion, or may be the result of a new mutation.

### Subjective Findings

The health history may reveal:

- Difficulty learning
- Pain, paresthesia, pruritis (plexiform neurofibromas cause pain due to size and impingement on nerves)
- Diffuse polyneuropathy due to multiple nerve root tumors (Gutmann et al., 2017)

### Risk Factors

The most common risk factors for NF1 are:

- NF1 is autosomal dominant and there is a 50% recurrence risk for each pregnancy if a parent is affected.
- About 50% of children with NF1 have a *de novo* or new mutation (not inherited; Miller et al., 2019).

### Review of Systems

The most common manifestations revealed during the review of systems include:

- **HEENT:** vision problems
- **Integumentary:** birthmarks
- **Cardiovascular:** stroke (due to vasculopathy)
- **Musculoskeletal**: skeletal problems (Gutmann et al., 2017)

### Objective Findings

The physical examination of the child with NF1 may reveal:

- Short stature and large head circumference (graph on NF growth charts)
- Optic gliomas (dilated eye examination) and Lisch nodules on slit-lamp examination

- Multiple café-au-lait spots (6+) and axillary/inguinal freckling (90%)
- Development of freckles where skin rubs against skin
- Cardiac issues such as valvular pulmonic stenosis and congenital heart defects
- Hypertension (renal arterial stenosis; rarely, pheochromocytoma)
- Reduced muscle strength
- Generalized osteopenia, dysplasia of long bones, scoliosis (Gutmann et al., 2017)

**PRO TIP** The number of café-au-lait macules does not predict the severity of NF1 (Miller et al., 2019).

## Laboratory/Diagnostic Testing

According to the National Institutes of Health, the diagnosis of NF1 is based upon the clinical findings in children with two or more of the following:

- Six or more café-au-lait macules >5 mm in greatest diameter in prepubertal individuals and 15 mm in greatest diameter in postpubertal individuals
- Two or more neurofibromas of any type or one plexiform neurofibroma
- Freckling in the axillary or inguinal regions
- Optic glioma
- Two or more Lisch nodules (iris hamartomas [benign tumor])
- A distinctive osseous lesion such as sphenoid dysplasia or tibial pseudarthrosis
- A first-degree relative (parent, sibling) with NF1 as defined by the preceding criteria (Miller et al., 2019)

## Differential Diagnosis

The differential diagnosis for NF1 includes:

- Legius syndrome
- McCune-Albright syndrome
- NS
- Silver-Russell syndrome
- Chromosomal mosaicism/ring chromosomes (can result in abnormal skin findings)
- PTEN hamartoma tumor syndrome
- Sotos syndrome
- Neurofibromatosis type 2 (NF2)
- Carney syndrome (Miller et al., 2019)

## Treatment/Management Plan

Recommendations for treatment and management of NF include:

- Annual monitoring of growth (including head circumference), blood pressure, signs of precocious or delayed puberty.
- Annual ophthalmologic examination in early childhood, less frequent examination in older children.
- Annual monitoring of the following systems: central nervous, musculoskeletal, cardiovascular, ophthalmologic, developmental and psychosocial, and dermatologic.
- Regular developmental assessment by screening questionnaire (in childhood).
- Diagnostic imaging (MRI) as needed with new symptoms or significant abnormalities (new-onset seizures, headaches, visual changes or disturbances, precocious puberty, accelerated growth, stroke-like symptoms, head and neck plexiform neurofibromas with change in growth or pain, encephalopathy or cognitive decline, signs of increased intracranial pressure, extremity asymmetry). Keep in mind that children with NF1 have a higher incidence of stroke due to cerebrovascular abnormalities.

▶ ALERT: Warning signs include vision loss, strabismus, and proptosis.

## Family Education

Teach the following:

- About genetic cause and recurrence risk
- Parents need an examination to rule out segmental or mosaic signs of NF1 in parents
- Health surveillance recommendations
- Support groups can be very helpful to the family:
  - Children's Tumor Foundation: www.ctf.org
  - Neurofibromatosis Network: www.nfnetwork.org
- About long-term planning, and sexual and reproductive planning

## Referral

Refer to the following:

- Refer to clinical geneticist for evaluation and counseling and subsequent annual physical examination
- See NF Clinic Network (NFCN) to find NF clinics in the United States: www.ctf.org/understanding-nf/find-a-doctor#nf-clinic-network
- Developmental pediatric specialist and/or early intervention as needed
- Pediatric ophthalmology, cardiology, neurology, dermatology, and orthopedics (as appropriate)

# X-LINKED SYNDROMES

## FRAGILE X SYNDROME

FXS is the second most common genetic cause of intellectual disability. It occurs in all racial and ethnic groups and in 1:5,000 to 1:7,000 males and 1:4,000 to 1:6,000 females (Ciaccio et al., 2017). FXS occurs in individuals with a trinucleotide repeat expansion (TNRE) mutation in the FMR1 gene (>200 CGG repeats) located on the X chromosome. The normal number of nucleotide bases (CGG, a DNA segment) is between 5 and 40. A premutation is a CGG repeat of 55 to 200 and a full mutation is more than 200 CGG repeats. An individual with a premutation may have normal intellect and appearance or have mild cognitive impairment, some physical signs of FXS, premature ovarian failure (females), and fragile X-associated tremor/ataxia syndrome (older males). Usually, the expansion of CGG repeats increases from generation to generation (anticipation effect) and results in increasing severity of FXS symptoms (Hunter et al., 2019).

FXS results in both intellectual and physical symptoms. Males with FXS are more severely affected due to having only one X chromosome. Females can also be affected, but symptoms are usually less severe due to having two X chromosomes (Hunter et al., 2019).

### Subjective Findings

The health history may reveal:

- Developmental delay, intellectual disability, or autism spectrum disorder
- A family history of FXS, premature ovarian failure, ataxia, or tremor (Hunter et al., 2019)

### Risk Factors

In females, the recurrence risk of FXS depends on the number of CGG repeats in the premutation on the X chromosome. The greater number of CGG repeats results in a larger risk of the expansion to a full mutation. There are several possible outcomes that occur with equal chance for each pregnancy for a mother with a premutation. These include the possibility of a male that is unaffected, a male with a premutation, a male with a full mutation (affected with FXS), an unaffected female, a female with a premutation, and a female with a full mutation (affected with FXS). Males with a premutation have a 50% chance of passing on the premutation to all of their daughters, but will not pass the premutation on to their sons (Firth & Hurst, 2017).

### Review of Systems

The most common manifestations revealed during the review of systems include:

- **Constitutional:** sleep disorders
- **HEENT:** strabismus, recurrent otitis media
- **Gastrointestinal:** gastroesophageal reflux disease
- **Neurological:** developmental delay, intellectual disability (mean IQ of 40–45), seizures, attention deficit hyperactivity disorder (ADHD), stereotypies (repetitive movements or sounds) or autism spectrum disorder
- **Psychological:** irritability, anxiety, behavioral problems (Hunter et al., 2019)

### Objective Findings

The physical examination of the child with FXS may reveal:

- Normal growth and often large (>50th percentile) occipitofrontal head circumference
- Facial features that are more obvious as child ages: long face, prominent forehead, large ears, prominent jaw (more obvious in adolescence)
- Soft and smooth skin
- Macro-orchidism in postpubertal males
- Hypotonia, joint laxity, scoliosis, pes planus
- Developmental delay/intellectual disability, poor eye contact, stereotypies (Hunter et al., 2019)

### Laboratory/Diagnostic Testing

The diagnosis of FXS is established through molecular genetic testing that confirms a CGG TNRE. An abnormal gene methylation of more than 200 repeats is diagnostic for FXS. Children with a history of developmental delay should also have a CMA completed to assess for microdeletions and duplications.

### Differential Diagnosis

The differential diagnosis for FXS includes:

- Developmental delay/intellectual disability
- Autism spectrum disorder
- ADHD
- Fragile XE syndrome (mild intellectual disability resulting from changes to the FRAXE gene on the X chromosome)
- Sotos syndrome
- Prader-Willi syndrome (PWS; Hunter et al., 2019)

## Treatment/Management Plan

Treatment is based on symptoms and is supportive (usually psychopharmacologic treatment and therapeutic services). Developmental and psychiatric/behavioral evaluations may be needed. Annual dental examinations should be performed. There should be baseline and surveillance evaluation of the musculoskeletal system (joint hypermobility, pes planus, scoliosis, hypotonia; Hunter et al., 2019).

▶ ALERT: Children with FXS are more sensitive to psychotropic medications and need to be treated with lower doses and gradual increases to achieve desired treatment effect. Avoid metoclopramide, as it can exacerbate parkinsonism. Use anticholinergics agents with caution due to possibility of exacerbating cognitive symptoms.

### Family Education

Teach the following:

- Provide information regarding recurrence risk.
- Refer family to support groups:
  - National Fragile X Foundation, https://fragilex.org
  - FRAXA Research Foundation, www.fraxa.org
- Educate about therapeutic services and individualized education plans (IEPs).
- Inform of increased risk for seizures, autism spectrum disorder, ADHD, behavioral problems, and sleep problems (GHR, 2020b).

### Referral

Refer the child with FXS to:

- Clinical genetics for evaluation, testing, and counseling regarding signs and symptoms related to FXS as well as recurrence risk
- Early intervention (up to 3 years of age); special education after 3 years of age
- Pediatric ophthalmology as needed for strabismus
- Pediatric cardiology if there are concerns with mitral valve prolapse or aortic root dilatation
- Pediatric pulmonology if the child demonstrates sleep apnea
- Pediatric gastroenterology if feeding problems exist or gastroesophageal reflux disease occurs
- Pediatric orthopedics for musculoskeletal concerns
- Pediatric neurology if seizures occur
- Pediatric psychiatry or developmental pediatrics as needed for behavioral or developmental concerns

# INBORN ERRORS OF METABOLISM

An inborn error of metabolism (IEM) occurs in about 1 in 1,000 live births; these errors are responsible for more than 500 different disorders (El-Hattab & Sutton, 2018). Most IEMs are inherited by an autosomal recessive pattern and involve a genetic defect in the enzyme or transporter required for the metabolism of proteins, lipids, or carbohydrates. Many IEM disorders are detected by state newborn screening programs, resulting in early diagnosis, treatment, and improved long-term outcomes. All states screen for phenylketonuria (PKU) in addition to other IEM disorders depending on the state's program. To see conditions screened by state, go to https://babysfirsttest.org. Newborn screening allows for early detection of patients with many, but not all, types of IEM disorders before signs and symptoms are clinically observed. Other IEM disorders include galactosemia, maple syrup urine disease (MSUD), biotinidase deficiency, homocystinuria, and lysosomal storage disorders such as Pompe disease.

## Subjective Findings

The health history may reveal:

- Developmental delay or developmental regression
- Acute sickness or frequent hospitalizations with routine childhood illnesses
- Abnormal body or urine odors (maple syrup odor in MSUD, cabbage odor in tyrosinemia; Rice & Steiner, 2016)

### Risk Factors

Parents who are both carriers of the autosomal recessive IEM disorder have a 25% chance of having an affected child with each pregnancy (Hoffmann et al., 2017). Some IEMs, such as ornithine transcarbamylase deficiency (OTC), Fabry disease, and mucopolysaccharidosis type II (Hunter syndrome) are X-linked. For X-linked disorders, if the mother is a carrier, there is a 50% chance of having an affected male child and a 50% chance of having a female child who is a carrier. If the father is affected, there is a 100% chance of having a carrier female child and no chance of having any affected male child. In some disorders, such as Fabry disease, females who are carriers can be affected due to skewed X-inactivation.

### Review of Systems

The most common manifestations revealed during the review of systems include:

- **Constitutional:** poor growth, lethargy, difficulty with feeding
- **Respiratory:** chronic hiccups
- **Cardiology:** cardiomyopathy
- **Gastrointestinal:** vomiting, diarrhea
- **Neurological:** seizures, developmental delay, coma
- **Endocrine:** history of hypoglycemia, acute metabolic acidosis, hyperammonemia, massive ketosis (Hoffmann et al., 2017)

### Objective Findings

The physical examination of the child with an IEM may reveal:

- Coarse facial features (lysosomal storage disorder)
- Abnormal skin or hair findings
- Hepatosplenomegaly (lysosomal or glycogen storage disorder)
- Skeletal abnormalities
- Encephalopathy, altered mental status, coma (Hoffmann et al., 2017)

**PRO TIP** Suspect an IEM disorder in an infant who is well and then has an acute life-threatening illness (Hoffmann et al., 2017).

## Laboratory/Diagnostic Testing

The child with an IEM who has a history of unusual symptoms may demonstrate unexplained findings in routine laboratory results. The diagnosis of an IEM is based on biochemical (ammonia, glucose, lactate, enzyme analysis, plasma amino acids, urine organic acids, acylcarnitine profiles, blood gases) and molecular results for the specific disorder. Many times the IEM disorder is diagnosed as a follow-up to abnormal findings on newborn screening results (Rice & Steiner, 2016).

### Differential Diagnosis

The differential diagnosis for an IEM may include:

- Sepsis
- Accidental ingestion
- Mitochondrial disorder (Hoffmann et al., 2017)

### Treatment/Management Plan

Treatment is specific to the specific IEM and is carefully managed by the genetics team in a tertiary care center that includes a clinician and metabolic dietitian experienced with IEMs. Depending on the disorder, dietary prescription, medications, and medical formulas may be appropriate to decrease the substrate that cannot be metabolized and minimize signs and symptoms. For example, in classic galactosemia, the infant's prescription diet consists of non-galactose–containing formula, such as a soy-based formula, and lifelong restriction of galactose-containing foods. In MSUD, the patient's prescription diet is carefully calculated to decrease branch chain amino acids (valine, leucine, and isoleucine), while supplying adequate amounts of all necessary amino acids for growth and development. It is important for the primary care provider to collaborate with the genetics team on questions related to how the specific IEM can affect the child's health. For a patient with an IEM, an illness such as a viral infection, pneumonia, or a tooth abscess can quickly result in a metabolic crisis (Rice & Steiner, 2016).

▶ ALERT: The genetic metabolic team should provide children/parents/primary care provider with acute care instructions with recommendations to follow during a time of illness. Routine sickness can result in acute illness (e.g., hyperammonemia, hypoglycemia) and metabolic emergency.

## Family Education

Teach the following:

- To seek care for routine childhood illnesses, because the child can quickly decompensate during times of illness.
- Explain that the metabolic dietitian will provide a dietary prescription, including medical formulas.
- Follow the prescribed dietary plan and avoid particular foods as instructed by the metabolic dietitian.
- A metabolic genetics specialist provides ongoing care, specific medications, and recommendations in times of illness.
- Refer the family to support groups for the specific disorder (e.g., NORD: www.rarediseases.org).

## Referral

Refer the child with an IEM to:

- Genetics (for counseling and clinical management of disorder)
- Early intervention
- Specific specialists as appropriate

▶ ALERT: Patients with IEM disorders can quickly decompensate with routine illnesses and require prompt intervention. Collaboration with genetics team is critical.

## NON-MENDELIAN INHERITANCE

Genetic syndromes that occur as a result of nonclassical inheritance are complex and do not follow the patterns of Mendelian inheritance. Syndromes that are a result of nonclassical inheritance can occur in several different ways, including deletion of a part of a chromosome, uniparental disomy (two copies of a chromosome or region on a chromosome are inherited from one parent and no copy from the other parent), mutations in the imprinting center that cause genes to be turned on or off during gamete formation, and other gene mutations (Nussbaum et al., 2016). An example of a syndrome involving nonclassical inheritance is Prader-Willi syndrome (PWS).

## PRADER-WILLI SYNDROME

PWS is a disorder that affects males and females equally and occurs in 1 in 10,000 to 1 in 15,000 individuals of all racial and ethnic groups (Firth & Hurst, 2017). It is the most common genetic cause of obesity. PWS results from several different types of mechanisms involving the paternal copy of the Prader-Willi critical region on chromosome 15, including:

- Deletion of the father's copy of the Prader-Willi critical region (15q11.2–q13) on chromosome 15 (70% of cases)
- Uniparental disomy, in which two copies of the Prader-Willi critical region are inherited from the mother instead of one from the mother and one from the father (20–30% of cases)
- Imprinting center defect, which involves the silencing of paternal genes in the PWS critical region, often by the biological mechanism of methylation (2.5% of cases)
- Mutations of the SNRPN gene (rare)

In general, patients with PWS only receive genomic information of maternal origin for the genetic information in the Prader-Willi critical region. This results in obesity, intellectual disability, short stature, neonatal hypotonia followed by excessive eating in young childhood, small hands and feet, and hypogonadism (Nussbaum et al., 2016).

### Subjective Findings

The health history may reveal:

- Normal birth weight
- Low muscle tone
- Feeding difficulties (often requiring hospitalization/feeding tube) in infancy
- Excessive eating in childhood
- Dry mouth
- Behavioral challenges and problems with sleeping
- Short stature in childhood/adolescence
- Compulsive behavior (skin picking; Driscoll et al., 2017)

### Risk Factors

The genetics of PWS are complex and the recurrence risk depends upon the mechanism that caused the syndrome in the child (Driscoll et al., 2017).

### Review of Systems

The most common manifestations revealed during the review of systems include:

- **Constitutional:** history of severe feeding problems in infancy followed by hyperphagia in childhood
- **Respiratory:** frequent respiratory infections (50%)
- **Musculoskeletal:** hypotonia in infancy
- **Neurological:** developmental delay, cognitive impairment, seizures (10%–20%)
- **Psychological:** behavioral problems, compulsive behaviors, psychosis in young adulthood (10%–20%; Driscoll et al., 2017).

### Objective Findings

The physical examination of the child with PWS may reveal:

- Short stature
- Obesity in childhood
- Narrow forehead, almond-shaped eyes, triangular mouth, small hands and feet
- Fair skin and light-colored hair and eyes
- Strabismus (60%–70%)
- Hip dysplasia (10%–20%)
- Hypotonia
- Signs of delayed or incomplete puberty
- Underdeveloped genitalia (in males: small penis, hypoplastic scrotum, unilateral or bilateral cryptorchidism; in females: smaller labia majora, minora, and clitoris; Driscoll et al., 2017).

### Laboratory/Diagnostic Testing

The diagnosis of PWS is based upon clinical findings and confirmed with molecular testing. DNA methylation testing detects 99% of deletions, imprinting defects, and uniparental disomy (Driscoll et al., 2017).

## Differential Diagnosis

The differential diagnosis for PWS includes disorders that overlap some parts of the phenotype:

- Craniopharyngioma
- Hyperphagic short stature
- Hypotonia in infancy
  - Neonatal sepsis
  - Central nervous system depression
  - Congenital myotonic dystrophy type 1
  - Severe myopathies and neuropathies such as spinal muscular atrophy
- Hypotonia/developmental delay
  - Angelman syndrome
  - FXS
- Developmental delay, obesity, +/− hypogonadism
  - Albright hereditary osteodystrophy
  - Bardet-Beidl syndrome
  - Cohen syndrome
- Other chromosomal abnormalities (Driscoll et al., 2017)

## Treatment/Management Plan

The treatment/management plan includes the following:

- For feeding difficulties and FTT in newborns/infants, consult a dietitian for feeding and caloric needs and speech therapist or occupational therapist for special feeding techniques.
- Closely monitor all growth parameters throughout childhood.
- Assess development and educational needs, and assess for behavioral problems at least annually.
- Evaluate for cryptorchidism.
- Yearly assessment for scoliosis (with x-rays in the presence of obesity).
- Special toothpastes, gels, mouthwash, and gum for treatment of dry mouth.
- Calcium and vitamin D supplement as needed.
- Evaluate for diabetes mellitus, hypothyroidism (including free T4 and TSH levels).

## Family Education

Teach the following:

- Counsel about genetic etiology, recurrence risk, and health surveillance and treatment.
- Discuss importance of early intervention and behavioral therapy.
- Refer the family to support groups:
  - Prader-Willi Syndrome Association (USA): www.pwsausa.org
  - Foundation for Prader-Willi Research: www.fpwr.org

## Referral

Refer the child with PWS to:

- Clinical genetics
- Pediatric endocrinology (growth hormone treatment can be started in infancy and helps to normalize lean body mass)
- Pediatric urology (for cryptorchidism)
- Nutritionist
- Pediatric ophthalmology (for strabismus)
- Pediatric orthopedics (for hip dysplasia or the development of scoliosis)
- Pediatric pulmonology (obstructive sleep apnea)
- Early intervention, special education, behavioral management programs

## KEY POINTS

- A karyotype is needed for confirmation of the diagnosis of DS. If karyotype is normal and suspicion for DS is high, additional cells should be evaluated to check for mosaicism.
- Refer all children with DS to genetics and to early intervention services as soon as possible.
- Karyotype and SRY testing are essential for the diagnosis of TS, with referral to endocrinology for evaluation for growth hormone treatment.
- Boys with KS need early diagnosis for appropriate intervention, identification of clinical changes, initiation of TRT, early sperm retrieval, and cryopreservation.
- For NS, positive genetic test results can confirm diagnosis, although negative test results cannot exclude diagnosis.
- Management of Marfan syndrome should be comprehensive and include regular follow-up with cardiology, cardiothoracic surgery, ophthalmology, orthopedics, and genetics (Dietz, 2017).
- NF1 presents with wide variability and is diagnosed when two or more features are present.
- Five or fewer café-au-lait macules is normal.
- Consider FXS for children with a history of developmental delay and/or autism spectrum disorder, as it is the most common single-gene cause for autism spectrum disorder.
- A negative newborn screening result does not eliminate the possibility of an IEM; IEMs may not

be diagnosed or obvious in the neonatal period but should be considered for any neonate with a sepsis-like illness.

- In children with PWS, early diagnosis and referral to pediatric endocrinology for growth hormone treatment is essential for best long-term outcomes.

## REFERENCES


Allanson, J. E., & Roberts, A. E. (2019). *Noonan syndrome.* https://www.ncbi.nlm.nih.gov/books/NBK1124

Bull, M. J., & Committee on Genetics. (2011). Health supervision for children with Down syndrome. *Pediatrics, 128*(2), 393–406. https://doi.org/10.1542/peds.2011-1605

Centers for Disease Control and Prevention. (2019). *Growth charts for children with Down syndrome.* https://www.cdc.gov/ncbddd/birthdefects/downsyndrome/growth-charts.html

Ciaccio, C., Fontana, L., Milani, D., Tabano, S., Miozzo, M., & Esposito, S. (2017). Fragile X syndrome: A review of clinical and molecular diagnoses. *Italian Journal of Pediatrics, 43*(1). https://doi.org/10.1186/s13052-017-0355-y

Clarke, A. (2020). *Harper's practical genetic counselling* (8th ed.). Taylor & Francis Group.

Defendi, G. L. (2020). *Klinefelter syndrome.* https://emedicine.medscape.com/article/945649-overview

Dietz, H. (2017). *Marfan syndrome.* https://www.ncbi.nlm.nih.gov/books/n/gene/marfan

Driscoll, D. J., Miller, J., Schwartz, S., & Cassidy, S. (2017). *Prader-Willi syndrome.* https://www.ncbi.nlm.nih.gov/books/NBK1330

El-Hattab, A. W., & Sutton, V. R. (2018). *Inborn errors of metabolism.* Elsevier.

Firth, H. V., & Hurst, J. A. (2017). *Oxford desk reference: Clinical genetics and genomics* (2nd ed.). Oxford University Press.

Genetics Home Reference. (2020a). *Down syndrome.* https://ghr.nlm.nih.gov/condition/down-syndrome#statistics

Genetics Home Reference. (2020b). *Fragile X syndrome.* https://ghr.nlm.nih.gov/condition/fragile-x-syndrome

Genetics Home Reference. (2020c). *Klinefelter syndrome.* https://ghr.nlm.nih.gov/condition/klinefelter-syndrome

Genetics Home Reference. (2020d). *Marfan syndrome.* https://ghr.nlm.nih.gov/condition/marfan-syndrome

Genetics Home Reference. (2020e). *Noonan syndrome.* https://ghr.nlm.nih.gov/condition/noonan-syndrome

Genetics Home Reference. (2020f). *Turner syndrome.* https://ghr.nlm.nih.gov/condition/turner-syndrome

Gutmann, D. H., Ferner, R. E., Listernick, R. H., Korf, B. R., Wolters, P. L., & Johnson, K. J. (2017). Neurofibromatosis type 1. *Nature Reviews Disease Primers, 3*(1). https://doi.org/10.1038/nrdp.2017.4

Hoffmann, G. F., Zschocke, J., & Nyhan, W. L. (2017). *Inherited metabolic diseases: A clinical approach.* Springer-Verlag.

Hunter, J. E., Berry-Kravis, E., Hipp, H., & Todd, P. K. (2019). *FMR1 disorders.* https://www.ncbi.nlm.nih.gov/books/NBK1384

Jones, K. L., Jones, M. C., & Campo, M. D. (2014). *Smith's recognizable patterns of human malformation* (7th ed.). Elsevier Saunders.

Miller, D. T., Freedenberg, D., Schorry, E., Ullrich, N. J., Viskochil, D., & Korf, B. R. (2019). Health supervision for children with neurofibromatosis type 1. *Pediatrics, 143*(5), e20190660. https://doi.org/10.1542/peds.2019-0660

Nussbaum, R. L., McInnes, R. R., & Willard, H. F. (2016). *Thompson & Thompson genetics in medicine.* Elsevier.

Radicioni, A. F., Ferlin, A., Balercia, G., Pasquali, D., Vignozzi, L., Maggi, M., Foresta, C., & Lenzi, A. (2010). Consensus statement on diagnosis and clinical management of Klinefelter syndrome. *Journal of Endocrinological Investigation, 33*(11), 839–850. https://doi.org/10.1007/BF03350351

Rice, G. M., & Steiner, R. D. (2016). Inborn errors of metabolism (metabolic disorders). *Pediatrics in Review, 37*(1), 3–17. https://doi.org/10.1542/pir.2014-0122

Romano, A. A., Allanson, J. E., Dahlgren, J., Gelb, B. D., Hall, B., Pierpont, M. E., Roberts, A. E., Robinson, W., Takemoto, C. M., & Noonan, J. A. (2010). Noonan syndrome: Clinical features, diagnosis, and management guidelines. *Pediatrics, 126*(4), 746–759. https://doi.org/10.1542/peds.2009-3207

Samson-Fang, L., & Goldman-Luthy, J. (2019). *Down syndrome.* https://www.medicalhomeportal.org/diagnoses-and-conditions/down-syndrome

Seibert, D. C., Edwards, Q. T., Maradiegue, A. H., & Tinley, S. T. (2016). *Genomic essentials for graduate level nurses.* DEStech Publications.

Shankar, R. K., & Backeljauw, P. F. (2017). Current best practice in the management of Turner syndrome. *Therapeutic Advances in Endocrinology and Metabolism, 9*(1), 33–40. https://doi.org/10.1177/2042018817746291

Tafazoli, A., Eshraghi, P., Koleti, Z. K., & Abbaszadegan, M. (2017). Noonan syndrome—A new survey. *Archives of Medical Science, 13*(1), 215–220. https://doi.org/10.5114/aoms.2017.64720

U.S. Food and Drug Administration. (2018). *FDA warns about increased risk of ruptures or tears in the aorta.* https://www.fda.gov/drugs/drug-safety-and-availability/fda-warns-about-increased-risk-ruptures-or-tears-aorta-blood-vessel-fluoroquinolone-antibiotics

World Health Organization. (2020). *Genes and human diseases.* https://www.who.int/genomics/public/geneticdiseases/en/index2.html

Wright, M. J., & Connolly, H. M. (2021). Genetics, clinical features, and diagnosis of Marfan syndrome and related disorders. *UpToDate.* https://www.uptodate.com/contents/genetics-clinical-features-and-diagnosis-of-marfan-syndrome-and-related-disorders

# Management of Neurodevelopmental Disorders

Elke Jones Zschaebitz and Kelly M. Henson

## Student Learning Outcomes

**Upon completion of the chapter the reader should be able to:**

1. Discuss pathophysiology and epidemiology of selected neurodevelopmental disorders in children.
2. Differentiate subjective and objective findings of selected neurodevelopmental disorders in children.
3. Choose appropriate laboratory or diagnostic tests for particular neurodevelopmental disorders in children.
4. Utilize the differential diagnosis process to determine neurodevelopmental diagnoses in children.
5. Determine treatment plan, child/family education, and need for referral in children with a neurodevelopmental disorder.

## INTRODUCTION

Neurodevelopmental disorders are a group of disorders that present during childhood and occur as a result of abnormal brain development. Deficits caused by neurodevelopmental disorders cause impairment in social, academic, personal, or occupational functioning, which may persist into adulthood. Co-occurrence of these disorders is common, and treatment often involves a multidisciplinary approach. Early intervention is associated with improved outcomes and routine developmental screening in the medical home can assist the pediatric nurse practitioner (PNP) in identifying children with developmental deficits. The severity of neurodevelopmental disorders ranges from mild limitations in learning or social functioning to profound intellectual disability (ID). Autism spectrum disorder (ASD), attention deficit hyperactivity disorder, learning disability (LD), fetal alcohol spectrum disorder (FASD), and intellectual disabilities are discussed in this chapter.

The content in this chapter maps to the following areas on the Pediatric Nursing Certification Board (PNCB) Pediatric Nurse Practitioner—Primary Care certification examination:

**CLINICAL PROBLEMS: DEVELOPMENTAL/ BEHAVIORAL/MENTAL HEALTH**

CONTENT AREAS:

**II. Assessment and Diagnosis**

**B. History and Physical Examination**

1. Obtain history of present illness
2. Obtain a comprehensive health history for new patients
3. Complete an interval history for established patients
4. Perform a review of systems
5. Perform a complete physical examination

**C. Diagnostic Testing and Screening**

1. Order and interpret office/clinic based screening tests
2. Order and interpret diagnostic laboratory tests

**D. Analyzing Information**

1. Integrate health history and physical examination findings into the plan of care
2. Assimilate findings from screening and diagnostic testing into plan of care

**E. Diagnosis**

1. Develop and prioritize differential diagnoses
2. Establish a diagnosis based on evaluation of patient data

## III. Management

**A. Child and Caregiver Counseling and Education**

1. Provide condition-specific counseling and education, including treatment options
2. Educate about benefits and potential adverse reactions of pharmacological interventions
3. Discuss non-pharmacological interventions
4. Counsel regarding the threshold for seeking follow-up care
5. Review the risks of non-adherence to recommended treatment

**B. Therapeutic Interventions**

1. Prescribe pharmacologic agents
2. Recommend the use of over-the-counter pharmacologic agents
3. Order or recommend non-pharmacologic treatments for the management of symptoms
4. Discuss use of complementary and alternative therapies as appropriate

**D. Collaboration and Referral**

2. Refer to specialists as indicated for evaluation, counseling, and/or treatment

**E. Care Coordination**

1. Facilitate patient and family-centered care for children of all ages with acute and chronic conditions

**F. Evaluation and Follow-up**

2. Establish a plan for follow-up care

## IV. Professional Role Responsibilities

**A. Leadership and Evidence-based Practice**

4. Develop, implement, and/or modify clinical practice guidelines

# INTELLECTUAL DISABILITY

ID is a neurodevelopmental disorder characterized by deficits in intelligence and adaptive functioning that presents prior to 18 years of age. ID affects approximately 1% of the population, frequently has coexisting medical and psychiatric disorders, and requires significant utilization of support services (Pivalizza & Lalani, 2018a). The American Psychiatric Association (APA) and the American Association of Intellectual and Developmental Disabilities (AAIDD) are consistent in defining ID; however, the severity categories differ between the two agencies. Intelligence quotient (IQ) testing is important for identifying intellectual deficits but is no longer used to classify severity of ID. Severity of ID is based on level of adaptive impairment and on the level of support services required for functioning within society (APA, 2013; Pivalizza & Lalani, 2018a). Adaptive functioning is measured across three domains—conceptual, social, and practical (personal care and daily living activities)—and affects individual participation in the community, home, and school (APA, 2013; Pivalizza & Lalani, 2018a). Intellectual functioning has an impact on learning, reasoning, problem solving, abstract thinking, and judgment, and individuals with ID generally have an IQ score below 70 (Pivalizza & Lalani, 2018a). Both intellectual and adaptive functioning should be assessed using standardized assessment tools.

The APA's *Diagnostic and Statistical Manual of Mental Disorders, 5th edition (DSM-5)* classifies ID severity as mild, moderate, severe, or profound (APA, 2013). The AAIDD's severity categories are based on the level of required services, and include intermittent, limited, extensive, or pervasive (Pivalizza & Lalani, 2018a). ID may be further described as syndromic or nonsyndromic. Syndromic ID occurs with physical features or other comorbid condition that are associated with a specific syndrome such as trisomy 21 (Down syndrome). Nonsyndromic ID is used to describe patients without a recognizable syndrome (Kaufman et al., 2010). According to the *DSM-5*, children who have not yet undergone comprehensive standardized testing or are too young to comply with testing may receive a *DSM-5* diagnosis of global developmental delay (GDD; APA, 2013). Not all children with GDD go on to qualify for a diagnosis of ID, and early intervention can significantly improve functionality. Mild ID is more prevalent than severe ID, and may not be diagnosed until school age, whereas children with severe ID are generally identified prior to 2 years of age (Pivalizza & Lalani, 2018b).

## Subjective Findings

The health history may reveal:

- Language delay, especially with GDD
- Immature behavior, play, and/or self-help skills
- Learning difficulties
- Failure to meet developmental milestones

The child's health history may also reveal associated conditions:

- Cerebral palsy
- Congenital heart disease
- Constipation, gastroesophageal reflux
- Dental caries
- Endocrine abnormalities, especially hypothyroidism
- Hearing or visual impairment
- Lead poisoning
- Obesity
- Seizures
- Sleep disorders
- Undescended testicles

Comorbid neurodevelopmental and mental health disorders are common with ID, affecting 30% to 70% of children with ID (Pivalizza & Lalani, 2018a). Associated disorders include:

- Autism (ASD)—28%
- Attention-deficit/hyperactivity disorder (ADHD)—44%
- Learning disabilities
- Feeding and eating disorders
- Depression and anxiety
- Injury, neglect, and abuse—14% to 30%
- Movement disorders
- Self-injurious behaviors (Pivalizza & Lalani, 2018a)

## Risk Factors

The most common risk factors for ID are genetic abnormalities. Other known causes for ID are metabolic disorders, neurologic abnormalities, and other congenital anomalies:

- Prenatal
  - Sequence variations or copy number variants
  - Chromosomal disorders (Trisomy 21)
  - Inborn errors of metabolism
  - Brain malformations
  - Maternal disease
  - Environmental influences (alcohol, drugs, toxins, teratogens)
- Perinatal
  - Labor and delivery-related events leading to neonatal encephalopathy
- Postnatal
  - Hypoxic ischemic injury
  - Traumatic brain injury
  - Infections
  - Demyelinating disorders
  - Seizure disorders
  - Severe and chronic social deprivation
  - Toxic metabolic syndromes
  - Intoxications

## Review of Systems

The most common manifestations revealed during the review of systems include:

- **Neurologic**: developmental delay, learning difficulties
- **Behavioral**: immature play or social interaction with same-aged peers

## Objective Findings

The physical examination of the child with ID may reveal:

- Dysmorphic features
- Micro- or macrocephaly
- Abnormal stature (short or tall)
- Cutaneous findings, including café-au-lait spots, ash-leaf spots, bruises (neurofibromatosis, tuberous sclerosis, physical abuse, or self-harm)
- Hyperactivity, impulsivity, abnormal social interaction
- Hearing or visual impairment
- Abnormal motor movements, tone, and reflexes

## Laboratory/Diagnostic Testing

The diagnosis of ID is based upon the clinical findings, as well as identification of significant impairment in both intellectual and adaptive functioning based on comprehensive, standardized evaluation (APA, 2013; Pivalizza & Lalani, 2018a). Consider blood lead testing if not previously obtained. Neuroimaging such as magnetic resonance imaging (MRI) should be performed based on concerning history of seizure disorder, progressive neurologic symptoms, focal neurologic deficits, or micro/macrocephaly (Pivalizza & Lalani, 2018b).

The American Academy of Pediatrics (AAP) recommends routine developmental and behavioral screening with a validated tool such as the Ages and Stages Questionnaire (ASQ) at 9, 18, and 24 or 30 months. Screen for ASD with a validated tool such as the Modified Checklist for Autism in Toddlers (M-CHAT) at 18 and 24 months. Also conduct screening at any time a parent or clinician has concerns about development.

**PRO TIP** PNPs should have a low threshold for referring children for further evaluation when parents express repeated concerns for developmental delay, as parental concern is highly sensitive. Standardized, validated screening tools such as the ASQ (https://agesandstages.com/asq-online) and M-CHAT (https://m-chat.org [free]) are accessible online and can be completed by parents prior to the appointment time to save valuable, limited time during wellness visits. Ensure that the ASQ being administered is valid for the child's age and is corrected for prematurity.

If screening suggests developmental delay, a comprehensive developmental-behavioral evaluation is warranted. The PNP should include the following components during evaluation for ID:

- Focused history with detailed family history (three generations)
- Birth history, including prenatal complications
- History of serious central nervous system (CNS) infection or trauma
- Developmental progress that includes stagnation or regression
- Physical examination—height, weight, head circumference, growth trajectory, neurologic examination, assessment of dysmorphic features
- Hearing and vision screening
- Sleep quality

Review results from previous evaluations completed by the school or other specialties. A comprehensive school-based evaluation is needed to determine individualized educational needs.

## Differential Diagnosis

The differential diagnosis for ID includes:

- Autism
- Cerebral palsy
- LD
- Hearing or visual impairment
- Hypothyroidism
- Lead poisoning
- Seizure disorder
- Posttraumatic stress disorder
- Reactive attachment disorder
- Severe language disorder

## Treatment/Management Plan

ID is a lifelong disorder, and the PNP should follow the chronic care and medical home models. Children with ID often require a significant amount of care coordination due to the high association of comorbidities. Planning for transition to adulthood is also critical and should begin at 12 years of age (White et al., 2018). If available, assigning a social worker or case manager to help families access community resources and to facilitate coordination among the primary care team and subspecialists can be of great value. Goals of treatment are to minimize the effects of the disability, prevent or limit deterioration, and optimize functioning (APA, 2013; Pivalizza, 2018). The PNP should prioritize treatment plans that establish effective communication, encourage independent function, and provide support to families. Most causes of ID do not have specific treatment recommendations; however, if a cause such as seizure disorder, congenital hypothyroidism, or inborn error of metabolism is identified, it should be promptly addressed (Pivalizza, 2018).

## Family Education

Teach the following:

- Cause, prognosis, and level of impairment.
- Most causes of ID cannot be prevented. Preventative strategies include:
  - Decreasing prenatal alcohol exposure
  - Folic acid supplementation
  - Reducing risk of congenital TORCH (toxoplasmosis, other, rubella, cytomegalovirus, and herpes) infection
  - Reducing lead exposure
  - Poverty reduction.
- Stress the potential need for genetic evaluation and counseling.
- Emphasize the importance of early intervention.
- Give anticipatory guidance based on developmental stage.
- Safety.
- Realistic expectations with interventions aimed to maximize independence and function in adaptive and intellectual domains.
- Available resources for both the child and the parents, to include respite care, behavior training, and stress management.
- Legal rights, to include access to special education and guardianship upon transition to adulthood.
- Planning for transition to adulthood should begin by age 12 (White et al., 2018).

### Referral

Evaluation for and management of ID require a multidisciplinary approach. Comprehensive neurodevelopmental evaluation with assessment of intellectual and adaptive functioning to establish a diagnosis of ID may require the following subspecialty referrals:

- Developmental pediatrician
- Pediatric neurologist
- Pediatric psychologist

Refer children 3 years and younger to early intervention specialists. Speech, occupational, and physical therapy referrals should be made for formal evaluation of functional levels and ongoing treatment if indicated. Referral for a genetic evaluation may be indicated to rule out and/or treat associated syndrome. A pediatric psychiatry referral may be indicated if the child has comorbid complex psychiatric conditions.

## LEARNING DISABILITIES

Assessment of a child's educational performance is an important component of the well child visit and should be routinely assessed by the primary care PNP. Educational status is a predictor of long-term health; preschool attendance, social-emotional status during elementary school, and completion of high school have been associated with positive health outcomes (Topitzes et al., 2009). Additionally, it is widely known that early intervention is most effective when addressing developmental delays and learning problems to prevent secondary emotional problems (von Hahn, 2019b). Approximately 10% of children in the United States are affected by learning disabilities (LDs; von Hahn, 2019a). An evaluation for LD should be initiated for any child whose parents are concerned about learning problems or academic failure (von Hahn, 2019c). Routine screening for LDs by the PNP may help to identify children whose problems may not yet have been detected by the school system. The medical evaluation for a child with LD is conducted by the primary care provider to identify any comorbid medical, behavioral, or neurologic conditions (Schulte, 2015). Most children's LDs do not have a medical cause; however, comorbid developmental and behavior disorders are common (von Hahn, 2019a).

LD is a neurodevelopmental disorder that affects the brain's ability to perceive or process information (APA, 2013). LDs are biologic in origin, and are a result of genetic, epigenetic, and environmental factors (APA, 2013). As a result, individuals with an LD experience lower levels of academic achievement than would be expected based on their intellectual potential (APA, 2013). LD is typically diagnosed by the education team or a psychologist through a comprehensive evaluation of:

- Intellectual ability
- Academic achievement
- Speech/language skills
- Gross and fine motor skills
- Psychological or emotional factors that affect learning
- Medical or neurologic conditions that require treatment or special accommodations

### Subjective Findings

The health history may reveal the following school-related problems:

- Academic failure or learning difficulties
  - Identify the age at which learning difficulties were first identified
  - Track progression over time
  - Review interventions that have improved or impeded learning
- Behavioral regulation
- Difficulty with peer interaction
- Difficulty with motor skills (handwriting, clumsiness)

Also include history related to the following:

- Speech delay
- Detailed developmental history, to include timing of milestone achievements and social development
- Pregnancy or birth complications, prematurity, fetal exposure to medications or illicit substances (especially alcohol)
- Social history, such as stressors (divorce, deployment, relocation), poverty, and trauma
- Conduct a thorough sleep history that includes:
  - Timing of onset and waking
  - Difficulty with sleep onset or maintenance
  - Waking up refreshed in the morning
  - Presence of snoring, enuresis, night terrors, or sleep walking

**PRO TIP** Multiple encounters may be required to conduct a comprehensive evaluation, identify a treatment plan, and provide education to the family. In established patients, it may be appropriate to obtain detailed developmental and educational history via telehealth, then schedule an office appointment to conduct physical examination, provide education, and establish a treatment plan.

## Risk Factors

The most common risk factors for LDs are:

- Family history of LD
- Poverty
- Premature birth
- Diagnosis of other developmental and/or mental health conditions (ADHD, disruptive behavior disorders, ASD, anxiety, and depression)
- Prenatal alcohol exposure
- Neurologic condition (seizure, neurofibromatosis, tuberous sclerosis complex, Tourette syndrome)
- Chromosomal disorders (fragile X syndrome, Turner syndrome, Klinefelter syndrome)
- Chronic medical conditions (type 1 diabetes, HIV)
- History of CNS infection, brain irradiation, or traumatic brain injury
- Lead toxicity

## Review of Systems

The most common manifestations revealed during the review of systems include:

- **Constitutional**: sleep disorder
- **Genitourinary**: nocturnal enuresis
- **Musculoskeletal**: difficulty with handwriting or other fine motor tasks, difficulty with coordination or other gross motor tasks
- **Neurologic**: staring spells, seizure disorder, tics, academic failure
- **Behavioral**: inattention, hyperactivity, behavior problems, difficulty with peer interaction
- **Psychiatric**: anxiety or depression

## Objective Findings

The physical examination of the child with LD may reveal:

- General observations—dysmorphic features (stigmata of genetic syndromes), behavior, overall ability to communicate (verbal, nonverbal, able to follow instructions, social engagement)
- Evidence of neurocutaneous disorders or reproductive anomalies associated with LD (neurofibromatosis, Turner syndrome, etc.)
- Abnormal tone, asymmetry (cerebral palsy), coordination problems (developmental coordination disorder), weakness (muscular dystrophy; von Hahn, 2019b)

## Laboratory/Diagnostic Testing

No routine clinic-based testing is indicated for LD; however, it is important to review report cards, evaluations completed by the educational system, and parent and teacher observations. Identify the child's abilities, strengths, and weaknesses (von Hahn, 2019b). Standardized questionnaires such as the Vanderbilt rating scale for ADHD (www.nichq.org/sites/default/files/resource-file/NICHQ_Vanderbilt_Assessment_Scales.pdf), the Conners (www.pediatricenter.com/assets/forms/Conners_Parent_Rating.pdf), or the Child Behavior Checklist (www.apa.org/depression-guideline/child-behavior-checklist.pdf) can be obtained from parents and teachers to provide information about behavior and academic performance (von Hahn, 2019b). It is recommended that primary care providers have a low threshold for referring children for evaluation if there is a family history of learning problems, prematurity, history of developmental delay (especially speech delay), neurologic or genetic condition, and behavior or mental health disorder (von Hahn, 2019c). Learning disabilities are diagnosed by psychometric testing conducted by the education team and/or psychologists.

Routine laboratory and/or diagnostic testing are not indicated in children with LD (von Hahn, 2019b). If a medical or genetic cause is suspected, refer to recommendations for evaluation of the specific disorder. If a co-occurring condition is identified, initiate treatment plans for LD and the co-occurring condition concurrently; do not delay the request for psychoeducational evaluation pending medical or genetic workup.

**PRO TIP** Comprehensive psychoeducational evaluations often take several months to be completed, and it may be up to 6 months before an individualized education plan (IEP) is put in place. Expedite referrals for speech, occupational, and physical therapy and subspecialty providers as indicated so that required outpatient services are not delayed awaiting formal diagnosis based on educational evaluations.

## FETAL ALCOHOL SPECTRUM DISORDER

Maternal alcohol consumption is known to cause irreversible damage to the CNS of the developing fetus, and effects may vary widely among individuals (Treit et al., 2020). Reduction in brain volume and abnormal brain functioning lead to impairment in cognition, impulse control, processing of information and emotions, goal-oriented behavior, and perception of space and time (Cobben et al., 2019; Weitzman & Rojmahamongkol, 2020a). A safe amount of alcohol intake during pregnancy has not been identified, and fetal damage due to alcohol exposure occurs during all stages of gestation.

Neurodevelopmental disorders that occur as a result of prenatal alcohol exposure are classified as FASD. FASD includes physical, cognitive, behavioral, and mental health effects that range from mild to severe impairment and persist into adulthood. FASD can be challenging to diagnose due to the broad range of signs and symptoms and reliance on accurate prenatal history. Prevalence in the United States ranges from 1.1% to 5% (Centers for Disease Control and Prevention [CDC], 2020a; May et al., 2018; Weitzman & Rojmahamongkol, 2020a). While children with FASD may be underdiagnosed among the general population due to a lack of standardization of diagnostic criteria, children who have been involved in the foster care system have been shown to be at increased risk for the disorder (Weitzman & Rojmahamongkol, 2020a). The role of the PNP in the primary care setting is to screen mothers for alcohol use during pregnancy, provide early identification of these disorders, and coordinate care under the chronic care and medical home models (Hagan et al., 2016; Hoyme et at., 2016; Turchi et al., 2018)

### Subjective Findings

The health history may reveal:

- Infancy
  - Prenatal exposure to drugs or alcohol
  - Irritability
  - Jitteriness
  - Autonomic instability
  - Difficult regulating state
  - Developmental delay
- Childhood
  - Hyperactivity
  - Inattention
  - Cognitive impairment
  - Emotional reactivity
  - Learning disabilities
  - Hypotonia
  - Auditory and visual impairment
  - Seizures
  - Deficits in memory and reasoning
- Adolescence and young adulthood
  - Deficits in social skills, adaptive function, and executive function

### Risk Factors

The most common risk factors for FASD are:

*Child risk factors:*

- Sibling with FASD
- Having ever lived in an orphanage or been placed in foster care
- Require psychiatric care
- Previous involvement in child protective services (CPS)
- Involvement in juvenile justice system

*Maternal factors:*

- Higher maternal age
- Higher gravidity and parity
- History of miscarriages and stillbirths
- Inadequate prenatal care
- Poor maternal nutrition during pregnancy
- History of FASD in previous children
- Substance use, including tobacco
- Mental health problems, including depression
- History of physical or sexual abuse
- Social isolation, including living in a rural area during pregnancy
- Intimate partner violence
- Alcohol and drug use by the mother's intimate partner at the time of pregnancy
- Other maternal family members with substance use at the time of pregnancy
- Poverty

### Review of Systems

The most common manifestations revealed during the review of systems include:

- **Neurologic**: seizures, developmental, learning, and cognitive problems, including school failure
- **Behavioral**: behavior problems

> **PRO TIP** Children with FASD often have a history of difficult behaviors, negative mood, and poor response to traditional treatment regimens (e.g., stimulant therapy). Consider FASD in children with treatment-resistant ADHD.

## Objective Findings

The physical examination of the child with FASD may reveal:

- Short palpebral fissures (see American Academy of Pediatrics [AAP, 2020] toolkit for instructions for measuring: www.aap.org/en-us/advocacy-and-policy/aap-health-initiatives/fetal-alcohol-spectrum-disorders-toolkit/Pages/default.aspx)
- Thin vermillion border and smooth philtrum (see University of Washington Lip Philtrum Guide: https://depts.washington.edu/fasdpn/htmls/lip-philtrum-guides.htm)
- CNS abnormalities (abnormal tone, abnormal reflexes, cranial nerve deficits)
- Growth retardation (height/weight less than or equal to 10th percentile)
- A variety of other minor congenital anomalies including structural birth defects

Physical features are absent in up to 75% of affected individuals. Also consider FASD in children with the following clinical features (Figure 39.1):

- Facial dysmorphism
- Intrauterine and/or postnatal growth retardation
- Microcephaly
- Structural brain anomaly
- Recurrent seizures
- Developmental, learning, and cognitive problems, including school failure
- Behavioral problems
- Social-emotional problems

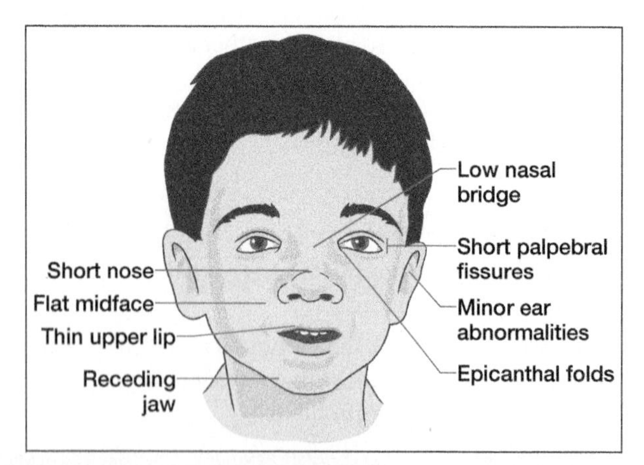


FIGURE 39.1 Characteristic facial features in a child with fetal alcohol spectrum disorder.

*Source*: Chiocca, E. M. (2020). *Advanced pediatric assessment* (3rd ed.). Springer Publishing Company.

## Laboratory/Diagnostic Testing

The diagnosis of FASD is based upon the clinical findings (APA, 2013). There are no universally accepted diagnostic criteria for FASD. The presence of prenatal alcohol exposure and two or three clinical features (facial dysmorphism, CNS involvement, and growth retardation) are used to make a clinical diagnosis. FASD is an umbrella term that describes a range of effects and disorders, including:

- FAS
- Partial FAS
- Alcohol-related neurodevelopmental disorder
- Neurobehavioral disorder associated with prenatal alcohol exposure
- Alcohol-related birth defects

## Differential Diagnosis

The differential diagnosis for FASD includes:

- Other genetic conditions with similar facial features
- Prenatal or postnatal growth retardation
- Microcephaly
- ADHD
- ASD
- Oppositional defiant disorder
- Conduct disorder
- Mood disorder or bipolar disorder
- Reactive attachment disorder
- Sleep disorder
- Trauma, poverty, abuse

## Treatment/Management Plan

Early diagnosis and treatment are associated with improved outcomes (Streissguth et al., 2004). Under the medical home model, the PNP provides comprehensive care for children with FASD, to include care coordination, monitoring of growth and nutrition, management of coexisting medical conditions, and preparation for transition to adulthood (Weitzman & Rojmahamongkol, 2020b). It is important to assess family members for substance use disorders and to screen for child abuse, neglect, and family violence. Maternal support services should be considered if the child remains with the birth parents. The PNP can help families access intervention services as indicated, including community resources and special education services. In the United States, a referral to CPS is required children under 3 years of age with a diagnosis of FASD (Burd & Edwards, 2019). Behavioral and environmental interventions are the primary treatment modalities for children with FASD. Medications may be required to treat comorbid conditions such as ADHD, mood disorders, and aggression. The AAP developed an algorithm and a toolkit to aid in the evaluation of FASD within the medical home (2020). The PNP is also integral to the process of preparing adolescents with FASD and their parents for the transition to adulthood (White et al., 2018).

### Family Education

Teach the following:

- The child's neurobehavioral symptoms are not intentional.
- Help parents develop realistic expectations for the child's functional level.
- Protective factors, including a stable, loving home.
- Behavior management techniques.
- Anticipatory guidance related to upcoming developmental stages.
- Help to reduce stigma and shame for parents of children with FASD.

### Referral

Referral to the FASD multidisciplinary team when FASD is suspected is recommended. Specialists are able to conduct a thorough assessment of physical features, neurobehavioral function, and cognitive function (Weitzman & Rojmahamongkol, 2020b). Referral to the following subspecialties may be warranted depending on clinical presentation:

- Early intervention
- Developmental pediatrician
- Pediatric psychiatrist and/or psychologist
- Pediatric neurologist
- Clinical geneticist
- Speech, occupational, and physical therapy
- Social worker
- Special education

## ATTENTION DEFICIT HYPERACTIVITY DISORDER

ADHD is a common pediatric neurodevelopmental disorder affecting approximately 10% of children from 4 to 17 years of age in the United States (Xu et al., 2018). According to the 2015 to 2016 National Health Interview Survey (NHIS), ADHD is more common in males than in females, with a prevalence of 14% in boys and 6% in girls (Xu et al., 2018). According to the *DSM-5*, the core symptoms of ADHD include hyperactivity, inattention, and/or impulsivity, and cause impairment in multiple settings (i.e., school and home; APA, 2013). Youth with ADHD also often have comorbid mental health disorders, substance abuse, learning difficulties, peer relationship difficulties, and difficulty with completion of activities of daily living (Wolraich et al., 2019). Individuals with ADHD have a higher incidence of injuries, suicide, motor vehicle accidents, drinking and driving, substance abuse, incarceration, and psychiatric comorbidities. The estimated U.S. economic burden of this disorder is between $36 and $52 billion annually (Wolraich et al., 2019).

The pathogenesis of ADHD is not well understood. Advances in neuroimaging and neuropsychological testing in children with ADHD identify difficulties with forward planning, abstract reasoning, mental flexibility, working memory, and response inhibition (Barkley, 2015). There appears to be genetically altered catecholamine metabolism in the cerebral cortex and limbic system based on findings from structural and functional brain imaging, animal studies, and drug trials (Krull, 2019b). These genetic alterations appear to cause decreased production of norepinephrine and dopamine in the prefrontal cortex and low tonic dopamine activity in the limbic system (Barkley, 2015; Krull, 2019b). As a result, children with ADHD experience impaired executive functions, forgetfulness, distractibility, impulsivity, difficulties with forward planning, abstract reasoning, mental flexibility, and hyperactivity (Barkley, 2015; Krull, 2019b). There is a strong genetic influence in the development of ADHD, with twin and first-degree relative association of approximately 75% (Krull, 2019b). A number of genes have been identified in association with ADHD, although these genetic variants are not specific for the disorder. Environmental factors also appear to play a role in development of this disorder, but their significance is poorly understood.

The primary care clinician should initiate an evaluation for ADHD in any child age 4 to 18 years presenting with academic or behavioral problems and symptoms of inattention, hyperactivity, or impulsivity. Also consider evaluation of children who have difficulty making and keeping friends and/or difficulty with team sports.

**PRO TIP** A complete ADHD evaluation may require several office and/or virtual visits. Consider scheduling the parents without the child (or over the phone) for younger children when providing lengthy education and discussing the treatment plan. Request that the parents drop off or email any relevant educational or psychological evaluations and ADHD rating scales prior to the appointment so that the provider has sufficient time to review and interpret these data.

## Subjective Findings

The health history may reveal:

- Difficulty staying on task or completing assignments, chores, etc.
- Difficulty with organization, frequently loses items
- Struggles to follow multiple-step directions, is forgetful
- Lacks attention to detail or makes careless mistakes
- Does not listen, mind wanders, distracted
- Constantly "on the go" or cannot sit still through a meal or in class
- Runs and climbs on things without thinking
- Interrupts, talks excessively
- Has trouble waiting for their turn
- Difficulty getting along with peers; bossy or intrusive of personal space

Assess duration and severity of symptoms, level of impairment, environments where symptoms are present, peer relationships, and school performance. Also note age of onset of concerning symptoms as well as their progression over time (Wolraich et al., 2019).

The health history should include prenatal exposure (e.g., tobacco, drugs, alcohol), perinatal complications, prematurity, trauma at birth, low birth weight, CNS infections, and developmental delays. Also assess for family history of ADHD or similar behaviors, substance abuse, incarceration, or difficulties with learning (Wolraich et al., 2019). Evaluate the family health history for the presence of palpitations, fatigue, syncope, rhythm disturbances, cardiomyopathy, sudden death or coronary artery disease prior to age 50, and seizures.

Obtain a psychosocial history to include recent stressors (moving, divorce), family stress, environmental exposures, and methods that parents have used to address behaviors. For adolescents, inquire about risky behaviors and substance use disorder (Wolraich et al., 2019).

## Risk Factors

Risk factors related to ADHD are largely unknown; however; there is a strong genetic component (CDC, 2020c). Other possible risk factors are:

- Brain injury
- Exposure to environmental toxins (e.g., lead) during pregnancy or at a young age
- Alcohol and tobacco use during pregnancy
- Premature delivery
- Low birth weight

Children with a genetic predisposition for developing ADHD may be more vulnerable to exhibiting core symptoms if their psychosocial environmental is one with high levels of stress and/or includes parents who are unable or unwilling to model coping techniques and self-regulation.

**PRO TIP** Inquire about status of parental deployment for youth in military families. Also include questions about sleep hygiene and use of technology (video games, smartphones, television in bedroom, etc.).

## Review of Systems

The most common manifestations revealed during the review of systems include:

- **Constitutional**: sleep problems, feeding difficulties such as picky eating
- **Cardiovascular**: palpitations, fatigue, syncope
- **Neurologic**: seizure disorder
- **Behavioral**: hyperactive, impulsive, inattentive, poor school performance, difficulty with peer interaction

Identify possible comorbidities; common coexisting disorders include:

- Learning disabilities—20% to 60%
- Anxiety—20% to 40%
- Depression—30%
- Oppositional defiant disorder—50% to 80%
- Conduct disorder—30%
- Tic disorders—20%
- Sleep disorders—30% to 50%
- Sensory processing difficulty
- ASD
- Language disorders
- Other neurodevelopmental disorders (e.g., developmental coordination disorder; Wolraich et al., 2019)

## Objective Findings

Complete a thorough physical and neurologic examination that includes hearing, vision, coordination, behavior, social engagement, and observation for tics. Note behavior and interaction between parent and child. The physical examination of the child with ADHD may reveal:

- Normal physical examination findings, including neurologic examination
- May have difficulty staying seated while in exam room; may be climbing on and off of table, grabbing things from siblings
- Parents may provide numerous reminders regarding expected behavior
- Older children may fidget with nails, clothing, or other items
- Normal eye contact, facial expressions, inflection of voice (age-appropriate) unless hyperactivity is severe
- Dysmorphic features
- Language or motor delays (Wolraich et al., 2019)

## Laboratory/Diagnostic Testing

Diagnosis of ADHD should be made based on *DSM-5* criteria, using a validated instrument such as the Vanderbilt ADHD Rating Scale completed by a caregiver or teacher in at least two separate settings (Wolraich et al., 2019). The primary care provider must also rule out any other alternative cause for symptoms. Initial and follow-up rating scales can be downloaded and printed from the website for the National Initiative for Children's Healthcare Quality (NICHQ) ADHD toolkit. For preschool-age children, the Conners Rating Scale and the ADHD Rating Scale-IV have been validated (Wolraich et al., 2019). It is common for adolescents to minimize their own behaviors, so self-reports in this age group often differ from rating scales completed by other individuals (teachers, parents, etc.).

Routine laboratory testing is not indicated when evaluating for ADHD unless warranted to evaluate for comorbid conditions or to rule out differential diagnoses (e.g., thyroid disorder, lead poisoning, genetic testing for fragile X syndrome). Diagnostic imaging is not routinely indicated for diagnosis or management of ADHD. Quantitative electroencephalography (qEEG), or brain mapping, is not recommended for evaluation of children with ADHD due to insufficient evidence to support its utility (Krull, 2019a). Neuropsychologic testing does not improve accuracy of diagnosis unless learning difficulties are also suspected (Wolraich et al., 2019). If concern for an LD exists, the family can request an educational evaluation with psychometric testing through the public school system.

**PRO TIP** Testing can also be conducted privately; however, services may not be covered by the child's insurance and may not be considered valid by the school system should educational intervention be recommended. Utilize services offered by the school system first when available. Resources for guiding parents through the process of requesting school services can be found at www.CHADD.org and www.ldaamerica.org.

Obtain reports from parents, teachers, other school personnel, and mental health professionals involved in the child's care. For adolescents, try to obtain reports from at least two teachers or other sources such as coaches or counselors (Wolraich et al., 2019). To meet *DSM-5* criteria for ADHD, the child must have six or more of the symptoms in either the inattention section or the hyperactivitye section, or from both sections. Symptoms must be causing significant impairment in more than one setting, have been present for more than 6 months, have occurred prior to 12 years of age, and must not be explained by another mental disorder (APA, 2013). A list of validated ADHD rating scales can be found at www.uptodate.com/contents/image?imageKey=PEDS%2F81675&topicKey=PEDS%2F624&source=outline_link&sp=0&search= (Krull, 2019a).

## Differential Diagnosis

The differential diagnosis for ADHD includes:

- Oppositional defiant disorder
- Conduct disorder
- Other neurodevelopmental disorders
- LD
- ID
- Reactive attachment disorder
- Anxiety disorders
- Depressive disorders
- Developmental coordination disorder
- ASD
- Sleep disorders
- Developmental variations (e.g., delays, intellectually gifted, ID)
- Neurodevelopmental disorders such as learning, language, visual-motor, or auditory processing problems
- Seizure disorders

- CNS trauma or infection (e.g., traumatic brain injury, meningitis)
- FASD
- Psychosocial or environmental factors (trauma, stress, parental separation)

Many children with ADHD have a separate comorbid condition as described in the review of systems section. Many comorbid conditions, such as oppositional defiant disorder, anxiety, or depression, will improve with treatment of ADHD; however, depending on the child, these conditions could require separate treatment or alter the course of treatment (Wolraich et al., 2019).

Most ADHD assessment tools also screen for common conditions such as oppositional defiant disorder, conduct disorder, anxiety, and depression. If a significant comorbid condition is suspected but is outside of the primary care clinician's level of expertise, further evaluation by a mental health professional may be warranted. Additionally, the Society for Developmental and Behavioral Pediatrics (SDBP) recently published clinical practice guidelines for the assessment and treatment of children and adolescents with complex ADHD (Barbaresi et al., 2020). Prioritize treatment of sleep disorders before diagnosing ADHD when possible, as disordered sleep often intensifies ADHD symptoms (Krull, 2019c).

**PRO TIP** Consider obtaining a sleep study if snoring, nocturnal enuresis, or other concerning sleep history findings exist. Provide education on sleep hygiene and regulated use of electronic devices for all children with concerns for inattention, hyperactivity, and impulsivity.

## Treatment/Management Plan

The treatment plan for ADHD includes a combination of behavioral/training therapy, educational support, and medication if indicated based on age and severity. Identify child- and family-centered treatment goals to be addressed and revised if needed at each subsequent visit.

Four dimensions of ADHD are identified by the *DSM-5*:

1. ADHD, combined presentation—314.01 (F90.2)
2. ADHD, predominately inattentive presentation—314.00 (F90.0)
3. ADHD, predominately hyperactive/impulsive presentation—314.01 (F90.1)
4. ADHD other specified and unspecified ADHD—413.01 (F90.8)

The treatment recommendations for each subtype are the same. Pharmacologic treatment for ADHD includes two primary drug classifications:

- Stimulant classes
  - Methylphenidate
  - Amphetamine
- Nonstimulant classes
  - Atomoxetine
  - Tricyclic antidepressants
  - Alpha agonists

Treatment with stimulants and/or behavior therapy has shown to be safe and effective, and treatment recommendations are guided by age range and severity of symptoms. A current list of U.S. Food and Drug Administration (FDA)-approved medications used to treat ADHD can be found for free download online at www.ADHDmedicationguide.com. Treatment recommendations based on age include:

- For preschool-age children (4–6 years), prescribe evidence-based parent training in behavior management (PTBM) and/or behavioral classroom interventions as the first line of treatment. Methylphenidate may be considered in preschoolers with moderate-to-severe ADHD that did not respond to PTBM, or if behavioral treatments are not available.
- Elementary and middle school-aged children (6–12 years) should be treated with medication (stimulant as first line, unless contraindicated) along with PTBM and/or behavior classroom intervention; it is preferable to include both parent and classroom intervention. Educational supports such as an individualized education plan or a 504 plan may be necessary.
- Adolescents (12–18 years) should be treated with medication (stimulant as first line, unless contraindicated) and evidence-based training and/or behavioral interventions if available. Educational supports such as an individualized education plan or a 504 plan may also be necessary (Wolraich et al., 2019).

Medication dosages should be adjusted to achieve a goal of maximum benefit with tolerable side effects. Young children tend to metabolize stimulant medications more slowly, so consider initiating therapy with lower doses. Medication dosing has not been shown to correlate with height and/or weight.

Additional considerations when prescribing stimulants to adolescents include monitoring for misuse and/or diversion and including coverage for driving. Adolescents of driving age may require a longer-acting formula or an immediate-release booster dose to take in the afternoons, depending on their schedules (Wolraich et al., 2019).

**PRO TIP** Many providers experienced in treating young children with ADHD prefer first prescribing an immediate-release formulation to assess response. This is also helpful in children who have not yet learned to swallow pills, because immediate-release methylphenidate is available in a very small chewable tablet.

Evidence is strong for stimulant medications, and sufficient but less strong for nonstimulants such as atomoxetine, extended-release guanfacine, and extended-release clonidine. Nonstimulants have not been FDA-approved for use in preschool-age children with ADHD. Although methylphenidate has not yet been FDA-approved for the preschool-age group, it has the strongest evidence for efficacy and safety at this age and should be considered first if medication is required (Wolraich et al., 2019). Amphetamines received FDA approval for use in children under 6 year of ages; however, the AAP states that the evidence is not adequate to recommend its use as first-line treatment for ADHD at this time (Wolraich et al., 2019).

The most common short-term side effects of stimulant medications include decreased appetite, abdominal pain, headaches, and difficulty sleeping. Very rarely, hallucinations and other psychotic symptoms may occur. Mild increases in heart rate and blood pressure may occur, but are typically clinically insignificant. Stimulant medications have not been shown to increase risk of sudden cardiac death in children; however, it is prudent to screen for cardiac risk factors prior to initiating stimulant therapy (Wolraich et al., 2019).

Ongoing follow-up is recommended to assess for medication efficacy and potential adverse effects, using a validated follow-up tool such as the Vanderbilt ADHD Follow-Up scale. Children with ADHD who are not receiving pharmacologic therapy should have follow-up at least every 6 months (Krull, 2019c). In children receiving pharmacologic therapy, prudent monitoring of treatment response, physiologic response via vital signs, weight, height, and neurologic examination, as well as assessing for side effects, is recommended 1 to 2 weeks after initiation, monthly until an effective dose has been determined, then every 3 to 6 months thereafter (Wolraich et al., 2019).

**PRO TIP** The 1 to 2 week follow-up is often conducted over the phone, via virtual telehealth, or a face-to-face visit to determine if an increase in the dose is indicated. Titration of stimulant dosing can occur every 7 days, or as frequently as every 3 days in the setting of severe behavior impairment (Jensen et al., 2001).

It is well established that ADHD is a chronic condition that is often present and impairing into adulthood (Friedman et al., 2010). Because long-term treatment adherence is a significant issue in this population, it is essential that the primary care manager maintain close communication with the family, school, and mental health team. The practitioner should use a chronic care and medical home model to improve the continuity of care provided. The chronic care model emphasizes that the community and the health organization work together to support an informed, involved patient with targeted goals as well as a prepared, proactive health care team (AAP, 2011). Target goals should be realistic, achievable, and measurable.

In an effort to reduce variability among providers, decrease cost, minimize harm, and produce optimal health outcomes, the AAP published evidence-based guidelines for the diagnosis and treatment of ADHD (AAP, 2011; Wolraich et al., 2019). Standardization of care and quality are promoted with the use of validated assessment tools and evidence-based interventions, which include assessment for comorbid conditions, medication management, behavior therapy, and recommendations for timing and focus of follow-up visits (Wolraich et al., 2019). Although the current guidelines have a strong evidence base, many barriers remain in addressing pediatric mental health concerns such as ADHD. Common barriers that have been identified by pediatric providers include lack of time and/or expertise, limited access to pediatric mental health specialists, stigma, and poor payment for services. Lack of time to interview children and families, communicate with the schools, and coordinate referrals, as well as insufficient reimbursement for time and effort, were additional identified barriers (Wolraich et al., 2019).

Melatonin can be used in children who have difficulty with sleep onset, including those with ADHD (Owens, 2020). Behavioral and/or training interventions may be offered by the public school system at no cost to the family depending on local resources.

Primary care providers should make every effort to become familiar with local support services. Referrals to private therapies can also be made, but may not be covered by all types of health insurance. An organization such as Children and Adults with Attention Deficit/Hyperactivity Disorder (CHADD) is also a good resource to obtain recommended services and support (www.chadd.org). At least 60 minutes of exercise each day is recommended for all children and has been shown to improve cognitive function and improvement in core ADHD symptoms in small trials (Krull, 2019c). Mindfulness training may be helpful as an adjunct to an evidence-based treatment program, although more robust clinical studies are needed (Krull, 2019c; Wolraich et al., 2019).

The following treatments for ADHD have either too little evidence to support use or have not shown any benefit:

- Elimination diets
- Fatty acid supplementation
- External trigeminal nerve stimulation
- Essential oils
- Cannabidiol oil
- EEG biofeedback
- Megavitamins and/or chelation (may have serious adverse effects; Krull, 2019c; Wolraich et al., 2019)

> ALERT: Caffeine is not recommended for treatment of ADHD symptoms.

## Family Education

Teach the following:

- Pathophysiology of ADHD.
- Long-term implications/prognosis.
- Diagnostic criteria.
- Pharmacologic treatment options with risks versus benefits.
- Resources for behavior and/or training therapy.
- Resources for educational support.
- Considerations for transition to adulthood in adolescents >14 years.
- Expected response and potential side effects associated with pharmacologic treatment.
- Safety, especially in impulsive subtypes.

Many parents may express fears that stimulant medications could cause personality changes, often described as hyperfocused or decreased socialized behavior (parents often refer to this as "zombie-like" behavior). Anecdotally, this effect is typically seen as a result of higher doses, and generally improves with a decreases in the prescribed dose. Parents are typically reassured when this is explained in advance as an unexpected response that can be addressed by adjusting the dose or changing to a different medication.

Nonstimulant medications may have a variety of adverse effects depending on their classification; the most common complaints include somnolence, gastrointestinal symptoms, dry mouth, dizziness, irritability, headache, bradycardia, and hypotension. Rarely, an increase in suicidal thoughts has been found in association with atomoxetine, leading to FDA black box labeling (Wolraich et al., 2019).

Behavioral and training interventions have been established to be effective in improving ADHD symptoms, although stimulant medications typically provide a greater degree of improvement over a shorter amount of time. Behavioral therapies train parents and teachers to adapt their response and/or the environment to improve the behavior of the child. Training interventions provide the children with skills to aid in coping with core ADHD symptoms. These interventions do not require a formal ADHD diagnosis, and it is recommended to refer parents for PTBM prior to diagnosing ADHD in preschool-age children when possible. Behavioral classroom interventions are also

> **PRO TIP** For parents or children who are hesitant to initiate treatment for ADHD, it often helps to explain that ADHD is a condition in which the brain developed with an imbalance of certain chemicals that help it to process information and control certain reactions. Help children and parents to understand that ADHD is not simply a problem with behaviors that are the child's choice; rather, the child's brain differences make it difficult to control the way they react to sensory information from their environment. Motivational interviewing techniques can be helpful when initiating the conversation about treatment options. For example, opening with as statement like "Tell me what you know about ADHD and how it is treated" can help identify and address common misperceptions held by many families. An explanation to help families understand how treatment may help is that parents, teachers, and children may notice a clear difference (like the "light being turned on"). It is also important to relay that ADHD symptoms may improve over time as the child matures, and that treatments are targeted to address the symptoms, and are not curative (Wolraich et al., 2019).

recommended for all ages, and parents can work with the public-school system to establish any additional required educational interventions and/or accommodations. While the improvement in ADHD symptoms may not be immediate, behavioral therapies may produce positive effects and teach coping strategies that persist over the long term (Wolraich et al., 2019).

Most common side effects of stimulant medications improve after 1 to 2 weeks of use. Recommend follow-up evaluation if abdominal pain, significant decrease in appetite, persistent headaches, new onset or worsening of motor tics, or sleep disturbances do not resolve after 2 weeks, or sooner if symptoms are severe.

ALERT: Seek immediate/emergent medical attention if suicidal thoughts, psychosis, concerning cardiac symptoms, or alterations in neurologic status occur.

It is important to educate children and families that ADHD is a chronic condition, and that there are significant risks associated with delaying or not adhering to treatment. Discontinuation of treatment has been associated with higher risk for criminality, violence, depression, substance abuse, interpersonal issues, and injuries (Wolraich et al., 2019). Routine follow-up to assess for side effects, efficacy of treatment, and adherence to treatment using a child/family-centered approach have been effective in other chronic conditions such as asthma. If families opt not to treat with medication due to religious or other beliefs or personal preference, those choices must be respected (Krull, 2019c).

### Referral

The primary care manager may consider referral to a specialist (pediatric psychiatrist, developmental-behavioral pediatrician, neurodevelopmentalist, pediatric neurologist, and/or child/school psychologist) if the diagnosis is unclear, there are significant comorbid conditions, or if there is not adequate response to treatment (Wolraich et al., 2019).

## AUTISM SPECTRUM DISORDERS

The word *autism* comes from the Greek word *autos*, which represents the meaning of *aloneness*. ASDs represent a broad range of developmental and neurologic disorders that can severely impair an individual's social interaction, communication, behaviors, and daily functioning. The etiology of these spectrum disorders is influenced by a combination of genetic and environmental factors, and currently has no cure. Autism formally entered the awareness of Western medicine largely in the middle of the 20th century. In the 1940s and 1950s two mental health practitioners, Hans Asperger and Bruno Bettelheim, sought to define a series of behavioral characteristics that ranged from mild, peculiar behavior (Asperger) to extreme social impairment and dysfunction. ASD was first described as a form of childhood schizophrenia marked by detachment from reality, was later categorized as a spectrum disorder, and to date is considered an all-inclusive diagnosis, ranging from mild to severe (Zeldovich, 2018).

ASD includes autistic disorder, pervasive developmental disorder, and Asperger syndrome (CDC, 2020c). Since May 2013, the *DSM-5* replaced all of these diagnoses, folding them into an umbrella diagnosis of ASDs with levels noted based on the amount of support needed. The requirement of a delay in language is no longer necessary for this diagnosis. Currently, there is no known single cause for ASD, but it is generally accepted that it is caused by abnormalities in brain structure or function. There is ongoing research into potential causes of ASD, which include genetics and genomics, triggers to include environmental factors, and theories regarding gut microbiota and associations to ASD. Autism occurs more frequently than expected among individuals with fragile X syndrome, tuberous sclerosis, congenital rubella syndrome, and untreated phenylketonuria (PKU). The Centers for Disease Control and Prevention's (CDC's) Study to Explore Early Development (SEED) is a multiyear U.S. study designed to identify factors that may put children at risk for ASD and other developmental disabilities (CDC, 2019).

The prevalence of ASD has been nationally tracked since 1996. By 2016 the CDC noted the prevalence of autism, as 1 in every 54 children has been diagnosed on the autism spectrum (2020b). Most children have been diagnosed after age 4, although ASD can be reliably diagnosed as early as age 2. Of children with ASD, 31% have an ID (IQ 85; Autism Speaks, 2020b). The latest findings from the CDC found no difference in prevalence rates between black and white children; however, a gap remains in prevalence among Hispanic children, indicating a need to expand screening and intervention in this group (2020b). As a disorder without a known etiology and a myriad of proposed treatment options, the challenge to healthcare practitioners is to recognize symptoms of pervasive developmental disorders and to screen for autism to link children to early intervention services.

## Subjective Findings

Because ASD occurs on a spectrum, behaviors can range from very mild to very severe and occur in all ethnic, socioeconomic, and age groups. It is important to remember to listen to parents when they describe behavior that seems atypical or delayed and to take your time with the history and physical examination to obtain a comprehensive assessment. Obtain a thorough history that includes key factors such as difficulties in childbirth, prematurity (in weeks), length in a neonatal intensive care unit with or without complications, and history of maternal substance abuse. The developmental history should be comprehensive, noting conditions such as deafness (which may cause speech delay) and other neurologic conditions known to impair fine and gross motor functioning. When obtaining the history, the PNP may find that some parents report that the child appeared to develop in a neurotypical range and then regressed, losing language or social skills previously gained (National Autism Association [NAA], n.d.).

Early symptoms of autism parents may report include:

- Not responding to their name (the child may appear deaf)
- Not pointing at objects or things of interest, or demonstrating interest
- Not playing "pretend" games
- Avoiding eye contact
- Wanting or preferring to be alone
- Having difficulty understanding, or demonstrating understanding of, other people's feelings or their own
- Having no speech, limited or delayed speech
- Repeating words or phrases over and over (echolalia)
- Giving unrelated answers to questions
- Getting upset by minor changes
- Having obsessive interests
- Flapping their hands, rocking their body, or spinning in circles
- Having unusual reactions (over- or undersensitivity) to the way things sound, smell, taste, look, or feel
- Having low to no social skills
- Demonstrating little safety or danger awareness
- Reversing pronouns (says "you" instead of "I")
- Lining up toys or other objects
- Playing with toys the same way every time
- Liking part of objects (e.g., the wheels)
- Becoming upset by minor changes
- Eating in unusual ways
- Sleeping in unusual ways, or not sleeping
- Reacting emotionally or demonstrating unusual moods
- Fearing more expected or lacking in fear
- Causing self-injury (head-banging or hitting head; NAA, n.d.)

### Risk Factors

The most common risk factors for autism are:

- Male gender
- Sibling or first-degree relative with autism or other atypical neurologic condition or genetic disorder

## Objective Findings

The physical examination of the child with ASD will likely be normal.

### Laboratory and Diagnostic Testing

The role of the primary care provider is to screen children appropriately for ASD. Developmental screening should take place at 9 months of age, 18 months of age, and at 24 or 30 months of age. The M-CHAT may be used from ages 16 to 30 months (https://m-chat.org). The M-CHAT is administered by the child's parent or caregiver and interpreted by the primary care provider. Additional screening might be needed if a child is at high risk for developmental delays due to preterm birth, low birth weight, having a sibling with ASD, or if behaviors associated with ASDs are present (NAA, n.d.). There are several free toolkits available to families who have concerns about their child's development or behavior. Two such toolkits are:

- NAA's *First Signs, Next Steps* (https://nationalautismassociation.org/first-signs-next-steps)
- Autism Speaks' *First Concern to Action Tool Kit* (www.autismspeaks.org/tool-kit/first-concern-action-tool-kit).

## Differential Diagnosis

The differential diagnosis for ASD includes:

- Angelman syndrome
- Chromosome disorder
- Epilepsy
- Habit disorder
- Hydrocephalus
- Infantile spasms
- Language disorder (mixed, phonologic, receptive, or stuttering)

- Minamata disease
- Moebius syndrome
- Nonketotic hyperglycinemia
- Tourette syndrome (Brasic et al., 2020)

ASD is a dyad of social *and* communication impairment as well as restricted repetitive and stereotyped patterns of behavior. The symptoms are present early on in development and affect daily functioning. The five persistent criteria noted at home and in a pediatric primary care setting are key to the diagnosis of ASD by a developmental specialist:

- **Criterion A:**
  - persistent social communication deficits and social interaction across multiple contexts such as social-emotional reciprocity, from abnormal social approach and failure of typical back-and-forth conversation to reduced sharing of interests, emotions, or affect as well as failure to initiate or respond to social interactions.
  - Deficits in nonverbal communicative behavior for social interaction ranging from poorly integrated verbal and nonverbal communication to abnormalities in eye contact and body language or deficits in understanding and use of gestures and total lack of facial expressions.
  - Deficits in the development, maintenance, and understanding of relationships to include social play, making friends, to absence of interest in peers.
- **Criterion B**: fixated interests and repetitive behaviors
- **Criterion C**: symptoms existing in early childhood
- **Criterion D**: symptoms impairing functioning
- **Criterion E**: impairments are not better explained by intellectual developmental disorder or GDD

In addition to these criteria, the diagnosing clinician measures the severity of these symptoms as very severe, severe, moderate, or mild in two symptom domains: social communication, and fixated interests and repetitive behaviors (APA, 2013).

## Treatment/Management

By identifying ASD as early as possible, maximal functioning of the child will be promoted. Treatment and intervention should be tailored to each individual child and be readjusted toward progress and goals of therapy. Applied behavior analysis (ABA) therapy is a therapy based on the science of learning and behavior. The main idea is to provide positive reinforcement for desired behavioral outcomes and rewards to repeat the behavior. Understanding the environment prior to behavior occurring or antecedents and consequences for desired or inappropriate behavior is rooted in rewards that are tailored to the child/adult with ASD. Those rewards can be praise, allowing time with a toy or book, access to a desired location like a playground or outing, and so on. Customizing behavioral outcomes involves a qualified and trained behavior analyst who designs and oversees programs to include skills, needs, interests, preferences, and family situation (Association for Science in Autism Treatment, 2020). In addition to ABA therapy, the provider should work with early intervention specialists, speech and language pathologists, occupational therapists, psychologists, psychiatrists, and/or developmental pediatricians to support interventions designed to improve outcomes in behavior, language, and socialization.

Monitor children with ASD for comorbidities including but not limited to:

- Gastrointestinal problems
- ADHD
- Anxiety
- Bipolar disorder
- Depression
- Disrupted sleep
- Epilepsy
- Feeding issues
- Obsessive compulsive disorder
- Schizophrenia

Of note for children with ASD are the well-documented issues around gut and dietary concerns. People with ASD have narrow diets and food jags, and often will only eat certain foods, all of which have profound effects on the microbiome and the bowel. The possible role of the microbiota-gut-brain correlation in ASD is in the forefront of research (Xiao et al., 2020). With the current pursuit of understanding of this neurodevelopmental condition, the possibility for a cure or therapies to mitigate the sequelae from this disorder can give hope to families and the healthcare communities caring for these individuals.

Provide follow-up with these children sooner rather than later to note subtle changes or persistent delays or abnormalities. Swift intervention with a multidisciplinary approach is paramount, and one must avoid excusing or downplaying the important role of early intervention with specialty care. Addressing questions and intentionally adding more time in your practice to allow for visual components and patience for these children will be key in avoiding behavioral issues and ensuring success when scheduling children for their assessments.

ASD is lifelong, and while services are available up to age 22, the implications for the increasing numbers of members of society with ASD are substantial. It is important to play a part in the individualized education plan process for families needing a 504 plan for their children in the school system. Also, teens with autism receive inadequate services and half as often as those with other special healthcare needs. In addition, the majority of autism's costs in the United States go toward for adult services: an estimated $175 to $196 billion a year (Autism Speaks, 2020b). One of the most meaningful ways to provide support is to ensure a warm hand-off for care from pediatric practice to adult family providers who will continue to provide quality care to adults with ASD.

**PRO TIP** Providing visual cues in the form of pictures, photographs, and lists (if the child has been taught to read) can help the child anticipate what their hour ahead and their day looks like, thus helping to ease anxiety of the unknown.

## Family Education

Teach the following:

- It can take many months to see a developmental specialist and get a confirmatory diagnosis of ASD. The assessment can take several hours for families and the office may be a lengthy driving distance for parents. Parents should NOT miss their appointment, as rescheduling can only further delay a diagnosis.
- Children and adults with ASD have splinter skill sets (abilities for certain tasks, not generalizing to other tasks). Some skills may be further developed than others and some may progress when other skill sets do not progress as rapidly as hoped or as desired. For poor fine and gross motor skills, the early interventionist as well as occupational or physical therapist can tailor a program to increase desired skill sets through intentional play or physical exercise to help with gait, eating, using a toothbrush, and the like.
- In all successful interventions, the physical organization and structured environment at home helps bring stability and anticipated outcomes for children and adults who become anxious when their environmental structure is altered. Children with ASD demand consistency, repetitive flow patterns, and structure in their daily lives. Any significant alterations can result in tantrums, meltdowns, or self-injurious behavior.
- Discuss myths related to autism and its treatment:
  - Treatments not demonstrated to cure autism (some may provide benefits to some children, others may pose health risks); these include chelation therapies, hyperbaric oxygen therapy, detoxifying clay baths, sensory-integration therapy, auditory enhancement, dietary or other supplements such as raw camel milk, or holding therapy (U.S. FDA, 2019).
  - Treatments for ASD behaviors vary widely and involve individual care plans for each child, with early behavioral interventions considered optimum for positive outcomes throughout a lifetime.
- Families should know that support is available. Autism Speaks provides valuable toolkits for both children and providers, with one of the most important toolkits being the 100 Day Toolkit (Autism Speaks, 2020a)

## Referral

If screening for an ASD is positive, refer for a comprehensive evaluation to a developmental pediatrician, a pediatric psychologist or psychiatrist, or pediatric neurologist. Once diagnosed, in addition to being followed by a pediatric developmental specialist, comprehensive services are provided through:

- Pediatric occupational, physical, and speech therapy.
- Registered dietitian or nutritional therapy.
- ABA therapy.
- Early intervention services.
- Special needs preschool programs.
- Counselors such as family therapists, licensed clinical social workers, or chaplains. Referral to pediatric gastroenterology may be needed for children demonstrating gastrointestinal issues.

## KEY POINTS

- ID is a neurodevelopmental condition that affects intellectual and adaptive functioning, with impairment ranging from mild to severe. It is a lifelong disorder, requires a multidisciplinary approach, and is highly associated with other neurodevelopmental and psychiatric disorders.
- FASD is a term that refers to a spectrum of physical, behavioral, cognitive, and mental health effects due to prenatal alcohol exposure ranging from mild to severe.
- The role of the PNP is to provide early identification, early intervention, and education, and to coordinate care with community resources, subspecialists, and educational services under the medical and chronic care models.

- PNPs in the primary care setting should initiate an evaluation for any child between ages 4–18 years presenting with academic or behavioral concerns and symptoms of inattention, hyperactivity, or impulsivity (Wolraich et al., 2019).
- Ensure that *DSM-5* criteria for ADHD have been met to make the diagnosis of ADHD, and rule out any alternative causes (Wolraich et al., 2019).
- Manage ADHD as a chronic condition under the chronic care model within the medical home (Wolraich et al., 2019).
- Titrate medication dosages for ADHD for maximum benefit with tolerable side effects (Wolraich et al., 2019).

## REFERENCES


American Academy of Pediatrics. (2020). *Fetal alcohol spectrum disorders program: Toolkit*. https://www.aap.org/en-us/advocacy-and-policy/aap-health-initiatives/fetal-alcohol-spectrum-disorders-toolkit/Pages/default.aspx

American Academy of Pediatrics, Subcommittee on Attention-Deficit/Hyperactivity Disorder and Steering Committee on Quality Improvement and Management. (2011). ADHD: Clinical practice guideline for the diagnosis, evaluation, and treatment of attention-deficit/hyperactivity disorder in children and adolescents. *Pediatrics, 128*(5), 1007–1022. https://doi.org/10.1542/peds.2011-2654

American Psychiatric Association. (2013). *Diagnostic and statistical manual of mental disorders: DSM-5* (5th ed.). American Psychiatric Publishing.

Autism Speaks. (2020a). *Autism speaks tool kits*. https://www.autismspeaks.org/autism-speaks-tool-kits

Autism Speaks. (2020b). *Autism statistics and facts*. https://www.autismspeaks.org/autism-statistics

Barbaresi, W. J., Campbell, L., Diekroger, E. A., Froehlich, T. E., Liu, Y. H., O'Malley, E., Pelham, W. E. J., Power, T. J., Zinner, S. H., & Chan, E. (2020). Society for Developmental and Behavioral Pediatrics clinical practice guideline for the assessment and treatment of children and adolescents with complex attention-deficit/hyperactivity disorder. *Journal of Developmental and Behavioral Pediatrics, 41*, S35–S57. https://doi.org/10.1097/DBP.0000000000000770

Barkley, R. A. (Ed.). (2015). *Attention-deficit hyperactivity disorder: A handbook for diagnosis and treatment* (4th ed.). Guilford Press.

Brasic, J. R., Farhadi, F., & Elshourbagy, T. (2020). Autism spectrum disorder. *eMedicine*. Retrieved October 4, 2002, from https://emedicine.medscape.com/article/912781-overview

Burd, L., & Edwards, W. (2019). *Fetal alcohol spectrum disorders: Implications for attorneys and the courts*. https://www.americanbar.org/groups/criminal_justice/publications/criminal-justice-magazine/2019/fall/fetal-alcohol-spectrum-disorders-implications-attorneys-courts

Centers for Disease Control and Prevention. (2019). *Study to explore early development (SEED)*. https://www.cdc.gov/ncbddd/autism/seed.html

Centers for Disease Control and Prevention. (2020a). *Data & statistics: Prevalence of FASDs*. https://www.cdc.gov/ncbddd/fasd/data.html

Centers for Disease Control and Prevention. (2020b). Prevalence of autism spectrum disorder among children 8 years—Autism and developmental disabilities monitoring network, 11 sites, United States, 2016. *Morbidity and Mortality Weekly Report, 69*(4), 1–12. https://www.cdc.gov/mmwr/volumes/69/ss/ss6904a1.htm?s_cid=ss6904a1_w

Centers for Disease Control and Prevention. (2020c). *What is autism spectrum disorder?* https://www.cdc.gov/ncbddd/autism/facts.html

Cobben, J. M., Krzyzewska, I. M., Venema, A., Mul, A. N., Polstra, A., Postma, A. V., Smigiel, R., Pesz, K., Niklinski, J., Chomczyk, M. A., Henneman, P., & Mannens, M. M. (2019). DNA methylation abundantly associates with fetal alcohol spectrum disorder and its subphenotypes. *Epigenomics, 11*(7), 767–785. https://doi.org/10.2217/epi-2018-0221

Friedman, L. S., Blaschke, G. S., Klam, W. P., & Stein, M. T. (2010). ADHD, medication, and the military service: A pediatrician's dilemma. *Journal of Developmental and Behavioral Pediatrics, 31*(3 Suppl.), S60–S63. https://doi.org/10.1097/DBP.0b013e3181d831b5

Hagan, J. F., Jr., Balachova, T., Bertrand, J., Chasnoff, I., Dang, E., Fernandez-Baca, D., Kable, J., Kosofsky, B., Senturias, Y. N., Singh, N., Sloane, M., Weitzman, C., Zubler, J., Neurobehavioral Disorder Associated with Prenatal Alcohol Exposure Workgroup, & American Academy of Pediatrics. (2016). Neurobehavioral disorder associated with prenatal alcohol exposure. *Pediatrics, 138*(4), e20151553. https://doi.org/10.1542/peds.2015-1553

Hoyme, H. E., Kalberg, W. O., Elliott, A. J., Blankenship, J., Buckley, D., Marais, A. S., Manning, M. A., Robinson, L. K., Adam, M. P., Abdul-Rahman, O., Jewett, T., Coles, C. D., Chambers, C., Jones, K. L., Adnams, C. M., Shah, P. E., Riley, E. P., Charness, M. E., Warren, K. R., & May, P. A. (2016). Updated clinical guidelines for diagnosing fetal alcohol spectrum disorders. *Pediatrics, 138*(2), e20154256. https://doi.org/10.1542/peds.2015-4256

Jensen, P. S., Hinshaw, S. P., Swanson, J. M., Greenhill, L. L., Conners, C. K., Arnold, L. E., Abikoff, H. B., Elliott, G., Hechtman, L., Hoza, B., March, J. S., Newcorn, J. H., Severe, J. B., Vitiello, B., Wells, K., & Wigal, T. (2001). Findings from the NIMH Multimodal Treatment Study of ADHD (MTA): Implications and applications for primary care providers. *Journal of Developmental and Behavioral Pediatrics, 22*(1), 60–73. https://doi.org/10.1097/00004703-200102000-00008

Kaufman, L., Ayub, M., & Vincent, J. B. (2010). The genetic basis of non-syndromic intellectual disability: A review. *Journal of Neurodevelopmental Disorders, 2*(4), 182–209. https://doi.org/10.1007/s11689-010-9055-2

Krull, K. R. (2019a). Attention deficit hyperactivity disorder in children and adolescents: Clinical features and diagnosis. *UpToDate*. Retrieved October 4, 2020, from https://www.uptodate.com/contents/attention-deficit-hyperactivity-disorder-in-children-and-adolescents-clinical-features-and-diagnosis

Krull, K. R. (2019b). Attention deficit hyperactivity disorder in children and adolescents: Epidemiology and pathogenesis. *UpToDate*. Retrieved October 4, 2020, from https://www.uptodate.com/contents/attention-deficit-hyperactivity-disorder-in-children-and-adolescents-epidemiology-and-pathogenesis

Krull, K. R. (2019c). Attention deficit hyperactivity disorder in children and adolescents: Overview of treatment and prognosis. *UpToDate*. Retrieved October 4, 2020, from https://www.uptodate.com/contents/attention-deficit-hyperactivity-disorder-in-children-and-

May, P. A., Chambers, C. D., Kalberg, W. O., Zellner, J., Feldman, H., Buckley, D., Kopald, D., Hasken, J. M., Xu, R., Honerkamp-Smith, G., Taras, H., Manning, M. A., Robinson, L. K., Adam, M. P., Abdul-Rahman, O., Vaux, K., Jewett, T., Elliott, A. J., Kable, J. A., … Hoyme, H. E. (2018). Prevalence of fetal alcohol spectrum disorders in 4 US communities. *JAMA, 319*(5), 474–482. https://doi.org/10.1001/jama.2017.21896

National Autism Association. (n.d.). *Signs of autism.* https://nationalautismassociation.org/resources/signs-of-autism

Owens, J. A. (2020). Pharmacotherapy for insomnia in children and adolescents: A rational approach. *UpToDate*. Retrieved October 4, 2020, from https://www.uptodate.com/contents/pharmacotherapy-for-insomnia-in-children-and-adolescents-a-rational-approach

Pivalizza, P. (2018). Intellectual disability in children: Management, outcomes, and prevention. *UpToDate*. Retrieved October 4, 2020, from https://www.uptodate.com/contents/intellectual-disability-in-children-management-outcomes-and-prevention

Pivalizza, P., & Lalani, S. R. (2018a). Intellectual disability in children: Definition, diagnosis, and assessment of needs. *UpToDate*. Retrieved October 4, 2020, from https://www.uptodate.com/contents/intellectual-disability-in-children-definition-diagnosis-and-assessment-of-needs

Pivalizza, P., & Lalani, S. R. (2018b). Intellectual disability in children: Evaluation for a cause. *UpToDate*. Retrieved October 4, 2020, from https://www.uptodate.com/contents/intellectual-disability-in-children-evaluation-for-a-cause

Schulte, E. E. (2015). Learning disorders: How pediatricians can help. *Cleveland Clinic Journal of Medicine, 82*(11, Suppl. 1), S24–S28. https://doi.org/10.3949/ccjm.82.s1.05

Streissguth, A. P., Bookstein, F. L., Barr, H. M., Sampson, P. D., O'Malley, K., & Young, J. K. (2004). Risk factors for adverse life outcomes in fetal alcohol syndrome and fetal alcohol effects. *Journal of Developmental and Behavioral Pediatrics, 25*(4), 228–238. https://doi.org/10.1097/00004703-200408000-00002

Topitzes, J., Godes, O., Mersky, J. P., Ceglarek, S., & Reynolds, A. J. (2009). Educational success and adult health: Findings from the Chicago longitudinal study. *Prevention Science, 10*(2), 175–195. https://doi.org/10.1007/s11121-009-0121-5

Treit, S., Jeffery, D., Beaulieu, C., & Emery, D. (2020). Radiological findings on structural magnetic resonance imaging in fetal alcohol spectrum disorders and healthy controls. *Alcoholism: Clinical Experimentation and Research, 44*(2), 455–462. https://doi.org/10.1111/acer.14263

Turchi, R. M., Smith, V. C., Committee on Substance Use and Prevention, & Council on Children with Disabilities. (2018). The role of integrated care in a medical home for patients with a fetal alcohol spectrum disorder. *Pediatrics, 142*(4), e20182333. https://doi.org/10.1542/peds.2018-2333

U.S. Food and Drug Administration. (2019). *Be aware of potentially dangerous products and therapies that claim to treat autism.* https://www.fda.gov/consumers/consumer-updates/be-aware-potentially-dangerous-products-and-therapies-claim-treat-autism

von Hahn, E. (2019a). Specific learning disabilities in children: Clinical features. *UpToDate*. Retrieved October 4, 2020, from https://www.uptodate.com/contents/specific-learning-disabilities-in-children-clinical-features?search=learning+disability

von Hahn, E. (2019b). Specific learning disabilities in children: Evaluation. *UpToDate*. Retrieved October 4, 2020, from https://www.uptodate.com/contents/specific-learning-disabilities-in-children-evaluation?search=learning+disability

von Hahn, E. (2019c). Specific learning disabilities in children: Role of the primary care provider. *UpToDate*. Retrieved October 4, 2020, from https://www.uptodate.com/contents/specific-learning-disabilities-in-children-role-of-the-primary-care-provider?search=learning+disability

Weitzman, C., & Rojmahamongkol, P. (2020a). Fetal alcohol spectrum disorder: Clinical features and diagnosis. *UpToDate*. Retrieved October 4, 2020, from https://www.uptodate.com/contents/fetal-alcohol-spectrum-disorder-clinical-features-and-diagnosis

Weitzman, C., & Rojmahamongkol, P. (2020b). Fetal alcohol spectrum disorder: Management and prognosis. *UpToDate*. Retrieved October 4, 2020, from https://www.uptodate.com/contents/fetal-alcohol-spectrum-disorder-management-and-prognosis

White, P. H., Cooley, W. C., & Transitions Clinical Report Authoring Group, American Academy of Pediatrics, American Academy of Family Physicians, American College of Physicians. (2018). Supporting the health care transition from adolescence to adulthood in the medical home. *Pediatrics, 142*(5), e20182587. https://doi.org/10.1542/peds.2018 -2587

Wolraich, M. L., Hagan, J. F., Jr., Allan, C., Chan, E., Davison, D., Earls, M., Evans, S. W., Flinn, S. K., Froehlich, T., Frost, J., Holbrook, J. R., Lehmann, C. U., Lessin, H. R., Okechukwu, K., Pierce, K. L., Winner, J. D., Zurhellen, W., & Subcommittee on Children and Adolescents with Attention-Deficit/Hyperactive Disorder. (2019). Clinical practice guideline for the diagnosis, evaluation, and treatment of attention-deficit/hyperactivity disorder in children and adolescents. *Pediatrics, 144*(4), e20192528. https://doi.org/10.1542/peds.2019-2528

Xiao, Y., Angulo, M. T., Lao, S., Weiss, S. T., & Yang-Yu, L. (2020). An ecological framework to understand the efficacy of fecal microbiota transplantation. *Nature Communications, 11*, 3329. https://doi.org/10.1038/s41467-020-17180-x

Xu, G., Strathearn, L., Liu, B., Yang, B., & Bao, W. (2018). Twenty-year trends in diagnosed attention-deficit/hyperactivity disorder among US children and adolescents, 1997–2016. *JAMA Network Open, 1*(4), e181471. https://doi.org/10.1001/jamanetworkopen.2018.1471

Zeldovich, L. (2018). *The evolution of 'autism' as a diagnosis, explained*. https://www.spectrumnews.org/news/evolution-autism-diagnosis-explained

## FURTHER READING

Individuals with Disabilities Education Improvement Act of 2004. (2004). Public Law No. 108-446. HYPERLINK "http://www.copyright" www.copyright.gov/legislation/pl108-446.pdf

Maki, K. E., Floyd, R. G., & Roberson, T. (2015). State learning disability eligibility criteria: A comprehensive review. *School Psychology Quarterly, 30*(4), 457–469. https://doi.apa.org/doi/10.1037/spq0000109

von Hahn, E. (2020). Definitions of specific learning disability and laws pertaining to learning disabilities in the United States. *UpToDate*. Retrieved October 4, 2020, from https://HYPERLINK "http://www.uptodate.com/contents/definitions-of-specific" www.uptodate.com/contents/definitions-of-specific-learning-disability-and-laws-pertaining-to-learning-disabilities-in-the-united-states?search=learning+disability

# Management of Mental Health Disorders

Rebecka Evans and Melody M. Avila

## Student Learning Outcomes

**Upon completion of this chapter the reader should be able to:**

1. Discuss pathophysiology and epidemiology of selected mental health disorders in children.
2. Differentiate subjective and objective findings of selected mental health disorders in children.
3. Choose appropriate laboratory or diagnostic tests for particular mental health disorders in children.
4. Utilize the differential diagnosis process to determine mental health diagnosis in children.
5. Determine treatment plan, child/family education, and need for referral for children with mental health diagnoses.

## INTRODUCTION

The goals of the clinical evaluation of a child with mental health concerns are to assess developmental progress and attainments; understand/clarify the presenting behavioral and emotional issues; assess current and previous functioning in various settings (i.e., school, home); and to assess the strengths of the child and the family (Srinath et al., 2019). Adolescents and older children should be interviewed without a parent/guardian present, as they will often disclose more information regarding their mental and social history and experiences in a confidential setting. The provider should also interview the parent for further information to support the child and adolescent's needs.

The content in this chapter maps to the following areas on the Pediatric Nursing Certification Board (PNCB) Pediatric Nurse Practitioner—Primary Care certification examination.

**CLINICAL PROBLEMS: DEVELOPMENTAL/ BEHAVIORAL/MENTAL HEALTH**

CONTENT AREAS:

**II. Assessment and Diagnosis**

**B. History and Physical Examination**

1. Obtain history of present illness.
2. Obtain a comprehensive health history for new patients.
3. Complete an interval history for established patients.
4. Perform a review of systems.
5. Perform a complete physical examination.

**C. Diagnostic Testing and Screening**

1. Order and interpret office/clinic-based screening tests.
2. Order and interpret diagnostic laboratory tests.
4. Select, utilize, and interpret developmental, behavioral, and mental health screening and assessment tools.

**D. Analyzing Information**

1. Integrate health history and physical examination findings into the plan of care.
2. Assimilate findings from screening and diagnostic testing into the plan of care.

3. Utilize information from consulting services in the plan of care.

**E. Diagnosis**

1. Develop and prioritize differential diagnoses.
2. Establish a diagnosis based on evaluation of patient data.

## III. Management

**A. Child and Caregiver Counseling and Education**

1. Provide condition-specific counseling and education, including treatment options.
2. Educate about benefits and potential adverse reactions of pharmacologic interventions.
3. Discuss nonpharmacologic interventions.
4. Counsel regarding the threshold for seeking follow-up care.
5. Review the risks of non-adherence to recommended treatment.

**B. Therapeutic Interventions**

1. Prescribe pharmacologic agents.
2. Recommend the use of over-the-counter pharmacologic agents.
3. Order or recommend nonpharmacologic treatments for the management of symptoms.
4. Discuss use of complementary and alternative therapies as appropriate.
5. Utilize communication techniques and brief cognitive interventions, including motivational interviewing and joint decision-making, to develop healthcare goals and facilitate change.

**D. Collaboration and Referral**

2. Refer to specialists as indicated for evaluation, counseling, and/or treatment.
3. Contact child protective services to report suspected maltreatment or neglect.

**E. Care Coordination**

1. Facilitate patient and family-centered care for children of all ages with acute and chronic conditions.

**F. Evaluation and Follow-up**

2. Establish a plan for follow-up care.

## IV. Professional Role and Responsibilities

**A. Leadership and Evidence-based Practice**

4. Develop, implement, and/or modify clinical practice guidelines.

# ANATOMY AND PHYSIOLOGY

Knowing typical growth patterns for cognitive, social, and emotional development in children and adolescents is critical for assessment of mental health concerns. Children and adolescents presenting with emotional and behavioral concerns may actually be within the parameters of expected growth and development. It is vital to differentiate between normal growth and development and those with developmental delays by obtaining a thorough and accurate history.

Brain development is a lifelong process; however, the rapid growth in the first 8 years of life is critical to prepare for the fountain of learning and long-term development (Centers for Disease Control and Prevention [CDC], 2020a). In the first years of life there is a rapid proliferation of neural connections followed by a process called pruning, where the connections are reduced and the brain becomes more efficient (Center on the Developing Child, 2020). There is an interaction between genes and experiences that shape cognitive, social, and emotional development.

The prefrontal cortex and the amygdala are the areas of the brain correlated with emotional development, planning, and problem-solving. These areas develop slowly, paralleling the development of emotion regulation (Tottenham, 2017). While the majority of the brain's physical growth is complete by age 8, the brain does not completely mature until the age of 25 (Arain et al., 2013).

There are many theories that explore cognitive and social emotional development. Stage theories, such as Piaget's theory, focus on qualitative changes in cognitive development and that these changes are due to biological maturation and interactions with their environment (Siegler, 2020). Sociocultural theories focus on how other people and the beliefs and values of the surrounding culture influence children's development, whereas information processing theories (i.e., David Klahr's theory) focus on one's ability to process and adapt information taken from the environment and store and alter this information based on continued learning (Siegler, 2020).

## Subjective Findings

The health history may reveal:

- Past history of behavioral concerns or medical issues: Note other emotional or development diagnoses, whether this issue is continuous or episodic, as well as the child's behavior in different situations/ environments (with family, friends, school)

- Fetal or maternal concerns during pregnancy or exposures to dangerous substances
- Concerns in the developmental history: Note at which age the child met developmental milestones. Are there any that have not yet been met for age or loss of any milestones? Any social, language, or learning delays? Any changes in development or learning? Note if there have been any interruptions (illness, surgery, etc.) that may have affected progress (such as hearing loss due to repeated ear infections affecting speech development).
- Temperament: What is the child's response/reaction to environmental situations? What way(s) does the child self-regulate or soothe themself? It is important to note parental perception of the behavior; parental personalities can lead to over- or underreporting of behavior.
- School history: academic or social challenges, child's strengths as related to school/learning, concerns with adjustments, transitions, teachers, or learning styles. Information should be obtained from parent, child, and teachers, if possible.
- Strengths, skills, and interests:
    - Asking about interests can help build rapport and connection with the child, such as what the child does for fun, extracurricular activities, and sports.
- When asking about family history, determine if there is any family history of mental health disorders including depression, anxiety, bipolar disorder (BPD), schizophrenia, learning disabilities, eating disorders, and if anyone else is the family has been on medication for these. Also determine family dynamics, perceptions, and influences.
- Social history: food insecurity, family dynamics, stressors, or parental discord (divorce, loss of job), development of friendships and relationships, if the adolescent is sexually active, gender and sexual identity, substance use (alcohol, marijuana, or other substances), and if the child has ever been trafficked for sex.

> **PRO TIP** Questions about the social history should be asked of the adolescent in private as well.

## Risk Factors

The most common risk factors for mental health disorders are adverse events associated with childhood experiences including (Oral et al., 2016):

- Abuse (physical, emotional, psychological, or sexual)
- Neglect (physical, emotional, basic needs)
- Insecure attachment to caregiver
- Divorce or separation of parents
- Intimate partner violence or domestic abuse
- Mother—a figure with history of abuse
- Caregiver with mental health illness, such as depression
- Household member in prison or with alcohol or substance use disorder
- Parental mental health problems are highly correlated to child or adolescent developing mental health concerns. This is due to genetic predisposition as well as parental reactivity to a child's temperament and needs. (Wlodarczyk et al., 2017).
- Lower socioeconomic status is associated with increased mental health issues. This increases with the child's age, so adolescents with parents with low socioeconomic status are at higher risk than young children (Wlodarczyk et al., 2017).
- Prolonged exposure to trauma and the biological stress response (toxic stress) affects early brain development and later brain function, including executive functions, control over emotions, and impulses (American Psychological Association, 2019).
- Hispanic and African American children, adolescents in particular, are at higher risk than their non-Hispanic white counterparts. Children who are racial and ethnic minorities are also more likely to have more persistent mental health problems. These differences are due to low socioeconomic status (which disproportionately affects minority children), increased likelihood of single parent or stepfamily homes, increased exposure to adverse childhood experiences, and disadvantages of neighborhood and social stressors (e.g., violence, access, mobility; American Psychological Association, 2019).
- Environmental risk factors include prenatal exposure to toxins including maternal nicotine and alcohol use, chemical contaminants, and maternal stress (American Psychological Association, 2019).
- Preschool children with more difficult, negative, or rigid temperaments are more likely to develop depressive and anxiety disorders. Difficult temperament is also associated with increased parental mental health issues (Wlodarczyk et al., 2017).
- Gender: Females are at increased risk of experiencing sexual abuse and assault at any age while males are at increased risk of experiencing physical violence and exposure to gang violence (American Psychological Association, 2019). Males have increased risk of externalizing symptoms while females are

more likely to experience internalized symptoms (internalized symptoms can take longer to diagnose due to underreporting and gender biases (American Psychological Association, 2019). Males are also less likely to seek care.

- Lesbian, gay, bisexual, transgender, and queer (LGBTQ+) children and adolescents are also at higher risk for mental health as compared with cisgender or heterosexual peers. They have higher rates of anxiety, depression, low self-esteem, self-injurious behaviors, suicide, substance use, and eating disorders (American Psychological Association, 2019). LGBTQ+ children and adolescents are more likely to be bullied or harassed and experience higher rates of dating violence. They are also less likely to access healthcare services due to provider discomfort or lack of knowledge to provide sensitive and comprehensive care (American Psychological Association, 2019).

## Review of Systems

The most common manifestations revealed during the review of systems include:

- **Constitutional**: fatigue, weight changes, irritability, chills, sweating
- **Integumentary:** rashes, scars, bruises, burns, lacerations, bald spots, missing eyelashes
- **HEENT:** changes in vision, earaches/infections, sinus infections
- **Pulmonary**: shortness of breath, cough, chest pain, smoking history
- **Cardiovascular**: pain, palpitations, syncope, tachycardia
- **Gastrointestinal:** nausea, vomiting, constipation, diarrhea, abdominal pain, acid reflux, urgency, encopresis (primary or secondary)
- **Genitourinary**: enuresis (primary or secondary), urgency and/or accidents, history of sexually transmitted infection, sexual dysfunction
- **Gynecological**: menarche, last menstrual period, cycle duration, dysmenorrhea, sexual dysfunction, breast changes (sensitivity, enlargement, pain, discharge)
- **Musculoskeletal**: muscle or joint pain, muscle cramping, weakness
- **Neurological**: headaches, migraines, history of concussion, coordination issues, chronic pain
- **Endocrine**: heat/cold intolerance
- **Psychiatric**: behavior concerns, irritability, depressed mood, anxiety, difficulty with sleep, attention and/or concentration issues, school concerns

## Objective Findings

The physical examination of the child with a mental health disorder may reveal:

- Signs of systemic illnesses as well as signs of self-injurious behaviors and/or abuse (scars, bruising, petechiae, abrasions, skin picking). Lesions on fingers/hands can be a sign of self-induced purging. Hair loss (particularly in patterns) or missing eyelashes can indicate compulsive behaviors.
- Signs of self-care and neglect of hygiene as these can be indicators of mental health concerns or parental abuse/neglect
- Dysmorphic facial features (which may indicate genetic disorders, such as Fragile X, Turner's, Angelman, or Prader-Willi syndrome)
- Dental hygiene and signs of self-induced vomiting. Assessment of vision and hearing rule out vision or hearing difficulties that may be contributing to behavioral and emotional symptoms.

Neurological assessment is critical for children presenting with mental health concerns. Assess cranial nerves, sensory and motor systems, balance and coordination, and reflexes. Asking a child to draw can help assess their fine motor skills as well as their cognition, attention, and emotional state. Knowing previous abilities aids in understanding if current presentation is a drastic change from previous level of functioning.

- **Mental Status Examination**
  - Attitude (cooperation, engagement, eye contact)
  - Appearance including hygiene and grooming
  - Mood (how does child/adolescent describe and rate)
  - Affect (emotional range [i.e., full, constricted, flat, labile])
  - Speech (rate, volume, rhythm, articulation)
  - Thought processes (are they logical, linear, concrete versus abstract?)
  - Thought content (MUST ask about these)
    - Suicidal and/or violent ideation
      - Assess for passive or active ideation both past and present
        - If having suicidal ideation it is important to assess for plan and intent:
          - Intent to harm
          - Protective factors (reason not to harm self or commit suicide)
    - Are they experiencing hallucinations, delusions, or paranoia?
    - Homicidal ideation (assess for child or adolescent's ideation for hurting someone else)

- Insight and judgment: Are they able to understand behaviors/emotions (generally rated as good, fair, poor)?
- Cognitive
  - Assess for orientation, working memory, attention and concentration, ability to abstract

▶ ALERT: Inform the child or adolescent that confidentiality is always secured with the provider unless the child or adolescent wants to hurt themselves or other people.

## EATING DISORDERS

The most common eating disorders include anorexia nervosa (AN), bulimia nervosa (BN), binge-eating disorder, and avoidant restrictive food intake disorder (ARFID). The primary age of onset of eating disorders is between 12 and 26 years of age, with the majority having onset between 14 and 18 years. The morbidity and mortality rates of eating disorders are 10 to 12 times higher than the typical adolescent rate for morbidity and mortality. Eating disorders have a long-term course of recovery.

### ANOREXIA NERVOSA

AN is characterized by refusal to maintain body weight at or above normal weight for age and height. Those with AN generally have an intense fear of gaining weight or being fat despite being underweight, and often have a distorted perspective of their weight and appearance (American Psychiatric Association, 2013).

There are two types of AN, restricting type and binge-eating and purging type. Those with restricting type only engage in restrictive eating behaviors. Those with binge-eating and purging type AN regularly engage in bingeing and purging behaviors, including self-induced vomiting, laxative and diuretic use/abuse, and exercise. These behaviors are used to reduce weight or limit weight gain.

AN has the highest mortality rate of all mental health disorders. Approximately 20% of those with AN will die without treatment and about 10% of those who receive treatment will die from complications related to their illness.

### BULIMIA NERVOSA

BN is characterized by recurrent episodes of binge eating, with recurrent and inappropriate behaviors to prevent weight gain. Binge eating is defined as eating an amount of food that is larger than what most people would eat in a similar period of time under similar circumstances. Individuals describe a lack of control over their eating during the episode. Binging and inappropriate weight control compensatory behaviors occur, on average, at least twice a week for at least 3 months. Compensatory behaviors include purging (self-induced vomiting); misuse of laxatives, diuretics, or enemas; fasting; and/or excessive exercise.

### BINGE-EATING DISORDER

Binge eating was first recognized as a distinct eating disorder in the *Diagnostic and Statistical Manual of Mental Disorders* (5th ed.; *DSM-5*; American Psychiatric Association, 2013). Binge eating disorder (BED) is the most common of all eating disorders, often presenting in subclinical form (National Eating Disorders Association [NEDA], 2018a). The peak prevalence of BED is ages 16 to 17 (Office on Women's Health, 2017). BED is defined as eating in a period of time an amount of food that is definitely larger than most people would eat in a similar period of time. Those with BED have a sense of lack of control over their eating during the episode. Binge eating episodes are also associated with eating rapidly, eating until uncomfortably full, eating a large amount of food without feeling hungry, eating alone because of embarrassment about the quantity of food, and feeling disgusted, depressed, or guilty after eating. Behaviors occur at least weekly for 3 months. There is no associated use of inappropriate compensatory behaviors (i.e., purging, exercising). While many with BED are overweight or obese, BED also occurs in normal weight individuals and is distinct from obesity. Most obese individuals do not engage in recurrent binge eating (American Psychiatric Association, 2013).

### AVOIDANT RESTRICTIVE FOOD INTAKE DISORDER

ARFID is characterized by highly selective eating and/or feeding patterns that often result in significant nutrition and energy deficiencies. In children and adolescents this can lead to failure to gain weight. The *DSM-5* defines ARFID as a feeding or eating disturbance due to lack of interest in eating or food; avoidance based on the sensory characteristics of food; or concern about aversive consequences of eating (i.e., fear of vomiting/choking, fear of nausea) with persistent failure to meet appropriate nutritional and/or energy needs associated with one (or more) of the following:

- Significant weight loss (or failure to achieve expected weight gain or faltering growth in children
- Significant nutritional deficiency
- Dependence on enteral feeding or oral nutritional supplements
- Significant interference with psychosocial functioning

In general, children and adolescents with ARFID do not have concerns with their weight or body shape. This diagnosis is made when there is not a better explanation of eating patterns, such as scarcity of food, cultural practices, or other condition. If the symptoms exist within the context of another condition, it is important to assess if the symptoms are more severe than would traditionally be expected. ARFID diagnosis is typically established at a younger age as compared with other eating disorders, such as AN and BN (Norris et al., 2016).

## Subjective Findings

The health history may reveal:

- Parental concern that there is something physically wrong with their child (due to weight loss, refusal to eat, complaints of discomfort when eating; AN, ARFID)
- Parental concern about their child's limited food choices, such as the child will only eat foods of certain consistency and texture (ARFID, AN), or the child has a history of being a "picky eater" (ARFID)
- Conflict around eating and meals, or the parent may notice the child/adolescent eating large amounts of food, or that food seems to disappear (BED, BN)
- Child or adolescent reports eating too much and not feeling like they can control their eating (BED, BN)
- Family history of diabetes, cardiovascular disease, eating disorders, obesity, metabolic disorders, celiac disease, food allergies/intolerance, or autism spectrum disorder (ASD)

## Risk Factors

The most common risk factors for eating disorders include:

*Biological:*

- Family history of disordered eating or eating disorder
- Female (3× higher rate than males)
- Males who identify as gay, bisexual, or transgender
- Transgender adolescents (rates of eating disorders are 5 times higher than gender conforming peers) (Diemer, et al 2015)
- Prader-Willi syndrome
- Childhood obesity (associated with the development of BED) Diemer et al., 2015; (Kornstein et al., 2016).

*Environmental:*

- Family conflict
- Change in family structure
- Death or severe illness of family member
- Abuse or neglect
- Parent or sibling with disordered eating or eating disorder, mental health concerns, or substance use

ARFID onset is typically at a younger age than other eating disorders and can also be a gradual progression of "picky eating" into disordered eating (Spicer et al, 2019). ARFID is more common in males than females, and at younger ages (NEDA, 2018b). Children and adolescents with an autism spectrum diagnosis and/or sensory hypersensitivity are at higher risk for ARFID and are more likely to have more severe symptoms than children and adolescents with typical social and emotional development (Dovey et al., 2019). Children and adolescents with anxiety around nausea and vomiting, fear of choking, or fears of food contamination are at risk for developing ARFID (NEDA, 2018a; Norris et al., 2016).

## Review of Systems

The most common manifestations revealed during the review of systems include:

- **Constitutional:** weight loss (AN), overweight, obese or significant weight gain (BED), abdominal discomfort or pain, "not hungry," "getting full too easily," weakness, fatigue, headache
- **HEENT:** gum sensitivity, caries (BN), swollen glands, specifically the salivary glands (BN)
- **Cardiovascular:** palpitations, chest pain
- **Gastrointestinal:** nausea, constipation, diarrhea, bloating, acid reflux, vague complaints of pain/discomfort, food allergies
- **Musculoskeletal:** muscle cramping, joint pain
- **Neurologic:** dizziness, syncope
- **Endocrine:** intolerance to cold
- **Reproductive:** menstrual irregularities, loss of menses, delayed menarche
- **Psychiatric/Behavioral:** restricted eating, fears around eating certain types of foods (especially carbohydrates and fats), mood disorders, ADHD, fear of choking, nausea, vomiting (ARFID), obsessive compulsive disorder or other anxiety disorder, ASD (ARFID)

## Objective Findings

The physical examination of the child with an eating disorder may reveal:

- Low body temperature, cold extremities (AN), dressing in layers to hide weight or to stay warm (AN), weight changes: loss, failure to meet expected growth and weight based on previous growth curves (AN, ARFID), weight may be normal or overweight (BN, BED), or overweight or obese (BED)
- Hypotension or orthostatic hypotension (AN, BN), bradycardia or tachycardia, arrhythmias
- Bruising, dry skin, lanugo (AN), hair loss, brittle nails, calluses on fingers/knuckles (signs of self-induced vomiting)
- Swelling/enlargement of salivary glands (BN), dental—cavities, tooth sensitivity, enamel erosion (BN), throat erythema (BN)
- Constipation (or diarrhea if laxative abuse), epigastric tenderness, decreased bowel sounds (AN, ARFID)
- Anxious or depressed mood/affect, suicidality.

▶ ALERT: Suicide attempts and completed suicide are relatively common among patients with eating disorders, especially in those with binge/purge or purging behaviors. Death from suicide is 50 times more likely in patients with AN, and 25% to 35% of patients with BN report a history of attempted suicide (Herpertz-Dahlmann, 2009; Keel et al., 2003).

## Laboratory/Diagnostic Testing

The diagnosis of an eating disorder is based primarily upon the clinical findings. Severity of the disorder is assessed by laboratory and diagnostic testing. For AN and BN, an electrocardiogram (ECG) should be obtained to assess for cardiovascular disturbances as well as orthostatic vital signs. The most common findings are sinus bradycardia and prolongation of the QT interval (Vargas & Gomez, 2015). Obtain a complete blood count (thrombocytopenia, anemia, leucopenia), urea and electrolytes (increased creatinine, low potassium, sodium, magnesium, calcium, phosphorus), glucose (low), and amylase level (BN). Follicle-stimulating hormone and luteal hormones may be suppressed. If these are markedly abnormal, the child may need oral or intravenous (IV) replacement and/or hospitalization to manage. If indicated (for AN or ARFID), testing should be done to rule out malabsorption issues and celiac disease. Bone density scan is often done to assess for osteoporosis or osteopenia as development of bone mass peaks between ages 11 to 14. Bone densitometry is recommended for adolescents who have not had a menstrual cycle for more than 6 to 12 months (Rosen & the Committee on Adolescence, 2010). There is a correlation between length of time a female is amenorrheic and level of bone loss.

**PRO TIP** Obtaining urine-specific gravity can be useful to determine if a child is water loading before being weighed to falsely elevate weight.

## Differential Diagnosis

The differential diagnosis for eating disorders includes (note that many of these can be comorbid or associated conditions):

- Inflammatory bowel disease, malabsorption, or celiac disease
- Diabetes mellitus, hyperthyroidism, hypopituitarism, or Addison disease
- Affective disorders, anxiety disorders, obsessive-compulsive disorder (OCD), posttraumatic stress disorder, or substance use/abuse
- Central nervous system (CNS) tumor
- Other chronic disease or chronic infections
- Superior mesenteric artery syndrome (can also be a consequence of AN)
- Stressful home environment, child abuse or neglect, or sexual abuse.

## Treatment/Management Plan

The level of care needed is determined by evaluation of vital signs, laboratory findings, weight, and psychiatric stability, as well as motivation for recovery and ability to restrain from using behaviors. There is often movement up and down in level of care during the course of treatment.

Inpatient medical or psychiatric hospitalization is needed with marked orthostatic hypotension, with an increase of pulse 20 bpm or a drop in blood pressure (BP) of 20 mmHg standing, bradycardia (heart rate <40 bpm), significant electrolyte imbalance (hypokalemia, hypophosphatemia, hyponatremia), inability to sustain body temperature, and refusal of fluids or food. Prepubertal children are at particular risk of becoming dehydrated and even small fluctuations in their weight can result in physiologic instability. Weight at less than 70% of ideal body weight requires medical stabilization. Many children and adolescents with ARFID who are admitted to hospital or residential treatment rely on enteral nutrition to gain weight and often require longer stays than for other eating disorders (Norris et al., 2016). If a child is medically stable, but under 85% of ideal body weight, residential level of care is recommended.

Intensive outpatient programs generally provide ~3 hours of program 3 to 5 days a week and participants are generally motivated for treatment. Partial hospital programs provide structure and support for 6 to 8 hours per day if participants are at least partially motivated for treatment. Residential programs are for those needing 24-hour monitoring to manage their eating disorder behaviors and other comorbid conditions.

For AN and BN, the first step in treatment is nutritional rehabilitation. The goals are to restore weight, normalize eating patterns, restore appropriate and more accurate perception of hunger and satiety, and to correct the sequelae of malnutrition. An individualized weight goal range is based on clinical data and considerations of current weight, restoration to previous growth curve, restoration of menses, and assessment of skeletal frame (determined by wrist x-ray) (Lenton-Brym et al., 2019). The expected weight gain in inpatient and residential treatment is 2 to 3 pounds/week while expected weight gain in outpatient treatment is 0.5 to –1 pound/week. Caloric intake is started at 30 to 40 kcal/kg per day (~1,000–1,600 kcal/day) and will progressively advance to 70 to 100 kcal/kg per day. Males require a larger number of calories to gain weight.

## Outpatient Monitoring

Outpatient monitoring by primary care includes:

- Weekly weight-checking (more frequent if needed). Weight is measured after the patient voids and while the patient is wearing a hospital gown or basic clothing. Blind weights (where the patient is looking away from the scale) are often recommended for outpatient monitoring in order to ensure the patient's weight is not known to them.
- Laboratory monitoring: monitor serum electrolyte and potassium regularly. Treat hypokalemia with oral potassium. For individuals with AN, magnesium and phosphorus are recommended during the refeeding and weight gain periods. Urine-specific gravity is useful to determine if a patient is water loading before weigh-in.
- Restrict physical activity while the individual needs to gain weight. Caloric expenditure is greater during the phase of recovery that requires weight gain. Once a patient has restored weight and is ready to return to activities/sports, it is important to adjust calorie intake so that weight can be maintained.

## Pharmacologic Treatments

There are no U.S. Food and Drug Administration (FDA)-approved pharmacologic treatments for AN, BED, or ARFID, though fluoxetine is approved for use in children 12 years of age and older with BN. Identifying and treating comorbid disorders is important for recovery.

Children and adolescents with AN are often started on calcium and vitamin D supplements to support bone growth and mineralization. There is evidence for use of medications to stimulate appetite (olanzapine, cyproheptadine [Brackett, 2017]), decrease obsessive thinking (olanzapine), decrease nausea (ondansetron), and increase gastrointestinal motility (metoclopramide). There is limited evidence regarding the use of benzodiazepines with meals to decrease anxiety around eating. Lisdexamfetamine dimesylate is approved by the FDA for the treatment of adults with BED. Selective serotonin reuptake inhibitors (SSRIs) and serotonin-norepinephrine reuptake inhibitors have been studied with variable results on improvement of binge-eating symptoms and weight reduction (Kornstein, 2016).

## Therapeutic Approach

A team approach is critical for children and adolescents with eating disorders. In addition to the primary care provider, the team should include a dietician, therapist, psychiatric medication management (if needed), and family therapist (if needed). Psychosocial and behavioral interventions are the most important and effective treatment tools for eating disorders.

**PRO TIP** Transition to high school, to college, or significant losses (death, relationship conflicts) can trigger behaviors that have been well controlled for a long time.

Cognitive behavior therapy (CBT) is the recommended treatment for eating disorders in adolescents. CBT focuses on changing thought processes and behaviors related to eating. There is also evidence that internet-based CBT can provide effective support for BED, especially when identified early. Online interventions may increase adolescent willingness to seek help and have increased accessibility, decreased cost, and time commitments (Marzille et al., 2018). Other therapeutic options are interpersonal therapy (short-term therapy focused on reducing interpersonal difficulties) and dialectical behavior therapy (DBT, which focuses on emotion dysregulation and learning how to recognize, tolerate, and regulate emotions and moods). For BED, behavioral weight loss treatments that focus on physical activity and modifying diet are best combined with CBT in adolescents to modulate potential negative impact on self-esteem and contribute to worsening of eating behaviors and psychiatric symptoms. There are no studies on the treatment of BED in adolescent males.

Currently there are no evidence-based treatment recommendations for ARFID; however, clinical experience suggests that treatment should be focused on the aspects that are contributing to the eating disturbances and distress/fear (Norris et al., 2016). For example, if an adolescent is presenting with restriction and weight loss due to fear of vomiting, it may be best to utilize CBT to address these fears, whereas a child with a long history of poor growth and "picky eating" that has intensified might need a combination of psychological and behavioral approaches. Despite some presentations of significant weight loss and restrictive eating, many eating disorder programs are not adequately equipped to manage ARFID patients, due to older age requirements (often over age 13) and limitations of programming to accommodate the gradual introduction of foods that have been avoided. Family-based therapy may also be utilized for ARFID.

### Family Education

Teach the following:

- Team approach is critical for long-term recovery.
- The entire family is affected, so education and support is needed for all of the family. Willingness to engage in family therapy and to be involved with the child who has been diagnosed with disordered eating increases likelihood of recovery.
- Remember that recovery is not a linear process. There are often setbacks, especially with transitions or life stressors.
- Family meals are a good way to reestablish good routines and healthy relationships with food.
- Regular and long-term follow-up is important due to the fluid nature of the illness.
- Treatment of comorbid and underlying disorders is important for long-term improvement.

## ANXIETY DISORDERS

Anxiety is a biochemical and maladaptive response to natural fears, worries, and concerns. The sense of unease and apprehension can be an adaptive and expected part of childhood development. This sensation is often useful to heighten the senses, drive motivation, and be protective in the perception of danger. Anxiety develops into a maladaptive response when it extends beyond practicality and becomes a notable distress that impairs daily activities.

Anxiety is one of the most prevalent psychiatric illnesses that often coincides with depression disorders, linking a possible neural and biochemical response in serotonin and norepinephrine (Żmudzka et al., 2018). The psychological stress of chronic anxiety can activate the sympathetic nervous system, resulting in a physical stress linked to multiple comorbidities when these children become adults such as hypertension, insomnia, and substance-use disorders.

The severity of anxiety varies based on degree of symptoms and existing protective factors. Protective factors for depression and anxiety in children and adolescents include:

- Increased resiliency
  - Good coping skills and problem-solving skills
  - Subjective sense of self-sufficiency
  - Optimism
- Secure attachment to an adult
- Sense of belonging
  - Participation in teams and clubs
  - Ability to make and sustain friendships
  - Developmentally appropriate peer relationships
- Healthy lifestyle choices
  - Healthy diet
  - Limiting caffeine
  - Limiting low-nutritional, high caloric foods
  - Regular exercise
- Emotional self- regulation and emotional intelligence
- Economic and financial security.

The maladaptation of anxiety can have several sources that can occur individually or simultaneously; these sources tend to stem from either a genetic or familial predisposition, temperamental disposition, or environmental and situational factors. Identifying the source may help to guide optimal treatment. This section will present a review of common anxiety disorders including separation anxiety disorder and generalized anxiety disorder (GAD).

### SEPARATION ANXIETY DISORDER

Separation anxiety disorder is an abnormal response to the perceived separation from a particular attachment such as a caregiver or familiar environment. There is a natural and expected level of uncertainty when a child is with an unknown individual or unfamiliar surroundings, but the separation anxiety disorder has an amplified and inconsolable response rather than the expected adaptation to the situation (Vaughan et al., 2017). This can be perceived as a morbid worry of threats or intense homesickness.

## Subjective Findings

The health history may reveal:

- Child becomes inconsolable while away from caregiver or familiar setting
- Excessive fear about harm to self or others in absence
- Fears of abandonment
- Socially withdrawn
- Nightmares
- Difficulty making friends
- Refusal to do things that may require separation
  - Refusal to go to school
- Poor school performance
- Temper tantrums.

## Risk Factors

The most common risk factors for separation anxiety disorder are:

- Unfamiliar caregiver or environmental setting
- Recent life-changing event or life stressors (such as moving to a new home or school, divorce of parent)
- Death of a loved one or pet
- Home dysfunction (parental dysfunction, maternal depression).

## Review of Systems

The review of systems may be negative and the most common manifestations revealed during the review of systems include:

*Infant and child:*

- **Constitutional:** crying, temper tantrums

*Adolescent:*

- **Psychiatric:** anxiety or depression

## Objective Findings

The physical examination of the child with separation anxiety disorder usually is unremarkable, but may reveal:

- Saddened affect
- Clinging to caregiver, calling for caregiver
- Violent, emotional temper tantrums when away from caregiver
- Severe or extreme crying without an organic cause
- Clear rhinorrhea, tearing eyes bilaterally, flushed face while crying or sadden affect
- Mild increased work of breathing while crying
- Mild, stable tachycardia while crying.

> **PRO TIP** Symptoms resolve with the comfort of attached caregiver.

## Laboratory/Diagnostic Testing

The diagnosis of separation anxiety disorder is based upon the clinical findings. No laboratory or diagnostic testing is needed, but may be ordered to rule in/out possible differential diagnoses such as anemia or thyroid disorder.

## Differential Diagnosis

The differential diagnosis for separation anxiety disorder includes:

- Developmentally appropriate separation anxiety
  - Between 7 months to 4 years; peaks between 18 to 36 months
- Bullying
- ASD
- Developmental delays
- GAD
- Panic disorder
- Posttraumatic stress disorder (PTSD)
- Social phobia
  - Stranger anxiety—developmentally appropriate age: 5 months to 2.5 years; peaks between 6 to 12 months
- Specific phobia
  - Nyctophobia—developmentally appropriate from 3 to 6 years
- Substance use disorder (alcohol, cocaine, psychedelics, withdrawal from opioids or benzodiazepines)
- Medication (caffeine, stimulants, steroids, albuterol)
- Medical conditions
  - Hyperthyroidism
  - Hypothyroidism
  - Anemia
  - Hypoglycemia
  - Asthma
  - Hypoxia
  - Dysthymia
  - Mitral valve prolapse
  - Irritable bowel syndrome.

## Treatment/Management Plan

Separation anxiety disorder is often treated similarly to GAD in children. Treatment is dependent on the degree of severity, impact on daily activities, school performance, and effect on family dynamics. Identifying a cause is often useful to guide treatment and may provide reassurance if it is self-limiting, such as adjustment to a new home. Developmentally appropriate separation anxiety does not warrant medical interventions other than supportive care and education to families that this is expected, natural, and often self-limiting.

Psychotherapy is the mainstay for many treatments for anxiety disorders. It can be used as a monotherapy or in conjunction with medications (Vaughan et al., 2017). Parent-child interaction therapy may be used for psychotherapy. A therapist interacts with the attached caregiver to teach techniques to help reinforce desired behaviors in the child (Vaughan et al., 2017). Pharmacologic treatment should be reserved for children who do not respond to nonpharmacologic treatment and when there is a noticeable negative impact on daily function. See GAD for the pharmacologic treatment.

### Family Education

Teach the following:

- Developmentally appropriate separation anxiety is usually self-limiting.
- For infants and younger children, teach techniques to diminishing separation anxiety such as spending time with an attached caregiver in a new setting such as daycare.
- For older children and adolescents, teach deep breathing and mindfulness techniques when among unfamiliar individuals or in unfamiliar settings.

### Referral

May refer to a pediatric psychopharmacologist (physician or nurse practitioner [NP]) for medication or pedatric therapist for psychotherapy.

## GENERALIZED ANXIETY DISORDER

GAD is the maladaptive response to fears and worries without a specific focus, such as an object or situation. This heightened sense of worry tends to have a negative impact on daily activities and functional performance. GAD tends to affect older children and adolescents but can be seen in younger children, especially those with a history of abuse (Oral et al., 2016). This disorder may have waxing and waning symptoms and differ from day to day (Bennett et al., 2016). In general, symptoms persist for longer than 6 months and occur more often than not. It is often linked with depressive symptoms due to a biochemical response to serotonin and norepinephrine. Children with GAD often have somatic symptoms that are either in conjunction with or absent of an underlying disease. There is a familial predisposition for GAD and parental mental health should be assessed.

### Subjective Findings

The health history may reveal:

- Excessive fear and worry
- Restlessness
- Irritability or easy fatigability
- Somatic complaints without an organic cause.

### Risk Factors

The most common risk factors for GAD are genetic or familial predisposition.

### Review of Systems

The most common manifestations revealed during the review of systems include:

- **Constitutional:** sleep disturbances
- **Respiratory:** sense of difficulty breathing
- **Cardiovascular:** chest pain or discomfort, sense of heart racing
- **Gastrointestinal:** discomfort or gastrointestinal issue
- **Musculoskeletal:** muscle tension
- **Neurologic:** headache
- **Psychiatric:** anxiety, depression
- **Behavioral:** crying or temper tantrums (infant, young child), difficulty concentrating, socially withdrawn, nightmares, difficulty making friends, poor school performance, lack of self-confidence

### Objective Findings

The physical examination of the child with GAD is generally unremarkable but may reveal:

- Saddened affect
- Fidgeting or repetitive movements such as bouncing leg.

### Laboratory/Diagnostic Testing

The diagnosis of GAD is based upon the clinical findings. No laboratory or diagnostic testing is needed but may be ordered to rule in/out possible differential diagnoses such as thyroid disorders or anemias.

### Differential Diagnosis

The differential diagnosis for GAD includes:

- Developmentally appropriate separation anxiety (7 months to 4 years; peaks between 18 to 36 months)

- Bullying
- ASD
- Developmental delays
- Panic disorder
- PTSD
- Separation anxiety disorder
- Social phobia
- Stranger anxiety (developmentally appropriate age: 5 months to 2.5 years; peaks between 6 to 12 months)
- Substance use disorder (alcohol, cocaine, psychedelics, withdrawals from opioids or benzodiazepines)
- Medication (caffeine, stimulants, steroids, albuterol)
- Medical conditions
  - Hyperthyroidism
  - Hypothyroidism
  - Anemia
  - Hypoglycemia
  - Asthma
  - Hypoxia
  - Dysthymia
  - Mitral valve prolapse
  - Irritable bowel syndrome.

### Treatment/Management Plan

Treatment for GAD is dependent on the degree of severity, impact on daily activities, school performance, and effect on family dynamics. Treatment for young children mainly focuses on behavioral and family interventions, such as CBT. Identifying a cause and risk factors is often useful to guide treatment. Identifying and recommending treatment for a primary caregiver can have a positive impact on the child's mental well-being and improve symptoms of GAD. As with most mental health concerns, treatment of GAD should include assessment of family and caregiver mental health needs. It is necessary to treat the family as a whole rather than as an individual to have the greatest impact on health (Bennett et al., 2016).

In older children and adolescents with mild to moderate GAD, the first-line treatment is also CBT. There should be an assessment of family needs, referral for parental/caregiver treatment, and recommendation to start psychotherapy (Bennett et al., 2016). When GAD is moderate to severe, the use of SSRIs is recommended in conjunction with psychotherapy in both children and adolescents. It has been shown that SSRIs are most efficacious when combined with psychotherapy (Bennett et al., 2016). Fluoxetine is an SSRI approved for ages 8 years and older for anxiety disorders. When prescribing fluoxetine, it is essential to educate about the possible side effects such as headache, nausea, diarrhea, insomnia, or sedation. Most gastrointestinal side effects peak around 2 weeks after starting, and it may take up to 6 weeks for the benefits of the medication to take effect. Duloxetine (Cymbalta), an SNRI, has also been approved for patients 7 and up. Grapefruit juice and alcohol should be avoided while on this medication. Benzodiazepines are not generally recommended in the treatment of GAD in pediatrics due to limited clinical trials of efficacy, cognitive impairment, and concerns of dependence (Bennett et al., 2016). It is vital that the patient and family be educated on the black box warning on all SSRI and SNRI medications and discuss that these medications have a 1% risk of potentially increasing suicidal thoughts and behaviors in patients under the age of 25. While this black box warning is controversial, it is important to discuss among your patients and their families.

Follow-up care is an important factor in GAD, as the disorder will have natural highs and lows of severity. Screening for depression and other mental health issues should be assessed as they are often linked; assessment for suicidal ideations, thoughts of self-harm, and harming others should be assessed for age-appropriate individuals.

### Family Education

Teach the following:

- Deep breathing and mindfulness techniques on a regular basis to help activate the paratympanic nervous system and diminish the autonomic responses to GAD

### Referral

May refer to a pediatric psychopharmacologist (physician or NP) or pediatric therapist for psychotherapy.

**PRO TIP** Assessment of GAD in adolescents should be kept confidential and not disclosed to parents and caregivers unless the adolescent requests otherwise.

## OBSESSIVE-COMPULSIVE DISORDER

OCD is the repetitive, ritualist thoughts or impulsive behaviors for which there is very little self-control. There is often a sense of distress and fear of consequences associated with this behavior. OCD has marked functional impairment of the child's social and academic performance and is time-consuming. The goal of performing these repetitive behaviors is to reduce anxiety. Children may have an obsession about contamination and cleanliness that may result in frequent or repetitive hand washing rituals. Most cases of OCD originate from childhood, but the exact etiology is unknown; it is suggested that there is a genetic risk factor (French et al., 2016). The onset for OCD appears to be between 9 and 11 years old in males and 11 to 13 years old in females (French et al., 2016).

There is a possible autoimmune subtype of OCD and Tourette syndrome that is known as pediatric autoimmune neuropsychiatric disorder associated with streptococcal infection (PANDAS). It is an autoimmune response to group A beta-hemolytic streptococci (GABHS). This a sudden onset of OCD or tic occurs after a GABHS infection (Chiarello et al., 2017).

## Subjective Findings

The health history may reveal:

- Observed rituals
- Sudden food or activity aversions
- Poor school performance
- Self-harm behavior
- Aggression
- Irritability
- Nightmares.

### Risk Factors

The most common risk factors for OCD are:

- Genetic predisposition
- Possible post GABHS infection if PANDAS.

### Review of Systems

The most common manifestations revealed during the review of systems include:

- **Constitutional:** headache
- **Gastrointestinal:** abdominal complaints
- **Psychiatric:** anxiety

## Objective Findings

The physical examination of the child with OCD may be unremarkable. However, there may be signs of repetitive rituals such as dry and cracked hands from excessive washing.

**PRO TIP** The clinician can receive training to administer the Children's Yale-Brown-Obsessive-Compulsive Scale (CY-BOCS) to rate the severity of OCD as well as monitor for changes.

### Laboratory/Diagnostic Testing

The diagnosis of OCD is based upon the clinical findings. No laboratory or diagnostic testing is needed.

## Differential Diagnosis

The differential diagnosis for OCD includes:

- PANDAS
- Trichotillomania (hair pulling or eyelash pulling)
- Phobia
- Body dysmorphic disorder
- ASD
- Early onset psychosis
- Tumors
- Encephalitis
- Traumatic brain injury
- Prader-Willi syndrome
- Compulsive eating
- Medication use such as stimulants.

## Treatment/Management Plan

Treatment is based on the severity of symptoms and impact on daily activities. First-line treatment for children with OCD is CBT. This provides the best long-term effectiveness for treating OCD. Individuals with severe OCD may benefit from CBT in conjunction with pharmacotherapy. SSRIs are the first-line pharmacologic treatment for severe symptoms or individuals who failed to respond to CBT. Fluoxetine, fluvoxamine, and sertraline are safe treatments for OCD in pediatrics. Exposure response prevention (ERP), which is a form of CBT, is a treatment of choice for children with OCD in which the child is exposed to their fears while refraining from compulsions. Unfortunately, ERP clinicians are limited and therefore poorly accessed by patients and their families.

### Family Education

Teach the following:

- Learn to recognize your child's OCD behaviors.
- Modify your expectations and create a supportive environment.
- Some days will go better than others. Avoid comparisons.

### Referral

May refer to a harmacologist (physician or NP) or a pediatric therapist for psychotherapy.

# MOOD DISORDERS

Mood disorders or affective disorders are characterized by persistent and intense changes in mood that affect a child's or adolescent's ability to manage thoughts and emotions. These changes can have an impact on a child's or adolescent's ability to function in daily life. The symptoms of a mood disorder in children and adolescents can differ from adult symptoms. It can be difficult for parents to recognize these differences, especially if the child or adolescent is not expressing their thoughts and feelings. One of the key differences between child and adolescent mood disorders and adult mood disorders is that children and adolescents often experience consistent episodes of irritability versus episodes of sadness.

Mood disorders are generally thought to be due to chemical imbalances in the brain, resulting from a combination of genetic and environmental factors such as chronic stress or unexpected life events. Rapid growth and hormonal shifts in adolescence are also contributing factors in the development of mood disorders. More recent research has identified brain gut peptides as having a role in mood disorders and advances in gene testing offer more insight into treatment and management of mood disorders (Li et al., 2017).

## MAJOR DEPRESSIVE DISORDER

Depression is one of the most prevalent mental health disorders in children. It is a chronic medical condition that is associated with a depressed mood and can be accompanied by changes in sleep, appetite, weight, poor concentration, decreased energy, and recurrent thoughts of worthlessness, guilt, self-harm, or even death (Walter & DeMaso, 2020). It can often coincide with anxiety disorders linking a possible neural and biochemical response in serotonin and norepinephrine (Żmudzka et al., 2018). The etiology of depression may be complex with a combination of genetic, environmental, and psychological factors. Adverse childhood events and significant life changes can influence the persistence of depression. Some adolescents with depression may have substance use disorder and may use illicit substances to maladaptively self-treat underlying depression symptoms, most commonly through the use of cannabis or alcohol (Wilkinson et al., 2016). Depression is often underdiagnosed and undertreated in pediatrics. Roughly 36% of children and adolescents have untreated depression (Soria-Saucedo et al., 2016). Furthermore adolescents that identify with LGBTQ may be at a greater risk for developing depression (Avenevoli et al., 2015). The risk for developing depression in females is greater than males (Avenevoli et al., 2015).

There is a varying degree of severity among children and adolescents with depression. Utilizing a validating screening tool is recommended (Siu, 2016). The Patient Health Questionnaire 9, modified for adolescents (PHQ-A), provides a scoring system for severity (see Figure 18.4). In mild to moderate depression, there is often the absence of suicidal ideations, psychotic features, and aggression. Severe depression may encompass those characteristics and require a more intensive treatment plan. Diagnosis is made with the support of the *DSM-5* criteria and the absence of other medical or psychiatric conditions.

### Subjective Findings

The health history may reveal:

- Feeling of sadness, helplessness, hopelessness, guilt, or feeling bad about one's self
- little interest in things that once interested the child or adolescent.

▶ ALERT: Children or adolescents may have thoughts about or attempts at self-harm. Always ask about suicidal ideation and take positive responses seriously.

### Risk Factors

The most common risk factors for major depressive disorder are:

- Genetic or familial predisposition
- Low birth weight
- Bullying
- Learning disabilities
- Chronic illnesses such as diabetes
- Substance use such as nicotine or alcohol
- Chronic sleep problems.

### Review of Systems

The most common manifestations revealed during the review of systems include:

- **Constitutional:** insomnia, difficulty sleeping, fatigue, changes in appetite
- **Gastrointestinal:** abdominal pain, constipation, diarrhea

- **Neurologic:** irritability, headaches
- **Psychiatric:** anxiety, verbalization of depression, irritability, thoughts of suicide, thoughts of or self-harm behaviors
- **Behavioral:** social withdrawal, poor school performance, difficulty concentrating

### Objective Findings

The child or adolescent with major depressive disorder may be withdrawn during the visit. The physical examination will likely be unremarkable. Some children may demonstrate a saddened affect, hygiene neglect, or signs of self-harm on the skin (such as cutting).

### Laboratory/Diagnostic Testing

The diagnosis of major depressive disorder is based upon the clinical findings. No laboratory or diagnostic testing is needed, but may be ordered to rule in/out possible differential diagnoses.

### Differential Diagnosis

The differential diagnosis for major depressive disorder includes:

- Bullying
- BPD
- Dysphoria (periods of sadness)
- Developmental delay
- GAD
- PTSD
- Specific phobia
- Substance use disorder (alcohol, withdrawal from opioids or benzodiazepines)
- Medical conditions
  - Hypothyroidism
  - Anemia
  - Hypoglycemia.

### Treatment/Management Plan

Treatment for depression begins with the assessment and evaluation of potential risk of self-harm or suicidal ideations. This will help determine if the child or adolescent is acutely appropriate to be treated in an outpatient setting and which interventions are most appropriate. If suicidal, referral to an inpatient setting may be needed.

When reviewing the interventions with child and family, it is important to review the risk and benefits of each recommendation and treatment is tailored to each child's needs. Depression can be treated in primary care or in collaboration with a psychiatrist. Education for the child and family is a key component for treatment of depression, noting a realistic time frame of 6 to 12 weeks for improvement of symptoms, particularly with pharmacotherapy. Distinct areas of treatment are psychotherapy, pharmacotherapy, and a combination of the two.

Initial treatment is dependent upon the severity of symptoms, duration, age, and complex psychosocial factors such as family conflict or bullying. For children/adolescents with mild depression, psychotherapy is often the initial treatment. If the depression is moderate to severe, the use of pharmacotherapy and psychotherapy may be appropriate. Combination treatment has an advantage to pharmacotherapy alone but pharmacotherapy may be useful with patients who decline psychotherapy. An SSRI, particularly fluoxetine, is often the first-line pharmacotherapy for adolescents and has been well-studied along with cognitive-behavioral therapy. Alternative SSRIs may include sertraline or escitalopram. There is a black box warning from the FDA about the concerns of suicidal ideation with administration of SSRIs. Therapeutic doses should be titrated at a minimum of 4 to 6 weeks.

### Family Education

Teach the following:

- Resources for suicide prevention hotlines and community resources. Advise to call 911 if impending thoughts of suicide or homicide.
- The benefits and advantages of psychotherapy alone or in combination with pharmacotherapy
- Potential risks and benefits of treatment therapies:
  - Potential risk of suicidal ideation with SSRIs.
  - SSRIs may take 4 to 6 weeks before noticing any benefits or change in dose.
  - Do not stop SSRIs abruptly without consultation of a provider.

### Referral

May refer to a pediatric psychiatrist for pharmacotherapy or a pediatric therapist for psychotherapy.

## DISRUPTIVE MOOD DYSREGULATION DISORDER

Disruptive mood dysregulation disorder (DMDD) was made a formal diagnosis in the most recent (5th) edition of the *DSM*. DMDD is a childhood illness that is characterized by an irritable angry mood as well as severe and recurrent behavioral outbursts that are inconsistent with developmental level. These behaviors and mood symptoms interfere with the child's functioning at home, school, and other environments. Many children now diagnosed with DMDD were previously categorized as having BPD, despite not meeting all criteria for BPD (American Academy of Child and Adolescent Psychiatry [AACAP], 2019a). Most children diagnosed with DMDD do not develop BPD, but are more prone to anxiety and depressive disorders as adults (Grohol, 2020).

The average age of diagnosis is 9 years, though 80% of these children met criteria at age 6 (Zepf et al., 2016). Children who are diagnosed by age 6 are at higher risk of developing attention deficit hyperactivity disorder (ADHD) and depressive disorders. The diagnosis is made when it cannot be better explained by another psychiatric disorder, such as major depressive disorder or BPD. The onset of symptoms needs to occur before the age of 10 and the diagnosis cannot be made before age 6 or after age 18 (Zepf et al., 2016).

## Subjective Findings

The health history may reveal:

- Concerns around behavioral outbursts and tantrums
- Issues with school performance and inappropriate behaviors
- Family history of mental health concerns
- Concerns around irritable and/or depressed mood, anger
- Difficulty with relationships—with peers, teachers, and/or family.

### Risk Factors

The most common risk factors for DMDD are:

- Parental history of a depressive disorder, ADHD, or anxiety. Children are unlikely to have a parent with BPD.
- Neurobiologic factors including poor motor inhibition, decreased cognitive flexibility, and cognitive deficits in the processing of emotional and social inputs.
- Environmental factors including parents who are more critical and irritable. This may be due to parental nature/mental illness or a result of a bidirectional parent-child process.
- Trauma (exposure, abuse, or neglect) is known to have an impact on affective disorders, but further research is needed to determine its impact on the development of DMDD (Zepf et al., 2016).

### Review of Systems

The most common manifestations revealed during the review of systems include:

- **Behavioral:** difficulty at school (behavior and performance), difficulty with relationships and peer interactions, irritability, trouble functioning at home

The irritability is persistent, often seen as tantrum or outbursts, and is observable by others (teachers, friends). The child appears irritable or angry most of the day, every day. The child's behavior is incongruent with the intensity of the situation.

## Objective Findings

The physical examination is important to rule out evidence of abuse. Although it is generally unremarkable, it may reveal:

- Irritable and/or depressed mood
- Disruptive or uncooperative behavior
- Outburst during visit.

### Laboratory/Diagnostic Testing

The diagnosis of DMDD is based upon the clinical findings. The outbursts typically occur at least three times per week. No laboratory or diagnostic testing is needed.

## Differential Diagnosis

The differential diagnosis for DMDD includes:

- Head injury
- Wilson disease
- Lead toxicity
- Intellectual disability
- BPD
- Intermittent explosive disorder (IED)
- Anxiety disorder
- ADHD
- Oppositional defiant disorder (ODD)
- Conduct disorder (CD)
- Attachment disorder
- Schizophrenia or schizoaffective disorder
- Substance abuse
- Emerging personality disorder
- Cyclothymia
- ASD
- Systemic lupus erythematosus
- Medication adverse reactions
- Meningitis
- Thyroid dysfunction
- Child abuse
- Trauma or exposure to trauma.

**PRO TIP** Many of the psychiatric diagnoses can be comorbid or associated conditions.

## Treatment/Management Plan

Treatment includes family education and support from the primary care setting on how to manage and move forward. Parent skills training, CBT, and involvement of the educational system are key components of an integrated, collaborative approach. Schools and teachers are important for development of strategies and meeting students' needs.

There is limited research on the use of medications for DMDD. Comorbid illnesses should be treated. There is no evidence for the use of antidepressants. Medication may be used to treat specific symptoms (angry outbursts, explosive behavior, and impulsivity). Antipsychotics such as risperidone are used off-label to reduce irritability and agitation. Sodium valproate/divalproex is used to reduce overall symptoms. Stimulants and guanfacine are used to reduce impulsivity and treat comorbid ADHD. These medications are generally started by a psychopharmacologist experienced with mood disorders in children.

Follow-up appointments with the primary care provider should include assessment for adverse effects of medications (even when not prescribing) as well as improvements in behavior and functioning. Continue to assess mood and suicidal thinking. Ensure that families have followed through with recommendations for support and continue to monitor family functioning. Additional interventions include family therapy, in home therapy, and neuropsychiatric assessment.

Children with DMDD often have comorbid illnesses and are at risk for suicidal thoughts and self-harming behaviors. They can also become extremely aggressive or out of control behaviorally. It is important that there is an emergency plan in place before it is needed. Safety planning includes solutions to deescalate behaviors and who to call in case of an emergency (i.e., crisis team if available, hospital, and/or police).

**PRO TIP** Educate parents/guardians that when a behavior happens at school, the school will follow its own safety protocols that may include emergency assessment before the child is allowed to return to school.

### Family Education

Teach the following:

- About the disorder, comorbid conditions, and strategies for managing behaviors and identifying triggers and stressors.
- Most families will benefit from referral to therapists for support with behavior management, lifestyle changes, understanding stressors and triggers, and evaluation and treatment of comorbid disorders.
- There can be long waits for therapy services, so families need to remember that school systems can be immediately available to support a child and provide them with services at school. This can include more structure, classroom support, extra time for assignments, and time with a school counselor.
- Current federal laws regarding appropriate resources for children with disabilities include psychiatric diagnoses.
- Encourage families to think of additional supports they might have (i.e., extended family, friends) and remind families to focus on what they can do rather than how they are limited (Evans, 2020).

### Referral

As appropriate for the individual, make referrals to school supports, neuropsychiatric testing, therapists, and psychiatric advanced practice nurses or psychiatrists with experience working with children and adolescents.

# BIPOLAR DISORDER

BPD is an affective disorder characterized by recurrent episodes of elevated mood that occur on a spectrum of severity. Symptoms can range from mild hypomania to severe mania, which can include suicidal ideation, dysphoria, and psychotic features (Bernstein, 2020; Birmaher, 2019). Although depression is not required for a diagnosis of BPD to be made, children and adolescents often have major depressive episodes. Retrospective studies have found that approximately 60% of adults with BPD had symptoms before the age of 20 and 20% before the age of 18 (Birmaher, 2019). Other studies have found that pediatric BPD often goes undiagnosed for 2 years from onset of symptoms (Birmaher, 2019). This is often due to underrecognition of symptoms as well as underreporting of symptoms by children, adolescents, and parents/guardians (Hirneth, et.al., 2014).

There are complex interactions between genetics, environment, and the risk of developing BPD in childhood or adolescence that are not yet fully understood. BPD is highly heritable; for offspring of parents with BPD, the risk for the child to develop it is 10 to 20 times greater than for the general population (Birmaher, 2019). Males are at higher risk than females. Biologic factors affected the development of BPD include:

- Hyperactivation of the amygdala, prefrontal cortex, and visual systems likely contributing to emotional dysfunction.
- Hypoactivation of the anterior cingulate cortex, which is linked to the cognitive deficits in children and adolescents with BPD.
- Altered neuronal ion channel function has also been identified in children and adolescents with a bipolar diagnosis. While BPD has a clear family heritability, it is unclear how much is genetic versus environmental stress.

Length of time to proper treatment and intervention is correlated to severity of illness; therefore, it is important to identify and refer children and adolescents with BPD to mental health providers with expertise in management of pediatric BPD. Additionally, when diagnosed in childhood there is typically a higher lifelong severity.

## Subjective Findings

The health history may reveal:

- Concerns around extreme mood swings, insomnia and/or restlessness, or sleeping too much. Insomnia is one of the classic symptoms for children and adolescents with BPD (National Institute of Mental Health, 2020).
- Issues with school performance and inappropriate or risky behaviors
- Child or adolescent may be very talkative, difficult to interrupt, or may talk about many different things.
- May be silly or very happy without context for mood.
- Concerns around irritable and/or depressed mood, anger
- Suicidal thinking
- Family history of mental health concerns, especially BPD.

## Risk Factors

The most common risk factors for BPD are:

- Parent with BPD
- Emotional disconnection between child and parents
- Drug or alcohol use
- Altered stress response in the child (Fletcher, 2017).

## Review of Systems

The most common manifestations revealed during the review of systems include:

- **Constitutional:** not sleeping, difficulty staying asleep, sleeping too much
- **Psychiatric:** irritability, anger, depressed or extremely elevated mood (often acting silly)
- **Behavioral:** difficulty with school or peers, getting in trouble at school or legal issues, risk-taking behaviors

## Objective Findings

The physical examination of the child with BPD may reveal:

- Psychomotor agitation or retardation
- Disheveled, unkempt appearance
- Talkativeness, difficult for other to interrupt talking, or slurred speech
- Irritability, depressed mood, overly happy or manic
- Affect may be labile, flat, or elevated
- Thought processes include flight of ideas or are difficult to follow/understand
- Suicidal or violent ideation, auditory or visual hallucinations, paranoia
- Impulsivity, poor judgment
- Impaired cognition.

Screening tools that are used for general assessment of mood, mania, and behavior are the Child Behavior Checklist (CBCL) and Child Symptom Inventory (CSI-4). The Mood Disorder Questionnaire (MDQ) is a brief self-administered questionnaire; if positive, further evaluation is needed. Other mania-specific screening tools are: General Behavior Inventory (P-GBI), Child Mania Rating Scale (P-CMRS), and the Young Mania Rating Scale (P-YMRS).

## Laboratory/Diagnostic Testing

The diagnosis of BPD is based upon the clinical findings. No laboratory or diagnostic testing is needed although it may be used to rule out physical disorders.

## Differential Diagnosis

The differential diagnosis for BPD includes:

- Head injury
- Wilson disease
- Lead toxicity
- Intellectual disability
- DMDD
- IED
- Anxiety disorder

- ADHD
- ODD
- CD
- Attachment disorder
- Schizophrenia, schizoaffective disorder
- Substance abuse
- Emerging personality disorder
- Cyclothymia
- ASD
- Systemic lupus erythematosus
- Medication adverse reactions
- Meningitis
- Thyroid dysfunction
- Child abuse
- Trauma or exposure to trauma.

As with DMDD, many of the psychiatric disorders can be comorbid or associated conditions. The diagnostic criteria for bipolar I disorder as outlined by the *DSM-5* requires at least one manic episode, defined as a distinct period of abnormal and persistently elevated mood. This may present as an irritable mood. There is persistently increased activity or energy. Mania lasts at least 1 week and is present most of the day every day during the episode. At least three of the following need to be present and need to be noticeably different from usual behavior: inflated self-esteem or grandiosity, decreased need for sleep, pressured speech or more talkative than usual, flight of ideas or racing thought, distractibility, increased activity (goal-directed or psychomotor agitation), excessive involvement in pleasurable or risky activities, or psychosis. These symptoms must also cause significant impairment of social, academic, or occupational functioning. Symptoms of depression or hypomania are often present but are not required for a diagnosis. A diagnosis of bipolar II disorder or mixed mood is made when depressed mood is present along with manic or hypomanic symptoms. Mixed mood is also referred to as rapid cycling.

## Treatment/Management Plan

When formulating the treatment plan, initial assessment of safety to self and others and level of functioning is needed. Determination of level of treatment needed (inpatient, partial hospital, or outpatient) is based on safety and level of functioning. If there are significant concerns regarding safety, the child or adolescent should be transported to an appropriate emergency facility (this can be via family or ambulance depending on the individual situation). If there is not an eminent safety concern and the primary care nurse practitioner is unable to begin treatment, immediate referral to an appropriate specialist is needed (i.e., advanced practice psychiatric nurse, pediatric psychiatrist, or emergency assessment team). Initial treatment goals are aimed at controlling and quickly stopping the current episode.

Although medication is the first-line treatment for BPD, there is limited evidence on pharmacologic treatment in children and adolescents. Despite this, use of medication decreases morbidity and mortality associated with BPD. Acute management is based on the presentation. A manic or mixed mood episode (initial presentation) has several first-line options including lithium, valproate, or atypical antipsychotics. Valproate is preferred over lithium for mixed mood presentation. Adjunct treatment with a benzodiazepine may be considered. Atypical antipsychotics are needed if psychosis is present and atypical antipsychotics are preferred over older typical psychotic agents due to their preferred side effect profiles. Lamotrigine is not used if the presentation is mania or hypomania, as it can be activating. Lamotrigine can be used as maintenance therapy (Wagner, 2016). If there is breakthrough mania or a mixed mood episode while on maintenance therapy, it is best to maximize the current medication(s) and then add or change the atypical antipsychotic. If the initial presentation is a depressive episode, first-line treatment is lamotrigine or lithium. Antidepressants (i.e., SSRIs) are not recommended for monotherapy due to risk of mania and/or agitation. As with a manic presentation, if there are psychotic features, an atypical antipsychotic is needed. For breakthrough depression, maximization of the initial medication is the best approach. Once an acute episode is managed, the risk of relapse is highest in the first 6 months. Baseline ECG and echocardiogram are indicated when starting medication for BPD, as many medications have potential cardiac impact; this is especially important if there is a family history of cardiac concerns related to structure or electrical conductivity.

Relapse, treatment nonadherence, and suicide/suicide attempts are most likely to occur after hospitalization and initial diagnosis. If appropriate mental healthcare providers have not been identified or appointments are not within a week of discharge from the hospital program, children should be seen in primary care weekly. Monitoring of weight, vital signs, and laboratory values are needed at least yearly, with higher frequency depending upon medications being used and presentation. Most commonly monitored laboratory tests are: metabolic panel (including glucose and kidney function), cholesterol, hemoglobin A1C, thyroid function, prolactin, complete metabolic panel, and pregnancy testing (when clinically indicated).

Follow-up appointments should include assessment for adverse effects of medications (even when not prescribing) as well as improvements in behavior and functioning. Medications used for the treatment of BPD carry the risk of adverse effects including hyperprolactinemia, polycystic ovary syndrome, weight gain, hypothyroidism (lithium), metabolic syndrome, diabetes mellitus, extrapyramidal side effects (antipsychotics), and Stevens-Johnson syndrome (lamotrigine). Stevens-Johnson syndrome is associated with human leukocyte antigen HLA-B*1502 allele, which is more common in Asian populations and specifically with Han-Chinese.

Continue to assess mood and suicidal thinking. Suicide and attempted suicide are risks inherent to a bipolar illness. Even when well-managed, there can be breakthrough episodes of mania, mixed mood episodes, or depression. Children and adolescents can have difficulties with family, school, and social relationships. They may experience educational delays and have cognitive impairment. It is important that there is an emergency plan in place before it is needed. Safety planning includes solutions to identify red flags and who to call in case of an emergency (i.e., crisis team if available, hospital, and/or police).

Ensure that families have followed through with recommendations for support and continue to monitor family functioning. Additional interventions include family therapy, in-home therapy, and neuropsychiatric assessment.

### Family Education

Teach the following:

- This is often a shocking and upsetting diagnosis, particularly for parents and guardians (as the child or adolescent is not always fully cognizant with initial presentation). Families need time and support to both acknowledge this is the diagnosis and learn to adjust to what their next weeks and years will look like for them and their child.
- BPD is a lifelong illness that will likely need treatment and support throughout life. There are often ups and downs, and life stressors can trigger symptoms.
- Medication adherence is an area that is often a struggle as many medications available for treatment have adverse effects. Children and adolescents may be resistant to taking medications for extended periods of time. The parent or guardian should be monitoring medications, including safe storage.
- Many medications used for BPD are not safe to use during pregnancy due to teratogenic effects. There need to be initial and ongoing discussions with family and individually with the adolescent regarding risks. If a female is on valproate, she needs effective and consistent contraception.
- Identify red flags, monitoring for breakthrough symptoms and adverse reactions to medications.
- There can be long waits for therapy services, so families need to remember that school systems can be immediately available to support a child and provide them with services at school.
- Current federal laws regarding appropriate resources for children with disabilities include psychiatric diagnoses.
- Encourage families to think of additional supports they might have (i.e., extended family, friends) and remind families to focus on what they can do rather than how they are limited (Evans, 2020).

### Referral

As previously noted, children, adolescents, and their families need continued support with skilled pediatric psychiatric providers. This can include the prescriber, individual therapist, family therapist, and support group.

# BEHAVIORAL DISORDERS

## CONDUCT DISORDER

CD is a psychiatric disorder that begins in childhood or adolescence and is characterized by antisocial behavior that violates the rules and rights of others. As defined in the *DSM-5*, these symptoms must be present for at least 3 months with one symptom having been present in the past 6 months and cause clinically significant impairment in social, academic, or occupational functioning. There is evidence that youth with CD have decreased activity of the noradrenergic system. High testosterone levels are also associated with aggression.

Behaviors generally are in four categories: aggression toward people or animals, destruction of property, lying and theft, and serious rule violations. Severity is rated mild, moderate, or severe and further characterized as child onset (at least one symptom before age 10) or adolescent onset. Earlier age of onset is associated with increased severity. Usually, disruptive behaviors stop during early adulthood, but in about one-third of cases, they persist. Many of these cases meet the criteria for antisocial personality disorder. Early onset is associated with a poorer prognosis (Elia, 2019).

## Subjective Findings

The health history may reveal:

- Parental concerns about aggressive behaviors, destruction of property, or lying/stealing
- Child or adolescent has had conflict with authorities (school, legal, parent).
- Parent may feel that child/adolescent is "out of control" with behaviors.
- School failure or difficulties
- There may be concern about substance use due to behavior or because of concurrent use.

**PRO TIP** It is important to ask about thoughts of harming others, as it will not likely be volunteered.

### Risk Factors

The most common risk factors for CD are:

- Biological factors including a moderate degree of heritability for antisocial behavior, impulsivity, temperament, aggression, and insensitivity to punishment (Mohan et al., 2019).
- Family history of mental illness or substance use
- Environmental factors including lack of structure, inadequate supervision, family/marital conflicts, parental discord, inconsistent discipline, emotional and physical abuse (between parents and/or toward child), substance use (alcohol especially) in parents, lower socioeconomic status, parental unemployment, financial instability, housing insecurity and school environments with large student to teacher ratios, and inadequate support staff (Mohan et al., 2019).
- Child sexual abuse (or neglect) may be directly associated with CD in both males and females, with increased occurrence when abuse is prolonged (Maniglio, 2015).

### Review of Systems

The most common manifestations revealed during the review of systems include:

- **Behavioral:** poor school performance, learning difficulties, inability to focus or complete tasks, defiance or disregard of rules at home and at school, risk-taking and/or aggressive behaviors (risky sexual encounters, substance use, driving while under influence of drugs or alcohol, shoplifting/stealing, destruction of property, getting into fights)

## Objective Findings

The physical examination of the child with CD may be unremarkable except for the mental health status that may reveal:

- Uncooperative, withdrawn, angry
- Hyperactive or fidgety
- Flat or depressed mood/affect
- Suicidal or homicidal thinking
- Perseveration around violence
- Poor insight, judgment.

Assessment scales are helpful for assessing for CD and other mental health disorders. Examples of evidence-based scales are the CBCL, the Disruptive Behavior Disorders Rating Scale, and the National Institute for Children's Health Quality Vanderbilt Assessment Scales (Lillig, 2018). The Vanderbilt Assessment Scales are used primarily to assess for ADHD, but they include screening questions for CD.

### Laboratory/Diagnostic Testing

The diagnosis of CD is based upon the clinical findings. Urine and blood serum laboratory testing should be done, including drug screen, to rule out any comorbid medical problems or substance abuse disorders.

## Differential Diagnosis

The differential diagnosis for CD includes:

- ADHD (comorbid 20%–50%)
- ODD (comorbid 50%–60%)
- Anxiety disorders
- Affective disorder
- Reactive attachment disorder
- Schizophrenia
- Substance use disorder (may be precursor)
- PTSD
- Learning disability
- Normal adolescent risk-taking behaviors
- Learning disability
- Normal adolescent risk-taking behaviors.

## Treatment/Management Plan

Evidence-based psychosocial treatments include:

- Parent management training (to train parents how to set consistent rules/discipline with appropriate rewards of positive and prosocial behaviors; Mohan et al., 2019). Parent management training is the most effective for having an impact on child coercive behavior (Berstein, 2018).

- Multisystems approach that targets family, school, and the individual, with a focus on improving family dynamics, academic functioning, and the child's behavior across systems. This has been found to be most useful if parent management training interventions have failed (Berstein, 2018).
- Individual therapy such as anger management training and CBT, although research has found this is not effective as a single treatment. Group treatment for adolescents with CD tends to worsen the behavior, particularly if the group participants engage in discussions of oppositional and illegal behaviors (Berstein, 2018).
- Community-based treatment includes therapeutic schools and residential treatment centers that can provide structured programs to reduce disruptive behaviors. Residential placement is needed for children and adolescents with extremely harmful behaviors (Elia, 2019).

### Pharmacologic Treatments

Pharmacologic interventions target the treatment of psychiatric comorbidities with appropriate medications. There is considerable overlap between CD and ADHD, so children and adolescents should be specifically evaluated for ADHD and treated appropriately (Berstein, 2018; Moyan, et al, 2020). Studies have shown that ADHD treatment reduces core ADHD symptoms as well as symptoms of comorbid disruptive behavior disorders (Saylor & Amann, 2016). Stimulants with less abuse potential or risk for diversion should be utilized (i.e., lisdexamfetamine, methylphenidate patch). There are no medications approved by the FDA for the specific treatment of CD. Anticonvulsants, such as carbamazepine and divalproex, as well as lithium can be used in nonspecific aggression (Berstein, 2018). There is weak evidence for use of lithium (Lillig, 2018). Guanfacine is used to treat ADHD, impulsivity, and aggressive behaviors. Atypical antipsychotics such as risperidone may be used to manage mood and behavior. If an atypical antipsychotic is prescribed, there is a need to monitor weight, BP, blood glucose, lipid profile, and hemoglobin A1C. When divalproex or lithium is used, there is a need to monitor drug levels, liver function, blood counts, and weight.

### Family Education

Teach the following:

- The prognosis of CD if not treated (development of antisocial personality disorder, escalation of behaviors, increased risk for substance use, high risk of school failure, and risk for criminal behavior and legal repercussions).
- There is need for clear communication of rules and expectations with appropriate rewards and consequences. Harsh discipline should be avoided (Lillig, 2018).
- Parental education on management is an effective treatment model for CD.
- Participation in sports and involvement with community groups exposes youth to positive and healthy activities. This can reduce the symptoms of CD as well as decrease the associated risk of developing antisocial personality disorder as an adult (Lillig, 2018).
- Coordination of care with all those involved in care, including school, is essential for management of CD.
- Seek treatment for parents' own mental health issues.

### Referral

As previously noted, referral to mental health providers with experience treating CD and comorbid illnesses is necessary for best outcomes. For severe cases, referral to a treatment facility or therapeutic school may be needed.

## OPPOSITIONAL DEFIANT DISORDER

ODD is defined by the *DSM-5* as a pattern of angry or irritable mood, argumentative/defiant behavior, or vindictiveness lasting at least 6 months. Angry or irritable mood is seen as losing temper, being easily annoyed, or being angry and resentful. Children or adolescents with ODD often argue with adults and authority figures or refuse to comply with requests from adults/authority figures. They may deliberately annoy others or blame others for their mistakes or misbehavior. They may be spiteful or vindictive toward others beyond family and siblings.

It is important to distinguish between normal child behavior and pathology. Persistence of the behaviors helps in that determination. For children younger than age 5, the behavior should occur most days for at least 6 months. For children over age 5, behaviors should occur at least weekly for at least 6 months. Other factors to consider when making this diagnosis include whether the behaviors are outside the range of what is considered developmentally appropriate given their age, gender, and culture and whether the behavior causes distress or negatively affects social, educational, or occupational functioning. ODD is classified as mild, moderate, or severe. Approximately 1% to 16% of children and adolescents have a diagnosis of ODD (AACAP, 2019c). Many of these children and adolescents have comorbid psychiatric disorders and some may go on to develop CD.

### Subjective Findings

The health history may reveal:

- Parental concerns about behavior such as temper tantrums, extreme irritability or anger, arguments with adults, refusal to comply with rules, being mean or hateful
- Issues at school due to behavior, conflict with adults, and/or mean and spiteful behavior.
- School failure or difficulties
- Concern about substance use due to behavior or because of concurrent use
- History of abuse or neglect
- Family history of mental illness, family conflict, parental discord, financial instability, or substance use.

### Risk Factors

The most common risk factors for ODD are as follows:

- Biological factors include nicotine use by parents, prenatal nutritional deficiencies, and developmental delay.
- Family history of mood disorder, ADHD, behavioral disorder, or personality disorder increases the risk of developing ODD. As ODD occurs in family clusters there is a suggestion of heritability, but this has been difficult to determine (Riley et al., 2016).
- Environmental risk factors correlated with ODD include history of abuse or neglect, parental psychiatric illness, and maternal aggression (Riley et al., 2016).
- Other risk factors correlated to the development with ODD are inconsistent or harsh discipline, instability such as relationship conflicts, divorce, frequent moves, and financial instability.

### Review of Systems

The most common manifestations revealed during the review of systems include:

- **Behavioral:** risk-taking and/or aggressive behaviors (risky sexual encounters, substance use, driving while under influence of drugs or alcohol, shoplifting/stealing, destruction of property, getting into fights)

### Objective Findings

The physical examination of the child with ODD may be unremarkable except in the area of mental status which may reveal:

- Uncooperative, withdrawn, angry
- Hyperactive, fidgety
- Mood/affect: depressed, flat mood/affect
- Suicidal or homicidal thinking
- Poor insight, judgment.

Assessment scales are helpful for assessing for ODD and other mental health disorders. See the tools mentioned in the section on CD for examples.

### Laboratory/Diagnostic Testing

The diagnosis of ODD is based upon the clinical findings. Urine and blood serum laboratory testing should be done, including drug screen, to rule out any comorbid medical problems or substance abuse disorders.

### Differential Diagnosis

The differential diagnosis for ODD includes:

- ADHD
- CD
- Anxiety disorders
- Affective disorder
- Reactive attachment disorder
- Schizophrenia
- Substance use disorder (may be precursor)
- PTSD.

### Treatment/Management Plan

Most of the research related to treatment of ODD focuses on general disruptive behavior in the early childhood years, with limited information on treating adolescents or ODD specifically (Burke & Loeber, 2016). Treatment for ODD is dependent on the individual child or adolescent and the severity of their presentation. As the behaviors often occur in both home and school settings, it is important for parents/guardians to collaborate with teachers and the team available at school.

Effective parenting techniques are essential for treating ODD. Parents/guardians need to understand that children and adolescents with ODD generally respond to nurturing and positive reinforcement with consistent and appropriate reward and consequence. Parents may not be able to implement management techniques without support due to unintentional reinforcement of negative behaviors or due to the severity of ODD (Burke & Loeber, 2016; Mitchell et al., 2018). Parent training can be individual or group-based.

Child-based therapy often focuses on problem-solving skills through CBT. Group CBT for children has also been found to decrease aggressive behaviors (Riley et al., 2016). Another effective technique for treating ODD is collaborative problem-solving, in which parents and children work together to prioritize and change behaviors. Collaborative problem-solving allows the parent and child to create an alliance within the family and can effectively improve behaviors (Cook, 2015).

Medications are not recommended as first-line treatment for ODD. There is limited evidence regarding the use of antipsychotics and mood stabilizers for children and adolescents with ODD. If needed for aggressive and extremely agitated behaviors, risperidone can be used short term in conjunction with behavioral therapy. Treatment of comorbid conditions often improves symptoms of ODD. For example, use of stimulants to treat ADHD can improve oppositional symptoms of ODD (Riley et al., 2016).

### Family Education

Teach the following:

- Children and adolescents with ODD often have comorbid mental health issues, most commonly ADHD.
- Follow-up with mental health providers for evaluation and treatment of comorbid disorders is important.
- Children and adolescents with ODD respond to positive parenting techniques. It is important to give praise and positive reinforcement when they show flexibility or concern.
- Choose your battles by prioritizing which expectations are most important. Be consistent with reinforcement, and set reasonable consequences (AACAP, 2019c).
- If parents/guardians struggle with implementation of effective strategies (or are simply overwhelmed at the task), they should be referred to parent training (either group or individual.)
- Caring for children and adolescents with ODD can be overwhelming. Parents/guardians need to utilize self-care and seek support of other adults such as partners, friends, teachers, and therapists.

### Referral

As previously noted, referral to mental health providers with experience treating ODD and comorbid illnesses is necessary for best outcomes.

## CHILD MALTREATMENT

Child maltreatment includes emotional, physical, and sexual abuse, as well as neglect. Emotional abuse occurs when the child is belittled or denigrated, or as a result of the child witnessing domestic violence. Intentionally inflicted injuries resulting in child morbidity or mortality is termed "physical abuse.' When a child is involved in any activity meant to provide sexual enjoyment to an adult, the label is sexual abuse. Neglect refers to failure to provide a child with appropriate food, clothing, shelter, medical care, or schooling (Chiesa & Sirotnak, 2020).

When family violence or child physical and sexual abuse occur, the perpetrator usually forces the victim into silence, making accurate statistics difficult to determine. Children usually do not want to admit that their parent or relative has hurt them, partly from feelings of guilt and partly because they do not want to lose that parent. In 2017, 4.1 million referrals to child protective services were made alleging child maltreatment in 7.5 million children, demonstrating an increase over prior years (Chiesa & Sirotnak, 2020). These shocking numbers may underestimate the prevalence of child abuse. Occurring across all socioeconomic levels, abuse and violence is more prevalent among the poor, with the largest percentage of affected children being under 3 years of age. Among confirmed cases of child maltreatment, nearly 75% were labelled as neglect (Chiesa & Sirotnak, 2020).

Child maltreatment has significant short-term and long-term negative effects on children. Child maltreatment may result in poor physical health, significant physical injury, and/or impaired brain development. Anxiety and depressive disorders, suicidal ideation and attempts, and alcohol and drug use are all associated with a history of childhood abuse. Being a victim of abuse places children at risk for developmental and behavioral problems, decreased cognitive functioning, poor academic achievement, and deficits in relationships (Kleinschmidt, 2018). Children who have been abused or neglected demonstrated significant cognitive delays and education failure in adolescence and adulthood. Children who have experienced emotional abuse demonstrate increased incidence of psychosis, injectable drug use, and harassment later in life, while childhood physical abuse is associated with externalizing behavior problems, delinquency, and substance abuse later in life. An increased incidence of cannabis abuse, having multiple sexual partners, and visual hallucinations occurs in the child who has experienced neglect (Strathearn et al., 2020).

### Subjective Findings

While obtaining the health history, note the appropriateness of parent-child attachment, which may be altered in the case of neglect. If an injury occurred, note the timing as well as the reported mechanism of injury. Determine whether the history provided seems to be consistent with the injury sustained.

Ask children if they are afraid of anyone at home or if anyone has hurt them or touched them in a way that made them feel uncomfortable. Ask parents/caregivers if they are afraid of anyone at home and if they have ever felt like they may hit or hurt the child when frustrated.

The health history may reveal:

- Vague or changing details related to the injury
- Report of an injury inconsistent with developmental stage or caused by a young sibling
- Report of orofacial injury in infant not yet cruising.

**PRO TIP** Avoid asking younger children to answer yes/no questions or to select answers from lists. Performance pressure leads to inaccurate answers.

## Risk Factors

The most common risk factors for child maltreatment include:

- Poverty
- Child who is a former premature infant, or has a chronic illness, cerebral palsy, or an intellectual disability
- Parents/caretakers with a history of being abused themselves, who abuse alcohol or other substances, or are undergoing extreme stress. Maternal physical abuse correlates with child physical abuse and neglect, and maternal depression only with child physical abuse (Yang et al., 2018).

## Review of Systems

The most common manifestations revealed during the review of systems include:

- **Constitutional:** sleep disturbance, headaches, stomachaches
- **HEENT:** difficulty swallowing, chronic sore throat (sexually transmitted infection or forced oral sex)
- **Genitourinary:** genital itching or burning (sexual abuse)
- **Psychiatric:** suicide attempt
- **Behavioral:** hypervigilance, hurting self or others (e.g., cutting), running away, involved in high-risk behaviors, inappropriate sexual behavior for developmental age (seductiveness may indicate sexual abuse)

**PRO TIP** History that changes over time, history of trauma inconsistent with the observed injury, and/or delay in seeking medical treatment all suggest child maltreatment.

## Objective Findings

Perform the physical examination gently, but thoroughly, using a calm voice and soft touch. Note how the child is dressed (appropriate for season, clean?). The most common manifestations revealed during the physical examination include:

- Parent-child interaction revealing fear in the child or an excessive desire to please
- Decreased level of consciousness (shaken baby syndrome)
- Bruises, abrasions, burns, contusions, cuts, scars, or any other unusual or suspicious marks
- Current or healed cuts or scratches on parts of the body ordinarily covered by clothing (child self-mutilation)
- Burns in a stocking (foot) or glove (hand) pattern, or only to the soles or palms (suspicious for inflicted burns)
- Injuries in various stages of healing
- Bruises on the head, neck, chest, or abdomen
- Retinal hemorrhage (shaken baby syndrome)
- Oropharyngeal inflammation (forced oral sex)
- Swelling or deformity
- Anal, penile, or vaginal bleeding or discharge (sexual abuse; Boos, 2020b; Chiesa & Sirotnak, 2020).

**PRO TIP** Nonambulatory children infrequently experience fractures or bruises.

## Laboratory and Diagnostic Testing

Some cases of child maltreatment will be based on the history and physical examination findings. Testing may include:

- Elevated serum alanine aminotransferase (ALT) and aspartate aminotransferase (AST), which suggest liver injury
- Skeletal survey or bone scan (current or past fractures)
- Computed tomography scan of the head (intracranial hemorrhage)
- Vaginal, urethral, rectal, or oral specimens, which may be tested for gonorrhea or chlamydia (sexual abuse).

▶ ALERT: Long bone fractures in children who do not yet walk and rib fractures in infants are highly correlated with child abuse.

## Differential Diagnosis

The differential diagnosis varies according to the clinical manifestations. Consultation with a multidisciplinary team experienced in child maltreatment will be helpful. The differential diagnosis for child abuse includes:

- Bruises
  - Vitamin K deficiency
  - Bleeding disorder
  - Mongolian spots
  - Immunoglobulin A vasculitis
  - Hemangiomas
  - Salicylate ingestion
  - Complementary or alternative therapy, cultural practice (cupping, coining, moxibustion, spooning)
- Fractures
  - Nonabusive trauma
  - Congenital insensitivity to pain
  - Osteogenesis imperfecta
  - Pathologic fracture from osteopenia of limited mobility, metabolic bone disease, rickets, neoplasm, copper or vitamin C deficiency
- Burns
  - Complementary or alternative therapy, cultural practice (cupping, coining, moxibustion, spooning)
  - Chemical or irritant nonintentional burn
  - Phytophotodermatitis
  - Impetigo (Boos, 2020a).

## Treatment/Management Plan

The management goals for child maltreatment include physical treatment of the injury and other interventions to restore or preserve the child's mental well-being, as well as family functioning. Management varies significantly depending upon the child's presentation.

### Family Education

Teach the following:

- Normal growth and development activities to be noted in the infant or child (parents may have unrealistic child behavior expectations based on the child's age, contributing to maltreatment).
- Parents may benefit from connecting with Parents Anonymous (https://parentsanonymous.org), an organization dedicated to strengthening of the family as a means for preventing child maltreatment.
- Follow through with all expectations set forth by child protective services.
- When psychological therapy is recommended, be sure to complete all sessions and activities as recommended.

### Referral

If abusive head trauma is suspected in any child younger than 5 years of age, immediate referral to pediatric ophthalmology for complete dilated indirect fundoscopic exam is warranted. Consult a multidisciplinary child maltreatment team for assistance with diagnosis and treatment. Depending upon local laws, refer suspected child maltreatment cases to child and family protective services, social services, and/or local law enforcement. Refer the child to a pediatric trauma center for inpatient management of serious injuries as appropriate.

▶ ALERT: All states (by law) require that healthcare professionals report suspected cases of child abuse or neglect (Child Welfare Information Gateway, 2019).

# MEDICAL CHILD ABUSE

Medical child abuse, formerly termed Munchausen syndrome by proxy, is a type of child abuse in which the parent or caregiver fictitiously creates psychological issues and/or symptoms of impairment or illness in the child, or induces illness in the child. In some cases, the child actually has a health problem, but the extent of symptoms and seeking of care is out of proportion to the usual. The attention provided by investigation of these symptoms and parenting of an "ill'"child permits the parent to meet their own psychological needs. Medical child abuse may remain hidden for many years as it is difficult to detect. In most cases, the biologic mother is the perpetrator (Roesler & Jenny, 2020).

## Subjective Findings

Obtain a detailed and thorough history of the child's symptoms and illness(es). When documenting parental responses, utilize quotations. During the history closely observe the mother's behavior with the child, and spouse or partner when also present. The report of subjective finding varies widely depending upon the individual parent's report of the child's symptoms.

The more commonly reported symptoms may be consistent with pseudo-seizure, sepsis, apnea, asthma, or pseudo-obstruction.

**PRO TIP** Medical child abuse warning signs include:

- ack of response to treatment
- iblings with similar history
- llness following a puzzling course
- ymptoms witnessed only by the caregiver
- hysical and laboratory findings that do not fit with the reported history
- epeated hospitalizations failing to produce a medical diagnosis, transfers to other hospitals, discharges against medical advice
- arent who refuses to accept that the diagnosis is not medical (Roesler & Jenny, 2018)

## Risk Factors

The most common risk factors for medical child abuse are as follows:

- Primary caregiver is biological mother (female).
- Maternal history exists of unfortunate childhood, somatoform or factitious disorder, substance abuse, self-harm, or criminal activity.

## Review of Systems

The review of systems may reveal:

- **Respiratory:** apnea
- **Gastrointestinal:** vomiting, diarrhea
- **Neurologic:** ataxia, seizure, coma
- **Immune:** allergic response

## Objective Findings

The physical examination is often normal. Note where reported health history differs from the physical examination findings. If the child has other medical conditions, the physical examination will reveal particular signs associated with that condition.

## Laboratory/Diagnostic Testing

Depending upon the subjective data presented by the caregiver and the physical examination findings, laboratory or diagnostic testing may be necessary. This will be very specific to each child's presentation.

## Differential Diagnosis

Early identification of medical child abuse is key. The differential diagnosis includes:

- Well child
- Complex pediatric condition (mitochondrial disease, postural orthostatic tachycardia syndrome, chronic Lyme disease, pain amplification syndromes).

**PRO TIP** Although not diagnostic of medical child abuse, caregiver qualities associated with medical child abuse include doctor shopping, insistence on painful procedure or hospitalization despite provider explanation of its lack of necessity, repeated office visits not yielding objective findings, and lack of respect for professional boundaries.

## Treatment/Management Plan

Treatment of medical child abuse is complex and requires consultation with a specialty multidisciplinary team. Management goals are ensuring the child's well-being and safety, and providing psychotherapy for the perpetrator. For mild cases of medical child abuse, exploring the reasons for amplification or fabrication of the child's symptoms may open the door for discussion of the parent's fears or possibly depression (parent psychology referral could be helpful). Maintaining an open, honest, nonjudgmental approach is critical. Moderate to severe medical child abuse necessitates referral (see the text that follows).

## Family Education

Teach the following:

- All actions taken by the provider are done in the best interests of the child.
- If the child indeed is not in need of further evaluation or hospitalization, provide truthful explanations to that effect.
- Follow through with all expectations set forth by child protective services and psychologic/psychiatric services.

## Referral

If moderate or severe medical child abuse is suspected, consultation with a multidisciplinary team is necessary. The team may include a child abuse specialist, psychologist, and legal counsel. Some instances of medical child abuse are revealed during covert video surveillance in the hospital. The surveillance may reveal maternal actions causing illness in the child or demonstrate complete lack of any symptoms the mother is reporting. Refer the perpetrator for psychiatric evaluation and treatment.

▶ ALERT: Suspicion of medical child abuse is mandated for reporting similar to other forms of child maltreatment.

## SUBSTANCE USE DISORDERS

Substance use disorders include use of alcohol, caffeine, cannabis, hallucinogens, inhalants, opioids, sedative, hypnotics, anxiolytics, stimulants, and tobacco. Teen substance use places adolescents at risk for substance use problems and addiction in adulthood. The earlier the age of onset of use, the higher the risk of addiction. Any use of nicotine, alcohol, or other drugs, including misuse of prescription drugs, is risky for children and adolescents. Alcohol is the most commonly abused substance, followed by nicotine and marijuana. In the United States, almost half of high school students report the use of addictive substances and over one million adolescents meet criteria for substance use disorder; however, less than 10% engage in treatment (Substance Abuse and Mental Health Services Administration [SAMHSA], 2018).

Diagnosis of a substance use disorder is based on behavioral manifestations and the severity of the disorder is based on the number of criteria present. There are four areas of criteria: impaired control, social impairment, risky use, and pharmacologic/physiological indicators or tolerance and withdrawal.

Impaired control includes using substances for longer than intended or in larger amounts than intended; inability to reduce use despite the desire to do so; excessive time getting, using, and/or recovering from drug use; and intense cravings that overwhelm thoughts. Social impairment includes problems with work, school, family, and friends. Risky use refers to use of substance without regard to the harm it may cause or continuing to use substance despite awareness of known harm. Tolerance and withdrawal are classic indicators of addiction. Tolerance is the need for an increased amount of a substance to achieve the desired effect. Withdrawal is the body's response to stopping a substance once tolerance has been developed.

The American Academy of Pediatrics (AAP) recommends that pediatric providers be knowledgeable about Screening, Brief Intervention, and Referral to Treatment (SBIRT). Screening tools are evidence-based and can identify, reduce, and prevent problematic use and abuse of alcohol and other substances. Brief intervention is used to engage an adolescent with a positive screening and give feedback and advice. Referral to treatment is for those with positive screening who are in need of additional services.

Screening tools can be self- or clinician-administered, depending on the tool used. There are multiple tools that have been developed and validated for use. The CRAFFT screening questionnaire is a widely available screening tool that is validated for use in 12- to 26-year-olds. The NIH Online Adolescent Screening Tools are brief screening and intervention tools that are validated for 12- to 17-year-olds. The Alcohol Screening and Brief Intervention for Youth (NIAAA and AAP joint publication) is a screening tool developed for early intervention and can be used for ages 9 to 18. There are many other tools available and providers need to take into account that there is evidence for use in the population they are screening.

### Risk Factors

The most common risk factors for substance use disorders are:

*Genetic predisposition:*

- Children and adolescents with a family history of substance use or psychiatric disorder and those with comorbid mental illnesses who are 60 to 75 are at higher risk; 188% of adolescents with substance use disorders have a comorbid mental illness (Bukstein, 2020).
- Alcoholism is known to be highly heritable.

*Environmental factors:*

- Parental influences (parents who use substances, including tobacco)
- Family structure including lower income, lower socioeconomic status, unstable income, divorce, single parenting, and marital discord
- Peer influence (having peers that use increases risk)
- Neglect and limited parental involvement
- Childhood sexual abuse (strong correlation to use and early age of first use)
- Availability of drugs in the community
- Drug laws (lower drinking age and legal use of substances results in increased use while higher taxes on alcohol results in decreased use by younger ages)
- Knowledge and beliefs around use, which can influence and increase risk; for example, the belief that moderate consumption is okay or beneficial increases likelihood of use

## ALCOHOL USE DISORDER

Alcohol use disorder is categorized as a chronic disease that is characterized by uncontrolled drinking and preoccupation with alcohol. Generally, there is the inability to control drinking due to physical and emotional dependence. Moderate drinking is defined as more than one drink per day for females and more than two drinks per day for males. Binge drinking is considered more than five alcoholic drinks at least once in the past 30 days. Heavy drinking is considered more than five drinks (on the same occasion) on 5 or more days in the past 30 days.

## TOBACCO USE DISORDER

Tobacco use disorder is diagnosed using the same criteria as other substance use disorders. There needs to be evidence of impaired control, social impairment, risky use, and pharmacologic or physiological indicators, or tolerance and withdrawal, in order to diagnose as a disorder (American Psychiatric Association, 2013). Nicotine, the addictive substance in tobacco, is available to smoke or chew.

Electronic cigarettes (e-cigarettes, vape pens) are battery-powered and can be rechargeable or disposable. Electronic cigarettes are used with propylene glycol synthetic, a syrupy liquid that is generally safe to consumers. The concentrations of nicotine are highly variable and unregulated (Wang et al., 2019). They are often marketed to youth and can be flavored. This masks odor and is often appealing to children and youth. The CDC reported that one of 10 middle school students and that more than one of every four high school students (27.5%) had used electronic cigarettes in the past 30 days (2020b).

The CDC found that cigarette use among children and adolescents has decreased from 2011 to 2019. In 2019, 2.3% (about two of 100 students) of middle schoolers reported smoking cigarettes in the last 30 days versus 4.3% in 2011, whereas 5.8% (six of 100 students) of high school students reported smoking cigarettes in 2019 versus 15.8% in 2011 (CDC, 2020b; CDC, 2020c). Use of smokeless tobacco also went down in both middle school and high school students from 2011 to 2019. Use of electronic cigarettes makes up for this difference rather than showing a downward trend in overall tobacco use in children and adolescents (CDC, 2019).

## CANNABIS (MARIJUANA) USE DISORDER

Cannabis is a plant that contains tetrahydrocannabinol (THC) and cannabidiol (CBD). THC is the psychoactive ingredient in marijuana. It can be made into an oil or dried and smoked. Oil is used in vape pens to be inhaled. When inhaled, it enters the bloodstream from the lungs and results in an immediate "high." Immediate effects include distorted perception, difficulty with thought processes and problem-solving, and decreased motor coordination. Cannabis use can have an impact on neurodevelopment, specifically the prefrontal cortex development in children and adolescents, even with infrequent use, leading to development of severe mental illness and decreased cognitive abilities. Cannabis and its forms are regulated in some states (AACAP, 2019b).

Cannabis use develops over time, with many youth using infrequently to begin with and then gradually increasing use to daily or multiple times per day. The disorder is identified when there is decreased functioning related to relationships, school and/or work, development of tolerance, cravings, and the development of withdrawal symptoms (such as insomnia, restlessness, anxiety, anger, depression) within a week of stopping heavy use (American Psychiatric Association, 2013). As with other substance use disorders, early identification is key to successful, long-term recovery.

## OPIOID USE DISORDER

Opioid use disorder is defined by impaired control of use, social impairment, and continued use despite interpersonal conflicts, known risks, and physiological indicators of tolerance and withdrawal. Opiates are derived from poppy plants, while opioids are synthetic drugs produced in a laboratory to mimic opiates. These chemicals attach to opioid receptors on nerve cells in the body and brain, reduce feelings of pain, and can cause euphoria. Prescription opioids are intended to treat acute pain, including oxycodone, codeine, hydromorphone, and morphine. Other synthetic opioids include fentanyl, methadone, tramadol, and carfentanil. Heroin is a synthetic opioid made from morphine. Opioids can be taken orally, injected, smoked, or snorted (Azadfard et al., 2020).

Fourteen percent of adolescents reported misusing opioid prescriptions, while 1.8% have used illicit injectable drugs (CDC, 2020d). Research has shown that high school students who are prescribed an opioid for any reason are at significantly higher risk of developing an opioid use disorder (33%) as compared with students who are never prescribed an opioid. As the onset of substance use disorders begins for a majority in adolescence and the growing availability of opioids, it is important for pediatric primary care providers to assess and be aware of the emerging data related to opioid use and abuse.

## OTHER SUBSTANCE USE DISORDERS

Other substance use disorders include hallucinogen use disorder, inhalant use disorder, sedative use disorder, hypnotic use disorder, anxiolytics use disorder, and stimulant use disorder.

Hallucinogen use disorder is diagnosed when there is continued use of hallucinogens despite impaired functioning. In the last decade, there has been an increase in presentation of adolescents to emergency care settings due to the effects of hallucinogens. Hallucinogens are dissociative drugs that distort sight and sound and produce feelings of detachment. There are several drugs that fall into the category of hallucinogens. Phencyclidine (PCP) is the most common and has many street names including Angel Dust, Supergrass, Boat, Tic-tac, Zoom, and Shermans. Ketamine is similar to PCP. It is available as powder, crystal, liquid, tablet, and capsules and it can be smoked, snorted, or swallowed. It will also dissolve in water or alcohol. Other hallucinogens available are lysergic acid diethylamide (LSD), morning glory seeds (concentrated LSD), mescaline, psilocybin (mushrooms, 'shrooms), 3,4-methylenedioxymethamphetamine (MDMA, Ecstasy, X, Adam, XTC, MDM), and N,N-Dimethyltryptamine (DMT, Snuff).

The most common effects of hallucinogens are sedation, analgesia, and immobility. Onset of action varies based on amount and how it is taken; smoking onset is 2 to 5 minutes, while oral ingestion is 30 to 60 minutes. The duration of effects generally lasts 4 to 8 hours with some reports of effects lasting 24 to 48 hours. Hallucinogens can trigger risk-taking behaviors, violence, and psychiatric consequences. Hallucinogen persisting perception disorder is diagnosed when an individual has vivid flashbacks and perceptual disturbances that last months or years after cessation.

Of note, some cultures (i.e., Native American tribes) use hallucinogens in religious or other rituals. When the hallucinogen is used only as part of a cultural ritual, it does not meet the criteria for a substance use disorder.

Inhalant use disorder refers to household products that contain hydrocarbons. Examples include glue, gasoline, paint thinners, cleaners, and aerosol sprays. Inhalants are often the first drugs used by youth as they are inexpensive and easily available. Intoxication is through inhaling the vapor (a paper bag may be used to disperse the vapor for inhalation). Inhalant use can be fatal on first use due to the toxic nature of the substance rather than dose-related issues.

Anxiolytic use disorder refers to use of CNS depressants. The most commonly used are benzodiazepines (i.e., Valium, Xanax, Ativan). Barbiturates (i.e., Amytal, Phenobarbital), sleeping medications, and other antianxiety medications are also included in this category. These can be deadly at higher doses due to CNS depression. When taken with alcohol (also a CNS depressant), a lower dose can be fatal. Anxiolytic use is often concurrent with other drug use as it is often used to counteract the effects of other drugs (i.e., "uppers").

Stimulant use disorder refers to the use of amphetamine-based drugs, both legal prescription medications (inappropriate use) and illegal drugs. Methamphetamine is the illegal substance known more commonly as meth, crystal meth, crank, speed, bennies, or dexies. Prescription amphetamines include Adderall (mixed amphetamine salts), Ritalin (methylphenidate) and Dexedrine (dextroamphetamine). When used appropriately and as prescribed for conditions such as ADHD, obesity and narcolepsy criteria for substance use disorder are not met. Stimulant use can be episodic or chronic. Overdose is rarely fatal. Longer-term consequences include weight loss, anemia, poor hygiene, skin-picking, and amphetamine-induced psychosis.

### Subjective Findings

The health history may reveal:

- Parents may present symptoms they notice in their child or adolescent after use
  - Poor judgment
  - Difficulty getting along with people
  - Impulsivity (aggression and risky sexual behavior)
  - Slurred speech, unsteady gait, lack of coordination, impaired attention/memory, loss of consciousness (alcohol)
- Withdrawal symptoms
  - Alcohol
    - Begins 4 to 12 hours after cessation or reduction of heavy use
    - Physical symptoms: sweating, tremor, nausea/vomiting, agitation, seizures
    - Psychological symptoms: hallucinations, agitation, insomnia, anxiety
  - Tobacco
    - Occurs after discontinuing or reduction of use when used at least daily for 3 to 4 weeks.
    - About one-half of tobacco users have withdrawal symptoms after 2 days of not using and symptoms typically last 2 to 3 weeks.
    - Physical symptoms: increased appetite, weight gain, and cravings
    - Psychological symptoms: depression, irritability, anger, anxiety, and difficulty concentrating

- Cannabis
  - Psychological symptoms: irritability, anxiety, depression, sleep issues
  - Physical symptoms: fever, chills, tremors, abdominal pain
  - Need to have at least one physical symptom to diagnose cannabis withdrawal
- Opioid
  - Psychological symptoms: irritability, anxiety, depression, mood alteration, sleep issues
  - Physical symptoms: fever, chills, tremors, abdominal pain, cravings
  - Withdrawal is not generally life-threatening (although use can be fatal).
- Other substances
  - Physical symptoms: sweating, heart rate changes, tremors
  - Psychological symptoms: sleep issues, irritability
- Speed and severity of withdrawal is dependent on the half-life of the drug used (Fluyau et al., 2018).
  - Shorter-acting drugs can have withdrawal within 6 to 8 hours and can last 7 or more days
  - Longer-acting drugs can have 5 to 7 days before withdrawal starts and withdrawal can last 3 to 4 weeks.

- Child/adolescent may admit using or parent/guardian may suspect or have found evidence of substance use. Child or adolescent may have found family member's prescription.

## Review of Systems

The most common manifestations revealed during the review of systems include:

- **Constitutional:** weight changes, sleep disturbance
- **Respiratory:** dry cough, shortness of breath (with inhaled/smoked substances)
- **Cardiovascular:** palpitations, BP changes
- **Gastrointestinal:** nausea, vomiting
- **Neurologic:** alteration in cognition, headache, irritability, decreased concentration
- **Psychiatric:** anxiety, mood disturbance
- **Behavioral:** poor school performance, isolating from family and peers, risky and/or disruptive behaviors, needing to smoke or use when wakes up (indicative of tolerance)

## Objective Findings

The physical examination of the child/adolescent with substance use disorder may reveal:

- Weight changes
- Poor personal hygiene
- Pallor, jaundice, track marks (IV use), scarring (IV use), cellulitis (IV use)
- Red/bloodshot eyes
- Decreased cough reflex (opioid), respiratory depression (opioid, benzodiazepine), increased respiratory rate, shortness of breath, dry cough (inhaled substances)
- Increased BP (alcohol), tachycardia
- Decreased bowel sounds (delayed gastric emptying, constipation)
- Pupil changes (dilated or constricted), decreased coordination, slower reaction times, increased sensitivity to pain (opioid), slowed reflexes, tremor (alcohol, other withdrawal)
- Personality change (i.e., adolescent who is usually quiet is now very talkative), suicidal thinking, depressed or anxious mood/affect, irritability.

Screening tools are an effective means of assessing and determining level of risk and severity of disorder. CRAFFT Brief Screening Questionnaire, Alcohol Screening and Brief Intervention, and NIH Online Adolescent Drug Screening are three evidence-based screening tools for older children and adolescents.

### Laboratory/Diagnostic Testing

The diagnosis of substance use disorder is based upon the clinical findings. Urine and/or serum screen for substances can be useful in assessing if any substances are being used. It is important that informed consent from the child or adolescent be obtained prior to performing drug testing unless for emergency needs. According to the AAP, informed consent and confidentiality should always be maintained in laboratory testing for drugs and alcohol (Levy et al., 2014). The AAP (2007) does not endorse at-home drug testing because the testing can be complex with potential for misinterpreted results and a potential risk to the parent-child relationship as well as poor evidence supporting home drug testing and reduction of substance use and abuse.

## Differential Diagnosis

The differential diagnosis for substance use disorders includes:

- Brain injury
- Sleep disorder
- Neurocognitive disorder
- Delirium
- Brain lesion
- Seizure disorder

- Anxiety disorder
- Mood disorder
- Psychotic disorder (schizophrenia or other)
- ADHD
- OCD
- CD
- Learning disability
- PTSD
- Diabetic ketoacidosis
- Uremia
- Hypoglycemia
- Hyperthyroidism
- Pheochromocytoma.

## Treatment/Management Plan

Any child or adolescent who meets the criteria for a substance use disorder should be evaluated by a professional who is familiar with treatment of adolescent addiction. If the youth screening indicates acute danger due to withdrawal, or exacerbation of psychiatric symptoms, immediate referral or transport to an appropriate emergency facility is indicated.

Treatment for substance use disorders generally begins with brief intervention and education regarding the risks of substance use. It is important to give clear medical advice and reinforcement regarding abstaining from and ceasing use. When the belief is that use is not harmful, use generally continues and can become more severe. For example, many children and adolescents believe that cannabis use is less harmful than use of alcohol or other substances (AACAP, 2019b).

Depending on the substance and intensity of use, more intensive and continued treatment may be required. Options for behavioral therapy include group therapy (outpatient and partial hospital program), CBT, Adolescent Community Reinforcement Approach (A-CRA), 12-step treatment such as Alcoholics Anonymous (AA) or Narcotics Anonymous (NA), and the family systems approach. Involving parents, family, and community and school resources provides for the most successful outcomes. There are also recovery-based schools to support adolescents in recovery. If the use is severe and is affecting the adolescent significantly, 24-hour residential or inpatient substance use-based treatment may be needed.

## Substance-Specific Treatments

Following are substance-specific treatments:

- Alcohol: There are no FDA-approved pharmacologic treatments for alcohol use disorder in children or adolescents. Naltrexone and disulfiram (Antabuse) can be used, but are not approved for use in children or adolescents.
- Tobacco: Goal of treatment and management of tobacco use disorder is to stop use. This can be done by abrupt discontinuation or more commonly to gradually taper nicotine intake. Assessing the type and amount of tobacco being used is essential for helping the youth decrease use. For electronic cigarettes and vape liquid, it is important to know the percent of and/or milligrams of nicotine per cartridge. Once this is determined, they can gradually decrease the number of times of using per day as well as decrease the concentration per cartridge.
  - The National Cancer Institute created the website smokefree.gov. This is a good resource for youth, parents, and clinicians for up-to-date information on helping and understanding cessation of tobacco use. There is a teen specific area: https://teen.smokefree.gov
  - Nicotine replacement therapies include patches, gum, lozenges, nasal spray, and inhalers. The only medication that is approved for tobacco use disorder is bupropion to reduce cravings and withdrawal symptoms. Bupropion is approved for use in children and adolescents for depression and ADHD, but not for nicotine cessation. Be aware that there is a black box warning for bupropion use in children and adolescents due to risk of increased mood symptoms, including suicidal thinking.
- Cannabis: There are no FDA-approved pharmacologic treatments for cannabis use disorder.
- Opioid: Pharmacologic treatment is available for older adolescents with opioid use disorder. Special training is required to administer and monitor these treatments. Buprenorphine (Subutex) and buprenorphine/naloxone (Suboxone) are not FDA-approved for pediatric use, but have been studied and shown to have a positive impact in older adolescents. Methadone decreases withdrawal symptoms and cravings; it can be used in 16- to 18-year-olds who have failed other trials and with parent/guardian signed consent. Naltrexone is used to help with cravings and to decrease euphoric effects, but is not FDA approved for use in adolescents. Naloxone (Narcan, Evzio) can be used to reverse an opioid overdose and restore breathing that has stopped or slowed due to an opioid overdose.
- Benzodiazepine: The treatment of benzodiazepine use disorder generally relies on gradual dose reduction as rapid decrease or cessation can be fatal. Use of

a long-acting benzodiazepine such as diazepam is the mainstay of treatment (Soyka, 2017).

- Hallucinogens, inhalants, and stimulants: There are no FDA-approved medications for treating the use/abuse of hallucinogens, inhalants, or stimulants.

## Family Education

Teach the following:

- In most states, adolescents have the right to confidentiality regarding treatment and disclosure of substance use. Know your state's laws and rights. Families and adolescents should be informed early on regarding rights to confidentiality, potential reasons to breach confidentiality, and areas where confidentiality might be affected (appointment notifications, billing, and result notification). Adolescents are less likely to disclose information if they believe it will not be confidential.
- Misuse can start with the child or adolescent finding and using medications that have been prescribed to family members. It is important to properly store and promptly dispose of leftover medications that have been prescribed. Encourage parents/guardians to engage their children early on regarding use and risk. Family history is important—when there is a history of close relatives with any substance abuse, a child needs to know they are also at increased risk of developing a substance use disorder. This is especially true of alcohol use disorder as alcoholism is known to be highly heritable.
- Give clear medical advice and reinforcement related to abstaining from and ceasing use of substances.
- Substance use in adolescents is often comorbid with psychiatric illnesses and families should follow up regarding their child's mental health.

## Referral

Referral to mental health providers who are experienced with children and adolescents with substance use disorders is important for successful treatment and recovery from substance use disorders.

## KEY POINTS

- AN is characterized by weight loss, failure to gain weight as expected in a child, amenorrhea in females, and distorted body image. People with AN restrict caloric intake, restrict types of food they eat and/or compulsively exercise, purge, and/or use laxatives or diuretics in order to maintain or lose weight. Onset is most commonly between the ages of 14 and 18.
- BN is characterized by recurrent episodes of binge eating, having the feeling of lack of control of overeating during the episode and then engaging in compensatory behaviors to prevent weight gain. Binge eating and inappropriate behaviors occur at least twice a week for at least 3 months. Compensatory behaviors include self-induced vomiting as well as misuse of laxatives, diuretics, or enemas (purging type) or fasting and/or excessive exercise (nonpurging type). BN is also correlated with a history of sexual abuse or trauma.
- BED is characterized by recurrent binge-eating episodes at least weekly for at least 3 months, during which a large amount of food is consumed and there is a lack of control of eating and associated distress. The primary goal of treating BED is to reduce binge-eating behaviors, not to promote weight management or weight loss. Focus on weight reduction can increase symptoms of disordered eating and psychiatric manifestations.
- ARFID is an eating disorder characterized by limited intake of food in terms of variety and/or quantity. This often impacts weight and growth and may become severe enough to require medical stabilization.
- ARFID often has an earlier onset than other eating disorders and may present initially as "picky eating." A key difference with ARFID as compared to other eating disorders is that there is not concern about weight or body shape. Many children and adolescents with ARFID have underlying or comorbid anxiety disorders. These need to be treated alongside of the eating disorder in order to normalize eating behaviors.
- For all eating disorders, intervention and treatment through a team approach, early intervention, and appropriate long-term monitoring and support are key factors in recovery.
- DMDD is characterized by a persistent irritable and/or angry mood and severe behavioral outbursts that are disproportional to the situation and developmental level of the child.
- There is no known prevention for DMDD, but early identification and implementations of supports and treatment for children and families provides the best outcomes.
- BPD is a mood disorder characterized by manic, hypomanic, or mixed mood episodes, although many children and adolescents experience a depressed mood.
- BPD is an episodic illness and children and adolescents will experience periods of stability along with exacerbations.
- Medication is needed for the management of bipolar illness and, as this is a lifelong illness, medication use

will be long-term. Children and families may struggle with the long-term need for medications. Nonadherence with medications is a common concern.

- CD is characterized by aggression toward people or animals, destruction of property, deceitfulness or theft, and serious violations of rules. Without treatment as many as 70% of children and adolescents with CD will develop antisocial personality disorder (Elia, 2019).
- A multifaceted approach is the most effective model for treatment of CD. It is important to treat comorbid mental health concerns, to support parents/guardians in effective parenting strategies, to involve children and adolescents in community and sports, and to have collaboration among all those involved in care.
- ODD is characterized by an angry or irritable mood, argumentative and defiant behavior, and may include vindictiveness.
- Left untreated, ODD can worsen and lead to CD as well as exacerbate other comorbid psychiatric illnesses. It is important to treat early for best long-term outcomes.
- Substance use disorder is defined by impaired control of use, social impairment, and continued use despite interpersonal conflicts, continued use despite known risks, and physiological indicators of tolerance and withdrawal. Withdrawal speed and severity are dependent on extent of use, drug used, and half-life of drug.
- Alcohol use disorder is a pattern of alcohol use that involves issues that control drinking, being preoccupied with alcohol, and continuing to use alcohol despite the problems that it causes.
- Tobacco use disorder is a pattern of tobacco use that involves issues controlling tobacco use and being preoccupied with tobacco and continuing to use it despite the problems that it causes. Not all youth using tobacco meet the criteria for the disorder; however, all youth who use tobacco need education about the risk.
- Cannabis use disorder occurs as a gradual progression. Use of cannabis in early adolescence results in a decline in cognitive abilities, most notably memory; increases risk of psychotic illnesses in adulthood; and may intensify symptoms of preexisting psychiatric illnesses.
- Opioid use disorder is defined by impaired control of use, social impairment and continued use despite interpersonal conflicts, continued use despite known risks, and physiological indicators of tolerance and withdrawal.
- The first 12 months of recovery for substance use disorders are the most tenuous. Relapse is preventable but also often part of the recovery process. Routine screening and early intervention are key to prevention and early treatment of substance use disorders.
- Child maltreatment may include physical, emotional, or sexual abuse, as well as neglect. All suspected cases of child abuse require mandatory reporting.
- Injuries inconsistent with the history or developmental capabilities are highly suspicious of child maltreatment.

## REFERENCES


American Academy of Child and Adolescent Psychiatry. (2019a). *Facts for families: Disruptive mood dysregulation disorder.* https://www.aacap.org/AACAP/Families_and_Youth/Facts_for_Families/FFF-Guide/Disruptive-Mood-Dysregulation-Disorder-_DMDD_-110.aspx

American Academy of Child and Adolescent Psychiatry. (2019b). *Marijuana and teens.* https://www.aacap.org/AACAP/Families_and_Youth/Facts_for_Families/FFF-Guide/Marijuana-and-Teens-106.aspx

American Academy of Child and Adolescent Psychiatry. (2019c). *Oppositional defiant disorder.* https//www.aacap.org/AACAP/Families_and_Youth/Facts_for_Families/FFF-Guide/Children-With-Oppositional-Defiant-Disorder-072.aspx

American Academy of Pediatrics, Committee on Substance Abuse, and Council on School Health. (2007). Testing for drugs of abuse in children and adolescents: Addendum—Testing in schools and at home. *Pediatrics, 119*(3), 627–630. https://doi.org/10.1542/peds.2006-3688

American Psychiatric Association. (2013). *Diagnostic and statistical manual of mental disorders* (5th ed.). https://doi.org/10.1176/appi.books.9780890425596.dsm10

American Psychological Association. (2019). *APA resolution on child and adolescent mental and behavioral health.* https://www.apa.org/about/policy/child-adolescent-mental-behavioral-health

Arain, M., Haque, M., Johal, L., Mathur, P., Nel, W., Rais, A., Sandhu, R., & Sharma, S. (2013). Maturation of the adolescent brain. *Neuropsychiatric Disease and Treatment, 9*, 449–461. https://doi.org/10.2147/NDT.S39776

Avenevoli, S., Swendsen, J., He, J.-P., Burstein, M., & Merikangas, K. (2015). Major depression in the national comorbidity survey-adolescent supplement: Prevalence, correlates, and treatment. *Journal of the American Academy of Child & Adolescent Psychiatry, 54*(1), 37–44.e2. https://doi.org/10.1016/j.jaac.2014.10.010

Azadfard, M., Huecker M., & Leaming J. (2020). *Opioid addiction.* https://www.ncbi.nlm.nih.gov/books/NBK448203/

Bennett, K., Manassis, K., Duda, S., Bagnell, A., Bernstein, G., Garland, E. J., Miller L., Newton, A., Thabane, L., & Wilansky, P. (2016). Treating child and adolescent anxiety effectively: Overview of systematic reviews. *Clinical Psychology Review, 50*, 84–90. https://doi.org/10.1016/j.cpr.2016.09.006

Bernstein, B. (2020). *Pediatric bipolar affective disorder.* https://emedicine.medscape.com/article/91 3464-overview

Berstein, B. E. (2018). *Conduct disorder.* https://emedicine.medscape.com/article/918213-overview#a1

Birmaher, B. (2019). Pediatric bipolar disorder. *UpToDate.* https://www.uptodate.com/contents/pediatric-bipolar-disorder-clinical-manifestations-and-course-of-illness#H6530592

Boos, S. C. (2020a). Differential diagnosis of suspected child physical abuse. *UpToDate.* Retrieved November 9, 2020, from https://www.uptodate.com/contents/differential

-diagnosis-of-suspected-child-physical-abuse? topicRef=6600&source=see_link#H7

Boos, S. C. (2020b). Physical child abuse: Diagnostic evaluation and management. *UpToDate*. Retrieved November 9, 2020, from https://www.uptodate.com/contents/physical-child-abuse-diagnostic-evaluation-and-management

Brackett, K. (2017). *Periactin to boost appetite*. Pediatric Feeding News. http://pediatricfeedingnews.com/using-periactin-to-boost-appetite/

Bukstein, O. (2020). Substance use disorder in adolescents: Epidemiology, pathogenesis, clinical manifestations and consequences, course, assessment, and diagnosis. *UpToDate*. Retrieved November 3, 2020, from https://www.uptodate.com/contents/substance-use-disorder-in-adolescents-epidemiology-pathogenesis-clinical-manifestations-and-consequences-course-assessment-and-diagnosis

Burke, J. D., & Loeber, R. (2016). Mechanisms of behavioral and affective treatment outcomes in a cognitive behavioral intervention for boys. *Journal of Abnormal Child Psychology, 44*(1), 179–189. https://doi.org/10.1007/s10802-015-9975-0

Center on the Developing Child. (2020). *Brain architecture*. https://developingchild.harvard.edu/science/key-concepts/brain-architecture/

Centers for Disease Control and Prevention. (2019). *2016 Surgeon General's report: E-cigarette use among youth and young adults*. https://www.cdc.gov/tobacco/data_statistics/sgr/e-cigarettes/index.htm

Centers for Disease Control and Prevention. (2020a). *Early brain development*. https://www.cdc.gov/ncbddd/childdevelopment/early-brain-development.html

Centers for Disease Control and Prevention. (2020b). *Teen substance use and risks*. https://www.cdc.gov/ncbddd/fasd/features/teen-substance-use.html

Centers for Disease Control and Prevention. (2020c). *YRBS data summary & trends*. https://www.cdc.gov/healthyyouth/data/yrbs/yrbs_data_summary_and_trends.htm

Chiarello, F., Spitoni, S., Hollander, E., Cerinic M. M., & Pallanti, S. (2017). An expert opinion on PANDAS/PANS: Highlights and controversies. *International Journal of Psychiatry in Clinical Practice, 21*(2), 91–98. https://doi.org/10.1080/13651501.2017.1285941

Chiesa, A., & Sirotnak, A. P. (2020). Child abuse & neglect. In W. W. Hay, M. J. Levin, M. J. Abzug, & M. Bunik (Eds.), *Current diagnosis & treatment: Pediatrics* (25th ed., Chapter 8). McGraw-Hill Education.

Child Welfare Information Gateway. (2019). *Mandatory reporters of child abuse and neglect*. https://www.childwelfare.gov/topics/systemwide/laws-policies/statutes/manda/?hasBeenRedirected=1

Cook, C. (2015). *Collaborative problem solving (CPS) in a nutshell summary*. http://www.pent.ca.gov/cdr/f15/cps.pdf

Diemer, E., Grant, J., Munn-Chernoff, M., Patterson, D., & Duncan, A. (2015). Identity, sexual orientation, and eating-related pathology in a national sample of college students. *Journal of Adolescent Health, 57*(2), 144–149. http://www.jahonline.org/article/S1054-139X(15)00087-7/pdf

Dovey, T., Kumari, V., & Blissett, J. (2019). Eating behaviour, behavioural problems and sensory profiles of children with avoidant/restrictive food intake disorder (ARFID), autistic spectrum disorders or picky eating: Same or different? *European Psychiatry, 61*, 56–62. https://doi.org/10.1016/j.eurpsy.2019.06.008

Elia, J. (2019). *Conduct disorder*. https://www.merckmanuals.com/professional/pediatrics/mental-disorders-in-children-and-adolescents/conduct-disorder

Evans, R. (2020). Mental health/behavioral guidelines. In M. Meadows-Oliver & N. Banasiak (Eds.), *Pediatric clinical guidelines* (pp. 367–410). Springer Publishing Company.

Fletcher, J. (2017). Bipolar disorder in children: Risk factors and symptoms. *Medical News Today*. https://www.medicalnewstoday.com/articles/319197.php

Fluyau, D., Revadigar, N., & Manobianco, B. (2018). Challenges of the pharmacological management of benzodiazepine withdrawal, dependence, and discontinuation. *Therapeutic Advances in Psychopharmacology, 8*(5), 147–168. https://doi.org/10.1177/2045125317753340

French, P., Boydston, L., & Varley, C. (2016). Obsessive compulsive disorders: A review. *Journal of Alternative Medicine Research, 8*(4), 431–439.

Grohol, J. (2020). *Symptoms of disruptive mood dysregulation disorder*. https://psychcentral.com/disorders/disruptive-mood-dysregulation-disorder/

Guerrier, K., Mitan, L., Wang, Y., & Czosek, R. J. (2016). Risk for prolonged QT interval and associated outcomes in children with early restrictive eating patterns. *Cardiology in the Young, 26*(4) 644 – 649. https://doi.org/10.1017/S1047951115000785

Herpertz-Dahlmann, B. (2009). Adolescent eating disorders: Definitions, symptomatology, epidemiology, and comorbidity. *Child and Adolescent Psychiatry Clinics of North America, 18*, 31–47. https://doi.org/10.1016/j.chc.2008.07.005

Hirneth, S. J., Hazell, P. L., Hanstock, T. L., & Lewin, T. J. (2015). Bipolar disorder subtypes in children and adolescents: demographic and clinical characteristics from an Australian sample. *Journal of Affective Disorders, 175*, 98–107. https://doi.org/10.1016/j.jad.2014.12.021

Keel, P. K., Dorer, D. J., Eddy, K. T., Franko, D., Charatan, D. L., & Herzog, D. B. (2003). Predictors of mortality in eating disorders. *Archives of General Psychiatry, 60*(2), 179–183.

Kleinschmidt, A. (2018). Child maltreatment red flags: Two cases of bruising in premobile infants. *Journal of Pediatric Health Care, 33*(1), 92–96. https://doi.org/10.1016/j.pedhc.2018.07.003

Kornstein, S. G., Kunovac, J. L., Herman, B. K., & Culpepper, L. (2016). Recognizing binge-eating disorder in the clinical setting: A review of the literature. *The Primary Care Companion for CNS Disorders, 18*(3). https://doi.org/10.4088/PCC.15r01905

Lenton-Brym, T., Rodrigues, A., Johnson, N., Couturier, J., & Toulany, A. (2019). A scoping review of the role of primary care providers and primary care-based interventions in the treatment of pediatric eating disorders. *Eating Disorders, 28*(1), 47–66. https://doi.org/10.1080/10640266.2018.1560853

Levy, S., Siqueira, L. M., & the Committee on Substance Abuse. (2014). Testing for drugs of abuse in children and adolescents. *Pediatrics, 133*(6), e1798–e1807. https://doi.org/10.1542/peds.2014-0865

Li, M., Yang, W., Ma, Q., Gopal, N., & Li, B. (2017) The role of brain-gut peptides in mood disorders. Biomedical Research, 28(13). https://www.alliedacademies.org/articles/the-role-of-braingut-peptides-in-mood-disorders-7822.html

Lillig, M. (2018). Conduct disorder: Recognition and management. *American Family Physician, 98*(10), 584–592. https://www.aafp.org/afp/2018/1115/p584.html

Maniglio, R. (2015). Significance, nature, and direction of the association between child sexual abuse and conduct disorder: A systematic review. *Trauma, Violence & Abuse, 16*(3), 241–257. https://psycnet.apa.org/doi/10.1177/1524838014526068

Marzille, E., Cerniglia, L., & Cimino, S. (2018). A narrative review of binging eating disorder in adolescence:

Prevalence, impact, and psychological treatment strategies. *Adolescent Health, Medicine and Therapeutics, 9*, 17–30. https://doi.org/10.2147/AHMT.S148050
Mitchell, Q., Pardini, D., & Lochman, J. (2018). Treatment of oppositional defiant disorder. In P. C. Kendall (Ed.), *Cognitive therapy with children and adolescents: A casebook for clinical practice* (pp. 122–143). The Guilford Press.
Mohan, L., Yilanli, M., & Ray, S. (2020). *Conduct disorder*. https://www.ncbi.nlm.nih.gov/books/NBK470238/
National Cancer Institute. (2020). *Become a smoke free teen.* https://teen.smokefree.gov/
National Eating Disorders Association. (2018a). *Avoidant restrictive food intake disorder (ARFID).* https://www.nationaleatingdisorders.org/learn/by-eating-disorder/arfid
National Eating Disorders Association. (2018b). *Statistics and research on eating disorders.* https://www.nationaleatingdisorders.org/statistics-research-eating-disorders
National Institute of Mental Health. (2020). *Bipolar disorder in children and teens.* https://www.nimh.nih.gov/health/publications/bipolar-disorder-in-children-and-teens/index.shtml
Norris, M. L., Spettigue, W. J., & Katzman, D. K. (2016). Update on eating disorders: Current perspectives on avoidant/restrictive food intake disorder in children and youth. *Neuropsychiatric Disease and Treatment, 12*, 213–218. https://doi.org/10.2147/NDT.S82538
Office on Women's Health. (2017). *Binge eating disorder.* https://www.womenshealth.gov/mental-health/mental-health-conditions/eating-disorders/binge-eating-disorder
Oral, R., Ramirez, M., Coohey, C., Nakada, S., Walz, A., Kuntz, A., Benoit, J., & Peek-Asa, C. (2016). Adverse childhood experiences and trauma informed care: The future of health care. *Pediatric Research, 79*(1–2), 227–233. https://doi.org/10.1038/pr.2015.197
Riley, M., Ahmed, S., &Locke A. (2016). Common questions about oppositional defiant disorder. *American Family Physician, 93*, 7, 586–591. https://www.aafp.org/afp/2016/0401/p586.html
Roesler, T. A., & Jenny, C. (2020). Medical child abuse (Munchausen syndrome by proxy). *UpToDate.* http://www.uptodate.com/contents/medical-child-abuse-munchausen-syndrome-by-proxy
Rosen, D., & the Committee on Adolescence. (2010). Identification and the management of eating disorders. *Pediatrics, 126*(6), 1240–1253. https://doi.org/10.1542/peds.2010-2821
Saylor, K., & Amann, B. (2016). Impulsive aggression as a comorbidity of attention-deficit/hyperactivity disorder in children and adolescents. *Journal of Child and Adolescent Psychopharmacology, 26*(1), 19–25. https://doi.org/10.1089/cap.2015.0126
Siegler, R. (2020). Cognitive development in childhood. In R. Biswas-Diener & E. Diener (Eds.), *Noba textbook series: Psychology*. DEF Publishers. http://noba.to/8uv4fn9h
Siu, A. L. (2016). Screening for depression in children and adolescents: U.S. Preventive Services Task Force recommendation statement. *Pediatrics, 137*(3), e20154467. https://doi.org/10.1542/peds.2015-4467
Soria-Saucedo, R., Walter, J., Cabral, H., England, J., & Kazis, E. (2016). Receipt of evidence-based pharmacotherapy and psychotherapy among children and adolescents with new diagnoses of depression. *Psychiatry Services, 67*(3), 316–323. https://doi.org/10.1176/appi.ps.201500090
Soyka, M. (2017). Treatment of benzodiazepine dependence. *The New England Journal of Medicine, 376*, 1147–1157. https://doi.org/10.1056/NEJMra1611832
Srinath, S., Jacob, P., Sharma, E., & Gautam, A. (2019). Clinical practice guidelines for assessment of children and adolescents. *Indian Journal of Psychiatry, 61*(Suppl. 2), 158–175. https://doi.org/10.4103/psychiatry.IndianJPsychiatry_580_18
Strathearn, L., Giannotti, M., Mills, R., Kisely, S., Najman, J., & Abajobir, A. (2020). Long-term cognitive, psychological, and health outcomes associated with child abuse and neglect. *Pediatrics, 146*(4), e20200438. https://doi.org/10.1542/peds.2020-0438
Substance Abuse and Mental Health Services Administration. (2018). *America's need for and receipt of substance use treatment in 2015.* https://www.hhs.gov/surgeongeneral/priorities/opioids-https://www.samhsa.gov/data/sites/default/files/report_2716/ShortReport-2716.html
Tottenham, N. (2017). *The brain's emotional development.*https://www.dana.org/article/the-brains-emotional-development/
Vargas, C. & Gómez, J. (2015). Alteraciones electrocardiográficas en anorexia nervosa: revisión crítica de la literatura [Electrocardiographic abnormalities in anorexia nervosa: a critical review of the literature]. *Revista Colombiana de Psiquiatría, 44*(1), 33-40. https://doi.org/10.1016/j.rcp.2014.10.003
Vaughan, J., Coddington, J., Ahmed, A., & Ertel, M. (2017). Separation anxiety disorder in school-age children: What health care providers should know. *Journal of Pediatric Health Care, 31*(4), 433–440. https://doi.org/10.1016/j.pedhc.2016.11.003
Wagner, K. (2016). Update on treatment of pediatric bipolar disorder. *Psychiatric Times.* https://www.psychiatrictimes.com/child-adolescent-psychiatry/update-treatment-pediatric-bipolar-disorder
Walter, H. J., & DeMaso, D. R. (2020). Chapter 39: Mood disorders. In R. M. Kliegman, J. W. St. Geme III, N. J. Blum, S. S. Shah, R. C. Tasker, K. M. Wilson, & R. E. Behrman (Eds.), *Nelson textbook of pediatrics* (21st ed.). Elsevier.
Wang, T., Gentzke, A., & Creamer, M. (2019). Tobacco product use and associated factors among middle and high school students—United States, 2019. *Morbidity and Mortality Weekly Report, 268*(12), 1–22. https://www.cdc.gov/tobacco/data_statistics/mmwrs/byyear/2019/ss6812a1/index.html
Wilkinson, A., Halper, C., & Herring, A. (2016). Directions of the relationship between substance use and depressive symptoms from adolescence to young adulthood. *Addictive Behaviors, 60*, 64–70. https://doi.org/10.1016/j.addbeh.2016.03.036
Wlodarczyk, O., Pawils, S., & Metzner, F. (2017). Risk and protective factors for mental health problems in preschool-aged children: Cross-sectional results of the BELLA preschool study. *Child and Adolescent Psychiatry and Mental Health, 11*, 12. https://doi.org/10.1186/s13034-017-0149-4
Yang, M.-Y., Font, S. Z., Ketchum, M., & Kim, Y. K. (2018). Intergenerational transmission of child abuse and neglect: Effects of maltreatment type and depressive symptoms. *Children and Youth Services Review, 91*, 364–371. https://doi.org/10.1016/j.childyouth.2018.06.036
Zepf, F., Biskup, C., Holtmann, M., & Runions, K. (2016). Disruptive mood dysregulation disorder. In J. M. Rey (Ed.), *IACAPAP e-textbook of child and adolescent mental health.*(Chapter E.3). International Association for Child and Adolescent Psychiatry and Allied Professions. https://iacapap.org/content/uploads/E.3-MOOD-DYSREGULATION-2016.pdf
Żmudzka, E., Sałaciak, K., Sapa, J., & Pytka, K. (2018). Serotonin receptors in depression and anxiety: Insights from animal studies. *Life Sciences, 210*, 106–124. https://doi.org/10.1016/j.lfs.2018.08.050

# Environmental Health and Toxicology

Vicky Fan, Priscilla Nakano, Samantha Colbert, and Meredith Kopp

## Student Learning Outcomes

**Upon completion of this chapter the reader should be able to:**

1. Discuss public health/legislation efforts to protect children from environmental and other hazards.
2. Distinguish prenatal exposures that may affect children's health.
3. Identify environmental hazards that have an impact on children's health and ways to mitigate their effects.
4. Discriminate among typical presentations of various toxidromes.
5. Develop a plan for treatment and/or prevention for children in relation to environmental hazards and toxic substances.

## INTRODUCTION

Environmental hazards encompass physical, chemical, social, and biological exposures that may have lasting impacts on children from prenatal development into adolescence. In 2019, the World Health Organization (WHO) stated that most of the 5.2 million deaths in children under 5 years of age were preventable and treatable (WHO, 2020a). Environmental hazards are indiscriminate to geography and continue to plague the lives of children with issues of pollution, access to clean water, and sanitation as well as newly emerging risks from a rapidly developing world. Each year there are over a million toxic exposures in children resulting in 250,000 healthcare facility visits (Gummin et al., 2019). This chapter aims to provide an introduction to common environmental hazards and toxicology as well as how to assess the risk of hazards to help clinicians advocate and create safer environments for their pediatric patients.

The content in this chapter maps to the following areas on the Pediatric Nursing Certification Board (PNCB) Pediatric Nurse Practitioner–Primary Care certification examination:

**CLINICAL PROBLEMS: ENVIRONMENTAL HEALTH/TOXICOLOGY**

CONTENT AREAS:

**I. Health Maintenance and Promotion**

**A. Partner with patients/caregivers to support growth and development from infancy to young adulthood.**

**E. Advise patients/caregivers about age-appropriate injury prevention and safety including but not limited to:**

1. Environmental exposure (e.g., animal and insect, weapons, toys, smoking, sun exposure, poisoning, disaster)

**II. Assessment and Diagnosis**

**B. History and Physical Examination**

1. Obtain history of present illness.
2. Complete an interval history for established patients.
3. Perform a complete physical examination.

**C. Analyzing Information**

1. Integrate health history and physical examination findings into the plan of care.

**D. Diagnosis**

2. Establish a diagnosis based on evaluation of patient data.

## III. Management

**A. Child and Caregiver Counseling and Education**

1. Provide condition-specific counseling and education, including treatment options.
2. Educate about benefits and potential adverse reactions of pharmacological interventions.

**B. Therapeutic Interventions**

1. Prescribe pharmacologic agents.

**E. Care Coordination**

1. Facilitate patient and family-centered care for children of all ages with acute and chronic conditions.

**C. Evaluation and Follow-Up**

2. Establish a plan for follow-up care.

## HOW CHILDREN ARE EXPOSED

When considering hazards to children, the provider must be thorough in their assessment and consider everywhere a child lives, learns, and plays, including their homes, schools, daycare facilities, the community around them, and the air they breathe. Some of the top household sources of exposure include water, diet, and environment. Air pollution has been associated with risk of low birth weight, prematurity, asthma, impaired neurocognitive development, obesity, and type 2 diabetes mellitus (Etzel & Balk, 2019). While there is legislation in place to provide safe drinking water, there is still the possibility for contamination. Well water can easily expose children to many chemicals, both natural and man-made, such as arsenic, copper, and manganese, as well as lead, pesticide run-off, perchlorates, and nitrates. Food in the home can also be a source of contamination, potentially exposing children to chemical residues such as bisphenols, metals, pesticides, and polychlorinated biphenyls (PCBs). Rice has been shown to have detectable levels of arsenic while fish can be a source of mercury. Herbal remedies and spices such as turmeric may also be a source of lead or mercury (Hauptman & Woolf, 2017).

The child's environment may also put them at risk. Children spend 80% to 90% of their time indoors, often in school or daycare. Air quality can be compromised indoors. Children may easily be exposed to second- and third-hand smoke, lead, mold, pesticides, and phthalates, as well as disinfectants and sanitizers. Another consideration of school and child-care settings is the condition of the school; if the school or daycare is older, the provider must consider exposure to asbestos, lead, and PCBs (Etzel & Balk, 2019).

Another aspect to consider is the design around the child's home. The community or area around the child's home could include areas of high traffic speeds, wide road lanes, and lack of safe walkways or bike paths. This easily puts children in the path of vehicles and bicycles. Where the home is located could put the child at risk for poor access to healthy foods, air pollution (traffic-induced or if close to a toxic waste site), or poor water quality due to many factors, including proximity to toxic waste site or depending on how storm water is managed (Etzel & Balk, 2019).

When considering possible hazard exposure in children, the provider must obtain a thorough history, as well as inquire about the age of the home, nearby airports, agriculture, toxic waste sites, and what is located in the area around the home. Ask about parents' occupations and consider if there may be additional exposures or objects around the house that could cause a threat to the child's health. Be sure to ask not only about diet and the water source in the home, but also about herbal remedies used, medications taken, and if there are any cultural treatments or supplements being used (Hauptman & Woolf, 2017).

## LAWS

In 1995, the United States Environmental Protection Agency (EPA) released its *Policy on Evaluating Risk to Children*. For the first time, the EPA was mandated directly to take into consideration the effects of all things in the environment, shining a light on risk assessment and characterization as well as setting public health standards in the United States. This was followed by the National Agenda to Protect Children's Health From Environmental Threats. The EPA was called upon to raise the standards of products to levels safe for children, as well as to enforce them. Additionally, it called for a scientific research strategy to be developed in order to identify the gaps in knowledge about the exposures of children (specifically at different ages), and to put legislation in place to address these exposures. This also tasked the agency with educating the community in order to better protect them as well as providing the funding needed to make children's environmental health a national priority (EPA, 2018). There had been several pieces of legislation leading to this national agenda, several of which have been amended multiple times and are still in use today. Refer to Table 41.1 for a review of other laws related to environmental health.

**TABLE 41.1 Laws Governing Environmental Health**

| Legislation/Date | Action/Meaning | Considerations/Comments | Citation |
|---|---|---|---|
| The Food and Drugs Act—1906 | Prohibited unsafe and contaminated products from being sold across state lines | Flawed: was easy to continue distributing products that had been outlawed<br>1937, public outcry about safety of pharmaceuticals (deaths from drugs recently, legally hitting market) | U.S. Food and Drug Administration [FDA] (2018a) |
| The Federal Food, Drug, and Cosmetic Act of 1938 (amended multiple times) | Regulates the amount of pesticide residue allowed to be in food | Toxicity of the pesticide exposure and its aggregates, poses risks to infants and children<br>To be marked safe, there must be a reasonable certainty that no harm will result from aggregate exposure to the pesticide residue | EPA (2019d) |
| The National Environmental Policy Act of 1969 | Basic framework to ensure the environment was considered when airports, buildings, highways, parks, and other federal actions are proposed | Under this act, agencies evaluate not only the economic effects of proposed plans, but also environmental and social aspects | EPA (2019f) |
| The Clean Water Act—1970 | Foundation for regulation of dumping pollutants into United States' waters | Also regulates the quality of surface waters<br>Illegal to dump any pollutant into surface waters without a permit | EPA (2019c) |
| The Clean Air Act (CAA)—1970 | To combat air pollution—air quality standards for particulate matter, ozone, sulfur dioxide, nitrogen dioxide, carbon monoxide, and lead were adapted to lower the amount of outdoor air pollutants that can cause smog and acid rain, cancer, and other serious health effects | It also aims to decrease and eventually stop use of chemicals that can destroy the ozone layer<br>Laws made by individual states.<br>These plans must control emissions that could cross state lines as well as combat pollution from motor vehicles and industrial plants, calling for use of the best available technology. | EPA (2020b) |
| The Federal Insecticide, Fungicide, and Rodenticide Act—1947 (transferred to EPA in 1972) | Called for the regulation of all pesticides including distribution, sale, and use | Applicants must demonstrate that their pesticides will not generally cause unreasonable adverse effects on the environment, defined as risk to man or the environment or human dietary risk from residues after use of the pesticide | EPA (2019e) |
| The Safe Drinking Water Act—1974 | Means to ensure drinking water was not contaminated | Ensured minimum standards to protect the quality of drinking water, from above and underground sources<br>Includes regulations on contaminants such as arsenic, lead, and microbials | EPA (2020c) |
| The Toxic Substances Control Act—1976 | Gave the EPA the authority to regulate chemical substances and mixtures—the EPA could now take action to assess risk to human health and the environment | An inventory was created with a review process of each chemical. In this process, chemical substances were tested to evaluate hazards to the human and the environment<br>Gave the authority to ban, as well as dispose of, certain chemical substances deemed unsafe<br>Allows for citizens to petition the EPA to take action against certain mixtures | EPA (2019g) |

*(continued)*

**TABLE 41.1 Laws Governing Environmental Health** *(continued)*

| Legislation/Date | Action/Meaning | Considerations/Comments | Citation |
|---|---|---|---|
| The Pollution Prevention Act of 1990 | Focused on reducing pollution through source reduction (reduces hazardous materials released in the environment before recycling, treatment, or disposal) | Required some technology and process modifications, substitution of materials, improvements in maintenance and inventory control<br>Aim was to work more efficiently with natural resources while protecting the environment | EPA (2017b) |
| The Endocrine Disruptor Screening Program (EDSP)—1998 | Two-tiered program to determine how pesticides, chemicals, and other environmental contaminants affect the endocrine system; constantly assesses risk under current laws to ensure the most up-to-date information | Tier 1 screens to identify chemicals that may interact with the endocrine system<br>Tier 2 tests and identifies objective data between dose and adverse effect of the chemical<br>These results are then combined with other risk assessments to determine regulatory measures | EPA (2017a) |

## ASSESSING RISK IN CHILDREN

Children are more susceptible to adverse effects from environmental toxins and exposures for several reasons, including but not limited to organ immaturity, their smaller size and relatively increased body water composition, behaviors (related to developmental status), diet, and even where they spend their time (Hauptman & Woolf, 2017). After discovering that certain chemicals and exposures can affect the development and later the health of a child (and adult), risk assessment was performed more broadly and led to increases in legislation, yet the current legislation is not comprehensive.

## RISK ASSESSMENT

Providers must consider a risk assessment on all children. Risk assessment is typically done in a four-step approach: (1) hazard identification/problem formulation, (2) dose-response assessment, (3) exposure assessment, and (4) risk characterization (Etzel & Balk, 2019).

### Hazard Identification

Hazard identification is used to gather data and determine what effects, if any, exist or are possibly associated with the exposure (Etzel & Balk, 2019). The EPA uses a lifestage problem formulation, assessing risks across different age groups. In this first stage, planning and scoping are used to identify the purpose of the study, the participants or stakeholders, the approach to be used, resources needed, and risk assessments. Next, a conceptual model is made to hypothesize why adverse effects happened from previous exposures or could possibly happen in the future. This analysis takes into account several aspects of the exposure such as the chemical properties and uses, sources of where the exposure may be, pathways, scenarios that include time frame of coming into contact with the exposure, and each potential effect at each life stage. The analysis plan then lays out methods, models, gaps in data, major variabilities, and uncertainties to consider as this assessment goes to a more in-depth analysis. This becomes the outline of the whole risk assessment. It is imperative to determine the most vulnerable age groups and key risk drivers relevant to the problem identified to help shape the assessment and decisions (EPA, 2006).

### Dose-Response and Exposure Assessment

The dose-response assessment determines the relationship of the dose and the health effect elicited. Chemicals are most often tested on laboratory animals. It is important to note there are multiple methods used to determine the maximum safe exposure. In many methods, a minimum safe exposure is not actually determined. In that case, the exposure assessment determines the likely human exposures to the hazard. It takes into further consideration and characterizes multiple sources of the toxicant or substance—ground water, surface water, air, soil, food, and so on. Exposure is determined in a quantified amount. Realistic scenarios must be considered such as at-risk populations, duration of exposure, route of exposure, and timing of exposure. More recently, blood and urine tests have become more readily available to determine levels and help better quantify effects of exposure (Etzel & Balk, 2019).

The EPA uses a lifestage-specific analysis using hazard characterization, dose-response characterization, and exposure characterization. In the hazard characterization, all data are analyzed both quantitatively and qualitatively. Toxicokinetics and toxicodynamics are considered across all life stages to determine the most critical windows of exposure. Several categories are evaluated, and the evidence is weighted, with human studies given the most weight. Hazard characterization leads to dose-response characterization in which conceptual data help scientists understand the mechanism of action, select-dose response models, and apply extrapolations and understand risk values. From here, exposure characterization occurs to further evaluate the human interaction with the environmental agent of concern. The primary purpose of this phase is to get a detailed description of the potential for exposure during all life stages, including preconception (EPA, 2006).

### Risk Characterization

Risk characterization is the final step and combines all the data collected and is usually expressed as a maximum acceptable exposure that ensures the health of an exposed population (Etzel & Balk, 2019). The EPA uses all the data into a summarization of the key conclusions. The risk characterization is often anticipated to provide an answer to the problem formulation, often detailing the evolution of the problem question. Scientific assumptions must be clearly stated; full discussion is to follow that includes other hypotheses, alternate potential mechanisms of action, and alternative risk estimates (EPA, 2006).

## ENVIRONMENTAL HAZARDS

In utero exposure to environmental toxins could interrupt neuronal maturation and brain development and lead to brain malformation as seen with fetal alcohol syndrome (FAS). Heavy metals, tobacco, and endocrine-disrupting chemicals (EDCs) that can lead to neurotoxicity will be discussed in greater depth later in the chapter.

## PRENATAL EXPOSURES

Worldwide in 2018, of the 5.3 million deaths that occurred in the first 5 years of life, 47% of those were neonatal deaths. Of the neonatal deaths, about a third of deaths occurred on the day of birth, and close to three-quarters of those deaths occurred prior to the first week of life (UNICEF, 2019). While the total number of neonatal deaths continues to decline yearly, recent data reveal that neonatal deaths continue to have the highest risk of death of all age groups, a slower decline in mortality rates compared with other age groups, and an overall increase in the contributed percentage of deaths under age 5 from 1990 to 2018 (UNICEF, 2019). The greatest contributors to death during the neonatal period include prematurity, intrapartum-related complications, neonatal sepsis, congenital anomalies, neonatal tetanus, and other perinatal and nutritional conditions.

Fetal growth is influenced by a multitude of interactions of maternal, placental, endocrine, and nutritional factors. Environmental exposure to various stimuli can have adverse effects on pregnancy, the placenta, and the fetus that increase the risk for pathological states and derangements to fetal development (Street & Bernasconi, 2020). Environmental factors during critical windows of cellular differentiation can alter fundamental processes that lead to functional and growth disturbances. For example, neural tube formation starts from day 18 until the fourth week of gestation. Exposure to toxins during this time could lead to severe birth defects of the brain and spinal cord if the neural tube fails to form (Moore et al., 2016). Environmental factors cause 7% to 10% of birth defects, but the details of mechanisms and causation remain largely to be determined (Moore et al., 2016, pp. 472–474).

### Organ Development

Organ development is based on the precisely choreographed timing of chemical messages and hormones. During the first 4 weeks of development, the formation of extraembryonic structures and organogenesis are particularly susceptible to environmental exposure. Limb defects caused by in utero exposure to thalidomide during critical periods of limb development is a well-known example illustrating the grave effects of exposure during embryonic development. Thalidomide was commonly used as an antiemetic and sedative in the 1950s by mothers during early pregnancy and is now contraindicated in women of childbearing age (Moore et al., 2016).

### Lung Development

Lung development is heavily controlled by signaling pathways regulated by gene expression. It begins at 4 weeks of gestation with the development of respiratory buds that will eventually divide and grow to form the main and secondary bronchi. All major lung elements not involved with gas exchange form by 16 weeks. By 24 weeks, respiratory bronchioles have developed. Surfactant production begins around weeks 20 to 22, but adequate vasculature and surfactant levels are not achieved until the late fetal period. Lung development continues postnatally and into adolescence with up to 95% of alveolar maturation developing postnatally (Moore et al., 2016).

## Maternal Smoking

Maternal smoking during pregnancy is associated with low birth weight, prematurity, birth defects, and sudden infant death syndrome (SIDS), as well as cognitive and developmental delays (Bhattacharya et al., 2020; Kuniyoshi & Rehan, 2019; U.S. Department of Health and Human Services [USDHHS], 2020). Nicotine crosses the placenta, enters into fetal circulation, and can remain at elevated levels in amniotic fluid. Exposure has been associated with upregulation and downregulation of gene expression, resulting in decreased lung volume and increased airway wall thickness and stiffness (Bhattacharya et al., 2020; Scherman et al., 2018). Smoking increases perinatal mortality by increasing the risk of placental abruption, placenta previa, preterm delivery, and premature and prolonged rupture of the membranes (PROM; USDHHS, 2020). Quitting at any point during pregnancy, but notably as early as possible, is associated with improvement to neonatal birth weights (Etzel & Balk, 2019).

Despite five decades of caution against smoking, 13 out of every 100 women in the United States are currently smoking. Approximately 9% to 10% of pregnant women reported smoking despite being aware of adverse effects to the fetus (Scherman et al., 2018; USDHHS, 2020). Barriers to cessation include continued targeted advertisements, the advent of flavor-filled electronic cigarette products marketed as safer alternatives, lack of follow-up inquiry on cessation, and lack of access to counseling, as well as socioeconomic disparities. Looking at data from the National Center for Health Statistics in 2017, demographic groups with the highest prevalence of prenatal smoking were 20- to 24-year-olds (9.9%), American Indian/Alaska natives (15%), and those with a high school diploma equivalent (General Educational Development or GED (12.2%; Azagba et al., 2020).

## Fetal Alcohol Spectrum Disorders

"Fetal alcohol spectrum disorders" (FASD) is a term collectively referring to the wide range of adverse effects resulting from prenatal exposure to alcohol. These can include milder symptoms from hyperactive behavior, difficulty with attention, and learning disabilities, to abnormal facial features, low body weight, poor growth, poor motor coordination, vision or hearing problems, or dysfunction of organs like the heart, kidney, or bones (Centers for Disease Control and Prevention [CDC], 2019c; Gupta et al., 2016). The features classically associated with FAS are microcephaly with short palpebral fissures, epicanthal folds, thin upper lip, abnormal palmar creases, joint defects, hypoplasia, and congenital heart defect (Etzel & Balk, 2019). Maternal alcohol consumption is one of the most common causes of mental deficiency with even moderate amounts of maternal alcohol consumption causing cognitive and behavioral impairments. In the United States, approximately 4 million infants are born with prenatal alcohol exposure yearly, and 1,000 to 6,000 infants are diagnosed with FAS (Etzel & Balk, 2019). Isolated and impoverished vulnerable populations such as American Indians and other racial minorities experience a rate of nine cases of FASD per 1,000 live births (Williams et al., 2015). While only 25% of children affected by in utero exposure to alcohol exhibit physical features, a majority of individuals with FASDs seem to have an IQ in the low average or borderline ranges (Hagan et al., 2016). Although full understanding of fetal transmission of alcohol is lacking, the metabolism of alcohol is not mature until later in fetal life. Consequently, concentrations of ethanol are higher and can remain in the system for longer periods of time. The breakdown of alcohol produces reactive oxygen species that cause damage to proteins and lipids, neurodegeneration of neurons, and alteration of brain matter and volume, which can lead to the aforementioned symptoms (Ehrhart et al., 2019)

The adverse effects of FASD in newborns is also the most preventable form of nongenetic birth defects related to neurocognitive deficits (Ehrhart et al., 2019). As front-line clinicians, comprehensive histories and assessments to recognize and identify potential exposures to alcohol and reduce drinking among pregnant women or women of childbearing age can help to reduce future exposures. In the most recent national data from the CDC, alcohol consumption during pregnancy is not rare, with 10.2% of pregnant women reporting consumption in the past 30 days and 3.1% reporting binge drinking in the past 30 days (Denny, 2019). In a prospective study interviewing women recruited from antenatal clinics in Australia, a majority of them ceased or significantly reduced their drinking after understanding the effects of their drinking (McCormack et al., 2017).

## AIR POLLUTION

Air pollution is an environmental hazard that all children are exposed to in both inside and outside environments. It can negatively affect a child's health and is even linked to increased mortality. Sources of air pollutants include automobiles, industrial facilities, gas appliances in the home, chemicals in paint and varnishes, asbestos in homes built between the 1940s and 1970s, and tobacco smoke. Air pollution can impair lung development and increase the likelihood of comorbidities like neurocognitive impairment, asthma, chronic lung disease, and other major noncommunicable diseases such as ischemic heart disease, cerebrovascular disease, and cancer (Lelieveld et al., 2015). Air pollution can come in many forms such as polycyclic aromatic hydrocarbons (PAHs), formed as a result of incomplete combustion of organic materials such as natural gas, vehicle exhaust, and burning of fossil fuels (Drwal et al., 2017). PAH compounds have been shown to reduce mitochondrial activity, alter lysosomal activity, and have endocrine-disrupting characteristics affecting maternal health. The effect on maternal health can, in turn, impair the environment on which the fetus is dependent for growth and maturation (Drwal et al., 2017, Drwal et al., 2019). Prenatally, PAHs can pass the placental barrier and lead to adverse outcomes such as preterm birth, low birth weight, organogenesis impairment, and intrauterine growth retardation (Drwal et al., 2017; Zajda et al., 2017). Negative effects of PAHs observed later in life include low IQ, behavioral issues, allergies, and asthma (Drwal et al., 2019).

Additional air pollutants include nitrogen dioxide, ozone, particulate matter, lead, sulfur dioxide, carbon monoxide (CO), and volatile organic compounds (Etzel & Balk, 2019; Schraufnagel et al., 2018). Inhalation of these pollutants can affect the cardiovascular and nervous systems, cause respiratory symptoms (particularly in those with underlying respiratory problems), and many of them are carcinogens (Etzel & Balk, 2019). Children are especially vulnerable to pollutants because they spend more time outdoors and breathe more air per body weight than adults (Etzel & Balk, 2019; Schraufnagel et al., 2018).

Carbon dioxide (CO) is an odorless gas that can be fatal, so it is important to educate families on what measures can be taken to prevent and detect exposures. Because CO has no odor or color, the primary method of detection is by CO detectors (Etzel & Balk, 2019). Families should be encouraged to have CO detectors near every sleeping area in the home (AAP, Council on Children and Disasters [CCD], n.d.). Sources of CO include gas-powered appliances, wood-burning fireplaces and stoves, space heaters, generators, and grills. It is important to ensure that these are installed correctly, in proper working condition, inspected per manufacturer recommendations, and used only for their intended purposes (Etzel & Balk, 2019). Vehicles are another source of CO exposure and are often the source of CO poisoning in suicide attempts. Symptoms of CO poisoning include headache, nausea, vomiting, confusion, and, in severe cases, coma, and death (AAP, CCD, n.d.; Etzel & Balk, 2019). CO poisoning should be considered when these symptoms are present, especially if multiple people in the household are experiencing symptoms. The primary treatment is removing the person from the environment where the CO poisoning occurred and providing 100% supplemental oxygen. In rare instances, hyperbaric oxygen therapy may be used (AAP, CCD, n.d.; Etzel & Balk, 2019).

Radon is a radioactive gas found in the ground that can enter houses and other buildings through cracks in the structure of the building (EPA, 2016a; Etzel & Balk, 2019). Although radon exposure does not cause symptoms, long-term exposure can cause lung cancer, so reducing exposure is important (EPA, 2016a). Testing homes for radon is essential in lowering the risk of radon exposure, as high levels of radon can be found in many different types of homes, regardless of age and condition of the home (EPA, 2016a). Families can purchase test kits or hire companies approved by the state radon division to test for radon (EPA, 2016a). If high levels of radon are detected, repairs should be made to reduce the radon levels.

Mold is a common source of health complaints and can be particularly bothersome when found inside the home. Mold can cause both upper and lower respiratory symptoms as well as headache and fatigue. Mold may be directly visualized or smelled, or there may be a history of water leaks or flood indicating mold in the home (CDC, 2016). If a child has symptoms that worsen at home and improve when they are away, this may indicate a home environmental cause and mold should be considered as a possible causative agent (Etzel & Balk, 2019). Generally, testing for mold is not recommended (CDC, 2016). The primary method for controlling mold in the home is to prevent conditions that enable mold growth. This includes keeping the humidity level low and ventilating areas that are prone to high humidity, such as bathrooms and laundry rooms (CDC, 2016). It is also necessary to fix any leaks to prevent water entry into the home. If items in the home become wet or damp from leaks or flooding, they should be thoroughly dried or removed to prevent mold growth (Etzel &

Balk, 2019; CDC, 2016). Once mold growth occurs on a surface that allows for water penetration, such as carpet or drywall, these items must be replaced to get rid of the mold (CDC, 2016).

### Educating Families

Although reducing outdoor air pollution is difficult on an individual level, there are a few steps that families can take to reduce their exposure. The air quality index is a numeric measure of the current air quality and can help guide when outside activities should be avoided (Etzel & Balk, 2019). Families can also be encouraged to avoid being around idling vehicles, particularly those producing diesel exhaust (Etzel & Balk, 2019). Families can help minimize indoor air pollution by making sure appliances and fireplaces are in proper working condition and well ventilated. Families should also be discouraged from using gas appliances in place of a heater. If chemicals such as paint, varnishes, and solvents are to be stored at home, they should be safely stored in a garage or shed (Etzel & Balk, 2019).

## HEAVY METALS

Metals are elements that are naturally occurring and found throughout the earth in various forms. Though some metals (copper, zinc, chromium) are necessary for daily life and normal physiologic function, some are toxic even at low levels. Lead, mercury, arsenic, and cadmium are among the WHO's 10 major chemicals of concern (WHO, n.d.). In most cases, acute exposure may cause detrimental organ damage that may progress to death. More recent research shows that heavy metal toxicity can occur at much lower levels of exposure than previously thought and suggests that chronic exposure may cause progressive or life-long consequences (Etzel & Balk, 2019). With these discoveries, legislation and policy changes have helped to mitigate the continued exposure to these metals both nationally and globally.

### Lead

Lead is a heavy metal found in the earth's crust. It has been used extensively throughout history in gasoline, paint, batteries, toys, plumbing, and ship building, among other uses. Its wide-ranging use has led to an abundance in the environment, resulting in continued sources of contamination. References to possible lead toxicity are documented as early as Egyptian scrolls in the second century BC. Despite early knowledge of possible lead toxicity, its use was not deterred until much more recently. In 1767, Sir George Baker described an array of symptoms that he linked to lead in the making of cider. Since that time, various hematologic, neurologic, gastrointestinal (GI), and teratogenic effects have been described at length throughout literature. Prior to the 1970s, lead toxicity was a clinical diagnosis. Once blood lead levels could be tested reliably, the association between toxicity and blood lead levels has become clear (Ettinger et al., 2019). Currently, there is no blood level of lead that has been shown to be "safe" or without toxicities in humans (American Academy of Pediatrics [AAP] Council on Environmental Health, 2016).

Recent literature describes the extent of lead toxicity to the fetal and pediatric populations. Lanphear et al. (2005) published a sentinel study presenting the correlation between lead and IQ deficits. Further studies have shown the correlation between both prenatal and postnatal lead exposure and toxicity. Evens et al. (2015) reported an association of lead levels less than 10 µg/dL with lower mathematics and reading scores on standardized tests in elementary school students. Nkomo et al. (2018) found significant association between elevated blood lead levels between 1 and 28 µg/dL with increased direct aggression in adolescents. Childhood blood levels are associated with decreased cognitive function and a negative impact on social mobility (Reuben et al., 2017). A mouse study established that low-level lead exposure during puberty can disrupt spermatogenesis. Although further human studies need to be performed, lead may adversely affect lifelong fertility if exposure is noted at the time of puberty (Xie et al., 2020). Higher lead blood levels are associated with higher adjusted odds of having asthma and associated wheezing (Wu et al., 2019). Studies are ongoing to determine the full realm of the health effects of lead on children.

Legislation has played an instrumental role in decreasing lead exposure in the United States. The National Health Center for Health Statistics (NCHS) at the CDC has shown that blood levels of lead in children in the United States have decreased significantly between 1960 and 2017, with the largest decrease between 1960 and 1980. This 20-year period correlates with the initial legislations that removed lead from paint, plumbing, and gasoline. Despite aggressive legislation, lead in soil and paint dust from homes built before 1978 remain the primary sources of lead exposure for children (Pediatric Environmental Health Specialty Units [PEHSU], 2016). Many homes that were built prior to the legislation have not been remediated; thereby, they continue to expose their inhabitants via paint dust and contaminated water. Data from NCHS shows that the median blood lead level in families above the poverty level is significantly lower than in those families below the national poverty level. Additionally, there is statistical significance between blood lead levels in black non-Hispanics versus white non-Hispanics and between Mexican Americans versus white non-Hispanics even when age, sex, and parental income are accounted for. This statistical significance demonstrates that socioeconomic factors such as race, income level, and immigrant status play a role in exposure to lead (EPA, 2019a).

Children younger than 6 years old are particularly vulnerable to lead ingestion because of their hand-to-mouth behaviors and the types of food they ingest. Infants that take formula can be exposed to lead from the water that is mixed with the formula. The EPA estimates that up to 20% of a person's total lead exposure is from drinking water and that this percentage is even higher in those infants that are formula-fed (EPA, 2019a). Both infants and children take in greater amounts of water per percentage body size than adults and thus they are at greater risk of elevated total exposure. Furthermore, children are more likely to play on the ground where they may have greater exposure to lead-containing dust particles. Given the higher hand-to-mouth behaviors in young children, these dust particles or chipped paint may find their ways into their mouths to be ingested (AAP, 2016; CDC, 2019b).

## Decreasing Lead Exposure

The AAP released a statement in 2016 that emphasized that the primary means to decrease lead toxicity is prevention of exposure. Practical recommendations were given to assist in the reduction of lead ingestion. First, homes need to be remediated with the removal of lead paint and plumbing if possible. If this is not possible, frequent wet mopping of the floors and other areas to reduce dust should be performed and any areas of paint chipping should be remediated. Toys with chipped paint, especially older or vintage toys, should be removed from the home. Private wells should be tested for lead levels. When using water to cook or drink, only cold water should be used, and faucets should be flushed for a few minutes prior to using them in an effort to move any settled contaminants. Additionally, faucet aerators should be cleaned frequently to ensure that any build-up of debris is removed. The primary care provider should ensure that a thorough history and risk assessment is performed. Additionally, they should educate families on the risk of lead exposure and provide these guidelines to families on reducing lead exposure risk. It is important that development is frequently assessed. If delays are noted, blood lead level should be obtained (AAP, 2016; PEHSU, 2016).

## Mercury

Mercury is naturally found in soil and rock and within breakdown of these elements from exposure to wind and water and from volcanic activity (New Hampshire Department of Environmental Services [DES], 2019). In its elemental form, mercury is a liquid at room temperature and can vaporize at low temperatures. Elemental mercury has been used in thermometers, fluorescent light bulbs, barometers, batteries, and in religious and cultural rituals. Mercury vapors can be inhaled and can accumulate to toxic levels. Inorganic mercury compounds occur when other elements combine with mercury to create a salt through a naturally occurring or industrial process. Organic mercury compounds are formed when mercury combines with carbon, with the most common forms being methylmercury and thimerosal. Methylmercury is easily dissolved into water and accumulates in water and sea life. Higher mercury levels are found as it bioaccumulates up the food chain; thus, ingestion of seafood is of concern. Thimerosal is also a well-known organic mercury compound that has been used as a preservative in vaccines and has been at the center of much debate about its effects in children leading to its removal in most childhood vaccines (EPA, 2019a). With increased industrialization, mining, and burning of fossil fuels, mercury spreads into the air and into water sources (DES, 2019; Agency for Toxic Substances & Disease Registry, 2021).

In 1956, the first large investigation into mercury toxicity began when a cluster of patients were noticed to have a variety of central nervous system complaints including, but not limited to, abnormal walking and talking, confusion, and convulsions. This led to many decades of investigation, which ultimately resulted in the discovery of the severe neurotoxic effects in humans and animals along with teratogenic effects. The Chisso Corporation released its industrial waste into the watershed, which contaminated the water source, increasing the mercury concentration in the fish, which then were consumed by the nearby residents. Ultimately, Minamata disease was named for the city where it was discovered and where many adults and children were found to have progressive neurological compromise and elevated rates of children born with cerebral palsy (Etzel & Balk, 2019). The lessons from Minamata have led to further research, campaigning, and, eventually, legislation surrounding mercury and how to reduce its use and overall exposure. The Minamata Convention in 2013 gathered 140 countries, who in 2017 released their international treaty to reduce and eliminate mercury from mining, control mercury emissions, phase-out mercury in use in commercial products, define disposal strategies, and promote awareness, research, and monitoring of mercury (United Nations Environment Programme, 2017).

Continued research post-Minamata has solidified the concerns of mercury to fetal and childhood development. The degree of methylmercury poisoning that happened in Minamata caused rapid progressive neurodegenerative disease and teratogenic effects. Mercury toxicity in Minamata caused cerebral palsy-like symptoms (cerebellar ataxia, altered primitive reflexes, mental retardation, and hyperkinesia) even with asymptomatic mothers (Harada et al., 2011). Maternal blood and cord blood levels have been associated with decreased verbal IQ and anxiety (Jeong et al., 2017; Patel et al., 2019). Childhood exposure to mercury can occur topically, and through ingestion or inhalation. A case study in 2018 reported symptoms of hypertension, fussiness, constipation, and arthralgias in a 17-month-old child diagnosed with mercury toxicity from a skin care product. The cream was being used as indicated to the face by the mother and grandmother who were unaware of the contents, and mercury was found throughout the house, exposing all family members (Ori et al., 2018). The Food and Drug Administration (FDA) limits the amount of mercury allowed in skin care products and cosmetics, but it does not regulate products that come from international channels and are sold in the United States (U.S. FDA, 2016). Controversial exposure of mercury for children are dental amalgams and thimerosal in childhood vaccines. Several studies have shown elevated levels of mercury in blood or urine of children after placement, but none have definitively demonstrated acute or chronic effects from the mercury in dental amalgams (Baek et al., 2016). Evidence-based meta-analyses have explored the association between thimerosal and its implications with autism in vaccinations and have found that there is no evidence to support any link (DeStefano et al., 2019). Regardless, thimerosal has been removed from most childhood vaccines in the United States, and there are campaigns to remove thimerosal from all vaccinations worldwide (U.S. FDA, 2018b).

## Reducing Mercury Exposure

Reduction of exposure is key to reducing mercury toxicity. Primary care practitioners should educate parents on the dangers of mercury toxicity. Education should be provided for parents to investigate the ingredients in skin care that they and their children use. Since some older thermometers and fluorescent lights may contain mercury, children should avoid direct contact with either product. A non-mercury-containing thermometer should be used. If one breaks, the Poison Control Center should be contacted for instructions on clean-up. The FDA now recommends that up to 8 ounces of seafood is safe for children (less for younger children) and pregnant women, and they provide a list of recommended options based on mercury content. Examples of seafood that are lower in mercury content are: salmon, shrimp, pollock, tilapia, and catfish; and some that are higher that should be avoided are: shark, swordfish, and king mackerel (U.S. Department of Health and Human Services and U.S. Department of Agriculture [USDHHS & USDA], 2020). Parents who work in industry such as mining or where fossil fuels are burned should take great caution to remove clothing and bathe prior to interacting with their children after returning from work to minimize exposure.

## Arsenic

Arsenic is naturally distributed in specific locations throughout the earth and is found to be in higher concentrations in certain locations in the United States. It can leach from the bedrock into ground water, contaminating well water and ocean water entering the food chain. Historically, arsenic was used in pesticides, termite wood treatment, and medications. Soil that was contaminated with arsenic from mining, hazardous sites, or agriculture from previous pesticide use can still be toxic when the soil is repurposed. Though arsenic-containing pesticides have been banned, it is still used in crops that are not used for direct human consumption, such as chicken feed. It is also no longer used as a termite wood treatment, but construction sites often expose previously treated wood, allowing the arsenic to seep into the soil or water. Inorganic arsenic is converted by the body into organic arsenic and is renally excreted in small quantities. Since children have reduced abilities to break down and excrete arsenic, it accumulates in their bodies for longer periods of time (Etzel & Balk, 2019).

Arsenic toxicity was documented in Taiwan, where in the mid-1950s there was widespread peripheral vascular disease found to be related to elevated levels from contaminated water in private drinking wells. The link between arsenic and cancer continues to increase with correlations between arsenic concentration and lung, bladder, skin, kidney, liver, prostate cancer, and breast cancer (American Cancer Society [ACS], 2019; Marciniak et al., 2020). Arsenic is related to negative effects on fetal growth in size, head circumference, and gestation (Claus Henn et al., 2016), and can be associated with respiratory symptoms, intellectual disability, and skin changes such as dyspigmentation and eczematous eruptions. Low dose chronic exposure is associated with hepatic dysfunction, bone marrow and immune suppression, and gastronintestinal upset (Etzel & Balk, 2019). The lowest level of arsenic exposure that may cause significant health effects is not known. The WHO recommends limiting drinking water to 10 µg/L, asserting that the lower level is preferred given that the recommendation is limited by measuring capabilities (WHO, 2018a).

The primary source of elevated arsenic levels in children is through ingestion (Etzel & Balk, 2019). In 2012, a Consumer Reports noted that there were elevated arsenic levels in apple juice (Hirsch, 2019). This was followed by a second report about the amount of arsenic found in rice cereal given to infants. Responding to the report, the Healthy Babies Bright Futures study (2019) showed that infant rice cereal contains on average 85 parts per billion (ppb) of arsenic compared with other infant cereals (multigrain, barley, quinoa, oatmeal, wheat, buckwheat) that contain 14 ppb. Additionally, children that are formula fed may be exposed to arsenic through the water that is used to mix the formula (Healthy Babies Bright Futures, 2019). There are several different agencies that monitor the arsenic content of consumed items, water, and food; thus, the cumulative amount of arsenic exposure must be coordinated and may not account for the entirety of the arsenic exposure to the population (Nachman et al., 2017). Arsenic exposure through seafood is present but not significant enough to cause adverse health side effects (Mania et al., 2015).

### Limiting Arsenic Exposure

Primary care providers should be vigilant and obtain a thorough environmental and exposure history during the examination. For parents who have infants, it is important to list food products (e.g., rice cereal and apple juice) that have been known to have possible levels of arsenic. Good alternatives for rice cereal include infant cereal made from other grains and soft vegetables. Parents should check for the use of rice syrup, which is often used as a sweetener, and eliminate those foods where possible. Well water should be tested frequently if it is utilized for cooking or consuming. Animal models have seen increased absorption of arsenic with iron deficiency; thus, iron levels should be monitored and kept within age-appropriate ranges (Etzel & Balk, 2019).

## Cadmium

Cadmium is a naturally occurring heavy metal found in the earth's crust. It is generally found with lead, zinc, and copper and is extracted as a byproduct of the mining of these other metals. The spread of cadmium occurs through mining, waste incineration, fires, erosion of rocks, and eruption of volcanos (Etzel & Balk, 2019). Airborne particles spread across agricultural lands into irrigation sources to contaminate water. Crops that are grown in those areas will accumulate the metal. Large accumulations have occurred in leafy and root vegetables, foods that contain chocolate, grains, and seeds. Despite the regulation of cadmium in water to 0.0005 mg/kg/day and maximum dietary exposure to 0.001 mg/kg/day (EPA, 2016b), it is estimated that the average childhood cadmium exposure is 0.38 to 0.44 µg/kg/day from the consumption of food (Spungen, 2019). The tobacco plant takes in large amounts of cadmium and widespread exposure occurs through the burning of the tobacco. In children, tobacco smoke inhalation occurs most frequently with exposure to secondhand smoke (Etzel & Balk, 2019). Metal jewelry and toys, specifically those made internationally or where there is less regulation, has been another source of exposure for children (Akimzhanova et al., 2020).

Concern for cadmium toxicity began in the 1950s when the Itai-Itai disease was discovered in a Japanese population that consumed large amounts of contaminated rice, leading to long-term exposure. The presenting symptoms of Itai-Itai were anemia, kidney damage, and brittle bones. Around the same time, a similar conglomeration of symptoms was found in industrial workers globally, but with the addition of respiratory tract symptoms and lung disease from inhalation exposure to fumes that contained cadmium (Mezynska & Brzóska, 2018). It is now known that cadmium is excreted by the kidneys, specifically the proximal tubular cells, and therefore elevated levels can lead to severe kidney injury. This kidney damage can lead to hypertension, artery disease, and end stage renal disease (Satarug et al., 2017). Since the half-life of cadmium elimination through the kidneys is 10 to 40 years, there is increased risk of bioaccumulation and chronic toxicity (Etzel & Balk, 2019). The oncologic risks of cadmium have been established in literature, and the EPA has labeled it as a chemical with probable human carcinogenic effects (EPA, 2016b). Direct links between cadmium exposure and breast, lung, pancreatic, nasopharyngeal, and thyroid cancers are known, and further research is concerning for other possible cancer associations (Buha et al., 2018; Chen et al., 2015; Nawrot et al., 2015; Peng et al., 2015a, 2015b). At even low levels of exposure, cadmium is thyroid-toxic and can play a role in immunodeficiencies (Buha et al., 2018). A meta-analysis of fetal exposure to cadmium has shown a significant relationship between cadmium exposure and low birth weight (Khoshali et al., 2020). The degree of cadmium exposure to child health is not known.

### Preventing Cadmium Exposure

As with all metals, preventing exposure is at the primary target. Parents should be counseled on the risks and health concerns relating to cadmium. This should include avoiding metal jewelry and toys around children, specifically those in ages with increased hand-to-mouth behaviors. The avoidance of tobacco smoke through secondhand smoke is essential as a lung protective strategy. Because iron deficiency has been linked with increased absorption of cadmium, iron levels should be checked regularly and maintained at age-appropriate levels. Batteries can contain cadmium, so children should never play with batteries and parents should ensure to dispose of batteries through appropriate recycling methods. Cadmium levels in water of those who use private wells or in those who live near industry should be tested (Etzel & Balk, 2019).

### Nickel

Nickel is found in the earth's crust, soil, and in volcano emissions. The hard metal is frequently combined with other metals such as iron and copper to form alloys used in jewelry, coins, and toys, among other metal objects. Though nickel mining is outlawed in the United States, nickel alloys are imported for use (Etzel & Balk, 2019). Sediment from metal waste incinerators or power plants is emitted and contaminates land, soil, and water sources. Although inhalation and ingestion of nickel can cause respiratory illness and acute toxicity, allergic reaction from exposure is the most common health effect from exposure (Das et al., 2019). Contact dermatitis is frequently observed with jewelry or belt buckles that contain alloys (Goldenberg et al., 2015). Dental and surgical implants may cause reactions confounding for postsurgical infections. Some testing of nickel allergies with skin has begun prior to higher risk surgeries, such as the Nuss procedure for pectus excavatum (Nuss et al., 2016; Zigante et al., 2020). Stainless steel cookware may leach nickel when filled with acidic contents at boiling temperatures (Etzel & Balk, 2019). Minimizing exposure to nickel alloys if one has demonstrated contact allergy is paramount in children.

## ENDOCRINE-DISRUPTING CHEMICALS

The evolution of the chemical industry has brought about the creation and refinement of a multitude of different chemicals pervasive in everyday life. Starting from the industrial revolution with the creation of the steam engine, to the development of concentrated acids and chemicals for explosive manufacturing, to the modification of polymers into synthetic products, humans have consistently searched to improve current materials in order to meet societal demands (Martín, 2016). While these chemicals have helped enrich our lives by providing a plethora of consumer goods, they do not come without consequences to human health.

The latest Toxic Substances Control Act inventory listing of the chemicals that are actively being manufactured, processed, and imported in the United States reveal that 86,228 chemicals are available for commercial production. Of those chemicals, 47% or 40,655 chemicals are currently in commerce (EPA, 2019b). Five cycles of the National Health and Nutrition Examination Survey (NAHES) sampled 4,299 children between the ages of 6–18 years for detectable levels of 36 specific chemical analytes, and an average of 93% of those children had detectable concentrations of the studied chemicals. Twenty-nine of 36 chemicals were detected in more than 90% of the children in the sampling (Hendryx & Luo, 2018).

EDCs are chemicals that adversely affect hormonal function. EDCs can alter the hypothalamic-pituitary-gonad, thyroid, and adrenal axes. Exposure to EDCs can alter hormonal systems and the trajectory of development, resulting in neurological impairments, disorders of sexual development, or even death (Etzel & Balk, 2019; Gore et al., 2015b). A classic example is diethylstilbestrol (DES), a synthetic nonsteroidal estrogenic compound given to women between 1940 and 1971 to prevent complications in pregnancy. It was later discovered that the drug caused a wide range of delayed effects in offspring exposed in utero. Female offspring with similar histories of DES exposure were noted to have developed clear cell adenocarcinoma of the vagina and congenital abnormalities (transverse vaginal ridges, cervical erosions, generalized glandular dysfunction). Male offspring exposed in utero had higher incidences of genital tract anomalies like epididymal cysts and hypoplastic testes (Di Renzo et al., 2015; Etzel & Balk, 2019; Moore et al., 2016). Exposure to EDCs can significantly influence the development of chronic and noncommunicable diseases like cardiovascular disease, stroke, and chronic respiratory disease as children develop into adults (Sly et al., 2016; WHO, 2017).

## Persistent Organic Pollutants

Persistent organic pollutants (POPs) are types of hydrocarbon compounds with carbon-halogen bonds that are resistant to biological degradation. Since they do not readily break down, they can bioaccumulate in humans via ingestion of contaminated meats in their diets. POPs include PCBs, perfluoroalkyl substances, polybrominated diphenyl ethers (PBDEs), and organochlorines. They are commonly known products such as pesticides and flame retardants that are found on furniture, textiles, and carpeting. They also make up nonstick cookware products, electronic products, and food packaging (Wang et al., 2016). Adverse health effects caused by POPs include cancer, reproductive disorders, immune disorders, allergies and hypersensitivity, central and peripheral nervous system effects, and alterations in normal development (Etzel & Balk, 2019). Consequently, many of these persistent pollutants have been removed from the market. In the United States, DDT was the first of the POPs to be banned. PCBs were removed under the Toxic Substances Control Act of 1977. However, despite being banned, several PCBs were still detectable in nearly 100% of women from the NHANES 2003 to 2004 study (Wang et al., 2016).

### Polychlorinated Biphenyls

PCBs were commonly used in industrial production as insulators and lubricants, but were also used as plasticizers added to paints, plastics, and rubber products. Although manufacture, sale, and use of PCBs were banned in the United States in 1979, ongoing detection of PCB can be attributed to previous years of high production as well as to its persistent nature (Dai et al., 2016; EPA, 2019a). PCBs can leak into the environment through the combustion of waste and fuel. They can be measured in the air in urban and industrial areas, especially near sites of electronic waste sites and recycling facilities (Dai et al., 2016). They can also be found in older schools and residential buildings that were built or renovated before the 1970s (Osemwengie & Morgan, 2019). It was estimated that the number of schools with PCB in building caulk in the United States ranged from 12,960 to 25,920 (Herrick et al., 2016). Because of their lipophilic nature, they can be found in fish, meat, poultry, dairy products, and breast milk (EPA, 2019a). Route of exposure occurs through ingestion, inhalation, and dermal absorption. PCBs are distributed and stored in adipose tissue with half-lives up to 15 years (Donat-Vargas et al., 2016). Fetal exposure can occur as PCBs can cross the placental barrier (Zou et al., 2019). Exposure to infants can occur through breastfeeding as well (Etzel & Balk, 2019). Concerns with PCB involve its portfolio of neurotoxicity, dermal and ocular effects, reproductive toxicity, hepatotoxicity, and increased risks for cancer (Dai et al., 2016; Osemwengie & Morgan, 2019). Researchers followed the acute effects of mothers and their children who lived through the historic mass Yusho food poisoning in Japan in 1968 as well as the Taiwanese cooking oil poisoning. It was caused by ingestion of rice bran oil contaminated with PCB, dioxin, and other compounds. In regard to reproductive function, there was an increase in induced abortions, preterm deliveries, and spontaneous abortion and pregnancy loss within the first 10 years after the incident. Low birth weight in male offspring was observed in babies delivered to mothers who were exposed to PCBs/dioxins with an inverse correlation. Other observed outcomes in newborn babies born to affected mothers from 1979 to 1983 included hyperpigmentation and increased PCB concentrations in umbilical cords compared with babies born to nonaffected mothers (Mitoma et al., 2015).

### Polybrominated Diphenyl Ethers

PBDEs are flame-retardant chemicals that are found in furniture, textiles, and electronics to help slow the rate of ignition and fire growth. Due to potential toxic effects and increasing environmental usage, PentaBDE and OctaBDE were phased out in 2004, but DecaBDE, the last of the three classes, remained in limited use until 2013 (EPA, 2019a; Parry et al., 2018). While use and manufacture has been strictly regulated and reduced around the world, human exposure to these persistent pollutants could remain an environmental challenge for an undetermined number of years to come (Fromme et al., 2016; Malliari & Kalantzi, 2017). Even though PBDEs have been phased out, their abundant detection in umbilical cord serum, breast milk, and maternal serum remain concerning for potential neurodevelopmental toxicity in exposed children (Shin et al., 2016). Child exposure to PBDEs can occur from inhalation of dust and particles, dermal absorption from hand to mouth behavior, and diet (Malliari & Kalantzi, 2017).

Because PBDEs accumulate in fat tissue, they can be found in fish, dairy, and meat products. The main concerns with PBDE exposure include liver, thyroid, endocrine, and neurodevelopmental toxicity (Fromme et al., 2016). Infants are a more susceptible demographic because body burden (total amount of chemical in the body) is three- to nine-fold higher compared with that of adults (Linares et al., 2015). Animal studies have correlated exposure to PBDEs with reductions in triiodothyronin (T3), increased pituitary rate, and reductions to circulating estradiol and testosterone in adult mice offspring. In addition to hormonal changes, changes in neurocognitive patterns involving learning and memory have also been noticed in mice studies (Lyche et al., 2015). The impact of PBDEs on hormone and neurodevelopment in humans remains scarce and difficult to assess in meta-analyses due to the heterogeneity of information. In a meta-analysis of PBDE exposure and neurodevelopmental effects in childhood, despite limited evidence for consistently reporting a relationship between PBDE exposure and attention deficit hyperactivity disorder (ADHD), the analysis found sufficient evidence to support an association of IQ reduction (3.7 points) with 10-fold increase in exposure (Lam et al., 2017).

### Organochlorine Pesticides

The advent of pesticides has helped to reduce transmission of disease and assist in sustaining crop yields from pesky organisms. These chemicals are widely ubiquitous, and exposure can occur in all environments (home, office, daycare, agriculture). Exposure for children can occur through inhalation and ingestion, as well as through dermal absorption. Breastfeeding infants can be at higher exposure since a portion of the lipophilic chemicals get transferred in the production of breast milk (Etzel & Balk, 2019). Concerns regarding pesticides include their association with adverse birth outcomes, disruption to endocrine and neurological systems, and the potential for carcinogenic effects. Dichloro-diphenyl-trichloroethane (DDT) is a well-known organochlorine that was first developed in the 1940s for insect control and reduction of vector-related diseases. However, it was banned in 1972 when the EPA ordered a stop on manufacturing due to its adverse environmental effects to wildlife and concerns for human health risks (EPA, 2020a).

## Less Persistent and Bioaccumulative Chemicals

Less persistent and bioaccumulative chemicals include the phenols (BPA, triclosan, parabens) and phthalates.

### Bisphenol A

Bisphenol A (BPA) is a high-volume phenolic chemical used to manufacture polycarbonate plastics and epoxy resins. It is commonly used to make plastic materials like bottles, dinnerware, eye glass lenses, toys, thermal paper for receipts, paints, floorings, and dental composites (CDC, 2019a; Gore et al., 2015a). The primary route of exposure is through diet and through migration of BPA from the container lining to food and liquids. Other possible sources include air, dust, water, and dental sealants (EPA, 2019a). Studies have demonstrated BPA detection through a variety of mediums including human plasma, urine, amniotic fluids, breast milk, and umbilical cord blood (Z. Zhou et al., 2019). Data from the Canadian Health Measures Survey indicates that more than 90% of youth 6 to 19 years of age have detectable levels of urinary BPA (Findlay & Kohen, 2015). BPA is frequently found in 80% to 100% of urine samples throughout pregnancy and postpartum. It is also detected in breast milk and maternal serum (Mitro et al., 2015). Interest in BPA as an endocrine disrupter focuses on its potential impact on early and adolescent development, neurocognitive and behavioral disruption, and likelihood of low birth weight (Hendryx & Luo, 2018). Animal studies have shown the correlation of BPA as a neuroendocrine disruptor (Palanza et al., 2016; Pivonello et al., 2020) with potential links for reproductive impairment (Müller et al., 2018), low birth weight with fetal exposure, and the development of insulin resistance (Fang et al., 2015; Li et al., 2016). However, effects of BPA in human studies are limited and inconsistent (Gore et al., 2015a). A meta-analysis review of 209 studies revealed a positive association between BPA exposure and birth weight, but not with birth length, head circumference, and gestational age (Z. Zhou et al., 2019), but these results were not consistent with a meta-analysis from 2018 revealing no correlation between BPA exposure and birth weight (Hu et al., 2018). A study investigating two cycles of results from the Canadian Health Measures Survey suggested an association between urinary BPA concentration and changes to external behavioral outcomes (Findlay & Kohen, 2015). More research is needed to better understand how BPA is absorbed, distributed, and metabolized, and the effects of exposure.

### Phthalates

Phthalates are added to plastics to create desired effects of flexibility and resilience. Phthalate-containing products include personal care products, car parts, plastic packaging film, polyvinyl chloride products

(PVCs), medical tubing, and blood storage containers (CDC, 2019d). They can be found on tablecloths, floor tiles, furniture upholstery, carpet, shower curtains, toys, and food packaging. Similar to BPA, exposure occurs mainly through eating and drinking foods from phthalate-containing containers. Exposure can also occur via ingestion of breast milk and inhalation of dust and dermal contact through hand-to-mouth activities. Phthalate metabolites are frequently detected in urine samples of pregnant women. They can also be detected in neonatal urine, as well as cord blood, amniotic fluid, breast milk, and meconium (Mitro et al., 2015). Phthalates are not covalent-bound polymers; thus, they can migrate into food when products are heated (EPA, 2019a; Etzel & Balk, 2019, p. 730). Concern for phthalate exposure comes from its demonstrated potential as endocrine disruptors. Di-2-ethylhexil phthalate (DEHP) and dibutyl phthalate (DBP) are the most toxic to the reproductive system (Etzel & Balk, 2019). They, along with butyl benzyl phthalate (BBzP), were banned by the Consumer Product Safety Improvement Act of 2008 (U.S. Consumer Product Safety Commission, 2016).

Animal studies have shown anti-androgenic effects in fetal and early postnatal development leading to male reproductive abnormalities, testicular lesions, and reduced sperm production (Di Nisio & Foresta, 2019). Male rodents exposed to prenatal doses of DEHP in utero displayed age- and dose-dependent signs of reduced fertility with low serum testosterone levels, higher serum estradiol levels, and higher luteinizing hormone levels (Barakat et al., 2017). Prenatal exposure in mice has also been shown to induce phthalate syndrome, characterized by malformations in the male reproductive organs, retention of nipples, and reduced anogenital distance. Female rodents exposed to relevant levels of phthalate mixtures were observed to have reproductive complications related to pathological changes to ovaries, loss of pregnancy, and failure to mate (C. Zhou et al., 2017).

Although literature remains inconsistent on phthalates, a wide range of human health effects have also been illustrated including preterm birth (Lenters et al., 2016), pregnancy duration (Polańska et al., 2016; Shoaff et al., 2016), adverse effects on child behavior, and reduced sperm quality and infertility in men (Chang et al., 2015; Thurston et al., 2016). Another area of research entails epigenetic changes possibly associated with phthalate exposure. Epidermal growth factor receptor was identified as a critical gene mediating exposure effects on placental function (Grindler et al., 2018). Additional studies are needed to confirm findings through repeat studies to determine if observed findings have negative potential health effects for children. Another area of research includes follow-up studies on exposed residents during the Taiwanese phthalate food crisis in 2011. A strong correlation of phthalate exposure during the second trimester was found with low birth outcomes, but also stated uncertainty in proving that prenatal phthalate exposure had adverse effects on newborns given that most of the newborns born to evaluated mothers in the study had normal birth weights, birth lengths, and head circumferences (Tsai et al., 2018). In addition, high levels of DEHP exposure from tainted food consumption was found to be negatively associated with body weight and height percentiles, bone age, and IGF-1 levels in children. However, extremely high levels of DEHP via tainted foods could still significantly affect the health of children by limiting their growth (Tsai et al., 2016).

## Parabens

Parabens are most commonly known for being preservatives in personal care products. They have been demonstrated to have weak estrogenic properties, and epidemiological surveys indicate potential endocrine-disrupting and obesogenic potential. While they are recommended as safe by the FDA, concerned consumers can avoid ingredients such as ethyl-paraben, propylparaben, butylparaben, isobutylparaben, isopropylparaben, and benzylparaben (Etzel & Balk, 2019; U.S. FDA, 2020). In a study quantifying amounts of paraben in maternal urine of 181 pregnant women, exposure to parabens were found to be 100% present in all urine samples at levels higher than method detectable levels, and certain types of parabens were also found to have transferred to fetal cord plasma (Pycke et al., 2015). Future biomonitoring studies will help determine exposure and potential health effects, but parabens currently have not been shown to have acute toxic effects and are not teratogenic. Health effects from environmental doses are unknown (CDC, 2019a).

## Prevention

Endocrine disruptors include chemicals that manipulate hormones that have the potential to cause adverse effects to reproductive and neurodevelopmental systems in children. Although many of the action mechanisms are not yet fully understood, epidemiological studies have shown correlations with many potentially concerning results related to decreased IQ, behavioral concerns, and fertility concerns. Heterogeneous as they are with multiple discrepancies due to multiple factors at play (different age groups, seasonal and geographical variability, measuring limitations), the overall evidence and increased general population issues of infertility and reproductive challenges bring attention to the need for future studies.

Clinically, it is imperative that front-line providers stay up-to-date on environmental agents that are endemic to their geographical areas to recognize, manage, and reduce the load of potentially toxic exposure on developing children. For example, North America and Europe had the highest concentrations of PBDEs with measured concentrations present in daycares, houses, and primary schools. In the United States, measurements of PBDEs seem to be higher in California compared with other states (Malliari & Kalantzi, 2017). Having up-to-date knowledge on local trends and environmental policies can help practitioners intervene as early as possible when risks are recognized. Assessment often takes place through questionnaires and a good pediatric environmental history to investigate where the child spends most of their time, learns, plays, or works. Household dust seems to be a common means of exposure of EDCs as they leech from their original materials into the environment. Frequent dusting, vacuuming, and discarding furniture and bedding containing chemicals like PBDEs are recommended. Evaluation of home environment, diet, and activities can help practitioners identify and correlate behaviors with potential environmental exposures. Although many EDCs can pass from mother to infant via breast milk, the advantages of breastfeeding still exceed the risk of exposure because of the immunologic and cognitive benefits. However, helping mothers recognize and modify their exposures can decrease exposure to the newborn. Lotions, sunscreens, and other personal care products contain chemicals that can be reduced by switching to safer alternative products. Evaluation of the work environment can also help identify disproportionately higher routes of exposure of EDCs compared with those of the average person (Etzel & Balk, 2019). Clinicians do not need to be experts in environmental toxicology but should be familiar with resources that can aid them in their pursuit of prevention.

## NOISE EXPOSURE

Noise exposure can have a negative impact on health. The loudness of sound is measured in decibels. Exposure to noise >85 decibels can cause permanent or temporary hearing loss and tinnitus, but prolonged exposure even at lower levels can also negatively affect health (Etzel & Balk, 2019). Exposure to loud noise has been linked to cardiovascular disease, cognitive impairment, sleep disturbances, and psychological stress (Etzel & Balk, 2019; WHO, 2018b). Many common noise exposures are within the range that can cause health problems, including noise from traffic, trains, airplanes, fireworks, music, and toys (Etzel & Balk, 2019; WHO, 2018b).

### Reducing Noise Exposure

Information should be provided to families about potential consequences from noise exposure and how to reduce noise exposure. Ways to decrease noise exposure include leaving noisy areas and decreasing the volume of noise-producing items. Headphones and earbuds are a common source of loud noise, and careful attention should be made to avoid having the volume too loud. Toys that produce loud noises should have the batteries removed or tape placed over the speakers to lower the volume (Etzel & Balk, 2019). If a child is going to be in a situation with unavoidable loud noises, hearing protection should be used (Etzel & Balk, 2019).

## SOCIAL AND BEHAVIORAL HAZARDS

Social and behavioral hazards encompass a growing field of study and have been found to be more hazardous to a child than previously imagined. The WHO defines social determinants of health as "the conditions in which people are born, grow, work, live and age, and the wider set of forces and systems shaping the conditions of daily life" (WHO, 2020b). Under this definition race and ethnicity, housing, neighborhood safety, access to care, exposure to violence, and social pressures are some of the elements to be considered in pediatric health. Often, the interplay between different components of social hazards create cumulative disparities.

Even when controlled for confounding variables, racial disparities still affect health outcomes in children. For example, black children are at higher risk for atopic and allergic conditions and asthma, with more frequent emergency department visits and worse outcomes (Sitarik et al., 2020). Inability to access care due to lack of insurance has a negative association with nonaccidental traumas in children. More children are victims of physical abuse if their families lack insurance (Jones et al., 2019). Food insecurity alone or having several compounding social risks, including household instability, low caregiver education, and caregiver unemployment, among others, puts children at increased risk for mental health conditions (Spencer et al., 2019).

The AAPs' policy on health equity and children's rights emphasizes screening and addressing social, economic, educational, environmental, and capital needs of children and families. It asserts that practitioners should be looking at food security, educational progress, family employment, health literacy, neighborhood safety, and adequate housing (Hughes et al., 2016). *Healthy People 2030* emphasizes assessing the level of economic stability, poverty, food insufficiency, education, access to early childhood education, the social and community context of the family unit, immigration status and social support, healthcare access, and neighborhood-built environments (Office of Disease Prevention and Health Promotion, 2020; also see https://health.gov/healthypeople/objectives-and-data for *Healthy People 2030* Objectives). Pediatric primary care practitioners must be active in screening for social determinants of health as there is significant interplay between health and social hazards.

Childhood and adolescence are dynamic periods where there are a multitude of influences on health and health behaviors. Bogl et al. (2020) confirm the interaction between peers and family on children's fast-food consumption and screen time. They found that children's food access is dependent on their family until about the age of 9, at which point peers and social pressures are the largest influences on pediatric behaviors related to food and screen time. Bogl et al. (2020) suggest that health interventions need to transition to community-based interventions for adolescents, possibly in schools or neighborhoods. Beck et al. (2016) show that primary practitioners must consider how to incorporate other practices to mitigate the risks of poverty in their patients. They suggest implementing home visitation programs, increasing care coordination services, and partnering with communities to increase access to health. Social and behavioral health are evolving as more research continues to show the disparities that are caused by social determinants of health and the effects of behaviors on health. Appropriate and thorough screening of these factors must occur at every intervention a child has with a healthcare provider.

## TOXICOLOGY

According to the Poison Control Center Database, over 2 million exposures to toxic substances are reported each year, a large number of which occur in children. In 2018, 59% of exposures were in children <20 years old (Gummin et al., 2019). Although 1.2 million children had exposures in 2018, only 127 resulted in death. The majority of exposures occurred in children 5 and under (44% of all exposures), but the children with the most fatalities were in the 13- to 19-year-old age group with 65 fatalities (4.8% of all fatalities; Gummin et al., 2019). Toxic exposures occur from both pharmaceuticals and nonpharmaceuticals. Pharmaceutical poisoning can be the result of accidental ingestion, improper dosing of medication, or intentional overdose. Nonpharmaceutical ingestions include cosmetics, cleaning supplies, and pesticides (Gummin et al., 2019). There are several different routes of exposure including ingestion, inhalation, enteral, and dermal. In 2018, 83% of exposures were by ingestion (Gummin et al., 2019). There are certain medications that are important to be aware of because they can cause death in small quantities. These include antipsychotics, tricyclic antidepressants, antimalarials, antiarrhythmics, calcium channel blockers, oral hypoglycemics, opioids, and imidazolines (Bar-Oz et al., 2004). Urgent medical referral should be made for these agents, as they can be fatal in as few as one pill (Bar-Oz et al., 2004).

## ASSESSMENT

When evaluating a child with a toxic exposure, it is important to obtain a thorough history and physical examination. Information should be obtained about the type of exposure, the route of exposure, the timing of the exposure, and the quantity of the exposure (Aki & Alessai, 2019). If the type of exposure is unknown, determining where the child was when the exposure took place and what possible toxins could be accessed by the child can be vital in determining the causative agent. For example, if a child was near a garage or shed where chemicals or pesticides are stored, they could have been exposed to fumes, ingested a toxin, or had dermal exposure. If a child was inside and there was medication within their reach, this could indicate a possible pharmaceutical ingestion. Bottles that are open, empty, or missing medication may provide insight into the type of exposure. It is important to ask about herbal medications and vitamins, as these may be initially overlooked (Aki & Alessai, 2019).

The majority of exposures are unintentional; however, there are also many cases of intentional overdoses. The highest number of deaths in children from the 2018 Poison Control Center Database were from suspected suicide in the 15- to 19-year-old age group (Gummin et al., 2019). Assessing for depression or a known history of depression can indicate a possible intentional exposure. Assessment for signs of child abuse is also important, since some exposures are intentional by caregivers. This includes forced ingestion which ranges from forcing a child to take medications that are not medically indicated to forced water or salt consumption. Poisonings with numerous different types of medications and substances have been reported and children may present with a broad range of symptoms including apnea, seizures, altered mental status, bleeding, GI symptoms, and rashes. One example is giving a child ipecac syrup to induce vomiting and then seeking medical attention for vomiting (Culotta & Thackeray, 2019).

### Physical Examination

The physical examination is important to determine the need for urgent intervention as well as to provide clues for the type of toxic exposure. Assess the child's ability to maintain their airway. Respiratory rate and effort should be noted, as well as signs of hypoxia. Cardiovascular status should be assessed with particular attention to vital signs, since many poisonings are characteristically associated with particular vital sign abnormalities (Mégarbane, 2014). A thorough neurologic examination should be performed, including assessment of mental status, reflexes, and pupil size. Assessment of mental status includes determining alertness and responsiveness as well as identifying any agitation, confusion, delusions, or hallucinations. Skin characteristics can provide information on the type of exposure. It is important to note if the skin is flushed, pale, cyanotic, diaphoretic, or dry. Hyperthermia or hypothermia may be present in various toxic exposures. Hyperactive or hypoactive bowel sounds should be noted, as this can help distinguish between anticholinergic and sympathomimetic syndromes (Mégarbane, 2014). Some poisonings are associated with a characteristic odor, so any odors should be noted (Aki & Alessai, 2019). For example, a smell of bitter almonds is associated with cyanide poisoning, garlic with arsenic poisoning, and gasoline with organophosphate poisoning (Mégarbane, 2014).

## TREATMENT

Treatment varies based on the availability of an antidote and severity of the toxic exposure. A call to the Poison Control Center is always warranted to ascertain appropriate treatment for an ingestion ([800] 222-1222). Treatment often involves supportive measures, which can include supplemental oxygen, endotracheal intubation and mechanical ventilation, fluid resuscitation, vasoactive medications for blood pressure support, dextrose administration, electrolyte correction, and benzodiazepine administration for seizures (Aki & Alessai, 2019). There are certain treatments specifically for ingested medications that aim to reduce the amount of medication that is absorbed. Gastric lavage and ipecac are no longer recommended. Gastric lavage involves placing a gastric tube and suctioning out gastric contents. This treatment is not recommended in children and very rarely recommended in adults. Ipecac induces vomiting and is no longer recommended as a treatment for ingestions (Schaider et al., 2015). There are several individual antidotes, and common ones are discussed in the text that follows.

### Activated Charcoal

One of the primary treatments is the administration of activated charcoal. Activated charcoal binds toxins and prevents absorption from the GI tract. To be effective, it must be given soon after the ingestion, ideally within 1 hour. There are certain substances that do not bind to activated charcoal, so it is not always an effective treatment. Generally, it is safe to administer activated charcoal, but there are certain situations where it should be avoided. If a child is not alert enough to protect their airway, activated charcoal should be avoided unless a secure airway is in place because of the risk of aspiration and subsequent pneumonia. Activated charcoal is contraindicated in ingestion of caustic agents, which are agents that cause tissue damage, primarily alkali or acids (Schaider et al., 2015). These are found in many cleaning products such as general cleaning products, drain cleaner, toilet bowel cleaner, and bleach (Hoffman et al., 2020). Lastly, activated charcoal should be avoided if a small bowel obstruction or ileus is present (Schaider et al., 2015).

### Cathartics

Cathartics are a class of drugs that increase gastric motility. The use of cathartics in toxic ingestions is controversial, and they have not been shown to be beneficial when used independently. There may be some benefit to administrating concurrently with activated charcoal, although there is not a consensus on whether this is truly beneficial and it is not routinely recommended (Schaider et al., 2015).

### Whole Bowel Irrigation

Whole bowel irrigation is another method to prevent absorption of toxic substances. It is achieved by giving polyethylene glycol at high doses until the bowels are cleared. This method can be used for sustained-release formulations of medications and for toxins that do not bind to activated charcoal. Like activated charcoal, it is contraindicated in bowel obstruction, ileus, and unprotected airways (Schaider et al., 2015).

## TOXIDROMES AND THEIR TREATMENTS

Often, the offending toxin is identified prior to seeking medical treatment; however, there are times when the specific agent is unknown. In these instances, toxidromes can be useful in identifying which toxin is likely responsible. A toxidrome is a group of signs and symptoms associated with a particular class of substances. There is some overlap in signs and symptoms between toxidromes and some drugs producing effects that fall into more than one toxidrome. In addition, some exposures involve more than one agent, so toxidromes may be less useful in these cases (Gummin et al., 2019).

### Cholinergic Toxidrome

The cholinergic toxidrome is caused by toxins that cause an accumulation of the neurotransmitter acetylcholine. This usually occurs from the inhibition of acetylcholinesterase but can also occur by directly increasing the amount of acetylcholine. Because acetylcholine is involved with the muscarinic receptors of the parasympathetic system, the nicotinic receptors of skeletal muscle, and the central nervous system, effects of toxicity can be seen in each of these areas (Carlson & Kraus, 2018). The effects are listed in Table 41.2.

The main causative agents are organophosphate and carbamate insecticides. The cholinergic toxidrome can also be seen in toxicity of cholinesterase inhibitors used to treat symptoms of Alzheimer's disease, sarin (a nerve gas), and mushrooms (Lott & Jones, 2020). Cholinergic agents can be treated with atropine followed by pralidoxime (Lott & Jones, 2020; Mégarbane, 2014).

### Anticholinergic Toxidrome

The anticholinergic toxidrome is caused by substances that block the effect of acetylcholine. Anticholinergic medications include:

- Antihistamines
- Tricyclic antidepressants
- Phenothiazines
- Antipsychotics
- Neuroleptics
- Cyclobenzaprine
- Antiparkinsonian drugs.

In addition, it can be caused by several plants that may be found in natural remedies (Broderick et al., 2020; Mégarbane, 2014). These substances work primarily on the muscarinic sites and have little effect on the nicotinic sites, thereby making many of the signs and symptoms present in the anticholinergic toxidrome opposite of the muscarinic effects in the cholinergic toxidrome. The effects are listed in Table 41.3.

Central effects include muscarinic effects. Hemodynamic changes can occur and, if associated with electrocardiogram changes, can point toward a tricyclic

TABLE 41.2 **Cholinergic Toxidrome**

| Type of Effect | Muscarinic Effects | Nicotinic Effects | Central Nervous System Effects |
|---|---|---|---|
| Clinical findings | Bradycardia<br>Hypotension<br>Miosis<br>Salivation<br>Rhinorrhea<br>Bronchorrhea<br>Bronchospasm<br>Lacrimation<br>Diaphoresis<br>Abdominal pain/cramping<br>Diarrhea<br>Incontinence of bladder and bowel | Tachycardia<br>Hypertension<br>Fasciculations<br>Weakness<br>Paralysis (including of respiratory muscles) | Headache<br>Confusion<br>Ataxia<br>Seizure<br>Coma<br>Respiratory depression |

*Sources*: Data from Lott, E. L., & Jones, E. B. (2020). Cholinergic toxicity. https://www.ncbi.nlm.nih.gov/books/NBK539783; Mégarbane, B. (2014). Toxidrome-based approach to common poisonings. *Asia Pacific Journal of Medical Toxicology*, 3, 2–12. https://doi.org/10.22038/APJMT.2014.2463.

**TABLE 41.3 Anticholinergic Toxidrome**

| Type of Effect | Muscarinic Effects | Central Nervous System Effects |
|---|---|---|
| Clinical findings | Mydriasis<br>Dry mucous membranes<br>Flushed skin<br>Hypoactive bowel sounds<br>Urinary retention | Confusion<br>Agitation<br>Hallucinations<br>Delirium<br>Seizures<br>Coma<br>Picking motion with the hands |

antidepressant toxicity (Broderick et al., 2020; Mégarbane, 2014). Treatment for anticholinergic syndrome usually involves supportive care, although physostigmine, a cholinergic agent, may be used in severe cases (Broderick et al., 2020).

## Sympathomimetic Toxidrome

The sympathomimetic toxidrome is caused by the inhibition of reuptake of norepinephrine and dopamine, causing activation of the sympathetic nervous system (Goldstein & Richards, 2019). This is caused by many illicit drugs such as cocaine, ecstasy, and methamphetamine (Goldstein & Richards, 2019; Mégarbane, 2014). Sympathomimetic syndrome shares many of the same symptoms as anticholinergic syndrome including:

- Agitation
- Confusion
- Seizures
- Mydriasis
- Hypertension
- Tachycardia (Goldstein & Richards, 2019; Mégarbane, 2014).

Two differentiating symptoms are diaphoresis and hyperactive bowel sounds (Mégarbane, 2014). Treatment is generally supportive. In particular, benzodiazepines can be used to treat agitation and seizures (Goldstein & Richards, 2019).

## Opioid/Narcotic Toxidrome

The opioid/narcotic toxidrome is caused by medications that act on the opioid receptors. There are three main types of opioid receptors (mu, delta, and kappa) located in both the central and peripheral nervous system. Medications classified as opioids are used to target the analgesia effects of the mu receptor (Stein, 2016). Examples of opioids include:

- Morphine
- Fentanyl
- Methadone
- Buprenorphine
- Codeine
- Tramadol
- Heroin (Ciejka et al., 2016).

Signs and symptoms of an opioid overdose include:

- Respiratory depression (bradypnea or apnea)
- Altered mental status
- Coma
- Bradycardia
- Hypotension
- Pinpoint pupils.

Naloxone can be used to treat an opioid overdose (Mégarbane, 2014; Stein, 2016).

## Sedative/Hypnotic Toxidrome

The sedative/hypnotic toxidrome is caused by medications that cause central nervous system depression and sedation such as:

- Barbiturates
- Benzodiazepines
- Insomnia z-drugs (e.g., zopiclone, zolpidem, zaleplon)
- Ethanol.

Signs and symptoms of sedative/hypnotic ingestion include:

- Behavior and memory impairment
- Coma
- Respiratory depression
- Hypotonia
- Hyporeflexia
- Nystagmus (Mégarbane, 2014; Weaver, 2015).

Supportive care is used for barbiturates and ethanol. Flumazenil is a benzodiazepine competitive antagonist and can be used to treat benzodiazepine and z-drug overdoses (Mégarbane, 2014; Weaver, 2015).

## Salicylate and Acetaminophen Ingestion

Salicylates and acetaminophen are agents commonly seen in both intentional and unintentional overdoses. Although they are not part of a specific toxidrome, they have signs and symptoms associated with toxicity. Salicylates, such as aspirin and oil of wintergreen, cause toxicity by disrupting aerobic metabolism leading to metabolic acidosis. In addition, they affect the respiratory center directly. Initially, this causes tachypnea, but in severe toxicity it causes bradypnea and hypoventilation. This disrupts the respiratory compensatory mechanism for the metabolic acidosis, thereby worsening the acidosis (Ciejka et al., 2016). A characteristic finding in salicylate toxicity is tinnitus. Hemorrhage can occur due to the antiplatelet properties of salicylates. Additional signs and symptoms include GI upset, headache, dizziness, confusion, hallucinations, seizures, and hypotension. Although there is not a specific antidote for salicylate overdoses, hemodialysis can remove the toxin from the blood and can be used in severe cases (Runde & Nappe, 2019).

Acetaminophen overdoses cause toxicity by damaging hepatocytes. During acetaminophen metabolism, there are multiple pathways that metabolize acetaminophen. One of the pathways results in a byproduct called N-acetyl-p-benzoquinone imine (NAPQI), which is toxic to the liver. Under normal therapeutic conditions, a small amount of NAPQI is produced and it is reduced by glutathione and renally cleared without causing toxic effects (Ciejka et al., 2016). In an acetaminophen overdose, the metabolism pathways become overwhelmed, and more NAPQI is produced. There is not enough glutathione to reduce the excess NAPQI, and the buildup of NAPQI can cause hepatic necrosis (Ciejka et al., 2016).

Although liver dysfunction is one of the prominent signs of severe acetaminophen overdose, it may not be present for 3 to 4 days after ingestion. Earlier signs and symptoms include vomiting and right upper quadrant pain (Agrawal & Khazaeni, 2020; Ciejka et al., 2016). If liver dysfunction occurs, signs and symptoms can include jaundice, altered mentation, metabolic acidosis, coagulopathies, and renal failure. Treatment of acetaminophen toxicity is with N-acetyl-cysteine. Not all overdoses require treatment and the Rumack-Matthew nomogram (readily available online) guides the need for treatment based on the serum acetaminophen level and time since ingestion (Agrawal & Khazaeni, 2020; Ciejka et al., 2016).

## PREVENTION

Reducing toxic exposures can be accomplished through both legislative measures and education. There have been several measures enacted in an attempt to prevent toxic exposures. In 1960, the Hazardous Substance Labeling Act was created so that substances that were toxic could easily be identified. In 1970, the Poison Prevention Packaging Act was enacted to try to reduce the number of unintentional toxic exposures in children. It provided regulations for the packaging of many toxic substances. It required most prescription medications, several over-the-counter medications, and many household products to be packaged in child-resistant containers (U.S. Consumer Product Safety Commission, 2005). After these regulations were put in place, child mortality from unintentional medication ingestion decreased (Rogers, 1996). In 2011, the FDA issued guidelines to help prevent medication administration errors by ensuring consistency between markings on dosage delivery devices and the medication administration instructions for over-the-counter liquid medications (U.S. Food and Drug Administration Center for Drug Evaluation and Research, 2011).

Education is another important aspect of prevention. Information should be provided to parents about safe storage of medication. It is recommended that medication is stored in the original child-resistant packaging and out of reach and sight of the child (AAP, 2020). If a medication is going to be used multiple times per day—for example, when a child is sick—it can be convenient to leave medications out; however, this practice should be avoided and medications should always be returned to a safe place of storage. Caregivers should share safe storage information with people who are visiting or who will be caring for the child to ensure a safe environment for the child (CDC, 2020b). Unused medications should be disposed of through a medication take-back program or through instructions provided on the medication information insert (AAP, 2020). Anticipatory guidance should also be provided to families about the risk of children accessing medications and household products as a result of normal child development, resulting in new milestones such as crawling, walking, and climbing. Medications that are stored in a previously safe location may become accessible as the child develops these new skills (Schwebel et al., 2017). Families should be given information on how to contact the Poison Control Center (800-222-1222), in the event that an exposure does occur (CDC, 2020b). Screening for depression and substance use and abuse can help reduce intentional toxic exposures. It is recommended that all adolescents be screened for substance use and depression (Committee on Substance Use and Prevention, 2016; Sui, 2016). Being aware of exposure risks, properly storing medications and household products, and identifying those who are at risk for intentional exposures can help reduce the risk of toxic ingestions and exposures.

## KEY POINTS

- Toxicity can cause disease and dysfunction in children, leading to chronic disease, increased hospital admissions, and reduced quality of life. Primary care providers play a pivotal role in screening and identification of exposures.

- Children are more susceptible to adverse effects from exposures for several reasons including size, behavior, diet, and metabolic pathway development.
- Environmental exposure during critical windows of prenatal development can alter fundamental processes leading to functional and growth disturbances.
- Determining social and behavioral hazards includes assessment of food insecurity, education progress, family employment, health literacy, neighborhood safety, and housing, while recognizing that social factors like race and ethnicity confound health outcomes.
- Recognition of toxicity to prevent, reduce, or remove exposure is key to most hazards discussed in this chapter.

## REFERENCES


Agency for Toxic Substances & Disease Registry. (2021). *Mercury*. https://wwwn.cdc.gov/TSP/substances/ToxSubstance.aspx?toxid=24

Agrawal, S., & Khazaeni, B. (2020). *Acetaminophen toxicity*. https://www.ncbi.nlm.nih.gov/books/NBK441917

Aki, E. S., & Alessai, J. (2019). *General approach to poisoned patient*. In O. Karcioglu & B. Aslan (Eds.), *Poisoning in the modern world—New tricks for an old dog?* IntechOpen. https://doi.org/10.5772/intechopen.84681

Akimzhanova, Z., Guney, M., Kismelyeva, S., Zhakiyenova, A., & Yogafarova, A. (2020). Contamination by eleven harmful elements in children's jewelry and toys from Central Asian market. *Environmental Science and Pollution Research, 27*, 21071–2108. https://doi.org/10.1007/s11356-020-08631-5

American Academy of Pediatrics, Committee on Substance Use and Prevention. (2020). *Poster on safe storage & disposal of medications*. https://www.aap.org/en-us/advocacy-and-policy/aap-health-initiatives/Substance-Use-and-Prevention/Pages/poster-safe-storage.aspx

American Academy of Pediatrics, Council on Children and Disasters. (n.d.). *Protecting children from carbon monoxide poisoning*. https://www.aap.org/en-us/advocacy-and-policy/aap-health-initiatives/Children-and-Disasters/Pages/Protecting-Children-from-Carbon-Monoxide-Poisoning.aspx

American Academy of Pediatrics Council on Environmental Health. (2016). Prevention of childhood lead toxicity. *Pediatrics, 138*(1). https://doi.org/10.1542/peds.2016-1493

American Cancer Society. (2019). *Arsenic and cancer risk*. https://www.cancer.org/cancer/cancer-causes/arsenic.html

Azagba, S., Manzione, L., Shan, L., & King, J. (2020). Trends in smoking during pregnancy by socioeconomic characteristics in the United States, 2010–2017. *BMC Pregnancy and Childbirth, 20*(1), 52. https://doi.org/10.1186/s12884-020-2748-y

Baek, H. J., Kim, E. K., Lee, S. G., Jeong, S. H., Sakong, J., Merchant, A. T., Im, S. U., Song, K. B., & Choi, Y. H. (2016). Dental amalgam exposure can elevate urine mercury concentrations in children. *International Dental Journal, 66*(3), 136–143. https://doi.org/10.1111/idj.12214

Barakat, R., Lin, P.-C. P., Rattan, S., Brehm, E., Canisso, I. F., Abosalum, M. E., Flaws, J. A., Hess, R., & Ko, C. (2017). Prenatal exposure to DEHP induces premature reproductive senescence in male mice. *Toxicological Sciences, 156*(1), 96–108. https://doi.org/10.1093/toxsci/kfw248

Bar-Oz, B., Levichek, Z., & Koren, G. (2004). Medications that can be fatal for a toddler with one tablet or teaspoon. *Pediatric Drugs, 6*, 123–126. https://doi.org/10.2165/00148581-200406020-00005

Beck, A. F., Tschudy, M. M., Coker, T. R., Mistry, K. B., Cox, J. E., Gitterman, B. A., Chamberlain, L. J., Grace, A. M., Hole, M. K., Klass, P. E., Lobach, K. S., Ma, C. T., Navsaria, D., Northrip, K. D., Sadof, M. D., Shah, A. N., & Fierman, A. H. (2016). Determinants of health and pediatric primary practice. *Pediatrics, 137*(3). https://doi.org/10.1542/peds.2015-3673

Bhattacharya, D., Fujihashi, A., Majrashi, M., Bloemer, J., Bhattacharya, S., Buabeid, M., Escobar, M., Moore, T., Suppiramaniam, V., & Dhanasekaran, M. (2020). Concurrent nicotine exposure to prenatal alcohol consumption alters the hippocampal and cortical neurotoxicity. *Heliyon, 6*(1). https://doi.org/10.1016/j.heliyon.2019.e03045

Bogl, L. H., Mehlig, K., Ahrens, W., Gwozdz, W., de Henauw, S., Molnar, D., Moreno, L., Pigeot, I., Russo, R., Solea, A., Veidebaum, T., Kaprio, J., Lissner, L., & Hebestreit, A. (2020). Like me, like me—Relative importance of peers and siblings on children's fast food consumption and screen time but not sports club participation depends on age. *International Journal of Behavioral Nutrition and Physical Activity, 17*(1), 50. https://doi.org/10.1186/s12966-020-00953-4

Broderick, E. D., Metheny, H., & Crosby, B. (2020). *Anticholinergic toxicity*. https://www.ncbi.nlm.nih.gov/books/NBK534798

Buha, A., Matovic, V., Antonijevic, B., Bulat, Z., Curcic, M., Renieri, E. A., Tsatsaki, A. M., Schweitzer, A., & Wallace, D. (2018). Overview of cadmium thyroid disrupting effects and mechanisms. *International Journal of Molecular Science, 19*(5), 1501. https://doi.org/10.3390/ijms19051501

Carlson, A. B., & Kraus, G. P. (2018). *Physiology, cholinergic receptors*. https://www.ncbi.nlm.nih.gov/books/NBK526134

Centers for Disease Control and Prevention. (2016). *Basic facts about mold and dampness*. https://www.cdc.gov/mold/faqs.htm

Centers for Disease Control and Prevention. (2019a). *Biomonitoring summary: Parabens*. https://www.cdc.gov/biomonitoring/Parabens_BiomonitoringSummary.html

Centers for Disease Control and Prevention. (2019b). *Childhood lead poisoning update*. https://www.cdc.gov/nceh/lead/prevention/default.htm

Centers for Disease Control and Prevention. (2019c). *FASDs*. https://www.cdc.gov/ncbddd/fasd/facts.html

Centers for Disease Control and Prevention. (2019d). *Phthalates factsheet*. https://www.cdc.gov/biomonitoring/Phthalates_FactSheet.html

Centers for Disease Control and Prevention. (2020a). *Health effects of secondhand smoke*. https://www.cdc.gov/tobacco/data_statistics/fact_sheets/secondhand_smoke/health_effects/index.htm

Centers for Disease Control and Prevention. (2020b). *Protect your children: Store & use medicines safely*. https://www.cdc.gov/patientsafety/features/safe-medicine-children.html

Chang, W.-H., Li, S.-S., Wu, M.-H., Pan, H.-A., & Lee, C.-C. (2015). Phthalates might interfere with testicular function by reducing testosterone and insulin-like factor 3 levels. *Human Reproduction, 30*(11), 2658–2670. https://doi.org/10.1093/humrep/dev225

Chen, C., Xun, P., Nishijo, M., Sekikawa, A., & He, K. (2015). Cadmium exposure and risk of pancreatic cancer: A meta-analysis of prospective cohort studies and case-control studies among individuals without occupational exposure history. *Environmental Science and Pollution Research, 22*, 17465–17474. https://doi.org/10.1007/s11356-015-5464-9

Ciejka, M., Nguyen, K., Bluth, M. H., & Dubey, E. (2016). Drug toxicities of common analgesic medications in the emergency department. *Clinics in Laboratory Medicine, 36*(4), 761–776. https://doi.org/10.1016/j.cll.2016.07.003

Claus Henn, B., Ettinger, A. S., Hopkins, M. R., Jim, R., Amarasriwardena, C., Christiani, D. C., Coull, B. A., Bellinger, D. C., & Wright, R. O. (2016). Prenatal arsenic exposure and birth outcomes among a population residing near a mining-related superfund site. *Environmental Health Perspectives, 124*(8), 1308–1315. https://doi.org/10.1289/ehp.1510070

Committee on Substance Use and Prevention. (2016). Substance use screening, brief intervention, and referral to treatment. *Pediatrics, 138*(1), e20161210. https://doi.org/10.1542/peds.2016-1210

Culotta, P., & Thackeray, J. (2019). Medical child abuse. In A. Laskey & A. Sirotnak (Eds.), *Child abuse: Medical diagnosis & management* (4th ed., pp. 673–701). American Academy of Pediatrics.

Dai, Q., Min, X., & Weng, M. (2016), A review of polychlorinated biphenyls (PCBs) pollution in indoor air environment. *Journal of the Air & Waste Management Association, 66*(10), 941–950. https://doi.org/10.1080/10962247.2016.1184193

Das, K. K., Reddy, R. C., Bagoji, I. B., Das, S., Bagali, S., Mullur, L., Khodnapur, J. P., & Biradar, M. S. (2019). Primary concept of nickel toxicity—An overview. *Journal of Basic and Clinical Physiology and Pharmacology, 30*(2), 141–152. https://doi.org/10.1515/jbcpp-2017-0171

Denny, C. H. (2019). Consumption of alcohol beverages and binge drinking among pregnant women aged 18–44 years—United States, 2015–2017. *MMWR. Morbidity and Mortality Weekly Report, 68*(16), 365–368. https://doi.org/10.15585/mmwr.mm6816a1

DeStefano, F., Bodenstab, H. M., & Offit, P. A. (2019). Principal controversies in vaccine safety in the United States. *Clinical Infectious Diseases, 69*(4), 726–731. https://doi.org/10.1093/cid/ciz135

Di Nisio, A., & Foresta, C. (2019). Water and soil pollution as determinant of water and food quality/contamination and its impact on male fertility. *Reproductive Biology and Endocrinology, 17*(4). https://doi.org/10.1186/s12958-018-0449-4

Di Renzo, G. C., Conry, J. A., Blake, J., DeFrancesco, M. S., DeNicola, N., Martin, J. N., McCue, K. A., Richmond, D., Shah, A., Sutton, P., Woodruff, T. J., van der Poel, S. Z., & Giudice, L. C. (2015). International Federation of Gynecology and Obstetrics (FIGO) opinion on reproductive health impacts of exposure to toxic environmental chemicals. *International Journal of Gynecology and Obstetrics, 131*(3), 219–225. https://doi.org/10.1016/j.ijgo.2015.09.002

Donat-Vargas, C., Åkesson, A., Berglund, M., Glynn, A., Wolk, A., & Kipple, M. (2016). Dietary exposure to polychlorinated biphenyls and risk of breast, endometrial and ovarian cancer in a prospective cohort. *British Journal of Cancer, 115*, 1113–1121. https://doi.org/10.1038/bjc.2016.282

Drwal, E., Rak, A., & Gregoraszczuk, E. L. (2019). Review: Polycyclic aromatic hydrocarbons (PAHs)-Action on placental function and health risks in future life of newborns. *Toxicology, 411*, 133–142. https://doi.org/10.1016/j.tox.2018.10.003

Drwal, E., Rak, A., Grochowalski, A., Milewicz, T., & Gregoraszczuk, E. L. (2017). Cell-specific and dose-dependent effects of PAHs on proliferation, cell cycle, and apoptosis protein expression and hormone secretion by placental cell lines. *Toxicology Letters, 280*, 10–19. https://doi.org/10.1016/j.toxlet.2017.08.002

Ehrhart, F., Roozen, S., Verbeek, J., Koek, G., Kok, G., van Kranen, H., Evelo, C. T., & Curfs, L. M. G. (2019). Review and gap analysis: Molecular pathways leading to fetal alcohol spectrum disorders. *Molecular Psychiatry, 24*(1), 10–17. https://doi.org/10.1038/s41380-018-0095-4

Environmental Protection Agency. (2006). *A framework for assessing health risks of environmental exposures to children*. https://cfpub.epa.gov/ncea/risk/recordisplay.cfm?deid=158363

Environmental Protection Agency. (2016a). *A citizen's guide to radon: The guide to protecting yourself and your family from radon*. https://www.epa.gov/radon/citizens-guide-radon-guide-protecting-yourself-and-your-family-radon

Environmental Protection Agency. (2016b). *Cadmium compounds (A)*. https://www.epa.gov/sites/production/files/2016-09/documents/cadmium-compounds.pdf

Environmental Protection Agency. (2017a). *Endocrine Disruptor Screening Program (EDSP) overview*. https://www.epa.gov/endocrine-disruption/endocrine-disruptor-screening-program-edsp-overview

Environmental Protection Agency. (2017b). *Pollution Prevention Act*. https://www.epa.gov/p2/pollution-prevention-act-1990

Environmental Protection Agency. (2018). *History of children's environmental health protection at EPA*. https://www.epa.gov/children/history-childrens-environmental-health-protection-epa

Environmental Protection Agency. (2019a). *America's children and the environment*. https://www.epa.gov/americaschildrenenvironment/americas-children-and-environment-october-2019

Environmental Protection Agency. (2019b). *EPA releases first major update to chemicals list in 40 years*. https://www.epa.gov/newsreleases/epa-releases-first-major-update-chemicals-list-40-years

Environmental Protection Agency. (2019c). *Summary of the Clean Water Act*. https://www.epa.gov/laws-regulations/summary-clean-water-act

Environmental Protection Agency. (2019d). *Summary of the Federal Food, Drug, and Cosmetic Act*. https://www.epa.gov/laws-regulations/summary-federal-food-drug-and-cosmetic-act

Environmental Protection Agency. (2019e). *Summary of the Federal Insecticide and Rodenticide Act*. https://www.epa.gov/laws-regulations/summary-federal-insecticide-fungicide-and-rodenticide-act

Environmental Protection Agency. (2019f). *Summary of the National Environmental Policy Act*. https://www.epa.gov/laws-regulations/summary-national-environmental-policy-act

Environmental Protection Agency. (2019g). *Summary of the Toxic Substances Control Act*. https://www.epa.gov/laws-regulations/summary-toxic-substances-control-act

Environmental Protection Agency. (2020a). *DDT—A brief history and status*. https://www.epa.gov/ingredients-used-pesticide-products/ddt-brief-history-and- status

Environmental Protection Agency. (2020b). *Overview of the Clean Air Act and air pollution*. https://www.epa.gov/clean-air-act-overview

Environmental Protection Agency. (2020c). *Safe Drinking Water Act*. https://www.epa.gov/sdwa

Ettinger, A. S., Leonard, M. L., & Mason, J. (2019). CDC's Lead Poisoning Prevention Program: A long-standing responsibility and commitment to protect children from lead exposure. *Journal of Public Health Management Practice, 25*, S5–S12. https://doi.org/10.1097/PHH.0000000000000868

Etzel, R. A., & Balk, S. J. (Eds.). (2019). *Pediatric environmental health* (4th ed.). American Academy of Pediatrics.

Evens, A., Hryhorczuk, D., Lanphear, B. P., Rankin, K. M., Lewis, D. A., Forst, L., & Rosenberg, D. (2015) The impact of low-level lead toxicity on school performance among children in the Chicago public schools: A population-based retrospective cohort study. *Environmental Health, 14*(21). https://doi.org/10.1186/s12940-015-0008-9

Fang, F., Chen, D., Yu, P., Qian, W., Zhou, J., Liu, J., Gao, R., Wang, J., & Xiao, H. (2015). Effects of bisphenol A on glucose homeostasis and brain insulin signaling pathways in male mice. *General and Comparative Endocrinology, 212*, 44–50. https://doi.org/10.1016/j.ygcen.2015.01.017

Findlay, L. C., & Kohen, D. E. (2015). Bisphenol A and child and youth behaviour: Canadian Health Measures Survey 2007 to 2011. *Health Reports, 26*(8), 3–9. https://www150.statcan.gc.ca/n1/en/pub/82-003-x/2015008/article/14215-eng.pdf?st=0ekXBtUu

Fromme, H., Becher, G., Hilger, B., & Völkel, W. (2016). Brominated flame retardants—Exposure and risk assessment for the general population. *International Journal of Hygiene and Environmental Health, 219*(1), 1–23. https://doi.org/10.1016/j.ijheh.2015.08.004

Goldenberg, A., Admani, S., Pelletier, J. L., & Jacob, S. E. (2015). Belt buckles—Increasing awareness of nickel exposure in children: A case report. *Pediatrics, 136*(3), e691–e693. https://doi.org/10.1542/peds.2015-0794

Goldstein, S., & Richards, J. R. (2019). *Sympathomimetic toxicity*. https://www.ncbi.nlm.nih.gov/books/NBK430757

Gore, A. C., Chappell, V. A., Fenton, S. E., Flaws, J. A., Nadal, A., Prins, G. S., Toppari, J., & Zoeller, R. T. (2015a). EDC-2: The Endocrine Society's second scientific statement on endocrine-disrupting chemicals. *Endocrine Reviews, 36*(6), E1–E150. https://doi.org/10.1210/er.2015-1010

Gore, A. C., Chappell, V. A., Fenton, S. E., Flaws, J. A., Nadal, A., Prins, G. S., Toppari, J., & Zoeller, R. T. (2015b). Executive summary to EDC-2: The Endocrine Society's second scientific statement on endocrine-disrupting chemicals. *Endocrine Reviews, 36*(6), 593–602. https://doi.org/10.1210/er.2015-1093

Grindler, N. M., Vanderlinden, L., Karthikraj, R., Kannan, K., Teal, S., Polotsky, A. J., Powell, T. L., Yang, I. V., & Jansson, T. (2018). Exposure to phthalate, an endocrine disrupting chemical, alters the first trimester placental methylome and transcriptome in women. *Scientific Reports, 8*, Article Number 6086. https://doi.org/10.1038/s41598-018-24505-w

Gummin, D. D., Mowry, J. B., Spyker, D. A., Brooks, D. E., Beuhler, M. C., Rivers, L. J., Hashem, H. A., & Ryan M. L. (2019). 2018 Annual report of the American Association of Poison Control Centers' National Poison Data System (NPDS): 36th annual report. *Clinical Toxicology, 57*(12), 1220–1413. https://doi.org/10.1080/15563650.2019.1677022

Gupta, K. K., Gupta, V. K., & Shirasaka, T. (2016). An update on fetal alcohol syndrome—Pathogenesis, risks, and treatment. *Alcoholism: Clinical and Experimental Research, 40*(8), 1594–1602. https://doi.org/10.1111/acer.13135

Hagan, J. F., Balachova, T., Bertrand, J., Chasnoff, I., Dang, E., Fernandez-Baca, D., Kable, J., Kosofsky, B., Senturias, Y. N., Singh, N., Sloane, M., Weitzman, C., & Zubler, J. (2016). Neurobehavioral disorder associated with prenatal alcohol exposure. *Pediatrics, 138*(4), e20151553. https://doi.org/10.1542/peds.2015-1553

Harada, M., Takashi, Y., & Tsuda, T. (2011). Epidemiology of congenital Minamata disease patients. *Epidemiology, 22*(1), S100. https://doi.org/10.1097/01.ede.0000391974.64822.d0

Hauptman, M., & Woolf, A. D. (2017). Childhood ingestions of environmental toxins: What are the risks? *Pediatric Annals, 46*(12), e466–e471. https://doi.org/10.3928/19382359-20171116-01.

Healthy Babies Bright Futures. (2019). *What's in my baby's food?* https://www.healthybabyfood.org/sites/healthy baby foods.org/files/2019-10/BabyFoodReport_FULLREPORT_ENGLISH_R5b.pdf

Hendryx, M., & Luo, J. (2018). Children's environmental chemical exposures in the USA, NHANES 2003–2012. *Environmental Science and Pollution Research, 25*(6), 5336–5343. https://doi.org/10.1007/s11356-017-0874-5

Herrick, R. F., Stewart, J. H., & Allen, J. G. (2016). Review of PCBs in US schools: A brief history, an estimate of the number of impacted schools, and an approach for evaluating indoor air samples. *Environmental Science and Pollution Research International, 23*(3), 1975–1985. https://doi.org/10.1007/s11356-015-4574-8

Hirsch, J. (2019). *Arsenic and lead are in your fruit juice: What you need to know*. https://www.consumerreports.org/food-safety/arsenic-and-lead-are-in-your-fruit-juice-what-you-need-to-know

Hoffman, R. S., Burns, M. M., & Gosselin, S. (2020). Ingestion of caustic substances. *New England Journal of Medicine, 382*, 1739–1748. https://doi.org/10.1056/NEJMra1810769

Hu, C.-Y., Li, F.-L., Hua, X.-G., Jiang, W., Mao, C., & Zhang, X.-J. (2018). The association between prenatal bisphenol A exposure and birth weight: A meta-analysis. *Reproductive Toxicology, 79*, 21–31. https://doi.org/10.1016/j.reprotox.2018.04.013

Hughes, L. S., Phillips, R. L., Jr., DeVoe, J. E., & Bazemore, A. W. (2016). Community vital signs: Taking the pulse of the community while caring for patients. *Journal of American Board of Family Medicine, 29*(3), 419–422. https://doi.org/10.3122/jabfm.2016.03.150172

Jeong, K. S., Park, H., Ha, E., Shin, J., Hong, Y.-C., Ha, M., Park, H., Kim, B.-N., Lee, B., Lee S.-J., Lee, K. Y., Kim, J. H., & Kim, Y. (2017). High maternal blood mercury levels is associated with low verbal—IQ in children. *Journal of Korean Medical Science, 32*(7), 1097–1104. https://doi.org/10.3346/jkms.2017.32.7.1097

Jones, R. E., Babb, J., Gee, K. M., & Beres, A. L. (2019). An investigation of social determinants of health and outcomes in pediatric nonaccidental trauma. *Pediatric Surgery International, 35*(8), 869–877. https://doi.org/10.1007/s00383-019-04491-4

Khoshali, M., Rafiei, N., Farajzadegan, Z., Shoshtari-Yeganeh, B., & Kelishadi, R. (2020). Maternal exposure to cadmium and fetal growth: A systemic review and meta-analysis. *Biological Trace Element Research, 195*(1), 9–19. https://doi.org/10.1007/s12011-019-01819-y

Kuniyoshi, K. M., & Rehan, V. K. (2019). The impact of perinatal nicotine exposure on fetal lung development and subsequent respiratory morbidity. *Birth Defects Research, 111*(17), 1270–1283. https://doi.org/10.1002/bdr2.1595

Lam, J., Lanphear, B. P., Bellinger, D., Axelrad, D. A., McPartland, J., Sutton, P., Davidson, L., Daniels, N., Sen, S., & Woodruff, T. J. (2017). Developmental PBDE exposure and IQ/ADHD in childhood: A systematic review and meta-analysis. *Environmental Health Perspectives, 125*(8). https://doi.org/10.1289/EHP1632

Lanphear, B. P., Hornung, R., Khoury, J., Yolton, K., Baghurst, P., Bellinger, D. C., Canfield, R. L., Dietrich, K. N., Bornschein, R., Green, T., Rothenberg, S. J., Needleman, H. L., Schnaas L., Wasserman, G., Graziano, J., & Roberts, R. (2005). Low-level environmental lead exposure and children's intellectual function: An international pooled analysis. *Environmental Health Perspective, 113*, 894–899. https://doi.org/10.1289/ehp.7688

Lelieveld, J., Evans, J. S., Fnais, M., Giannadaki, D., & Pozzer, A. (2015). The contribution of outdoor air pollution sources to premature mortality on a global scale. *Nature, 525*(7569), 367–371. https://doi.org/10.1038/nature15371

Lenters, V., Portengen, L., Rignell-Hydbom, A., Jönsson, B. A. G., Lindh, C. H., Piersma, A. H., Toft, G., Bonde, J. P., Heederik, D., Rylander, L., & Vermeulen, R. (2016). Prenatal phthalate, perfluoroalkyl acid, and organochlorine exposures and term birth weight in three birth cohorts: Multi-pollutant models based on elastic net regression. *Environmental Health Perspectives, 124*(3), 365–372. https://doi.org/10.1289/ehp.1408933

Li, J., Wang, Y., Fang, F., Chen, D., Gao, Y., Liu, J., Gao, R., Wang, J., & Xiao, H. (2016). Bisphenol A disrupts glucose transport and neurophysiological role of IR/IRS/AKT/GSK3β axis in the brain of male mice. *Environmental Toxicology and Pharmacology, 43*, 7–12. https://doi.org/10.1016/j.etap.2015.11.025

Linares, V., Bellés, M., & Domingo, J. L. (2015). Human exposure to PBDE and critical evaluation of health hazards. *Archives of Toxicology, 89*(3), 335–356. https://doi.org/10.1007/s00204-015-1457-1

Lott, E. L., & Jones, E. B. (2020). *Cholinergic toxicity*. https://www.ncbi.nlm.nih.gov/books/NBK539783

Lyche, J. L., Rosseland, C., Berge, G., & Polder, A. (2015). Human health risk associated with brominated flame-retardants (BFRs). *Environment International, 74*, 170–180. https://doi.org/10.1016/j.envint.2014.09.006

Malliari, E., & Kalantzi, O.-I. (2017). Children's exposure to brominated flame retardants in indoor environments—A review. *Environment International, 108*, 146–169. https://doi.org/10.1016/j.envint.2017.08.011

Mania, M., Rebeniak, M., Szynal, T., Wojciechowska-Mazurek, M., Starska, K., Ledzion, E., & Postupolski, J. (2015). Total and inorganic arsenic in fish, seafood and seaweed—Exposure assessment. *Roczniki Panstwowego Zakladu Higieny (Annals of the National Institute of Hygiene), 66*(2), 203–210. https://pubmed.ncbi.nlm.nih.gov/26400115/

Marciniak, W., Derkacz, R., Muszynska, M., Baszuk, P., Gronwald, J., Huzarski, T., Cybulski, C., Jakubowska, A., Fal, M., Debniak, T., Lener, M., Oszurek, O., Pullella, K., Kotsopoulos, J., Sun, P., Narod, S. A., & Lubinski, J. (2020). Blood arsenic levels and the risk of familial breast cancer in Poland. *International Journal of Cancer, 146*(10), 2721–2727. https://doi.org/10.1002/ijc.32595

Martín, M. M. (2016). *Industrial chemical process analysis and design*. Elsevier.

McCormack, C., Hutchinson, D., Burns, L., Wilson, J., Elliott, E., Allsop, S., Najman, J., Jacobs, S., Rossen, L., Olsson, C., & Mattick, R. (2017). Prenatal alcohol consumption between conception and recognition of pregnancy. *Alcoholism, Clinical and Experimental Research, 41*(2), 369–378. https://doi.org/10.1111/acer.13305

Mégarbane, B. (2014). Toxidrome-based approach to common poisonings. *Asia Pacific Journal of Medical Toxicology, 3*, 2–12. https://doi.org/10.22038/APJMT.2014.2463

Mezynska, M., & Brzóska, M. M. (2018). Environmental exposure to cadmium—A risk for health of the general population in industrialized countries and preventive strategies. *Environmental Science and Pollution Research, 25*, 3211–3232. https://doi.org/10.1007/s11356-017-0827-z

Mitoma, C., Uchi, H., Tsukimori, K., Yamada, H., Akahane, M., Imamura, T., Utani, A., & Furue, M. (2015). Yusho and its latest findings—A review in studies conducted by the Yusho Group. *Environment International, 82*, 41–48. https://doi.org/10.1016/j.envint.2015.05.004

Mitro, S. D., Johnson, T., & Zota, A. R. (2015). Cumulative chemical exposures during pregnancy and early development. *Current Environmental Health Reports, 2*(4), 367–378. https://doi.org/10.1007/s40572-015-0064-x

Moore, K. L., Persaud, T. V. N., & Torchia, M. G. (2016). *The developing human: Clinically oriented embryology* (10th ed.). Elsevier.

Müller, J. E., Meyer, N., Santamaria, C. G., Schumacher, A., Luque, E. H., Zenclussen, M. L., Rodriguez, H. A., & Zenclussen, A. C. (2018). Bisphenol A exposure during early pregnancy impairs uterine spiral artery remodeling and provokes intrauterine growth restriction in mice. *Scientific Reports, 8*(1), 9196. https://doi.org/10.1038/s41598-018-27575-y

Nachman, K. E., Ginsberg, G. L., Miller, M. D., Murray, C. J., Nigra, A. E., & Pendergrast, C.B. (2017). Mitigating dietary arsenic exposure: current status in the United States and recommendations for an improved path forward. *Science of the Total Environment, 581–582*, 221–236. https://doi:.org/10.1016/j.scitotenv.2016.12.112

Nawrot, T. S., Martens, D. S., Hara, A., Plusquin, M., Vangronsveld, J., Roels, H. A., & Staessen, J. A. (2015). Association of total cancer and lung cancer with environmental exposure to cadmium: The meta-analytical evidence. *Cancer Causes & Control, 26*, 1281–1288. https://doi.org/10.1007/s10552-015-0621-5

New Hampshire Department of Environmental Services. (2019). *Environmental fact sheet: Mercury sources, transport, deposition and impacts.* https://www.des.nh.gov/organization/commissioner/pip/factsheets/ard/documents/ard-28.pdf

Nkomo, P., Naicker, N., Matthew, A., Galpin, J., Richter, L. M., & Norris, S. A. (2018). The association between environmental lead exposure with aggressive behavior, and dimensionality of direct and indirect aggression during adolescence: Birth to twenty plus cohort. *Science of the Total Environment, 612*, 472–479. https://doi.org/10.1016/j.scitotenv.2017.08.138

Nuss, D., Obermeyer, R. J., & Kelly, R. E. (2016). Nuss bar procedure: Past, present and future. *Annals Cardiothoracic Surgery, 5*(5), 422–433. https://doi.org/10.21037/acs.2016.08.05

Office of Disease Prevention and Health Promotion. (2020). Social determinants. *Healthy People.* https://www.healthypeople.gov/2020/leading-health-indicators/2020-lhi-topics/Social-Determinants

Ori, M. R., Larsen, J. B., & Shirazi, F. M. (2018). Mercury poisoning in a toddler from home contamination due to skin-lightening cream. *Journal of Pediatrics, 196*, 314–317. https://doi.org/10.1016/j.jpeds.2017.12.023

Osemwengie, L. I., & Morgan, J. (2019). PCBs in older buildings: Measuring PCB levels in caulk and window glazing materials in older buildings. *Environments, 6*(2), 15. https://doi.org/10.3390/environments6020015

Palanza, P., Nagel, S. C., Parmigiani, S., & Vom Saal, F. S. (2016). Perinatal exposure to endocrine disruptors: Sex, timing and behavioral endpoints. *Current Opinion in Behavioral Sciences, 7*, 69–75. https://doi.org/10.1016/j.cobeha.2015.11.017

Parry, E., Zota, A. R., Park, J.-S., & Woodruff, T. J. (2018). Polybrominated diphenyl ethers (PBDEs) and hydroxylated PBDE metabolites (OH-PBDEs): A six-year temporal trend in Northern California pregnant women. *Chemosphere, 195*, 777–783. https://doi.org/10.1016/j.chemosphere.2017.12.065

Patel, N. B., Xu, Y., McCandless, L. C., Chen, A., Yolton, K., Braun, J., Jones, R. L., Dietrich, K. N., & Lanphear, B. P. (2019). Very low-level prenatal mercury exposure and behaviors in children: The HOME Study. *Environmental Health, 18*(4). https:/doi.org/10.1186/s12940-018-0443-5

Pediatric Environmental Health Specialty Units. (2016). *Lead and drinking water: Information for health professionals around the United States*. https://www.pehsu.net/_Library/facts/LeadandDrinkingWater_62116_final.pdf

Peng, L., Huang, Y., Zhang, J., Peng, Y., Lin, X., Wu, K., & Chou, X. (2015a). Cadmium exposure and the risk of breast cancer in Chaoshan population of southeast China. *Environmental Science and Pollution Research, 22*(24), 19870–19878. https://doi.org/10.1007/s11356-015-5212-1

Peng, L., Wang, X., Huo, X., Xu, X., Lin, K., Zhang, J., Huang, Y., & Wu, K. (2015b). Blood cadmium burden and the risk of nasopharyngeal carcinoma: A case-control study in Chinese Chaoshan population. *Environmental Science and Pollution Research, 22*(16), 12323–12331. https://doi.org/10.1007/s11356-015-4533-4

Pivonello, C., Muscogiuri, G., Nardone, A., Garifalos, F., Provvisiero, D. P., Verde, N., de Angelis, C., Conforti, A., Piscopo, M., Auriemma, R. S., Colao, A., & Pivonello, R. (2020). Bisphenol A: An emerging threat to female fertility. *Reproductive Biology and Endocrinology: RB&E, 18*(1), 22. https://doi.org/10.1186/s12958-019-0558-8

Polańska, K., Ligocka, D., Sobala, W., & Hanke, W. (2016). Effect of environmental phthalate exposure on pregnancy duration and birth outcomes. *International Journal of Occupational Medicine and Environmental Health, 29*(4), 683–697. https://doi.org/10.13075/ijomeh.1896.00691

Pycke, B. F. G., Geer, L. A., Dalloul, M., Abulafia, O., & Halden, R. U. (2015). Maternal and fetal exposure to parabens in a multiethnic urban U.S. population. *Environment International, 84*, 193–200. https://doi.org/10.1016/j.envint.2015.08.012

Reuben, A., Caspi, A., Belsky, D. W., Broadbent, J., Harrington, H., Sugden, K., Houts, R. M., Ramrakha, S., Poulton, R., & Moffitt, T. E. (2017). Association of childhood blood lead levels with cognitive function and socioeconomic status at age 38 years and with IQ change and socioeconomic mobility between childhood and adulthood. *JAMA, 317*(12), 1244–1251. https://doi.org/10.1001/jama.2017.1712

Rogers, G. B. (1996). The safety effects of child-resistant packaging for oral prescription drugs. Two decades of experience. *Journal of the American Medical Association, 275*(21), 1661–1665. https://doi.org/10.1001/jama.1996.03530450051032

Runde, T. J., & Nappe, T. M. (2019). *Salicylates toxicity*. https://www.ncbi.nlm.nih.gov/books/NBK499879/

Satarug, S., Vesey, D. A., & Gobe, G. C. (2017). Kidney cadmium toxicity, diabetes and high blood pressure: The perfect storm. *Tohoku Journal of Experimental Medicine, 241*(1), 65–87. https://doi.org10.1620/tjem.241.65

Schaider, J. J., Barkin R. M., Hayden, S. R., Wolfe, R. E., Barkin, A. Z., Philip, S., & Rosen, P. (2015). *Rosen & Barkin's 5-minute emergency medicine consult* (5th ed.). Lippincott Williams & Wilkins.

Scherman, A., Tolosa, J. E., & McEvoy, C. (2018). Smoking cessation in pregnancy: A continuing challenge in the United States. *Therapeutic Advances in Drug Safety, 9*(8), 457–474. https://doi.org/10.1177/2042098618775366

Schraufnagel, D. E., Balms, J. R., Cowl, C. T., De Matteis, S., Jung, S., Mortimer, K., Perez-Padila, R., Rice, M. B., Riojas-Rodriguez, H., Sood, A., Thurston, G. D., To, T., Vanker, A., & Wuebbles, D. J. (2018). Air pollution and noncommunicable diseases. *CHEST Journal, 155*(2), 409–416. https://doi.org/10.1016/j.chest.2018.10.042

Schwebel, D. C., Evans, W. D., Hoeffler, S. E., Marlenga, B. L., Nguyen, S. P., Jovanov, E., Meltzer, D. O., & Sheares, B. J. (2017). Unintentional child poisoning risk: A review of causal factors and prevention studies. *Children's Health Care, 46*(2), 109–130. https://doi.org/10.1080/02739615.2015.1124775

Shin, M.-Y., Lee, S., Kim, H.-J., Lee, J. J., Choi, G., Choi, S., Kim, S., Kim, S. Y., Park, J., Moon, H.-B., Choi, K., & Kim, S. (2016). Polybrominated diphenyl ethers in maternal serum, breast milk, umbilical cord serum, and house dust in a South Korean birth panel of mother-neonate pairs. *International Journal of Environmental Research and Public Health, 13*(8), 767. https://doi.org/10.3390/ijerph13080767

Shoaff, J. R., Romano, M. E., Yolton, K., Lanphear, B. P., Calafat, A. M., & Braun, J. M. (2016). Prenatal phthalate exposure and infant size at birth and gestational duration. *Environmental Research, 150*, 52–58. https://doi.org/10.1016/j.envres.2016.05.033

Sitarik, A., Havstad, S., Kim, H., Zoratti, E. M., Ownby, D., Johnson, C. C., & Wegienka, G. (2020). Racial disparities in allergic outcomes persist to age 10 years in black and white children. *Annals of Allergy, Asthma & Immunology, 124*(4), 342–349. https://doi.org/10.1016/j.anai.2020.01.001

Sly, P. D., Carpenter, D. O., Van den Berg, M., Stein, R. T., Landrigan, P. J., Brune-Drisse, M.-N., & Suk, W. (2016). Health consequences of environmental exposures: Causal thinking in global environmental epidemiology. *Annals of Global Health, 82*(1), 3–9. https://doi.org/10.1016/j.aogh.2016.01.004

Spencer, A. E., Baul, T. D., Sikov, J., Adams, W. G., Tripodis, Y., Buonocore, O., Jellinek, M., Murphy, J. M., & Garg, A. (2019). The relationship between social risks and the mental health of school-age children in primary care. *Academic Pediatrics, 20*(2), 208–215. https://doi.org/10.1016/j.acap.2019.11.006

Spungen, J. H. (2019). Children's exposure to lead and cadmium: FDA total diet study 2014–2016. *Food Additives and Contaminants: Part A, 36*(6), 893–903. https://doi.org/10.1080/19440049.2019.1595170

Stein, C. (2016). Opioid receptors. *Annual Review of Medicine, 67*, 433–451. https://doi.org/10.1146/annurev-med-062613-093100

Street, M. E., & Bernasconi, S. (2020). Endocrine-disrupting chemicals in human fetal growth. *International Journal of Molecular Sciences, 21*(4). https://doi.org/10.3390/ijms21041430

Sui, A. L. (2016). Screening for depression in children and adolescents: US Preventive Services Task Force recommendation statement. *Pediatrics, 137*(3), e20154467. https://doi.org/10.1542/peds.2015-4467

Thurston, S. W., Mendiola, J., Bellamy, A. R., Levine, H., Wang, C., Sparks, A., Redmon, J. B., Drobnis, E. Z., & Swan, S. H. (2016). Phthalate exposure and semen quality in fertile US men. *Andrology, 4*(4), 632–638. https://doi.org/10.1111/andr.12124

Tsai, Y.-A., Lin, C.-L., Hou, J.-W., Huang, P.-C., Lee, M.-C., Chen, B.-H., Wu, M.-T., Chen, C.-C., Wang, S.-L., Lee, C.-C., Hsiung, C. A., & Chen, M.-L. (2016). Effects of high di(2-ethylhexyl) phthalate (DEHP) exposure due to tainted food intake on pre-pubertal growth characteristics in a Taiwanese population. *Environmental Research, 149*, 197–205. https://doi.org/10.1016/j.envres.2016.05.005

Tsai, Y.-A., Tsai, M.-S., Hou, J.-W., Lin, C.-L., Chen, C.-Y., Chang, C.-H., Liao, K.-W., Wang, S.-L., Chen, B.-H., Wu, M.-T., Hsieh, C.-J., & Chen, M.-L. (2018). Evidence of high di(2-ethylhexyl) phthalate (DEHP) exposure due to tainted food intake in Taiwanese pregnant women and the health effects on birth outcomes. *Science of the Total Environment, 618*, 635–644. https://doi.org/10.1016/j.scitotenv.2017.07.175

UNICEF. (2019). *Levels and trends in child mortality 2019*. https://www.unicef.org/reports/levels-and-trends-child-mortality-report-2019

United Nations Environment Programme. (2017). *Minamata Convention on Mercury: Text and annexes*. http://www.mercuryconvention.org/Portals/11/documents/Booklets/COP1%20version/Minamata-Convention-booklet-eng-full.pdf

U.S. Consumer Product Safety Commission. (2005). *Poison prevention packaging: A guide for healthcare professionals*. https://www.cpsc.gov/s3fs-public/384.pdf

U.S. Consumer Product Safety Commission. (2016). *Phthalates business guidance & small entity compliance guide*. https://www.cpsc.gov/Business--Manufacturing/Business-Education/Business-Guidance/Phthalates-Information

U.S. Department of Health and Human Services. (2020). *Smoking cessation: A report of the Surgeon General*. https://www.cdc.gov/tobacco/data_statistics/sgr/2020-smoking-cessation/index.html

U.S. Department of Health and Human Services and U.S. Department of Agriculture. (2020). *2015–2020 dietary guidelines for Americans* (8th ed.). http://health.gov/dietaryguidelines/2015/guidelines/

U.S. Food and Drug Administration. (2016). *Mercury poisoning linked to skin products*. https://www.fda.gov/consumers/consumer-updates/mercury-poisoning-linked-skin-products

U.S. Food and Drug Administration. (2018a). *How did the Food and Drug Administration come about?* https://www.fda.gov/about-fda/fda-basics/how-did-federal-food-drug-and-cosmetic-act-come-about

U.S. Food and Drug Administration. (2018b). *Thimerosal in vaccines questions and answer*. https://www.fda.gov/vaccines-blood-biologics/vaccines/thimerosal-vaccines-questions-and-answers

U.S. Food and Drug Administration. (2020). *Parabens in cosmetics*. https://www.fda.gov/cosmetics/cosmetic-ingredients/parabens-cosmetics

U.S. Food and Drug Administration Center for Drug Evaluation and Research. (2011). *Guidance for industry: Dosage delivery devices for orally ingested OTC liquid drug products*. https://www.fda.gov/media/78087/download

Wang, A., Padula, A., Sirota, M., & Woodruff, T. J. (2016). Environmental influences on reproductive health: The importance of chemical exposures. *Fertility and Sterility, 106*(4), 905–929. https://doi.org/10.1016/j.fertnstert.2016.07.1076

Weaver, M. F. (2015). Prescription sedative misuse and abuse. *Yale Journal of Biology and Medicine, 88*(3), 247–256. https://www.ncbi.nlm.nih.gov/pmc/articles/PMC4553644

Williams, J. F., Smith, V. C., & the Committee on Substance Abuse. (2015). Fetal alcohol spectrum disorders. *Pediatrics, 136*(5), e1395–e1406. https://doi.org/10.1542/peds.2015-3113

World Health Organization. (n.d.). *Ten chemicals of public health concern*. https://www.who.int/ipcs/assessment/public_health/chemicals_phc/en

World Health Organization. (2017). *Inheriting a sustainable world: Atlas on children's health and the environment*. http://www.who.int/ceh/publications/inheriting-a-sustainable-world/en

World Health Organization. (2018a). *Arsenic*. https://www.who.int/news-room/fact-sheets/detail/arsenic

World Health Organization. (2018b). *Environmental noise guidelines for the European region*. https://www.euro.who.int/__data/assets/pdf_file/0008/383921/noise-guidelines-eng.pdf

World Health Organization. (2020a). *Children: Improving survival and well-being*. https://www.who.int/news-room/fact-sheets/detail/children-reducing-mortality

World Health Organization. (2020b). *Social determinants of health*. https://www.who.int/social_determinants/sdh_definition/en

Wu, K. G., Chang, C. Y., Yen, C. Y., & Lai, C. C. (2019). Associations between environmental heavy metal exposure and childhood asthma: A population based study. *Journal of Microbiology, Immunology, and Infection, 52*(2), 352–362. https://doi.org/10.1016/j.jmii.2018.08.001

Xie, J., Yu, J., Fan, Y., Zhao, X., Su, J., Meg, Y., Wu, Y., Uddin, M. B., Wang, C., & Wang, Z. (2020). Low dose lead exposure on the onset of puberty disrupts spermatogenesis-related gene expression and causes abnormal spermatogenesis in mouse. 2020. *Toxicology Applied Pharmacology, 393*, 114942. https://doi.org/10.1016/j.taap.2020.114942

Zajda, K., Ptak, A., Rak, A., Fiedor, E., Grochowalski, A., Milewicz, T., & Gregoraszczuk, E. L. (2017). Effects of human blood levels of two PAH mixtures on the AHR signaling activation pathway and CYP1A1 and COMT target genes in granulosa non-tumor and granulosa tumor cell lines. *Toxicology, 389*, 1–12. https://doi.org/10.1016/j.tox.2017.07.003

Zhou, C., Gao, L., & Flaws, J. A. (2017). Prenatal exposure to an environmentally relevant phthalate mixture disrupts reproduction in F1 female mice. *Toxicology and Applied Pharmacology, 318*, 49–57. https://doi.org/10.1016/j.taap.2017.01.010

Zhou, Z., Lei, Y., Wei, W., Zhao, Y., Jiang, Y., Wang, N., Li, X., & Chen, X. (2019). Association between prenatal exposure to bisphenol A and birth outcomes. *Medicine, 98*(44). https://doi.org/10.1097/MD.0000000000017672

Zigante, M., Peternel, S., Muhvic Urek, M., Rincic Mlinaric, M., Pop Acev, D., & Spalj, S. (2020). Smell and taste in titanium and nickel allergic sensitization in orthodontic patients: Cross-sectional study. *Orthodontics & Craniofacial Research, 23*, 517–522. https://doi.org/10.1111/ocr.12379

Zou, H., Lin, Y., Yang, L., Ou, C., Geng, F., Wang, Y., Chen, W., Niu, Y., Liang, R., Su, Q., & Sun, Y. (2019). Neonatal weight and prenatal exposure to polychlorinated biphenyls: A meta-analysis. *Asian Pacific Journal of Cancer Prevention, 20*(11), 3251–3258. https://doi.org/10.31557/APJCP.2019.20.11.3251

# Newborn Concerns

Lani A. Kajihara-Liehr

## Student Learning Outcomes

**Upon completion of this chapter the reader should be able to:**

1. Discuss pathophysiology and epidemiology of selected disorders of the newborn.
2. Differentiate subjective and objective assessment findings of selected disorders of the newborn.
3. Choose appropriate laboratory or diagnostic tests for selected disorders of the newborn.
4. Utilize the differential diagnosis process to determine a common diagnosis of the newborn.
5. Determine treatment plan, child/family education, and need for referral for newborns with a specific diagnosis.

## INTRODUCTION

The newborn goes through many physiologic changes as it transitions from intrauterine life to extrauterine (or to being a neonate). As these changes occur, several serious health problems can arise, and the primary care provider must be prepared to recognize and manage these health complexities. In addition, providers must be abreast of current medical knowledge in order to provide education and support to families with children.

The content in this chapter maps to the following areas on the Pediatric Nursing Certification Board (PNCB) Pediatric Nurse Practitioner—Primary Care certification examination:

CONTENT AREAS:

**II. Assessment and Diagnosis**

**B. History and Physical Examination**

1. Obtain history of present illness.
2. Obtain a comprehensive health history for new patients.
3. Complete an interval history for established patients.
4. Perform a review of systems.
5. Perform a complete physical examination.

**C. Diagnostic Testing and Screening**

1. Order and interpret office/clinic-based screening tests.
2. Order and interpret diagnostic laboratory tests.
3. Order and interpret the results of diagnostic imaging tests.

**D. Analyzing Information**

1. Integrate health history and physical examination findings into the plan of care.
2. Assimilate findings from screening and diagnostic testing into plan of care.

**E. Diagnosis**

1. Develop and prioritize differential diagnoses.
2. Establish a diagnosis based on evaluation of patient data.

## III. Management

**A. Child and Caregiver Counseling and Education**

1. Provide condition-specific counseling and education, including treatment options.
2. Educate about benefits and potential adverse reactions of pharmacologic interventions.
3. Discuss nonpharmacologic interventions.
4. Counsel regarding the threshold for seeking follow-up care.
5. Review the risks of non-adherence to recommended treatment.

**B. Therapeutic Interventions**

1. Prescribe pharmacologic agents.
3. Order or recommend nonpharmacologic treatments for the management of symptoms.

**C. Procedures**

1. Perform procedures in accordance with diagnostic guidelines and plan of care.

**D. Collaboration and Referral**

2. Refer to specialists as indicated for evaluation, counseling, and/or treatment.

**E. Care Coordination**

1. Facilitate patient and family-centered care for children of all ages with acute and chronic conditions.

**F. Evaluation and Follow-Up**

2. Establish a plan for follow-up care.

## IV. Professional Role and Responsibilities

**A. Leadership and Evidence-Based Practice**

4. Develop, implement, and/or modify clinical practice guidelines.

# ANATOMY AND PHYSIOLOGY

The most significant changes occurring at birth involve the cardiovascular and pulmonary systems, as the infant takes its first breaths and transitions from fetal to newborn circulation. Understanding the basics of fetal anatomy and the transition of the newborn allows the practitioner to be prepared to recognize common newborn concerns.

## Transition From Fetal to Newborn Circulation

In utero, the placenta plays a crucial role in fetal circulation; gas exchange and diffusion occur through the umbilical blood vessels. Fetal oxygenated blood leaves the placenta through the umbilical vein, which passes through the liver into the ductus venosus. This oxygenated blood in the ductus venosus joins the inferior vena cava and enters into the right atrium of the heart. In the fetal heart, the blood is shunted from the right atrium to the left atrium through the foramen ovale. The blood flow is prevented from flowing backwards by the septum primum.

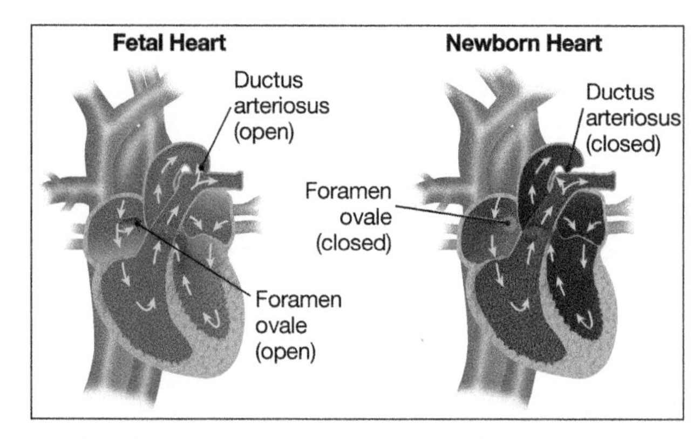


FIGURE 42.1 Comparison between fetal and newborn hearts and circulation.

*Source*: From Gawlik, K. S. (2020). *Evidence-based physical examination*. Springer Publishing Company.

When the umbilical cord is severed at birth and placental circulation ceases, the heart is required to function as a four-chamber system by creating constant back pressure on the septum primum holding it closed, over time closing it permanently. During fetal development, the fetal alveoli are filled with fluid instead of air and pulmonary vessels are constricted; therefore, blood cannot be oxygenated by fetal lungs. Blood flowing within the heart chambers flows through the pulmonary artery, bypassing the lungs for oxygenation. The blood crosses from the right-side of the heart into the left-side through the foramen ovale and/or from the pulmonary artery into the aorta through the ductus arteriosus. After birth, the pulmonary vessels relax, allowing increased blood flow through the lungs and opening of the alveoli (Hoffman et al., 2019; Figure 42.1).

## Bilirubin Metabolism

The newborn's metabolism of bilirubin is essential to understanding and managing hyperbilirubinemia. After birth, the liver and kidneys start to filter the blood within the body. As fetal erythrocytes are broken down and filtered, bilirubin is released and transported into the liver cells where it binds to cytosolic glutathione S-transferase. It is then conjugated by the enzyme bilirubin UDP-glucuronosyl transferase (BUGT). In the newborn, BUGT activity is low, allowing deconjugation of bilirubin and increased difficulty with bilirubin excretion. In addition, bilirubin reabsorption from the intestine occurs due to the lack of bacterial intestinal flora which, when present, produces urobilinoids needed for bilirubin excretion from the gastrointestinal tract (Pan & Rivas, 2017).

## HYPERBILIRUBINEMIA

Jaundice is one of the most common newborn conditions faced by primary care providers and often results in re-hospitalization of the newborn within the first week of life (Akpan et al., 2019). Hyperbilirubinemia occurs when there are elevated bilirubin levels in the neonate's blood (Bhutani, Wong, & Stevenson, 2016). The majority of normal newborns will experience a total serum bilirubin of >1 mg/dL (near the upper limit of the adult normal). When the total serum bilirubin is above 25 mg/dL (428 µmol/L), severe hyperbilirubinemia exists. Severe hyperbilirubinemia places the infant at risk of neurological damage from either acute bilirubin encephalopathy or chronic bilirubin encephalopathy (CBE, formerly termed kernicterus) and leads to risk of death or permanent neurodevelopmental disabilities (Bertini & Dani, 2018; Wong & Bhutani, 2019).

Hyperbilirubinemia in the newborn may be classified as either physiologic or pathologic. Both result in jaundice and icterus. All newborns should be screened for jaundice using an hour-specific nomogram after birth (Bhardwaj et al., 2017). Determining the bilirubin level according to gestational age and post-birth age assists the provider with determining the next course of evaluation and/or treatment.

### UNCONJUGATED HYPERBILIRUBINEMIA

Mild unconjugated hyperbilirubinemia is also known as physiologic jaundice. Unconjugated hyperbilirubinemia may occur as physiologic jaundice or pathologic jaundice. Physiologic jaundice is a mild, unconjugated hyperbilirubinemia and is termed "physiologic" as the healthy newborn has:

- A relatively high red blood cell load with shorter life span with hemolysis of excess cells (increased bilirubin release)
- Low BUGT enzyme activity (so that the bilirubin that is easily deconjugated is reabsorbed in the intestine)
- Slow intestinal mobility
- Absence of intestinal flora to help metabolize the bilirubin
- Increased enterohepatic circulation of bilirubin in the newborn (Pan & Rivas, 2017).

In healthy term or near-term infants, physiologic hyperbilirubinemia occurs without any underlying conditions, beginning on day 2 to 4 of life. The total serum bilirubin is greater than 1.2 mg/dL (usually between 5 and 10 mg/dL before jaundice is noticeable), and the bilirubin returns to normal by age 5 to 8 days (Morris & Omecene, 2021). Additional nonpathologic types of neonatal hyperbilirubinemia are as follows:

- Breastfeeding jaundice may appear in the early neonatal period due to inadequate intake of breast milk (failure to establish an adequate milk supply), increased weight loss, and dehydration.
- Breast milk jaundice occurs later after the first week and lasts longer than breastfeeding jaundice (as long as 2 to 3 months). Compounds in breast milk inhibit the BGUT enzyme and increase the enterohepatic circulation of bilirubin (Pan & Rivas, 2017).

In contrast, pathologic unconjugated hyperbilirubinemia may result from a number of underlying issues that include immune hemolytic disorders and nonimmune hemolytic causes.

Immune hemolytic causes:

- ABO incompatibility: One of the most common causes of hemolytic disease in the newborn. Hemolysis occurs when the mother's blood type (typically O) creates antibodies against the baby's blood type (type A or B), resulting in increased bilirubin release from the hemolyzed cells. ABO incompatibility is seen in approximately 15% of all pregnancies but only results in hemolytic disease in 3% of newborns (Pan & Rivas, 2017).
- Rh incompatibility: Less common but can be more severe in the newborn (Smith, 2020). An Rh-positive fetus is exposed to a Rh-negative mother during pregnancy or delivery. These newborns are often anemic at birth, there is in increase in hepatosplenomegaly, and the hemolysis that occurs can cause severe hyperbilirubinemia. In severe cases, fetal hydrops can occur where there is intrauterine fetal hemolysis. Most Rh disease can be prevented by administering Rho (D) immune globulin to the Rh-negative mother.

Nonimmune hemolytic causes:

- Hereditary spherocytosis: Defects in the red cell membrane cause hemolysis of the cells

- G6PD deficiency: Most common red cell enzyme defect causing hemolysis in neonates of African, Mediterranean, and Asian descent
- Enclosed hemorrhage: Such as cephalohematoma, subgaleal hemorrhage, or extensive bruising
- Gilbert syndrome: Mild autosomal disorder resulting in a defect in the UDPGT gene; more likely to have prolonged neonatal jaundice and breast milk jaundice
- Criglar-Najjar syndrome (UDPGT deficiency): Type I (complete deficiency) results in severe nonhemolytic jaundice early in life, often requiring prolonged phototherapy or liver transplant. Type II (partial deficiency) is usually less severe. Both types place the newborn at increased risk for CBE.

## Subjective Findings

Explore the health history for symptoms such as poor feeding or excessive weight loss (>10% from birth).

The maternal history may reveal:

- Diabetes
- Infection
- Use of medications or herbal preparations.

The birth history may reveal:

- Traumatic delivery
- Preterm delivery

### Risk Factors

The most common risk factors for jaundice are:

- Traumatic birth or birth trauma (significant bruising, cephalohematoma, or subgaleal hematoma)
- Delayed cord clamping
- Blood group incompatibilities (ABO, Rh factor)
- Prematurity
- East Asian or American Indian race
- Prior siblings required phototherapy
- Sepsis
- Maternal blood type O in infant with blood type A, B, or ABO (ABO incompatibility)
- Rh-negative mother with a Rh-positive infant (Rh incompatibility)

### Review of Systems

The most common manifestations revealed during the review of systems include:

- **Constitutional:** inadequate oral intake, breastfeeding difficulties, poor or painful latch.
- **Integumentary:** jaundice after 24 hours of age (physiologic jaundice), jaundice before 24 hours of age (pathologic jaundice)
- **HEENT:** yellow sclerae
- **Gastrointestinal:** loss of stool color, inadequate number of stools
- **Genitourinary:** decreased number of wet diapers
- **Neurological:** changes in mental status—sleepy baby, hard to arouse, irritability

## Objective Findings

The physical examination of the newborn with unconjugated hyperbilirubinemia may reveal:

- Excessive weight loss (>10% of birth weight)
- Yellow color of the skin progressing in a cephalocaudal progression, beginning after 24 hours of age with physiologic jaundice, before 24 hours of age with pathologic jaundice
- Icteric sclerae
- Lethargic, difficult to arouse.

### Laboratory/Diagnostic Testing

A transcutaneous bilirubin reading can be obtained by using a handheld transcutaneous bilirubinometer. While this is more accurate than visual assessment of jaundice, the gold standard remains a total serum bilirubin level. At least one total and direct bilirubin level should be obtained in the newborn if there is any suspicion of jaundice. ABO direct antiglobulin test (DAT) in the newborn also needs to be obtained A direct Coombs test and testing for Rh incompatibility is also important to detect pathologic hyperbilirubinemia (Patel, Desai, & Patel, 2017). Hemoglobin and hematocrit levels may also be useful (Smith, 2020).

## Differential Diagnosis

The differential diagnosis for jaundice includes:

- Physiologic hyperbilirubinemia:
  - Breastfeeding jaundice
  - Breast milk jaundice
- Pathologic hyperbilirubinemia
  - ABO incompatibility
  - Rh incompatibility
  - Hereditary spherocytosis
  - G6PD deficiency
  - Gilbert syndrome

## Treatment/Management Plan

Supportive care for newborns with jaundice includes close follow-up and monitoring. Following serial bilirubin levels prior to discharge and requiring close follow-up with the outpatient practitioner is imperative. According to the updated American Academy of Pediatrics guidelines on the management of hyperbilirubinemia, all pregnant women should be tested for ABO and Rh blood types. The infant's cord blood should be tested for blood type and Rh as well as a direct antibody test (Coombs test), especially if the mother has not had any prenatal blood grouping or is Rh-negative. In any baby that is at risk for ABO incompatibility, obtain a transcutaneous or serum total bilirubin level in the first 24 hours of life and then follow the nomogram for hour-specific bilirubin levels to predict which infants are at risk for hyperbilirubinemia prior to and after discharge from the hospital (Smith, 2020). The BiliTool™ provides this calculation automatically (available: https://bilitool.org)

Phototherapy (bilirubin lights and/or biliblanket) is the initial treatment recommended when the serum total bilirubin falls above the high-risk range according to the infant's age in hours. Infants with Rh incompatibility require phototherapy in the nursery shortly after birth. If there is continued hemolysis, then an exchange transfusion is needed (Smith, 2020). Another intervention that can be provided is giving the infant intravenous (IV) immunoglobulin (IVIG, 0.5–1.0 g/kg) soon after the diagnosis of Rh disorder is confirmed. This can reduce the need for exchange transfusion (Smith, 2020).

### Family Education

Teach the following:

- Signs and symptoms of increasing jaundice.
- Importance of feeding newborn every 2 to 3 hours, not allowing longer than 4 hours in between feedings. Wake the baby to feed if necessary.
- Reassure parents that waking up baby to feed is important.
- Discuss importance of counting number of dirty or wet diapers.
- Importance of keeping the baby's skin exposed to the phototherapy lights and keeping blindfolds over the eyes while under the bili lights. Blindfolds are not required for home bili blankets.

### Referral

Most infants with physiologic hyperbilirubinemia recover without incident. For newborns with pathologic hyperbilirubinemia, referral to a pediatric liver specialist is needed if the bilirubin level does not decrease despite intervention.

## CONJUGATED HYPERBILIRUBINEMIA

Conjugated hyperbilirubinemia is always pathologic and occurs when more than 15% of the total bilirubin is direct. This is also known as cholestasis and is caused by the interrupted flow of bile into the intra- or extrahepatic biliary system or there is impaired bile formation in the liver (Pan & Rivas, 2017). Obstructive causes of conjugated hyperbilirubinemia include total parenteral nutrition administration, infections, metabolic disease and inborn errors of metabolism, and biliary atresia. Conjugated hyperbilirubinemia is caused by total parenteral nutrition administration in the neonatal intensive care unit (NICU) and quickly resolves with oral feeding.

Nonobstructive causes of cholestasis include hepatitis infections such as inflammation of the hepatocytes from herpes, rubella, syphilis, cytomegalovirus, toxoplasmosis, or HIV (Weiss & Vora, 2018). Bacterial infections, such as a urinary tract infection (UTI) or blood sepsis, can result in cholestasis and conjugated hyperbilirubinemia in the neonatal period (Weiss & Vora, 2018). Cholestasis should be considered in the differential diagnosis for any newborn that presents with temperature instability and jaundice.

## BILIARY ATRESIA

The most common type of conjugated hyperbilirubinemia is from biliary atresia. Between 30% and 50% of all neonatal cholestasis is due to biliary atresia (Weiss & Vora, 2018). It is important to diagnosis biliary atresia in newborns because early diagnosis is key to a better prognosis. Biliary atresia occurs when there is inflammation and progressive destruction of intrahepatic and extrahepatic bile ducts that leads to scarring and biliary cirrhosis (Pan & Rivas, 2017). This leads to end-stage liver disease by 6 to 9 months of age and is the most common cause for the need of a liver transplant (Weiss & Vora, 2018). Early diagnosis can lead to surgical repair to re-establish biliary flow and is best when performed before 8 weeks after birth (Pan & Rivas, 2017). Alagille syndrome is the most common genetic cause of obstructive conjugated hyperbilirubinemia. This syndrome is characterized by a paucity of interlobular bile ducts and is associated with the following clinical features: chronic cholestasis, vascular and cardiac anomalies, peculiar facies, butterfly vertebrae, ophthalmologic anomalies, and renal issues (Weiss & Vora, 2018).

Other causes of biliary obstruction include metabolic disease, inborn errors of metabolism, and genetic disorders such as gestational alloimmune liver disease (GALD; Pan & Rivas, 2017). Biliary cysts, gallstones, biliary sludge, tumors, congenital hepatic fibrosis, neonatal sclerosing cholangitis, and bile plug syndrome (inspissated bile) may also be seen (Weiss & Vora, 2018).

## Subjective Findings

The health history may reveal:

- Dark yellow-greenish skin
- Weight loss
- Stools without color (white clay stool)

### Risk Factors

The most common risk factors for biliary atresia are:

- History of maternal infection
- Family history of metabolic disease, inborn errors of metabolism, or liver disease

### Review of Systems

The most common manifestations revealed during the review of systems include:

- **Constitutional:** feeding difficulties including inadequate intake, breastfeeding difficulties, poor or painful latch
- **Integumentary:** jaundice within the first 24 hours of life.
- **HEENT:** changes in scleral color
- **Neurologic:** changes in mental status—sleepy baby, hard to arouse, irritable

## Objective Findings

The physical examination of the child with conjugated biliary atresia may reveal:

- Small for gestational age
- Dark yellow greenish skin color
- Prolonged jaundice (>2 weeks of age)
- Skin rash
- Unusual facies
- Possible murmur
- Enlarged liver and/or spleen
- Possible intra-abdominal mass or ascites
- Acholic stools (lack of color in stool)

### Laboratory/Diagnostic Testing

In the infant with biliary atresia, total bilirubin is moderately elevated and direct bilirubin is significantly elevated. Complete blood count and blood culture rule out infectious causes of cholestasis. Aspartate aminotransferase, alanine aminotransferase, and γ-glutamyl transpeptidase assess for hepatocyte injury. Abdominal ultrasound may reveal hepatobiliary tract structural abnormalities and hepatobiliary iminodiacetic acid scintigraphy (HIDA scan) provides information about biliary obstruction.

▶ ALERT: A conjugated bilirubin greater than 1.0 mg/dL in a child with a total bilirubin less than or equal to 5.0 mg/dL is always pathologic and warrants further investigation (Weiss & Vora, 2018).

## Differential Diagnosis

The differential diagnosis for biliary atresia includes:

- Metabolic diseases
- Inborn errors of metabolism
- TORCH infection
- Alagille syndrome
- Cystic fibrosis
- Gestation alloimmune liver disease (GALD)
- Gallstones
- Hepatitis

## Treatment/Management Plan

Management of newborns with biliary atresia includes following up on the laboratory tests including newborn screening. A common complication for children with biliary atresia includes malabsorption of fat and fat-soluble vitamins, so a diet higher in medium chain triglycerides (MCTs) is important to promote growth (Pan & Rivas, 2017). Specialized prescribed formulas that are higher in MCTs are often advised, such as Alimentum (Abbott), Pregestimil (Mead Johnson), or Enfaport (Mead Johnson; Pan & Rivas, 2017). Supplementation of the fat-soluble vitamins is also necessary with frequent follow-up to monitor their vitamin levels because these infants often continue to have deficiencies despite supplementation (Pan & Rivas, 2017).

### Family Education

Teach the following:

- Advise on the importance of keeping all appointments.
- Monitor signs of increasing jaundice.
- Emphasize the importance of feeding and monitoring intake.
- Monitor the amount and color of stools.
- Adhere to medication regimen as directed.

### Referral

Refer the infant with likely biliary atresia immediately to a pediatric gastroenterologist for appropriate management. These infants will require surgical correction early in life.

# UMBILICAL GRANULOMA

Umbilical granuloma is one of the most common umbilical findings in a newborn. On average, the umbilical cord separates from the umbilicus within 2 weeks after birth. This gives time for the umbilical ring to contract, close, and allow skin to grow over its surface (Beasley, 2017). A localized, mild infection can impair the healing process and a granuloma can form, causing the tissue to become overgrown. Umbilical granuloma is a soft 3- to 10-mm lesion that occurs in the umbilical ring after separation of the umbilical cord (Ogawa et al., 2019). The granuloma is pink, dull red in color, and has a seropurulent secretion. It may be a round, or pedunculated pin-mushroom-shaped lesion in the umbilicus. There is usually no pain or fever.

## Subjective Findings

The health history may reveal:

- Delayed release of umbilical stump
- Discharge from umbilicus after stump has separated (can last for months)
- Redness in and around the umbilicus

### Risk Factors

The risk factor for development of an umbilical granuloma is delayed release of the umbilical stump.

### Review of Systems

The most common manifestations revealed during the review of systems include:

- **Constitutional:** healthy infant who is growing well
- **Integumentary:** umbilical irritation, persistent discharge from umbilicus

## Objective Findings

The physical examination of the child with umbilical granuloma may reveal:

- 3- to 10-mm pink, moist lesion in the umbilical ring
- Erythema in umbilical ring
- Discharge that may be clear or mucopurulent.

## Laboratory/Diagnostic Testing

The diagnosis of umbilical granuloma is based upon the clinical findings; no laboratory or diagnostic testing is needed. If the granuloma does not resolve despite several rounds of silver nitrate, further testing may be indicated. In this case, ultrasound or contrast-enhanced radiography may be useful to identify urachal or omphalomesenteric abnormalities.

## Differential Diagnosis

The differential diagnosis for umbilical granuloma includes:

- Umbilical polyp
- Omphalitis
- Ectopic small bowel mucosa
- Patent urachus
- Urachal cyst
- Omphalomesenteric duct
- Umbilical adenoma
- Umbilical hernia (Beasley, 2017; Ogawa et al., 2019)

## Treatment/Management Plan

- Silver nitrate cauterization—most common treatment
- Table salt
- Topical steroids
- Alcohol wipe use
- Suture ligation
- Excision (Ogawa et al., 2019)

### Family Education

Teach the following:

- Good handwashing
- Importance of keeping diaper below umbilicus until healed
- To not place umbilicus in bath water until healed
- Signs of infection

### Referral

Pediatric surgery may be needed if abnormalities are identified.

### Procedure: Umbilical Cord Cauterization

**Materials:**

- Gloves
- Silver nitrate sticks
- Alcohol swabs
- Gauze
- Saline
- Sterile water

**Steps in the Procedure:**

1. Discuss the procedure with the family, proceeding with their consent.
2. Wash and dry hands well.

3. Put on gloves.
4. Clean umbilicus with alcohol swabs, allowing the area to dry (or dry off with gauze).
5. Moisten one silver nitrate stick with one drop of distilled or de-ionized water.
6. Apply the silver nitrate stick to the umbilical granuloma.
   - Caution should be used as silver nitrate burns and can cause black staining of the periumbilical and abdominal skin; some recommend applying petroleum jelly around the umbilical site to protect the skin.
7. Repeat if necessary.
8. Use saline to clean the skin around the umbilicus (saline neutralizes silver nitrate) then rinse area with water (Jakhar et al., 2018).
9. Advise parents to keep area clean and dry until healed.
10. Repeat if not completely healed in 1 week.

## CIRCUMCISION

Male circumcision is not just a medical decision but a parental choice that is performed mostly for cultural or religious traditions (Freedman, 2016). The decision to circumcise a newborn baby is multifactorial and parents factor religion, culture, aesthetic preference, familial identity, and personal experience into their decision (Freedman, 2016). Existing evidence demonstrates circumcision protects against certain medical conditions such as UTI, penile and prostate cancers, and various sexually transmitted infections including HIV (Starzyk et al., 2015). In August 2012, the American Academy of Pediatrics published an updated policy statement explaining that the benefits associated with circumcision outweigh the risks (Starzyk et al., 2015), also noting that the benefits were not great enough to recommend routine circumcision (Freedman, 2016). There are several reasons that circumcision may not be an option directly after a baby is born, including a premature or ill neonate; small penis size; any phallic abnormality, such as hypospadias, penile torsion, chordee, or mega urethra; or history of bleeding disorder (Starzyk et al., 2015). This procedure is a parental decision. Healthcare providers are to inform parents of the benefits and the risks of circumcision.

▶ ALERT: If hypospadias is suspected, do not perform circumcision without consultation with a pediatric urologist; the foreskin is used in the repair of hypospadias.

### Treatment/Management Plan

Newborn circumcision (performed within the first month of life) is typically performed under local anesthesia with one of three methods (Plastibell method, use of the Gomco, or Mogen clamp). With the Plastibell method, a plastic device is placed directly on the glans of the phallus, but underneath the foreskin. A tied piece of suture holds the Plastibell in place. The foreskin is excised, and the plastic tip of the device is removed, leaving a plastic ring around the glans of the phallus. As the skin heals, the plastic ring will naturally fall off of the glans. In either clamp method, the metal clamp is applied to the glans penis, with the foreskin threaded through the base plate. Tension is applied with the clamp and the excise foreskin is then excised. Observe for bleeding and for first urinary void after the procedure.

### Family Education

Teach the following:

- Use petrolatum jelly and gauze on the tip of the penis with each diaper change for the first few days after circumcision.
- Change diaper frequently.
- Reassure that yellow crusting on the tip of the penis is normal and should resolve in a few days. Advise on signs and symptoms of infection.
- Use of antipyretics and pain medication is not recommended.

## BIRTH TRAUMA

Several types of injury may occur to the infant during delivery (Table 42.1). Many of these are fairly benign in nature, such as caput succedaneum, cephalohematoma, clavicular fracture, and facial nerve palsy. Caput succedaneum and cephalohematoma result from pressure on the newborn's skull as it passes through the birth canal or application of a vacuum to assist with the birthing process. Clavicular fracture typically occurs in larger newborns or those having experienced shoulder dystocia during delivery. Facial nerve injury may result from forceps use or from in utero pressure of the newborn's head against the mother's sacrum. Brachial plexus injury can be slightly more involved and is discussed in the text that follows.

▶ ALERT: Newborns with intracranial hemorrhage may present with irritability, altered tone, altered level of consciousness, seizure, respiratory depression, or apnea.

TABLE 42.1 **Objective Findings and Management of Common Types of Birth Trauma**

| Type of Birth Trauma | Objective Findings | Management |
|---|---|---|
| Caput succedaneum | Diffuse edema of the soft tissues of the scalp, crossing suture lines, possible bruising | No treatment necessary; resolves within a few days |
| Cephalohematoma | Edema of the scalp (from subperiosteal collection of blood) that does not cross suture lines; may increase in size several hours after birth | No treatment necessary; typically resolves within 6 to 8 weeks, though it may leave a small calcified area on the scalp (the brain is unaffected) |
| Clavicular fracture | Decreased movement of the affected arm; tenderness and crepitus over the affected clavicle | Gentle handling and immobilization on the affected side by aligning the humerus alongside the chest with the elbow flexed |
| Facial nerve palsy | Asymmetrical eye closure and mouth movements with decreased facial movement on the affected side | No treatment necessary; resolves spontaneously in a few days to weeks |

*Source*: Data from Smith, D. (2020). The newborn infant. In W. W. Hay, M. J. Levin, M. J. Abzug, & M. Bunik (Eds.), *Current diagnosis & treatment: Pediatrics* (25th ed., pp. 10–65). McGraw-Hill Education.

## BRACHIAL PLEXUS INJURY

Brachial plexus injury is a rare neonatal injury, only occurring in up to 0.3% of births (Russman, 2020). Brachial plexus injury results in flaccid paresis of the arm of a newborn. Bilateral involvement only occurs in about 5% of cases (Russman, 2020). This injury was thought to result from birth trauma, when there is traction on the brachial plexus nerve at delivery, such as seen with shoulder dystocia. More recently, it has been suggested that this injury may result from abnormal infant positioning or from an abnormal uterine environment.

The types of brachial plexus injury that occur at birth include the following:

- Erb palsy involves cervical nerve root five and six (C5, C6) and occurs in 50% of cases.
- Erb palsy plus involves cervical nerve roots five through 7 (C5, C6, C7) and occurs in 35% of cases.
- Complete brachial plexus involves all the nerve roots in the plexus cervical root 5 through thoracic 1 (CN5-T1).
- Klumpke palsy involves cervical nerve root eight and thoracic nerve one (CN8 and T1) and occurs least frequently (Russman, 2020).

### Subjective Findings

The health history may reveal decreased or lack of use of an upper extremity.

### Risk Factors

The only true established risk factor for brachial nerve palsy is shoulder dystocia, although brachial nerve palsy has been known to occur in macrosomic infants, as well as those who have a maternal history of diabetes mellitus or excessive gestational weight gain, have labor abnormalities, or undergo an operative vaginal birth (forceps or vacuum extraction).

### Review of Systems

The most common manifestations revealed during the review of systems include:

- **Musculoskeletal:** decreased movement in upper extremity, poor tone in one upper extremity
- **Neurological:** weak Moro reflex, pain

### Objective Findings

The physical examination of the child with brachial plexus injury may reveal:

- Poor muscle tone in one upper extremity or asymmetric Moro reflex
- Erb palsy
  - Upper arm adduction with internal rotation, and extended forearm (hand and wrist movement are preserved)
- Erb palsy plus
  - Upper arm adduction with internal rotation, extended and pronated forearm with flexed wrist and fingers ("waiter's tip" posture)
- Klumpke palsy
  - Isolated hand paralysis, decreased pupil size and drooping eyelid on affected side (Horner syndrome)
- Complete brachial palsy: no movement of affected arm.

### Laboratory/Diagnostic Testing

The diagnosis of brachial plexus injury is based upon the clinical findings. Ultrasound may prove useful for visualization of the brachial plexus and cervical nerves 5 to 8. If associated fracture is suspected, obtain x-rays.

### Differential Diagnosis

The differential diagnosis for brachial plexus injury includes:

- Humerus fracture
- Clavicle fracture
- Shoulder dislocation
- Cerebral injury
- Lower cervical injury
- Amyoplasia congenita

### Treatment/Management Plan

Conservative management is recommended with gentle handling. No improvement in function by 1 month of age is concerning and specialty referral needs to be considered.

### Family Education

Teach the following:

- Perform gentle handling; immobilization is not needed.
- Position the affected arm appropriately; mimic action with the affected arm.
- Place a wrist rattle on the affected arm.
- With time, function is likely to return.

### Referral

Refer to an occupational therapist if deficits are present at 7 to 10 days of age. If there is lack of function in the affected arm by 1 month of age, refer to a pediatric neurosurgeon or pediatric orthopedist. Reconstructive surgery may be needed if there is no deltoid or bicep activity noted at 3 months of age.

## NEONATAL ABSTINENCE SYNDROME

As many as 13% of women over age 18 report use of illicit (federally illegal drug or misuse of prescription opioids) drugs annually (Wright, 2019). The incidence of opioid-exposed infants has risen fivefold in the United States (Winkelman et al., 2018). Any newborn that is born to a mother who has a substance use disorder is at risk for withdrawal. More clinically significant is if the infant is exposed to opioids in utero. These newborns need to be screened for neonatal abstinence syndrome (NAS). NAS is a very costly, complex syndrome in which the newborn exhibits symptoms of withdrawal shortly after birth (Khan, 2020). Newborns with NAS have prolonged hospital stays (often in the NICU) and have higher rates of readmission to the hospital. Different types of opioids lead to different types of withdrawal symptoms. According to Khan (2020), methadone withdrawal presents with tremors, hypertonia, exaggerated reflexes, and myoclonic jerks, whereas withdrawal from buprenorphine more often presents with temperature instability, sneezing, sweating, and mottling. Knowing what substances the newborn has been exposed to can help the provider anticipate the newborn's needs and can allow for more thorough anticipatory guidance and education for all caregivers (Khan, 2020).

Other factors that contribute to the well-being of the opioid-exposed newborn are how healthy the mother was during the pregnancy; the type, amount, and extent of opioid exposure to the neonate; metabolism of the mother and neonate; genetic variabilities; whether there was exposure to more than one substance; and other comorbidities such as infection (Khan, 2020). These infants are at higher risk for congenital anomalies. Infants with exposure to multiple substances (polysubstance use), along with cigarette exposure and male gender, have been known to have more severe symptoms, while premature infants are more likely to have a milder course. They may also be a genetic factor that influences the severity of symptoms (Anbalagan & Mendez, 2020).

### Subjective Findings

The maternal health history may reveal:

- Irritability, poor sleep, tremors, poor feeding, respiratory distress, even seizures
- Documented or reported maternal history of use of alcohol, drugs (prescribed or recreational), and/or tobacco
- Poor or no prenatal care
- Psychiatric disease or substance abuse
- Unexplained fetal demise, repeated spontaneous abortion, or precipitous labor.

The newborn history may reveal:

- Poor tone after delivery
- Poor feeding
- High pitched cry
- Frequent yawning

- Irritability
- Difficult to console
- Sweating (Khan, 2020).

### Risk Factors

The risk factors for NAS are:

- Maternal history of substance use or abuse
- Maternal psychiatric disorder

### Review of Systems

The most common manifestations revealed during the review of systems include:

- **Constitutional:** poor feeding, dehydration, excessive weight loss, temperature instability
- **Gastrointestinal:** diarrhea, vomiting
- **Neurologic:** high-pitched cry, irritability (Anbalagan & Mendez, 2019; Khan, 2020)

## Objective Findings

Timing of the physical examination findings is multifaceted and is dependent on the timing of and type of substance(s) to which the newborn was exposed prior to delivery. In heroin exposure, the withdrawal is short-acting and presents in the first 24 to 48 hours of life, whereas long-acting buprenorphine withdrawal may present at 36 to 60 hours from birth, and with methadone withdrawal may present at 48 to 72 hours from birth (Anbalagan & Mendez, 2020). Infants with exposure to multiple substances, along with cigarette exposure, and male gender have been known to have more severe symptoms, while premature infants are more likely to have a milder course (Anbalagan & Mendez, 2020).

When neonatal exposure of substances is suspected, it is important to monitor the newborn closely. There are multiple tools that are available for use. The most widely used is the modified Finnegan NAS (FNAS) scoring system. The FNAS scores 21 different symptoms of withdrawal in three different categories to guide the user to initiate, titrate, or terminate therapy (Khan, 2020). The scoring is performed every 4 hours after feedings; a score of eight or above advised initiation of treatment or escalation of therapy (Anbalagan & Mendez, 2020). Another approach that is currently being researched is the Eat, Sleep, Console (ESC) method that assesses the ability of the newborn to function after birth. This approach advises that if the newborn can eat more than 1 ounce per feeding, sleep for longer than 1 hour, and be consoled within 10 minutes, then pharmacologic treatment is not needed. This method has been shown to decrease the amount of pharmacologic intervention required for withdrawal (Khan, 2020).

The physical examination of the infant with NAS may reveal:

- Triad of increased muscle tone, tremors when undisturbed, and exaggerated Moro reflex
- Excessive sneezing, stuffy nose, or yawning
- Seizures
- Sweating/poor temperature control
- Diaper rash

## Laboratory/Diagnostic Testing

NAS is based on pertinent clinical findings in an infant with a high suspicion of exposure. There are several ways to test for substance exposure in the newborn, including testing the newborn's urine, meconium, cord blood, and hair for evidence of a particular substance. Testing the newborn's urine and meconium for illicit substances is the most practiced because of the ease of collection and obtaining results (Anbalagan & Mendez, 2020). Urine testing can be variable in that it is dependent on the type of substance used, amount, and timing of the last dose. It is also dependent on when the urine is collected: the first void is preferred (Anbalagan & Mendez, 2020). Meconium testing is the most sensitive because it can identify the substance exposure from back to 20 weeks of gestation (Anbalagan & Mendez, 2020). All testing can have false negatives and positives depending on timing and method of collecting the specimens, so interpretation needs to be done with care. The more accurate way of testing for substances is a combination of testing the newborn's meconium and the maternal urine (Anbalagan & Mendez, 2020).

## Differential Diagnosis

The differential diagnosis for NAS includes:

- Infection
- Hypoglycemia
- Hyperthyroidism
- Intracranial hemorrhage
- Hypoxic-ischemic encephalopathy
- Seizure disorder

## Treatment/Management Plan

Utilize a standardized NAS scoring tool to determine the severity of opioid withdrawal in the newborn. One such tool, the modified FNAS tool, is available for use online (www.mdcalc.com/modified-finnegan-neonatal-abstinence-score-nas).

## Nonpharmacologic Therapies

Treatment for newborns with NAS should always start with nonpharmacologic therapies. It should be noted that each newborn with NAS has neurobehavioral dysfunction with disorganized behavior so the provider must adapt to the individual newborn's needs (Anbalagan & Mendez, 2020). Encourage the family to be a part of the newborn's care if possible. Changes to the physical environment to decrease stimuli include darkening the room to reduce visual stimuli, quieting the surrounding environment to decrease auditory stimuli, and clustering of care to reduce tactile stimulation. Swaddling, swaying, vertical rocking, and a side-lying C-position can help reduce irritability. Kangaroo care by allowing the parent to hold the baby skin to skin has also shown to be helpful (Khan, 2020). Pacifier use helps to decrease oral hypersensitivity.

Encourage mothers to breastfeed, unless contraindicated (i.e., HIV infection, IV drug use, or polysubstance abuse). Breast milk from mothers in treatment programs utilizing methadone or buprenorphine has been shown to help with withdrawal symptoms in their newborns because these medications do cross over into the breast milk and decrease the need for pharmacologic support (Anbalagan & Mendez, 2020; Khan, 2020). Some infants may require the use of calorie-dense formula (150 Kcal/kg/day) in small, frequent feedings (Anbalagan & Mendez, 2020).

Caregiver participation is essential in the discharge planning process. Essential components include include creating a safe plan of care that includes: responsive care giving, providing a safe and secure environment, providing adequate and appropriate nutrition, and promoting healthy behaviors in the parents (Bordelon et al., 2020)

## Pharmacologic Therapies

Pharmacologic therapy is started only when the newborn has sustained high withdrawal scores or there are more serious symptoms that occur (e.g., seizures or vomiting and diarrhea), which have led to dehydration (Khan, 2020). Medications include:

- *Methadone*: This is a long-acting synthetic opioid. It is given twice daily and allows for better control of symptoms with less frequent disruptions to the infant but limits the frequency of titration. Methdone is metabolized by cytochrome 450 enzymes, so it can interact with many different medications such as phenobarbital and antivirals (Anbalagan & Mendez, 2020).
- *Buprenorphine*: This is a partial agonist opioid that has shown shorter lengths of hospitalizations than with methadone or morphine. It is administered sublingually, which makes it easier to give (Anbalagan & Mendez, 2020).
- *Morphine*: This is the most used short-acting opioid; however, it is associated with longer lengths of stay in the hospital due to its need for slower weaning. Dosing varies based on severity of symptoms and withdrawal scores, generally starting at 0.04 mg/kg/dose (maximum 0.2 mg/kg/dose) and is given every 3 to 4 hours. This allows for easy titration but disturbs the infant frequently (Anbalagan & Mendez, 2020).
- *Adjunct medications*: Phenobarbital and clonidine may also be utilized (Khan, 2020).

Most of these infants who require pharmacologic therapy are managed as inpatients for the entire length of therapy until their symptoms are well under control off therapeutic medication(s). However, there are some infants who may be managed as inpatients, then as outpatients to complete the weaning process. Outpatient management has been shown to increase the days on pharmacotherapy, and there are concerns about management in parents who are at risk of relapse (Anbalagan & Mendez, 2020).

▶ ALERT: Naloxone hydrocholoride (Narcan) is an opioid antagonist and is not recommended in the management of NAS. Its safety profile has not been studied in neonates and it can accelerate withdrawal symptoms (Anbalagan & Mendez, 2020).

## Family Education

Teach the following:

- Causes and treatment of NAS including medication administration
- How to identify and respond to the newborn's cues
- How to handle the newborn, including swaddling, swaying, vertical C-position
- Breastfeeding

**PRO TIP** Ensure that a safety plan is in place with the hospital's department of family and children services' involvement prior to discharge.

## Referral

Newborns with NAS and their families should be referred to social work, case management, the department of human services or child and family services, and early intervention.

# NEONATAL HERPES SIMPLEX INFECTION

In the United States, neonatal herpes simplex virus (HSV) affects about 1,500 to 2,200 infants per year with about 75% of cases caused by infection with HSV-2, and 25% of cases associated with HSV-1 (Grossman & Ivan, 2017). Neonatal transmission may occur in utero, during the peripartum period, or postnatally. Infection occurs most commonly during vaginal delivery as the neonate moves through the birth canal; however, uncommon transplacental and postnatal transmissions have been documented. Symptoms usually arise during the first week of life but have also presented at 3 or 4 weeks of age. The infection is classified based on the extent of involvement. Infection of the skin, eyes, or mouth may occur. Central nervous infection is a major complication of neonatal HSV and has the highest morbidity involving the brain. Disseminated disease is the most serious, involves multiple organs (lung, liver, adrenal glands, brain, and skin), and often causes death (Kabani & Kimberlin, 2018).

## Subjective Findings

The health history may reveal:

- Skin rash
- Fever or hypothermia

### Risk Factors

The most common risk factors for neonatal HSV infection are:

- Maternal history of first HSV infection during third trimester or open labial lesions at the time of birth
- Invasive monitoring of the fetus
- Delivery earlier than 38 weeks of gestation
- Maternal age less than 21 years

### Review of Systems

The most common manifestations revealed during the review of systems include:

- **Constitutional:** temperature instability, poor feeding, weight loss
- **Integumentary:** rash
- **Respiratory:** respiratory distress, apnea
- **Gastrointestinal:** vomiting
- **Neurologic:** irritability, lethargy, seizure

## Objective Findings

The physical examination of the child with neonatal HSV may reveal:

- Hyper- or hypothermia
- Weight loss
- Vesiculopapular or vesiculoulcerative lesions on an erythematous base
- Purpura
- Cyanosis, tachypnea, respiratory distress
- Hepatomegaly
- Bulging fontanel
- Cranial nerve abnormalities

### Laboratory/Diagnostic Testing

Neonatal HSV infection may be diagnosed based upon clinical presentation and confirmed with viral culture (isolated from skin, urine, blood, stool, or mucous membranes), immunofluorescence, or polymerase. Cerebrospinal fluid should be obtained if disseminated or central nervous system HSV is suspected. Obtain alanine aminotransferase if hepatic involvement is suspected (Kabani & Kimberlin, 2018).

## Differential Diagnosis

The differential diagnosis of neonatal HSV infection includes:

- Neonatal sepsis
- Cytomegalovirus
- Erythema toxicum
- Transient neonatal pustular melanosis
- Scabies
- Herpes zoster

## Treatment/Management Plan

Neonatal HSV infection requires hospitalization and treatment with IV acyclovir. Treatment of infants younger than 3 months must be continued for 21 days, and for infants older than 3 months old treatment should continue for 14 to 21 days (Grossman & Ivan, 2017). Ocular infection is treated with vidarabine, trifluridine, or iododeoxyuridine.

### Family Education

Teach the following:

- Importance of good handwashing
- Maintenance of hydration
- Completion of medications upon discharge from hospital
- Close developmental follow-up after discharge
- Any family member with open lesion on lips, mouth, or fingers should avoid contact with newborn.

## Referral

Neonatal HSV infection requires hospitalization for IV acyclovir treatment and intensive monitoring by critical care, neonatology, and infectious disease staff. With suspected central nervous system involvement, also consult a pediatric neurologist. Refer to a pediatric developmental care team for postdischarge follow-up.

## KEY POINTS

- Jaundice commonly occurs in newborns.
- Physiologic hyperbilirubinemia is treated with phototherapy, frequent feeding, and serial bilirubin measurements.
- Pathologic hyperbilirubinemia manifests as jaundice within the first 24 hours of life and requires prompt recognition and treatment.
- Circumcision is a cultural and/or religious decision with both risks and benefits. It may be accomplished via the Plastibell or clamp method.
- Birth trauma such as caput succedaneum, cephalohematoma, clavicular fracture, and facial nerve palsy usually resolve without incident and only require supportive care.
- The treatment of brachial plexus injury is gentle handling and referral to pediatric occupational therapy.
- With NAS it is very important to provide supportive care to baby, mother, and extended family in a nonjudgmental manner, reserving pharmacologic treatment for infants with high withdrawal scores.
- Neonatal HSV infection requires hospitalization for IV acyclovir therapy and intensive care.

## REFERENCES


Akpan, U., Orth, E., Moore, R., Timoney, P. M., Cavaliere, T. A., Davila, R. C., & Calhoun, D. A. (2019). The hematopoietic system. In A. J. Jnah & A. N. Trembath (Eds.), *Fetal and neonatal physiology for the advanced practice nurse* (pp. 191–238). Springer Publishing Company.

Anbalagan, S., & Mendez, M. D. (2020). *Neonatal abstinence syndrome*. https://www.ncbi.nlm.nih.gov/books/NBK551498

Beasley, S. W. (2017). Umbilicus and its extensive clinical repertoire. *Journal of Paediatrics and Child Health, 53*(11), 1123–1126. https://doi.org/10.1111/jpc.13760

Bertini, G., & Dani, C. (2018). Bilirubin metabolism, unconjugated hyperbilirubinemia, and physiologic neonatal jaundice. In G. Buonocore, R. Bracci, & M. Weindling (Eds.), *Neonatology: A practical approach to neonatal diseases* (2nd ed., pp. 1143–1149). Springer.

Bhardwaj, K., Locke, T., Biringer, A., Booth, A., Darling, E. K., Dougan, S., Harrison, J., Hill, S., Johnson, A., Makin, S., Potter, B., Lacaze-Masmonteil, T., & Little, J. (2017). Newborn bilirubin screening for preventing severe hyperbilirubinemia and bilirubin encephalopathy: A rapid review. *Current Pediatric Reviews, 13*(1), 67–90. https://doi.org/10.2174/1573396313666170110144345.

Bhutani, V. K., Wong, R. J., & Stevenson, D. K. (2016) Hyperbilirubinemia in Preterm Neonates, *Clinics in Perinatology, 43*(2), 215–232. https://doi.org/10.1016/j.clp.2016.01.001

Bordelon, C., Wood, T., Johnson, M., & Fogger, S. (2020). Transition home. *Journal of Addictions Nursing, 31*(1), 60–65. https://doi.org/10.1097/jan.0000000000000325

Freedman, A. L. (2016). The circumcision debate: Beyond benefits and risks. *Pediatrics, 137*(5). https://doi.org/10.1542/peds.2016-0594

Grossman, L. K., & Ivan, Y. (2017). Herpes infections. In T. K. McInerny, H. M. Adam, D. E. Campbell, T. G. DeWitt, J. M. Foy, & D. M. Kamat (Eds.), *American Academy of Pediatrics textbook of pediatric care* (2nd ed., Chapter 266). American Academy of Pediatrics.

Hoffman, J., Thompson-Bowie, N., & Jnah, A. J. (2019). The cardiovascular system. In A. J. Jnah & A. N. Trembath (Eds.), *Fetal and neonatal physiology for the advanced practice nurse* (pp. 119–158). Springer Publishing Company.

Jakhar, D., Tandon, N., Makkar, R., Kaur, I., & Chilana, A. S. (2018). Pre-activated silver nitrate for umbilical granuloma. *Research in Clinical Dermatology, 1*(1), 12–13. https://doi.org/10.35841/clinical-dermatology.1.1.12-13

Kabani, N., & Kimberlin, D. (2018). Neonatal herpes simplex virus infection. In J. Cantey (Ed.), *Neonatal infections: Pathophysiology, diagnosis, and management* (pp. 119–126). Springer.

Khan, L. (2020). Neonatal abstinence syndrome. *Pediatric Annals, 49*(1), e3–e7. https://doi.org/10.3928/19382359-20191211-01

Morris, M., & Omecene, N. E. (2021). Liver: Pediatrics considerations. In N. C. Tkacs, L. L. Herrmann, & R. L. Johnson (Eds.), *Advanced physiology and pathophysiology: Essentials for clinical practice* (pp. 530–532). Springer Publishing Company.

Ogawa, C., Sato, Y., Suzuki, C., Mano, A., Tashiro, A., Niwa, T., Hamazaki, S., Tanahashi, Y., Suzumura, M., Hayano, S., Hayakawa, M., Tsuji, T., Hoshino, S., Sugiyama, Y., Kidokoro, H., Kawada, J., Muramatsu, H., Hirakawa, A., Ando, M., ... Kojima, S. (2019). Correction: Treatment with silver nitrate versus topical steroid treatment for umbilical granuloma: A non-inferiority randomized control trial. *PLoS ONE, 14*(6), e0192688. https://doi.org/10.1371/journal.pone.0192688

Pan, D. H., & Rivas, Y. (2017). Jaundice. In T. K. McInerny, H. M. Adam, D. E. Campbell, T. G. DeWitt, J. M. Foy, & D. M. Kamat (Eds.), *American Academy of Pediatrics textbook of pediatric care* (2nd ed., Chapter 170). American Academy of Pediatrics.

**Patel, A., Desai, D., & Patel, A. (2017).** Association of ABO and Rh incompatibility with neonatal hyperbilirubinaemia. *International Journal of Reproduction, Contraception, Obstetrics and Gynecology, 6*(4), 1368–1375. http://doi.org/10.18203/2320-1770.ijrcog20171393

Russman, B. (2020). Neonatal brachial plexus injury. *UpToDate.* Retrieved September 13, 2020, from https://www.uptodate.com/contents/neonatal-brachial-plexus-palsy

Smith, D. (2020). The newborn infant. In W. W. Hay, M. J. Levin, M. J. Abzug, & M. Bunik (Eds.), *Current diagnosis & treatment: Pediatrics* (25th ed., pp. 10–65). McGraw-Hill Education.

Starzyk, E. J., Kelley, M. A., Caskey, R. N., Schwartz, A., Kennelly, J. F., & Bailey, R. C. (2015). Infant male circumcision:

Healthcare provider knowledge and associated factors. *PLoS ONE, 10*(1). https://doi.org/10.1371/journal.pone.0115891

Weiss, A. K., & Vora, P. V. (2018). Conjugated hyperbilirubinemia in the neonate and young infant. *Pediatric Emergency Care, 34*(4), 280–283. https://doi.org/10.1097/pec.0000000000001467

Winkelman, T. N., Villapiano, N., Kozhimannil, K. B., Davis, M. M., & Patrick, S. W. (2018). Incidence and costs neonatal abstinence syndrome among infants with Medicaid: 2004–2014. *Pediatrics, 141*(4), e20173520. https://doi.org/10.1542/peds.2017-3520

Wright, M. E. (2019). *Perinatal substance exposure*. The 4th Annual SC NAPNAP Conference, Charleston, SC.

# Children With Special Healthcare Needs

Shelby R. Boone, Elizabeth P. Elliott, Donna Lisa Evans,
Wendy Quiroz Nasser, and Theresa Kyle

## Student Learning Outcomes

**Upon completion of this chapter the reader should be able to:**

1. Describe the unique healthcare and developmental needs experienced by the medically fragile child and their family.
2. Identify skills needed by families caring for the technology-dependent child at home.
3. Distinguish particular medical and developmental needs of the former premature infant.
4. Describe strategies for the successful transition to adulthood for the adolescent with special healthcare needs.
5. Discuss the role of the nurse practitioner in caring for the child undergoing chemotherapy, the childhood cancer survivor, and the terminally ill child.

## INTRODUCTION

The number of children with a diagnosis of at least one chronic illness (a long-lasting or recurrent illness) is increasing, with 30% of children having a chronic illness (Hall et al., 2019). A subset of this group, children and youth with special healthcare needs (CYSHCN), is comprised of those who are at particular risk due to their illness(es) and require significantly more care than other children. Twenty percent of the child population in the United States (U.S.) is considered to be CYSHCN (Health Resources and Services Administration [HRSA], Maternal and Child Health Bureau, n.d.). Among these children, larger numbers are living with the assistance of high-tech treatments and equipment.

As continued medical advances are made, more children will be living with chronic illnesses and technological dependencies. These children will be cared for by the primary care provider (PCP), and many disease-specific symptoms and complications will be managed in the outpatient setting. The PCP should be familiar with surveillance methods, management strategies, and complications for CYSHCN.

The content in this chapter maps to the following areas on the Pediatric Nursing Certification Board (PNCB) Pediatric Nurse Practitioner—Primary Care certification examination:

### CONTENT AREAS:

#### II. Assessment and Diagnosis

**B. History and Physical Examination**

1. Obtain history of present illness.
2. Obtain a comprehensive health history for new patients.
1. Complete an interval history for established patients.
2. Perform a review of systems.
3. Perform a complete physical examination.

**C. Diagnostic Testing and Screening**

1. Order and interpret office/clinic-based screening tests.
2. Order and interpret diagnostic laboratory tests.

**D. Analyzing Information**

1. Integrate health history and physical examination findings into the plan of care.
2. Assimilate findings from screening and diagnostic testing into the plan of care.

**E. Diagnosis**

1. Develop and prioritize differential diagnoses.
2. Establish a diagnosis based on evaluation of patient data.

### III. Management

**A. Child and Caregiver Counseling and Education**

1. Provide condition-specific counseling and education, including treatment options.
2. Educate about benefits and potential adverse reactions of pharmacologic interventions.
4. Counsel regarding the threshold for seeking follow-up care.
5. Review the risks of non-adherence to recommended treatment.

**B. Therapeutic Interventions**

2. Recommend the use of over-the-counter pharmacologic agents.
3. Order or recommend nonpharmacologic treatments for the management of symptoms.

**D. Collaboration and Referral**

2. Refer to specialists as indicated for evaluation, counseling, and/or treatment.

**E. Care Coordination**

1. Facilitate patient and family-centered care for children of all ages with acute and chronic conditions.

**F. Evaluation and Follow-Up**

2. Establish a plan for follow-up care.

### IV. Professional Role and Responsibilities

**A. Leadership and Evidence-Based Practice**

4. Develop, implement, and/or modify clinical practice guidelines.

## THE MEDICALLY FRAGILE CHILD

CYSHCN may have functional limitations requiring therapy and may need medications, medical care, and educational or mental health services more than other children of their same age. The multiple needs of CYSHCN present challenges for families in navigating the system and obtaining the services the child requires. When a child is injured and requires long-term rehabilitation and special care, when an infant is born very prematurely, or when a child is diagnosed with a complex chronic health condition, the parents may be initially devastated. Yet they learn to adapt and become experts in the care of their child. Education is of the utmost importance, should begin as early in the hospitalization as possible, build on the family's strengths, and empower families to care for their medically fragile infant or special needs child (Cincinnati Children's Hospital Medical Center [CCHMC], 2020b).

## EFFECTS ON THE CHILD

CYSHCN and those who are dependent on technology usually progress through stages of growth and development just as other children do, though possibly at a slower pace. The child with significant psychomotor retardation may not do so, although some developmental progression may occur. CYSHCN desire to and should be treated as normal, and experience the same events that other children do.

The medically fragile child may experience altered coping as a result of the illness effects and family stressors. CYHSCN experience alterations based on the developmental level. Infants may not appropriately attach with the parents or develop a sense of trust. Their sensorimotor abilities may be impaired, negatively affecting their learning abilities. Increased dependency or parent overinvolvement may interfere with the toddler's autonomy development. When the toddler is not provided opportunities to test limits and abilities, motor and language skills may be delayed. The sense of initiative in the preschooler may also be reduced due to limited opportunity. In the typical preschooler, magical thinking may result in guilt (Boyse et al., 2020).

Lack of socialization for a child of any age limits their ability to form peer relationships. With school absence and the inability to participate in activities or competitive events, the school-age child may have difficulty achieving a feeling of industry. When adolescents feel they are different from their peers because of differences in their skills, abilities, or appearance, they may have difficulty forming a sense of personal identity. Without significant support from their parents, adolescents with special healthcare needs have difficulty achieving independence (Boyse et al., 2020). Additionally, reaching the level of abstract thinking, which usually occurs in adolescence, may be blocked when earlier stages of cognitive development have been delayed (American Academy of Child and Adolescent Psychiatry [AACAP], 2015).

The child or youth with special healthcare needs may have a positive outlook that leads to effective coping and may experience as much independence as possible. Some children may withdraw, be irritable, or act out. Other children may simply comply, or seek the support they need. Coping patterns may change over time or with certain situations, such as repeat hospitalization, relapse, or worsening of the condition. Marked dependence and fearfulness may be observed in children with overprotective parents. Independent streaks and defiance may be noted in children whose parents have been overly protective (Fortin & Downes, 2019).

## EFFECTS ON THE FAMILY

All family members experience effects related to the child having special needs. Their experiences and responses to the child's illness directly influence each other. Generally, parents did not expect their lives to include raising a child with special needs. Parents may adapt over time, demonstrate hopefulness, or experience denial or chronic sorrow. Parents of children with special needs face numerous changes and emotions in their lives. They experience worry, the burden of continual care, feeling overwhelmed, and grief. Emotions may fluctuate on a day-to-day basis and may include anger, fear, frustration, guilt, or resentment (Bally et al., 2018).

Life is experienced differently in families with CYHSCN. Their housing arrangements may need to change to accommodate the child's needs, parental sleep is affected, and the family identity and parents' employment may change drastically. A balance must be achieved to successfully manage basic household activities, care of other children, medical and technical care, and potentially constant supervision of a technology-dependent child. Family life is also disrupted due to healthcare provider visits. Holidays and vacations are affected, as it is difficult to plan activities. Nursing and other healthcare professional visits are disruptive to family life. Marital and relationship stress often occurs affecting the primary caretaker and partner. Even relationships with extended family and friends may be affected, leading to feelings of isolation. Additional stress is experienced during times of transition in the child's care such as at initial diagnosis or change in prognosis, when increased symptoms occur or the child moves to a new setting and during a parent's absence or the child's periods of developmental change

Siblings of CYSHCN may also experience effects such as a difference in their relationship with their parents. Emotional and psychological responses to their sibling's long-term needs may occur. Siblings may face challenges with peers, as their family is not viewed as "normal." The sibling's adjustment is affected by their knowledge about the illness, their attitude toward and adjustment to it, their own self-esteem, the parents' awareness of the sibling's feelings, and the degree of social support for the sibling (Boyse, 2020).

### Financing Care

These children and their families are often insured inadequately, have financial needs and/or unmet family support needs, or have difficulty obtaining the specialty care that the child requires (Kuo & Turchi, 2020). The Children's Health Insurance Program (CHIP) provides low-cost health insurance to eligible children, and many families with CYSHCN who have the financial need may be eligible for CHIP. CHIP is administered and eligibility and benefits may vary by each state (Centers for Medicare and Medicaid Services, n.d.). Some children may be eligible for Supplemental Security Income (SSI). SSI, a cash assistance program, was created in 1972 through Public Law 92-603. Accompanying SSI qualification is state-administered Medicaid, with benefits varying slightly from state to state (Social Security Administration [SSA], n.d.-a). The Maternal and Child Health Bureau Block Grant program provides Title V programs, which issue funds to the individual states for administration of services such as community-based, comprehensive service coordination for children with special needs (SSA, n.d.-b).

## FAMILY-CENTERED CARE

The PCP should provide family-centered care when caring for the CYSHCN and their families, as family-centered care provides the ideal context, minimizing the impact of chronic illness while maximizing the child's developmental potential. While providing this care it is essential to incorporate the family's preferences as well as cultural beliefs and values into planning (de Leon Siantz et al., 2018). CYSHCN require coordinated and comprehensive services from multiple professionals working collaboratively to address the child's health, educational, psychological, and social service needs. While raising children is universally challenging, parents of a CYSHCN may find it exhausting and overwhelming. The trust established with a consistent PCP allows for efficient two-way flow of information.

### The Role of the Medical Home

The PCP and the medical home provide ongoing care coordination and follow-up. The PCP in the outpatient medical home will develop written health plans as well as modify office routines to promote child and family comfort. Additional activities include:

- Coordinating and collaborating with specialists in other disciplines, early intervention, schools, and other public agencies
- Assisting parents with childcare decisions and educating childcare providers on child health needs
- Addressing needs for prior authorization for treatments, medications, or specialist referrals
- Helping parents get involved with parent support networks and community resources available to children with special healthcare needs.

## Education

To reach their developmental potential later in life, CYSHCN often require multiple developmental interventions and special education in the early years. Early intervention programs exist for the purpose of enhancing the development of infants and toddlers with, or who are at risk for, disabilities. When successful, education costs and special education are minimized and family capacity for meeting their child's needs is enhanced, maximizing the likelihood of independent living. Government-funded care coordination and special education for children up to 3 years of age is mandated through the Individuals With Disabilities Education Improvement Act of 2004 (IDEA, formerly called Public Law 99-457), and the early intervention program is administered through each state. This law guarantees eligible children access to services for enhancing their development. Children receive care coordination and an individualized family service plan, with services being provided in the natural environment (the home or day care center). Home visits by the service coordinator and maintenance of regular contact with the family ensure the success of the program.

IDEA provides for the education of children with special needs through the public school system, from age 3 to 21 years. Each special-needs student is entitled to an individualized education program. The individualized education plan is a written plan designed to meet the student's individual needs, and is established by a committee including the child's parent, a regular teacher, a special education teacher, and various other specialists (U.S. Department of Education, n.d.). The PCP may be called upon to provide information to this committee. Additionally, the PCP will work with the parents on strategies for advocating for their child in the educational system.

## Complementary Therapies

The PCP should be aware that families of CYSHCN often use adjuvant and complementary therapies but do not always notify the provider. In search of palliation or a cure, many families seek out natural or Eastern medicine. During the health history, specifically ask about homeopathy, supplements, or herbal medications the child may be taking. Families may use pet therapy as a component of psychotherapy or simply as a way to decrease stress. Hippotherapy (the use of equine movement for the engagement of the sensory, neuromuscular, and cognitive systems) may be utilized as a means for achieving functional outcomes (American Hippotherapy Association, 2019). Positive behavioral changes and reduction of pain or stress may be achieved through music therapy (American Music Therapy Association, 2020). Reduction of pain, relaxation promotion, or a specific positive effect related to the child's particular medical condition may be sought through the use of massage therapy (Provenzi et al., 2016).

# TECHNOLOGY DEPENDENCY

Discharge readiness is initiated the moment a child is admitted to the inpatient setting. It involves the constant reassessment of the child's condition and evaluation of the future provider's readiness to transition care outside of the hospital. To achieve a successful discharge, when the child has a new health baseline identified involving technology dependence, the child then will qualify for discharge with modifications. Modifications may include new equipment, new therapies, altered medication regimens, changes to or addition of outpatient nursing hours, or assertion of new expectations. In all of the scenarios, discharge planning and education must begin early as parents will need detailed instructions for the technology-dependent child at home (CCHMC, 2020b). The inpatient provider will coordinate these activities to maximize the possibility of the child's safe transition away from the hospital, while avoiding unnecessary readmissions.

Discharge destinations for technology-dependent children who require complex medical care include tertiary care facilities, foster care, group homes, and private homes, and can include plans for inpatient or outpatient hospice. The destination dictates the amount of education that must be provided to future caregiver(s). Even for children who are technologically dependent, home is the most developmentally appropriate environment for children as it provides a socially stimulating and emotionally nurturing environment (Hosley et al., 2018). Advances in technology permit children with extensive medical and developmental needs to be cared for at home even when requiring assisted enteral or parenteral feeding, parenteral medication administration, supplemental oxygen, tracheostomy care, or assisted ventilation. Deciding on home care is a serious consideration for the family and the healthcare team (Hanks & Carrico, 2017).

When medically complex children are discharged to a group or private home, the home must be adapted. Upon inspection, it must be capable of functioning as the equivalent of a remote intensive care unit. It must be well-appointed with specialty medical equipment, backup electrical generators (if the child is ventilator dependent), readily available medications, and knowledgeable personnel.

The discharge transition places high expectations on caregivers and support personnel. Establishment of an outpatient medical home is an important factor that can reinforce education provided prior to discharge from the hospital. Depending on the amount of support the child qualifies for, support personnel may include the primary caregiver(s), home-healthcare nurses, and physical/occupational/speech therapists.

## FINANCIAL IMPLICATIONS

Providing care for medically complex children can place a financial burden on families and result in high medical bills. Prior to 1981, in order to qualify for Medicaid benefits, most technology-dependent children from middle class families remained hospitalized instead of being discharged home. This was largely due to government regulations that deemed middle class incomes too high to qualify for federal aid and made them ineligible for Medicaid benefits. The adoption of the Katie Beckett Waiver granted Medicaid availability to qualifying technology-dependent children and enabled them to receive financial aid while being cared for at home. Today, the Medically Dependent Children's Program is available to better support families caring for these children from birth to 20 years of age (Kids' Waivers, n.d.). The program promotes deinstitutionalization of children and provides flexible support services, minor home modifications, respite care for providers, home care nursing, and other services for families.

The cost of medications can also be prohibitive for many families. Private insurance companies and Medicaid utilize lists of preferred medications. While Medicare is a national program, Medicaid is a state-managed program. Therefore, variability does occur among services covered from state to state. For example, one state may approve reimbursement of generic drugs over more expensive, name-brand drugs. Additionally, some states require pre-authorization before patients can have more than six medications filled at the time of discharge. Others limit the maximum amount of medication or volume that can be prescribed over a 30-day period. Therefore, it is imperative that providers become familiar with state limitations and regulations in order to provide accurate information and resources to families of technology-dependent children.

## MAXIMIZING THE SUCCESS OF CAREGIVERS

Primary caregiver(s), often the child's parent(s), must commit to becoming proficient caretakers. They are required to learn daily medication schedules and administration techniques. Caregivers must also be deemed proficient with equipment management and common troubleshooting techniques in order to identify and intervene during medical emergencies that could occur at home. Medical providers, in turn, must be able to answer caregivers' questions regarding the most commonly encountered equipment utilized by technology-dependent children.

### Oxygen

It is important to prioritize the education of caregivers on signs of respiratory distress and impending failure (i.e., nasal flaring, tachypnea, bradypnea, retractions, grunting). Oxygen ($O_2$) is a medication that can be titrated based on the child's need. However, the overall goal is to provide the least amount of oxygen necessary to achieve adequate gas exchange. Volumes from one-fourth to 4 liters of oxygen can be delivered via nasal cannula. Furthermore, oxygen delivery can be increased as the modality is transitioned to simple face masks (accommodating 5–10 L $O_2$/min). Venturi masks (capable of delivering 4–8 L $O_2$/min), nonrebreather masks (accommodating 10–15 L $O_2$/min), and more advanced rescue measures are reserved for inpatients. Noninvasive ventilation delivered via CPAP or BiPap differs from invasive ventilation. No matter the mode of oxygen supplementation, families must educate in its safe use, including avoidance of flames.

### Tracheostomy

Children with difficulty maintaining a patent airway and/or requiring chronic ventilation may have a tracheostomy tube. Caregivers must be familiar with the parts of a tracheostomy, and use of the tracheostomy humidity collar (if not ventilated). They must also become proficient at cleaning the tracheostomy tube site, exchanging the tube, suctioning, and utilizing the Ambu® bag (i.e., the manual resuscitator or self-inflating bag) to ventilate the child.

Humidification for the prevention of tracheostomy occlusion from dry secretions may be achieved with a humidified trach collar or heat moisture exchanger. The humidified trach collar allows administration of heated mist directly to the tracheostomy. The heat moisture exchanger is a filter that, once attached to the end of a tracheostomy, provides humidification. The heat moisture exchanger can be left on for a maximum of 8 hours or when it becomes saturated. The caregiver must monitor work of breathing and for signs of intolerance (Johns Hopkins Medicine, n.d.).

The Passy Muir valve is a speaking valve that can be placed over a tracheostomy to allow phonation. It can also help improve secretion management and swallowing abilities. Its use requires practice and is best taught by a speech therapist. Children should not sleep with the Passy Muir valve in place (Passy Muir, n.d.).

## Ventilators

There are many kinds of ventilators and ventilation modalities prescribed to address specific medical needs. Recognition of normal functioning is an important aspect of ventilation safety. Caregivers must learn how to connect the child to the ventilator, how to utilize the Ambu® bag and suction the airway, and how to respond to ventilator alarms. The caregiver should become familiar with basic settings required by their child. Settings vary depending on whether the goal is to deliver noninvasive ventilation (via CPAP/BiPap) or invasive ventilation. Settings vary depending on the type of machine used and can include ventilator mode, $FiO_2$, rate, peep, pressure support, tidal volume, and inspiratory time.

## Monitors

There are a variety of monitors available for home use. Simple ones monitor heart rate and oxygenation via pulse oximetry. More complicated monitors include ECG strips, respirations, blood pressure (BP), and so on. Regardless of the model, the caregiver must understand the meaning of set alarm limits.

## Feeding Tubes

A variety of feeding tubes (gastrostomy, jejunostomy, gastrojejunostomy) may be used to provide enteral feeding to the child with technological dependency. Enteral feedings may be provided in an intermittent (bolus) or continuous fashion depending upon the type of tube and the child's individual needs. Caregivers should monitor for granulation tissue, leaking of infused volumes, and irritation around the stoma. Noting that the water-filled balloon remains inflated verifies proper tube positioning (CCHMC, 2020a). Refer to Table 43.1 for a comparison of the various types of feeding tubes. Signs of feeding intolerance may manifest as abdominal distention, constipation, or emesis (Berman, 2019).

## Aspiration Precautions

The caregiver should utilize proper upright positioning when feeding to decrease the incidence of reflux leading to aspiration. Medical management of

**TABLE 43.1 Comparing Permanent Enteral Feeding Tubes**

| Type of Tube | Location | Replacement |
|---|---|---|
| Gastrostomy tube (GT) | Allows for delivery of food or medications to the stomach | After initial healing of insertion site, can be performed by trained caregivers, without the need for x-ray confirmation |
| Jejunostomy tube (JT) | Terminates in the jejunum, bypassing the stomach. Use of the JT is restricted to continuous feedings. | Must be performed by a medical provider under fluoroscopy or x-ray verification for proper placement |
| Gastrostomy-jejunostomy tube (GJ) | Placed into the stomach with a distal portion extending into the jejunum. Continuous feedings are administered into the jejunum, while the gastrostomy portion can be vented or have medications administered through the gastric port. | Must be performed by a medical provider under fluoroscopy or x-ray verification for proper placement |

*Sources:* Data from Cincinnati Children's Hospital Medical Center. (2020a). *Gastrostomy-jejunostomy tube care.* http://www.cincinnatichildrens.org/health/g/gastro-jejuno-tube; Children's Hospital of Philadelphia. (2020). *Jejunostomy tube (j-tube).* https://www.chop.edu/treatments/jejunostomy-tubes.

secretion control may be needed to prevent aspiration. If medical management is unsuccessful, the child may be evaluated for botulinum toxin injection or surgical correction per an otolaryngologist. A formal swallow study may be used to diagnose the residual severity of the problem and rule out the need for food thickeners to minimize ongoing risk of aspiration.

### Respite Care

Caring for a special needs or technology-dependent child can be very exhausting, both physically and emotionally. Many parents never really experience a break from caregiving and may be overwhelmed. A variety of respite care services are available and vary significantly from region to region. Parents may want to participate in monthly community-based partnerships featuring monthly events for special needs children that allow the child to be safely cared for while the parent(s) experience a few hours of much-needed respite. The PCP should be familiar, with services available in the local area, and refer families as needed (Whitmore & Snethen, 2018).

## THE FORMER PREMATURE INFANT

The former premature infant is very often a child with special healthcare needs. Premature birth is defined as delivery of the infant before completion of 37 weeks' gestation. Preterm birth may be further described according to gestational age as follows:

- Late preterm birth: 34 to 36 6/7 weeks
- Moderate preterm birth: 32 to 33 6/7 weeks
- Very preterm birth: 28 to 31 6/7 weeks
- Extremely preterm birth: less than 28 weeks (Wilson-Costello & Payne, 2020).

Preterm infants may be further classified according to their birth weight:

- Low birth weight (LBW): < 2,000 gm
- Very low birth weight (VLBW): < 1,500 gm
- Extremely low birth weight (ELBW): < 1,000 gm (Wilson-Costello & Payne, 2020).

Improvements in the care of premature infants in the neonatal intensive care unit (NICU) over the past several decades have led to improved survival rates for these infants (Chung et al., 2020). Yet prematurity is associated with a spectrum of neurodevelopmental morbidity. Additionally, many of these infants are discharged from the NICU with significant ongoing medical needs and up to 40% of premature infants are re-hospitalized in the first year of life (American Academy of Pediatrics [AAP], 2015).

## NEURODEVELOPMENTAL OUTCOME

Being born early and missing the opportunity for the fetus' organ systems to mature in utero places the premature infant at risk for a multitude of illnesses that may develop in the NICU. Once stabilized and discharged home, the former premature infant is at increased risk for both major and minor disabilities. Major disabilities include cerebral palsy, intellectual disability, blindness, and deafness. These major disabilities are usually noted early in life (1–3 years of age) and have a significant impact on a child's quality of life. Gestational age and birth weight are inversely related to development of a major disability, with extremely preterm infants experiencing the highest rates of neurodevelopmental impairment (Adams-Chapman et al., 2018; Pappas et al., 2018). Infants born at the borderline of viability (22 to 24 weeks) are experiencing an increasing survival rate, yet only 20% survive without a neurodevelopmental impairment (Younge et al., 2017).

Minor disabling conditions are more subtle in progression, can be diagnosed at the age of 3 to 6 years (often later), and are not as clearly defined. Minor disabilities include learning disabilities, sensory integration issues, and behavioral, emotional, or social issues. Additionally, many former premature infants are medically fragile, have multiple developmental needs, and require the services of multiple specialists. Traditionally, their healthcare has been fragmented, so this special population would benefit greatly from the care coordination received through the medical home.

The criteria for discharge from the NICU for the premature infant include:

- Maintain normal temperature: In an open crib with room temperature between 68 °F and 72 °F, must maintain axillary temperature between 36.5 °C and 37.5 °C (97.0 °F and 100.3 °F).
- Have mature respiratory control: Be free from episodes of apnea and bradycardia for at least 5 to 8 days (off of caffeine if the neonate had been given caffeine).
- Feed orally in a mature manner: Breast and/or bottle feed sufficiently to demonstrate consistent weight gain: if the neonate is less then 2 kg it should gain 15 to 20 g/daily; if greater than 2 kg it should gain 20 to 30 g/daily.
- Remain stable while sleeping supine: Head of bed must be flat.

**PRO TIP** The high-risk infant visit is *not* your routine visit. Allow time to address the many needs of the child and family.

## PROVIDING ROUTINE WELL-CHILD CARE

Similar to other infants, former premature infants need routine well-child appointments with additional visits for management of multiple complex medical issues and developmental screening and intervention. Schedule the initial primary care visit for within 48 to 72 hours after NICU discharge (Stewart, 2020). Schedule all visits for primary care follow-up based on the infant's chronologic age. As with typical infants, teach families routine newborn care, including bathing, dressing, and avoidance of passive cigarette smoke, as well as infectious exposures. In order to remain safe, a former premature infant must ride in an approved car seat for travel, just as other infants do. The infant will be tested for oxygen desaturation while seated in the car seat prior to discharge from the NICU (Smith & Stewart, 2020). Some infants may need to continue with cardiac/apnea monitoring while in the car seat. For the infant to ride in the car safely, the parents may require assistance with padding the car seat or adding an additional semi-firm cushion inside the seat in order for the infant to fit and be properly secured. As with other infants, former premature infants should be placed on their backs to sleep unless they have gastroesophageal disease (Stewart, 2020). Follow up on newborn screening results. Additional testing requiring follow-up includes:

- Vision screening—Infants born at less than 30 weeks' gestation are at increased risk for retinopathy of prematurity.
- Hearing screening—Determine results of auditory brainstem evoked response.
- Head imaging—Close to term postmenstrual age; prior to discharge, ultrasound or magnetic resonance imaging (MRI) may be performed to detect periventricular leukomalacia or white matter injury in certain at-risk infants.
- Other blood laboratory tests—See the following: anemia of prematurity, metabolic bone disease.

### Immunizations

Give all recommended immunizations according to the immunization schedule, based on the infant's chronologic age. Provide the usual doses for each vaccine. The same immunization contraindications exist for former premature infants. For inactivated polio vaccine, opt to give the third dose at age 6 months rather than later, as this may help extremely premature infants to achieve adequate antibody levels within the first year of life. Former premature infants, particularly those with chronic lung disease (CLD), are at high risk for increased morbidity and mortality related to bronchiolitis caused by respiratory syncytial virus (RSV). RSV prophylaxis is important for certain groups of premature infants and palivizumab (Synagis) vaccine should be administered according to the recommended schedule (Stewart, 2020). Former premature infants for whom RSV prophylaxis is recommended include:

- Less than 12 months of age, born at less than 29 weeks' gestation
- Less than 12 months of age, born at less than 32 weeks' gestation, having CLD (requiring oxygen supplementation for at least the first 28 days of life)
- Less than 24 months of age, born at less than 32 weeks' gestation, having CLD (requiring oxygen supplementation for at least the first 28 days of life; second RSV season; AAP, 2014).

Begin the monthly vaccine series in November with an intramuscular injection of 15 mg/kg/dose and the last dose being provided in April (Lexicomp, 2020). Discontinue monthly prophylaxis in any child who experiences a breakthrough RSV infection. Florida and Alaska residents should consult local authorities about seasonality and start/stop dates in their local area (AAP, 2015).

### Parental Concerns

Parents of former premature infants are often quite concerned with highly visible differences in their infants as compared with other infants. They are often concerned with the head shape, the hair (or lack of it), how the skin looks, and the way the infant's hips turn out. They also may express concern that the infant is a noisy breather and notice that the infant has a grooved palate.

Since premature infants are born early, they often do not have much hair on their head when they are born as compared with term infants. Additionally, the head may be shaved in the NICU to accommodate intravenous access. Reassure the parents that eventually the hair will grow (often not until the second year of life). The premature infant's head is quite malleable and, due to positioning in the NICU, may develop a narrow appearance (dolichocephaly). The head continues to have adequate space for appropriate brain growth and the shape will resolve somewhat over time, although it might never be quite as round in appearance as it could have been. Preemies may have loss of skin pigmentation in some areas from long-term exposure to tape, scarring from intravenous injections or procedures, and epidermal inclusion cysts from multiple needle sticks. The appearance of the skin will improve somewhat over time as the infant matures.

Additional concerns involve the mouth. Infants that experienced oral endotracheal intubation for a period of time may have a grooved palate. It may flatten somewhat over time, but having the groove in it will not affect the infant's ability to speak eventually. The primary teeth when they emerge may be discolored or damaged. This should not affect the permanent teeth and the important thing is that the primary teeth do emerge (but this may be quite late in some infants). Former premature infants are small; thus, their airways are also smaller, resulting in noisy breathing. This improves over time as the infant's airway grows. Positioning in the NICU may have led to hip abduction (a somewhat frog-legged appearance of the lower extremities). Parents may exercise the hips and encourage adduction by gently rotating the hips upward with diaper changes and flexing the hips with the knees bent. Additionally, after lengthy NICU stays, parents often fear the infant may become sick or have complications when home, which leads to further stress on the family (see earlier discussion of having CYSHCN effects on the family).

### Provider Concerns

The provider has other concerns to monitor for in the former premature infant. Carefully measure head circumference to determine adequacy of brain growth. Assess the fontanels. If the anterior fontanel closes earlier than expected, craniosynostosis (early fusion of the skull sutures) may be an issue. On the other hand, an enlarged fontanel and splitting of sutures may indicate hydrocephalus or benign ventriculomegaly. Both genders of former premature infants are at increased risk for the development of inguinal hernia; be sure to assess the inguinal/femoral area carefully with each examination. Lastly, leg length discrepancies are not uncommon in the former premature infant related to umbilical catheterization for vascular access. Carefully assess the lower extremities, gently pulling them into full extension to evaluate the lengths in comparison with each other.

## NUTRITION AND GROWTH

Poor growth occurs with increased frequency in very preterm infants as compared with those born at or near full term, and may persist into school age for those with ELBW. These infants tend to be shorter, lighter, and have lower body mass index and head circumference (Mandy, 2020). In most cases the body will preferentially provide for brain growth over increases in length or weight gain. As with other infants, optimal head growth occurs over the first 6 months of life. Adequate brain growth is dependent upon sufficient and appropriate nutrition. Most of the premature infant's catch-up growth will occur in the first 2 years, with little catch-up occurring after age 3. When assessing the former premature infant's growth, always plot the measurements on the growth chart according to the infant's adjusted age, rather than chronological age.

Breast milk is the preferred form of nutrition for former premature infants, similar to term infants. Yet many preemies require special nutritional supplementation to foster catch-up growth (Stewart, 2020). Additional calories are necessary for increased growth needs, while extra calcium and phosphorus are needed for appropriate bone mineralization. Breast milk may be fortified with additional nutrients or a commercially prepared formula specific for premature infants may be used. Premature infant postdischarge formulas such as NeoSure® or EnfaCare® are more nutrient dense, appropriate for infants > 36 weeks postconceptual age, can easily be concentrated to 20, 22, or 24 cal/oz., and can be used up to 12 months adjusted age. In infants older than 36 weeks post-conceptual age, with adequate bone mineralization, term infant formulas such as Similac® or Enfamil® may be used. Soy formulas are NOT recommended due to decreased calcium and phosphorus absorption as well as decreased nitrogen retention. Pregestimil or casein hydrolysate formulas are not recommended unless necessary (i.e., history of necrotizing enterocolitis) and should be used as transition formula only.

Determine the infant's ability to suck efficiently. If the infant is a slow feeder, has difficulty feeding, or has an oral aversion, refer to occupational or speech therapy for additional assistance. Tips for intervening for feeding concerns are provided in Table 43.2.

Base all anticipatory guidance related to feeding on the infant's adjusted age. Until 4 months adjusted age, the infant needs only breast milk or formula (24–32 ounces per day). As the tongue extrusion reflex disappears around 6 months adjusted age, introduce solid food with a spoon. Additional signs that the former premature infant may be ready to attempt spoon feeding include interest in feeding and adequate head control. The first solid food should be rice cereal mixed with breast milk or formula (1 teaspoon cereal with ½ ounce formula). After the infant has established taking the

TABLE 43.2 **Interventions for Premature Infant Feeding Concerns**

| Concern | Interventions |
|---|---|
| Sleepy, quickly becomes sleepy<br>Poor waking cues<br>Fussy with feeding<br>Difficulty initiating sucking or focusing on feeding<br>Apnea/bradycardia<br>Shuts down | Watch for subtle/early hunger cues<br>Quiet alert state is best time to begin feeding<br>Decrease excess environmental stimulation<br>Alerting techniques<br>Change diaper<br>Frequently burp<br>Unswaddle |
| Endurance | |
| Sleepy baby—poor waking for feeding<br>Pokey feeder<br>Requires longer than 30 to 45 minutes<br>Increased loss of liquid<br>Disorganization of sucking as feeding progresses | Limit feeding to 20 min.<br>Discontinue when infant is fatigued<br>Reduce environmental stimulation<br>Support flexed position, head aligned with body, chin support<br>Consultation |
| Cannot suck/swallow/breathe | |
| Takes 1 to 2 sucks then pulls away<br>Gulping<br>Coughing/choking<br>Gasping for breath<br>Excessive liquid loss<br>Apnea and/or bradycardia | Swaddle in flexed position, head aligned with body<br>Begin nursing after initial let down<br>Pace feeding—give breathing breaks<br>Slow flow of milk<br>Consultation<br>If takes pacifier but not bottle, may need swallow study |

rice cereal well, add strained fruits and vegetables (one new food every 4–7 days). At 8 to 10 months adjusted age, strained meats, egg yolks, and soft mashed table foods may be introduced. Soft, mashed table foods and soft finger foods may be started at 10 to 12 months adjusted age. Do not provide juice or water until after 12 months adjusted age. Extra fluids fill the stomach, displacing much-needed caloric intake. Whole milk may be provided after 12 months adjusted age.

**PRO TIP** Some infants have sensory issues and may not tolerate the addition of textures in foods. Be mindful of this, and consider obtaining a swallow study and/or refer to occupational or speech therapy as needed.

## MONITORING DEVELOPMENTAL PROGRESSION

Prior and current medical problems place former premature infants at high risk for developmental delay. Compared with other infants, former premature infants are at higher risk of developing cognitive delay, cerebral palsy, attention deficit disorder, learning disabilities, and difficulties with socialization (Mandy, 2020; Stewart, 2020). Additionally, alterations in muscle tone at or shortly after discharge from the NICU occur in many former premature infants and may require physical therapy intervention. Careful assessment will discern subtle changes in former premature infants that may affect their long-term physical, cognitive, emotional, and/or social outcome.

Screen development in all former premature infants at each well-child visit. Early identification of developmental issues allows for earlier developmental intervention and is critical for the attainment of optimal development (Scharf et al., 2016). Developmental screening tools may be used, although they do not always identify children at risk. Parent-report questionnaires are simple to use and demonstrate fairly accurate estimations of developmental problems. Determine integration of primitive reflexes followed by emergence of postural reactions (this is a critical step in the child's development). Evaluate the infant's or toddler's gross motor skills. Of utmost importance, compare the child's development based on adjusted age until the child is 3 years old. Refer any child with delay in gross motor, fine motor, or language skills based on adjusted age to physical therapy, occupational therapy, and/or speech therapy for evaluation and possible treatment. Also refer to local early intervention services.

## UNIQUE MEDICAL PROBLEMS

Many former premature infants suffer from numerous medical and developmental problems throughout infancy and childhood. Upon or following discharge, one or many of the following medical or developmental problems may be present:

- Transient dystonia
- Retinopathy of prematurity, strabismus, decreased visual acuity
- CLD (bronchopulmonary dysplasia)
- apnea of prematurity, gastroesophageal reflux disease, bradycardia
- Cardiovascular changes such as right ventricular hypertrophy and pulmonary arterial hypertension (PAH)
- Metabolic bone disease
- Growth retardation, poor feeding, anemia of prematurity, or other nutrient deficiencies
- Hydrocephalus, ventriculomegaly, abnormal head MRI results, ventriculoperitoneal shunt
- Inguinal or umbilical hernias
- Hearing deficits
- Gross motor, fine motor, and language delay
- Oral aversion or sensory integration issues (Stewart, 2020).

### Transient Dystonia

Premature infants usually display hypotonia while in the NICU and may have hypertonia once they are home. For many infants, this is simply transient dystonia, but others may have cerebral palsy. Typically, the shoulders are retracted (from lying supine in the NICU). The hips, legs, and heel cords may be tight. Gentle stretching exercises and placing of the infant in a swaddled position with the shoulders slightly rotated forward and the hips/knees flexed can be helpful. Physical therapy may be warranted if the hypertonia is more severe. If the hypertonia persists, primitive reflexes are retained, and there is a delay in the emergence of the protective reflexes, cerebral palsy may be considered.

Perform a thorough neurologic examination. Assess the infant's muscle tone through palpation, range of motion, and angle measurement (adductor angle, popliteal angle, heel-to-ear maneuver, dorsiflexion, and the scarf sign) (Salandy et al., 2019). Refer to Table

**TABLE 43.3 Angle Measurement for Adjusted Age**

| Angles | Birth to 3 Months | 4 to 6 Months | 7 to 9 Months | 10 Months & Older |
|---|---|---|---|---|
| Adductor angle | 40° to 80° | 70° to 110° | 100° to 140° | 130° to 150° |
| Popliteal angle | 80° to 100° | 90° to 120° | 110° to 160° | 150° to 170° |
| Heel-to-ear | 80° to 100° | 90° to 130° | 120° to 150° | 140° to 170° |
| Dorsiflexion | 60° to 70° | 60° to 70° | 60° to 70° | 60° to 70° |
| Scarf sign | 1 | 2 | 3 | 4 |

43.3 for illustrations of the angle measurements at various adjusted ages. Assess deep tendon reflexes (they may be brisk if hypertonia is present). Due to positioning in the NICU, many former premature infants have tight shoulder and hip muscles. To promote appropriate shoulder muscle tone, teach parents to swaddle the younger infant with the shoulders brought forward, the elbows bent, and the hands at midline. To facilitate improvement in hip muscle tone, teach parents to exercise the hips at each diaper change, moving the hips through full range of motion, then after rediapering, adduct the hips with knees bent and swaddle in that position. These gentle stretches of the shoulder and hip muscles help the infant's muscle to return to normal tone, permitting motor skill attainment.

▶ ALERT: Persistent hypertonia, brisk deep tendon reflexes, persistent primitive reflexes, and delays in gross motor skill attainment are associated with cerebral palsy.

## Retinopathy of Prematurity

As is true with all infants, it is important to assess for strabismus, evaluate the Hirschberg reflex, and grossly screen vision with every well-child visit. Infants with a history of retinopathy of prematurity may need additional follow-up with pediatric ophthalmology. Retinopathy of prematurity is common in VLBW infants and results in retinal vascular proliferation that may lead to visual acuity deficit and blindness if unresolved. In the majority of infants, it advances until about 45 weeks postmenstrual age, then eventually resolves spontaneously in the majority of infants with some infants requiring surgical correction (Coats, 2020). After discharge from the NICU, ensure infants with retinopathy of prematurity receive ongoing screening by pediatric ophthalmology until the retinopathy of prematurity has regressed or surgical treatment is needed.

## Chronic Lung Disease

Infants born very or extremely prematurely are at risk for the development of bronchopulmonary dysplasia (CLD). CLD in infancy increases the risk for reduced exercise capacity and asthma as the child ages, with increased respiratory problems into childhood and adulthood (Mandy, 2020). Because of changes in the lungs with CLD, some infants also develop PAH (evidenced on echocardiogram). Infants may be discharged on supplemental oxygen (often very small amounts), aerosol medications, or diuretics such as spironolactone or furosemide. For the infant with CLD it is important to carefully assess work of breathing (at rest and with feeding or activity), oxygen saturation, and adequacy of growth.

When the baby is stable and has been growing adequately for some time, the baby may be weaned off medications and oxygen. As the infant's weight has increased over time, the diuretic doses are often outgrown, at which time they may be discontinued. When opting to wean the baby off supplemental oxygen, maintain routine and as-needed aerosol medications. The infant is ready for attempted weaning off when all of the following are true:

- Has been medically stable for several weeks
- Gains weight adequately
- Feeds efficiently
- Tolerates activity
- Oxygen saturation remains >95% at all times
- Tolerates respiratory infections without increased oxygen need
- PAH is resolved.

At that time, at 3- to 4-week intervals, decrease continuous oxygen by half at each weaning until down to 1/16 liter/minute. Then transition to 1/16 liter/minute at night only, then stop oxygen. Prior to, during, and after weaning, reassess each of the previously listed parameters. Pediatric pulmonology may be consulted for assistance with management of CLD.

## Apnea of Prematurity

Some former premature infants are discharged home on a cardiac/apnea monitor, either due to continued episodes of apnea or because the infant has demonstrated episodes of bradycardia. Continuous use of the cardiac/apnea monitor should continue for approximately 2 months. In that time, if there are no significant alarms use may be decreased with sleep and when in a car seat. At least 90 days should pass since the last significant event prior to complete discontinuation of monitor use.

## Cardiovascular Changes

Measure BP at each well-child examination. Former premature infants are at increased risk for hypertension related to potential renal or vascular damage from treatments or health status in the NICU. Infants with CLD may have right ventricular hypertrophy and/or PAH. These infants will require repeat echocardiogram to determine resolution of PAH as the infant's lungs heal. Pediatric cardiology should be consulted for echocardiogram interpretation.

### Metabolic Bone Disease

Premature infants are born with a calcium deficit and have difficulty taking in adequate amounts of calcium (either parenterally or enterally) during their initial NICU stay. As a result, they may have metabolic bone disease (also called rickets or osteopenia of prematurity). In the exclusively breastfed infant, measure the alkaline phosphatase level 2 to 4 weeks after discharge, then monthly until the alkaline phosphatase level is less than 600 international units/L. All breastfed premature infants require vitamin D supplementation. In the formula-fed infant to ensure optimum calcium/phosphorus balance, provide Similac Special Care until the infant's weight reaches 3.6 kg. The infant weighing greater than 3.6 kg may be transitioned to NeoSure®. In either the breastfed or formula-fed infant, if the alkaline phosphatase is >800 international units/L and the phosphorus is low, prescribe:

- Calcium glubionate 20 mg/kg/day divided q12h
- Sodium phosphate 10–20 mg/kg/day divided q12h (give at opposite times from calcium; Abrams, 2019).

### Anemia of Prematurity

Premature infants experience an earlier decrease in erythropoiesis as compared with term infants who usually reach a hemoglobin nadir of 11 g/dL by 2 to 3 months of age. In premature infants, this nadir is more pronounced (9.5 g/dL), occurs earlier (age 6 weeks), and results from impaired erythropoietin production, reduced red blood cell life span, iron depletion, and blood loss from phlebotomy. In some infants, the hemoglobin will be 7 g/dL or lower. It may resolve by 6 months of age (Abrams, 2019). Anemia of prematurity may result in poor weight gain, tachycardia, increased supplemental oxygen requirement, or increased episodes of apnea or bradycardia. Supplement the exclusively breastfed infant with 2 to 4 mg/kg of iron daily through the first year of life. Recheck hemoglobin per the AAP periodicity schedule, unless the infant continues to have other medical problems after NICU discharge such as CLD, necessitating early laboratory monitoring.

## ASSISTING THE ADOLESCENT WITH TRANSITION

During adolescence, numerous physical changes and psychosocial challenges occur while the youth is initiating independence from the parents. The youth with a chronic illness or one who is technology dependent may experience this period differently from other adolescents and may find it more difficult making the transition to adulthood. With a special health condition, the adolescent may be experiencing significant dependence at a time when the youth should be developing independence from the parents. The adolescent with special healthcare needs may require increased amounts of support during this complex time of transition (White et al., 2018).

The nurse practitioner is in a prime position for meeting the psychosocial and physical care needs of adolescents with special healthcare needs as they transition into young adulthood. Transition planning is of utmost importance for this special population and will also include education and support. Comprehensive support processes will assist the adolescent or young adult with moving in a coordinated fashion from a child-centered to an adult-centered healthcare system (National Association of Pediatric Nurse Practitioners [NAPNAP], 2019).

## BARRIERS TO SUCCESSFUL TRANSITION

Despite the importance of successful transition planning, numerous barriers to transition exist. These barriers may include:

- Adolescent and family lack of readiness to let go
- Adolescent and family attachment to pediatric providers
- Difficulty recognizing the adolescent's ability to advocate and care for self
- Family stress and lack of cohesion or communication
- Poverty or otherwise disadvantaged environment.

When young adults experience these barriers during transition from pediatric to adult care, an increased utilization of acute medical care services and a high rate of mortality from disease complications may occur (Health Transition Wisconsin, 2020).

## TRANSITION PLANNING

Making a successful transition to adult care for an adolescent with special healthcare needs should ultimately result in the young adult's seamless transition to adult providers and fostering of adult competencies for independent, productive, and inclusive living within the community (Betz et al., 2018). Advance planning leads to a smoother transition. Successful transition begins with acknowledging the changing roles among the youth, family, and healthcare professionals. It then moves on to fostering the adolescent's self-determination skills and involves multidisciplinary care coordination. The nurse practitioner will have ongoing conversations about transition with the adolescent as well as review of a written plan for transition (Letishock et al., 2018).

It is recommended to begin transition planning in early adolescence, around age 12. Ensure that the adolescent is aware of the facility's transition process and reinforce this concept on subsequent visits. Tracking the adolescent's transition progress via registry can be very helpful. In collaboration with the adolescent and family, identify the adult provider. Also plan with and support the youth and family in regard to healthcare goals, legal changes (including insurance coverage), and emergency preparation. The youth should understand the treatments and their rationales, symptoms of worsening condition, and, especially, danger signs. At transition, verbally collaborate with the care coordinator or advanced practice nurse, then provide a detailed written plan to ensure a seamless transfer. As needed, consult with the transition services coordinator or other service agency as available in the local community as well as the adult provider. For online resources related to transition, as well as education opportunities, visit https://healthtransitionwi.org.

**PRO TIP** Some adolescents will not be able to become independent due to their physical or mental disabilities. In these cases, refer parents to legal counsel related to maintaining responsibility for the child past the age of majority.

# THE CHILD UNDERGOING CANCER TREATMENT

Cancer diagnosis in children younger than 20 is a relatively uncommon occurrence, with the incidence ranging from approximately 120 to 170 per million in developed countries (Peikert et al., 2018). In the last decade, diagnostic and treatment methods have vastly improved the childhood cancer 5-year survival rate, with overall survival rates at 83% (Asselin, 2020). Survival rates are best for acute lymphocytic leukemia and Hodgkin lymphoma and can be much lower for inoperable tumors such as brainstem glioma.

Additionally, after the first shock of a cancer diagnosis, each member of the family adapts to new situations, roles, and responsibilities (Peikert et al., 2018). Achieving normalcy during treatment and transitioning after treatment can be a major challenge (yet should be a goal) for the child, parents, siblings, and even the extended family. Childhood cancer treatment is a family challenge that extends way beyond cancer treatment, with family routines disrupted, emotional and financial resources strained, and with an impact on the quality of life (Wengenroth et al., 2015). During the diagnosis and treatment phases, children often have to undergo procedures and tests that can be new, painful, and scary. While these are unpleasant for the child and often upsetting to the families, waiting for test results and treatment options are additional stressors for children and families (Santacroce et al., 2018). The child and family often endure repeated long hospital stays away from home, family, friends, school, and work, and the family must adjust to a new normal while undergoing painful and stressful therapies. The burden on children and their families changes over time as therapies continue, and children will have developmentally specific needs such as keeping up in school, connecting with friends and peers, coping skills, and changes to family relationships (Peikert et al., 2018).

## TREATMENT MODALITIES AND THEIR SIDE EFFECTS

Treating cancer is complex and often multimodal with combinations of radiation therapy, chemotherapy, surgical interventions, immunotherapy, targeted biotherapies, and/or hematopoietic stem cell transplant (National Cancer Institute [NCI], 2020). All of these can have adverse effects on a child's development, and can result in serious long-term medical, physical, and psychosocial effects. The majority of children with cancer are treated in children's hospitals or university medical centers by pediatric oncologists and multidisciplinary oncology teams that follow protocols as part of the worldwide Children's Oncology Group (COG). COG is a large national organization committed to improving treatment and outcomes in childhood cancers by conducting disease-specific research. There are often several supportive and adjunct groups involved with the child and caregivers in both the inpatient and outpatient areas such as respiratory therapy; physical, occupational, and speech therapies; music and pet therapy; dietary support; religious belief partners; and child life specialists.

During therapy, children are encouraged to stay in contact with local PCPs and continue to get routine physicals along with anticipatory guidance education. Scheduled vaccines are placed on hold until completion of therapy due to the variable response of vaccine when immunosuppressed (Horton & Steuber, 2019). Once therapy is complete, the oncology team will work with PCPs on immunization catch-up or revaccination.

Children with cancer, while enduring its treatment, can develop short- and long-term effects including difficulties with physical function, emotional health and social integration, the need to minimize the adverse effects, increasing morbidities for the child, and family challenges (Grimshaw et al., 2018). Children often feel a loss of control, which may lead to food refusal or adherence issues as a means to exert some control over some aspect of their lives. Some of the treatment-related side effects that directly affect physical functioning include cardiotoxicity, nausea and vomiting, peripheral neuropathy, steroid myopathy, and loss of muscle mass and bone density (Grimshaw et al., 2018).

As advances in treatment for childhood cancers continue to improve survival, it is important for providers to optimize quality of life, function, emotional health, and help to manage side effects. The child and caregiver should be educated about complications, side effects of therapies, and signs and symptoms, as well as how to treat and when to call the oncology team for further care or come to the emergency department for further care. Some of the more severe symptoms can require an inpatient hospital admission, while many others can be managed as an outpatient or at home. The timing of these side effects can vary with each treatment modality and can involve any body system.

## Chemotherapy

Side effects of chemotherapy are addressed by the oncology team. Chemotherapy side effects may occur while it is being administered up to hours, days, weeks, or years later, and the severity also varies based on the agent used (Gillard et al., 2019). Common side effects include neutropenia, anemia, thrombocytopenia (bleeding), mucositis, nausea and vomiting, and pain. The most common and problematic complication of children undergoing chemotherapy is infection. Fever may be the first indicator of an infection and in the setting of neutropenia should be treated as an oncologic emergency (Ahmed & Flynn, 2019). Psychological and emotional support should be ongoing and can be provided within the community.

Some of the side effects are mild and some are transient (such as hair loss); others such as hearing loss are often permanent and some are severe, like myelosuppression, and may be significant enough to change the treatment plan (Gillard et al., 2019). It is important to educate caregivers and children as appropriate about how to evaluate potential side effects and toxicities, how to manage symptoms at home, and when to notify their healthcare team about concerns (Gillard et al., 2019).

### Pulmonary Effects

Chemotherapy may have toxic effects on the pulmonary system, with damage being restrictive or obstructive. During treatment, interstitial lung injury may occur in the initial phase and more significant disease such as pulmonary fibrosis can develop months or even years later. Pneumonitis is an acute, localized inflammation caused by an infectious or irritation process related to chemotherapy or radiation, which can cause direct damage to endothelium with resulting inflammation and capillary permeability. Symptoms such as dyspnea, crackles, nonproductive cough, low-grade fever, and fatigue may occur. Upon physical examination, the provider may note crackles, or a friction rub with continued deteriorating pulmonary function, tachypnea, desaturation, and cyanosis. Children may also develop noncardiac-related pulmonary edema from infection or trauma from cytokines, damaging the alveolar endothelium and resulting in an excess of fluids in the alveoli. This can be triggered by an inflammatory response within a few hours to days after exposure to chemotherapy. Children and caregivers should be educated about respiratory changes in respiratory status and instructed to promptly report any new cough, dyspnea, or puffiness (Gillard et al., 2019).

### Cardiac Effects

Chemotherapy may also have toxic effects on the cardiovascular system, resulting in a long QT interval and other arrhythmias. These may occur simply as cardiotoxic effects of particular chemotherapeutic medications or related to other factors such as cumulative chemotherapy doses, electrolyte imbalances, radiation therapy of the chest, iron overload, and history of preexisting cardiac disease. Cardiomyopathy can also occur as acute, early, or later in onset. Child and family education should include how to recognize potential arrhythmias, such as fast heartbeat or skipping beats, chest pain, syncope, lightheadedness, and dizziness and also encourage regular physical examinations and long-term follow-up (Gillard et al., 2019).

## Neurologic System

Neurologic effects of chemotherapy include cranial nerve deficits; peripheral motor, autonomic, or sensory neuropathies; pain; visual disturbances; cognitive and behavioral changes; and emergencies such as posterior reversible encephalopathy syndrome, which is related to disordered cerebral autoregulation. These neurologic symptoms can be very distressing to children and caregivers. The disabilities and symptoms can be temporary or may result in permanent disability (such as with posterior reversible encephalopathy syndrome, which can prove to be acutely fatal). Some children may have neurologic symptoms prior to diagnosis (causing the child and caregiver to seek treatment). An example is pain, which is present in 50% of children as a presenting symptom (Ritchey & Friehling, 2020).

Cognitive deficits are reflected by changes in intellect, learning, and memory. Symptoms may include personality changes, depression, poor impulse control, mood swings, fatigue, psychosis, and changes in social functioning and personality. These changes may result from the disease or the treatment regimen, and be temporary or long-term, affecting childhood development, behavior, and intellectual ability (Gillard et al., 2019). Some children may have decreased intelligence quotient, lowered standardized test scores, loss of developmental milestones, poor school performance, inattentiveness, difficulty with math and visual–spatial skills, decreased processing speeds, and short-term memory problems. Additionally, there is an increase in poor peer relationships, lower self-esteem, and the risk of self-harm (Peikert et al., 2018). The management of cognitive issues is stressful for the child and family, requiring anticipatory guidance and education about promoting healthy, attainable lifestyles for the child. Encouraging self-care and maximization of potential, helping caregivers to advocate for their child at school and in the community, and working collaboratively with a multidisciplinary team (child life specialist, psychiatry, psychologists, social services, occupation therapy, physical therapy, speech therapy) is needed (COG, 2018b, Gillard et al., 2019). The educational process for the child may be affected by prolonged absences, decreased energy levels, and effects on memory, learning, emotional, and cognitive abilities. Caregivers, educators, and the healthcare team need to be aware of the potential educational and emotional problems for this at-risk population so they can be closely monitored and given extra support and help as the need arises (COG, 2018a).

**PRO TIP** Early support and school plans are important in the overall success of survivors with neurocognitive issues.

## Gastrointestinal Effects

Children often experience gastrointestinal (GI) side effects including nausea and vomiting, diarrhea, constipation, and drug-induced liver injury such as hepatitis, pancreatitis, and altered nutrition (Gillard et al., 2019). Children who receive chemotherapy frequently experience chemotherapy-induced nausea and vomiting despite being treated with proper antiemetics (Flank et al., 2016). For children receiving chemotherapy, prophylactic antiemetics should be prescribed. Other interventions for nausea and vomiting include aromatherapy, acupuncture, acupressure, biofeedback, cognitive behavioral therapy, hypnosis, and pet therapies (Gillard et al., 2019).

Children often develop altered feeding, which can include a lack of calories and resulting malnutrition or obesity, often as side effects of the type of cancer or the chemotherapy/radiation treatment. For the child who has difficulty in achieving adequate nutrition, they may require oral supplements, initiation of enteral feed, or total parental nutrition (although enteral is preferred given the risk for infection). Adequate nutrition with appropriate calories is important to the well-being of the child as well as to overall healing. To help achieve adequate nutrition, the child should have appropriate symptom management and may need an appetite stimulant and meal planning assistance. It may help the child to have small, frequent meals, while avoiding strong smells and overly sweet foods (Gillard et al., 2019).

Constipation is a common childhood problem, with prevalence as high as 50% in children with cancer (Gillard et al., 2019). The etiology is multifactorial and may be primary due to external issues (such as decreased fluid intake), secondary due to issues such as vomiting or anorexia, or due to pharmacologic causes (narcotic or chemotherapy use). Constipation may be managed with a high fiber diet, adequate hydration, and as needed with medications. Diarrhea may also occur and can quickly lead to dehydration and/or electrolyte imbalances. The need to rule out infectious causes for diarrhea and to provide hydration may result in hospital admission.

### *Mucositis*

Given that mucosa is made of rapidly dividing cells that are significantly affected by cancer treatment, the child may develop mucositis, stomatitis, and esophagitis. This mucositis may occur anywhere along the GI tract and results directly from therapies or indirectly from immunosuppression. Interventions for prevention and care include proper oral care with soft toothbrushes, oral rinses, flossing, good oral hydration, using a sponge toothbrush when oral lesions are present, avoiding irritating oral medications, discouraging carbonated drinks, encouraging soft, bland foods (while discouraging spicy, acidic, salty, or sharp foods), the use of straws for drinks, and lesion culture for the presence of infection (Gillard et al., 2019).

When the child has braces or orthodontic appliances that may harbor organisms, these should be removed prior to initiation of therapy with a moderate-to-high risk of mucosal changes (COG, n.d.-a). Cutaneous alterations from chemotherapy effects include changes in pigmentation, alopecia and other hair changes, rashes, painful cracks and fissures, acne, dermatitis, nail bed changes, urticaria, pruritis, and photosensitivity (Gillard et al., 2019). These changes are distressing to children and families and can lead to secondary infection for opportunistic organisms with the break of natural barriers to infection.

### Immunosuppression

The hematopoietic system is responsible for the production of the following cell lines: white blood cells, red blood cells, and platelets. Normal function of bone marrow can be altered by certain cancers and suppressed by chemotherapy, radiation, and biotherapy. Myelosuppression (the reduction of bone marrow activity) is the most common cause of dose-limiting toxicity of many regimens and can result in anemia, neutropenia, or thrombocytopenia (Gillard et al., 2019).

Neutropenia is a decrease in the number of circulating neutrophils that serve as first line of defense against infection. This leads to significantly elevated risk for infection, which is greatest when severe neutropenia occurs (the absolute neutrophil count is less than 500/μL; Michniacki & Walkovich, 2020). Monitor children for signs of infection and fever. Instruct children and caregivers about infection prevention such as good handwashing, avoiding crowds and sick contacts, not sharing drinks or utensils, not performing rectal temperatures or medications, not caring for pets, having no birds or reptile contact, and not receiving live vaccinations. Provide specific instruction to children and families about surveilling for infectious symptoms including: temperature parameters for notification of providers, chills, rapid or shallow breathing, altered level of consciousness, erythema, rashes, headaches, and bone pain, as well as generalized pain, cramping abdominal pain, and diarrhea (Lehrnbecher et al., 2017). The child with neutropenia and fever will usually require hospital admission to receive appropriate treatment for infection, as the infections can be life threatening in these children.

▶ **ALERT:** The child undergoing chemotherapy who develops fever and neutropenia should have antibiotics administered within 60 minutes of presentation to the facility. Prompt initiation of antibiotics showed improved outcomes (Ahmed & Flynn, 2019).

### Ototoxicity

Ototoxicity can be associated with chemotherapy, radiation, or tumors affecting cranial nerve VIII. Ototoxicity is often associated with high frequency hearing loss, which is often progressive and may be temporary or permanent, partial, or total (Gillard et al., 2019). Children should have periodic hearing evaluations to assess for deficits, while educating children and caregivers about ototoxic effects of therapies, subtle signs of loss, and that hearing loss can occur years after therapy is completed, with the need for long-term periodic hearing evaluations. Assess children for nausea, vomiting, tinnitus, vertigo, and ataxia as well as other causes of hearing loss, such as increased cerumen or increased tympanic membrane fluid.

## THE CHILDHOOD CANCER SURVIVOR

Childhood cancer cure rates have increased through the years and now 84% of children will be cured (NCI, 2020). As cure rates rise, more and more children with cancer are becoming cancer survivors and living normal lives into adulthood. However, these positive outcomes bring associated risks related to treatment toxicities that can occur months to years after treatment has ended.

Whether undergoing chemotherapy, radiation, surgery, or stem cell transplantation, these children often have lasting effects, both physical and psychological. Between 60% and 90% of childhood cancer survivors will develop one or more chronic health conditions (Constine et al., 2020). It is important for the PCP to recognize these complications and treat accordingly.

Childhood cancer survivors are at an increased risk for many diseases including cardiovascular disease, diabetes, osteopenia, learning problems, obesity, secondary

**TABLE 43.4 Common Late Side Effects Based on Cancer and Treatment**

| Diagnosis | Common Therapy/Known Late Effects | Management |
|---|---|---|
| Leukemia | *Intrathecal chemotherapy:* neurotoxicity<br>*Cranial radiation*: SN, neurotoxicity, and endocrine<br>*Steroids:* bone health, obesity<br>*Anthracycline:* cardiomyopathy<br>*Tyrosine kinase inhibitors:* endocrine<br>*Alkylating agents:* fertility<br>*Topoisomerase inhibitors and alkylating agents*: SN | Inquire about school grades: neuropsychologic testing<br>Routine echocardiograms<br>Monitor Tanner staging, growth percentile<br>Menstrual history<br>Monitor for obesity and provide necessary education, monitor cholesterol and lipid |
| Lymphoma | *Radiation:* SN, endocrine, pulmonary dysfunction<br>*Alkylating agents*: fertility<br>*Bleomycin:* pulmonary toxicity<br>*Steroids:* bone health<br>*Anthracycline:* cardiomyopathy | Routine pulmonary function tests<br>Inquire about school grades: neuropsychologic testing<br>Routine echocardiograms<br>Monitor Tanner staging/growth percentiles<br>Menstrual history |
| Sarcoma | *Anthracycline:* cardiomyopathy<br>*Surgery:* musculoskeletal<br>*Radiation:* SN, endocrine, pulmonary dysfunction, strictures<br>*Topoisomerase inhibitors and alkylating agents*: SN | Routine echocardiograms<br>Routine pulmonary function<br>Monitor Tanner staging/growth percentiles<br>Menstrual history<br>Activity restrictions |
| CNS | *Radiation:* SN, neurotoxicity, musculoskeletal, and endocrine<br>*Surgery:* seizures, visual/auditory impairment<br>*Platinum:* ototoxicity, nephrotoxicity | Inquire about school grades: neuropsychologic testing<br>Routine echocardiograms<br>Routine pulmonary function<br>Monitor Tanner staging/growth percentiles<br>Menstrual history<br>Activity restrictions |
| Neuroblastoma | *Anthracycline:* cardiomyopathy<br>*Platinum:* ototoxicity, nephrotoxicity<br>*Surgery:* strictures<br>*Radiation:* SN, musculoskeletal, endocrine<br>*I-MIBG:* endocrine, including fertility<br>*Cis-retinoic acid:* endocrine<br>Busulfan: pulmonary toxicity | Routine echocardiograms<br>Routine pulmonary function<br>Routine hearing tests<br>Monitor Tanner staging/growth percentiles<br>Menstrual history<br>Activity restrictions |

CNS, central nervous system; SN, secondary neoplasm

*Sources*: Data from Applebaum, M. A., Henderson, T. O., Lee, S. M., Pinto, N., Volchenboum, S. L., & Cohn, S. L. (2015). Second malignancies in patients with neuroblastoma: The effects of risk-based therapy. *Pediatric Blood & Cancer, 62*(1), 128–133. https://doi.org/10.1002/pbc.25249; Children's Oncology Group. (2018a). *Educational issues after cancer treatment, version 5.0.* http://www.survivorshipguidelines.org/pdf/2018/English%20Health%20Links/14_educational_issues%20(secured).pdf; Children's Oncology Group. (2018b). *Emotional issues after cancer treatment, version 5.0.* http://www.survivorshipguidelines.org/pdf/2018/English%20Health%20Links/15_emotional_issues%20(secured).pdf; Phelan, R., Eissa, H., Becktell, K., Bhatt, N., Kudek, M., Nuechterlein, B., Pommert, L., Tanaka, R., & Baker, K. S. (2019). Upfront therapies and downstream effects: Navigating late effects in childhood cancer survivors in the current era. *Current Oncology Reports, 21*(104). https://doi.org/10.1007/s11912-019-0861-8; Pui, C.-H., Yang, J. J., Hunger, S. P., Pieters, R., Schrappe, M., Biondi, A., Vora, A., Baruche, A., Silverman, L. B., Schmiegelow, K., Escherich, G., Horibe, K., Benoit, Y. C. M., Izraeli, S., Yeoh, A. E. J., Liang, D.-C., Downing, J. R., Evans, W. E., Relling, M. V., & Mullighan, C. G. (2015). Childhood acute lymphoblastic leukemia: Progress through collaboration. *Journal of Clinical Oncology, 33*(27), 2938–2948. https://doi.org/10.1200/JCO.2014.59.1636

cancers, and other endocrine abnormalities (Hunger & Mullighan, 2015). Specialized clinics have been established to monitor toxicities in childhood cancer survivors. Although survivorship clinics are increasing, community providers should have some knowledge of potential complications. Table 43.4 gives some of the common late side effects based on cancer type and treatment. It also provides some surveillance education for PCPs based on treatment. As cure rates continue to increase, more and more cancer survivors will be seen at their primary care clinics. The most common treatment-related late effects are discussed in Table 43.4.

## CHEMOTHERAPY-INDUCED CARDIOTOXICITY

Many of the chemotherapeutic agents used as part of treatment regimens for malignancy can have cardiotoxic side effects. These can be either an acute finding while the child is actively undergoing chemotherapy or a late finding years after receiving chemotherapy. The class of chemotherapeutic agents called anthracyclines are typically the cause for this often progressive and irreversible form of cardiac damage or cardiomyopathy, and more than 50% of childhood cancer survivors will have been treated with some type of anthracycline (Bansal et al., 2017). Doxorubicin, daunorubicin, idarubicin, and epirubicin are members of the anthracycline class (McGowan et al., 2017).

Some data suggest that the incidence of cardiotoxicity may be dose-related, thus providing the current recommendation to limit lifetime anthracycline dosage to 450 mg/m$^2$ or less (Bansal et al., 2017). It is important to know the child's cumulative dosage of anthracycline in order to provide the appropriate amount of surveillance for cardiotoxicity. An echocardiogram including corrected QT segment measurement (QTc) should be performed at the initial onset of long-term follow-up and repeated as clinically indicated, as well as the following timepoint as recommended by the COG:

- Anthracycline dose <250 mg/m$^2$: every 5 years if no or <15 Gy radiation, or every 2 years if ≥15 Gy radiation
- Anthracycline dose ≥250 mg/m$^2$: every 2 years (York, 2018).

If QTc is prolonged, medication known to further prolong the segment should be avoided (e.g., tricyclic antidepressants, antifungals, macrolide antibiotics, metronidazole; York, 2018).

Children that have received anthracycline therapy should be counseled on maintaining a heart-healthy diet, BP, and appropriate body mass index. Exercise is safe and should be encouraged for all children with normal systolic cardiac function. Cardiology consultation can be considered for high-risk survivors who participate in strenuous exercise (York, 2018). Prior to becoming pregnant, cardiology consultation is recommended for any child that received >250 mg/m$^2$ anthracycline dosage, >35 Gy chest radiation, or any dosage of anthracycline combined with chest radiation (>15 Gy). These children are at high risk of developing pregnancy-associated cardiomyopathy and should be monitored frequently throughout pregnancy and delivery given risk for cardiac failure (York, 2018).

## SECONDARY MALIGNANCY

After completing cancer treatment with radiation, chemotherapy, or a combination of both, it is important for these children to have close follow-up and screening for secondary malignancies that can be caused by their cancer treatment. The greatest rates of secondary malignancies have been seen in children who have previously undergone radiation treatment. Radiation treatment for childhood malignancies has steadily decreased over the last few decades, and with that decrease there has been a concomitant increase in the use of chemotherapeutic agents. Despite having a lower risk for causing secondary malignancies, chemotherapeutic agents are contributing factors. Alkylating agents, epipodophyllotoxins, anthracyclines, and platinum agents are the typical contributors to secondary malignancies in childhood cancer survivors (Turcotte et al., 2019). Presentation of secondary leukemia typically occurs within 10 years of treatment, whereas secondary sarcomas typically present 10 years or later after treatment is complete (COG, n.d.-c). Table 43.5 lists the most common drugs in the previously noted categories.

All childhood cancer survivors should have an annual comprehensive health check-up. The COG (n.d.-c) recommends specific screening for the signs and symptoms that may indicate a secondary malignancy (Box 43.1).

Survivors should receive counseling on environmental factors that can help to avoid secondary malignancies, including smoking avoidance or cessation, wearing sunscreen when outside, avoiding alcohol or using in moderation only, and having a healthy diet (COG, n.d.-c).

## PERIPHERAL NEUROPATHY

Peripheral neuropathy may be caused by very common chemotherapeutic agents such as vincristine, vinblastine, cisplatin, and carboplatin (COG, n.d.-b). Children that have received one of these drugs as part of their chemotherapy regimen should be screened for numbness in their extremities, tingling sensation, sensitivity to touch, muscle weakness, or nerve-related pain. Although there is no cure for peripheral neuropathy, great strides can be made when working with physical therapy and making environmental changes. In addition to a physical therapy referral, these children should be counseled to wear loose fitting clothing, avoid hot temperatures, leave feet uncovered in

**TABLE 43.5 Chemotherapeutic Drugs By Category**

| Alkylating Agents | Epipodophyllotoxins | Anthracyclines | Platinum-based |
|---|---|---|---|
| Busulfan<br>Carmustine<br>Cyclophosphamide<br>Dacarbazine<br>Ifosfamide<br>Lomustine<br>Melphalan<br>Temozolomide<br>Thiotepa | Etoposide<br>Teniposide | Daunorubicin<br>Doxorubicin<br>Epirubicin<br>Idarubicin | Carboplatin<br>Cisplatin<br>Oxaliplatin |

*Source*: Crean, D., & Jones, E. (n.d.). *Types of chemotherapy drugs*. https://chemoth.com/medicines; Oun, R., Moussa, Y. E., & Wheate, N. J. (2018). The side effects of platinum-based chemotherapy drugs: A review for chemists. *Dalton Transactions*, 47(19), 6645–6653. https://doi.org/10.1039/C8DT00838H

**BOX 43.1 Signs and Symptoms of a Secondary Malignancy**

- Persistent bruising/bleeding
- Pallor
- Fatigue
- Bone pain
- Mole changes
- Delayed healing
- Lumps
- Difficulty swallowing
- Persistent abdominal pain
- Hematuria or hematochezia
- Dysuria
- Shortness of breath
- Persistent cough
- Hemoptysis
- Persistent headaches
- Vision changes
- Early morning emesis

bed, and use cool soaks or massage to the area, which may alleviate symptoms (COG, n.d.-b).

## FERTILITY

Issues with fertility, premature ovarian failure, and inability to enter puberty are all possible late effects of cancer treatment. Both radiation and certain chemotherapies may have these effects on children. Recent studies report rates of post-treatment infertility ranging from 11% to 66%, and those survivors with a history of bone marrow transplant can have rates as high as 90% (Lehmann et al., 2017). Cancer survivors should have an annual comprehensive health check-up including menstrual history, hormonal status (can consider testing FSH, LH, testosterone, and/or estradiol) and progression through puberty. Common chemotherapeutic agents that may cause fertility are listed in Box 43.2.

If any issues arise or are detected, the PCP may refer these children to an endocrinologist who can determine whether hormonal replacement therapy is warranted.

## PSYCHOLOGICAL CONSIDERATIONS

The diagnosis of cancer as well as the treatment strategies and side effects to achieve remission (painful procedures, multiple hospitalizations, hair loss) can be traumatic for a child. The treatment and its aftermath can have long-lasting psychological effects on not only the child, but each member of the family. The PCP should be aware of this and provide developmentally appropriate support, counseling, and referral if

**BOX 43.2 Common Chemotherapeutic Agents That May Cause Fertility Problems**

- Busulfan
- Carboplatin
- Carmustine
- Chlorambucil
- Cisplatin
- Cyclophosphamide
- Dacarbazine
- Ifosfamide
- Nitrogen mustard
- Lomustine
- Melphalan
- Procarbazine
- Temozolomide
- Thiotepa

necessary. Cancer treatment is incredibly challenging and disruptive to a child, and can lead to increased rates of depression and suicide (Constine et al., 2020). The childhood cancer survivor should be screened for depression, posttraumatic stress disorder, and suicidal ideation, and referred to a psychologist if applicable. Throughout treatment, most children with cancer will have to be taken out of school and enrolled in home school or a homebound program; reintroduction into the school system can be especially challenging and psychologically difficult for the cancer survivor. Many times, there are physical sequelae of treatment such as alopecia, amputation, scarring, and so on, which can make it difficult for the child to feel comfortable or accepted in the school environment. It may be helpful to refer these children to various organizations dedicated to children with cancer in order to link them with other cancer survivors, thus making these treatment-related sequelae the social norm among these children. There are many local and national organizations that serve this purpose.

All in all, it is the role of the PCP to be aware of these possible psychological sequelae, screen children often, and support the family. Many times, there are siblings involved that may begin acting out given the decreased level of attention being received due to their sibling's cancer treatment or due to fear of their sibling's death. Studies show that siblings of children with cancer and childhood cancer survivors have higher rates of anxiety, depression, and posttraumatic distress. The risk of anxiety and/or depression in siblings of cancer children increases with younger child age, longer duration of treatment, and whether the child with cancer dies. Support services such as sibling groups and summer camps appear to lessen this risk and help these siblings have increased self-esteem and decreased anxiety (Constine et al., 2020).

## TERMINALLY ILL CHILDREN

Terminal illness is defined as a disease or condition that cannot be cured or adequately treated and is expected to result in death. A terminal illness can result from a long-standing chronic condition, or an acute injury or illness. In the pediatric population, terminal illness is less common than in the adult population, and pediatric PCPs are often unfamiliar with how to deal with the death of a child (Wender et al., 2012, reaffirmed, 2016). However, dealing with terminal illness in children is a challenge faced at some point by all pediatric providers. The challenges are different, but no less important, than in the adult population. These situations are fraught with difficulty. Delivering age-appropriate care and support for both the child and the family differs based on the child's age, the presence of other children in the family, and pediatric options for end of life care and support available in the community.

## CHILD'S UNDERSTANDING OF DEATH AND DYING

Just as in other areas of pediatrics, children's developmental understanding of the concept of death and dying varies greatly. Understanding the child's developmental age is crucial to providing care that is appropriate and connecting the family to age-appropriate resources. In addition to the child, there may be other family members (siblings, cousins, etc.) whose developmental understanding of death and dying may be different from that of the child. When considering referrals for resources, the entire family should be considered as well as the child.

The AAP discusses children's developmental understanding of death from the standpoint of four main concepts: irreversibility (death is permanent), finality (all functioning stops with death), inevitability (death is universal for all living things), and causality (causes of death; Salek & Ginsburg, 2014). For infants and toddlers, they do not understand death or any of the four main concepts. However, they do understand and sense feelings from their caregivers. In this age group, routines are important, as they are a source of comfort for infants and toddlers. Also, increasing physical contact provides a sense of security (Salek & Ginsburg, 2014).

For preschoolers, death is often viewed as something temporary. They are concrete thinkers and do not understand phrases commonly used to describe death such as "passed away" or "gone to sleep." They should be told in clear, plain terms the finality of death. Preschoolers will often repeatedly ask questions to clarify this concept. And you will often see it in their play, acting out their feelings and the situation. They may have developmental regression or anger outbursts in response to a death, as they do not know yet how to express their emotions adequately with words (Salek & Ginsburg, 2014).

School-age children are starting to understand the finality of death. Experiencing a death may cause a school-age child to fear the death of their parents or a loved one. They may have feelings of guilt surrounding death, or believe they contributed to the situation. They can easily become anxious surrounding death, especially if they are taking cues from the anxious adults around them. School-age children need plenty of time to be heard and to express their feelings. They need reaffirmation and time spent with caring adults in order to process these feelings. In response to experiencing a death, school-age children may display new somatic complaints such as a headache or stomachache (Salek & Ginsburg, 2014).

Teenagers have more or less an adult understanding of death and dying, although they may be resistant to express their feelings around the subject. They are becoming more abstract thinkers, and this subject will often have them contemplate broader questions, like the purpose of life. They often feel guilty if they are the survivor and can easily become angry over their lack of control of life and death. They need healthy outlets to express their emotions, such as talking to a trusted individual or journaling. Teens may respond to death by engaging in risky behaviors or withdrawing from social groups. These behaviors are their attempt to regain control of the situation (Salek & Ginsburg, 2014).

## EFFECT ON THE FAMILY

Terminal illness and death in children defies the natural order; parents and families are not meant to bury their children. Siblings of children with terminal illnesses also experience their own sense of loss when death occurs. As noted earlier, a child's developmental response to death and dying varies; the reaction also varies for adults. In some situations, the death is expected or known well before it occurs. In others, it results from an acute injury or illness. Some parents feel a profound sense of guilt with a diagnosis of a terminal illness or experiencing the death of their child. Many will not function following the event for some time, even with the most basic of life skills such as eating and sleeping (Wender et al., 2012, reaffirmed, 2016).

## PALLIATIVE CARE AND HOSPICE

Palliative care and hospice care are integral components of the treatment of children with terminal conditions. The International Children's Palliative Care Network (ICPCN) offers an explanation on the difference between the two. While they both focus on emotional, physical, social, and spiritual care of the child, hospice care is usually reserved for when death is imminent in the next 6 months. Palliative care is used throughout the treatment of a terminal illness while the child is receiving active treatment (International Children's Palliative Care Network [ICPCN], 2015). Its main goal is to provide comfort to the child due to the side effect of their illness or injury. Hospice care can be provided in a facility or in the child's own home. Additionally, hospice care can provide 24 -hour care at the end of life and bereavement resources for the family. Depending on your community resources, pediatric palliative and hospice care is an excellent option for children and families during this difficult time. While this will not take the place of a primary caregiver, organizations providing this care have a wealth of other resources for the family, including caregiver respite care, sibling respite care, and social workers (ICPCN, 2015).

### Do Not Resuscitate and Allow Natural Death

Do Not Resuscitate (DNR) and Allow Natural Death (AND) orders are ways that children and their families can direct the medical team surrounding end-of-life care. Generally, children, parents, and healthcare providers agree that continued suffering is not desirable for any child suffering with a terminal illness. Survival is no longer possible when all potential curative efforts have been made (Bortz, 2018). While AND orders have not gained the popularity of DNR orders, there is a growing body of evidence that the softer terminology of AND orders might be beneficial in some cases. A DNR instructs the medical team caring for the child to withhold cardiopulmonary resuscitation in the event that a child's breathing stops or their heart stops beating. Some states allow for DNR orders to be utilized in the out-of-hospital setting (Weise et al., 2017).

**PRO TIP** Families may change their minds about a DNR order. Respect their decisions and provide support as needed.

The National Hospice and Palliative Care Organization (NHPCO) has established standards in pediatric care that all children have "a right to open and honest communication of age-appropriate information about his or her illness, as well as potential treatments and outcomes" and "to be given the opportunity to participate in decision affecting his or her care, according to age, understanding, capacity, and parental support" (Weise et al., 2017). Within these guidelines, pediatric providers need, when appropriate, to seek assent (usually in the child age 7 or above) and consider dissent when decision-making capacity has been demonstrated (Weise et al., 2017).

In children, DNR orders are commonly utilized in the inpatient setting, particularly in critical care and emergency units of hospitals (Weise et al., 2017). But, the PCP also plays an important role. As the provider with a long-standing relationship with the child and family, a pediatric PCP can help families navigate these discussions, particularly in the case of terminal illness. Determining what the child's and family's wishes would be in the case of needed resuscitation at a time away from the setting of acute decompensation can provide clarity for those who will need to make the decision in a less-threatening environment.

## THE ROLE OF THE PRIMARY CARE PROVIDER

The role of the PCP in supporting the family through these times varies depending on each family's individual needs. In the case of primary care, the provider is often not acutely involved in the child's care at the time of the death or diagnosis of a terminal illness. Rather, the PCP usually has had a long-standing relationship with the family and child in the case of a chronic medical condition or a sudden unexpected illness or injury. Because of this long-standing relationship, PCPs are often a touchpoint or source of continued comfort for the family leading up to and following the death (Wender et al., 2012, reaffirmed, 2016). With a terminal diagnosis or death, many PCPs fear that reaching out will only make the situation worse. And, many providers feel ill-equipped to discuss terminal diseases with their children and families. PCPs should always contact the family when they learn of a child's terminal diagnosis or death. The provider should make time to meet in person with the parents in order to allow the parents to freely express their emotions (Wender et al., 2012, reaffirmed, 2016). Family support during these challenging times takes on many forms. Providing the family with resources for support groups for the child, the parents, and any siblings will give those affected the ability to freely express emotions and be around others experiencing similar losses. In the case of a sibling, the provider may continue to be that child's provider. The provider should closely monitor the sibling's emotional development and intervene when necessary if issues are noted (Wender et al., 2012, reaffirmed, 2016). Individual therapy is also often needed, although medication is rarely prescribed. Other resources can include the family's religious community or social groups, such as through the child's school.

Pediatric PCPs are well-equipped to deal with terminal illness and death in children. The benefit of their long-standing relationship with both the family and child make them a powerful advocate in these cases, including resource referral for the child and family, as well as discussion of end-of-life and resuscitation care.

## KEY POINTS

- The medically fragile child experiences unique healthcare and developmental needs that affect not only the child, but the family as well.
- The nurse practitioner is in a unique position to provide family-centered care and become the medical home for children and youth with special healthcare needs.
- When families take care of a technology-dependent child at home, they may need to learn about oxygen supplementation, tracheostomies, ventilators, and feeding tubes.
- The former premature infant is at increased risk for a poor neurodevelopmental outcome and may also be discharged with ongoing particular medical needs including transient dystonia, developmental delays, CLD, retinopathy of prematurity, and apnea, among others. Care is focused on maximizing the infant's potential.
- Overcoming the barriers to and assisting the adolescent with special healthcare needs with transition to adult care can be successfully achieved with significant advanced planning and the support of the nurse practitioner.
- The nurse practitioner caring for the child undergoing chemotherapy should monitor and intervene for pulmonary, cardiovascular, GI, and neurologic system adverse effects as well as immunosuppression and ototoxicity.
- The survivor of childhood cancer may experience chemotherapy-induced cardiotoxicity, peripheral neuropathy, fertility issues, or secondary malignancy, as well as have psychosocial concerns.
- When caring for the terminally ill child, it is important to understand developmental understanding of death and dying, and to support the child and family's desires for palliative care or hospice and allowing natural death.

## REFERENCES

Abrams, S. A. (2019). Management of neonatal bone health. *UpToDate*. https://www.uptodate.com/contents/management-of-neonatal-bone-health

Adams-Chapman, I., Heyne, R. J., DeMauro, S. B., Duncan, A. F., Hintz, S. R., Pappas, A., Vohr, B. R., McDonald, S. A., Das, A., Newman, J. E., & Higgins, R. D. (2018). Neurodevelopmental impairment among extremely preterm infants in the Neonatal Research Network. *Pediatrics, 141*(5), e20173091. https://doi.org/10.1542/peds.2017-3091

Ahmed, N., & Flynn, P. (2019). Fever in children with chemotherapy-induced neutropenia. *UpToDate*. https://www.uptodate.com/contents/fever-in-children-with-chemotherapy-induced-neutropenia

American Academy of Child and Adolescent Psychiatry. (2015). *Chronic illness and children*. https://www.aacap.org/aacap/families_and_youth/facts_for_families/fff-guide/The-Child-With-A-Long-Term-Illness-019.aspx

American Academy of Pediatrics. (2014). Updated guidance for palivizumab prophylaxis among infants and young children at increased risk of hospitalization for respiratory syncytial virus infection. *Pediatrics, 134*, 415–420. https://doi.org/10.1542/peds.2014-1665

American Academy of Pediatrics. (2015). *Common reasons for rehospitalization*. https://www.healthychildren.org/English/ages-stages/baby/preemie/Pages/Common-Reasons-for-Rehospitalization.aspx

American Hippotherapy Association. (2019). *Use of hippotherapy in occupational therapy, physical therapy and speech therapy*. https://www.americanhippotherapyassociation.org/assets/docs/Present-Use-of-HPOT-final-proposed-revision-February-2019-2.pdf

American Music Therapy Association. (2020). *What is music therapy?* http://www.musictherapy.org

Applebaum, M. A., Henderson, T. O., Lee, S. M., Pinto, N., Volchenboum, S. L., & Cohn, S. L. (2015). Second malignancies in patients with neuroblastoma: The effects of risk-based therapy. *Pediatric Blood & Cancer, 62*(1), 128–133. https://doi.org/10.1002/pbc.25249

Asselin, B. L. (2020). Epidemiology of childhood and adolescent cancer. In R. M. Kliegman, J. W. St. Geme III, N. J. Blum, S. S. Shah, R. C. Tasker, K. M. Wilson, & R. E. Behrman (Eds.), *Nelson textbook of pediatrics* (21st ed., Chapter 518). Elsevier.

Bally, J., Smith, N., Holtslander, L., Duncan, V., Hodgson-Viden, H., Mpofu, C., & Zimmer, M. (2018). A metasynthesis: Uncovering what is known about the experiences of families with children who have life-limiting and life-threatening illnesses. *Journal of Pediatric Nursing, 38*, 88–98. https://doi.org/10.1016/j.pedn.2017.11.004

Bansal, N., Amdani, S., Lipshultz, E. R., & Lipshultz, S. E. (2017). Chemotherapy-induced cardiotoxicity in children. *Expert Opinion on Drug Metabolism & Toxicology, 13*(8), 817–832. https://doi.org/10.1080/17425255.2017.1351547

Berman, L. (2019). *Gastrostomy tube (g-tube)*. https://kidshealth.org/en/parents/g-tube.html

Betz, C. L., Smith, K., Van Speybroeck, A., Jacobs, R. A., Rivera, N., Lee, J., Saghhafi, S., Nguyen, B., & Tu, H. (2018). Descriptive analysis of profile of health care transition services provided to adolescents and emerging adult in the Movin' On Up health care transition program. *Journal of Pediatric Health Care, 32*(3), 273–284. https://doi.org/10.1016/j.pedhc.2017.11.006

Bortz, K. (2018). *AAP: Special considerations to be made for pediatric DNRs*. https://www.healio.com/pediatrics/practice-management/news/online/%7B16d61aaf-86a0-492e-a3c4-b0a225de7e85%7D/aap-special-considerations-to-be-made-for-pediatric-dnrs

Boyse, K. (2020). *Siblings of kids with special needs*. http://www.med.umich.edu/yourchild/topics/specneed.htm

Boyse, K., Boujaouse, L., & Laundy, J. (2020). *Children with chronic conditions*. http://www.med.umich.edu/yourchild/topics/chronic.htm

Centers for Medicare and Medicaid Services. (n.d.). *Children's Health Insurance Program (CHIP)*. https://www.medicaid.gov/chip/index.html

Children's Hospital of Philadelphia. (2020). *Jejunostomy tube (j-tube)*. https://www.chop.edu/treatments/jejunostomy-tubes

Children's Oncology Group. (2018a). *Educational issues after cancer treatment, version 5.0*. http://www.survivorshipguidelines.org/pdf/2018/English%20Health%20Links/14_educational_issues%20(secured).pdf

Children's Oncology Group. (2018b). *Emotional issues after cancer treatment, version 5.0*. http://www.survivorshipguidelines.org/pdf/2018/English%20Health%20Links/15_emotional_issues%20(secured).pdf

Children's Oncology Group. (n.d.-a). *Dental health*. https://www.childrensoncologygroup.org/index.php/sensory/dentalhealth

Children's Oncology Group. (n.d.-b). *Peripheral neuropathy*. https:www.childrensoncologygroup.org/index.php/peripheralneuropathy

Children's Oncology Group. (n.d.-c). *Secondary cancers*. https://www.childrensoncologygroup.org/index.php/secondarycancer

Chung, E. H., Chou, J., & Brown, K. A. (2020). Neurodevelopmental outcomes of preterm infants: A recent literature review. *Translational Pediatrics, 9*(Suppl. 1), S3–S8. https://doi.org/10.21037/tp.2019.09.10

Cincinnati Children's Hospital Medical Center. (2020a). *Gastrostomy-jejunostomy tube care*. http://www.cincinnatichildrens.org/health/g/gastro-jejuno-tube

Cincinnati Children's Hospital Medical Center. (2020b). *Special needs resource directory*. https://www.cincinnatichildrens.org/patients/child/special-needs/getting-started

Coats, D. K. (2020). Retinopathy of prematurity: Pathogenesis, epidemiology, classification, and screening. *UpToDate*. https://www.uptodate.com/contents/retinopathy-of-prematurity-pathogenesis-epidemiology-classification-and-screening

Constine, L. S., Hudson, M. M., & Seibel, N. L. (Eds.). (2020). *Late effects of treatment for childhood cancer (PDQ®)—Health professional version*. https://www.cancer.gov/types/childhood-cancers/late-effects-hp-pdq

Crean, D., & Jones, E. (n.d.). *Types of chemotherapy drugs*. https://chemoth.com/medicines

de Leon Siantz, M. L., Kilanowski, J. F., & Thomas, T. L. (2018). Cultural values, beliefs, and preference are integral to family-centered care. In C. L. Betz, M. J. Krajicek, & M. Craft-Rosenberg (Eds.), *Guidelines for nursing excellence in the care of children, youth, and families* (2nd ed., pp. 57–76). Springer Publishing Company.

Flank, J., Robinson, P. D., Holdsworth, M., Phillips, R., Portwine, C., Gibson, P., Maan, C., Hons, N. S., Sung, L., & Dupuis, L. L. (2016). Guideline for the treatment of breakthrough and the prevention of refractory chemotherapy-induced nausea and vomiting in children with cancer. *Pediatric Blood and Cancer, 63*(7), 1144–1151. https://doi.org/10.1002/pbc.25955

Fortin, K., & Downes, A. H. (2019). Psychosocial issues. In K. J. Marcdante & R. M. Kliegman (Eds.), *Nelson's essentials of pediatrics* (8th ed., Section 5). Elsevier.

Gillard, M. A., Herring, R. A., & Hesselgrave, J. (2019). Toxicity and symptom management. In R. A. Herrin, J. O. Curry, J.

Hesselgrave, C. Nixon, M. L. Rae, & the APHON Chemotherapy and Biotherapy Provider Program Committee (Eds.), *The pediatric chemotherapy and biotherapy curriculum* (4th ed., Chapter 8). Association of Pediatric Hematology/Oncology Nurses.

Grimshaw, S. L., Taylor, N. F., Mechinaud, F., & Shields, N. (2018). Assessment of physical function in children: A systematic review. *Pediatric Blood and Cancer, 65*(12). https://doi.org/10.1002/pbc.27369

Hall, C. A., Donza, C., McGinn, S., Rimmer, A., Skomial, S., Todd, E., & Vaccaro, F. (2019). Health-related quality of life in children with chronic illness compared to parents: A systematic review. *Pediatric Physical Therapy, 31*(4), 315–322. https://doi.org/10.1097/PEP.0000000000000638

Hanks, H., & Carrico, C. A. (2017). Evaluating the use of a stability guideline for long-term ventilator-dependent children discharging to home: A quality improvement project. *Journal of Pediatric Health Care, 31*(6), 648–653. http://doi.org/10.1016/j.pedhc.2017.04.018

Health Resources and Services Administration, Maternal and Child Health Bureau. (n.d.). *Children with special health care needs.* https://mchb.hrsa.gov/maternal-child-health-topics/children-and-youth-special-health-needs

Health Transition Wisconsin. (2020). *Welcome to Wisconsin's youth health transition initiative!* https://healthtransitionwi.org

Horton, T. M., & Steuber, C. P. (2019). Overview of the treatment of acute lymphoblastic leukemia lymphoma in children and adolescents. *UpToDate.* https://www.uptodate.com/contents/overview-of-the-treatment-of-acute-lymphoblastic-leukemia-lymphoma-in-children-and-adolescents

Hosley, S., Zeno, F., Harrison, T. M., & Steward, D. (2018). Supporting families when a child has a complex chronic condition. In K. F. Pridham, R. Limbo, & M. M. Schroeder (Eds.), *Guided participation in pediatric nursing practice: Relationship-based teaching and learning with parents, children, and adolescents* (pp. 133–154). Springer Publishing Company

Hunger, S., & Mullighan, C. (2015). Acute lymphoblastic leukemia in children. *New England Journal of Medicine, 373*(16), 1541–1552. https://doi.org/10.1056/NEJMra1400972

International Children's Palliative Care Network. (2015). *What is children's palliative care?* http://www.icpcn.org/about-icpcn/what-is-childrens-palliative-care

Johns Hopkins Medicine. (n.d.). *Tracheostomy humidification.* https://www.hopkinsmedicine.org/tracheostomy/living/humidification.html

Kids' Waivers. (n.d.). *Welcome to Kids' Waivers.* https://www.kidswaivers.org

Kuo, D. Z., & Turchi, R. M. (2020). Children and youth with special health care needs. *UpToDate.* https://www.uptodate.com/contents/children-and-youth-with-special-health-care-needs#topicContent

Lehmann, V., Keim, M. C., Nahata, L., Schultz, E. L., Klosky, J. L., Tuinman, M. A., & Gerhardt, C. A. (2017). Fertility-related knowledge and reproductive goals in childhood cancer survivors: Short communication. *Human Reproduction, 32*(11), 2250–2253. https://doi.org/10.1093/humrep/dex297

Lehrnbecher, T., Robinson, P., Fisher, B., Alexander, S., Ammann, R. A., Beauchemin, M., Carlesse, F., Groll, A. H., Haeusler, G. M., Santolaya, M., Steinbach, W. J., Castagnola, E., Davis, B. L., Dupuis, L. L., Gaur, A. H., Tissing, W. J. E., Zaoutis, T., Phillips, R., & Sung, L. (2017). Guideline for the management of fever and neutropenia in children with cancer and hematopoietic stem-cell transplantation recipients: 2017 update. *Journal of Clinical Oncology, 35*(18), 2082–2094. http://ascopubs.org/doi/abs/10.1200/JCO.2016.71.7017

Letishock, L., Daly, A. M., & White, P. (2018). Pediatric nurse practitioners' perspectives on health care transition from pediatric to adult care. *Journal of Pediatric Health Care, 32*(3), 263–272. https://doi.org/10.1016/j.pedhc.2017.11.005

Lexicomp. (2020). *Lexicomp clinical drug information* (version 5.7.1) [Mobile app]. App store. https://apps.apple.com/us/app/lexicomp/id313401238

Mandy, G. T. (2020). Long-term complications of the preterm infant. *UpToDate.* https://www.uptodate.com/contents/long-term-complications-of-the-preterm-infant

McGowan, J. V., Chung, R., Maulik, A., Piotrowska, I., Walker, J. M., & Yellon, D. M. (2017). Anthracycline chemotherapy and cardiotoxicity. *Cardiovascular Drugs and Therapy, 31*(1), 63–75. https://doi.org/10.1007/s10557-016-6711-0

Michniacki, T. F., & Walkovich, K. J. (2020). Leukopenia. In R. M. Kliegman, J. W. St. Geme III, N. J. Blum, S. S. Shah, R. C. Tasker, K. M. Wilson, & R. E. Behrman (Eds.), *Nelson textbook of pediatrics* (21st ed., Chapter 157). Elsevier.

National Association of Pediatric Nurse Practitioners. (2019). NAPNAP position statement on age parameters for pediatric nurse practitioner practice. *Journal of Pediatric Health Care, 33*, A11–A13. https://doi.org/10.1016/j.pedhc.2018.10.007

National Cancer Institute. (2020). *Childhood cancers.* https://www.cancer.gov/types/childhood-cancers

Oun, R., Moussa, Y. E., & Wheate, N. J. (2018). The side effects of platinum-based chemotherapy drugs: A review for chemists. *Dalton Transactions, 47*(19), 6645–6653. https://doi.org/10.1039/C8DT00838H

Pappas, A., Adams-Chapman, I., Shankaran, S., McDonald, S. A., Stoll, B. J., Laptook, A. R., Carlo, W. A., Van Meurs, K. P., Hintz, S. R., Carlson, M. D., Brumbaugh, J. E., Walsh, M. C., Wyckoff, M. H., Das, A., & Higgins, R. D. (2018). Neurodevelopmental and behavioral outcomes in extremely premature neonates with ventriculomegaly in the absence of periventricular-intraventricular hemorrhage. *JAMA Pediatrics, 172*(1), 32–42. https://doi.org/10.1001/jamapediatrics.2017.3545

Passy Muir. (n.d.). *What is a Passy Muir speaking valve?* https://www.passy-muir.com

Peikert, M. L., Inhestern, L., & Bergelt, C. (2018). Psychosocial interventions for rehabilitation and reintegration into daily life of pediatric cancer survivors and their families: A systematic review. *PLoS ONE, 13*(4), e0196151. https://doi.org/10.1371/journal.pone.0196151

Phelan, R., Eissa, H., Becktell, K., Bhatt, N., Kudek, M., Nuechterlein, B., Pommert, L., Tanaka, R., & Baker, K. S. (2019). Upfront therapies and downstream effects: Navigating late effects in childhood cancer survivors in the current era. *Current Oncology Reports, 21*(104). https://doi.org/10.1007/s11912-019-0861-8

Provenzi, L., Saettini, F., Barello, S., & Borgatti, R. (2016). Research paper: Complementary and alternative medicine (CAM) for children with special health care needs: A comparative usage study in Italy. *Special Issue on Paediatric Integrative Medicine, European Journal of Integrative Medicine, 8*(2), 115–121. https://doi.org/10.1016/j.eujim.2015.06.005

Pui, C.-H., Yang, J. J., Hunger, S. P., Pieters, R., Schrappe, M., Biondi, A., Vora, A., Baruche, A., Silverman, L. B., Schmiegelow, K., Escherich, G., Horibe, K., Benoit, Y. C.

M., Izraeli, S., Yeoh, A. E. J., Liang, D.-C., Downing, J. R., Evans, W. E., Relling, M. V., & Mullighan, C. G. (2015). Childhood acute lymphoblastic leukemia: Progress through collaboration. *Journal of Clinical Oncology, 33*(27), 2938–2948. https://doi.org/10.1200/JCO.2014.59.1636

Ritchey, A. K., & Friehling, E. (2020). Principles of cancer diagnosis. In R. M. Kliegman, J. W. St. Geme III, N. J. Blum, S. S. Shah, R. C. Tasker, K. M. Wilson, & R. E. Behrman (Eds.), *Nelson textbook of pediatrics* (21st ed., Chapter 520). Elsevier.

Salandy, S., Rai, R., Gutierrez, S., Ishak, B., & Tubbs, R. S. (2019). Neurological examination of the infant: A comprehensive review. *Clinical Anatomy, 32*(6), 770–777. https://doi.org/10.1002/ca.23352

Salek, E. C., & Ginsburg, K. R. (2014). *How children understand death & what you should say*. https://www.healthychildren.org/English/healthy-living/emotional-wellness/Building-Resilience/Pages/How-Children-Understand-Death-What-You-Should-Say.aspx

Santacroce, S. J., Tan, K., & Killela, M. (2018). A systematic scoping review of the recent literature (~2011–2017) about the costs of illness to parents of children diagnosed with cancer. *European Journal of Oncology, 35*, 22–32. https://doi.org/10.1016/j.ejon.2018.04.004

Scharf, R. J., Scharf, G. J., & Stroustrup, A. (2016). Developmental milestones. *Pediatrics in Review, 37*(1), 25–47. https://doi.org/10.1542/pir.2014-0103

Smith, V. C., & Stewart, J. (2020). Discharge planning for high-risk newborns. *UpToDate*. https://www.uptodate.com/contents/discharge-planning-for-high-risk-newborns

Social Security Administration. (n.d.-a). *Supplemental security income (SSI): Child recipient fact sheet*. https://www.ssa.gov/news/press/factsheets/ss-customer/ssi-children.pdf

Social Security Administration. (n.d.-b). *Title V—maternal and child health services block grant*. http://www.ssa.gov/OP_Home/ssact/title05/0500.htm

Stewart, J. (2020). Care of the neonatal intensive care unit graduate. *UpToDate*. https://www.uptodate.com/contents/care-of-the-neonatal-intensive-care-unit-graduate#H6

Turcotte, L. M., Liu, Q., Yasui, Y., Henderson, T. O., Gibson, T. M., Leisenring, W., Arnold, M. A., Howell, R. M., Green, D. M., Armstrong, G. T., Robison, L. L., & Neglia, J. P. (2019). Chemotherapy and risk of subsequent malignant neoplasms in the childhood cancer survivor study cohort. *Journal of Clinical Oncology, 37*(34), 3310–3319. https://doi.org/10.1200/JCO.19.00129

U.S. Department of Education. (n.d.). *IDEA*. https://sites.ed.gov/idea

Weise, K. L., Okun, A. L., Carter, B. S., Christian, C. W., & Committee on Bioethics, Section on Hospice and Palliative Medicine, and Committee on Child Abuse and Neglect. (2017). Guidance on forgoing life-sustaining medical treatment. *Pediatrics, 140*(3), e20171905. https://doi.org/10.1542/peds.2017-1905

Wender, E., & the Committee on Psychosocial Aspects of Child and Family Health. (2012, reaffirmed 2016). Supporting the family after the death of a child. *Pediatrics, 130*(6), 1164–1169. http://pediatrics.aappublications.org/content/130/6/1164

Wengenroth, L., Gianinazzi, M., Rueegg, C., Lüer, S., Bergstraesser, E., Kuehni, C., & Michel, G. (2015). Health-related quality of life in young survivors of childhood cancer. *Quality of Life Research, 24*(9), 2151–2161. http://www.jstor.org/stable/44849311

White, P. H., Cooley, W. C., & Transitions Clinical Report Authoring Group, American Academy of Pediatrics, American Academy of Family Physicians, American College of Physicians. (2018). Supporting the health care transition from adolescence to adulthood in the medical home. *Pediatrics, 142*(5), e20182587. https://doi.org/10.1542/peds.2018-258

Whitmore, K., & Snethen, J. (2018). Respite care services for children with special healthcare needs: Parental perceptions. *Journal for Specialists in Pediatric Nursing, 23*(3), e12217. https://doi.org/10.1111/jspn.12217

Wilson-Costello, D., & Payne, A. (2020). Long-term neurodevelopmental outcome of preterm infants: Epidemiology and risk factors. *UpToDate*. https://www.uptodate.com/contents/long-term-neurodevelopmental-outcome-of-preterm-infants-epidemiology-and-risk-factors

York, J. M. (Ed.). (2018). *Children's oncology group long term follow-up guidelines*. http://www.survivorshipguidelines.org/pdf/2018/COG_LTFU_Guidelines_v5.pdf

Younge, N., Goldstein, R. F., Bann, C. M., Hintz, S. R., Patel, R. M., Smith, P. B., Bell, E. F., Rysavy, M. A., Duncan, A. F., Vohr, B. R., Das. A., Goldberg, R. N., Higgins, R. D., & Cotton, C. M. (2017). Survival and neurodevelopmental outcomes among periviable infants. *New England Journal of Medicine, 376*(7), 617–628. https://doi.org/10.1056/NEJMoa1605566

# Approach to the Care of Children in Special Populations

Sara Rose McClelland

## Student Learning Outcomes

**Upon completion of this chapter the reader should be able to:**

1. Recognize patients who may be in a societal minority group.
2. Modify assessment to be culturally sensitive while still getting key information.
3. Recognize social determinants of health that are significant for your patient.
4. Assess for signs and symptoms of physical and psychological trauma.
5. Recognize what community resources are available for specific populations.
6. Identify which professionals in the community you should coordinate and collaborate with to provide high levels of interdisciplinary, holistic care.

## INTRODUCTION

As a primary care advanced practice provider, you will come in contact with a diverse array of patients and families. Whether you work in a public or private office, an emergency room, a family practice or a pediatric-specific office, health department, military sector, or internationally, your patient population may contain children or families that are not included in the societal majority. Each of these children comes with a specific set of challenges, needs, risks, and strengths that varies from the child that came before or after them. The following chapter will discuss several types of children who fall outside of the societal majority.

The content in this chapter maps to the following areas on the Pediatric Nursing Certification Board (PNCB) Pediatric Nurse Practitioner—Primary Care certification examination:

**CLINICAL PROBLEMS: DEVELOPMENTAL/BEHAVIORAL/MENTAL HEALTH, SEXUAL IDENTITY**

CONTENT AREAS:

### I. Health Maintenance and Promotion

**A. Partner with patients/caregivers to support growth and development from infancy to young adulthood.**

### II. Assessment and Diagnosis

**B. History and Physical Examination**

1. Obtain history of present illness.
2. Obtain a comprehensive health history for new patients.
3. Complete an interval history for established patients.
4. Perform a review of systems.
5. Perform a complete physical examination.

**D. Analyzing Information**

1. Integrate health history and physical examination findings into the plan of care.

### III. Management

**A. Child and Caregiver Counseling and Education**

1. Provide condition-specific counseling and education, including treatment options.

**B. Therapeutic Interventions**

5. Utilize communication techniques and brief cognitive interventions, including motivational interviewing and joint decision-making, to develop healthcare goals and facilitate change.

**C. Collaboration and Referral**

1. Collaborate with other health professionals to meet patient care needs.
2. Refer to specialists as indicated for evaluation, counseling, and/or treatment.
3. Refer children, adolescents, or caregivers to community resources as indicated.
4. Contact child protective services to report suspected maltreatment or neglect.

**E. Care Coordination**

1. Facilitate patient and family-centered care for children of all ages with acute and chronic conditions.

**F. Evaluation and Follow-Up**

2. Establish a plan for follow-up care.

### IV. Professional Role and Responsibilities

**A. Leadership and Evidence-Based Practice**

4. Develop, implement, and/or modify clinical practice guidelines.

**C. Legal and Ethical Issues**

2. Incorporate cultural awareness and inclusiveness into all aspects of practice.

## LESBIAN, GAY, BISEXUAL, TRANSGENDER, QUEER POPULATION

In this section, we will be discussing the process of gender identity formation, the assessment of the Lesbian, Gay, Bisexual, Transgender, and Queer or Questioning (LGBTQ+) youth (rainbow spectrum), unique challenges facing this population, health maintenance and anticipatory guidance, and reasons for referral. As the pediatric patient grows and develops, one integral part of physical, mental, and social maturity is the development of gender identity and sexual orientation. While children are born with a biologic sex, their behaviors and identity are not bound by the societal "norms" of their physical characteristics. The subjects of gender and sexuality beyond what has been considered the "norm" in society have been controversial for many years. Regardless, research has been increasing steadily in this area regarding the health and wellness of a population that pushes the established norms. *Healthy People 2020* named physical and mental care of the LGBTQ population as one of their priorities (Snyder et al., 2017). Nationally, governments are ruling in favor for marriage equality and protection of rights for members of the LGBTQ community, but this has been faced with significant backlash in many states who institute laws and policies that further discriminate and negatively affect against those on the rainbow spectrum. The medical community has the opportunity to be at the forefront of medical and emotional support, education, and normalization to remove the stigma experienced by many members of the sexual minority population.

Collecting statistics regarding the incidence of children and youth that identify as part of the LGBTQ community is challenging due to multiple factors. Reasons for this may include fear of disclosure or that their private information will not be kept confidential. For other children, their developmental stage and understanding may not be sufficiently mature for them to truly correlate their feelings or desires to something that can be labeled (Perron et al., 2017a). The 2019 Youth Behavioral Risk Survey (YRBS) indicated 84.4% of youths self-identified as heterosexual, 8.7% reported being bisexual, 2.5% stated they were gay or lesbian, while 4.5% of youths reported being unsure of their sexual identity (Underwood et al., 2020). In regard to sexual contact, 47.6% of youths reported they had had no sexual contact, 45.4% indicated sexual contact with only the opposite sex, 4.8% reported sexual contact with both sexes, and 2.2% indicated sexual contact with only those of the same sex (Underwood et al., 2020). These numbers indicate that while LGBTQ youth remain in the sexual minority, their preferences are far from uncommon.

## ANATOMY, GENDER IDENTIFICATION, AND GENDER EXPRESSION

Shortly after fertilization (approximately 7 weeks), the fetus forms sex organs and the biological sex is developed. Based on hormonal influences, the fetus will develop male or female external genitalia and reproductive organs. If there are hormonal inconsistencies during this critical period, the fetus may develop ambiguous genitalia. Children born with ambiguous genitalia are often labeled "intersex." It is important to identify the differences between gender identity (what gender the patient feels they are) and gender expression (how the patient expresses their gender identity) and to recognize how these either correlate or conflict with their biological sex (strictly which reproductive organs the child is born with).

Gender identification begins as early as toddlerhood. Around age 2, children are able to recognize that males and females are different and have different body parts; by age 3, they are typically able to label themselves as "boy" or "girl," and over the next few years that identification solidifies for some children (Rafferty, 2018). Current thought indicates that gender identity does not automatically become stable at a particular developmental age. Rather, it is considered more fluid in nature. This thinking then allows for valuing of children for who they are, even at younger ages (Rafferty et al., 2018).

Gender identity and gender expression do not necessarily correlate with sexual orientation, and sexual orientation does not necessarily correlate with partners with whom the patient is sexually active. Unrelated to gender identity and expression is the child's sexual orientation, or which gender the patient is attracted to. This can also fall on a spectrum where the patient may be attracted to those of the opposite biological sex (heterosexual), the same biological sex (homosexual/gay or lesbian), or a mixture of the two (bisexual). This will present special considerations for the practitioner as they assess the sexual practices and also educate on safe sex practices.

## ASSESSMENT

There are many important things to remember as a practitioner caring for a child or youth regardless of gender identity or sexual orientation. Before walking into the examination room, it is vital that the care provider do their own self-assessment of beliefs, prejudices, and preconceived notions. Those need to be checked and left outside the door. Healthcare providers need to be aware of their own biases and prejudices prior to caring for patients. A good practitioner will examine their own beliefs and ideas prior to practicing and will be open to caring for a variety of patients. Providing culturally competent care begins with self-examination and a willingness to practice cultural humility. This attitude is no different when caring for patients who identify on the rainbow spectrum of gender identity and sexual orientation.

The following sections will describe the challenges, associated comorbidities, and health risks that LGBTQ+ youth may experience. These youth need a safe, nondiscriminatory ally in their healthcare provider to support them as they go through what may be a confusing and isolating process of navigating their gender identity and sexuality. Identifying as LGBTQ should not be considered a potential health hazard. However, individuals who identify on the rainbow spectrum still need to have the knowledge, tools, and support to make responsible decisions for their own health and well-being.

Sensitive care first begins in the waiting room. Paperwork should have a place for the child or adolescent to state their legal name, their preferred name, and their preferred pronouns. For some individuals with gender dysphoria, even though their physical body looks like one gender, it may cause them emotional distress to be referred to by pronouns associated with that gender. It is vital to honor the pronoun that the patient prefers. The provider should review the paperwork prior to initiating contact with the individual to ensure that the correct pronouns are being used (Earnshaw et al., 2017).

When assessing any adolescent, time should be saved during the appointment or interaction to converse with them without a family member in the room. While some providers find it helpful to do this at the end of the visit, doing so at the beginning of the assessment can help lay a foundation of knowledge and establish rapport between the adolescent and provider. This discussion can serve as a time for the adolescent to disclose valuable information about their comfort level and the involvement of the parents, particularly when the conversation may be about sexuality or gender identity. In setting this boundary at the beginning of the appointment, the adolescent may be more at ease during the remainder of the assessment. Some individuals will not disclose to their provider the challenges they are facing with their identity formation or sexual orientation, and it is vital that the advanced practice provider does not label the child until the child labels themself.

Individuals whose gender identity does not correlate with their biological sex may opt to use different ways to express their gender identity. Recognizing, acknowledging, and carrying out the physical examination around this can be helpful when building a rapport and making the examination room a safe place. Examples of how individuals may use different materials to express their gender identity may include chest binders to hide breast tissue, bra inserts to give the appearance of breast tissue, and inserts to give the impression of male genitalia (House et al., 2019). Typically, these are seen in adolescents who are more open about their gender dysphoria (the mismatch between assigned sex and gender identity). Asking judgment-free questions about how the patient uses gender identity supportive materials, if they are currently wearing them, and what they are provides the practitioner with important information. By providing nonjudgmental support, the practitioner can either work around the materials during the physical assessment or ask the patient to remove them in privacy. Creating this sense of support and honesty with the patient will facilitate a more sensitive and caring environment during an assessment (House et al., 2019).

## Health Disparities and Risks

As previously stated, the healthcare professional should not automatically assume a youth who identifies as LGBTQ is also at high risk without first assessing behaviors, challenges, supports, and strength (Rafferty et al., 2018). While most members of the LGBTQ community are able to grow and develop and become functioning, content adults, the prevalence of risk-associated comorbidities is associated with stigmatization and discrimination leading to feelings of rejection and isolation (Rafferty et al., 2018).

### Sexual/Reproductive Health Risks

As previously mentioned, there is not necessarily a correlation between gender, gender identification, and sexual orientation to the gender of partners that youth may have. In the 2019 YRBS study, 2.5% of youth polled characterized themselves as being gay or lesbian, but nearly twice that revealed having sex with partners of both genders (Underwood et al., 2020). In earlier YRBS data, as compared with reports from heterosexual high school students, sexual/gender minority youth (SMY) indicated:

- A higher percentage of earlier initiation of sexual intercourse (before 13 years old)
- A larger partner pool (females: over four partners)
- Decreased percentage of using condoms with most recent sexual intercourse
- Decreased percentage of pregnancy prevention use with most recent sexual intercourse (Rasberry et al., 2018).

These increased risk behaviors among SMY places them at increased risk for unintended pregnancy, sexually transmitted infection (STI), and human immunodeficiency virus infection (Rasberry et al., 2018).

When talking with the adolescent about sexual health, it is vital to remember that it is not identifying as an LGBTQ member that puts them in danger of STIs and unintended pregnancy; it is risk behaviors that do. Individuals who engage in protected, monogamous sex, with no history of drug misuse, should be tested for STIs yearly. The more risk factors that are present, the more frequently testing should be done. Females should also be tested for a variety of STIs due to the possible previous incidence of intercourse with biological males (Table 44.1).

**TABLE 44.1 Sexually Transmitted Infection Testing by Gender**

| Female | Male |
|---|---|
| Chlamydia<br>Syphilis<br>HSV (serum for high risk)<br>HIV | Chlamydia<br>Syphilis<br>HSV<br>HIV<br>Hep C (if HIV +)<br>Hepatitis B (serum)<br>Gonorrhea (urethral, rectal, pharyngeal) |

### Psychological/Social

Depression rates among teens are increasing, and among them gender and sexual minority youths experience increased rates of loneliness, anxiety, and depression as compared with heterosexual youths (Perron et al., 2017b). Forty-two percent of SMY report suicidal ideation as compared with 14% in non-LGBTQ youth. In the same study, while 9% of non-LGBTQ youth reported a past suicide attempt, 29% of SMY had attempted to take their own life in the past 6 months (Hatchel et al., 2019).

One causative factor behind the depression, anxiety, conduct disorder, and substance abuse risks among LGBTQ adolescents is the presence of bullying at home, school, and in the community. The presence or perception that an individual is a sexual minority youth is sometimes all that is needed to prompt bullying and harassment (both physical and emotional; Perron et al., 2017b). LGBTQ youth experience double the amount of bullying as compared to their heterosexual peers and each time the youth experiences this bullying, they are 2.5 times more likely to inflict self-harm (Mental Health America [MHA], 2020). Additionally, LGBTQ youth are twice as likely to experiment with drugs and alcohol as their heterosexual peers (MHA, 2020).

For LGBTQ youth without supportive homes or supportive adults in their lives, being kicked out or running away can lead to homelessness. Nearly 40% of homeless teens may be sexual minorities, and their risk for homelessness is 120% higher than heterosexual youths' risk. Homelessness may lead to risky behaviors, sexual abuse, and exploitation, as well as increased stigmatization and discrimination (Dashow, 2017). Lastly, the stress of victimization and the struggle with sexual identity development may place SMY at increased risk for disordered eating and problems related to weight. Studies have shown an increase in restrictive dieting and purging in sexual minority males (Miller & Luk, 2019). Sexual minority females may struggle with overweight or obesity and some will experience disordered eating (Miller & Luk, 2019).

## HEALTH MAINTENANCE

The human papillomavirus (HPV) 9-valent recombinant vaccine (Gardasil 9®) is recommended for all youth regardless of their sexual orientation or gender beginning at 11 to 12 years of age. The vaccine protects against HPV infection, which is known to cause cancer (anal, cervical, vaginal, vulvar) and genital warts and is most effective if given prior to any sexual exposure to HPV. The vaccine is given in a two-dose series if started before age 15 years, and a three-dose series if started at 15 years of age or older, and may be given to all males and females until the age of 26 years (Centers for Disease Control and Prevention [CDC], 2019).

Conversion/reparative therapy is contraindicated in every case of LGBTQ youth. These are programs, therapies, and facilities whose goal is changing the patient's gender identification or sexual orientation, therefore "fixing" them. These interventions have been found to be immensely dangerous to the mental and sometimes physical health of the youth. The American Academy of Child & Adolescent Psychiatry (AACAP) has determined these therapies lack clinical utility and may harm the individual; thus, they should not be included in behavioral health treatment of children and adolescents (AACAP, 2018).

### Anticipatory Guidance

Anticipatory guidance is an important part of the care that the provider offers in the office. These are tools that you offer the child and family to make the most informed, empowered, healthy decisions that can lead them to a richer and more healthy relationship with their body, their family/friends, and themselves.

Refer to Chapter 29 for anticipatory guidance on safe sex practices. Most importantly, condoms should be encouraged and the use of dental dams in oral sex should be taught and made available. Birth control options need to be discussed when females anticipate sex with males and vice versa. The difference between birth control and STI prevention should also be discussed and the different methods for both made available.

One of the many benefits of primary care clinics is the provision for continuity of care across childhood. Gender identification and sexual health should be discussed with families from early on in childhood when sexual behaviors first arise. Having these conversations will build the rapport between the provider and the family so that the parent/parental figure may see the provider as a resource for discussion of gender identity development. It is important to remind parents that sexual orientation and gender identity are individual for each child and adolescent. Some parents may view heterosexuality as the norm, while others may be accepting of different gender and sexual orientations. Giving families the space and safety to discuss this with the pediatric provider is imperative, as is reinforcing that their child needs love, acceptance, and support as they navigate being a minority in their sexual orientation or gender identity. It may be helpful to remind families that having good family and community support is protective against the risks and risk behaviors that the parents may fear for their child. Resources should be given to both the family and the youth.

## MILITARY FAMILIES

The United States (U.S.) has a large and esteemed military sector that has grown and strengthened in the years since 2001, when we entered back into wartime. There are approximately 2.2 million active-duty and reserve service members in all branches of the military (Rossiter et al., 2016). A large portion of the military includes families with children of all ages, but predominantly a majority are under 5 years old (Sullivan et al., 2019). With frequent moves, stress over parent safety, possible distance from family/friends, deployments, ever-changing roles in the family, and new schools, the military child may present with a specific toolset of strengths as well as a unique array of challenges. Children of active-duty military service members are typically easy to identify and therefore have greater access to support. However, children of reserve military members may have the same challenges but without the supports that come with active duty, making it important to identify them early in order that they may receive the support they need.

# ASSESSMENT

Military life is a culture in itself. It includes long hours with low pay and the understanding that the service member's time belongs to the military branch (Sullivan et al., 2019). Even when not deployed, training and classes can take a service member away from the home for extended periods (Sullivan et al., 2019). For active-duty members, bases and assignments may change every couple of years, resulting in kids being moved to different homes and schools multiple times through their lives.

The family makeup for military members can vary. Members of the service may marry at a relatively early age, and mixed with the marital stresses that come with frequent separations and an ever-shifting lifestyle with possible distance from developed support systems, families may experience divorce, remarriage, blended families, and custodial stresses (Sullivan et al., 2019).

For active-duty and reserve service members, there is also the unique expectation for certain behavior from youth to prevent any negative attention to the parent or family (Huebner et al., 2019). For reserve service members, however, children and youth typically live in a civilian culture where the challenges and stresses they are under are not well-understood or shared with peers (Panton, 2018).

Active-duty families have universal healthcare coverage through age 21, or age 23 if enrolled in college through TRICARE (Sullivan et al., 2019). This coverage does not necessarily pertain to reserve service members or to families who are no longer in the military, so it is important to ask as part of the intake paperwork or assessment if a parent has ever or currently serves in any branch of the military. This will help to identify children who may have risk factors that are different than those of their civilian peers.

If a deployment is imminent, it is crucial to know the stage of the deployment cycle for the family. There are five main stages of the deployment cycle: predeployment, deployment, sustainment, redeployment, and postdeployment (Sullivan et al., 2019). Each of these stages brings unique concerns:

- Predeployment is the period prior to the deployment when there is an increase in training and education for the upcoming mission. While this brings a sense of bonding to the members of the unit it also brings stress, concern, and confusion at home owing to the unknown nature of what is ahead (Sullivan et al., 2019).
- Deployment is the period when the service member leaves and is away from home (possibly overseas) for an extended period of time. This again is marked by a sense of stress as the initial grief of missing the family member sets in as does the uncertainty and unreliability of communication between the deployed parent and their family (Sullivan et al., 2019).
- Sustainment begins as a new sense of normalcy arises; families are able to find their new temporary normal for the time-being.
- Redeployment comes as the deployment nears its end; this is a period marked by the excitement and preparation for the deployed parent's return.
- Postdeployment ends the cycle. It is a period of reintegration of the deployed family member, realigning roles, and navigating the collective experiences of both the deployed member of the family and the ones left at home (Sullivan et al., 2019).

If a parent has served in the military, an important follow-up question is whether they have experienced an injury or death, for these are also predictive of certain risk factors. With the start of combat warfare in 2001, there have been over 50,000 significant physical injuries recorded with results including amputation, blindness, loss of hearing, and chronic functional impairments (Sullivan et al., 2019). In addition to that, traumatic brain injuries may not be diagnosed until later, and posttraumatic stress disorder (PTSD) may also take time to be recognized. It is thought that upwards of 15% of Iraq and Afghanistan War veterans have PTSD. In addition, from 2001 to 2011 there were around 16,000 deaths of active-duty military members, resulting in a large number of bereaved children (Sullivan et al., 2019).

## Health Disparities and Risks

The frequent moves and culture of the military make military children both resilient and vulnerable (Huebner et al., 2019). Service members and their families with TRICARE may receive their healthcare on the military installation or via network (civilian) providers (Huebner et al., 2019). Utilizing healthcare in the nonmilitary setting, paired with frequent moves, can cause a breakdown in continuity of care. Both the experiences of the child and the experiences of the family can play into the emotional and physical well-being of the child. With frequent parental absence because of deployments and trainings combined with the risk of injury, especially to the deployed family member, and physical distance from extended family with breaks in social support for people who do not live on base, there are multiple threats to the stability of the family (Sullivan et al., 2019). Over the years as children age, the way they show stress may be different, but the impact of deployments tends to accumulate (Huebner et al., 2019). The effects of deployment and separation will affect each gender and age group differently, with younger children being more vulnerable to the effects (Sullivan et al., 2019). Preschool-age children experience increased anxiety associated with deployment, school-age children have more problems with behavior and peer relations, and adolescents find it increasingly difficult to deal with deployment (Huebner et al., 2019).

### Social

Bonds between each parent and child may change throughout the deployment cycle. The military child is at a higher risk of child maltreatment than their civilian peers, especially at deployment and reunification (Panton, 2018). During deployment, the risk of abuse would be associated with the nondeployed parent as the abuser (more commonly physical abuse). At reunification, maltreatment would be associated with both the nondeployed parent and the deployed parent who has returned, and most commonly manifests as neglect (Panton, 2018). Those are two of the most intense phases in the deployment cycle with an increase in stress levels.

### Psychological

There is a common misunderstanding that the frequent and regular moving in a military family is detrimental to children growing up in that family, when in fact it actually in the long-term may result in a high resilience level (Huebner et al., 2019). This is not the case during deployments, however, when the psychological risks of acute stress disorder, adjustment issues, depression, and anxiety are highest for military kids (Sullivan et al., 2019). Especially during this time, youth in military families are more likely to experience more severe depression and suicidal ideation than their civilian peers (Sullivan et al., 2019). Toddlers may experience developmental regression, changes in eating patterns and voiding patterns, and emotional outbursts (Sullivan et al., 2019). Other behavioral issues and declining academic performance also may occur (Huebner et al., 2019).

For children whose parent(s) have been wounded, the possibility of an unplanned relocation to a home closer to a treatment facility; the feelings of loss, isolation, and loneliness; and possible change of role to a caregiver can increase the emotional toll taken (Sullivan et al., 2019). Increases in child maltreatment and use of mental healthcare providers have been found in children of wounded service people (Sullivan et al., 2019). For children whose parents have been killed, they not only suffer the loss of their parent, but they also suffer the loss of military status, housing, and community, resulting in very complicated grief (Sullivan et al., 2019).

While decreases in primary care visits have been seen during deployments, there is a sharp increase in outpatient visits for mental health and behavioral issues as well as emergency room and urgent care visits. Children of servicemen and servicewomen have an increased risk for increases in emotional, relational, and psychosocial challenges, especially during deployments with as many as one in four children having a behavioral or emotional challenge associated with deployment (Huebner et al., 2019).

### Physical

The primary effects of being raised in a military family are psychological in nature, yet somatic expressions of these effects may occur. When assessing the child, keep in mind that physical complaints such as abdominal discomfort, headache, and other pain may be a somatic expression of emotional struggle. While it is important to rule out possible physical causes, it is also important to assess thoroughly for psychological triggers when making a differential diagnosis. School-age children experience somatic symptoms most frequently (Sullivan et al., 2019).

## HEALTH MAINTENANCE

As with any health visit, it is important that you reiterate that, as a primary care provider, you are there as a resource to the child and family. It will be important for resources to be given to the caregiver who will be home during the deployment to give them the tools to care for their own physical and emotional health. There is a correlation between poor emotional health of the parent with increased emotional distress in the child/youth as well as decreases in academic and social functioning (Sullivan et al., 2019).

The American Association of Nurse Practitioners recommends the use of the ICARE Support Strategy for Military Children: Identify, Correlate, Ask, Ready Resources, and Encourage and Educate (Rossiter et al., 2018). This can be used throughout the relationship with the child and family (Figure 44.1).

- *Identify* refers to being able to recognize children of military families, their risk factors, their personal strengths, and important dates of moves or deployments.

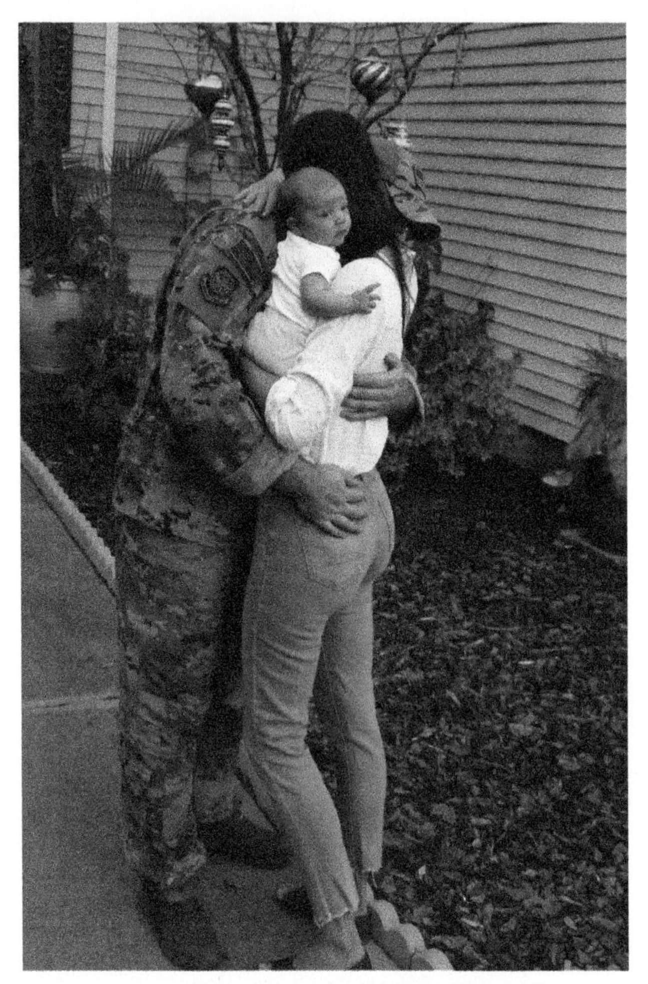

FIGURE 44.1 Deployment photograph of airman and family.

- *Correlate* means to attempt to link behaviors and challenges of children to the phase of deployment or the life stage.
- *Ask* is the investigation into the things going on, feelings they are having, and thoughts that they experience.
- *Ready Resources* is making sure that your toolkit is full of online and in-person resources that may benefit the child and family.
- *Encourage and Educate* is being a member of their team, advocating and praising the very hard work that they do day in and day out (Rossiter et al., 2018).

If you are able to interact with the family before deployment, you will be able to build rapport and recognize strengths and vulnerabilities that may affect future stresses. When deployment does arrive, helping plan primary care needs to address them prior to the family being reduced to one parent may be helpful. Especially in multiple child homes, going from having two parents present to one will bring many challenges, including coordinating getting to appointments. School physicals, immunizations, and well-child checks planned while both parents are still present is ideal.

TABLE 44.2 **Anticipatory Guidance: Online Resources for the Military Family**

| Resource | URL |
|---|---|
| Military One Source | www.militaryonesource.mil |
| Give An Hour | https://giveanhour.org |
| Military Family Association | www.militaryfamily.org |
| Military Child Education Coalition | www.militarychild.org |
| Sesame Street for Military Families | https://sesamestreetformilitaryfamilies.org |
| FOCUS Project | https://focusproject.org |

Prior to deployments, having an opportunity to prepare the parents for challenges that may arise, and alerting them to warning signs of depression or anxiety in the children, can help educate ahead of the stress of deployment. Also, discussing ways of reintegration postdeployment can help normalize the challenges that will come up. Normalization of thoughts and feelings during these incredibly hard periods of transition can help empower the family instead of isolating them.

The greatest predictor for emotional and behavioral well-being is whether or not counseling was done prior to deployment (Sullivan et al., 2019). To help equip the family, resources can be given and referrals made for both individual and family counseling (Table 44.2).

## INTERNATIONAL ADOPTEES

While the numbers surrounding adoption are growing, the rate of international adoptions is significantly decreasing due to changes in policies and procedures in both the United States and partnering countries (Crist, 2019). From 2004 to 2015 alone, there was a 77% decrease in children coming into the United States owing to international adoptions (Crist, 2019). Even with these numbers, the United States has the highest rate of international adoptions (Totaro et al., 2018).

The top three areas where children are being adopted from are China, The Democratic Republic of the

Congo, and Ukraine. Each of these areas, as well as other sites where adoptions occur, pose different risks for the child. While many of the challenges, disparities, and interventions are similar to the care of the foster child, we will discuss those that are more individualized to children adopted from international locations in this section.

## ASSESSMENT

Assessment of the adopted child will come in several parts, starting before the child even comes to the United States. The advanced practice provider should perform a thorough chart review of whatever paperwork is available, however fragmented or incomplete it is, keeping in mind it may also be in another language. The provider should also prepare by doing research on the home country and province to learn what risk factors the child may have because of the physical location, such as exposure to specific infectious diseases, exposure to war/trauma, or risk for nutritional deficits.

The child should be seen within a week of arrival to the United States for a comprehensive evaluation. With the extensive amount of assessment, testing, and screening that needs to be done for the newly arrived child, it may not be feasible to complete it all within one visit; rather, it may need to be spread out over multiple visits (Jones et al., 2019). The multivisit approach, if planned correctly, can also help the provider build a relationship and rapport with the child, making screening more reliable. Prior to the child's arrival, a medical provider with the U.S. Department of State does an examination to make sure there are not any major infectious/health risks for the child coming into the country. While these examinations are helpful, they are not comprehensive and all assessments should be repeated. Most children adopted from outside of the United States will be underimmunized (Staat et al., 2019). Refer to the CDC catch-up schedule to plan and administer the necessary immunizations.

If the child is able to communicate verbally, a translator should be available to facilitate the child's understanding, allowing them to interact more during the visit (Jones et al., 2019). It is also important to take time on the visit and perform functions slowly, following the child's cues for when they are feeling afraid and when they may be emotionally triggered, and taking breaks as needed (Jones et al., 2019).

A complete examination should be done, including an unclothed assessment. All testing that was done in the home country should be repeated, including testing for HIV, hepatitis B infection, and STIs. Lead levels should also be monitored. Infectious diseases are typically at the forefront of risk stratification, so assessing blood and stool for parasites and ova, as well as Zika virus, trypanosoma cruzi, strongyloides, schistosoma, toxocara, and lymphatic filariasis should also be considered (Staat et al., 2019).

Developmental and mental health screening should be performed utilizing a validated screening tool, keeping in mind that the initial screening may be difficult if a language barrier is present. International adoptees experience increased incidence of developmental delays and mental health disorders, so continue to monitor these children and screen as needed in addition to the routinely recommended schedule. On arrival, screen hearing and vision due to the increased risk of deficits that international adoptees have over their domestic counterparts (Jones et al., 2019).

### Health Disparities and Risks

As with other children who come into a family in nontraditional ways, children who are adopted come into the new home with a higher risk of physical, developmental, and mental health concerns that may be diagnosed prior to placement or discovered later (Jones et al., 2019).

#### Physical

The physical risks that international adoptees may face start before birth. Sometimes, information about the parents and prenatal care are available, but not in all situations. Prenatal care may have been fragmented or nonexistent. Maternal poverty and poverty early in the child's life may contribute to nutritional deficits. Depending on the location, the child may have been exposed to environmental toxins prenatally or early in life in addition to possible exposure to drugs, alcohol, and/or smoking. All of these factors can increase the risk for poor physical growth. Internationally adopted children have higher rates of vision and hearing impairments, and children raised in an institution have a higher risk for strabismus and should be provided with early intervention to prevent the progression of developmental delays (Jones et al., 2019).

#### Psychological

Children who do not have stable home environments and are placed up for adoption may have an increased risk of physical, emotional, and sexual abuse prior to their arrival to the United States (Jones et al., 2019). Whether or not they experienced violence in life can determine if they are at risk for toxic stress reactions, which are hugely detrimental as a child grows and develops and may lead to further behavioral and developmental issues. The combination of what their life was prior to adoption with the stress of travel, moving to a new country, language barriers, and a new family in a new culture can bring along any combination of adjustment issues that can include tantrums, emotional withdrawal, aggressive behavior, regression, sleep or eating problems, and autistic-like behaviors (Jones et al., 2019).

### Developmental

The combination of nutritional deficits, trauma, and possible institutionalization at an early age can affect the child's current and long-term development. There appears to be a correlation between the age of adoption and the amount of time the child spent in a facility with whether or not they are meeting developmental milestones (Jones et al., 2019). It is helpful to know whether or not a child was placed with a family or in a group home/orphanage prior to arrival to the United States.

## HEALTH MAINTENANCE

The partnership with the adoptee's family should start during the planning phases of adoption. Building a rapport with the family and instituting a medical home (a primary care provider who will serve as the coordinator/manager of the child's medical and developmental needs) will help prepare the family for challenges that they know are coming, anticipate possible needs and challenges in the future, and set up a network of resources to give the child and family the best possible chance to thrive (Jones et al., 2019).

The relationship and anticipatory guidance starts pre-adoption. During these visits the advanced practice provider should sit with the family and share information about the child and area. This is a great time to build rapport and then set expectations. While families may have an understanding of what they may experience in the first months of parenting, assessing their understanding of possible added challenges after arrival is helpful. Discussing the known medical and emotional needs (if any) and the interventions available will help lessen the information load after the child's arrival (Jones et al., 2019). Also, discussing the area the child is coming from and other health risks is imperative.

The first several weeks of parenthood will be overwhelming for families, so talking through what the medical visits will look like prior to the child arriving can help lay a foundation for the family on what to expect. Educating the family on trauma and trauma responses can help equip them to differentiate between the child being triggered versus having other unmet needs. Prepare parents for the fact that it may take longer than they would like for attachment to form. Reiterate this through the post-arrival visits to help decrease the emotional stress of parents who may feel that they are doing something wrong if the relationship does not work straight away. To promote attachment, encourage parents to spend a great deal of quiet, uninterrupted time with their new child (Springer, 2017).

Depending on the age of the child and number of deficits they had prior to adoption, families will need to be educated on their child's need for increased food, sleep, and family security (Crist, 2019). If a child has grown up only knowing what it is to experience hunger, exhaustion, and lack of love, it will take time for them to feel safe in their new home.

While the child is going to be coming to the United States to live, it is also important to remember that they will recognize that they are different than their family and peers and to embrace their culture of origin (Jones et al., 2019). Especially early on, having pictures of people they know from home (if available), room decorations, and music that they are used to may help ease the stress of settling. As they age, being open to answering questions and exposing them to that culture will help remove shame that may be associated with coming into the family in a non-traditional way and let them recognize acceptance and belonging.

Parenting is challenging for any family but adopting a child who is from a different country and culture with a possible extensive list of medical needs takes the support of a group of dedicated and invested teammates throughout the process.

## REFUGEES AND IMMIGRANT FAMILIES

The United States has long been a safe harbor for those facing turmoil, hunger, war, and abuse at the hands of their government or those who overthrew the government. The poem by Emma Lazarus on the Statue of Liberty, "The New Colossus," says "Give me your tired, your poor, your huddled masses yearning to breathe free...." Since 1975, there have been over 3 million refugees in the United States and 65 million people worldwide who were forcibly displaced from their home country (Mishori et al., 2017). Half of the people seeking asylum and safety around the world are under the age of 18 (Pohl et al., 2017). There are times that young children are traveling with older children who have taken over the task of parenting and safety. Currently, about one-quarter of the children in the United States live in immigrant families (Kan et al., 2015).

## ASSESSMENT

Assessment and treatment of the refugee can be challenging and share many similarities with those of the international adoptee. Language barriers are frequently present, and if the patient or family is undocumented, they may also withhold information out of fear. Similar to international adoptees, documented immigrants have been screened prior to their arrival to the United States and then again within 30 days of arrival (Mishori et al., 2017). Both documented and undocumented refugees each come with stories of resilience and survival. Displaced people often come with their own set of beliefs and understanding. Assessing throughout the visit can help remove barriers to care, especially if an illness is linked with tribal or spiritual causes. The provider should be nonjudgmental when approaching the family regarding cultural beliefs.

### Health Disparities and Risks

Refugee and immigrant children experience health disparities based upon events occurring in their country of origin. Commonly occurring health concerns in this population are pain, mental health issues, nutritional disorders, and chronic health conditions (possibly previously undiagnosed; Mishori et al., 2017).

### Psychological

Three of the countries with the most prevalent movement to the United States and European countries are Syria, Afghanistan, and Somalia (Pohl et al., 2017). These countries have intense histories of civil war, government oppression, and forced displacement. In the United States, there is a growing population of undocumented arrivals from areas south of the United States where drug cartels and government oppression are also common. An estimated 50% of immigrants have experienced torture (Mishori et al., 2017). This torture, and other histories of trauma through their life span, as well as events experienced during their displacement, migration, and resettlement can contribute to high levels of PTSD, mood disorders, chronic pain, and anxiety, some of which does not emerge until later in life (Mishori et al., 2017).

### Physical

The examination of refugee and immigrant children should also take into consideration high-prevalence diseases in their country of origin and where they passed through to get to the United States (Mishori et al., 2017). Children should be assessed for communicable diseases, dental problems, and nutrition status and growth, as well as lead levels (Mishori et al., 2017). Immunizations are often missing as well (Mishori et al., 2017).

## HEALTH MAINTENANCE

Refugees and immigrants, both documented and undocumented, have very unique physical and emotional needs. Being aware of resources in the area to assist with food and housing is helpful. This population of patients has faced an unprecedented amount of adversity in life and will have continued care needs through the life span.

# FOSTER CHILDREN

The United States has an extensive welfare system set up to remove a child from unsafe situations and place them into what is hoped to be a more stable, physically and emotionally safe environment. The most recent data show that there are currently nearly 440,000 children in the foster care system (Child Welfare Information Gateway, 2020). These children come with incomplete primary care as well as medical, dental, and mental healthcare needs and often have a history of trauma and abuse.

Children and youth may enter into an emergency placement and then be shifted from one home to another home. Kinship placements are done when a family member or family friend takes custody of the child. These kinship placements make up approximately one-quarter of foster care scenarios and come with positive outcomes but also risks that nonkinship placements may not have (Jones et al., 2019). While there may be greater stability in transferring care to a person who is connected to the family, where there is less risk of moving, there is also a risk that this will increase contact between the child and the potentially abusive situation from which they were rescued. Also, there may not be economic stability present in those scenarios (Jones et al., 2019). States also have

"Safe Haven" laws allowing for the drop-off of infants in designated areas with no questions asked. Each state varies but these infants will also enter into the foster care system after medical clearance. Group homes are another type of placement, with approximately 60% of teens in the foster care system living in those settings (Lewis & Beatty, 2018).

## ASSESSMENT

There are multiple barriers to the care for children in foster care. First, there may be a lack of information related to the child's health if it is not passed along from the previous caregiver. Children who move from home to home may either not have been followed by a practitioner in the past, or there may be no written documentation of immunizations, social history, and medical history. When children are removed from the home, there may be little gleaned from the person with whom they were living at the time of removal and may also be a lack of medical records (Lewis & Beatty, 2018). There are also often multiple layers of adult involvement in the child's life, including the biological parent, the foster parent, workers from the child welfare agency, private agencies if they are involved, and the court system, so coordination among all the stakeholders, as well as communication and consent, can be complicated and ever-dynamic (Lewis & Beatty, 2018). In addition to those challenges is the fact that a child's living situation may change multiple times in a short span of time if placements are temporary or do not work out for a number of reasons (Lewis & Beatty, 2018).

### Health Disparities and Risks

Children who are in foster care face a significant amount of disparities that are not necessarily shared with their peers who have stable family environments. Physical and mental illness are higher for the child who has spent time in the foster care system and, if not treated, can persist into adulthood causing crisis through the entire life span (Dunnigan et al., 2017).

#### Physical

Studies have shown that 35% of children who enter the foster care system have some sort of chronic or medical need that has not been adequately treated (Bennett et al., 2020). Twenty percent have dental conditions requiring a specialist's care (Bennett et al., 2020). Medical conditions can be related to nutritional deficits or excess food intake as well as sedentary lifestyles (Jones et al., 2019). Asthma is twice as common among children who have spent time in the foster care system than those children who have not, with a very high risk of decreased control and symptom exacerbation (Dunnigan et al., 2017).

#### Psychological

Children and youth only enter into the foster care system if there is a history of neglect or abuse, so it is no surprise that children can come in with extensive emotional health repercussions. Around 80% of parents of children who are removed from the home also have some sort of mental illness or habit that affects prospective foster parenting (Lewis & Beatty, 2018). What is surprising is the true extent of that and the way that a trauma history manifests. Upwards of 90% of children in the foster system have some sort of mental health condition (Bennett et al., 2020). Toxic trauma that they have experienced can affect development and future behavior as well. Manifestations of mental health challenges include attention deficit hyperactivity disorder (ADHD), depressive disorders, anxiety disorders, personality manifestations such as oppositional defiant disorder or conduct disorders, and disorders of eating and elimination (Jones et al., 2019). Lack of support and coping skills in the midst of mental health crisis leads to an increased risk of self-mutilation, risky behaviors, suicide attempts, and substance dependency.

Many of these children come from backgrounds with high levels of stress, abuse, and neglect, which may often lead to psychological issues being triggered in the patient. The way that stress reactions manifest, even once the child is in a more stable environment, can often be mislabeled, making it more difficult to treat or successfully provide interventions for the child (Lewis & Beatty, 2018). A history of trauma can be exacerbated as children may also experience trauma in their foster care experience. With housing insecurity, sometimes negative interactions with the court system, and foster siblings or parents, children may have a continued feeling of rejection and instability, leading to further behavioral challenges.

#### Developmental

Lack of consistent healthcare, history of trauma, and a background of abuse and neglect are all contributory to a high incidence of developmental delays among children in the foster care system. It is estimated that 60% of foster children under the age of 5 show some sort of delay in their developmental milestones (Bennett et al., 2020).

## HEALTH MAINTENANCE

One of the most beneficial interventions for a child in the foster care system is the development of a consistent medical home that they will belong to regardless of placement (Bennett et al., 2020). The medical home model provides care coordination for children with chronic or extensive healthcare needs. Children in foster care often have numerous risk factors, comorbidities, and challenges to intervention, making having a medical home essential to their health. A medical home is like the hub of a wheel; it is the foundation around which all the spokes (specialists) come together, making it possible for the wheel to function and transport. A medical home for a child in foster care can be one of the few places of consistency through their childhood. As specialists get involved to care for the different, extensive medical, emotional, and developmental needs of the child, the medical home is present to collect data and close the loop, making sure that the child does not fall through any cracks and has the resources needed to pursue improved health as well as a healthcare provider during times of crisis.

Children in the foster care system not only get admitted to the hospital more frequently, but they also have higher length of stays than their peers who are not in the system (Bennett et al., 2020). Medical homes have been shown to decrease the utilization of the emergency room, thus lowering healthcare costs and helping to encourage continuity and consistency of care instead of the fragmented care caused by use of the emergency departments and urgent care centers (Bennett et al., 2020).

The provider in the medical home should be well versed in trauma-informed care and able to share information with both the child and foster family. All aspects of trauma care, screening, treatment, and education are severely underutilized (Lewis & Beatty, 2018).

Care of the foster child is challenging for the advanced practice provider in a multitude of ways. Inconsistent care, missing information, and a potentially resistant child or foster parent, paired with multiple physical and emotional health issues, can be both mentally and emotionally demanding. The advanced practice provider has the unique and unparalleled opportunity to be an advocate at the forefront of the child's team moving forward. In some situations, the child in the foster care system has deeply felt the lack of care and encouragement, and the advanced practice provider can help empower families to overcome the struggles and fill that void.

# HOMELESS CHILDREN/YOUTH

Homelessness or housing insecurity is a prevalent but often hidden problem in the United States. While there are multiple working definitions for homelessness, the definition we use here is that homelessness is a situation in which a child does not have a stable, consistent place to eat and sleep outside of school or daycare facilities. The United States has the highest homeless rate among any developed country, including 2.5 million children without adequate housing (Chatterjee et al., 2017).

There are two main types of homeless children/youth: (1) children who are homeless but still under the care of parents or guardians and (2) unaccompanied youth. Housing insecurity is higher in younger children, with twice as many children being preschool aged and under versus high school age, plus another 2 million young adults under the age of 25 (Anderson & Adams, 2018). The challenges that these different groups face are diverse, but sometimes interconnected.

Homelessness can look very different depending on the situation and children may face multiple scenarios of homelessness. While some families live on the streets, in their cars, and in tent cities, other children may be found "couch surfing" or staying at different homes for short amounts of time, in hotels/motels, or in shelters. (Schifalacqua et al., 2019). All of the previously noted scenarios are unstable and ever changing.

A variety of situations can bring families and youth into an unstable housing situation. Parents may lose housing because of job loss or debt as a result of lifestyle, medical bills, or unforeseen circumstances. One-third of homeless youth stated they chose homelessness to escape domestic violence in their homes (Anderson & Adams, 2018). Youth may attempt to escape abusive homes or may be kicked out owing to relationships, sexual orientation, or gender identity.

Minority families make up the majority of the homeless population (Anderson & Adams, 2018). While housing instability is seen to be an issue in cities and urban areas, homelessness in rural areas is growing as well (Anderson & Adams, 2018).

## ASSESSMENT

As with every interaction with a child and family, it is important to approach the patient with lack of judgment, with empathy, and with understanding in their care. It is not uncommon for patients and families to try to hide their housing situation out of fear of judgment, stigmatization, and legal intervention (Schifalacqua et al., 2019). One way to look further into their housing while not making assumptions is to ask if the address they presented on their assessment paperwork is permanent or temporary (Schifalacqua et al., 2019). If the child seems communicative, you can ask further questions about who lives at home with them and what their housing is like, while using open-ended questions.

## Health Disparities and Risks

Before addressing the health disparities experienced by homeless children and youth, it is important to discuss the risks and experiences of their parents. While many comorbidities are shared among generations, so are social disparities. People who experienced homelessness as children have an increased risk of repeat homelessness as adults. When young men witness violence as children or youth they are four times more likely to have violent tendencies as adults, while females who bear witness to assault are three times more likely to be victims later in life (Anderson & Adams, 2018).

Multiple factors can lead to homelessness in adults. Many reliable employment opportunities require a permanent address, which a homeless person may be unable to provide. The amount of mental illness among homeless adults is higher. While family makeup can vary, among the population of people lacking housing security, mothers with small children are common. Homeless mothers are less likely to have a high school diploma, and are therefore not equipped to compete for more secure jobs. Violence against women is also increased both before women become homeless and then again on the streets, with 92% of mothers experiencing physical attack, sexual violence, or both. Lack of adequate support can lead to higher rates of mental illness, recreational drug use, or other substance abuse (Anderson & Adams, 2018).

### Prenatal Care

Infants born to homeless families are at risk for adverse outcomes even before birth. Lack of food security and access to healthcare, and the possibility of smoking, drug, and alcohol abuse can lead to any number of complications in a developing fetus. Homeless mothers have a higher incidence of giving birth to low birth weight babies (Anderson & Adams, 2018). Fetal alcohol syndrome and neonatal abstinence syndrome may also occur.

### Nutritional

Housing insecurity can correlate with food insecurity, so infants and children may suffer from nutritional deficits (both under- and overnutrition; Chatterjee et al., 2017). Children with a lack of reliable nutrition or food early in life are two-thirds more likely to show developmental delays later in life (Anderson & Adams, 2018). With a lack of reliable and regular screening and care, along with decreased access to hygiene products such as toothbrushes and toothpaste, dental decay is common and may require follow-up by a specialist.

### Psychological

Just as mental health concerns are common among parents, they are also common among the children and youth who lack secure and reliable housing. Violence and toxic stress prior to homelessness is common, with many children retreating to the streets due to domestic violence. Prior abuse combined with the violence so often experienced on the streets can lead to unresolved trauma responses. One study shows that one-third of children and youth on the streets show similar levels of PTSD as experienced by combat veterans, with 40% to 80% experiencing suicidal ideation and two-thirds making suicide attempts (Schifalacqua et al., 2019).

Children who are homeless may also experience behavior problems as well as other mental and emotional health issues (Anderson & Adams, 2018). With transient attendance, frequently switched schools, or no formal education at all, developmental delays and learning disabilities are not reliably recognized or addressed. These students are less likely than their peers to receive special education and individualized education programs (IEPs) (Anderson & Adams, 2018). Shelters and other unsafe environments can often be unsupportive of children. Children may appear withdrawn, insecure, lacking trust for those around them, anxious, depressed, and irritable.

### Sexual Health

Homeless youth are at a higher risk and have a higher incidence for STIs, pregnancy, and sexual violence (Schifalacqua et al., 2019). Forty percent of homeless youth identify as LGBTQ members, in stark contrast with less than 10% of youth with stable housing (Anderson & Adams, 2018). This difference may be a result of youth being kicked out of their homes when they come out to their families, or an attempt to escape violence and bullying.

## HEALTH MAINTENANCE

During a visit with a family who expresses they are experiencing homelessness, it is important to ask if they need any assistance with housing, food, or clothing (hidden healthcare). While there are many assistance programs available, few children or parents know about them or how to access them. Without an address or a place to access the Internet, they may not have the ability to complete paperwork or start the process of applying. For example, even with nutritional assistance programs widely available, less than half of children in the homeless community were enrolled in those programs (Anderson & Adams, 2018).

One challenge for the practitioner is deciding if and when to contact social services or child protective services (CPSs). While children who have unstable housing are most definitely at risk for other forms of neglect, states differ on whether homelessness alone warrants a CPSs consult. According to the U.S. Health and Human Services Administration for Children and Families, "homelessness is considered neglect when the inability to provide shelter is the result of mismanagement of financial resources or when spending rent, resources on drugs or alcohol results in frequent evictions" (User & DePanfilis, 2006, p. 12). Helping to partner the family or youth with appropriate resources can help create a connection with social workers and other team members with the goal of keeping the family together while providing the resources they need.

Recognizing barriers to adequate care can help the practitioner make a plan for further follow-up and monitoring of the child and family. Guardians and children who lack housing often lack transportation and funds for living essentials such as food and gas (Schifalacqua et al., 2019). They may also be unaware of resources available for their basic needs of food, clothing, housing, and gas and how to access them. For unaccompanied youth, fear of forced return to the situation that they sought to leave may also hinder the child-practitioner relationship. In a life where they may never have the feeling of safety and security, their time with you may be some of the only interactions that they have with a caring adult.

### Anticipatory Guidance

Caring for the homeless family and child is challenging for the pediatric provider. Often they come with complex social, medical, and mental healthcare needs while navigating a trauma-filled past. Without intervention, homeless children may continue the pattern of homelessness and enter into adulthood without stable housing, resources, or knowledge of how to overcome their circumstances. Supporting these families or youth will take a multifaceted and interdisciplinary approach including assessing needs, empowering families, equipping them with resources, and following up in aftercare. For both the child and family, having lived a life that may include trauma and violence, they may enter into your care untrusting and defensive. Building a rapport and helping them see that you are there to help as part of a team may take time, multiple visits, and continued interaction. This process can be frustrating, but as their provider, you are at the forefront of their team, helping to equip them with the gaining of knowledge, resources, and empowerment to seek healthier options and, one hopes, break the cycle of homelessness.

## HUMAN TRAFFICKING

Human trafficking is a growing problem worldwide and is often invisible in the United States. It can be called "modern slavery" because it literally steals freedom from the victim, forcing sexual or labor exploitation via force, fraud, or coercion (United Against Human Trafficking, 2020). Commercial sexual exploitation (CSE) is when a sex act is exchanged for money. When the person in question is under 18 years old, CSE of children is considered human trafficking even when there is no force, fraud, or coercion present (United Against Human Trafficking, 2020). While trafficking victims are challenging to identify and quantify, it is estimated that there are 25.9 million victims of human trafficking worldwide (United Against Human Trafficking, 2020).

Trafficking victims are both male and female, with 33% of those trafficked being children (Greenbaum & Crawford-Jakubiak, 2015). The average age of entrance into the human trafficking industry is 12 to 16 years old (Greenbaum & Crawford-Jakubiak, 2015). Children and youth are targeted because of their vulnerability to manipulation and underdevelopment of their prefrontal cortex, which is responsible for critical thinking, analysis of situations, and impulse control (Greenbaum & Crawford-Jakubiak, 2015).

Healthcare providers have a unique opportunity to recognize, support, empower, and intervene when there is a concern about possible trafficking. Eighty-eight percent of human trafficking victims will come in contact with the healthcare system, whether in a clinic, an urgent care center, an emergency room, a family planning clinic, or via emergency medical service, yet they are often not being identified by the healthcare workers in those systems (United Against Human Trafficking, 2020).

Multiple government and anti-trafficking organizations use the Action-Means-Purpose (AMP) Model to help understand what is and is not human trafficking (United Against Human Trafficking, 2020). Traffickers take action by recruiting and soliciting their victims, then harbor or transport them via means of force, fraud, or coercion for the purpose of either sexual or labor exploitation (United Against Human Trafficking, 2020). Force, fraud, and coercion can look very differently depending on the situation. Force can include beating, chaining a victim somewhere, choking, and other forms of physical abuse. Fraud includes things like threats against the person or their family, blackmailing, or stealing papers or personal identification (IDs; United Against Human Trafficking, 2020). Coercion may be false promises, wooing, or offering something the person needs or desires such as a safe home, a modeling or acting job, or a romantic relationship (United Against Human Trafficking, 2020).

Not all victims of sex and labor trafficking in the United States come from international locales. Misconception exists that the United States is a destination country for trafficking, but 88% of sex-trafficking victims in the United States are typically U.S. citizens, while the majority of labor-trafficking victims are female foreign nationals (Greenbaum et al., 2017). The federal Trafficking Victims Protection Act (TVPA) originated in 2000 and was reauthorized in 2019 (Wells, 2019). The act includes prevention initiatives, victim protection, and offender enforcement and accountability programs. Despite the TVPA, human trafficking continues in the United States.

## ASSESSMENT

The most important part of the assessment of the human trafficking survivor is recognition. Risk factors for human trafficking include:

- Homelessness
- Young people with a history of abuse or interaction with CPSs
- Youth who identify as an LGBTQ person
- Family history of intimate partner violence
- Family history of psychiatric issues and drug use
- Having a psychiatric history
- Learning disabilities or cognitive disabilities
- Living in areas with a pimp culture (Greenbaum & Crawford-Jakubiak, 2015).

If a life situation leaves a youth ostracized or not accepted, they are at risk for being taken advantage of because of that need and desire for belonging. Even if a youth does not self-identify as a victim, it should not be ruled out.

Conditions that you may find in a victim of human trafficking may be associated with incidental findings such as STIs, evidence of assault, and complications of substance abuse and reproductive care (Greenbaum & Crawford-Jakubiak, 2015). There may be evidence of genital or anal trauma or injury. Other red flags include branding tattoos, tension headaches, exacerbations of chronic conditions, dental neglect, and gastrointestinal symptoms (United Against Human Trafficking, 2020). While performing the health history, the youth may lie about their age, provide false information, or seem very guarded in their responses to you. The propensity of being a poor historian during intake as well as clothing that may be inappropriate for the current weather or season can serve as a red flag for concern regarding potential human trafficking (United Against Human Trafficking, 2020).

Prior to the health interview, it is important to build a rapport. Upon arrival, if the youth is accompanied by another person, try to remove that person from the room in a nonthreatening manner. No standard screening tools exist, and youth rarely recognize that they are victims in the situation, so pointed questions may be met with hostility as youth may want to protect their traffickers (Greenbaum & Crawford-Jakubiak, 2015). Let them know that they are in control, that they may choose which questions to answer or consent to an examination. Transparency regarding your role as a mandated reporter (one who, by state law, must report abuse) is very important. Being honest will help build long-term trust (Greenbaum & Crawford-Jakubiak, 2015).

Trauma-informed care is imperative when approaching the sex and human trafficking survivor. This means understanding the toll that physical and psychological trauma can take on a victim, physical manifestations of that trauma, and knowledge of how to perform the care the patient needs without provoking further trauma. Medical offices and hospital settings may be a source of anxiety and may trigger a trauma response in a survivor. Triggers may include smells like rubbing alcohol, other scents, sounds like sirens, and white lab coats (United Against Human Trafficking, 2020). Watch the youth closely for signs of distress (e.g., panicked look, hand-wringing, increase in heart rate or respiratory rate, sweating, hypervigilance, fearfulness, or aggression). When signs of distress are noted, adjusting or slowing your examination as needed may be time-consuming but will ultimately serve the complex needs of the youth.

**PRO TIP** Signs of distress can look different for different people; be alert and vigilant during the history and physical examination.

While these youth may be hesitant to share information, the use of open-ended questions regarding their life, school, jobs, and living situation may assist in getting more information than close-ended questions requiring a "yes" or "no" response. Multiple resources have webinars and trainings to help you learn how to modify the care you provide to victims of trafficking. One resource, United Against Human Trafficking (2020), has a webinar for healthcare professionals that recommends asking questions like "tell me about (relationships, jobs)" as well as "where do you sleep at night?"

### Health Disparities and Risks

Human trafficking victims often become victims due to manipulation and lies by the trafficker. Often they are also victims of intense physical and sexual abuse (Greenbaum & Crawford-Jakubiak, 2015).

#### Physical

The bodies of human trafficking victims may show visible scars or other signs of abuse (bruising, scrapes, cigarette burns, ligature markings). They may have chronic pain from the physical and sexual abuse. They may also experience complications from STIs and multiple abortions.

#### Psychological

Victims of human trafficking have deep psychological effects from forced slavery. Since rarely do well-resourced, well-supported youth end up in human trafficking, the victims may enter into the life with extensive histories of abuse, parental drug use, being in foster care, and/or parental trauma even before the experience of trafficking, multiplying the adverse psychological effects. Trauma responses vary, and people manifest the effects in very different ways. While some people may become meeker and withdrawn, others may be more aggressive and angry. Depression and PTSD are common among people who have experienced human trafficking, as are episodes of dissociation, fear, and intense shame (United Against Human Trafficking, 2020). People may experience problems sleeping and concentrating or may find that they are plagued by nightmares or flashbacks (Greenbaum et al., 2017). Both substance use and suicide attempts (higher in victims of trafficking) are presumed to be sought for escape from abuse they have experienced (Greenbaum et al., 2017).

## HEALTH MAINTENANCE

One of the most important parts of caring for a trafficking victim is to be nonjudgmental and to recognize the person as a survivor. After being used, oftentimes abused, and manipulated, these young people may not even see themselves as victims.

Working with victims of human trafficking requires community outreach and education. As a healthcare provider, it is part of your responsibility to take part in policy changes to help ensure that these people are seen as victims, not perpetrators. You should be aware of the community resources available, which law enforcement agencies or departments have trafficking workgroups, which social services are available, and which behavioral health organizations can be partnered with, as well as the existence of other nonprofit service organizations who may serve the many needs of survivors (Greenbaum & Crawford-Jakubiak, 2015). Reaching out to law enforcement before a crisis arises will help you build a rapport with the agencies and law enforcement officers, further building a team dynamic to better serve the victims and patients. Human trafficking can sometimes be disguised as free-will prostitution, where victims are actually seen as perpetrators. Explaining how the child victim is in fact a victim by describing the physical, mental, and emotional developmental levels of children and youth and how they are vulnerable to manipulation and coercion can help reframe the oftentimes incorrect societal view and serve law enforcement and the youth (Greenbaum & Crawford-Jakubiak, 2015).

Reporting a case of suspected human trafficking may feel complicated for the healthcare professional. Since many of these children and youth may come in alone or with a very controlling counterpart, you may be unsure of what you are allowed and not allowed to do. Follow up with your specific state regarding policies, but for the most part reporting human trafficking is the same as reporting abuse or neglect: you are a mandated reporter. This is not the same for patients over 18 years old for whom you must have consent to report. Reporting a case for a victim over the age of 18 without their consent is considered a violation of the Health Insurance Portability and Accountability Act (HIPAA; United Against Human Trafficking, 2020). Reports should be made to your state's department of family and protective services as well as to the National Human Trafficking Hotline (call 1-888-373-7888 or text BEFREE 233733).

Human trafficking survivors have a wide variety of acute and chronic, physical and emotional, short-term and long-term needs. Meeting their immediate medical needs while also educating them on the resources available will help empower them while providing them with necessary services. Exiting "the life" as a victim of human trafficking is incredibly challenging and something that many people will not understand. It may require many attempts of breaking away from their captor before they are able to successfully leave their perpetrator (Greenbaum & Crawford-Jakubiak, 2015). It takes patience, compassion, and resolve to help young people who are victims of human trafficking, but you are in a unique position to serve their extensive needs (see https://humantraffickinghotline.org).

## KEY POINTS

- Children in societal minority groups come with a unique set of challenges in assessment and treatment. It is imperative that the advanced practice provider is able to cater their assessment and treatment plan to the specific needs of the child and family to provide the most thorough and holistic care possible.
- Every advanced practice provider comes to their setting with a set of beliefs, experiences, and understandings that drives their practice and behavior. It is important to recognize beliefs and biases and leave them at the door, to provide a judgment-free and safe place for the child and family being served.
- Children may experience trauma in their home or in their community. Being able to identify the risk factors, signs, symptoms, and possible repercussions of traumatic experiences or settings and having the awareness of what community resources there are available to the family will serve both the short-term and long-term psychological, physical, and emotional needs of the child and family.

## REFERENCES

American Academy of Child & Adolescent Psychiatry. (2018). *Conversion therapy*. https://www.aacap.org/aacap/policy_statements/2018/Conversion_Therapy.aspx

Anderson, D., & Adams, M. (2018). Chapter 3: Who are homeless children? In A. D. Hunter, D. Heise, & B. H. Johns (Eds.), *Art for children experiencing psychological trauma* (pp. 15–36). Routledge. https://dl.uswr.ac.ir/bitstream/Hannan/32609/1/9781138236943.pdf#page=36

Bennett, C. E., Wood, J. N., & Scribano, P. V. (2020). Healthcare utilization for children in foster care. *Academic Pediatrics, 20*(3), 341–347. https://doi.org/10.1016/j.acap.2019.10.004

Centers for Disease Control and Prevention. (2019). *Human papillomavirus (HPV): For healthcare professionals*. https://www.cdc.gov/hpv/hcp/index.html

Chatterjee, A., So, M., Dunleavy, S., & Oken, E. (2017). Quality health care for homeless children: Achieving the AAP recommendations for care of homeless children and youth. *Journal of Health Care for the Poor and Underserved, 28*(4), 1376–1392. https://doi.org/10.1353/hpu.2017.0121

Child Welfare Information Gateway. (2020). *Foster care statistics 2018*. U.S. Department of Health and Human Services, Administration for Children and Families, Children's Bureau.

Crist, C. (2019, May 3). Newly adopted children need specialized health exams. *Reuters*. https://www.reuters.com/article/us-health-pediatrics-adoption/newly-adopted-children-need-specialized-health-exams-idUSKCN1S9204

Dashow, J. (2017). *New report on youth homeless affirms that LGBTQ youth disproportionately experience homelessness*. https://www.hrc.org/news/new-report-on-youth-homeless-affirms-that-lgbtq-youth-disproportionately-ex

Dunnigan, A. E., Thompson, T., Jonson-Reid, M., & Drake, F. B. (2017). Chronic health conditions and children in foster care: Determining demographic and placement-related correlates. *Journal of Public Child Welfare, 11*(4–5), 586–598. https://doi.org/10.1080/15548732.2017.1339655

Earnshaw, V. A., Reisner, S. L., Juvonen, J., Hatzenbuehler, M. L., Perrotti, J., & Schuster, M. A. (2017). LGBTQ bullying: Translating research to action in pediatrics. *Pediatrics, 140*(4), e20170432. https://doi.org/10.1542/peds.2017-0432

Greenbaum, J., Bodrick, N., & the Committee on Child Abuse and Neglect, Section on International Child Health. (2017). Global human trafficking and child victimization. *Pediatrics, 140*(6), 20173138. https://pediatrics.aappublications.org/content/pediatrics/140/6/e20173138.full.pdf

Greenbaum, J., & Crawford-Jakubiak, J. E. (2015). Child sex trafficking and commercial sexual exploitation: Health care needs of victims. *Pediatrics, 135*(3), 566–574. https://doi.org/10.1542/peds.2014-4138

Hatchel, T., Ingram, K. M., Mintz, S., Hartley, C., Valido, A., Espelage, D. L., & Wyman, P. (2019). Predictors of suicidal ideation and attempts among LGBTQ adolescents: The roles of help-seeking beliefs, peer victimization, depressive symptoms, and drug use. *Journal of Child and Family Studies, 28*, 2443–2455. https://doi.org/10.1007/s10826-019-01339-2

House, H., Gaines, S., & Hawkins, L. A. (2019). Sexual and gender minority adolescents: Meeting the needs of our LGBTQ patients and their families. *Clinical Pediatric Emergency Medicine, 20*(1), 9–16. https://doi.org/10.1016/j.cpem.2019.02.004

Huebner, C. R., & the Section on Uniformed Services and Committee on Psychosocial Aspects of Child and Family Health. (2019). Health and mental health needs of children in US military families. *Pediatrics, 143*(1), e20183258. https://doi.org/10.1542/peds.2018-3258

Jones, V. F., Schulte, E. E., & the AAP Council on Foster Care, Adoption, and Kinship Care. (2019). Comprehensive health evaluation of the newly adopted child.

*Pediatrics, 143*(5), e20190657. https://doi.org/10.1542/peds.2019-0657

Kan, K., Choi, H., & Davis, M. (2015). Immigrant families, children with special health care needs, and the medical home. *Pediatrics, 137*(1), e20153221. https://doi.org/10.1542/peds.2015-3221

Lewis, J. M., & Beatty, A. E. (2018). Meeting the health-care challenges for children in foster care: A survey of West Virginia pediatricians. *West Virginia Medical Journal, 114*(2). link.gale.com/apps/doc/A539648353/EAIM?u=pens49866&sid=EAIM&xid=c90bbdd8.

Mental Health America. (2020). *Bullying: LGBT youth.* https://www.mhanational.org/bullying-lgbt-youth

Miller, J. M., & Luk, J. W. (2019). A systematic review of sexual orientation disparities in disordered eating and weight-related behaviors among adolescents and young adults: Toward a developmental model. *Adolescent Research Review, 4*(2), 187–208. https://doi.org/10.1007/s40894-018-0079-2

Mishori, R., Aleinikoff, S., & Davis, D. M. (2017). Primary care for refugees: Challenges and opportunities. *American Family Physician, 96*(2), 112–120. https://www.aafp.org/afp/2017/0715/p112.html

Panton, J. (2018). Caring for military children: Implications for nurse practitioners. *Journal of Pediatric Healthcare, 32*(5), 435–444. https://doi-org.resource.ahu.edu/10.1016/j.pedhc.2018.02.007

Perron, T., Kartoz, C., & Himelfarb, C. (2017a). LGBTQ Youth Part 1: Cultural competence for school nurses caring for LGBTQ youth—Learning the culture and the language. *NASN School Nurse, 32*(2), 106–115. https://doi.org/10.1177/1942602x16689327

Perron, T., Kartoz, C., & Himelfarb, C. (2017b). LGBTQ Youth part 2: Examining the health disparities and psychological struggles experienced by LGBTQ youth. *NASN School Nurse, 32*(2), 116–121. https://doi.org/10.1177%2F1942602X16689263

Pohl, C., Mack, I., Schmitz, T., & Ritz, N. (2017). The spectrum of care for pediatric refugees and asylum seekers at a tertiary health care facility in Switzerland in 2015. *European Journal of Pediatrics, 176*(12), 1681–1687. https://doi.org/10.1007/s00431-017-3014-9

Rafferty, J. (2018). *Gender identity development in children.* https://www.healthychildren.org/English/ages-stages/gradeschool/Pages/Gender-Identity-and-Gender-Confusion-In-Children.aspx

Rafferty, J., & Committee on Psychosocial Aspects of Child and Family Health, Committee on Adolescence, and Section on Lesbian, Gay, Bisexual, and Transgender Health and Wellness. (2018). Ensuring comprehensive care and support for transgender and gender-diverse children and adolescents. *Pediatrics, 142*(4), e20182162. https://doi.org/10.1542/peds.2018-2162

Rasberry, C. M., Lowry, R., Johns, M., Robin, L., Dunville, R., Pampati, S., Dittus, P. J., & Balaji, A. (2018). Sexual risk behavior differences among sexual minority high school students—United States, 2015 and 2017. *Morbidity and Mortality Weekly Report, 67,* 1007–1011. http://dx.doi.org/10.15585/mmwr.mm6736a3external icon

Rossiter, A. G., Dumas, M. A., Wilmoth, M. C., & Patrician, P. A. (2016). "I serve 2": Meeting the needs of military children in civilian practice. Nursing Outlook, *64*(5), 485–490. https://doi.org/10.1016/j.outlook.2016.05.011

Rossiter, A. G., Patrician, P. A., Banton, D. B., Dumas, M. A., Ling, C. G., Johnson, H. L., & Wilmoth, M. C. (2018). I serve 2. Journal of the American Association of Nurse Practitioners, *30*(11), 614-618. https://doi.org/10.1097/JXX.0000000000000084

Schifalacqua, M., Ghafoori, A., & Jacobowitz, M. (2019). A hidden healthcare crisis: Youth homelessness. *Nurse Leader, 17*(3), 193–196. https://doi.org/10.1016/j.mnl.2019.03.005

Snyder, B. K., Burack, G. D., & Petrova, A. (2017). LGBTQ youth's perceptions of primary care. *Clinical Pediatrics, 56*(5), 443–450. https://doi.org/10.1177/0009922816673306

Springer, S. H. (2017). Adoption. In T. K. McInerny, H. M. Adam, D. E. Campbell, T. G. DeWitt, J. M. Foy, & D. M. Kamat (Eds.), *American Academy of Pediatrics textbook of pediatric care* (2nd ed., Chapter 70). American Academy of Pediatrics.

Staat, M. A., Wien, S., & Jentes, E. (2019). Family travel, international adoption. In G. W. Brunette, J. B. Nemhauser, & the Centers for Disease Control and Prevention (Eds.), *CDC yellow book 2020: Health information for international travel* (Chapter 7). Oxford University Press.

Sullivan, R. M., Cozza, S. J., & Dougherty, J. G. (2019). Children of military families. *Child and Adolescent Psychiatric Clinics of North America, 28*(3), 337–348. https://doi.org/10.1016/j.chc.2019.02.004

Totaro, C., Bortone, B., Putignano, P., Sollai, S., Galli, L., de Martino, M., & Chiappini, E. (2018). Internationally adopted children: Not only infectious diseases! *Journal of Travel Medicine, 25*(1). https://doi.org/10.1093/jtm/tay036

Underwood, J. M., Brener, N., Thornton, J., Harris, W. A., Bryan, L. N., Shanklin, S. L., Deputy, N., Roberts, A. M., Queen, B., Chyen, D., Whittle, L., Lim, C., Yamakawa, Y., Leon-Nguyen, M., Kilmer, G., Smith-Grant, J., Demissie, Z., Jones, E., Clayton, H., & Dittus, P. (2020). Overview and methods for the youth risk behavior surveillance system—United States, 2019. *Mortality and Morbidity Weekly Reports, 69*(Suppl. 1), 1–10. http://dx.doi.org/10.15585/mmwr.su6901a1

United Against Human Trafficking. (2020). *Human trafficking & health professionals: Look beneath the surface and H.E.A.R. your patients* [Video]. YouTube. https://www.youtube.com/watch?v=DO9ub66a0_s&t=10s

User, M., & DePanfilis, D. (2006). *Child neglect: A guide for prevention, assessment and intervention.* https://www.childwelfare.gov/pubPDFs/neglect.pdf

Wells, K. (2019). *The 2019 Trafficking Victims Protection Reauthorization Act: A topical summary and analysis of four bills.* https://polarisproject.org/wp-content/uploads/2020/01/Polaris-TVPRA-2019-Analysis.pdf

# Index